MW01169547

Return to Play in Football

Volker Musahl • Jón Karlsson
Werner Krutsch • Bert R. Mandelbaum
João Espregueira-Mendes
Pieter d'Hooghe
Editors

Return to Play in Football

An Evidence-based Approach

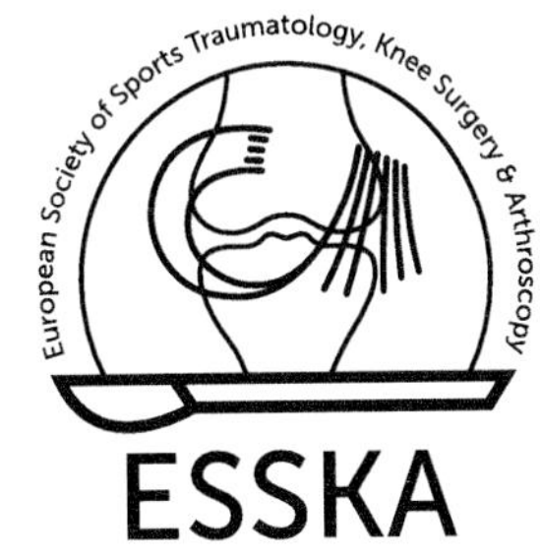

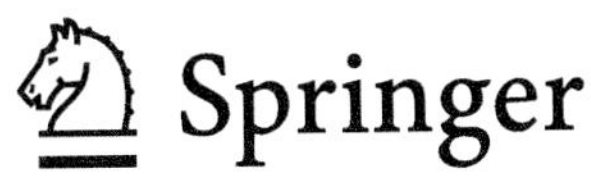

Editors
Volker Musahl
UPMC Rooney Sports Complex
University of Pittsburgh
Pittsburgh, Pennsylvania, USA

Werner Krutsch
Department of Trauma Surgery
University Medical Centre Regensburg
Regensburg, Germany

João Espregueira-Mendes
Clínica do Dragão
Espregueira-Mendes Sports Centre
Porto, Portugal

Jón Karlsson
Department of Orthopaedics
University of Gothenburg
Gothenburg, Sweden

Bert R. Mandelbaum
Santa Monica, California, USA

Pieter d'Hooghe
Orthopaedic Surgery
Aspetar Hospital
Doha, Qatar

ISBN 978-3-662-55712-9   ISBN 978-3-662-55713-6 (eBook)
https://doi.org/10.1007/978-3-662-55713-6

Library of Congress Control Number: 2017964012

Printed on acid-free paper

This Springer imprint is published by Springer Nature
The registered company is Springer-Verlag GmbH Berlin Heidelberg
The registered company address is: Heidelberger Platz 3, 14197 Berlin, Germany

Foreword

Many recent innovations, particularly in the field of biotechnology, informatics, artificial intelligence, nanotechnology, and cognitive sciences, create a new vision upon the different aspects of football medicine.

They find their applications as well in the prevention, the diagnosis, and the therapy.

But at the end of all that comes the most difficult decision: the return to play.

Our English friends say: "The proof of the pudding is the eating."

In my experience, "return to play" decisions are among the most difficult challenges for us, football doctors, whereby we must, of course, make good use of the classical criteria, without underestimating our clinical judgment and our personal experience.

The "return to play" moment is an important moment, in the first place for the player himself, reaching the end of a dark medical tunnel, but also for his medical and technical surrounding.

The surgeon, the team doctor, and the physiotherapist are concerned: they take the responsibility of giving the green light to the player, being under a constant pressure of coaches, directors, and fans, who consider every rehabilitation as too long, but knowing that the most frequent reason for a new injury is an old injury.

Also concerned is the technical staff, particularly the fitness coach, responsible for a progressive evolution of the intensity and pressure of trainings and matches.

The "return to play" moment opens the door of the medical and paramedical infrastructure and allows the player, at last, to enjoy again the smell of the grass.

It is the moment where medical and technical collaborators join their efforts, proving that only their perfect symbiosis reaches the best result.

Michel d'Hooghe
Medical Committee of UEFA and FIFA, Nyon, Switzerland

Contents

About the Editors

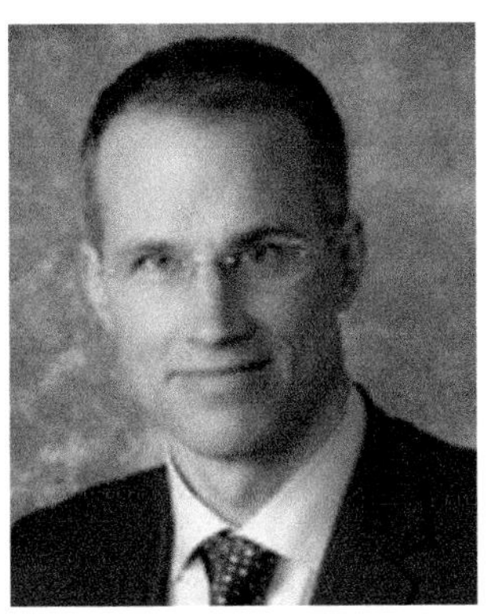

Volker Musahl, M.D., is associate professor of orthopedic surgery at the University of Pittsburgh School of Medicine, associate professor of bioengineering at the University of Pittsburgh's Swanson School of Engineering, program director of the sports medicine fellowship program, and medical director of the UPMC Center for Sports Medicine. In addition to his work as a University of Pittsburgh associate professor and a leading orthopedic surgeon, he is cohead team physician for the University of Pittsburgh football team. Dr. Musahl has received various honors and awards and in 2015 was appointed assistant editor-in-chief of *Knee Surgery, Sports Traumatology, Arthroscopy* (KSSTA). His research interests include knee and shoulder biomechanics. He is a member of ESSKA ISAKOS, AAOS, ORS, AOSSM, AANA, and AGA.

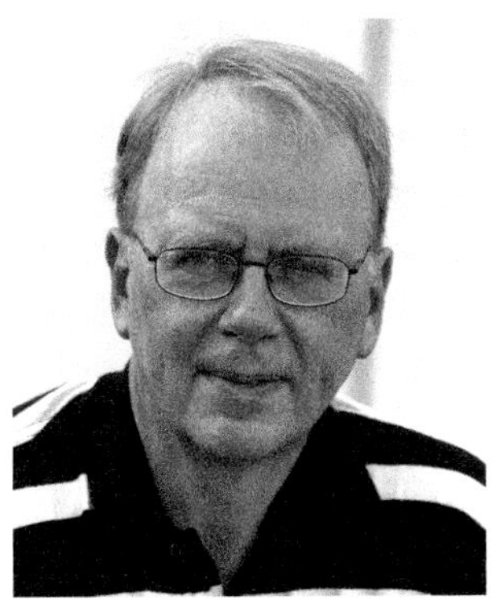

Jon Karlsson, M.D., Ph.D., is professor of orthopedics and sports traumatology at Sahlgrenska Academy, mainly related to knee and foot and ankle injuries, including tendon injuries. Dr. Karlsson graduated from the medical school in Reykjavik, Iceland. He then moved to Sweden for orthopedic training, becoming a specialist in orthopedics in 1986. He has worked at the Sahlgrenska University Hospital ever since and is currently senior consultant and full-time professor. He has been clinical head of the Orthopaedic Department and is now its academic head. He has published more than 300 papers and 30 textbooks in orthopedics and sports traumatology. He has held important positions in both ESSKA and ISAKOS and is currently editor-in-chief of *Knee Surgery, Sports Traumatology, Arthroscopy* (KSSTA), the official clinical journal of ESSKA.

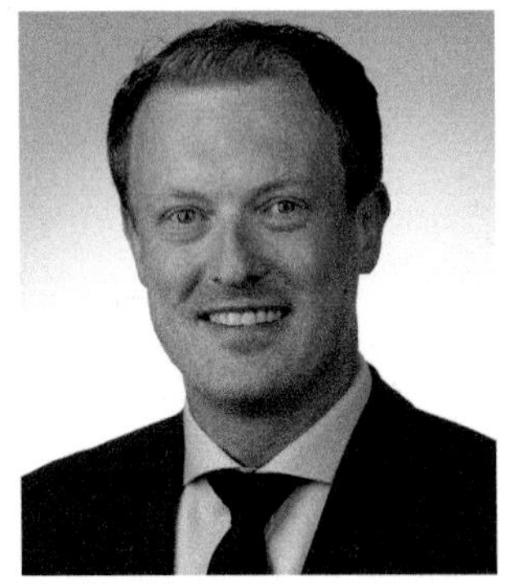

Werner Krutsch, M.D., is associate professor of orthopaedic and trauma surgery and head of sports traumatology and knee surgery in the Department of Trauma Surgery at the University Medical Centre, Regensburg, Germany. He is deputy director of the FIFA Medical Centre of Excellence, Regensburg, and medical director of the Football Association Bayern. Dr. Krutsch is head of the AO Clinical Study Center of the University of Regensburg, member of the knee ligament committee of the AGA, and education secretary of ESMA-ESSKA. He has had an active professional football career with clubs including VFB Stuttgart and 1. FC Nürnberg. He is currently the captain of the German national football team of medical doctors. The focus of the scientific work of Dr. Krutsch is football medicine and injury prevention.

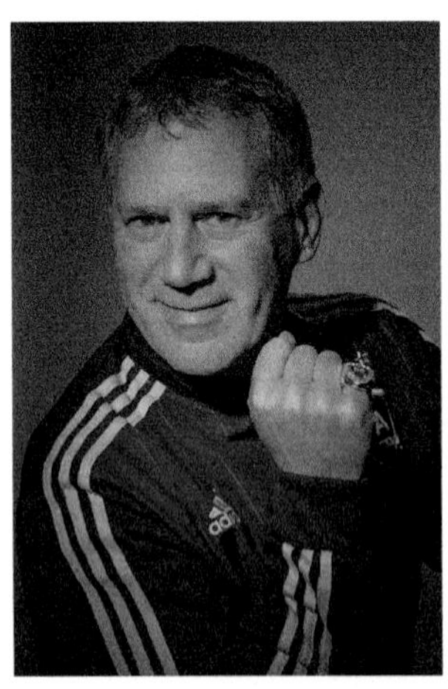

Bert R. Mandelbaum, M.D., practices with the Santa Monica Orthopaedic & Sports Medicine Group, where he serves as director of the sports medicine fellowship program and of the Research and Education Foundation and as medical director for the FIFA Medical Center of Excellence in Santa Monica. He was appointed as chief medical officer for the World Special Olympic Games 2015 in LA. Dr. Mandelbaum is a past president of the International Cartilage Repair Society. He was the chief medical officer for Women's World Cup Soccer in 1999 and 2003 and has been assistant medical director for Major League Soccer since 1996. He served as US team physician for the football World Cups from 1994 to 2010 and was FIFA medical officer for the Brazil World Cup in 2014. He has published over 100 journal articles and several books.

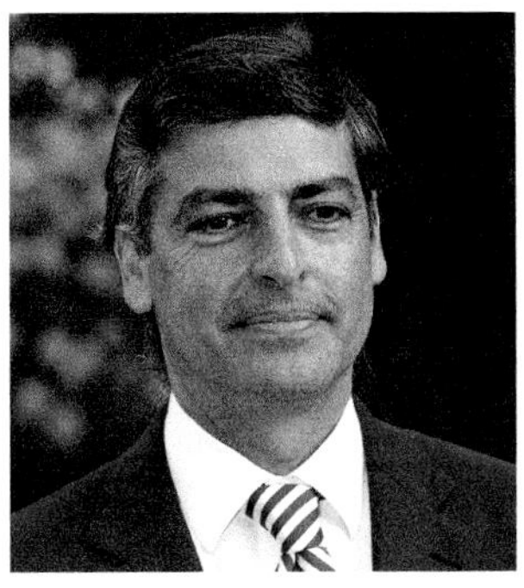

João Espregueira-Mendes, M.D., Ph.D., has been professor of orthopedic traumatology and chairman of the Orthopaedic Department at Minho University, Portugal, since 2005. In addition, he is director of Clínica do Dragão–Espregueira-Mendes Sports Centre–FIFA Medical Centre of Excellence, FC Porto Dragão Stadium, Porto, Portugal. His further posts include orthopedic surgeon of FC Porto and senior researcher in biomaterials, biodegradables, and biomimetics in the Department of Polymer Engineering at Minho University. Dr. Espregueira-Mendes was president of the European Society of Sports Traumatology, Knee Surgery and Arthroscopy (ESSKA) from 2012 to 2014, and he is treasurer and chairman of the Publication Committee of ISAKOS. He is a member of the editorial board of *Knee Surgery, Sports Traumatology, Arthroscopy*.

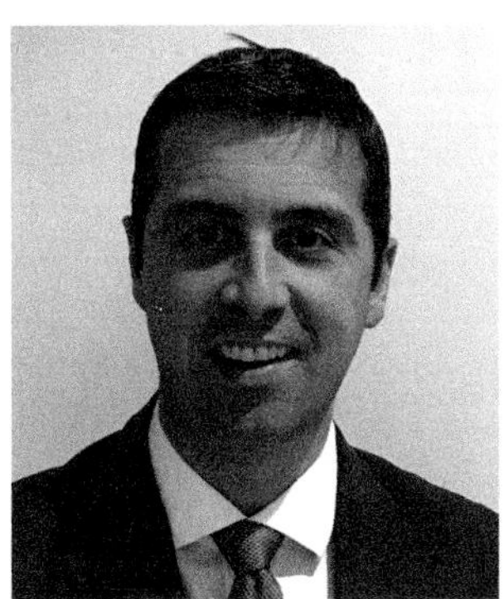

Pieter d'Hooghe M.D., MSC, MBA is Assistant Professor at the Weill Cornell University and previous football captain of FC Bruges. He is an orthopedic sports surgeon with special interest in lower limb biosurgery at Aspetar Orthopaedic and Sports Medicine Hospital in Doha, Qatar. As ISAKOS LAF Chair, he is heading a global group of experts, active in the field of research and education on foot and ankle injuries. He is a passionate member of the International Sports Medical Family.

List of Associate Editors

Marcin Kowalchuk Department of Orthopaedic Surgery, University of Pittsburgh, Pittsburgh, PA, USA

Christopher D. Murawski Department of Orthopaedic Surgery, University of Pittsburgh School of Medicine, Pittsburgh, PA, USA

List of Contributors

Leonard Achenbach Department of Trauma Surgery, University Medical Centre Regensburg, Regensburg, Germany

Andrea Achtnich Sportorthopädie, Munich, Germany

Marcio Bottene Villa Albers Department of Orthopaedic Surgery, University of Pittsburgh, Pittsburgh, PA, USA

Eduard Alentorn-Geli Artroscopia GC, SL, Hospital Quirón, Barcelona, Spain

Fundación García-Cugat, Barcelona, Spain

Mutualidad Catalana de Futbolistas – Federación Española de Fútbol, Barcelona, Spain

Thor Einar Andersen Department of Sports Medicine, Oslo Sports Trauma Research Center, Norwegian School of Sport Sciences, Ullevaal Stadion, Oslo, Norway

Morgan Anderson Department of Health, Human Performance and Recreation, Office for Sport Concussion Research, University of Arkansas, Fayetteville, AR, USA

Renato Andrade Clínica do Dragão, Espregueira-Mendes Sports Centre—FIFA Medical Centre of Excellence, Porto, Portugal

Dom Henrique Research Centre, Porto, Portugal

Faculty of Sports, University of Porto, Porto, Portugal

Peter Angele Department of Trauma Surgery, University Medical Centre Regensburg, Regensburg, Germany

Sporthopaedicum Regensburg, Regensburg, Germany

Elizabeth A. Arendt Department of Orthopaedic Surgery, University of Minnesota, Minneapolis, MN, USA

Gustavo Gonçalves Arliani Centro de Traumatologia do Esporte (CETE)/ Universidade Federal de São Paulo, São Paulo, Brazil

Justin Arner Department of Orthopaedic Surgery, UPMC Center for Sports Medicine, University of Pittsburgh, Pittsburgh, PA, USA

Daniel Arvidsson Department of Food and Nutrition, and Sport Science, Center for Health and Performance (CHP), University of Gothenburg, Gothenburg, Sweden

Isam Atroshi Department of Clinical Sciences—Orthopaedics, Lund University, Lund, Sweden

Olufemi R. Ayeni Division of Orthopaedic Surgery, Department of Surgery, McMaster University, Hamilton, ON, Canada

Khatija Bahdur Department of Human Movement Science, University of Zululand, Kwadlangezwa, South Africa

Simon Ball Fortius Clinic, London, UK

Chelsea and Westminster Hospital, London, UK

Adad Baranto Department of Orthopaedics, Institute of Clinical Sciences at the Sahlgrenska Academy, University of Gothenburg, Gothenburg, Sweden

Sahlgrenska University Hospital, Gothenburg, Sweden

Ricardo Bastos Clínica do Dragão, Espregueira-Mendes Sports Centre – FIFA Medical Centre of Excellence, Porto, Portugal

Dom Henrique Research Centre, Porto, Portugal

Universidade Federal Fluminense, Niterói, Rio de Janeiro, Brazil

Cécile Batailler Orthopedic Surgery, Centre Albert Trillat – Croix-Rousse Hospital, Lyon, France

Philip Batty Isokinetic Medical Centre, London, UK

University College, London, UK

Asheesh Bedi Domino's Farms – MedSport, University of Michigan Health System, Ann Arbor, MI, USA

Håkan Bengtsson Football Research Group, Division of Physiotherapy, Department of Medical and Health Sciences, Linköping University, Linköping, Sweden

Raymond Best Department of Sports Orthopaedics and Sports Traumatology, Sportklinik Stuttgart, Stuttgart, Germany

Mario Bizzini Schulthess Clinic, Zurich, Switzerland

John Bjørneboe Department of Sports Medicine, Oslo Sports Trauma Research Center, Norwegian School of Sport Sciences, Ullevaal Stadion, Oslo, Norway

Hendrik Bloch VBG, German Social Accident Insurance Institution for the Administrative Sector, Hamburg, Germany

Mats Börjesson Department of Food and Nutrition, and Sport Science, Center for Health and Performance (CHP), University of Gothenburg, Gothenburg, Sweden

Department of Neuroscience and Physiology, Sahlgrenska Academy and Sahlgrenska University Hospital/Östra, Göteborg, Sweden

Thomas P. Branch University Orthopedics, Decatur, GA, USA

ERMI Inc., Atlanta, GA, USA

Robert H. Brophy Department of Orthopaedic Surgery, Washington University School of Medicine, St. Louis, MO, USA

Jeremy M. Burnham Department of Orthopaedic Surgery, UPMC Center for Sports Medicine, University of Pittsburgh, Pittsburgh, PA, USA

Tyrrell Burrus Domino's Farms – MedSport, University of Michigan Health System, Ann Arbor, MI, USA

Atakan Çağlayan Sports Sciences, School of Sports Sciences, Duzce University, Duzce, Turkey

Daniele Caminati Education and Research Department, Isokinetic Medical Group, FIFA Medical Centre of Excellence, Bologna, Italy

Jacob J. Capin Biomechanics and Movement Science, University of Delaware, Newark, DE, USA

Michael R. Carmont Department of Orthopaedic Surgery, Princess Royal Hospital, Shrewsbury & Telford Hospital NHS Trust, Shrewsbury, UK

Department of Neurosciences, Biomedicine and Movement Science, University of Verona, Verona, Italy

Livia Carrai Laboratory of Applied Biomechanics, Department of Biomedical Sciences for Health, University of Milan, Milan, Italy

U.O.C. 1° Divisione, Azienda Socio Sanitaria Territoriale Centro Specialistico Ortopedico Traumatologico Gaetano Pini-CTO, Milan, Italy

Etienne Cavaignac Département de Chirurgie Orthopédique, CHU Toulouse, Toulouse, France

Jorge Chahla Steadman Philippon Research Institute—The Steadman Clinic, Vail, CO, USA

Allison A. Chan Michael G. DeGroote School of Medicine, McMaster University, Hamilton, ON, Canada

Daniel Charek Sports Concussion Program, Department of Orthopedic Surgery, University of Pittsburgh Medical Center, Pittsburgh, PA, USA

George Chiampas Department of Orthopaedics, Northwestern University, Chicago, IL, USA

Hema N. Choudur Department of Radiology, Hamilton General Hospital, East Hamilton, ON, Canada

Moises Cohen Centro de Traumatologia do Esporte (CETE)/ Universidade Federal de São Paulo, São Paulo, Brazil

Michael W. Collins Sports Medicine Concussion Program, Department of Orthopaedic Surgery, University of Pittsburgh Medical Center, Pittsburgh, PA, USA

Riccardo Compagnoni U.O.C. 1° Divisione, Azienda Socio Sanitaria Territoriale Centro Specialistico Ortopedico Traumatologico Gaetano Pini-CTO, Milan, Italy

Christopher Connaboy Neuromuscular Research Laboratory/Warrior Human Performance Research Center, Department of Sports Medicine and Nutrition, School of Health and Rehabilitation Sciences, University of Pittsburgh, Pittsburgh, PA, USA

Tracey Covassin Department of Kinesiology, Michigan State University, East Lansing, MI, USA

Ilaria Cucurnia Clinica Ortopedica e Traumatologica II, Istituto Ortopedico Rizzoli, Bologna, Italy

Laboratorio di Biomeccanica e Innovazione Tecnologica, Istituto Ortopedico Rizzoli, Bologna, Italy

Nathan D'Amico Department of Health, Human Performance and Recreation, Office for Sport Concussion Research, University of Arkansas, Fayetteville, AR, USA

Pieter d'Hooghe Department of Orthopaedic Surgery, Aspetar Orthopaedic and Sports medical Hospital, Aspire Zone, Doha, Qatar

Matthew E. Darnell Neuromuscular Research Laboratory/Warrior Human Performance Research Center, Department of Sports Medicine and Nutrition, School of Health and Rehabilitation Sciences, University of Pittsburgh, Pittsburgh, PA, USA

Richard E. Debski Departments of Bioengineering and Orthopaedic Surgery, University of Pittsburgh, Pittsburgh, PA, USA

Francesco Della Villa Education and Research Department, Isokinetic Medical Group, FIFA Medical Centre of Excellence, Bologna, Italy

Stefano Della Villa Education and Research Department, Isokinetic Medical Group, FIFA Medical Centre of Excellence, Bologna, Italy

Pete Draovitch The Hip, James M. Benson Sports Rehabilitation Center, New York, NY, USA

Jonathan Drezner Department of Family Medicine, University of Washington, Washington, DC, USA

Hugo Duarte Hospital Riviera Chablais, Vaud-Valais, Switzerland

Shawn Eagle Neuromuscular Research Laboratory/Warrior Human Performance Research Center, Department of Sports Medicine and Nutrition, School of Health and Rehabilitation Sciences, University of Pittsburgh, Pittsburgh, PA, USA

Klaus Eder Eden Reha Rehabilitation Centre, Eden-Reha, Donaustauf, Germany

Seper Ekhtiari Michael G. DeGroote School of Medicine, McMaster University, Hamilton, ON, Canada

Jan Ekstrand Football Research Group, Division of Community Medicine, Department of Medical and Health Sciences, Linköping University, Linköping, Sweden

Robert J. Elbin Department of Health, Human Performance and Recreation, Office for Sport Concussion Research, University of Arkansas, Fayetteville, AR, USA

Lars Engebretsen Oslo Sport Trauma Research Center, The Norwegian School of Sport Sciences, Oslo, Norway

Department of Orthopaedic Surgery, Oslo University Hospital, Faculty of Medicine, University of Oslo, Oslo, Norway

Zoe Englander Department of Orthopedics, Duke University, Durham, NC, USA

Department of Biomedical Engineering, Duke University, Durham, NC, USA

David Espinoza Department of Orthopaedics, University of Pittsburgh, Pittsburgh, PA, USA

João Espregueira-Mendes Clínica do Dragão, Espregueira-Mendes Sports Centre – FIFA Medical Centre of Excellence, Porto, Portugal

Dom Henrique Research Centre, Porto, Portugal

3B's Research Group – Biomaterials, Biodegradables and Biomimetics, University of Minho, Headquarters of the European Institute of Excellence on Tissue Engineering and Regenerative Medicine, Barco, Guimarães, Portugal

ICVS/3B's – PT Government Associate Laboratory, Braga/Guimarães, Portugal

Department of Orthopaedics, Minho University, Braga, Portugal

Maurizio Fanchini Department of Neurosciences, Biomedicine and Movement Science, University of Verona, Verona, Italy

Julian A Feller OrthoSport Victoria, Epworth HealthCare, Richmond, Australia

Mario Ferretti Hospital Israelita Albert Einstein, São Paulo, Brazil

Giuseppe Filardo I Clinic – Nano-Biotechnology Lab, Rizzoli Orthopedic Institute, Bologna, Italy

Christian Fink Research Unit of Orthopaedic Sports Medicine and Injury Prevention, ISAG/UMIT, Hall in Tirol, Austria

FIFA Medical Centre of Excellence, Innsbruck/Tirol, Austria

Gelenkpunkt – Sport and Joint Surgery, Innsbruck, Austria

Felix Fischer Research Unit of Orthopaedic Sports Medicine and Injury Prevention, ISAG/UMIT, Hall in Tirol, Austria

FIFA Medical Centre of Excellence, Innsbruck/Tirol, Austria

Magnus Forssblad Stockholm Sports Trauma Research Center, Karolinska Institutet, Stockholm, Sweden

Freddie H. Fu Department of Orthopaedic Surgery, University of Pittsburgh, Pittsburgh, PA, USA

Michael Fuchs 1.FC Nürnberg, Nürnberg, Germany

Jacopo Gamberini Education and Research Department, Isokinetic Medical Group, FIFA Medical Centre of Excellence, Bologna, Italy

Greg Gasbarro Department of Orthopaedic Surgery, UPMC Center for Sports Medicine, University of Pittsburgh, Pittsburgh, PA, USA

Pablo E. Gelber Orthopaedic Surgery, Hospital de la Santa Creu i Sant Pau, ICATME-Hospital Universitari Dexeus, ReSport Clinic, Universitat Autònoma de Barcelona, Barcelona, Spain

Peter Gföller FIFA Medical Centre of Excellence, Innsbruck/Tirol, Austria

Gelenkpunkt – Sport and Joint Surgery, Innsbruck, Austria

Peter B. Gifford University College Hospital, London, UK

Brandon Gillie Sports Concussion Program, Department of Orthopedic Surgery, University of Pittsburgh Medical Center, Pittsburgh, PA, USA

Alberto Gobbi Orthopaedic Arthroscopic Surgery International (OASI) Bioresearch Foundation, NPO, Milan, Italy

Jonathan A. Godin Steadman Philippon Research Institute—The Steadman Clinic, Vail, CO, USA

Alli Gokeler University of Groningen, University Medical Center Groningen, Center for Human Movement Sciences, Groningen, The Netherlands

Sérgio Gomes International Sports Traumatology Centre of Ave, Taipas Termal, Caldas das Taipas, Portugal

Clínica do Dragão, Espregueira-Mendes Sports Centre—FIFA Medical Centre of Excellence, Porto, Portugal

Vincent Gouttebarge World Players' Union (FIFPro), Hoofddorp, The Netherlands

Academic Center for Evidence based Sports Medicine (ACES), Academic Medical Center, Amsterdam, The Netherlands

Department of Orthopaedic Surgery, Academic Medical Center, University of Amsterdam, Amsterdam Movement Sciences, Amsterdam, The Netherlands

Alberto Grassi Clinica Ortopedica e Traumatologica II, Istituto Ortopedico Rizzoli, Bologna, Italy

Laboratorio di Biomeccanica e Innovazione Tecnologica, Istituto Ortopedico Rizzoli, Bologna, Italy

Jonathan A. Gustafson Department of Bioengineering, University of Pittsburgh, Pittsburgh, PA, USA

Fares S. Haddad University College Hospital, London, UK

Martin Hägglund Football Research Group, Department of Medical and Health Sciences, Linköping University, Linköping, Sweden

Michael Hantes Department of Orthopedic Surgery, University of Thessalia, Larissa, Greece

Mirco Herbort Clinic for Trauma-, Hand- and Reconstructive Surgery, University Clinic Muenster, Muenster, Germany

Elmar Herbst FIFA Medical Centre of Excellence, Innsbruck/Tirol, Austria

Gelenkpunkt – Sport and Joint Surgery, Innsbruck, Austria

Helmut Hoffmann Eden Reha, Private Clinic for Orthopaedic/ Traumatologic Rehabilitation, Donaustauf, Germany

Nolan S. Horner Division of Orthopaedic Surgery, Department of Surgery, McMaster University, Hamilton, ON, Canada

Christian Hoser FIFA Medical Centre of Excellence, Innsbruck/Tirol, Austria

Gelenkpunkt – Sport and Joint Surgery, Innsbruck, Austria

Yuichi Hoshino Department of Orthopaedic Surgery, Kobe University Graduate School of Medicine, Chuo-ku, Kobe, Hyogo, Japan

Jonathan Hughes Department of Orthopaedic Surgery, University of Pittsburgh, Pittsburgh, PA, USA

Kenneth Hunt Department of Orthopaedic Surgery, University of Colorado School of Medicine, Aurora, CO, USA

José F. Huylebroek Sportsmed Orthopaedic Centre, Parc Leopold, Brussels, Belgium

James J. Irrgang Department of Physical Therapy, University of Pittsburgh, Pittsburgh, PA, USA

Department of Orthopaedic Surgery, University of Pittsburgh, Pittsburgh, PA, USA

Caleb D. Johnson Neuromuscular Research Laboratory/Warrior Human Performance Research Center, Department of Sports Medicine and Nutrition, School of Health and Rehabilitation Sciences, University of Pittsburgh, Pittsburgh, PA, USA

Ross Julian Institute of Sports and Preventive Medicine, Saarland University, Saarbrücken, Germany

Mustafa Karahan Department of Orthopedic Surgery, Acibadem University, Istanbul, Turkey

Jon Karlsson The Department of Orthopaedic Surgery, Institute of Clinical Sciences, Sahlgrenska Academy, University of Gothenburg, Gothenburg, Sweden

John G. Kennedy Hospital for Special Surgery, New York, NY, USA

Gino M.M.J. Kerkhoffs Department of Orthopaedic Surgery, Academic Medical Center, Amsterdam, The Netherlands

Academic Center for Evidence-based Sports Medicine (ACES), Amsterdam, The Netherlands

Amsterdam Collaboration for Health and Safety in Sports (ACHSS), AMC/VUmc IOC Research Center, Amsterdam, The Netherlands

Christoph Kittl Clinic for Trauma-, Hand- and Reconstructive Surgery, University Clinic Muenster, Muenster, Germany

Christian Klein VBG, German Social Accident Insurance Institution for the Administrative Sector, Hamburg, Germany

Mariann Gajhede Knudsen Football Research Group, Linköping, Sweden

Matthias Koch Department of Trauma Surgery, University Medical Centre Regensburg, Regensburg, Germany

Elizaveta Kon Department of Biomedical Sciences – Humanitas Clinical and Research Center, Knee Joint Reconstruction Center - 3rd Orthopaedic Division, Humanitas Clinical Institute, Humanitas University, Milan, Italy

Anthony P. Kontos Department of Orthopaedic Surgery, University of Pittsburgh, Pittsburgh, PA, USA

UPMC Rooney Sports Complex, Pittsburgh, PA, USA

Marcin Kowalczuk Department of Orthopaedic Surgery, University of Pittsburgh, Pittsburgh, PA, USA

Volker Krutsch Department of Otorhinolaryngology, Nuremberg General Hospital, Paracelsus Medical University, Nürnberg, Germany

Werner Krutsch Department of Trauma Surgery, University Medical Centre Regensburg, FIFA Medical Centre of Excellence, Regensburg, Germany

A.J. Krych Department of Orthopedic Surgery and the Sports Medicine Center, Mayo Clinic and Mayo Foundation, Rochester, MN, USA

Ryosuke Kuroda Department of Orthopaedic Surgery, Kobe University Graduate School of Medicine, Chuo-ku, Kobe, Hyogo, Japan

John G. Lane Orthopaedic Arthroscopic Surgery International (OASI) Bioresearch Foundation, NPO, Milan, Italy

Musculoskeletal and Joint Research Foundation, San Diego, CA, USA

Robert F. LaPrade Steadman Philippon Research Institute—The Steadman Clinic, Vail, CO, USA

Simon Lee University of Michigan Health System, Ann Arbor, MI, USA

F. Lemmens Paediatrics ZOL, Genk, Belgium

Bryson Lesniak Division of Sports Medicine, University of Pittsburgh Medical Center, Pittsburgh, PA, USA

Hanna Lindblom Division of Physiotherapy, Department of Medical and Health Sciences, Linköping University, Linköping, Sweden

Frank G.J. Loeffen Department of Orthopaedic Surgery, Academic Medical Center, Amsterdam, The Netherlands

Academic Center for Evidence-based Sports Medicine (ACES), Amsterdam, The Netherlands

Amsterdam Collaboration for Health and Safety in Sports (ACHSS), AMC/VUmc IOC Research Center, Amsterdam, The Netherlands

Oliver Loose Department of Pediatric Surgery, Hospital St. Hedwig, Regensburg, Germany

Patrick Luig VBG, German Social Accident Insurance Institution for the Administrative Sector, Hamburg, Germany

Matilda Lundblad Football Research Group, Department of Medical and Health Sciences, Linköping University, Linköping, Sweden

Department of Orthopaedics, Sahlgrenska University, Gothenburg, Sweden

Sébastien Lustig Orthopedic Surgery, Centre Albert Trillat – Croix-Rousse Hospital, Lyon, France

Jacques Ménétrey Department of Surgery, University of Geneva, Geneva, Switzerland

Luca Macchiarola Clinica Ortopedica e Traumatologica II, Istituto Ortopedico Rizzoli, Bologna, Italy

Laboratorio di Biomeccanica e Innovazione Tecnologica, Istituto Ortopedico Rizzoli, Bologna, Italy

Robert Magnussen Department of Orthopaedics, OSU Sports Medicine, The Ohio State University, Columbus, OH, USA

Bert R. Mandelbaum Santa Monica Orthopaedic Group, Santa Monica, CA, USA

Aaron V. Mares Department of Orthopaedics, University of Pittsburgh, Pittsburgh, PA, USA

Vincent Marot Département de Chirurgie Orthopédique, CHU Toulouse, Toulouse, France

Hermann Mayr Schoen Clinic Munich-Harlaching, Munich, Germany

Tamara Valovich McLeod Athletic Training Programs, School of Osteopathic Medicine in Arizona, A.T. Still University, Mesa, AZ, USA

Alessandra Menon Laboratory of Applied Biomechanics, Department of Biomedical Sciences for Health, University of Milan, Milan, Italy

U.O.C. 1° Divisione, Azienda Socio Sanitaria Territoriale Centro Specialistico Ortopedico Traumatologico Gaetano Pini-CTO, Milan, Italy

Tim Meyer Institute of Sports and Preventive Medicine, Saarland University, Saarbrücken, Germany

Håvard Moksnes Oslo Sport Trauma Research Center, The Norwegian School of Sport Sciences, Oslo, Norway

The Norwegian Olympic Training Center, Oslo, Norway

The Norwegian Sports Medicine Center (Idrettens Helsesenter), Oslo, Norway

Hauke Mommsen Endo-Reha Zentrum, Hamburg, Germany

Caroline Mouton Department of Orthopedic Surgery, Centre Hospitalier de Luxemburg, Luxembourg City, Luxembourg

Sports Medicine Research Laboratory, Department of Population Health, Luxembourg Institute of Health, Luxembourg City, Luxembourg

Hans-Wilhelm Mueller-Wohlfahrt MW Center of Orthopedics and Sports Medicine, Munich, Germany

Conor Murphy Department of Orthopaedic Surgery, University of Pittsburgh, Pittsburgh, PA, USA

Volker Musahl Department of Orthopaedic Surgery, UPMC Center for Sports Medicine, University of Pittsburgh, Pittsburgh, PA, USA

Annica Näsmark Capio Artro Clinic, Swedish Football Association, Stockholm, Sweden

Philippe Neyret Orthopedic Surgery, Centre Albert Trillat – Croix-Rousse Hospital, Lyon, France

Bradley C. Nindl Neuromuscular Research Laboratory/Warrior Human Performance Research Center, Department of Sports Medicine and Nutrition, School of Health and Rehabilitation Sciences, University of Pittsburgh, Pittsburgh, PA, USA

John A. Norwig Pittsburgh Steelers Football Club, Pittsburgh, PA, USA

Luke O'Brien Howard Head Sports Medicine, Vail, CO, USA

Joaquim Miguel Oliveira 3B's Research Group–Biomaterials, Biodegradables and Biomimetics, University of Minho, Headquarters of the European Institute of Excellence on Tissue Engineering and Regenerative Medicine, Barco, Guimarães, Portugal

ICVS/3B's–PT Government Associate Laboratory, Braga, Guimarães, Portugal

Department of Orthopedic, Centro Hospitalar Póvoa de Varzim, Vila do Conde, Portugal

Ripoll y De Prado Sports Clinic—FIFA Medical Centre of Excellence, Murcia, Madrid, Spain

International Sports Traumatology Centre of Ave, Taipas Termal, Caldas das Taipas, Portugal

Dom Henrique Research Centre, Porto, Portugal

Francesco Perdisa I Clinic – Nano-Biotechnology Lab, Rizzoli Orthopedic Institute, Bologna, Italy

Hélder Pereira 3B's Research Group–Biomaterials, Biodegradables and Biomimetics, University of Minho, Headquarters of the European Institute of Excellence on Tissue Engineering and Regenerative Medicine, Barco, Guimarães, Portugal

ICVS/3B's–PT Government Associate Laboratory, Braga, Guimarães, Portugal

Department of Orthopedic, Centro Hospitalar Póvoa de Varzim, Vila do Conde, Portugal

Ripoll y De Prado Sports Clinic—FIFA Medical Centre of Excellence, Murcia, Madrid, Spain

International Sports Traumatology Centre of Ave, Taipas Termal, Caldas das Taipas, Portugal

Dom Henrique Research Centre, Porto, Portugal

Rogério Pereira Clínica do Dragão, Espregueira-Mendes Sports Centre – FIFA Medical Centre of Excellence, Porto, Portugal

Dom Henrique Research Centre, Porto, Portugal

Faculty of Sports, University of Porto, Porto, Portugal

Faculty of Health Science, University Fernando Pessoa, Porto, Portugal

Wolf Petersen Martin Luther Hospital, Berlin, Germany

Thomas Pfeiffer Department of Orthopaedic Surgery, Traumatology, and Sports Medicine, Kliniken der StadtKoelngGmbH, Köln, Germany

Pelin Pişirici Private Pendik Regional Hospital, Istanbul, Turkey

Adam J. Popchak Department of Physical Therapy, University of Pittsburgh, Pittsburgh, PA, USA

Ricard Pruna FC Barcelona Medical Services, FIFA Medical Centre of Excellence, Barcelona, Spain

Luca Pulici Laboratory of Applied Biomechanics, Department of Biomedical Sciences for Health, University of Milan, Milan, Italy

U.O.C. 1° Divisione, Azienda Socio Sanitaria Territoriale Centro Specialistico Ortopedico Traumatologico Gaetano Pini-CTO, Milan, Italy

Pietro Randelli Laboratory of Applied Biomechanics, Department of Biomedical Sciences for Health, University of Milan, Milan, Italy

U.O.C. 1° Divisione, Azienda Socio Sanitaria Territoriale Centro Specialistico Ortopedico Traumatologico Gaetano Pini-CTO, Milan, Italy

Rui L. Reis 3B's Research Group – Biomaterials, Biodegradables and Biomimetics, University of Minho, Headquarters of the European Institute of

Excellence on Tissue Engineering and Regenerative Medicine, Barco, Guimarães, Portugal

ICVS/3B's – PT Government Associate Laboratory, Braga/Guimarães, Portugal

Christa Janse Van Rensburg Faculty of Health Sciences, Section Sports Medicine, Sport, Exercise Medicine and Lifestyle Institute (SEMLI), University of Pretoria, Pretoria, South Africa

Margherita Ricci Education and Research Department, Isokinetic Medical Group, FIFA Medical Centre of Excellence, Bologna, Italy

Helge Riepenhof BG Clinic Hamburg, Hamburg, Germany

Pedro L. Ripoll Ripoll y De Prado Sports Clinic—FIFA Medical Centre of Excellence, Murcia, Madrid, Spain

Sérgio Rodrigues-Gomes Clínica do Dragão, Espregueira-Mendes Sports Centre—FIFA Medical Centre of Excellence, Porto, Portugal

SMIC Serviço Médico de Imagem Computorizada, Porto, Portugal

Dani Romero-Rodríguez EUSES (University School of Health and Sport, University of Girona), Barcelona, Spain

Sonia Ruef Pittsburgh Steelers Football Club, Pittsburgh, PA, USA

Jaakko Ryynänen University of Helsinki, Helsinki, Finland

Kristian Samuelsson Department of Orthopedics, Institute of Clinical Sciences, The Sahlgrenska Academy, University of Gothenburg, Göteborg, Sweden

Natalie Sandel Sports Medicine Concussion Program, Department of Orthopaedic Surgery, University of Pittsburgh Medical Center, Pittsburgh, PA, USA

K. Sas Urgentist AZ Glorieux, Ronse, Belgium

Philip Schatz Saint Joseph's University, Philadelphia, PA, USA

Laura C. Schmitt Division of Physical Therapy, School of Health and Rehabilitation Sciences, Ohio State University, Columbus, OH, USA

Tobias Schweinsteiger FC Bayern München e.V., Munich, Germany

Martin Schwellnus Faculty of Health Sciences, Section Sports Medicine, Sport, Exercise Medicine and Lifestyle Institute (SEMLI), University of Pretoria, Pretoria, South Africa

Romain Seil Department of Orthopedic Surgery, Centre Hospitalier de Luxemburg, Luxembourg City, Luxembourg

Sports Medicine Research Laboratory, Department of Population Health, Luxembourg Institute of Health, Luxembourg City, Luxembourg

Elvire Servien Orthopedic Surgery, Centre Albert Trillat – Croix-Rousse Hospital, Lyon, France

Andrea Sessa I Clinic – Nano-Biotechnology Lab, Rizzoli Orthopedic Institute, Bologna, Italy

Yoshiharu Shimozono Hospital for Special Surgery, New York, NY, USA

Jason Shin Department of Orthopaedic Surgery, University of Pittsburgh, Pittsburgh, PA, USA

Division of Sports Medicine, University of Pittsburgh Medical Center, Pittsburgh, PA, USA

Cecilia Signorelli Laboratorio di Biomeccanica e Innovazione Tecnologica, Istituto Ortopedico Rizzoli, Bologna, Italy

Karin Grävare Silbernagel The Department of Physiotherapy, University of Delware, Newark, DE, USA

The Department of Orthopaedic Surgery, Institute of Clinical Sciences, Sahlgrenska Academy, University of Gothenburg, Gothenburg, Sweden

Holly J. Silvers-Granelli Biomechanics and Movement Science, University of Delaware, Newark, DE, USA

Velocity Physical Therapy, Los Angeles, CA, USA

Thomas Sisk Department of Orthopaedics, University of Pittsburgh, Pittsburgh, PA, USA

Mia Smucny Department of Orthopaedic Surgery, Cleveland Clinic Foundation, Garfield Heights, OH, USA

Lynn Snyder-Mackler Biomechanics and Movement Science, University of Delaware, Newark, DE, USA

Department of Physical Therapy, University of Delaware, Newark, DE, USA

Duarte Sousa Orthopedic Department, Centro Hospitalar Póvoa de Varzim, Vila do Conde, Portugal

Kurt P. Spindler Department of Orthopaedic Surgery, Cleveland Clinic Foundation, Garfield Heights, OH, USA

Amelie Stöhr Orthopaedic Surgery Munich OCM, Munich, Germany

Shaun K. Stinton University Orthopedics, Decatur, GA, USA

ERMI Inc., Atlanta, GA, USA

Heiko Striegel Department of Sports Medicine, University Hospital Tübingen, Tuebingen, Germany

M.J. Stuart Department of Orthopedic Surgery and the Sports Medicine Center, Mayo Clinic and Mayo Foundation, Rochester, MN, USA

Alicia Sufrinko Sports Concussion Program, Department of Orthopedic Surgery, University of Pittsburgh Medical Center, Pittsburgh, PA, USA

David Sundemo Department of Orthopedics, Institute of Clinical Sciences, The Sahlgrenska Academy, University of Gothenburg, Göteborg, Sweden

Tetsuya Takenaga Department of Orthopaedic Surgery, University of Pittsburgh, Pittsburgh, PA, USA

Matthew A. Tao Hospital for Special Surgery, New York, NY, USA

Athol Thomson Department of Sports Podiatry, Aspetar Orthopaedic and Sports medical Hospital, Aspire Zone, Doha, Qatar

Chris Thompson Institute of Sports and Preventive Medicine, Saarland University, Saarbrücken, Germany

Peter Ueblacker MW Center of Orthopedics and Sports Medicine, Munich, Germany

Markus Waldén Football Research Group, Department of Medical and Health Sciences, Linköping University, Linköping, Sweden

Dean Wang Hospital for Special Surgery, New York, NY, USA

Johannes Weber Department of Trauma Surgery, University Medical Centre Regensburg, Regensburg, Germany

Kate E Webster School of Allied Health, La Trobe University, Bundoora, Melbourne, Australia

Jonas Werner Football Research Group, Department of Orthopaedics, Vrinnevisjukhuset, Norrköping, Sweden

Suzanne Werner Stockholm Sports Trauma Research Center, Karolinska Institutet, Stockholm, Sweden

Nathan White Fortius Clinic, London, UK

Chelsea and Westminster Hospital, London, UK

Graeme P. Whyte Orthopaedic Arthroscopic Surgery International (OASI) Bioresearch Foundation, NPO, Milan, Italy

Cornell University, Weill Medical College, New York Presbyterian Hospital/Queens, New York, NY, USA

Andy Williams Fortius Clinic, London, UK

Riley J. Williams Hospital for Special Surgery, New York, NY, USA

J.M. Woodmass Department of Orthopedic Surgery and the Sports Medicine Center, Mayo Clinic and Mayo Foundation, Rochester, MN, USA

Frank Wormuth Deutscher Fußball-Bund, Frankfurt am Main, Germany

Mohammad A. Yabroudi Department of Rehabilitation Sciences, Jordan University of Science and Technology, Irbid, Jordan

Stefano Zaffagnini Clinica Ortopedica e Traumatologica II, Istituto Ortopedico Rizzoli, Bologna, Italy

Laboratorio di Biomeccanica e Innovazione Tecnologica, Istituto Ortopedico Rizzoli, Bologna, Italy

Beatrice Zanini U.O.C. 1° Divisione, Azienda Socio Sanitaria Territoriale Centro Specialistico Ortopedico Traumatologico Gaetano Pini-CTO, Milan, Italy

Christian Zantop Return to Play, Straubing, Germany

Thore Zantop Sporthopaedicum, Straubing, Germany

Jennifer A. Zellers The Department of Physiotherapy, University of Delware, Newark, DE, USA

Johannes Zellner Department of Trauma Surgery, University Medical Centre Regensburg, Regensburg, Germany

Part I

Introduction

Basic Concepts in Functional Biomechanics

1

Jonathan A. Gustafson, Tetsuya Takenaga, and Richard E. Debski

Contents

J.A. Gustafson, Ph.D.
Department of Bioengineering, University of Pittsburgh, 408 Center for Bioengineering, 300 Technology Drive, Pittsburgh, PA, 15219, USA

T. Takenaga, M.D., Ph.D.
Department of Orthopaedic Surgery, University of Pittsburgh, Pittsburgh, PA, USA

R.E. Debski, Ph.D. (✉)
Departments of Bioengineering and Orthopaedic Surgery, University of Pittsburgh, 408 Center for Bioengineering, 300 Technology Drive, Pittsburgh, PA, 15219, USA
e-mail: genesis1@pitt.edu

1.1 Introduction

Sports-related injuries in pediatric and adolescent athletes are common and provide challenges in determining the best course of care and appropriate criteria for the athletes return to sport. Injuries to adults are also significant in that they can permanently impair function and severely limit activities of daily living. In football, the knee joint is one of the most common sources of both contact and noncontact injuries. Current work in the field of sports medicine aims to diagnose injuries accurately, implement appropriate surgical/nonsurgical treatment solutions and, ultimately, develop the best criteria for early return to sport. In order to best achieve these goals, it is important to understand the normal function of the body in response to daily loading. Functional biomechanics plays a large role in evaluating the body's response to both normal and excessive loading, such as in an injury event.

Biomechanics is an interdisciplinary field that utilizes principles of mechanics applied to the human body in order to improve function through design and development of equipment, as well as analysis of systems and therapies. Applied biomechanics can provide additional knowledge of the effect of loading on the musculoskeletal system and the mechanical responses of the body to these loads, which can be used to assess both normal and abnormal function, as well as predict changes and propose interventions. Additionally,

V. Musahl et al. (eds.), *Return to Play in Football*, https://doi.org/10.1007/978-3-662-55713-6_1

basic biomechanics explores the effects of external forces and moments required for movement and, in effect, the consequence of internal loads on soft tissue deformation. This chapter will explore important, sports-related biomechanics concepts and is divided into four different topics: statics, dynamics, mechanics of materials, and applications. Throughout the chapter are examples of applying these biomechanical principles to sports medicine problems and improving return to play following injury.

Functional biomechanics allows one to appreciate the relationships and interactions that various systems, segments, and body parts have with one another that contribute to its ability to perform. These relationships are the foundation for understanding the complexities of human function.

1.2 Statics

Statics analysis of structures evaluates the effect of external loads on a rigid body at rest or in motion at a constant velocity. When applied to the body, statics analysis allows for the determination of the magnitudes and directions of passive, soft tissue forces (e.g., ligaments), muscle forces, and joint reaction forces. In order to perform a statics analysis, a basic principle of physics must be applied.

1.2.1 Newton's Law of Static Equilibrium

Newton's law of static equilibrium states that a body at rest remains at rest and a body in motion tends to stay in motion at a constant speed and in the same direction unless acted on by an unbalanced force. Additionally, every force of action has an opposite and equal reaction in order to maintain this balance. An example of this concept is the ground reaction force. Every time a person places his/her foot on the ground, there is an equal and opposite force exerted from the ground up through the foot. This ground reaction force is transmitted through the kinetic chain of the body (foot, ankle, knee, hip, back, etc.), which loads our joints. As the body prefers a state of equilibrium, drastic changes in the ground reaction force, in terms of magnitude and direction, can lead to potential injury. Similarly, within joints, there are muscles and connective tissues that create a joint reaction force in order to maintain proper joint stability.

When considering a state of static equilibrium, the forces and moments acting on the body must equate to zero (i.e., no motion). The resulting equations for force and moment equilibrium in three dimensions are:

$$\sum Fx = 0; \sum Mx = 0$$
$$\sum Fy = 0; \sum My = 0$$
$$\sum Fz = 0; \sum Mz = 0$$

Forces provide both mobility and stability to the body but can also introduce the potential to deform and injure the body. Healthy tissue can typically withstand the deformations caused by these action and reaction forces; however, injured or diseased tissue may not be able to sustain the same loads required to perform activities of daily living. Statics analysis allows the researcher to represent the complex interactions of the forces and moments acting on the body through the use of vectors and free-body diagrams.

1.2.2 Free-Body Diagrams

To better evaluate a biomechanical system, such as forces or moments being applied to a specified part of the body, free-body diagrams are an effective tool to simplify a complex analysis. Free-body diagrams provide a "snapshot" that represent the interaction between body and environment and allow for visualization and ease of calculation by properly identifying all the forces and moments acting on the body of interest in order to successfully achieve equilibrium.

Force vectors generate the "push and pull" to a system and can originate from internal sources (i.e., muscle forces and joint contact forces) as well as external sources (i.e., friction forces and gravitational forces). A moment (or torque) is a force applied at a distance from a fixed point that tends to cause the rigid segment to rotate.

The magnitude of the moment is a product of the force applied and the perpendicular distance from the applied force to the fixed point. This distance is commonly defined as the moment or lever arm. A larger moment arm requires less force to achieve equivalent angular motion about the axis of rotation. Although a moment can be calculated about any point, typically when performing biomechanical analyses, it is calculated about a joint axis of rotation.

Using the example of a leg extension exercise (Fig. 1.1a) in evaluating the forces about the knee joint, a free-body diagram can assess the change in tension in the quadriceps muscles when adding a weight to the ankle (Fig. 1.1b). The applied forces (both external and internal forces) throughout the system are drawn in order visualize the problem. External forces in the leg extension problem are represented by the weight of the leg and the ankle weight, and internal forces are represented by the force in the quadriceps and the joint reaction force (Fig. 1.1c). The external weight, combined with the weight of leg, causes the leg to experience a flexion moment, while the force from the quadriceps acts in extension in order to balance these external moments (Fig. 1.1d). It is important to note the significant difference in the moment arm between the quadriceps force and the external forces. It is not uncommon for muscle forces to exhibit force magnitudes several times greater than the applied external loads for balance, due to the significantly shortened moment arm of the muscle. Once all of the forces in the free-body diagram have been defined, the laws of static equilibrium are applied to solve for the unknown muscle forces and joint reaction forces.

Reducing the joint reaction force is a common strategy in rehabilitation programs aimed at preventing further joint degeneration in persons with

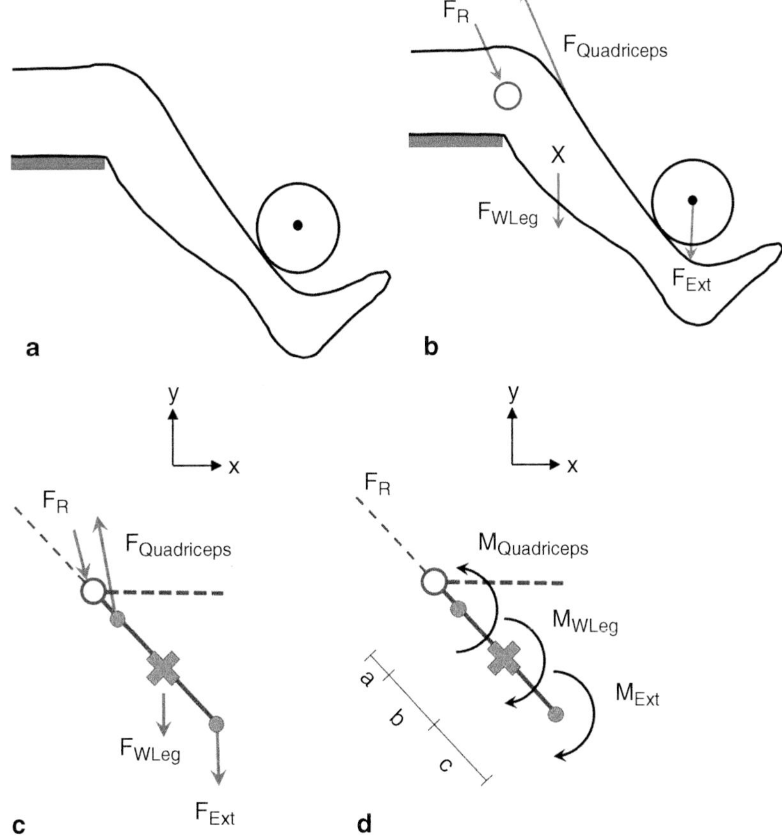

Fig. 1.1 (**a**) Simulation of a person performing a leg extension. (**b**) The ankle weight applies an external force (F_{Ext}) downward in addition to the gravitational force due to the weight of the lower leg (F_{WLeg}). The quadriceps muscle generates a force ($F_{Quadriceps}$) to the lower leg and causes a joint reaction force (F_R) at the knee to keep the joint stabilized. (**c**) A free-body diagram of the lower leg representing each force as an *arrow*, with the *head of the arrow* pointing in the direction of the applied force. (**d**) The quadriceps muscle creates a counterclockwise moment ($M_{Quadriceps}$) to resist the clockwise moments due to the weight of the lower leg (M_{WLeg}) and ankle weight (M_{Ext})

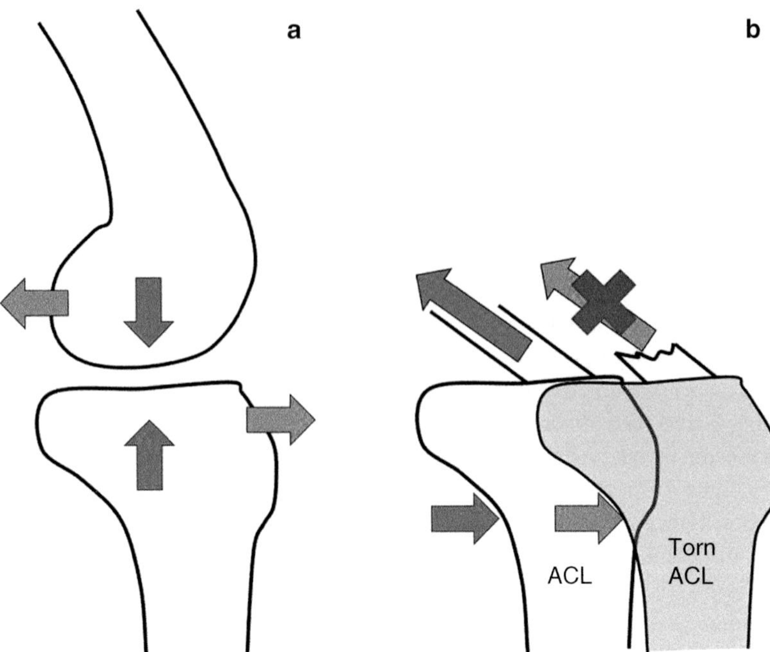

Fig. 1.2 (**a**) At the joint surface, the knee can undergo compressive forces (*blue arrows*), which act in the direction perpendicular to both surfaces, or shear forces (*orange arrows*), which act in the tangential direction to both surfaces. (**b**) Forces applied to the knee joint are transmitted through the ACL (*solid tibia*; *blue arrows*), which resist anterior motion. Rupture of the ACL (*shaded tibia*; *orange arrow*) leads to excessive anterior motion and instability as the forces are unable to be transmitted properly

arthritis. This is commonly achieved by changing the magnitudes of muscle forces or reducing external loads transmitted through the body. For example, a person with medial tibiofemoral osteoarthritis may use a cane on their contralateral side in order to reduce the joint reaction forces in the painful/affected knee joint. When obesity is a factor, a weight reduction program may be implemented to reduce the joint reaction forces. Alternatively in sports rehabilitation, statics analysis can be implemented to improve strengthening programs tailored to best target the proper muscles for the recovering athlete and expedite return to play.

1.2.3 Ligament and Joint Contact Forces

These concepts of statics analysis can be applied not only to whole-body analyses but also at the joint and tissue level. For the typical joint, forces can be related to compression and shear. The tibial plateau and femoral condyles experience compressive forces in the direction perpendicular to each articular surface while standing with the knee in full extension (Fig. 1.2a). Shear forces are experienced in the tangential direction along the surface of interest (Fig. 1.2a), such as when performing an anterior drawer test. Forces can also be transmitted through the soft tissue structures. During a pivoting maneuver, the anterior cruciate ligament (ACL) can become significantly loaded to resist anterior tibial translation and provide stability for the joint. This represents functional loading of the joint and soft tissue. However, after an injury such as an ACL rupture, opposing shear forces cannot be transferred through the ligament, resulting in anterior laxity (Fig. 1.2b).

Fact Box 1 Statics

- Statics analysis assumes state of equilibrium.
- Utilizes Newton's laws of static equilibrium and action-reaction.
- Free-body diagrams aid to simplify complex systems to understand net external and internal forces and moments.

1.3 Dynamics

Dynamics is the study of systems in motion, where the laws of equilibrium have been violated and the net forces and moments of a system do not equate to zero. Analysis of bodies in motion can be subdivided into two subgroups: kinematics and kinetics. Kinematics describes the motion of the bodies without regard to the forces causing the motion. This is typically done by characterizing the geometric and time-dependent aspects of motion. Conversely, kinetics utilizes concepts from kinematics but additionally includes the effects of the forces and moments within a system. Both kinematic and kinetic analyses are commonly performed in sports biomechanics for evaluating motion. This section will primarily focus on kinematics.

1.3.1 Kinematics

As previously stated, kinematics studies motion without regard to the forces and moments causing the motion, which include translations and rotations. Translations are simply the linear motions in which all the points of a rigid body move simultaneously in the same direction and at the same velocity. Rotations are the angular motions of a rigid body along a circular path and about an axis of rotation. During passive knee flexion, the tibiofemoral joint undergoes both linear and angular motions, and both of these motions can occur in multiple planes, such as combined flexion-extension with internal-external tibial rotation.

Motion at an articular surface can be described in terms of three motions that exist resulting from a convex surface moving on a concave surface (Fig. 1.3). Rolling motion occurs when the convex surface rotates. This causes a change in the point of contact for both articular surfaces. A sliding motion is experienced when one articular surface translates across the other with no rotation and progressively changes the point of contact. Lastly, spinning motion occurs at a single point of contact on the fixed surface, where the point of contact changes on the rotating surface and no linear motion occurs. At the tibiofemoral

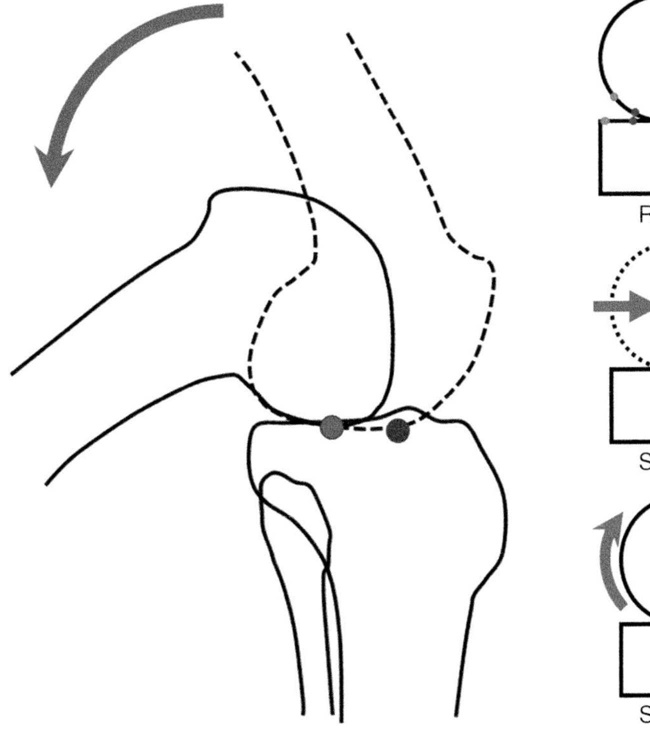

Fig. 1.3 Three fundamental motions that occur between articular surfaces. The point of contact changes on both articular surfaces during rolling motion. The point of contact on the moving surface remains constant during sliding motion. A single point of contact occurs on the fixed surface during a spinning motion. Some joints, such as the tibiofemoral joint, experience up to all three of these motions simultaneously

joint during flexion, the femur (convex surface) will roll in the posterior direction but slide in the anterior direction along the tibial plateau. This type of convex-concave motion encompasses all three motions (rolling, sliding, and spinning) of the femur relative to the tibia through flexion rotation, anterior translation, and external rotation, respectively.

Clinically, it is important to understand these joint motions when performing a pivot-shift maneuver for evaluating the knee joint for stability and assessing potential injury. The pivot-shift maneuver is performed through the combination of compressive and valgus forces, as well as internal rotational torques applied to the lower leg. These forces and torques generate simultaneous sliding (translational), spinning (rotational), and rolling (flexion) motions at the joint surface, which elicit the integrity of the ACL and its ability to stabilize these joint motions. Objective quantification of the pivot-shift maneuver can allow clinicians to track the changes in these joint motions post-surgery and throughout a rehabilitation program in order to make the most informed decision about the athlete's knee state and function. This objective quantification has been an ongoing research topic [1], with studies using inertial sensors [2], electromagnetic tracking sensors [3], and tablet computer software programs [1] to track the complex rolling, sliding, and spinning motion of the knee joint during clinical exams.

In football, noncontact tears of the ACL are common, and injury is 3–4 times higher particularly among female athletes [4]. Studies have shown significant changes in the joint motions after ACL tears in terms of increased rotations (spinning) and joint translations (sliding). The choice of the surgical technique and graft type can significantly impact the restored motion of the joint and, ultimately, the athlete's ability to return to play. For example, it has been shown that drilling a femoral tunnel via an anteromedial portal improves anterior-posterior translation and external femoral rotation during gait compared to transtibial techniques [5]. Additionally, a recent study found significant improvements in rotatory kinematics during gait when using a double-bundle ACL reconstruction compared to a single-bundle ACL reconstruction [6]. It should be noted that neither the single-bundle nor double-bundle ACL reconstructions were able to fully restore rotational kinematics during gait after 14 weeks of postoperative physiotherapy. In order to improve outcomes from these surgeries, it is important to understand the forces within structural tissue, such as ligaments, and how the properties of the tissue can affect its function.

Fact Box 2: Kinematics

- Kinematics studies motions without regard to the forces and moments causing motion.
- Motion of the human body can occur simultaneously in multiple planes.
- Understanding and measuring changes in joint motion are important for developing appropriate treatment strategies and developing criteria for return to sport.

1.4 Mechanics of Materials

Mechanics of materials is the study of forces and their effects on motion within rigid and deformable systems. When examining the behavior of solid bodies, such as the forces acting on joint limbs and their resulting motions, rigid body mechanics may apply. When examining the effect of forces and motions on the internal stresses of the body, deformable mechanics may apply. Both rigid body mechanics and deformable mechanics provide information about the behavior of the body and tissue structures (i.e., ligaments) when exposed to loads, particularly when these loads can lead to injury.

1.4.1 Rigid Body Mechanics

Rigid body mechanics assumes that any deformations caused by forces acting on a body are negligible. While this assumption can aid in simplifying biomechanical analyses, it should be noted that no

Table 1.1 Structural properties of common ACL graft choices for reconstruction

	Native ACL	Hamstring tendon [7]	Patellar tendon [8]	Quadriceps tendon [9]
		Doubled ST + GT	10 mm graft	
Load-to-failure (N)	2160	2831	2977	2353
Stiffness (N/mm)	242	456	455	326

ST semitendinosus tendon, *GT* gracilis tendon

material in the human body can truly be considered a rigid body, as all tissues undergo some degree of deformation. Therefore, it is important to clearly understand when the rigid body assumption is applicable. If one material is much stiffer than the other or the deformations experienced by a body are much smaller than the translations or rotations of that body, then the rigid body principle can be applied. Branches of statics and dynamics are forms of analyses that utilize the principle of rigid body mechanics. For example, when analyzing gait, the translations and rotations of the lower extremity will be much greater than any deformations experienced by the segments of the lower extremity, allowing it to be treated as a rigid body. This assumption is also applicable when performing mechanical testing of a joint complex, such as the femur-ACL-tibia complex, where the bones can be considered a rigid body since it is much stiffer than the ligament tissue. Traditional approaches to evaluate both static and dynamic systems assume that each object in the system is a rigid body. The following section better accounts for the realistic deformations that occur in the musculoskeletal system as a result of loads applied at the tissue level. This includes both soft (articular cartilage, tendons, ligaments, capsular tissues) and hard (bone) tissues.

1.4.2 Structural Properties of a Complex

Mechanics of materials when applied to a structure that may incorporate multiple materials or tissue types (termed complex) can provide information about the structural properties of the complex when exposed to different forms of loading (i.e., tensile, compressive, shear). For example, the structural properties of the femur-ACL-tibia complex can be determined in response to a tensile load to assess its load-elongation behavior. To do this, a tensile force is applied to the bone-ligament-bone complex, causing the tissue to become stretched until the complex ruptures. While loading is applied, the corresponding increase in length in the complex is measured. The resulting nonlinear load-elongation curve that is typical of biologic soft tissues provides information about the structural properties of the tissue complex, such as its stiffness and ultimate load at failure. These parameters are important to define for healthy tissue as, clinically, they can factor into the graft choice for a reconstruction surgery. Table 1.1 clearly shows the differences between the structural properties of different tissue complexes that are commonly used as graft types for ligament reconstruction [1]. These properties can significantly affect the function of the joint and should be carefully considered prior to reconstruction.

In the biomechanics field, it has been well established that factors such as age, injury, and healing can significantly affect the structural properties of a bone-ligament-bone complex as well as the failure mode of the complex [10, 11]. Tensile failure tests in a rabbit femur-medial collateral ligament (MCL)-tibia complex demonstrated significant increases in tensile strength as a result of maturation. Additionally, failure modes in these models progressed from tibial avulsions in the younger tissue to failure in the midsubstance of ligament [11]. It has also been shown in a recovering femur-MCL-tibia complex that the recovering tissue complex exhibits significantly decreased stiffness (53%) and ultimate load (29%) compared to an uninjured joint state [10]. These classic studies have provided evidence as to how the structural properties of tissue complexes change as a result of aging, injury, and throughout recovery. These concepts are important when evaluating the rehabilitation choice (surgical vs. nonsurgical) for an injured athlete and the timeline for return to play.

1.4.3 Mechanical Properties of Tissue

It is also important to understand the mechanical response of an individual tissue or material, which is independent of specimen geometry, by using normalized load and deformation parameters. Measuring the mechanical properties of tissues, such as ligaments, can be used to evaluate the quality of the tissue when making comparisons between normal, injured, and healing states and are represented by the stress-strain relationship. Stress is defined as the amount of force applied per unit area and is one of the most basic engineering principles. Strain is considered as a dimensionless measure of the degree of deformation in the tissue, which is defined as the change in length per unit length. Stress-strain relationships are obtained experimentally during tensile, compressive, or shear loading of the excised tissue.

A typical stress-strain curve for biologic tissues consists of four distinct regions (see Fig. 1.4). The first noticeable region is a nonlinear toe region (region 1), where significant stretch

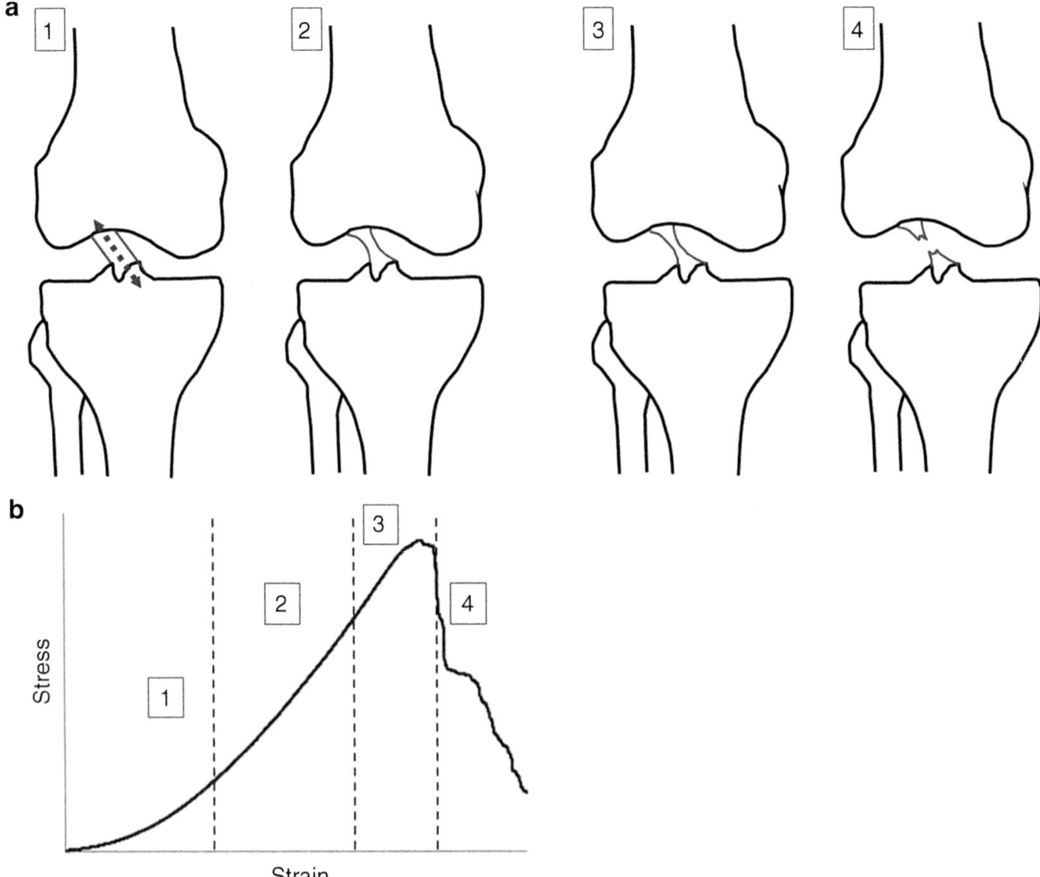

Fig. 1.4 (**a**) Conceptual example of load-to-failure test in the ligament consisting of four regions of loading: (*1*) initial recruitment of the collagen fibers; (*2*) increased load bearing through the ligament; (*3*) continued loading and deformation of the ligament; (*4*) ultimate rupture of the ligament. (**b**) Stress-strain curve of the ligament substance that characterizes the mechanical properties during a load-to-failure test. Regions *1*, *2*, *3*, and *4* correspond to the toe region, linear region, partial failure of the material, and complete rupture of the material, respectively

of the material occurs with a minimal increase in stress. This is a direct result from stretching of the crimped collagen fibrils as the fibers are being drawn taut in the material and before significant tension occurs within the material. Strain becomes linearly proportional to stress in region 2, and the slope of the curve in this region can be calculated to determine the tangent modulus of the tissue. The tangent modulus defines the threshold of the material beyond which permanent deformation (plastic) can begin to occur. The area under the curve within this linear region can be referred to as the strain energy density. This region is commonly reached during daily activities, where the tissue undergoes a form of "elastic" deformation, meaning the tissue will return to its original length or shape upon unloading. Furthermore, the energy used to deform the tissue is released when the applied stress is removed. When the tissue experiences abnormally large levels of strain, the tissue undergoes only a marginal increase in corresponding stress (region 3). It is at this point that the tissue begins experiencing microscopic failures. The area under this region of the curve represents plastic deformation energy. Once the tissue undergoes this amount of deformation, the tissue does not recover and return to its original state in its entirety upon release of the deforming stress. If the tissue continues to deform, it will eventually experience complete failure (region 4). Common mechanical properties of tissues derived from mechanical tests include modulus, ultimate strength, ultimate strain, and strain energy density. These properties describing the mechanical properties of tissue can be used to evaluate injured and healing states.

Clinically, the mechanical properties of tissue can be significantly influenced by not only injury but also during recovery [10, 12]. The detrimental effects of disuse injuries have been well documented. Specifically, immobilization of tendons and ligaments can significantly reduce the mechanical properties of the tissue as well as the mass of the structure [12]. Additionally, the long-term effects of disuse have been shown to require up to 12 months of time for complete recovery of ligament strength parameters [13]. Classic studies have had a major impact on the decision hierarchy for return to play that has evolved in sports medicine/sports traumatology over time.

1.4.4 Viscoelasticity

Viscoelastic materials exhibit both solid-like characteristics, such as strength and elasticity, and fluidlike characteristics, like flow, which are dependent on time and rate of loading. Most tissues within the musculoskeletal system demonstrate at least some degree of viscoelasticity. When plotting a load-elongation curve during a nondestructive tensile test, unloading of a viscoelastic material will leave a region between the loading and unloading curves known as hysteresis, a common viscoelastic property of all biologic tissues (Fig. 1.5). This region of hysteresis is created due to energy lost (heat) when unloading the material. Preconditioning with repeated loading and unloading of the tissue decreases this area of hysteresis and maximizes elongation of the tissue, which is why athletes precondition the tissue in their bodies to maximize performance by completing repetitive stretching activities prior to competition.

A viscoelastic material experiences two common phenomena known as creep and stress relaxation. Creep describes a progressive increase in elongation of a material when exposed to a constant load over time (Fig. 1.6a). Simply, creep can be considered the tendency of

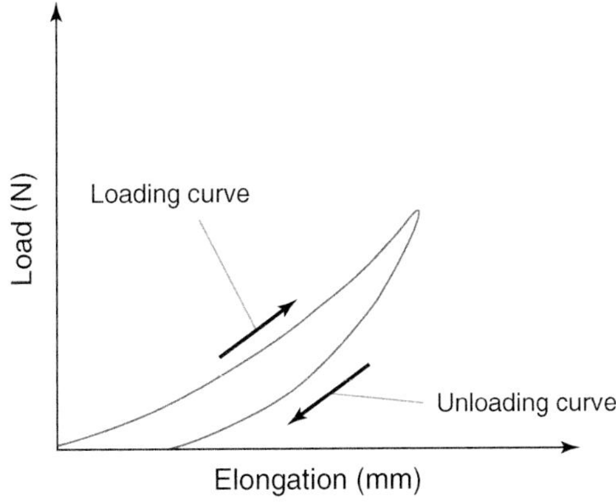

Fig. 1.5 Load-elongation curve of a biological soft tissue in response to an applied tensile load. The area between the loading and unloading curves represents the energy absorbed by the tissue during this loading regimen, which is known as hysteresis

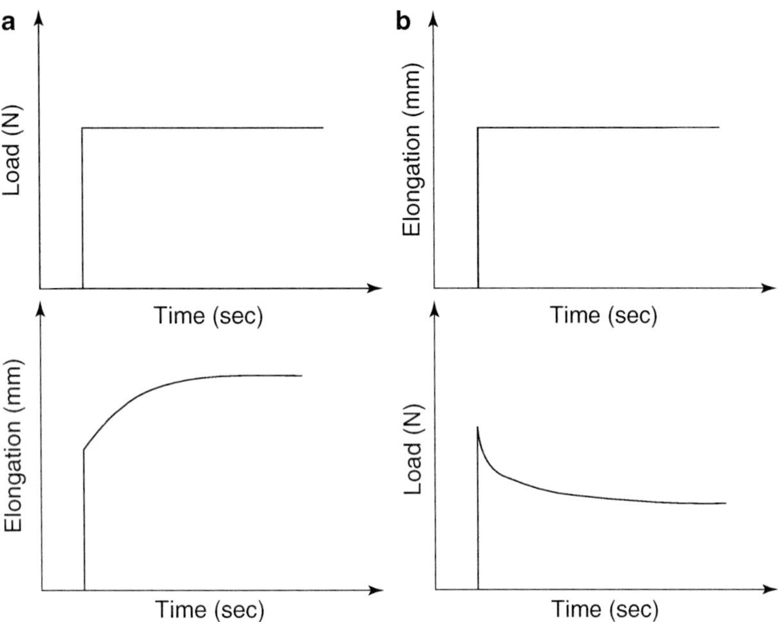

Fig. 1.6 Viscoelastic phenomena exhibited by biologic tissues include (**a**) creep response due to a constant applied load and (**b**) stress relaxation response due to a constant applied elongation over some time

a material to move or deform in response to a constant stress. Conversely, with stress relaxation, a decrease in load occurs over time upon application of a constant elongation (see Fig. 1.6b). Stress relaxation is the phenomenon that occurs in a material to relieve stress under a constant elongation due to the fluidlike characteristic of viscoelasticity. For both creep and stress relaxation, the tissue will reach a state of equilibrium after a period of time.

A practical observation of creep in the clinic is demonstrated when the length of a graft from a tendon or ligament reconstruction inevitably increases from its original length. Applying both tension and circumferential compression of hamstring ACL grafts has been shown to elongate the graft while reducing the average diameter by as much as 0.7–0.8 mm [14]. Foregoing this preconditioning could potentially lead to instability due to creep-related elongation over time as well as a mismatch of graft diameter within the bone tunnel. This is clinically relevant as surgeons may be able to reduce the size of their bone tunnel for operation, thus reducing the amount of bone removal.

Fact Box 3: Mechanics of Materials

- Mechanics of materials studies forces and their effect on motion.
- Mechanics of materials can be used to understand structural properties of whole tissue complexes and mechanical properties of individual tissue, such as ligaments.
- Biomechanical properties are important for understanding changes in the native tissue when injured, as well as important to choosing the best surgical graft for repair.

1.5 Applications

The concepts presented throughout this chapter provide a methodology to understand and quantify how the human body performs activities of daily living. This information can be used in orthopedic sports medicine to improve injury diagnosis, advance surgical reconstruction techniques, and monitor rehabilitation programs to aid the player in return to play.

1.5.1 Injury Diagnosis

Functional biomechanics can be used when evaluating and improving the diagnosis of potential injuries by conceptualizing the forces and moments (i.e., free-body diagrams) applied during an activity and identifying the appropriate tissues supporting these loads. For example, understanding the magnitude and direction of the loads applied during an anterior drawer test can aid in identifying the state of the ACL, as it is the primary restraint to anterior tibial load. Applications of biomechanics has led to the development of tools and devices capable of providing objective quantification of the pivot shift test, which can be used to identify the function and injury state of the ACL. Improving the accuracy and clinical utility of these applications will one day allow athletic programs to implement these tools in establishing a baseline measurement of each athlete's joint motions upon entering the program, thus improving diagnosis when an athlete has suffered an injury.

1.5.2 Surgical Reconstruction

The purpose of surgical reconstruction is to restore function by replacing nonfunctional tissue with a replacement, such as a graft or other implant. However, in order to adequately restore function, it is important to understand the mechanics and biomechanical properties of the original tissues and whatever material is being used to replace them. Any materials being used to replace natural tissues, such as tendons or ligaments, must be able to function under the same range of motion experienced by those connective tissues while maintaining adequate strength and stiffness. For example, the ACL is part of a complex loading environment experiencing both shear and longitudinal stresses during normal gait. The primary function of the ACL is to resist anterior translation of the tibia with respect to the femur. The graft choice for ACL reconstruction must match the stiffness of the original tissue in order to sufficiently resist anterior translation of the tibia due to the forces and moments experienced during gait. However, the graft must also be compliant enough to allow for the normal range of knee motion. Time-dependent viscoelastic properties of the graft must also be taken into account, since any amount of creep occurring after the surgical reconstruction can result in increased translations at the joint.

1.5.3 Improving Rehabilitation

Principles of biomechanics are important to consider when developing rehabilitation programs for individuals after injury and/or surgery. Statics analysis can aid the clinician in developing the best rehabilitation treatment exercise that will optimize the muscular/soft tissue activity for earlier recovery.

Designing a rehabilitation protocol that maintains range of motion and muscle strength is advantageous to the long-term healing of the patient. However, overaggressive rehabilitation could lead to failure of the repair. For example, it is common for limited weight bearing and range of motion exercises to be prescribed within the first week after an ACL reconstruction. These exercises are meant to provide functional levels of preconditioning in order to minimize the viscoelastic effects within the graft and prevent degenerative changes associated with immobilization. Knowledge of normal biomechanical properties can be used to design a regimen that would maintain motion and muscle tone while also protecting the graft used for repair, which would ultimately expedite recovery.

Conclusions

Despite the advances in diagnostic tools, surgical treatments, rehabilitations techniques, and injury prevention programs, ligament tears, particularly of the ACL, are still common in sports. The field of biomechanics will continue to explore each of these aspects of sports injury in order to improve existing treatment methods or develop newer modalities to prevent injury and expedite the players' return to play. This chapter introduced the basic terminology and concepts of statics, dynamics, and mechanics of materials using examples relevant to sports medicine and return to sport. The concepts discussed provide a guideline to approaching both static and dynamic systems to estimate unknown forces and moments experienced on the body by use of a free-body diagram. A description of biologic materials within the musculoskeletal system has been presented. Although biomechanics has great depth and breadth to it, the concepts presented should allow the reader to begin making the link between sports medicine and biomechanics.

Take-Home Message

- Newton's laws of motion are used to describe the relationship between the forces applied to the body and the results of those forces on human motion.
- Statics analysis evaluates the external effects of forces on a rigid body at rest or during motion with a constant velocity.
- Dynamic analyses evaluate bodies in motion and can be divided into two subgroups: kinematics (motion without regard to forces and moments) and kinetics (includes the effect of forces and moments).
- Mechanics of materials can be utilized to evaluate biologic materials, including both soft and hard tissues, under different forms of loading and characterize the tissue based on two categories: structural properties of whole tissue complexes (i.e., bone-ligament-bone) and mechanical properties of tissue (i.e., ligaments).
- Structural properties of tissue complexes provide the mechanics of a structure that incorporates multiple materials or tissue types and the response of this complex to tensile, shear, and compressive loading.
- Mechanical properties of tissue are evaluated by the stress-strain relationship and can be used to evaluate the quality of the tissue when making comparisons between normal, injured, and healing states.
- Understanding the biomechanical properties of tissue is important for improving injury diagnosis, generating new therapies through surgical reconstruction, and designing functional rehabilitation strategies.

Top Five Evidence Based References

Guilak F (2003) Functional tissue engineering. Springer, New York

Jung HJ, Fisher MB, Woo SL (2009) Role of biomechanics in the understanding of normal, injured, and healing ligaments and tendons. Sports Med Arthrosc Rehabil Ther Technol 1:9

Maquet PGJ (1984) Biomechanics of the knee: with application to the pathogenesis and the surgical treatment of osteoarthritis, vol 2nd, expand and rev. Springer, New York

Nissan M (1980) Review of some basic assumptions in knee biomechanics. J Biomech 13:375–381

Nordin M, Frankel VH (1989) Basic biomechanics of the musculoskeletal system, vol Vol 2. Lea & Febiger, Philadelphia

References

1. Naendrup JH, Zlotnicki JP, Chao T, Nagai K, Musahl V (2016) Kinematic outcomes following ACL reconstruction. Curr Rev Musculoskelet Med 9:348–360
2. Borgstrom PH, Markolf KL, Wang Y, Xu X, Yang PR, Joshi NB et al (2015) Use of inertial sensors to predict pivot-shift grade and diagnose an ACL injury during preoperative testing. Am J Sports Med 43:857–864
3. Kuroda R, Hoshino Y (2016) Electromagnetic tracking of the pivot-shift. Curr Rev Musculoskelet Med 9:164–169
4. Engstrom B, Johansson C, Tornkvist H (1991) Soccer injuries among elite female players. Am J Sports Med 19:372–375
5. Wang H, Fleischli JE, Zheng NN (2013) Transtibial versus anteromedial portal technique in single-bundle anterior cruciate ligament reconstruction: outcomes of knee joint kinematics during walking. Am J Sports Med 41:1847–1856
6. Czamara A, Markowska I, Krolikowska A, Szopa A, Domagalska Szopa M (2015) Kinematics of rotation in joints of the lower limbs and pelvis during gait: early results-SB ACLR approach versus DB ACLR approach. Biomed Res Int 2015:707168

7. Hamner DL, Brown CH Jr, Steiner ME, Hecker AT, Hayes WC (1999) Hamstring tendon grafts for reconstruction of the anterior cruciate ligament: biomechanical evaluation of the use of multiple strands and tensioning techniques. J Bone Joint Surg Am 81:549–557
8. Cooper DE, Deng XH, Burstein AL, Warren RF (1993) The strength of the central third patellar tendon graft. A biomechanical study. Am J Sports Med 21:818–823. discussion 823–814
9. Staubli HU, Schatzmann L, Brunner P, Rincon L, Nolte LP (1996) Quadriceps tendon and patellar ligament: cryosectional anatomy and structural properties in young adults. Knee Surg Sports Traumatol Arthrosc 4:100–110
10. Abramowitch SD, Yagi M, Tsuda E, Woo SL (2003) The healing medial collateral ligament following a combined anterior cruciate and medial collateral ligament injury--a biomechanical study in a goat model. J Orthop Res 21:1124–1130
11. Woo SL, Orlando CA, Gomez MA, Frank CB, Akeson WH (1986) Tensile properties of the medial collateral ligament as a function of age. J Orthop Res 4:133–141
12. Woo SL, Gomez MA, Woo YK, Akeson WH (1982) Mechanical properties of tendons and ligaments. II. The relationships of immobilization and exercise on tissue remodeling. Biorheology 19:397–408
13. Noyes FR (1977) Functional properties of knee ligaments and alterations induced by immobilization: a correlative biomechanical and histological study in primates. Clin Orthop Relat Res:210–242
14. Cruz AI Jr, Fabricant PD, Seeley MA, Ganley TJ, Lawrence JT (2016) Change in size of hamstring grafts during preparation for ACL reconstruction: effect of tension and circumferential compression on graft diameter. J Bone Joint Surg Am 98:484–489

Emerging Concepts in Human Performance Optimization

2

Christopher Connaboy, Matthew E. Darnell, Shawn Eagle, Caleb D. Johnson, and Bradley C. Nindl

Contents

2.1 Overview

Human performance optimization is a broad term used to refer to maximizing the potential for success in occupational and competitive athletes who fall into a wide range of populations. In the context of football, human performance optimization falls to a number of disciplines, including coaches, trainers, physiotherapists, and dieticians. Further, the modalities for improving human performance align with these professions and can include optimizing physical characteristics (strength, power, speed, aerobic capacity, fatigue resistance), technical skills (passing, shooting, tackling), nutrition, and injury risk profiles. Given the highly competitive arena that football clubs operate in globally, the aforementioned disciplines are always looking for a way to give their player's the smallest edge over other clubs.

C. Connaboy, Ph.D. (✉) • M.E. Darnell, Ph.D.
S. Eagle • C.D. Johnson • B.C. Nindl, Ph.D.
Neuromuscular Research Laboratory/Warrior Human Performance Research Center, Department of Sports Medicine and Nutrition, School of Health and Rehabilitation Sciences, University of Pittsburgh, 3860 South Water Street, Pittsburgh, PA, 15203, USA
e-mail: connaboy@pitt.edu

V. Musahl et al. (eds.), *Return to Play in Football*, https://doi.org/10.1007/978-3-662-55713-6_2

While many concepts around human performance optimization in football are well known and developed, the field is ever evolving. Old practices are shown to be ineffective, and new practices are tested and implemented to replace them. Therefore, staying in tune with the latest developments and ideas in human performance optimization is key for clinicians charged with its practice. This chapter will outline emerging concepts, both in football literature and clinical practice, related to training, injury prevention, nutrition, and technologies used for monitoring and tracking human performance characteristics.

Incorporation of resistance training into a fitness regimen has been widely recommended for maintaining or improving overall health, as well as athletic performance [1]. Resistance training has been shown to decrease blood pressure, improve glucose tolerance and insulin sensitivity, and reduce osteoporosis, among a myriad of other potential benefits [2–5]. Reductions in total body fat, local adipose tissue, and increased basal metabolic rate have also been noted previously in those performing resistance training [6] Relative to athletic performance, a specific resistance training program can increase muscular strength, power, speed, muscle size, endurance, balance, and coordination [7]. The health benefits of resistance training are widely noted, and improvements in athletic characteristics, like muscular strength, are often seen as a result of resistance training [8].

2.2 Guiding Principles of Training Adaptation

2.2.1 Progressive Overload

Progressive overload refers to gradually increasing the stress placed on the body during a resistance training program [9]. The human body has an innate ability to adapt to increasing levels of stress; thus, it is necessary to incrementally increase the force output demand to elicit continuous adaptations to resistance training over an extended period of time [6]. Increasing "stress" during a resistance training program should be highly individualized and could include increasing the load, manipulations of frequency or duration of training, changing the speed with which a repetition is completed, altering rest periods between sets, or increasing training volume (number of repetitions completed in a single session) [9–11]. Applying overload should be specific to the desired adaptations one is trying to elicit from the resistance training program [9, 11].

2.2.2 Specificity

Specificity refers to the body's response and adaptations to an applied stimulus [6, 9, 10]. A resistance training program should be individualized, and the exercises chosen should mimic the specific demands of the individual's sport (see Fact Box 3 for a football-specific needs analysis) [11, 12]. Physiological adaptations are specific to the exercises that are completed and include movement velocity, range of motion, energy systems utilized, and muscle actions involved [6, 9–11].

2.2.3 Variation

Resistance training variation is a systematic altering of the training stimulus [6, 9–11]. Application of this principle is crucial for obtaining continual adaptations, especially over long-term training programs [6, 9]. Further, variety can help limit "staleness" in those being trained and can enhance adherence to training programs [9, 11]. Altering training volume and intensity have been shown to best optimize training adaptations in athletic populations [10, 11]. Indeed, a recent systematic review concluded that varying the stimulus, relative to the individual's training history, is of greater importance than the type of periodization chosen to design the program [13].

2.3 Basics of Program Design

The American College of Sports Medicine recommends using periodized over non-periodized training in healthy adults [14]. Periodization, at its core, has three fundamental goals: (1) to provide an outline for maintaining a certain level of physical fitness pertinent to success in sport, (2) to reduce the potential for overtraining, and (3) to reach maximum physical fitness at the most appropriate time, i.e., competition [15, 16]. The concept can be divided into two overarching categories: linear, or "traditional," and nonlinear. Both methods have been shown to elicit significant adaptations, but according to the current evidence, there is no difference in the magnitude of fitness gains between the two [13]. Still, arguments for and against each type of periodization remain highly debated.

2.3.1 Linear Periodization

Linear periodization is a design where the initial training load is characterized as high volume/low intensity and gradual progression through the training program leads to lower-volume but higher-intensity exercises [9, 11]. The end goal is preparation for a competition, so the high-intensity exercises would ideally peak near the competition date. The linear periodization model can be broken down into cycles; weekly, monthly, and multi-monthly cycles have been previously described [9, 11]. Comprehensive descriptions of micro- (weekly), meso- (monthly), and macrocycles (multi-monthly) can be found elsewhere and are beyond the scope of this work [9, 11]. Linear periodization can be viewed as the "traditional" model, as it has a well-established record of success for increasing physical fitness adaptations [13]. However, modifications have been proposed that suggest linear periodization may not be optimal for training advanced athletes.

2.3.2 Nonlinear Periodization

Nonlinear periodization, sometimes referred to as "undulating" periodization, uses shorter cycles (daily, weekly, or biweekly) to add more variety to the training stimulus [9, 11, 13]. Stone and colleagues [17] have suggested that this type of periodization may be more appropriate for advanced athletes, whereas linear may be best suited for novice athletes due to the likelihood of gradual intensity increases still able to induce adaptations in the novice nervous system. Further, it has been suggested that nonlinear periodization may be more applicable to train athletes with multiple in-season contests [9]. Given that most football leagues have an 11-month season and that the top teams in the most competitive European leagues compete in three separate competitions during one season [18], a strong case could be made for using undulating periodization in elite football.

2.4 Progressive Concepts in Football Human Performance Training

2.4.1 The Volume Conundrum

A professional player in top leagues has an off-season period of ~4–6 weeks per year. Coupled with the volume of matches during the season, this insufficient detraining period makes for a mentally and physically demanding season. The grueling pace of the schedule and the physiological demand of a single match are often reasons cited for lesser volume of training, during the off-season and season alike. This strategy may place players at a disadvantage in the early part of their season, as they try to readjust to the demands of play. For example, top-level professional soccer players, following typical off-season training guidelines (2 weeks rest, 4 weeks with moderate training load), have demonstrated a decrease in aerobic performance accompanied by an increase in body fat mass and reduction of fat-free mass in the lower limbs [18]. A 2-week period of rest can have considerable negative effects on aerobic capacity, especially in highly trained athletes [18, 19]. These results suggest the importance of a well-designed year-long program to limit physiological losses, so that a 2-week rest period is not necessary to mitigate concerns of overtraining.

2.4.2 Individualized Training

Responses to training stimuli can be highly variable between players and relative to a number of individual physiological and psychological factors [20, 21]. While the gap between research and application needs to be more limited, taking an individual's intrinsic and extrinsic factors into account while balancing training schedules is where the "art" of strength and conditioning meets the science. Even the highest level of athlete has week-to-week variation in their performance [20, 22]. Simple statistical measures, such as coefficient of variation, smallest worthwhile change, and accumulation of marginal gains can provide a practitioner with highly useful tools to individualize a player's training and understand if their current practices are making useful adaptations (see Fact Boxes 1 and 2) [22, 23].

Fact Box 1

An emerging concept in training athletes is repurposing the concept of prehabilitation. Once limited to a pre-surgical exercise prescription designed to encourage quicker and more successful outcomes post-surgery [24], prehabilitation has been applied to training programs for injury prevention purposes in healthy athletes [2, 25, 102]. Strictly speaking, prehabilitation programs are designed to optimize function and pain measures before injury and should be used as an adjunct to a broader strength and conditioning program [24, 25]. Thus, prehabilitation can be usefully applied in athletes who are participating in sports with high incidence of specific injuries (see below for an example), or they can be useful in correcting functional deficiencies that are causing pain, as in an overuse condition like patellofemoral pain syndrome [1].

For example, hamstring strains are one of the most common injuries reported in football [3, 69]. Factors such as inadequate warm-up, fatigue, muscular imbalances, muscular weakness, and lack of flexibility have been indicated as important contributors to suffering a hamstring strain [62]. Applying a specific prehabilitation strategy could be useful in mitigating injury risk based on these factors. Eccentric strength training has been demonstrated repeatedly to be a superior method to increase strength in the hamstrings as well as lower injury risk in football players [26, 40, 47, 71, 89, 103]. A combination of warm-up stretching and eccentric strength training has been shown to decrease hamstring injury risk in elite football players, compared to flexibility training alone [89]. Side-to-side hamstring strength imbalances have also been shown to increase injury risk in football players, and, importantly, risk can be lowered when imbalances are normalized after an eccentric strength training intervention [47]. Therefore, based on the evidence, the following prehabilitation program could be applied in warm-up to limit hamstring strain incidence:

Exercise	Description	Prescription		
		Sets	Reps per set	Rest (min)
Alternating toe touches	Take a step forward with right leg and bend from the waist: to touch ground with left hand in front of right foot. Keep slight bend (~30°) in the stepping foot. Alternate legs until 50 yards have been covered	2	50 yards	1
Single leg squats	Descend until the thigh is near parallel to the ground by bending at the knee and stand up. Focus on pushing hips back during decent and keep upper body upright. Use partner for support if necessary	1	10/side	1

360° lunge[a]	(1) Step into a forward lunge with right foot and return to standing position. (2) Step ~45° forward into a lunge and return. (3) Step right into a side lunge and return. (4) Step backwards ~135° into a lunge and return. (5) Step right leg 180° back into a reverse hinge and return. That sequence is one rep; repeat five times per side	2	5/side	1
Nordic lowers	Kneel on the ground and use a partner to stabilize at the ankles. Keep the body in a straight line from the head down through the knees. Slowly lower upper body down to ground and push back to the starting position	2	5	2
Partner hamstring stretch	Lie supine on the ground and use a partner to raise a straight leg in hip flexion until resistance is met. Hold at sticking point for 1 min and repeat with leg slightly bent (~30°)	1	1/side	None
Hip flexor stretch	Lie prone on the ground and use a partner to raise a bent knee into hip extension until resistance is met. Hold at sticking point for 1 min and repeat on other side	1	1/side	None

[a]360° Lunge Diagram

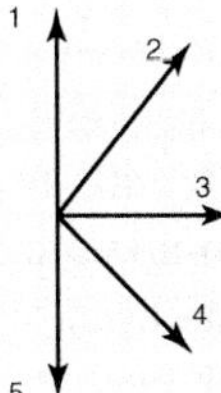

Fact Box 2

An athlete's performance level can vary from day to day. This variation can be thought of as **noise** that clouds interpretation of the **signal**, or actual performance value. Moreover, the instruments used to measure performance carry a certain amount of noise, as well. This reality necessitates the need for practitioners to evaluate an individual's performance variation for a given measurement as well as the error ("noise") that the measuring instrument possesses, in order to determine a real and meaningful change. Variation in performance is described as the **coefficient of variation (CV)** whereas meaningful changes are discussed as **smallest worthwhile change**, or the minimum value needed to demonstrate change in that individual's performance. Implementation of these methods can provide crucial information about how an athlete is responding to training at an individual level. Understanding and applying these principles can be especially beneficial in training elite footballers, with extensive training history. Highly trained individuals will not be capable of obtaining large "gains'" in physical performance, compared to novice footballers. As such, an interesting new training ideology has emerged in training elite athletes called **aggregation of marginal gains**. While novice athletes may observe fitness improvements at or greater than 30% in the early stages of training, elite athletes may struggle to improve on performance levels. However, small improvements

(~1–2%) in performance may be satisfactory to create a competitive edge at the highest level of competition. Further, accumulating these small improvements over several seasons may separate professional athletes from the truly elite. A football-specific example is offered below.

Repeated sprint ability (RSA) is a seminal test in football that evaluates a combination of neuromuscular and metabolic fitness. RSA test performance can even discriminate between amateur and professional footballers. Let's take a look at how to apply progressive statistics to human performance within the RSA.

Table 1. Repealed RSA tests for one professional player throughout their rookie season						**Mean ± SD (95% CI)**
RSA (secs)	6.35	6.28	6.31	6.25	6.24	6.29 ± 0.05 (6.23–6.34)

So, 0.05 s is the noise (error) within the signal (individual test performance) in the RSA. The smallest worthwhile change for this individual then is 0.06 s. You can think of this as reliable change in performance: the smallest change that is greater than the athlete's individual CV.

Table 2. Repeated RSA tests for one professional player over their next five seasons						**Mean ± SD (95% CI)**
RSA (secs)	6.26	6.25	6.23	6.23	6.21	6.24 ± 0.02 (6.21–6.26)

So, this player's mean RSA performance from their rookie season to the end of their sixth season improved by 5%. When training a novice athlete, this would be a terrible result, given their capacity for adaptation. However, in a top-level, highly trained athlete, improving a skill by 5% is likely to be a noticeable improvement. This example illustrates the concept of **aggregation of marginal gains**, as minor improvements were made year to year (~1–2%), but the end result is a worthwhile aggregate improvement over time.

2.4.3 Injury Prevention

The future of football training may place less emphasis on enhancing fitness and more on preventing injuries. Preventing injuries has been documented to have a significant, positive effect on *team performance*. Lower injury rates strongly correlate with final league ranking and team success in major professional leagues [24–26]. Unfortunately, however, there is still a significant gap between cutting-edge sports medicine research and implementation in practice [27]. A survey of premier league soccer teams and their medical staff found that a majority of injury perceptions and interventions in current practice had a low level of evidence [28]. While this does not imply that the practices are not effective, it highlights the gap between research and practice. Given the high level of injury rates in football (~1000× greater than other occupations [25]) and the magnitude of cost (i.e., individual long-term health, club finances, and team performance [28]), injury prevention should be critical in football training.

2.5 Emerging Concepts in Sports Performance Optimization: Nutrition

To achieve optimal performance, an athlete needs both appropriate training and nutrition. Without adequate nutrition, it is difficult for the body to fully recover and adapt to a training stimulus, decreasing an athlete's performance and increasing risk for overtraining and injury [29–31]. One emerging concept in the field of sports nutrition includes individualized and periodized nutrition programs to match energy and macronutrient needs of training and competition [31, 32] (see Fact Box 3).

Fact Box 3 Football needs analysis

Physiology

Football is a physiologically demanding sport, characterized by continual, intermittent bursts of high-intensity activity (e.g., sprinting, jumping, cutting, changing direction) followed by lower intensity activity. As a result, unique demands are placed on an athlete's physiological system, as both the *aerobic and anaerobic systems* are taxed throughout a match. Footballers have demonstrated high aerobic capacities, which is a necessity to endure the lengthy matches and is crucial to buffer lactate buildup from the bursts of anaerobic activity. For success in football, high levels of anaerobic and aerobic fitness will be necessary.

Neuromuscular

Explosive actions, such as kicking, jumping, and sprinting, are crucial for success in football. In fact, it has been reported that 83% of goals are preceded by at least one "powerful action" in the sequence leading up to the score. Thus, training that incorporates *power* through enhancing rate of force development is necessary. Furthermore, since football is a highly strenuous physiological activity, improving *power endurance* may be paramount, as well. The capacity to generate force quickly is diminished when fatigued, so limiting the difference between a footballer's power output when unfatigued versus after strenuous activity may give a team the edge late in matches.

Musculoskeletal

Muscular strength is an important component of a successful footballer, both in performance and prevention of injury. Musculoskeletal injuries are still quite pervasive in all levels of football. While important strides have been made, such as a documented decline in ligamentous injuries, injuries to muscle (i.e., strains) have not declined. Injury prevention programs, such as "the 11" or "FIFA 11+" have decreased injury incidence in football teams. An enhanced version that targets maintaining muscular integrity specifically may help decrease this continuous issue within the sport.

2.5.1 Periodized Nutrition

The field of sports nutrition applies to a broad range of individuals participating in a variety of different athletic activities, each with unique physiological demands depending on the sport. Even more, the physiological demands can also vary within a particular sport (i.e., a goalie vs. a midfielder in football). Add in individual athlete's weight goals (lose/gain weight, decrease body fat, or increase lean mass) and these variations can make it easy to understand why blanket nutrition recommendations are not appropriate for athletes. In addition to nutrition plans matching individual goals, they also need to match the intensity and level of training the athlete is currently participating in. The foundation of a well-planned nutrition program focuses on matching energy intake to the energy demands of the athlete and their training. From there, carbohydrate, protein, and fat needs can be determined to meet caloric needs as well as to fuel the specific metabolic demands and goals of the current training plan.

2.5.2 Energy Needs

Calorie needs and requirements for athletes vary depending on training and athlete goals. In periods of weight maintenance, the goal for optimal performance should be for the athlete to achieve equilibrium between energy intake and total energy expenditure (TEE). TEE is the sum of basal metabolic rate (BMR), the thermic effects of food, and the thermic effect of activity (which includes planned, spontaneous, and non-exercise activity). When accurate measures of body composition are available, the Cunningham equation is a reliable formula to estimate basal metabolic rate in an athletic population [33, 34]. The Cunningham equations uses fat-free mass (FFM) to predict resting energy expenditure ($22 \times FFM + 500$). Total daily energy expenditure can then be estimated by multiplying the BMR by an activity factor or by using a physical activity compendium to determine metabolic cost during training activities [35]. For athletes engaged in moderate-heavy training, an activity factor of 1.6–1.9 is recommended [36, 37].

2.5.3 Carbohydrate Needs

The importance of carbohydrates for team sport athletes is often overshadowed by the overwhelming focus on protein consumption. However, carbohydrates especially in the form of glycogen provide the main energy sources for these athletes during competition and training [38]. Resistance training has been shown to reduce glycogen stores as much as 40% [39] and single or repeated sprint exercise has been shown to reduce glycogen stores in the muscle by 14% [40] and 47% [41] respectively. In order to maintain energy and intensity levels during training (especially when training multiple times per day), carbohydrates should be consumed in adequate amounts to restore and replenish glycogen losses from activity [31, 42]. Evidence suggests that during moderate training lasting about 1 h carbohydrate intake should be between 5 and 7 g/kg of body weight and between 6 and 10 g/kg body weight for moderate- to high-intensity exercise lasting 1–3 h [31, 43]. Adequate carbohydrate consumption is important for maximizing training potential, allowing athletes to train at higher intensities or for longer duration before fatigue [44]. In addition to maintaining energy levels, carbohydrate intake has also been suggested to aid in muscle recovery. Carbohydrate intake combined with protein provides the right type of environment for muscles to repair and restore glycogen levels [45, 46].

2.5.4 Protein Needs

Inadequate protein intake is seldom a concern for athletes. The majority of football players reports protein intakes that easily meet or exceed the recommendations for athletes [47]. Protein recommendations for athletes range from 1.2 to 2.0 g per kg of body weight [48]. Previous protein recommendations were set ranges based on athlete categories (strength versus endurance), with strength-trained athletes having higher recommended intakes than endurance trained [37]. However, recent research indicates that protein needs should be determined instead by training loads, training experience, and energy availability [31]. Protein is in greater demand when training intensities increase, training frequency increases, or if a new training stimulus is introduced. Similarly, novice athletes have a greater need for high amounts of protein. The increased demand is due largely to the increased muscle protein breakdown that results in all of these scenarios [45]. In athletes that are following a calorie-restricted diet in efforts to lose weight, higher levels of protein may be beneficial. In a study conducted by Mettler et al., athletes who followed a calorie-restricted diet and consumed approximately 2.3 g protein per kg body weight lost significantly less lean body mass than those who consumed a diet consisting of 1.0 g protein per kg of body weight [49].

2.5.5 Fat Needs

After determining carbohydrate and protein needs for athletes, the remainder of the calories needed should come from fat. In most cases, fat intake should be between 20 and 35% of total calories [31]. Diets containing less than 10% of calories from fat may lead to nutrient deficiencies and hormonal imbalances [36, 50], and higher fat diets (>60% of calories) have not shown to be beneficial for improved performance in intermittent high-intensity-type activities [51]. Some resources provide fat recommendations in grams per kilogram of body weight similar to the protein and carbohydrate recommendations. Generally 0.8–1.0 g of fat per kg of body weight would be deemed appropriate for team sport athletes [52]. For long-term health, athletes should limit amounts of saturated fat intake to no more than 10% of total calories while aiming to consume more mono- and polyunsaturated fats [53].

2.5.6 Nutrient Timing: Recovery

Determining total daily macronutrient and energy needs for athletes in relation to training demands is the fundamental base for developing a periodized nutrition plan. The next phase in developing a periodized plan focuses on proper frequency and timing of these nutrients to maximize performance and physical adaptation to training. A handful of nutrition strategies have been researched for pre-, during, and post-event fueling for optimizing performance during competition or specific training sessions [38, 43, 54, 55]. Although both before and during event nutrition strategies are important, a particular amount of attention has been given to recovery or post-training/competition strategies for optimizing performance and adaptations to training [56]. Similar to determining total energy and macronutrient needs per day, recovery nutrition needs should also be periodized to match the demands of the training bout or event (Table 2.1) [31, 32, 56].

A key element of producing and monitoring a periodized nutrition and training program is the quantification of an athlete's training volume and intensities. Traditionally quantification of training volume and intensities are usually calculated by monitoring the length of training as well as the athletes' and/or coaches' subjective perceptions of the difficulty of the training. Recently, new technologies and products have been developed that may aid in more objectively monitoring training intensities.

Table 2.1 Periodized nutrition recovery

Intensity	Description	Nutrition recovery recommendations
Hard	High volume/ intensity Competition Multi-session training days	Refuel immediately after training for best recovery 1.0–1.2 g/kg body weight carbohydrate 0.25–0.4 g/kg body weight protein 1.3 L of fluid for every kg lost (consider electrolyte replacement)
Moderate	Medium volume/ intensity Single sessions (18–24 h between sessions)	Refuel within 30–60 min 0.5–1.0 g/kg body weight carbohydrate 0.25 g/kg body weight protein 1–1.3 L fluid for every kg lost
Light	Single session (>24 h between sessions) "Easy" or "recovery" days	Timing less critical Eat a balanced snack or meal within 2 h

2.6 Emerging Concepts: Technological Developments

Player monitoring is an important concept in the modern game, as clubs, coaches, and players themselves seek to optimize individual player performance. Player monitoring has many goals, including identifying training need(s), tracking performance across multiple physiological/psychological/biomechanical domains, monitoring adherence to training programs, determining response(s) to training programs, measuring and classifying quality and quantity of sleep, identifying possible overtraining/overreaching, detecting injury risk potential, benchmarking key performance markers, and providing data to inform the return to play decision-making process. Ensuring that players receive an optimal training stimulus, maximize their rest and sleep, maintain optimal nutritional intake and hydration status, and return to play in a timely manner requires the collection, processing, and management of an extensive amount of information. In view of the complexity and multifactorial nature of human performance optimization, it is important that the information gathered when monitoring the players provides the coaching staff and performance optimization team with appropriate data to inform their decision-making processes. Therefore, the validity, availability, accuracy, organization, and management of the all data collected to monitor the player status are integral to the process of performance optimization.

2.7 Player Monitoring Using Wearable Technology

Recently, there has been a large increase in the amount of commercially available, wearable player monitoring technologies. This plethora of available technologies raises numerous questions for the coaching, performance, and sports medicine team overseeing the performance optimization process (see Table 2.2). Addressing questions surrounding the selection, determination of the cost/benefit, and implementation of such technologies to successfully monitor the players becomes an important challenge. Indeed, McCall et al. [20] highlight the contention between the performance optimization teams' desire to be innovative and early adopters of "cutting-edge" technology in the pursuit of a competitive advantage, balanced against the need to retain an evidence-based practice approach to player performance enhancement. There is a requirement for any player monitor technology to add value and provide a level of reliability and validity to enable the assessments of real and meaningful changes in performance over a requisite time frame [20].

To explore some of the emerging concepts related to optimizing football performance, two areas will be discussed in detail: one from a technology-based point of view, examining the utility and employment of existing technology with respect to player monitoring in football, and a second examining player monitoring from a research focus (its associated technology) and its potential utility within the process of player performance optimization.

2.7.1 Catapult Sensors in Football Training

Player tracking technology, such as the Catapult system (Catapult Innovations, Canberra Australia: Fig. 2.2), utilize Global Positioning System (GPS) technology, integrated with a triaxial accelerometer, 3D gyroscope, 3D magnetometer, and heart rate monitor. Contained in a unit small and light enough to be worn with a tight-fitting harness during normal training and athletic play, this integration of technologies allows for the automated calculation of a number of variables related to the physical demands of training and match play in football. With extensive literature demonstrating their validity and reliability, the Catapult system is the most widely used of this type of sensor among most field-based sports, including football [57–61]. Football coaches and trainers using the Catapult system range from English Premier League and German Bundesliga clubs to US collegiate squads.

The number of player-specific variables capable of being calculated by the Catapult system sensors are wide-ranging, including distance traveled, maximal and average speeds, time spent at different exercise intensities (i.e., high, middle, low) or movement velocities (i.e., jogging, running, sprinting), total distance covered at different exercise intensities or movement velocities, training load, and magnitude and frequency of impacts. Of particular interest for football clubs is training load, termed "Body Load" in the Catapult software, which is calculated by summing the duration of activities at different exercise intensities across a given period of training or match play. Impacts are measured through accelerometer and gyroscope data and are a measurement of contact with players or other external forces. Generally this has been applied more toward Australian Rules Football and rugby; however, it may have some applicability for sports medicine professionals working with football athletes [62].

The practical applications for Catapult-collected data in football are many. Some of the well-researched applications include quantifying the differences in physical demand between types of training (small- vs. large-sided games, drills vs. gameplay) and training and competition, quantifying differences in demand between positions, and comparing methods of quantifying training load [63–66]. Applications of the Catapult system that have yet to be explored include tracking the effects

Table 2.2 Player Monitoring Technology

Equipment name	Variables measured	Validation and reliability	Research in football
Integrated wearable technologies			
EquiVital™—TnR model (Fig. 2.1)	Acceleration, velocity, distance, heart rate (HR) (2-lead ECG), breathing rate, skin temperature, galvanic skin response, energy expenditure (EE)	*Team sports:* Unknown *General:* [77, 78]	Impellizzeri [79]
Catapult—OptimEye and MinimaxX models	Acceleration, velocity, distance, HR, impacts, training intensity, training load, EE	*Team sports*: [58, 60, 61]	Casamichana [63, 64] Hill-Haas [66] Harley [65]
Catapult—GPSports models (Fig. 2.2)	Acceleration, velocity, distance, HR, impacts, training intensity, training load, EE	*Team sports*: [57–59]	Hill-Haas [66] Castagna [80]
Garmin—Forerunner and Vivoactive® HR models	Acceleration, velocity, distance, HR, elevation change, training intensity	*Team sports*: Unknown *General*: [81]	Brandes [82] Hennig [83]
ActiGraph	Acceleration, velocity, energy expenditure, sleep latency and time	*Team sports*: Unknown *General:* [84–86]	Briggs [87] Robey [81] Sæther [88]
Polar Team Pro models	Acceleration, velocity, distance, HR, training intensity, training load	*Team sports*: Unknown *General*: [89, 90]	Owen [91] Castagna [92] Kelly [93]
Sport Performance Tracker (SPT™)	Distance, velocity, training intensity (estimated w/o HR)	*Team sports*: Unknown *General*: Unknown	Unknown
Strength and power			
Handheld dynamometry (number of manufacturers)	Isometric and eccentric strength: peak force, time to peak force, average force	Thorborg [94, 95] Stark [96] Piva [97] Stoll [98]	Nilstad [99] Thorborg [100, 101] Engebretesen [102]
Tendo Sports—Tendo Unit models	On weighted lifts: average/peak power, partial average power, average/peak bar velocity, peak force, eccentric average velocity	Garnacho-Castaño [103] Sato [104] Stock [105]	Palmer [106] Jajtner [107]
Body composition			
Intelametrix®—BodyMetrix™	Body fat %, muscle cross-sectional area	Wagner [108] Cain [109]	Unknown
Heart rate monitor systems			
Firstbeat—Sports models	HR and HR variability, estimations of: O_2 consumption, EE	Smolander [110] Montgomery [111]	Luhtanen [112] Vanttinen [113]
Agility and response time			
FitLight trainer™	Response/movement time and accuracy to a visual stimulus	N/A	Unknown
Movement screenings			
Functional Movement Screen (FMS™)	Subjective ratings of movement deficiencies and asymmetries	*Validity*: Questionable [114, 115] *Reliability*: [116]	Smith [117] Chorba [118]

of fatigue throughout a match relative to decrements in running velocity and overall activity. Further, this data on the progression of fatigue could be combined with data on technical performance (shots on target, percentage of passes completed, etc.), enabling coaches and trainers to track a player's training load and its impact, negative or positive, on performance in matches. Probably the most significant applications yet to be fully explored are related to tracking a player's training load, physical performance, and potential fatigue and utilizing these variables to individualize their training, return to play after an injury, or substitution strategy during matches.

2.7.2 Monitoring Players' Sleep

Sleep plays a critical role in the recovery process of elite athletes, providing essential physiological and psychological functions to recover from the neurometabolic costs associated with the waking state [67, 68]. Disturbances (deprivation, dysregulation, and/or disruption) to sleep are suggested to be detrimental to post-football match recovery, as a consequence of factors such as diminished muscle glycogen replenishment, increased mental fatigue, reduction in muscle damage repair [68], autonomic nervous system imbalance, and increases in pro-inflammatory cytokines potentially promoting immune system dysfunction [69]. Recent research [70] has highlighted the extent to which sleep is already recognized by football players as an important and vital recovery modality, and further research has suggested, albeit anecdotally, that sleep is the most efficacious recovery strategy [71]. Given the recognition of the requirement for optimal levels of recovery to balance the stresses of training and competition [69], it would be expected that the importance of good sleep hygiene is a priority for both practitioners and researchers in the athletic arena. However, the sleep needs of athletes in general, and in football players specifically, has not been extensively researched or routinely monitored [72].

While there are many factors which are thought to influence sleep quantity and quality in football players, including both acute (arousal level, exposure to bright polychromatic lights (floodlights), mood, caffeine/alcohol consumption, etc.) and chronic (inconsistencies in playing schedule, individual chronotype (i.e., night owls), early morning training schedule, etc.) stressors, the individual player's response(s) needs to be determined in order to generate data to provide actionable information and make informed decisions. Indeed, Nédélec et al. [68]

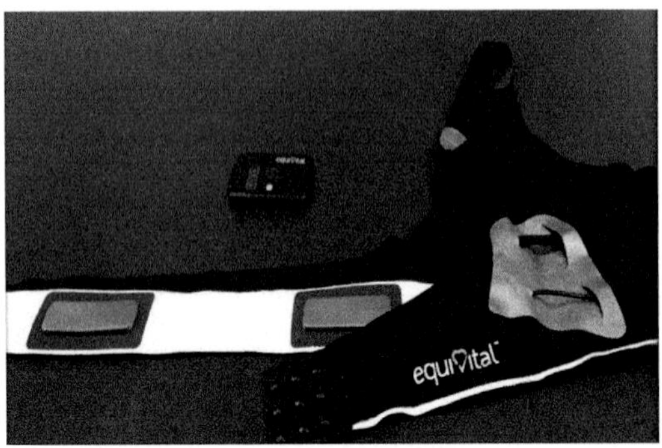

Fig. 2.1 The Equivital™ EQ02 LifeMonitor

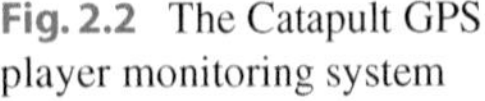

Fig. 2.2 The Catapult GPS player monitoring system

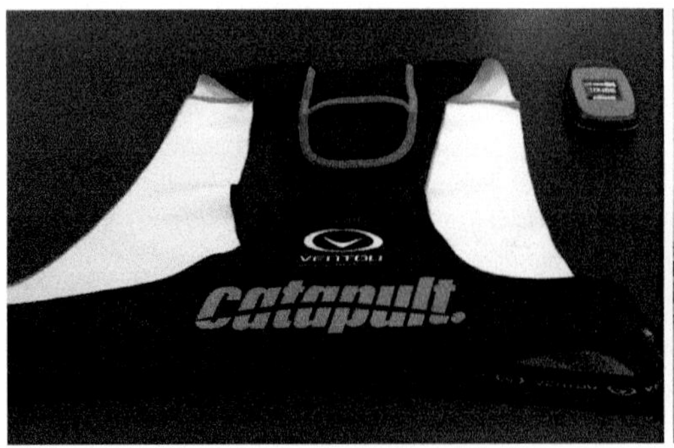

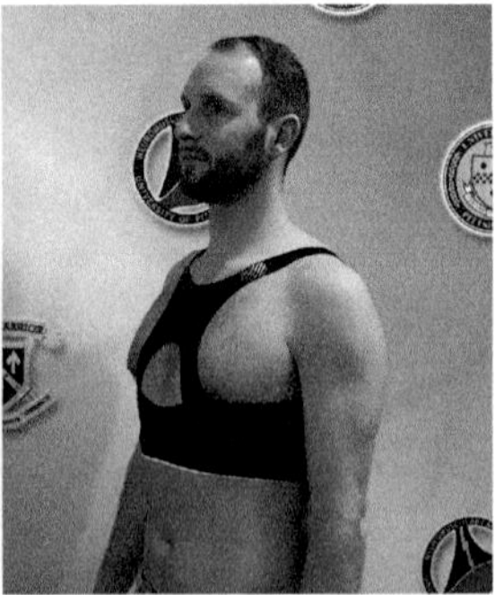

suggest that the complexity and multifactorial nature of the interactions between sleep, recovery, training, and performance requires the capture of detailed sleep quality and quantity data in conjunction with the monitoring of exposure to acute and chronic stressors to further understand their relationships and enable efficient and individualized solutions to promote optimal recovery.

2.7.3 Actigraphy

In response to this need to monitor players' sleep and examine their reactions to the many factors which may influence sleep quality and quantity, valid, cost-effective, and nonintrusive solutions have been sought. Wristwatch actigraphy, such as the ActiGraph™, represents a potential solution and is able to capture several measures of sleep quality and quantity from the raw actigraphy data collected (time in bed, time asleep, time awake, percentage time sleeping when in bed, sleep efficiency, sleep latency, moving minutes, percentage moving time, and sleep restlessness (fragmentation index)). Wristwatch actigraphy is widely utilized in sleep studies [73, 74] and has been shown to produce accurate and reliable measures of sleep when compared to the gold standard polysomnography [75]. Thus, the actigraphy measures are extremely useful for identifying potential issues with a player's sleep, which may then be acted upon to ameliorate any of the factors/stressors which may have led to the sleep disturbance/disruption.

While the validity, reliability, and utility of the actigraphy technology are not in question for the assessment of sleep behavior, the adoption of the wrist-worn technology to aid in the monitoring of player recovery may not be guaranteed. The acceptability and adoption of any wearable technology, such as player tracking systems or wristwatch actigraphy to monitor player performance, are critically dependent on "buy in" from key stakeholders (coaches, players, members of the sports medicine team, and club officials). It has recently been recognized that, in the fast-moving player-focused environment, key decision-makers are concerned with simple "yes/no" answers to questions such as can the player train/play and/or will they suffer recurrent injury [20]? The large quantity of data produced, its quality, data accessibility, and its ease of analysis to produce actionable information, all combine to challenge the utility and adoption of a specific technology. This is further challenged when you consider the vast amounts of data from multiple data sources contained within the variety of wearable technologies that may be employed to capture the required data to effectively monitor player performance. This represents the challenge of "big data," where the abundance of information that can be collected when monitoring a player can be both a blessing and a curse. When attempting to make informed and evidence-based decisions related to the optimization of a player's performance, the abundance of available data can overwhelm and hinder the decision making process.

The promise of a wealth of data to monitor and better understand the complexity and multifactorial nature of human performance optimization via wearable technologies is extremely tempting. However, the potential value and utility of the data have to be balanced against the challenges and costs associated with processing, managing, and interpreting the large amounts of information available from these wearable player monitoring technologies into actionable information. In addition, the principal caveat to consider before employing any technology to monitor and assess players is the reliability and validity of the data it produces. Halson et al. [76] highlight the importance of and requirement for scientific rigor and careful analysis of the data produced from these wearable technologies to enable the generation of truly meaningful data, and also notes that the majority of these wearable devices have not been adequately assessed in terms of accuracy, reliability and validity.

Several challenges are still facing the successful adoption and utilization of these technologies to monitor the training and performance of football players. There is a requirement for more detailed empirical research to establish the reliability, validity, and efficacy of each of the individual technologies to satisfy the evidence-based practice approach employed in effective performance optimization programs. As these technologies continue to develop, and multiple, accurate data sources become available to measure and monitor player performance, additional work will be required to analyze and interpret the interactions between variables, in order to satisfy the ultimate goal of providing reliable, easy to use, cost-effective, valid, and actionable information to the players, coaches, and sports medicine team.

Take-Home Message

What becomes abundantly clear during the process of human performance optimization is the need to accurately acquire, extract, and operationalize relevant data from numerous sources into actionable information in an effort to effectively guide the process of optimization. That information may refer to factors such as the duration, total volume, or intensity of training undertaken, the amount and quality of sleep experienced, changes in power production occurring as a consequence of a training intervention, players' perception of the difficulty of training, the coaches' perception of the players' current form, etc. Fundamental to success is the ability to distill and integrate all the available information to effectively inform and optimize practice and performance, irrespective of which domain of player health and/or performance the player and coaches of sports medicine team are focusing on.

One challenge still remains. As new training techniques, nutritional strategies, and/or player monitoring technologies emerge, decisions regarding adoption and embedding of these new options to inform the process optimization are required. While evidence-based practice is a compelling goal, assessing the efficacy and utility of each of the emerging technologies and/or strategies before adoption may result in late adopters sacrificing potential competitive advantage offered as a consequence of their use [20]. Conversely, time wasted attempting to integrate these may effectively serve to dilute the effort of those involved and limit the effective time directed toward the goal of performance optimization, if the new technologies/strategies do not work out. Therefore, individual managers need to consider and implement their own decision-making processes for the adoption and integration of these emerging concepts to ensure the players' performance optimization.

Top Five Evidence-Based References

Casamichana D, Castellano J, Castagna C (2012) Comparing the physical demands of friendly matches and small-sided games in semiprofessional soccer players. J Strength & Cond Res 26:837–843

Ekstrand J (2013) Keeping your top players on the pitch: The key to football medicine at a professional level. Br J Sports Med 47:723–724

McCall A, Carling C, Nedelec M, Davison M, Le Gall F, Berthoin S, Dupont G (2014) Risk factors, testing and preventative strategies for non-contact injuries in professional football: current perceptions and practices of 44 teams from various premier leagues. Br J Sports Med 48((18)):1352–1357. https://doi.org/10.1136/bjsports-2014-093439

Thomas DT, Erdman KA, Burke LM (2016) Position of the academy of nutrition and dietetics, dietitians of Canada, and the American College of Sports Medicine: Nutrition and athletic performance. J Acad Nutr Diet 116:501–528

Venter RE (2014) Perceptions of team athletes on the importance of recovery modalities. European J Sport Sci 14:S69–S76

References

1. Evetovich TK (2009) Progression models in resistance training for healthy adults (vol 41, pg 687, 2009). Med Sci Sports Exerc 41:1351–1351
2. Evans WJ (1996) Reversing sarcopenia: how weight training can build strength and vitality. Geriatrics 51(46–47):51–43. quiz 54
3. Feigenbaum MS, Pollock ML (1999) Prescription of resistance training for health and disease. Med Sci Sports Exerc 31:38–45
4. Kelley GA, Kelley KS (2000) Progressive resistance exercise and resting blood pressure a meta-analysis of randomized controlled trials. Hypertension 35:838–843

5. Winett RA, Carpinelli RN (2001) Potential health-related benefits of resistance training. Prev Med 33:503–513
6. Kraemer WJ, Ratamess NA, French DN (2002) Resistance training for health and performance. Curr Sports Med Rep 1:165–171
7. Kraemer W, Ratamess N (2000) Physiology of resistance training: current issues. Orthopaedic Phys Ther Clin N Am 9:467–514
8. Hubal MJ, Gordish-Dressman H, Thompson PD, Price TB, Hoffman EP, Angelopoulos TJ et al (2005) Variability in muscle size and strength gain after unilateral resistance training. Med Sci Sports Exerc 37:964–972
9. Baechle TR, Earle RW (2008) Essentials of strength training and conditioning. Human kinetics, Champaign
10. Hass CJ, Feigenbaum MS, Franklin BA (2001) Prescription of resistance training for healthy populations. Sports Med 31:953–964
11. Hoffman J (2012) Association C. NSCA's guide to program design. Human Kinetics, Champaign, IL
12. Speirs DE, Bennett M, Finn CV, Turner AP (2015) Unilateral vs bilateral squat training for strength, sprints and agility in academy rugby players. J Strength Cond Res 30:386–392
13. Harries SK, Lubans DR, Callister R (2015) Systematic review and meta-analysis of linear and undulating periodized resistance training programs on muscular strength. J Strength Cond Res 29:1113–1125
14. Stand P (2009) Progression models in resistance training for healthy adults. Med Sci Sports Exerc 41:687–708
15. Stone M, O'bryant H, Schilling B, Johnson R, Pierce K, Haff GG et al (1999) Periodization: effects of manipulating volume and intensity. Part 1. Strength Cond J 21:56
16. Stone M, O'bryant H, Schilling B, Johnson R, Pierce K, Haff GG et al (1999) Periodization: effects of manipulating volume and intensity. Part 2. Strength Cond J 21:54
17. Stone MH, O'Bryant HS (1987) Weight training: a scientific approach. Burgess International Group, Edina, MN
18. Requena B, García I, Suárez-Arrones L, de Villarreal ES, Orellana JN, Santalla A (2017) Off-season effects on functional performance, body composition and blood parameters in top-level professional soccer players. J Strength Cond Res 31:939–946
19. Coyle EF, Wr M, Sinacore DR, Joyner MJ, Hagberg JM, Holloszy JO (1984) Time course of loss of adaptations after stopping prolonged intense endurance training. J Appl Physiol 57:1857–1864
20. McCall A, Davison M, Carling C, Buckthorpe M, Coutts AJ, Dupont G (2016) Can off-field 'brains' provide a competitive advantage in professional football? Br J Sports Med 50:710–712
21. McCall A, Lewin C, O'driscoll G, Witvrouw E, Ardern C (2016) Return to play: the challenge of balancing research and practice. Br J Sports Med 51:702–703
22. Hopkins W, Marshall S, Batterham A, Hanin J (2009) Progressive statistics for studies in sports medicine and exercise science. Med Sci Sports Exerc 41:3
23. Durrand J, Batterham A, Danjoux G (2014) Prehabilitation (i): aggregation of marginal gains. Anaesthesia 69:403–406
24. Eirale C, Tol J, Farooq A, Smiley F, Chalabi H (2013) Low injury rate strongly correlates with team success in Qatari professional football. Br J Sports Med 47:807–808
25. Ekstrand J (2013) Keeping your top players on the pitch: the key to football medicine at a professional level. Br J Sports Med 47:723–724
26. Hägglund M, Waldén M, Magnusson H, Kristenson K, Bengtsson H, Ekstrand J (2013) Injuries affect team performance negatively in professional football: an 11-year follow-up of the UEFA champions league injury study. Br J Sports Med 47:738–742
27. McCall A, Carling C, Davison M, Nedelec M, Le Gall F, Berthoin S et al (2015) Injury risk factors, screening tests and preventative strategies: a systematic review of the evidence that underpins the perceptions and practices of 44 football (soccer) teams from various premier leagues. Br J Sports Med 49:583–589
28. McCall A, Carling C, Nedelec M, Davison M, Le Gall F, Berthoin S et al (2014) Risk factors, testing and preventative strategies for non-contact injuries in professional football: current perceptions and practices of 44 teams from various premier leagues. Br J Sports Med 48:1352–1357. bjsports-2014-093439
29. Eichner ER (1995) Overtraining: consequences and prevention. J Sports Sci 13:S41–S48
30. Schlabach G (1994) Carbohydrate strategies for injury prevention. J Athl Train 29:244
31. Thomas DT, Erdman KA, Burke LM (2016) Position of the academy of nutrition and dietetics, dietitians of Canada, and the American college of sports medicine: nutrition and athletic performance. J Acad Nutr Diet 116:501–528
32. Jeukendrup AE (2017) Periodized nutrition for athletes. Sports Med 47:51–63
33. Cunningham JJ (1991) Body composition as a determinant of energy expenditure: a synthetic review and a proposed general prediction equation. Am J Clin Nutr 54:963–969
34. Thompson J, Manore MM (1996) Predicted and measured resting metabolic rate of male and female endurance athletes. J Am Diet Assoc 96:30–34
35. Ainsworth BE, Haskell WL, Herrmann SD, Meckes N, Bassett DR Jr, Tudor-Locke C et al (2011) 2011 compendium of physical activities: a second update of codes and MET values. Med Sci Sports Exerc 43:1575–1581
36. Io M (2005) Dietary reference intakes for energy, carbohydrate, fiber, fat, fatty acids, cholesterol, protein, and amino acids (Macronutrients). The National Academies Press, Washington, DC. Doi: 10.17226/10490

37. Rodriguez NR, DiMarco NM, Langley S (2009) Position of the American dietetic association, dietitians of Canada, and the American College of Sports Medicine: nutrition and athletic performance. J Am Diet Assoc 109:509–527
38. Burke LM, Kiens B, Ivy JL (2004) Carbohydrates and fat for training and recovery. J Sports Sci 22:15–30
39. Knuiman P, Hopman MT, Mensink M (2015) Glycogen availability and skeletal muscle adaptations with endurance and resistance exercise. Nutr Metab (Lond) 12:59
40. Gaitanos GC, Williams C, Boobis LH, Brooks S (1993) Human muscle metabolism during intermittent maximal exercise. J Appl Physiol 75:712–719
41. Hargreaves M, Finn JP, Withers RT, Scroop GC, Mackay M, Snow RJ et al (1997) Effect of muscle glycogen availability on maximal exercise performance. Eur J Appl Physiol Occup Physiol 75:188–192
42. Zehnder M, Rico-Sanz J, Kuhne G, Boutellier U (2001) Resynthesis of muscle glycogen after soccer specific performance examined by 13-magnetic resonance spectroscopy in elite players. Eur J Appl Physiol 84:443–447
43. Burke LM, Hawley JA, Wong SH, Jeukendrup AE (2011) Carbohydrates for training and competition. J Sports Sci 29:S17–S27
44. Achten J, Halson SL, Moseley L, Rayson MP, Casey A, Jeukendrup AE (2004) Higher carbohydrate content during intensified running training results in better maintenance of performance and mood state. J Appl Physiol (1985) 96:1331–1340
45. Morton RW, McGlory C, Phillips SM (2015) Nutritional interventions to augment resistance training-induced skeletal muscle hypertrophy. Front Physiol 6:245
46. Zawadzki K, Yaspelkis B, Ivy J (1992) Carbohydrate-protein complex increases the rate of muscle glycogen storage after exercise. J Appl Physiol 72:1854–1859
47. Garcia-Roves PM, Garcia-Zapico P, Patterson AM, Iglesias-Gutierrez E (2014) Nutrient intake and food habits of soccer players: analyzing the correlates of eating practice. Forum Nutr 6:2697–2717
48. Phillips SM, Van Loon LJ (2011) Dietary protein for athletes: from requirements to optimum adaptation. J Sports Sci 29:S29–S38
49. Mettler S, Mitchell N, Tipton KD (2010) Increased protein intake reduces lean body mass loss during weight loss in athletes. Med Sci Sports Exerc 42:326–337
50. Brownell KD, Steen SN, Wilmore JH (1987) Weight regulation practices in athletes: analysis of metabolic and health effects. Med Sci Sports Exerc 19:546–556
51. Havemann L, West SJ, Goedecke JH, Macdonald IA, Gibson ASC, Noakes T et al (2006) Fat adaptation followed by carbohydrate loading compromises high-intensity sprint performance. J Appl Physiol 100:194–202
52. Seebohar B. 2014 Metabolic Efficiency Training: Teaching the Body to Burn More Fat. Fuel4mance
53. Health UDo, Services H (2015) 2015–2020 dietary guidelines for Americans. USDA, Washington (DC)
54. Jeukendrup AE (2008) Carbohydrate feeding during exercise. Eur J Sport Sci 8:77–86
55. Kerksick C, Harvey T, Stout J, Campbell B, Wilborn C, Kreider R et al (2008) International Society of Sports Nutrition position stand: nutrient timing. J Int Soc Sports Nutr 5:17
56. Beck KL, Thomson JS, Swift RJ, von Hurst PR (2015) Role of nutrition in performance enhancement and postexercise recovery. Open Access J Sports Med 6:259
57. Coutts AJ, Duffield R (2010) Validity and reliability of GPS devices for measuring movement demands of team sports. J Sci Med Sport 13:133–135
58. Johnston RJ, Watsford ML, Kelly SJ, Pine MJ, Spurrs RW (2014) Validity and interunit reliability of 10 Hz and 15 Hz GPS units for assessing athlete movement demands. J Strength Cond Res 28:1649–1655
59. Koklu Y, Arslan Y, Alemdaroglu U, Duffield R (2015) Accuracy and reliability of SPI ProX global positioning system devices for measuring movement demands of team sports. J Sports Med Phys Fitness 55:471–477
60. Portas MD, Harley JA, Barnes CA, Rush CJ (2010) The validity and reliability of 1-Hz and 5-Hz global positioning systems for linear, multidirectional, and soccer-specific activities. Int J Sports Physiol Perform 5:448–458
61. Varley MC, Fairweather IH, Aughey RJ (2012) Validity and reliability of GPS for measuring instantaneous velocity during acceleration, deceleration, and constant motion. J Sports Sci 30:121–127
62. Gabbett TJ (2013) Quantifying the physical demands of collision sports: does microsensor technology measure what it claims to measure? J Strength Cond Res 27:2319–2322
63. Casamichana D, Castellano J, Calleja-Gonzalez J, San Roman J, Castagna C (2013) Relationship between indicators of training load in soccer players. J Strength Cond Res 27:369–374
64. Casamichana D, Castellano J, Castagna C (2012) Comparing the physical demands of friendly matches and small-sided games in semiprofessional soccer players. J Strength Cond Res 26:837–843
65. Harley JA, Barnes CA, Portas M, Lovell R, Barrett S, Paul D et al (2010) Motion analysis of match-play in elite U12 to U16 age-group soccer players. J Sports Sci 28:1391–1397
66. Hill-Haas SV, Dawson B, Impellizzeri FM, Coutts AJ (2011) Physiology of small-sided games training in football: a systematic review. Sports Med 41:199–220
67. Beersma DG (1998) Models of human sleep regulation. Sleep Med Rev 2:31–43
68. Nédélec M, Halson S, Abaidia A-E, Ahmaidi S, Dupont G (2015) Stress, sleep and recovery in elite soccer: a critical review of the literature. Sports Med 45:1387–1400

69. Fullagar HH, Skorski S, Duffield R, Hammes D, Coutts AJ, Meyer T (2015) Sleep and athletic performance: the effects of sleep loss on exercise performance, and physiological and cognitive responses to exercise. Sports Med 45:161–186
70. Venter RE (2014) Perceptions of team athletes on the importance of recovery modalities. Eur J Sport Sci 14:S69–S76
71. Halson SL (2008) Nutrition, sleep and recovery. European J Sport Sci 8:119–126
72. Roky R, Herrera CP, Ahmed Q (2012) Sleep in athletes and the effects of Ramadan. J Sports Sci 30:S75–S84
73. Miller NL, Shatluck LG. Sleep patterns of young men and women enrolled at the United States Military Academy: results from year 1 of a 4-year longitudinal study. DTIC Document 2005
74. Stanley N (2003) Actigraphy in human psychopharmacology: a review. Hum Psychopharmacol Clin Exp 18:39–49
75. Kushida CA, Chang A, Gadkary C, Guilleminault C, Carrillo O, Dement WC (2001) Comparison of actigraphic, polysomnographic, and subjective assessment of sleep parameters in sleep-disordered patients. Sleep Med 2:389–396
76. Halson SL, Peake JM, Sullivan JP (2016) Wearable technology for athletes: information overload and pseudoscience? Int J Sports Physiol Perform 11:705–706
77. Liu Y, Zhu SH, Wang GH, Ye F, Li PZ (2013) Validity and reliability of multiparameter physiological measurements recorded by the Equivital LifeMonitor during activities of various intensities. J Occup Environ Hyg 10:78–85
78. Weippert M, Stielow J, Kumar M, Kreuzfeld S, Rieger A, Stoll R (2013) Tri-axial high-resolution acceleration for oxygen consumption estimation: validation of a multi-sensor device and a novel analysis method. Appl Physiol, Nutr, Metabol 38:345–351
79. Impellizzeri FM, Bizzini M, Dvorak J, Pellegrini B, Schena F, Junge A (2013) Physiological and performance responses to the FIFA 11+(part 2): a randomised controlled trial on the training effects. J Sports Sci 31:1491–1502
80. Castagna C, Impellizzeri F, Cecchini E, Rampinini E, Alvarez JC (2009) Effects of intermittent-endurance fitness on match performance in young male soccer players. J Strength Cond Res 23:1954–1959
81. Schutz Y, Chambaz A (1997) Could a satellite-based navigation system (GPS) be used to assess the physical activity of individuals on earth? Eur J Clin Nutr 51:338–339
82. Brandes M, Heitmann A, Müller L (2012) Physical responses of different small-sided game formats in elite youth soccer players. J Strength Cond Res 26:1353–1360
83. Hennig EM, Sterzing T (2010) The influence of soccer shoe design on playing performance: a series of biomechanical studies. Footwear Sci 2:3–11
84. Brage S, Brage N, Franks P, Ekelund U, Wareham N (2005) Reliability and validity of the combined heart rate and movement sensor actiheart. Eur J Clin Nutr 59:561–570
85. Sadeh A (2011) The role and validity of actigraphy in sleep medicine: an update. Sleep Med Rev 15:259–267
86. Steeves JA, Bowles HR, McClain JJ, Dodd KW, Brychta RJ, Wang J et al (2015) Ability of thigh-worn actigraph and activPAL monitors to classify posture and motion. Med Sci Sports Exerc 47:952–959
87. Briggs MA, Cockburn E, Rumbold PL, Rae G, Stevenson EJ, Russell M (2015) Assessment of energy intake and energy expenditure of male adolescent academy-level soccer players during a competitive week. Forum Nutr 7:8392–8401
88. Sæther SA, Aspvik NP (2017) Descriptive analysis of objectively assessed physical activity among talented soccer players–a study of 3 Norwegian professional football clubs. Br J Sports Med
89. Gamelin FX, Berthoin S, Bosquet L (2006) Validity of the polar S810 heart rate monitor to measure RR intervals at rest. Med Sci Sports Exerc 38:887
90. Hurst HT, Atkins S (2006) Agreement between polar and SRM mobile ergometer systems during laboratory-based high-intensity, intermittent cycling activity. J Sports Sci 24:863–868
91. Owen AL, Wong DP, McKenna M, Dellal A (2011) Heart rate responses and technical comparison between small-vs. large-sided games in elite professional soccer. J Strength Cond Res 25:2104–2110
92. Castagna C, Impellizzeri FM, Chaouachi A, Bordon C, Manzi V (2011) Effect of training intensity distribution on aerobic fitness variables in elite soccer players: a case study. J Strength Cond Res 25:66–71
93. Kelly DM, Strudwick AJ, Atkinson G, Drust B, Gregson W (2016) The within-participant correlation between perception of effort and heart rate-based estimations of training load in elite soccer players. J Sports Sci 34:1328–1332
94. Thorborg K, Bandholm T, Hölmich P (2013) Hip- and knee-strength assessments using a hand-held dynamometer with external belt-fixation are inter-tester reliable. Knee Surg Sports Traumatol Arthrosc 21:550–555
95. Thorborg K, Petersen J, Magnusson SP, Holmich P (2010) Clinical assessment of hip strength using a hand-held dynamometer is reliable. Scand J Med Sci Sports 20:493–501
96. Stark T, Walker B, Phillips JK, Fejer R, Beck R (2011) Hand-held dynamometry correlation with the gold standard isokinetic dynamometry: a systematic review. PM R 3:472–479
97. Piva SR, Fitzgerald K, Irrgang JJ, Jones S, Hando BR, Browder DA et al (2006) Reliability of measures of impairments associated with patellofemoral pain syndrome. BMC Musculoskelet Disord 7:33
98. Stoll T, Huber E, Seifert B, Michel BA, Stucki G (2000) Maximal isometric muscle strength: normative values and gender-specific relation to age. Clin Rheumatol 19:105–113

99. Nilstad A, Andersen TE, Bahr R, Holme I, Steffen K (2014) Risk factors for lower extremity injuries in elite female soccer players. Am J Sports Med 42:940–948
100. Thorborg K, Couppé C, Petersen J, Magnusson P, Holmich P (2009) Eccentric hip adduction and abduction strength in elite soccer players and matched controls a cross-sectional study. Br J Sports Med 45:10–13. 2009.061762
101. Thorborg K, Serner A, Petersen J, Madsen TM, Magnusson P, Hölmich P (2011) Hip adduction and abduction strength profiles in elite soccer players: implications for clinical evaluation of hip adductor muscle recovery after injury. Am J Sports Med 39:121–126
102. Engebretsen AH, Myklebust G, Holme I, Engebretsen L, Bahr R (2010) Intrinsic risk factors for groin injuries among male soccer players a prospective cohort study. Am J Sports Med 38:2051–2057
103. Garnacho-Castaño MV, López-Lastra S, Maté-Muñoz JL (2015) Reliability and validity assessment of a linear position transducer. J Sports Sci Med 14:128
104. Sato K, Beckham GK, Carroll K, Bazyler C, Sha Z, Haff G (2015) Validity of wireless device measuring velocity of resistance exercises. J Trainol 4:15–18
105. Stock MS, Beck TW, DeFreitas JM, Dillon MA (2011) Test–retest reliability of barbell velocity during the free-weight bench-press exercise. J Strength Cond Res 25:171–177
106. Palmer TB, Thompson BJ, Hawkey MJ, Conchola EC, Adams BM, Akehi K et al (2014) The influence of athletic status on the passive properties of the muscle-tendon unit and traditional performance measures in division I female soccer players and nonathlete controls. J Strength Cond Res 28:2026–2034
107. Jajtner AR, Hoffman JR, Scanlon TC, Wells AJ, Townsend JR, Beyer KS et al (2013) Performance and muscle architecture comparisons between starters and nonstarters in National Collegiate Athletic Association Division I women's soccer. J Strength Cond Res 27:2355–2365
108. Wagner DR, Cain DL, Clark NW (2016) Validity and reliability of A-mode ultrasound for body composition assessment of NCAA division I athletes. PLoS One 11:e0153146
109. Cain DL (2015) Validity and reliability of A-mode ultrasound for body composition assessment of lean, division I athletes. Utah State University, Logan, Utah
110. Smolander J, Juuti T, Kinnunen M-L, Laine K, Louhevaara V, Männikkö K et al (2008) A new heart rate variability-based method for the estimation of oxygen consumption without individual laboratory calibration: application example on postal workers. Appl Ergon 39:325–331
111. Montgomery PG, Green DJ, Etxebarria N, Pyne DB, Saunders PU, Minahan CL (2009) Validation of heart rate monitor-based predictions of oxygen uptake and energy expenditure. J Strength Cond Res 23:1489–1495
112. Luhtanen P, Nummela A, Lipponen K (2008) 24 Physical loading, stress and recovery in a youth soccer tournament. Science and Football VI 143
113. Vanttinen T, Blomqvist M, Lehto H, Hakkinen K (2008) 20 Heart rate and match analysis of Finnish junior football players. Science and Football VI 119
114. Dorrel BS, Long T, Shaffer S, Myer GD (2015) Evaluation of the functional movement screen as an injury prediction tool among active adult populations: a systematic review and meta-analysis. Sports Health 7:532–537
115. Koehle MS, Saffer BY, Sinnen NM, MacInnis MJ (2016) Factor structure and internal validity of the functional movement screen in adults. J Strength Cond Res 30:540–546
116. Cuchna JW, Hoch MC, Hoch JM (2016) The interrater and intrarater reliability of the functional movement screen: a systematic review with meta-analysis. Phys Ther Sport 19:57–65
117. Smith PD, Hanlon M (2017) Assessing the effectiveness of the functional movement screen (FMS (TM)) in predicting non-contact injury rates in soccer players. J Strength Condition Res. https://doi.org/10.1519/JSC.0000000000001757
118. Chorba RS, Chorba DJ, Bouillon LE, Overmyer CA, Landis JA (2010) Use of a functional movement screening tool to determine injury risk in female collegiate athletes. N Am J Sports Phys Ther 5:47

3 How to Predict Injury Risk

David Sundemo, Eduard Alentorn-Geli, and Kristian Samuelsson

Contents

3.1 Introduction

One possible subtitle of this chapter could be—how can we avoid football players sustaining injuries? The reliable prediction and understand of injury mechanisms and etiology are crucial steps in effective injury prevention [1]. For sports teams to be successful the athletes need to be healthy, since injury load is clearly correlated to team performance [2, 3]. Injuries in high-level football players are common and occur about twice a season, causing a mean absence of 37 days or 12% of the season [4]. Serious injuries, such as injury to the anterior cruciate ligament (ACL), can ruin more than one season. Interest focus heavily on surgery and the rehabilitation of football injuries, but the optimal scenario is to avoid injury in the first place. It is therefore important to investigate risk factors to predict the risk of injury in athletes. Knowledge of the risk factors that significantly predict a specific injury has led to the development and implementation of prevention programs that mitigate the risk of injury. For example, prior research has led to knowledge of the increased risk of ACL rupture in female players with impaired neuromuscular control [5]. The development of prevention programs and neuromuscular training has reduced the risk of injury substantially [6]. The Swedish Football Association, among others, has popularized the subject by constructing a smartphone application that is free for all players to download.

There are different categories of factors influencing the risk of injury. Depending on the type of injury, different systems are used to categorize factors [7, 8]. One common method for dividing factors is based on intrinsic

D. Sundemo (✉) • K. Samuelsson
Department of Orthopedics, Institute of Clinical Sciences, The Sahlgrenska Academy, University of Gothenburg, Göteborg, Sweden
e-mail: David.Sundemo@Outlook.com

E. Alentorn-Geli
Artroscopia GC, SL, Hospital Quirón, Barcelona, Spain

Fundación García-Cugat, Barcelona, Spain

Mutualidad Catalana de Futbolistas – Federación Española de Fútbol, Barcelona, Spain

V. Musahl et al. (eds.), *Return to Play in Football*, https://doi.org/10.1007/978-3-662-55713-6_3

Table 3.1 Risk factors for lower extremity injury

Risk factors for lower extremity injury	
Intrinsic	**Extrinsic**
Age	Level of competition
Gender	Shoe type
Phase of menstrual cycle	Ankle bracing
Previous injury	Playing surface
Inadequate rehab	Climate
Aerobic fitness	
Body size and composition	
Limb dominance	
Generalized joint laxity	
Joint specific laxity	
Muscle tightness	
Range of motion	
Muscle strength, imbalance	
Muscle reaction time	
Muscular fatigue	
Limb girth	
Postural and core stability	
Anatomical alignment	
Foot morphology	
Skill level	
Genetic predisposition	

(individual) or extrinsic (environmental) origin (Table 3.1) [8, 9]. Risk factors can be either non-modifiable, such as gender or anatomical alignment, or modifiable, like body mass index or muscle strength. It is important to be aware of the non-modifiable, risk factors; however, knowledge of the modifiable risk factors is perhaps more crucial, since they vary and their influence can be reduced.

In this chapter, the etiology of sports injuries and the utilization and the implementation of screening tools to predict injuries will be discussed. Further, the predictive ability of certain important risk factors will be assessed in relation to specific and common injuries that affect football players. A study assessing players in the top 50 clubs in Europe revealed that 87% of football injuries affect the lower extremities. The hip/groin, thigh, knee, and ankle were the most commonly injured sites, and they will be the focus of this chapter [4]. Lastly, a section discussing study design in the construction of injury prediction studies is included.

3.2 Sports Injury Etiology

The etiology of sports injuries is multifactorial and it is often influenced by both harmful and protective factors (Fig. 3.1). The categorization of risk factors has been discussed above. However, intrinsic and extrinsic risk factors do not exclusively explain sports injury etiology. A model for presenting the intricate network of contributory factors was presented by Meeuwisse et al. in 1994 and was later refined by Bahr and Krosshaug [10, 11]. The reader can follow the model, starting with the predisposed athlete with individual intrinsic risk factors. When practicing a specific sport, the athlete is affected by the extrinsic factors increasing the susceptibility of injury. Lastly, the injury occurs, caused by the mechanism at the time of the injury [10]. It has been suggested that, with regard to injury mechanism, not only should the biomechanical movements be included, but the skill performed (shot, pass, and so on), player-to-player interaction or the position on the field of play, for example, should also be investigated [10, 12]. Understanding the influence of risk factors alone is therefore not sufficient. Injury mechanisms are equally important. However, injury mechanisms are difficult to investigate, since this often relies on the history of the

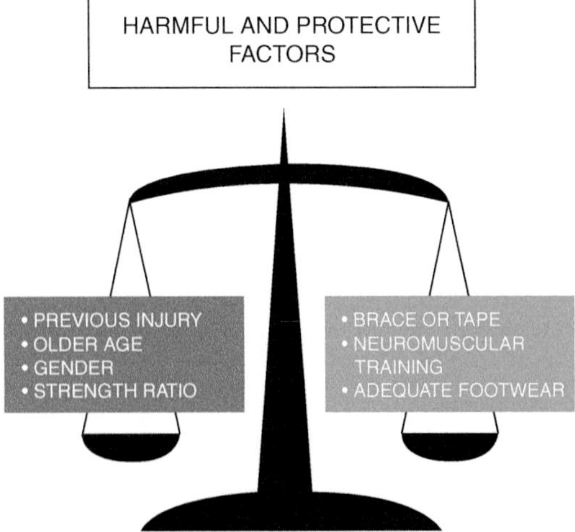

Fig. 3.1 Examples of harmful and protective factors seen in different types of sports injuries

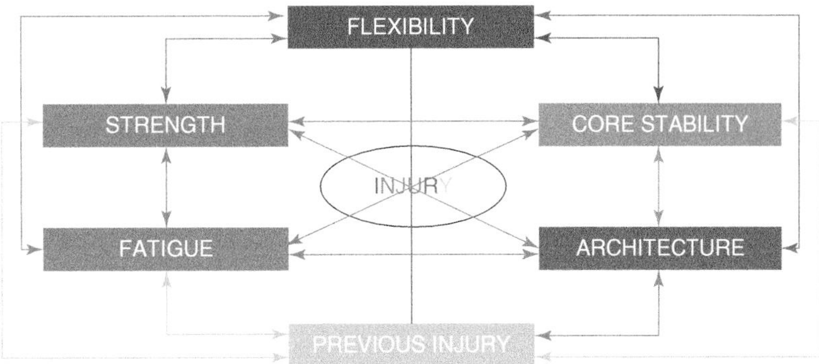

Fig. 3.2 Non-linear multifactorial model for the risk of hamstring muscle injuries

individual trying to reproduce the, often emotionally charged, turn of events. To increase precision and objectivity in the assessment of injury mechanisms, novel studies are utilizing video analysis [12]. Deciphering the etiology of sports injuries is complicated due to their diverse origin, but considerable research has been conducted in the last few decades to elucidate this.

There is a current tendency to consider multifactorial models for the risk of injury, with a non-linear relationship between factors; i.e. there would not be a causal-effect relationship between a single risk factor and injury but, instead, an interaction between several factors, which would lead to the final risk of injury (Fig. 3.2) [13].

3.3 Prediction of Specific Injuries to the Lower Extremities

3.3.1 Hip/groin Injury

Diagnosing injury to the hip or groin is complicated, due to the number of involved structures and potential culprits (e.g., hip fracture, cartilage lesion, femoroacetabular impingement, muscles and so on). The adductors of the hip are the most commonly injured muscles in the groin. In a recent comprehensive study, the majority of injuries to the groin were considered severe, and the mean absence from play was determined as 15 days [14]. The reoccurrence of sprains in the groin adductors is not uncommon, causing the further disruption of player and team development. Previous injury to the groin as a risk factor for reinjury was previously the subject of debate due to the lack of good prospective studies [15], but a high-quality prospective cohort study assessing 508 football players identifies previous injury as a significant predictor [16]. This has been verified in a recent systematic review assessing field-based sports [17]. Further, male gender is a significant predictor of injury. An aggregated analysis of relevant studies, controlling for exposure, has revealed a more than two-fold increase in the risk in comparison with females [18]. Moreover, strength deficit in the adductor muscles is also regarded as a risk factor for groin injury [16, 17, 19]. However, a recent meta-analysis investigating the prevention of groin injury by adductor muscle training did not find a significant reduction in sports-related injuries [20]. Age as a predictor of injury is the subject of debate. The systematic review assessing field-based sports, which includes football, stated that it was of significance. The authors referred to two studies showing that age was a significant predictor: a single football-specific study and a study examining rugby players [17]. In contrast, a more general systematic review published in 2015 deemed age to be an insignificant factor. Of the 12 studies (including one randomized, controlled trial and eight cohort studies) analyzing the age factor in the general systematic review, all but 2 found no association between age and hip/groin injury [19]. It is evident that there is a lack of football-specific research on this risk factor, but, based on the abundance of high-quality evidence found in the

Table 3.2 Potential predictors for hip/groin injury in football

Evidence relating to potential predictors of hip/groin injury in football		
Likely predictive	Unlikely predictive	Insufficient evidence
Previous injury Male gender Weak hip adductor muscles Lower level of sports-specific training	Age BMI Performance in fitness tests	Early maturation Hip abduction ROM Level of play

general review, age must be regarded as an unlikely predictor. Further, the significance of BMI was assessed in the same general review cited above, presenting data where all four football-specific studies analyzing soccer showed that this factor was not predictive of injury [19].

As a result, a few significant predictors have been identified (Table 3.2). In spite of this, prevention programs do not produce satisfactory results, and more research is needed, both in the identification of additional potential risk factors and in improvement of prevention.

3.3.2 Thigh Injury

Injuries sustained in the thigh when playing football predominantly affect the hamstrings or the quadriceps. The muscles of the thigh are commonly injured in football players, due to the pattern of movement, performing fast accelerations and decelerations, causing the muscles to over-stretch. Risk factors for hamstring injury are the subject of debate, and many studies investigating potential predictors have been performed. A systematic review assessing high-quality prospective studies of football players recognized previous injury as the only significant risk factor [21]. Further, the authors concluded that, among other things, BMI, height, weight, and player exposure were probably insignificant factors. In a previous study, players with a previous injury to the hamstring ran twice the risk of reinjury [22]. Additionally, there is evidence supporting age as a potential risk factor for hamstring injury in football players [23, 24]. There is conflicting evidence regarding the influence of muscle strength, although a high-quality prospective study determined hamstring and quadriceps strength deficit as weak risk factors for hamstring injury [25].

Nevertheless, the authors of this study doubted its clinical relevance and do not recommend screening isokinetic strength to identify patients at risk [25]. Quadriceps peak torque was regarded as a risk factor in a recent systematic review and meta-analysis. This marker was found in four studies of which one involved football and three involved Australian football. Consequently, quadriceps peak torque can be regarded as a likely predictive factor in football, although further football-specific studies are warranted for a conclusive statement [26]. A large number of potential predictors of hamstring injury have been investigated, but there is currently insufficient evidence to draw conclusions. The most important factors have been listed below (Table 3.3). For a complete list, readers can be recommended the following reviews [21, 26].

The quadriceps constitutes four individual muscles, the vastus medialis, vastus lateralis, vastus intermedius, and rectus femoris, of which the latter is the most commonly injured [27]. Quadriceps injuries may not be as common as injuries to the groin or the hamstrings, but they cause more missed matches than any other muscle injury in football [28]. Age does not appear to be a significant predictor of quadriceps injury, since two prospective studies assessing football players did not identify this, and an additional study examining Australian football players verified these results [28–30]. A study analyzing 1401 football players demonstrated that previous injury was a significant risk factor [31]. Similarly, in Australian football, previous ipsilateral injury to the quadriceps, but also to the hamstrings, was a significant predictor of injury to the quadriceps [30]. Short stature and higher weight have been suggested as risk factors, but studies assessing football have not identified a statistically significant link, perhaps due to an underpowered study design [32]. Conversely, a study examining English Premier League football players found no connection between weight and injury incidence, but this was

Table 3.3 Potential predictors for hamstring injury in football

Evidence relating to potential predictors of hamstring injury in football		
Likely predictive	Unlikely predictive	Insufficient evidence
Previous injury Older age Increased quadriceps peak torque Sprinting and kicking sports	BMI Limb dominance Height Weight Player exposure	Weather conditions Dominance Playing surface Hamstring/quadriceps and hip flexor flexibility Player position strength imbalance, and so on

in a small study with no more than 36 players [29]. Further, isokinetic strength as a risk factor has been investigated. A study published in 2011 claimed that there was a trend towards significance between quadriceps injury and preseason eccentric strength, but the results did not reach statistical significance [32]. According to one study, male players run a greater risk of sustaining injury to the quadriceps when playing on artificial turf as opposed to natural grass [33]. This might be due to the higher degree of shoe-surface friction during kicking. This theory was supported by Orchard et al. who found that quadriceps injuries were more frequent in dry weather where the surface friction component is stronger, but this study assessed Australian football players [30]. Muscle flexibility has also been reported to predict quadriceps injury. Two prospective studies examining football players identified a connection of this kind [32, 34]. Regarding flexibility, a recent study did not identify this as a significant risk factor, although in that study comprising 36 players only six players sustained an injury, indicating that insignificant power may be an issue. The current evidence relating to quadriceps injury predictors is listed below (Table 3.4).

Table 3.4 Potential predictors for quadriceps injury in football

Evidence relating to potential predictors of quadriceps injury in football		
Likely predictive	Unlikely predictive	Insufficient evidence
Previous injury Sprinting and kicking sports Quadriceps muscle flexibility Playing surface	Age	Weight Height Weather conditions Limb dominance Strength abnormalities or imbalance

3.3.3 Knee Injury

Injuries to the knees can include sprains in the medial or lateral collateral ligaments, lesions of the menisci, or—perhaps the most severe of the common injuries attained during football—injury to the anterior cruciate ligament (ACL). This section will focus primarily on injuries to the ACL. Risk factors for sustaining an injury to the ACL have been thoroughly investigated. A return to high-level football after an ACL injury normally takes six to 12 months and, in a considerable number of player's, stability and functionality is never restored. A recent study revealed that, 3 years after reconstruction, only 65% of football players still compete at the same level, and a meta-analysis including other sports demonstrated that as few as 55% return to competitive level [35, 36]. Prediction and prevention are therefore of the utmost importance.

Gender is a strong and relevant predictive factor in understanding ACL pathology and functions as a watershed in the assessment of several risk factors. Women run a greater risk of injury [37, 38] than their male counterparts, and the influence of other risk factors varies between the sexes. In one study, women had an incidence rate of 0.1 per 1,000 h of football as compared to 0.057 for males [38]. Another study reported a sixfold increase in the risk for ACL rupture in females [37]. The exact numbers vary between studies, although there is substantial evidence of a significant difference in relative risk with regard to gender [38–41].

One factor considered to contribute to increased risk in females is inferior neuromuscular control [42]. A study by Hewett et al. targeted young female athletes to examine the influence of valgus joint load on ACL injury risk. Two hundred and five athletes participating in volleyball, basketball, or football were prospectively screened. An analysis identified knee abduction moment as a significant predictor of ACL injury with 73% specificity and 78% sensitivity [5]. However, a prospective study published in 2016 assessing 782 elite female football players revealed that knee abduction moment was not predictive of ACL injury in this large cohort [43].

The influence of the relationship between height and weight, measured using BMI, is uncertain, since there is both supportive [44, 45] and contradictory evidence [46, 47]. Further, the effect of joint laxity on the relative risk of ACL injury is the subject of debate. Generalized joint laxity has been related to an increased risk of leg injuries in female football players [48], and an augmented risk of ACL injury specifically has been found in non-football-specific groups [49, 50]. Increased knee joint laxity, specifically, was significantly related to a higher risk of ACL injury in female football and basketball players in a recent case-control study [51]. Large prospective cohort studies assessing football players exclusively are lacking. Future studies with this design would further elucidate the influence of joint laxity further.

Several modifiable extrinsic risk factors have been discussed with regard to football and knee injuries. One interesting factor is the choice of footwear. In a systematic review from 2015, the authors concluded that increased rotational traction, depending on the design and number of shoe cleats, augmented the risk of lower extremity injury [52] in American football. The authors believed that this postulation could be transferred to all other kinds of football. Moreover, a recent study found a 3.4 times higher risk of ACL injury in American football players using cleats with the highest level of rotational traction. However, clinical football-specific studies are lacking, and laboratory studies performed in this particular field do not reveal differences in knee loading [53, 54]. As a result, there is still insufficient evidence to draw any definite conclusion.

Male Champions League players in countries in the north of Europe, with a cooler climate and more precipitation, are less prone to ACL injury

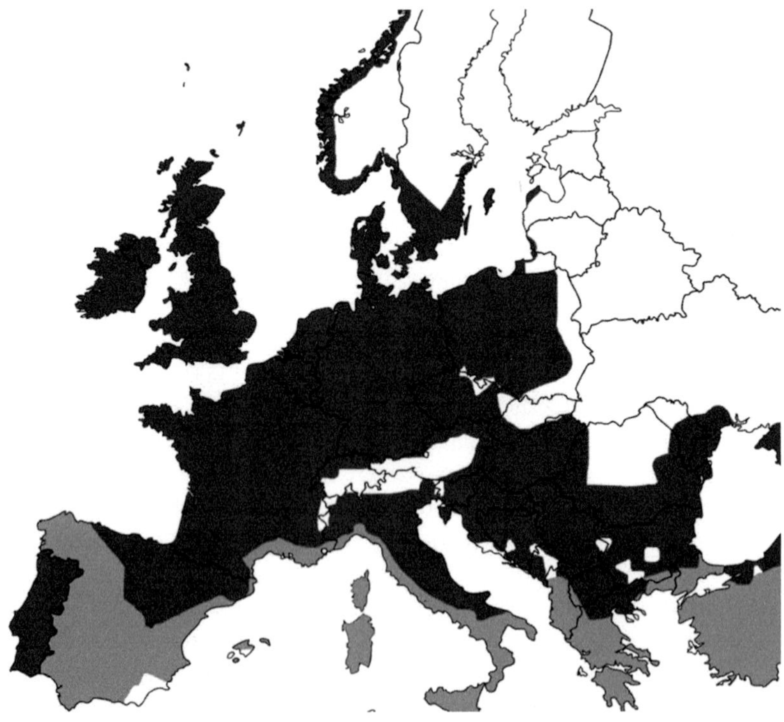

Fig. 3.3 A simplified version of the climate zones used in a recent study [55]. *Dark green* indicates the northern zone with a cooler climate, in contrast to the southern zone colored *light green. White land areas* indicate other climate zones not used in this study

Table 3.5 Potential predictors for ACL injury in football

Evidence relating to potential predictors of ACL injury in football		
Likely predictive	Unlikely predictive	Insufficient evidence
Female gender Abnormal neuromuscular control Altered biomechanics Generalized joint laxity Playing surface Anatomics Footwear	BMI Leg dominance Sports level Player position	Genetics Age Knee joint laxity Climate

than players in Mediterranean countries in the south (Fig. 3.3) [55]. Although the difference in incidence was statistically significant, the climate itself is probably not the sole explanation for this. As mentioned by the authors, potential sources of bias could be differences in style or the intensity of play or playing surface between the two groups.

Regrettably, research aiming to understand the influence of playing surface on ACL ruptures in football is lacking. A recent systematic review found that there is a higher risk of ACL rupture in players participating in American football when playing on artificial turf [56] and in Australian football playing on Bermuda grass when compared with ryegrass [57]. It was hypothesized that artificial grass (compared with natural grass) and Bermuda grass (compared with ryegrass) produce a higher degree of shoe-surface friction. However, in football, no such difference has been seen [56]. A summary of relevant risk factors is presented below (Table 3.5).

3.3.4 Ankle Injury

As football is a fast-paced game with quick changes of direction, it predisposes to ankle injuries, making them one of the most common traumatic injuries, in football, in both male and female players [58, 59]. Fractures to the ankle occur and can be troublesome, but the main problem causing absence from play is ankle sprains [60]. One debated extrinsic risk factor is the influence of artificial turf when compared with natural grass. In a prospective study of 290 male football players, the authors found more ankle sprains related to artificial turf [61]. In line with this, a recent systematic review investigating the influence of playing surface concluded that football players run a greater risk of ankle sprain on artificial turf and preventive strategies were advised [62]. Contradictory studies exist [63], but in conclusion, harmful effects have been seen in both males and females, although the current evidence is stronger in the case of male players.

There appears to be substantial evidence to indicate that previous injury is a risk factor for ankle sprain in male football players. Three large, recently conducted prospective cohort studies with a total of 1,132 players revealed that it was a significant predictor [23, 64, 65], and there is further evidence in the literature [58, 66, 67]. In two contradictory studies, fewer participants were recruited, which may have caused a type 2 error, and the studies did not exclusively assess football players [68, 69]. Other plausible causes of discrepancy in the results are the influence of and differences in rehabilitation regimens across studies and the utilization of external stabilizers, such as tape or braces [70]. In females, a study by Faude et al. did not find that previous injury was a predictor, but there is still insufficient evidence to draw any definite conclusions in female players [71].

Gender does not appear to have a predictive ability in ankle sprain in general [70], and a study analyzing football specifically supports that notion [72]. Furthermore, anatomical foot type (pronated, neutral, or supinated) or the level of generalized joint laxity do not appear to predict a risk of ankle sprain [70]. The body mass index was found to be predictive of ankle sprain in a recent football-specific study [73], and a general systematic review and meta-analysis of ankle sprain risk factors support the results [74].

Postural sway, measured with various balance tests, has been suggested as a risk factor, since neuromuscular training has been effective in preventing ankle injuries [75]. Two studies using the single-leg balance test did not find a connection

Table 3.6 Potential predictors of ankle injury in football

Evidence relating to potential predictors of ankle injury in football		
Likely predictive	Unlikely predictive	Insufficient evidence
Artificial turf Previous injury BMI	Gender Anatomical foot type Generalized joint laxity	Balance/postural sway Age Slow eccentric inversion strength Fast concentric plantar flexion strength Low inversion proprioception

between balance and risk of injury, as opposed to another study that was able to predict injury [64, 68, 69]. However, only one of the studies assessed football players exclusively [64]. Additionally, in a study using a different method to measure postural sway, the authors were able to predict the risk of injury in a group of male football players [76]. There is therefore controversy about the influence of balance in football, but, as a predictor or ankle injury in sports in general, there is more evidence [77, 78]. Recent reviews and meta-analyses have identified markers, such as slow eccentric inversion strength, fast concentric plantar flexion strength, and lower inversion proprioception, as being predictive of ankle sprain, but the studies have primarily examined non-footballing athletess which makes these factors uncertain at present [74, 78]. The quality of evidence for each predictor can be seen in the below list (Table 3.6).

3.4 Screening Tools to Predict Injury

Screening tools are utilized to identify players, or groups of players, at risk of injury. Consequently, the goal of the preseason screening of players is to obtain information for the medical staff to aid in injury prevention. In football, screening tools implement the use of known risk factors either to predict unspecific injuries, such as lower extremity injuries or knee injuries [47, 79], or they are used to predict specific injuries, such as rupture of the ACL [80] or patellofemoral pain [81]. Screening tools focus mainly on modifiable risk factors, and only factors that are of known significance and that can be prevented are of interest in this respect. A few examples will be provided in this section, but the complexity of screening tool development needs to be discussed first. A recently published article on the subject presents three crucial steps in this regard. First, using prospective studies, a strong correlation between markers from a screening test and injury risk needs to be demonstrated. Second, the properties of the test need to be examined in relevant populations using appropriate statistical methods. Third, an implemented intervention program (preferably undertaken using a randomized controlled trial study design) needs to show superior results for the individuals at high risk in comparison to the program being given to all athletes. According to the author, there is currently no intervention study providing support for the screening of sports injuries that complies with these guidelines. One of the main difficulties is the overlap of risk factor markers between individuals that suffer or do not suffer injury. This results in complexity in the determination of cut-off values where continuous risk factor marker values need to be dichotomized in order to provide support for the individuals who will benefit from intervention [82].

Fact Box 1 High Knee Abduction Moment

High knee abduction moment is measured by a player dropping from a 31-cm box to the floor and then performing a jump at maximum height. Imagery in two dimensions is obtained using two video cameras capturing the frontal and sagittal aspects of the legs. Using a freeware application, values from knee valgus motion and knee flexion range of motion were determined. These values were combined with three other predictors (tibia length, body mass, and quadriceps-to-hamstring strength ratio), and a nomogram was used to interpret the results. Points from the respective predictors are summarized and can easily be compared with the corresponding probability of a high knee load. High knee abduction moment has been shown to be predicted with 77% sensitivity and 71% specificity [58].

An example of a well-known screening tool has been presented by Myer et al. The authors developed a simplified, affordable setup for their intricate method of using high knee abduction moment to predict ACL injury in young female athletes as an alternative to the more expensive 3D motion analysis [83]. Since knee abduction moment, as mentioned above, has been regarded as being predictive of ACL injury, the authors recommended the use of this method in the preseason screening of young female athletes. The aim was to prevent ACL injury by reducing knee abduction moment in high-risk athletes [84]. To summarize, using this method to measure knee abduction moment is appealing, but questions have been raised recently as to the predictive ability of high knee abduction moment following the results of the recent negative publication of the abovementioned prospective cohort study [43].

Balance is a modifiable factor, and a common assessment test is the Star Excursion Balance Test. The Star Excursion Balance Test was first described by Gray in 1995 as a rehabilitative tool [85]. The test measures balance by placing the participant in the center of a star of lines. The participant is instructed to stand on one foot and achieve maximum reach with the other foot along one of eight lines. The test has been used for more than two decades, and there are accumulated data suggesting that it is reliable in detecting dynamic balance deficit [86]. In addition, it has been shown that it is possible to improve the performance by following a neuromuscular training program [87]. The question still remains of whether the improvement in balance that was observed results in a reduced risk of lower extremity injury. Further, 235 youth basketball players were examined prospectively, and a 2.5 fold increase in the risk of lower extremity injury in players with poor results using the Star Excursion Balance Test was demonstrated. Predictive studies using the test in assessments of football players are few in number, although one previous study has implemented the test in its cohort study [88].

Take-Home Message

During the last few decades, we have seen extensive and ambitious research designed to enhance our understanding of injury predictors in football. It is obvious that a combination of risk factors and injury mechanisms contributes to an increased risk of injury. There is sufficient evidence to conclude that female gender, for example, is a predictor of ACL rupture or that previous injury is a significant risk factor for an increased risk of ankle sprain. Based on previous research, screening tools have been developed to aid the medical team to prevent future injuries in the squad. The implementation of screening tools requires modifiable risk factors with preventive methods that produce a scientifically significant reduction in injury risk. The emergence of screening tools constitutes a promising field. However, there are scientific pitfalls, and vigilance is required when interpreting the results of novel studies assessing this. Moreover, there is still controversy about several potential predictors that require additional data from large, high-quality studies.

Top Five Evidence-Based References

Arnason A, Sigurdsson SB, Gudmundsson A, Holme I, Engebretsen L, Bahr R (2004) Risk factors for injuries in football. Am J Sports Med 32:5s–16s. [23] (Ankle injury)

van Dyk N, Bahr R, Whiteley R, Tol JL, Kumar BD, Hamilton B et al (2016) Hamstring and quadriceps isokinetic strength deficits are weak risk factors for hamstring strain injuries: a 4-year cohort study. Am J Sports Med 44:1789–1795. [25] (Hamstrings injury)

Engebretsen AH, Myklebust G, Holme I, Engebretsen L, Bahr R (2010) Intrinsic risk factors for groin injuries among male soccer players: a prospective cohort study. Am J Sports Med 38:2051–2057. [16] (Hip/groin injury)

Hagglund M, Walden M, Ekstrand J (2013) Risk factors for lower extremity muscle injury in professional soccer: the UEFA Injury Study. Am J Sports Med 41:327–335. [31] (Quadriceps injury)

Krosshaug T, Steffen K, Kristianslund E, Nilstad A, Mok KM, Myklebust G et al (2016) The vertical drop jump is a poor screening test for ACL injuries in female elite soccer and handball players: a prospective cohort study of 710 athletes. Am J Sports Med 44:874–883. [43] (Knee injury)

References

1. van Mechelen W, Hlobil H, Kemper HC (1992) Incidence, severity, aetiology and prevention of sports injuries. A review of concepts. Sports Med 14:82–99

2. Eirale C, Tol JL, Farooq A, Smiley F, Chalabi H (2013) Low injury rate strongly correlates with team success in Qatari professional football. Br J Sports Med 47:807–808
3. Hagglund M, Walden M, Magnusson H, Kristenson K, Bengtsson H, Ekstrand J (2013) Injuries affect team performance negatively in professional football: an 11-year follow-up of the UEFA Champions League injury study. Br J Sports Med 47:738–742
4. Ekstrand J, Hagglund M, Walden M (2011) Injury incidence and injury patterns in professional football: the UEFA injury study. Br J Sports Med 45:553–558
5. Hewett TE, Myer GD, Ford KR, Heidt RS Jr, Colosimo AJ, McLean SG et al (2005) Biomechanical measures of neuromuscular control and valgus loading of the knee predict anterior cruciate ligament injury risk in female athletes: a prospective study. Am J Sports Med 33:492–501
6. Michaelidis M, Koumantakis GA (2014) Effects of knee injury primary prevention programs on anterior cruciate ligament injury rates in female athletes in different sports: a systematic review. Phys Ther Sport 15:200–210
7. Griffin LY, Albohm MJ, Arendt EA, Bahr R, Beynnon BD, Demaio M et al (2006) Understanding and preventing noncontact anterior cruciate ligament injuries: a review of the Hunt Valley II meeting, January 2005. Am J Sports Med 34:1512–1532
8. Williams JGP (1971) Aetiological classification of injuries in sportsmen. Br J Sports Med 5:228–230
9. Murphy DF, Connolly DA, Beynnon BD (2003) Risk factors for lower extremity injury: a review of the literature. Br J Sports Med 37:13–29
10. Bahr R, Krosshaug T (2005) Understanding injury mechanisms: a key component of preventing injuries in sport. Br J Sports Med 39:324–329
11. Meeuwisse WH (1994) Athletic injury etiology: distinguishing between interaction and confounding. Clin J Sport Med 4:171–175
12. Andersen TE, Larsen O, Tenga A, Engebretsen L, Bahr R (2003) Football incident analysis: a new video based method to describe injury mechanisms in professional football. Br J Sports Med 37:226–232
13. Mendiguchia J, Alentorn-Geli E, Brughelli M (2012) Hamstring strain injuries: are we heading in the right direction? Br J Sports Med 46:81–85
14. Werner J, Hagglund M, Walden M, Ekstrand J (2009) UEFA injury study: a prospective study of hip and groin injuries in professional football over seven consecutive seasons. Br J Sports Med 43:1036–1040
15. Maffey L, Emery C (2007) What are the risk factors for groin strain injury in sport? A systematic review of the literature. Sports Med 37:881–894
16. Engebretsen AH, Myklebust G, Holme I, Engebretsen L, Bahr R (2010) Intrinsic risk factors for groin injuries among male soccer players: a prospective cohort study. Am J Sports Med 38:2051–2057
17. Ryan J, DeBurca N, Mc Creesh K (2014) Risk factors for groin/hip injuries in field-based sports: a systematic review. Br J Sports Med 48:1089–1096
18. Walden M, Hagglund M, Ekstrand J (2015) The epidemiology of groin injury in senior football: a systematic review of prospective studies. Br J Sports Med 49:792–797
19. Whittaker JL, Small C, Maffey L, Emery CA (2015) Risk factors for groin injury in sport: an updated systematic review. Br J Sports Med 49:803–809
20. Esteve E, Rathleff MS, Bagur-Calafat C, Urrutia G, Thorborg K (2015) Prevention of groin injuries in sports: a systematic review with meta-analysis of randomised controlled trials. Br J Sports Med 49:785–791
21. van Beijsterveldt AM, van de Port IG, Vereijken AJ, Backx FJ (2013) Risk factors for hamstring injuries in male soccer players: a systematic review of prospective studies. Scand J Med Sci Sports 23:253–262
22. Engebretsen AH, Myklebust G, Holme I, Engebretsen L, Bahr R (2010) Intrinsic risk factors for hamstring injuries among male soccer players: a prospective cohort study. Am J Sports Med 38:1147–1153
23. Arnason A, Sigurdsson SB, Gudmundsson A, Holme I, Engebretsen L, Bahr R (2004) Risk factors for injuries in football. Am J Sports Med 32:5s–16s
24. Hagglund M, Walden M, Ekstrand J (2006) Previous injury as a risk factor for injury in elite football: a prospective study over two consecutive seasons. Br J Sports Med 40:767–772
25. van Dyk N, Bahr R, Whiteley R, Tol JL, Kumar BD, Hamilton B et al (2016) Hamstring and quadriceps isokinetic strength deficits are weak risk factors for hamstring strain injuries: a 4-year cohort study. Am J Sports Med 44:1789–1795
26. Freckleton G, Pizzari T (2013) Risk factors for hamstring muscle strain injury in sport: a systematic review and meta-analysis. Br J Sports Med 47:351–358
27. Mendiguchia J, Alentorn-Geli E, Idoate F, Myer GD (2013) Rectus femoris muscle injuries in football: a clinically relevant review of mechanisms of injury, risk factors and preventive strategies. Br J Sports Med 47:359–366
28. Ekstrand J, Hagglund M, Walden M (2011) Epidemiology of muscle injuries in professional football (soccer). Am J Sports Med 39:1226–1232
29. Bradley PS, Portas MD (2007) The relationship between preseason range of motion and muscle strain injury in elite soccer players. J Strength Cond Res 21:1155–1159
30. Orchard JW (2001) Intrinsic and extrinsic risk factors for muscle strains in Australian football. Am J Sports Med 29:300–303
31. Hagglund M, Walden M, Ekstrand J (2013) Risk factors for lower extremity muscle injury in professional soccer: the UEFA injury study. Am J Sports Med 41:327–335
32. Fousekis K, Tsepis E, Poulmedis P, Athanasopoulos S, Vagenas G (2011) Intrinsic risk factors of non-contact quadriceps and hamstring strains in soccer: a prospective study of 100 professional players. Br J Sports Med 45:709–714

33. Ekstrand J, Hagglund M, Fuller CW (2011) Comparison of injuries sustained on artificial turf and grass by male and female elite football players. Scand J Med Sci Sports 21:824–832
34. Witvrouw E, Danneels L, Asselman P, D'Have T, Cambier D (2003) Muscle flexibility as a risk factor for developing muscle injuries in male professional soccer players. A prospective study. Am J Sports Med 31:41–46
35. Ardern CL, Taylor NF, Feller JA, Webster KE (2014) Fifty-five per cent return to competitive sport following anterior cruciate ligament reconstruction surgery: an updated systematic review and meta-analysis including aspects of physical functioning and contextual factors. Br J Sports Med 48:1543–1552
36. Walden M, Hagglund M, Magnusson H, Ekstrand J (2016) ACL injuries in men's professional football: a 15-year prospective study on time trends and return-to-play rates reveals only 65% of players still play at the top level 3 years after ACL rupture. Br J Sports Med. https://doi.org/10.1136/bjsports-2015-095952
37. Arendt E, Dick R (1995) Knee injury patterns among men and women in collegiate basketball and soccer. NCAA data and review of literature. Am J Sports Med 23:694–701
38. Bjordal JM, Arnly F, Hannestad B, Strand T (1997) Epidemiology of anterior cruciate ligament injuries in soccer. Am J Sports Med 25:341–345
39. Quisquater L, Bollars P, Vanlommel L, Claes S, Corten K, Bellemans J (2013) The incidence of knee and anterior cruciate ligament injuries over one decade in the Belgian Soccer League. Acta Orthop Belg 79:541–546
40. Roos H, Ornell M, Gardsell P, Lohmander LS, Lindstrand A (1995) Soccer after anterior cruciate ligament injury--an incompatible combination? A national survey of incidence and risk factors and a 7-year follow-up of 310 players. Acta Orthop Scand 66:107–112
41. Volpi P, Bisciotti GN, Chamari K, Cena E, Carimati G, Bragazzi NL (2016) Risk factors of anterior cruciate ligament injury in football players: a systematic review of the literature. Muscles Ligaments Tendons J 6:480–485
42. Ford KR, Myer GD, Hewett TE (2003) Valgus knee motion during landing in high school female and male basketball players. Med Sci Sports Exerc 35:1745–1750
43. Krosshaug T, Steffen K, Kristianslund E, Nilstad A, Mok KM, Myklebust G et al (2016) The vertical drop jump is a poor screening test for ACL injuries in female elite soccer and handball players: a prospective cohort study of 710 athletes. Am J Sports Med 44:874–883
44. Hewett TE, Myer GD, Ford KR (2006) Anterior cruciate ligament injuries in female athletes: part 1, mechanisms and risk factors. Am J Sports Med 34:299–311
45. Yund CB. A longitudinal study of injury rates and risk factors in 5 to 12 year old soccer players. 1999
46. Kucera KL, Marshall SW, Kirkendall DT, Marchak PM, Garrett WE Jr (2005) Injury history as a risk factor for incident injury in youth soccer. Br J Sports Med 39:462
47. Ostenberg A, Roos H (2000) Injury risk factors in female European football. A prospective study of 123 players during one season. Scand J Med Sci Sports 10:279–285
48. Soderman K, Alfredson H, Pietila T, Werner S (2001) Risk factors for leg injuries in female soccer players: a prospective investigation during one out-door season. Knee Surg Sports Traumatol Arthrosc 9:313–321
49. Ramesh R, Von Arx O, Azzopardi T, Schranz PJ (2005) The risk of anterior cruciate ligament rupture with generalised joint laxity. J Bone Joint Surg Br 87:800–803
50. Uhorchak JM, Scoville CR, Williams GN, Arciero RA, St Pierre P, Taylor DC (2003) Risk factors associated with noncontact injury of the anterior cruciate ligament: a prospective four-year evaluation of 859 west point cadets. Am J Sports Med 31:831–842
51. Myer GD, Ford KR, Paterno MV, Nick TG, Hewett TE (2008) The effects of generalized joint laxity on risk of anterior cruciate ligament injury in young female athletes. Am J Sports Med 36:1073–1080
52. Thomson A, Whiteley R, Bleakley C (2015) Higher shoe-surface interaction is associated with doubling of lower extremity injury risk in football codes: a systematic review and meta-analysis. Br J Sports Med 49:1245–1252
53. Gehring D, Rott F, Stapelfeldt B, Gollhofer A (2007) Effect of soccer shoe cleats on knee joint loads. Int J Sports Med 28:1030–1034
54. Kaila R (2007) Influence of modern studded and bladed soccer boots and sidestep cutting on knee loading during match play conditions. Am J Sports Med 35:1528–1536
55. Walden M, Hagglund M, Orchard J, Kristenson K, Ekstrand J (2013) Regional differences in injury incidence in European professional football. Scand J Med Sci Sports 23:424–430
56. Balazs GC, Pavey GJ, Brelin AM, Pickett A, Keblish DJ, Rue JP (2015) Risk of anterior cruciate ligament injury in athletes on synthetic playing surfaces: a systematic review. Am J Sports Med 43:1798–1804
57. Orchard JW, Chivers I, Aldous D, Bennell K, Seward H (2005) Rye grass is associated with fewer non-contact anterior cruciate ligament injuries than bermuda grass. Br J Sports Med 39:704–709
58. Ekstrand J, Tropp H (1990) The incidence of ankle sprains in soccer. Foot Ankle 11:41–44
59. Gaulrapp H, Becker A, Walther M, Hess H (2010) Injuries in women's soccer: a 1-year all players prospective field study of the women's Bundesliga (German premier league). Clin J Sport Med 20:264–271
60. Robertson GA, Wood AM, Aitken SA, Court Brown C (2014) Epidemiology, management, and outcome

of sport-related ankle fractures in a standard UK population. Foot Ankle Int 35:1143–1152

61. Ekstrand J, Timpka T, Hagglund M (2006) Risk of injury in elite football played on artificial turf versus natural grass: a prospective two-cohort study. Br J Sports Med 40:975–980
62. Williams S, Hume PA, Kara S (2011) A review of football injuries on third and fourth generation artificial turfs compared with natural turf. Sports Med 41:903–923
63. Kristenson K, Bjorneboe J, Walden M, Andersen TE, Ekstrand J, Hagglund M (2013) The Nordic football injury audit: higher injury rates for professional football clubs with third-generation artificial turf at their home venue. Br J Sports Med 47:775–781
64. Engebretsen AH, Myklebust G, Holme I, Engebretsen L, Bahr R (2010) Intrinsic risk factors for acute ankle injuries among male soccer players: a prospective cohort study. Scand J Med Sci Sports 20:403–410
65. Kofotolis ND, Kellis E, Vlachopoulos SP (2007) Ankle sprain injuries and risk factors in amateur soccer players during a 2-year period. Am J Sports Med 35:458–466
66. Chomiak J, Junge A, Peterson L, Dvorak J (2000) Severe injuries in football players. Influencing factors. Am J Sports Med 28:S58–S68
67. Ekstrand J, Gillquist J (1983) The avoidability of soccer injuries. Int J Sports Med 4:124–128
68. McHugh MP, Tyler TF, Tetro DT, Mullaney MJ, Nicholas SJ (2006) Risk factors for noncontact ankle sprains in high school athletes: the role of hip strength and balance ability. Am J Sports Med 34:464–470
69. Trojian TH, McKeag DB (2006) Single leg balance test to identify risk of ankle sprains. Br J Sports Med 40:610–613. discussion 613
70. Beynnon BD, Murphy DF, Alosa DM (2002) Predictive factors for lateral ankle sprains: a literature review. J Athl Train 37:376–380
71. Faude O, Junge A, Kindermann W, Dvorak J (2006) Risk factors for injuries in elite female soccer players. Br J Sports Med 40:785–790
72. Beynnon BD, Vacek PM, Murphy D, Alosa D, Paller D (2005) First-time inversion ankle ligament trauma: the effects of sex, level of competition, and sport on the incidence of injury. Am J Sports Med 33:1485–1491
73. Fousekis K, Tsepis E, Vagenas G (2012) Intrinsic risk factors of noncontact ankle sprains in soccer: a prospective study on 100 professional players. Am J Sports Med 40:1842–1850
74. Kobayashi T, Tanaka M, Shida M (2016) Intrinsic risk factors of lateral ankle sprain: a systematic review and meta-analysis. Sports Health 8:190–193
75. Tropp H, Askling C, Gillquist J (1985) Prevention of ankle sprains. Am J Sports Med 13:259–262
76. Tropp H, Ekstrand J, Gillquist J (1984) Stabilometry in functional instability of the ankle and its value in predicting injury. Med Sci Sports Exerc 16:64–66
77. Dallinga JM, Benjaminse A, Lemmink KA (2012) Which screening tools can predict injury to the lower extremities in team sports?: a systematic review. Sports Med 42:791–815
78. Witchalls J, Blanch P, Waddington G, Adams R (2012) Intrinsic functional deficits associated with increased risk of ankle injuries: a systematic review with meta-analysis. Br J Sports Med 46:515–523
79. Engebretsen AH, Myklebust G, Holme I, Engebretsen L, Bahr R (2011) Intrinsic risk factors for acute knee injuries among male football players: a prospective cohort study. Scand J Med Sci Sports 21:645–652
80. Alentorn-Geli E, Myer GD, Silvers HJ, Samitier G, Romero D, Lazaro-Haro C et al (2009) Prevention of non-contact anterior cruciate ligament injuries in soccer players. Part 1: mechanisms of injury and underlying risk factors. Knee Surg Sports Traumatol Arthrosc 17:705–729
81. Myer GD, Ford KR, Foss KD, Rauh MJ, Paterno MV, Hewett TE (2014) A predictive model to estimate knee-abduction moment: implications for development of a clinically applicable patellofemoral pain screening tool in female athletes. J Athl Train 49:389–398
82. Bahr R (2016) Why screening tests to predict injury do not work-and probably never will...: a critical review. Br J Sports Med 50:776–780
83. Myer GD, Ford KR, Hewett TE (2011) New method to identify athletes at high risk of ACL injury using clinic-based measurements and freeware computer analysis. Br J Sports Med 45:238–244
84. Myer GD, Ford KR, Brent JL, Hewett TE (2007) Differential neuromuscular training effects on ACL injury risk factors in "high-risk" versus "low-risk" athletes. BMC Musculoskelet Disord 8:39
85. Gray GW (1995) Lower extremity functional profile. Wynn Marketing Inc, Adrian, Mich
86. Gribble PA, Hertel J, Plisky P (2012) Using the star excursion balance test to assess dynamic postural-control deficits and outcomes in lower extremity injury: a literature and systematic review. J Athl Train 47:339–357
87. Filipa A, Byrnes R, Paterno MV, Myer GD, Hewett TE (2010) Neuromuscular training improves performance on the star excursion balance test in young female athletes. J Orthop Sports Phys Ther 40:551–558
88. Nilstad A, Andersen TE, Bahr R, Holme I, Steffen K (2014) Risk factors for lower extremity injuries in elite female soccer players. Am J Sports Med 42:940–948

4 How to Predict Knee Kinematics During an ACL Injury

Zoe Englander, Shaun K. Stinton, and Thomas P. Branch

Contents

Z. Englander, M.S.
Department of Orthopedics, Duke University, Durham, NC, USA

Department of Biomedical Engineering, Duke University, Durham, NC, USA

S.K. Stinton, Ph.D. • T.P. Branch, M.D. (✉)
University Orthopedics, Decatur, GA, USA

ERMI Inc., 441 Armour Place NE, Atlanta, GA, USA
e-mail: doctorbranch@yahoo.com

4.1 Introduction

To accurately predict knee kinematics during an anterior cruciate ligament (ACL) injury, a full understanding of three-dimensional knee structure and function is required. The concept of joint stability as a "system" must be fully understood. Unique features of bone morphology, overall body posture, and ligament function interplay to allow a healthy knee to remain stable during sports activities. In addition, knowledge of the impact of forces in a kinetic chain will allow the surgeon to conceptualize how whole body movement and posture impacts knee function. The development of a prediction algorithm requires both identification of patients with high-risk knee characteristics, as well as the situations that put an individual at risk for an ACL injury. While much research has been dedicated to understanding ACL injury, there is no absolute consensus in the literature regarding high-risk knee joint characteristics or motions [1–4].

One key to predicting which individuals are most likely to sustain an ACL injury is the identification of the at-risk population. ACL injuries affect a relatively young, active population [5, 6] and are more common in females than in males [7, 8]. Non-contact ACL injuries (without direct external impact) account for more than 70% of ACL tears [6], with women more likely to have a non-contact ACL injury than men [9]. Sports requiring sudden pivot or cutting

V. Musahl et al. (eds.), *Return to Play in Football*, https://doi.org/10.1007/978-3-662-55713-6_4

maneuvers, such as football (soccer), are at a higher risk for an ACL injury than pattern sports such as track and field or swimming [9–13]. Contact ACL injuries are likely to be high energy and have a more unpredictable knee kinematic pattern at the time of ACL rupture. Therefore, for simplicity, the focus of this chapter will be on identifying factors that will allow the clinician to predict knee kinematics at the time of a non-contact ACL injury. In this chapter, we will attempt to guide the reader through the complexity of papers into an insightful understanding of how the leg works as a "system" with certain characteristics that can put it at risk for an ACL injury and how these characteristics suggest specific knee kinematics in a non-contact ACL injury. This will help the clinician to decide which patients require more time for recovery of full protective function and which patients are likely to readily handle early return to play for soccer.

4.2 The Concept of Stability

When a patient refers to the stability of their joint, it is described as either stable or unstable. This concept can be difficult to understand and deserves clarification. Is "instability" a symptom felt only by the patient or is it a condition of the joint as a system? "Instability" as a symptom can be misleading. The patient describes an unpredictable event that causes the knee to buckle suddenly. It is the sudden and unpredictable nature of the event that causes the knee to be described as "unstable." Treating surgeons spend time trying to understand the true nature of the event; is it mechanical subluxation or give way weakness from sudden knee pain? Mechanical subluxation occurs when a joint is in a non-anatomical position for a finite period of time. Loading the joint while in this non-anatomical position is unpredictable in nature. In this situation, the knee joint as a system is seen as "unstable." A joint, in an anatomical position, is considered "stable."

The concept of stability in a mechanical system is described in the book *Modern Control Systems* [14]. Consider a right circular cone on its base (Fig. 4.1). Notice that even though each cone is currently balanced in a "stable" state, the potential for each to become "unstable" increases as your eyes move toward the right. Progressively cutting the tip of the cone makes it "more stable" as the cut gets closer to the base. For the knee, the size and shape of the bone combined with ligament function interplay to maintain the tibia in an anatomical position under the femoral condyles. These ligaments form an envelope of "joint play" which can increase in size at the time of a knee injury. It is this increase in size or volume that allows the potential for a "non-anatomical or unstable event" to occur. Remember that the joint remains "stable" if it never experiences a force that puts it into an "unstable" position or state. This becomes very important to understand when determining the timing of return to play. If the athlete has an inherently stable knee due to bone morphology/postural positioning or the knee can be protected from dangerous outside forces or activities with low risk force production are chosen, return to play can be accelerated.

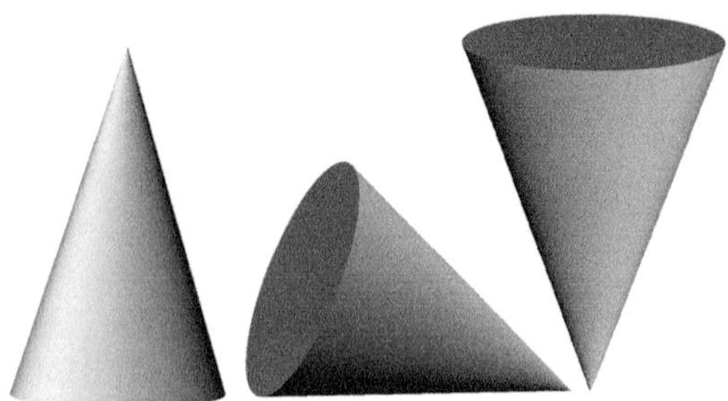

Fig. 4.1 These cones represent a stable condition. The one on its base is the most stable, the one on its side is moderately stable, and the one balanced on its tip is the least stable. It is the amount of force necessary to cause the cones to become unstable that helps categorize them. Once pushed they will become unstable until they settle back into a stable position

Fact Box 1

A joint remains "stable" if it never experiences a force that puts it into an "unstable" state.

4.3 Bone Morphology

The shape of the distal femur and the proximal tibia is important in predicting which knee joint is more likely to have an ACL injury. Multiple studies have evaluated bone morphology and its impact on predicting ACL injury. Some have looked at the femoral notch; specifically, a narrow notch has been suggested as an indication of a smaller ACL [15–18]. Others have surmised that the narrow notch allows for lateral wall impingement increasing load on the ACL with tibial rotation [19]. On the tibial side, the posterior slope of the lateral tibial plateau has been associated with an increased risk of ACL failure [20–23]. The biomechanical concept put forward is that an increased posterior slope contributes to more anterior tibial subluxation with weight bearing. The combination of BMI and posterior slope of the lateral tibial plateau was identified as a predictor for risk of ACL injury [24, 25].

Another concept to consider is the femur to tibial size mismatch. Consider for a moment the golf ball on a tee (Fig. 4.2). The size of the tee has influence on the "stability" of its accompanied golf ball. During the performance of a Pivot Shift Test, it would require more rotation and/or translation for a positive test if, like the small golf ball and the large tee, the tibial plateau was much larger than the distal femur. In one study, the size of the distal femur as measured by its AP dimension plus the height of the lateral femoral condyle divided by its lateral tibial plateau AP dimension produced a "mismatch" ratio, such that a value greater than 1.4 could identify those with a positive pivot shift [26]. This suggests that patients with a large femur and a small tibia are at increased structural risk for a positive pivot shift after ACL injury. Similarly, it was found that the medial/lateral dimension of the tibial plateau correlated with pivot shift grade in women only, not men [27]. Clinicians should use this data to help select the ACL at-risk athlete.

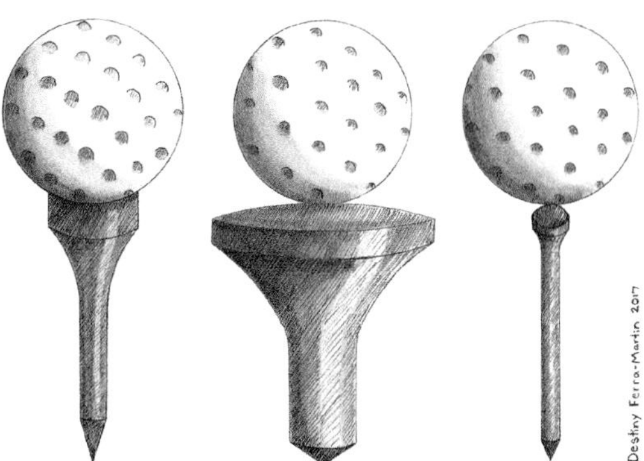

Fig. 4.2 The size of the tee contributes to the stability of the golf ball. The larger surface area of contact allows the ball to move farther before falling off. Similarly, if the tee is leaning with a particular slope, one can imagine that it is harder to balance the golf ball on the tee. A larger lip on the tee might have an additional constraining effect

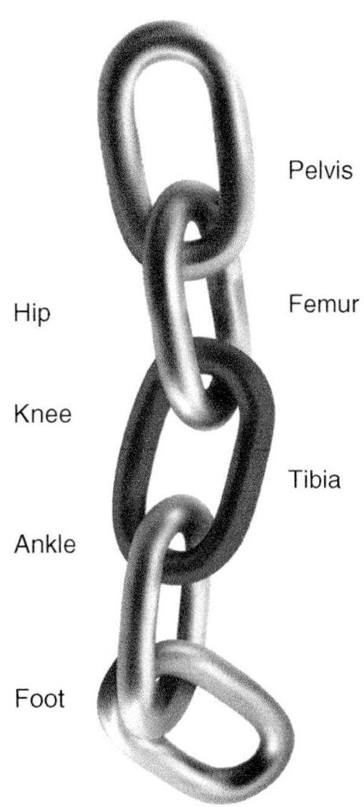

Fig. 4.3 The kinetic chain considers the lower extremity to be like a formal chain where each link is attached to and influences its adjoining link and other links distant to it. Therefore, it is important to know where each link is in space and how each link influences the two that are directly linked to it

Fact Box 2

A small tibial plateau with a posterior slope may indicate bone morphology at risk for ACL injury.

4.4 The Kinetic Chain

The lower extremities are like links of a chain (Fig. 4.3). The position of each link in space influences the adjoining links. Forces applied at one link can propagate up and down the entire chain. For example, if one link is damaged resulting in a limitation of motion between two links, then to achieve full normal motion, the collection of healthy connections in the chain must necessarily increase their motion to make up for the loss in one connection. There are conditions of the foot/ankle and/or hip that will cause the knee to be subjected to pathological forces through the concepts of this "kinetic chain." Ligaments have inherent flexibility and are more like "ropes" than they are like "bars."

The femur "floats" on top of the tibia such that contact forces are minimized in all positions of the kinetic chain. For instance, if you are standing on the side of a hill, the femur is going to position itself on top of the tibia in a way to optimize the balance of the kinetic chain. Specifically, the downhill leg may be in valgus with forces predominantly through the lateral femoral condyle, and the uphill leg may be in varus with the forces predominantly through the medial femoral condyle. This suggests that the knee, to function optimally, must have a certain amount of "joint play" to accommodate all positions of the femur with respect to the tibia and maintain function as a linkage between the two bones. This is particularly true when the knee joint within the kinetic chain acts more like a puppet's knee connected by strings, i.e., wobbly and dependent upon position during load application. Therefore, consideration of a patient's posture during a normal or athletic activity is important in describing the kinetic chain in the clinical world.

4.5 The Knee as a Self-Contained System

Every knee is unique in its bone morphology and ligament construct. It is this combination of passive features interacting together that allows it to perform as an optimal linkage system and maintain system stability. As such, each knee can and should be evaluated separately for its degree of stability as opposed to relying upon side-to-side comparison. Use of the opposite knee as a means for comparison to the injured knee for diagnosis of ligament injury is fraught with danger due to significant anatomical side-to-side variability [28–33]. One study showed that side-to-side differences in 18 paired specimens fell within 1.1 degrees (0–3.0) for adduction/abduction rotation, 2.8 degrees (1.0–8.3) for external/internal tibial axial rotation, and 1.5 mm (0.3–3.9) for anterior/posterior translation [31]. If possible, each knee should be evaluated individually.

> **Fact Box 3**
> It is best to evaluate each knee individually for stability as side-to-side comparison can be misleading.

The shape of each bone combined with the "envelope of joint play" can be used to predict the degree of stability enjoyed by a specific knee. The only clinical knee examination test that does not rely upon side-to-side comparison for the determination of potential instability is the Pivot Shift Test [34–46]. While there is a system for grading the Pivot Shift Test, the clinician is more interested in whether it is present or not present as an indication of a possible "unstable" state. Either the lateral femoral condyle can be subluxed in front of the lateral tibial plateau and forcibly reduced or the knee cannot find that position. The Pivot Shift Test evaluates the knee as its own "self-contained system" by trying to put the femur and the tibia into a non-anatomical position and then cause them to slip back into an anatomical position. When considering return to play, each knee should be evaluated for its potential to slip into a non-anatomic or unstable position and the amount of force it takes to do so. The clinician can then decide whether that knee is at-risk for ACL injury or re-injury when determining return to play.

4.6 Evidence-Based Decision Making for Return to Play

4.6.1 In Vitro Cadaveric Studies

The first task in predicting the kinematics during an ACL injury is the characterization of the "joint play envelope." Cadaveric studies take the knee separate from the limb and cement/lock the tibia and the femur in a pot for placement into a testing device. This technique has been used with sequential cutting of ligaments to provide this information [31, 48–58]. Either a load is applied along a specific direction with the resultant new position recorded or the tibia is moved to a new position relative to the femur with a change in the load recorded (Fig. 4.4). Information about the extent of the "joint play envelope" and its load-deformation characteristics are gathered in accordance with the specific criteria defined by the researcher. The normal values for the "joint play envelope" are compiled in Table 4.1. The idea is to provide the clinician with a range of normal based upon current research. Athletes with motion outside these normal ranges may represent post-injury changes that put the knee at increased risk for re-injury. The well-reconstructed and rehabilitated knee includes an honest evaluation of the current "joint play envelope" with provisions made for unacceptable increases.

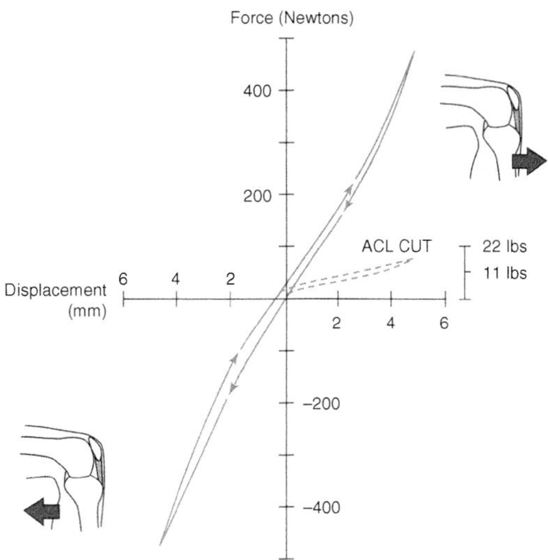

Fig. 4.4 This is a typical load-deformation curve seen in a cadaveric study [47]. This represents the "toe region" of the combined anterior and posterior load-deformation curves

Table 4.1 Envelope of passive motion between the femur and the tibia. Note that there may be some discrepancies between studies as to the zero position of the motion. In some cases, zero position/rotation is taken based upon the shape of the curve, and in other cases, it is based upon a preset coordinate system

Envelope of joint play			
Anterior translation at 30 degree	*Force*	*Intact knee*	*ACLDK*
Rassmussen AM J Sports Med 2015	88 N	33 ± 0.8 mm	12.3 ± 3.7 mm
Aims JBJS(Br) 2002	By hand	4.5 ± 1.3 mm	16.0 ± 4.0 mm
Noyes/Harms Arthrocopy 2015	100 N	5.4 ± 1.1 mm	15.7 ±4.5 mm
Markolf/Sherman Clin Orthop Rel Res 1987	89 N	3.4 ±1.4 mm	6.8 ± 23 mm
UCLA Device->	200 N	5.0± 1.8 mm	10.2 ± 2.6 mm
KT-1000->	89 N	5.6 ± 2.0 mm	12.1 ± 2.6 mm
Lewis			
Daniels Am J Sports Med 1985	89 N	7.3 ± 2.4 mm	11.4 ± 29 mm
Amis JBJS (Br) 1993	150 N	8 mm	25 mm
Espregueira-Mendes KSSTA 2012	88 N	5.1 ± 0.6 mm	10.5 ± 19 mm
Roth ASME Bioengineering Conf (2013)	45 N	Ant—5 mm	n/a
		Post—3 mm	n/a
Internal rotation at 30 degree	*Torque*	*Intact knee*	*ACLDK*
Rassmussen Am J Sports Med 2015	5 Nm	15.7 ± 5.1 degree	163 ±5.1 degree
Alam Am J Sports Med 2012	4 Nm	4.1 ± 0.2 degree	n/a
	6 Nm	6.1 ± 0.3 degree	n/a
Nest of birds->	8 Nm	10.3 ± 0.6 degree	n/a
Rotational measurement device ->	4 Nm	7.3 ± 0.4 degree	n/a
	6 Nm	11.3 ± 0.8 degree	n/a
	8 Nm	14.8 ± 1.0 degree	n/a
Musahl KSSTA 2007	6 Nm	21.9 ± 0.83 degree	n/a
Noyes/Harms Arthroscopy 2015	5 Nm	18.8 ± 3.4 degree	203 ± 4.0 degree

(continued)

Table 4.1 (continued)

Envelope of joint play			
Roth ASM Bioengineering Conf (2013)	3 Nm	15 degree	n/a
External rotation at 30 degree	*Torque*	*Intact knee*	*ACLDK*
Alam Am J Sports Med 2012	4 Nm	4.3 ± 0.1 degree	n/a
	6 Nm	6.9 ± 0.4 degree	n/a
Nest of birds->	8 Nm	103 ± 0.5 degree	n/a
Rotational measurement device ->	4 Nm	7.8 ± 0.5 degree	n/a
	6 Nm	11.8 ± 0.8 degree	n/a
	8 Nm	15.5 ± 1.1 degree	n/a
Roth ASIUE Bioengineering Conf (2013)	3 Nm	19 degree	n/a
Abduction/adduction at 30 degree	*Torque*	*Intact Knee*	*ACLDK*
Shultz J Orthop Res 2007 (20 degree flex)	10 Nm	Valgus-5.35 degree	n/a
		Varus-4.4 degree	n/a
Amis JBJS(Br) 1993	10 Nm	13 degree	14 degree
Markolf JBJS (Am) 1976 (20 degree flex)	29 Nm	Valgus-5.4 ± 2.1 degree	n/a
		Varus-5.4 ± 2.1 degree	n/a
Roth ASME Bioengineering Conf (2013)	5 Nm	Valgus-:1.8 degree	n/a
		Varus-2.2 degree	n/a

4.6.2 In Vivo Gait/Posture Studies

To return an athlete to play, the clinician must understand at-risk sports posture and muscle activity. Gait analysis and/or postural analysis studies are useful as they allow for quantitative analysis of the three-dimensional trajectories of the joints, as well as the forces and moments experienced throughout activity. This allows researchers to investigate the extrinsic factors that may play a role in ACL injury, such as altered motor control strategies during movement [59]. These studies are particularly advantageous as they allow the body to position itself without interference, which may provide clues to "ACL at-risk" postures [1, 22, 59–62]. Furthermore, muscle timing and function can be studied using EMG, which may help us understand the role of muscle contraction on the ACL. For instance, using this technique, hamstring co-contraction has been suggested to have a protective effect on the ACL [63].

Given higher rates of ACL injury in females as opposed to males, posture used by females may provide clues for at-risk knee motions. For instance, it has been suggested that female recreational athletes have smaller knee flexion angles and greater knee valgus angles during the stance phases of running and cutting tasks and may experience greater anterior tibial shear force and have less knee flexion and greater valgus moments during jump and landing tasks than males [59, 61]. One group showed that of 205 athletes evaluated pre-season for jump-landing characteristics, the nine subjects who ultimately sustained an ACL injury had a significantly higher average knee abduction (valgus) angle as well as a 2.5 times higher knee abduction moment and 20% higher ground reaction force [1]. Analysis of videographic footage at the time of injury showed that female players landed with significantly more knee and hip flexion and had a much higher relative risk of sustaining a postural "valgus collapse" than did male players [64], while another videographic study implicated valgus loading at a low flexion angle as a key causative factor for ACL injury [65]. These studies would suggest that loading on a valgus knee, or landing with the knee positioned at a low flexion angle, may increase the risk of ACL injury. The clinician should be aware that patients demonstrating these postural mechanics may be at higher risk for injury and require more strength and postural training than other post-injury or post-surgery patients before return to playing soccer.

The definition of "valgus collapse" used in these studies includes such criteria as increased femoral anteversion, genu valgum, and hindfoot pronation. It is important to understand that the "valgus collapse" described in the literature is a postural only event. There is a fundamental difference between the "valgus collapse" as identified via videographic studies and "valgus overlap" as seen when the lateral tibial plateau falls in front of the radius of curvature of the femur resulting in a "non-anatomical" position. This "valgus overlap" is the non-anatomical position described during the Pivot Shift Test and is the result of the joint losing stability due to the ACL rupture, rather than the mechanism of ACL rupture itself. While there are studies suggesting that a form of a positive pivot shift, known as the pivot glide, might occur in a healthy knee, it is generally understood that a positive pivot shift is associated with an absent ACL [34–46]. Therefore, the authors would like to make a note of this difference; "valgus collapse" is not the same as "valgus overlap." By combining information from in vitro studies with in vivo studies, it appears that axial loading on a valgus knee may be an example of an "ACL at-risk posture." However, what remains important to consider are the other factors associated with gender and kinetic chain morphology that may magnify forces in the ACL seen with axial loading on a valgus knee. Still it may be important to consider additional physical training to change these postural behaviors prior to return to sport.

Fact Box 4
"Valgus overlap" is not the same as "valgus collapse."

4.6.3 Perturbation Studies

There is a need to identify the athlete with at-risk motions within the knee. To study these motions, the interaction between the tibia and the femur must be allowed to have unimpeded limb segment motion, in a precise environment for measurement of rotations/translations and exposed forces. The use of these techniques could be considered "perturbation" studies. There are several examples of in vitro and in vivo "perturbation" studies in the literature [18, 34–36, 40, 66–73]. These studies allow the investigation of system-based interactions that couple together to increase load on the ACL and its risk for injury. It is these "coupling" events that give insight into the knee kinematics at the time of non-contact ACL injury.

Current optical tracking systems during gait or postural testing fail to provide accuracy at the level necessary to distinguish the subtle knee kinematics associated with knee ligament injury. Typically, changes in femur/tibia juxtaposition after injury involve translations and/or rotations that are on the order of millimeters or single digit degrees. Therefore, techniques that provide higher accuracy that can be obtained from traditional gait analysis studies are necessary. A unique system for evaluating knee kinematics and ligament function in vivo has been developed using three-dimensional models of the knee joint created from MR images [49, 74–77]. The joint models represent the structure of the femur and tibia, as well as the origin and insertion points of ligaments. By mapping these models onto dynamic biplanar fluoroscopy images obtained during postural tasks or dynamic activity, the relative positions of the femur and tibia, as well as ligament strains, can be calculated for various knee positions. Thus, the in vivo kinematics of the ACL in the uninjured knee, as well as kinematic changes due to ACL injury, can be quantified. For example, it was found that the length of the ACL decreased and tibial insertion of the ACL twisted internally relative to the femoral insertion as knee flexion angle increased in the uninjured knee [74]. Another study found that ACL strain peaked just prior to landing during a jump-landing task [76], and that ACL strain peaked when the knee was near full extension, with a second local maximum near the end of swing phase just prior to heel strike during gait [75]. Furthermore, a subsequent study demonstrated that in males subjected to various postural positions, the "valgus collapse" posture resulted lowest ACL strain, while the maximum ACL strain occurred at full knee extension [77]. ACL-deficient knees have also been studied using this technique. It was demonstrated that loss of the ACL resulted in a mean medial (1.4 mm) and anterior (3.8 mm) shift of the tibia relative to the femur during lunge loading at 15 degrees of knee flexion [52]. Furthermore, it was found that the ACL-deficient knee demonstrated an anterior shift (1.9 mm), medial shift (1.2 mm), and internal rotation (2.2 deg) compared to the intact knee [78].

In the clinical world, the physical examination of the knee provides significant information to the surgeon. The classic clinical knee examination includes the AP Lachman Test, Tibial Axial Rotation Test, and the Varus/Valgus Stress Test. Each test is characterized by the clinician's application of a force or torque in a primary direction, e.g., anterior/posterior force in the AP Lachman Test. During the test, motion of the knee in the direction of primary force application along with motion in the other 5 degrees of freedom is felt by the clinician. To aid in making each test more objective, measurement systems like the KT-1000, KT-2000, Stryker KT, Rolimeter, and Vermont Laxity Tester have been developed. Recently, a standardized and automated robotic (STAR) clinical knee examination system was devised to allow the application of a standard force/torque to the foot/leg while measuring 3D motion between the femur and the tibia using an electromagnetic system. Objective load-deformation curves can demonstrate all "coupled" 3D motions during each clinical knee examination test. These motions are "coupled" to the "primary motion." This "coupling effect" in the knee was first described as the presence of internal and external rotation of the tibia in response to an anterior/posterior translational force during the AP Lachman Test (see Fig. 4.5) [79]. The "coupling effect" between the primary and all secondary directions is shown in Fig. 4.6. For instance, the loss of the anterior cruciate ligament results in, not only, increased anterior translation (Fig. 4.6d) but increased tibial flexion (Fig. 4.6a), loss of coupled internal rotation (Fig. 4.6e), and joint distraction (Fig. 4.6f). The

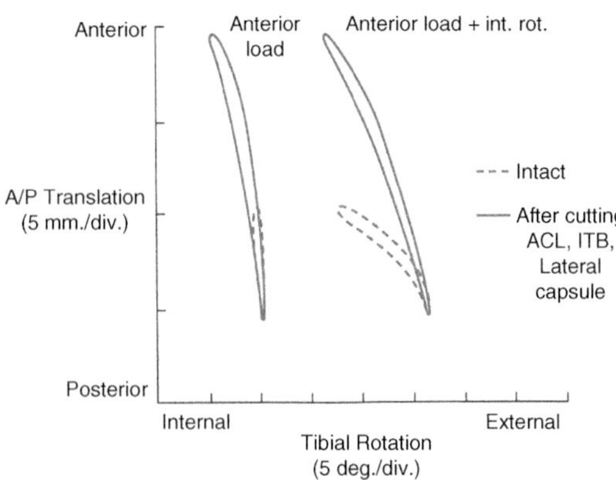

Fig. 4.5 Note that in the first example, only a direct anterior load is applied, while in the second example, combined anterior and internal rotation loads are applied. In this example, the entire hysteresis curve in a single cadaver is shown (modified from [79])

loss of coupled internal rotation and the increased medial translation of the tibia after cutting the ACL with anterior loading previously described is confirmed in this Fig. 4.6 [52, 53, 78]. These results are similar to those reported by Noyes et. al [48 and Table 4.2].

The application of a knee abduction moment has been of great interest [1, 2]. This same moment is applied during the Varus/Valgus Stress Test. The "coupled" primary and secondary motions are seen in Fig. 4.7. The most important of these coupled motions is anterior translation (Fig. 4.7b) and internal rotation (Fig. 4.7c) of the tibia with respect to the femur during a knee abduction moment. In addition, there is a "valgus overlap" that occurs during the knee abduction moment as seen by relative joint compression (Fig. 4.7d) only with complete loss of the ACL. For the test, the foot is internally rotated making the second toe perpendicular to the floor. This internally rotated foot helps to create the coupled anterior translation/internal rotation during application of the knee abduction moment. It is the tibial position at application of the knee abduction moment that has influence on lateral compartment translation during valgus force application. It is important to see that this "valgus overlap" does not occur even if all the secondary stabilizers to internal rotation are cut. "Valgus overlap" only occurs after the ACL is cut.

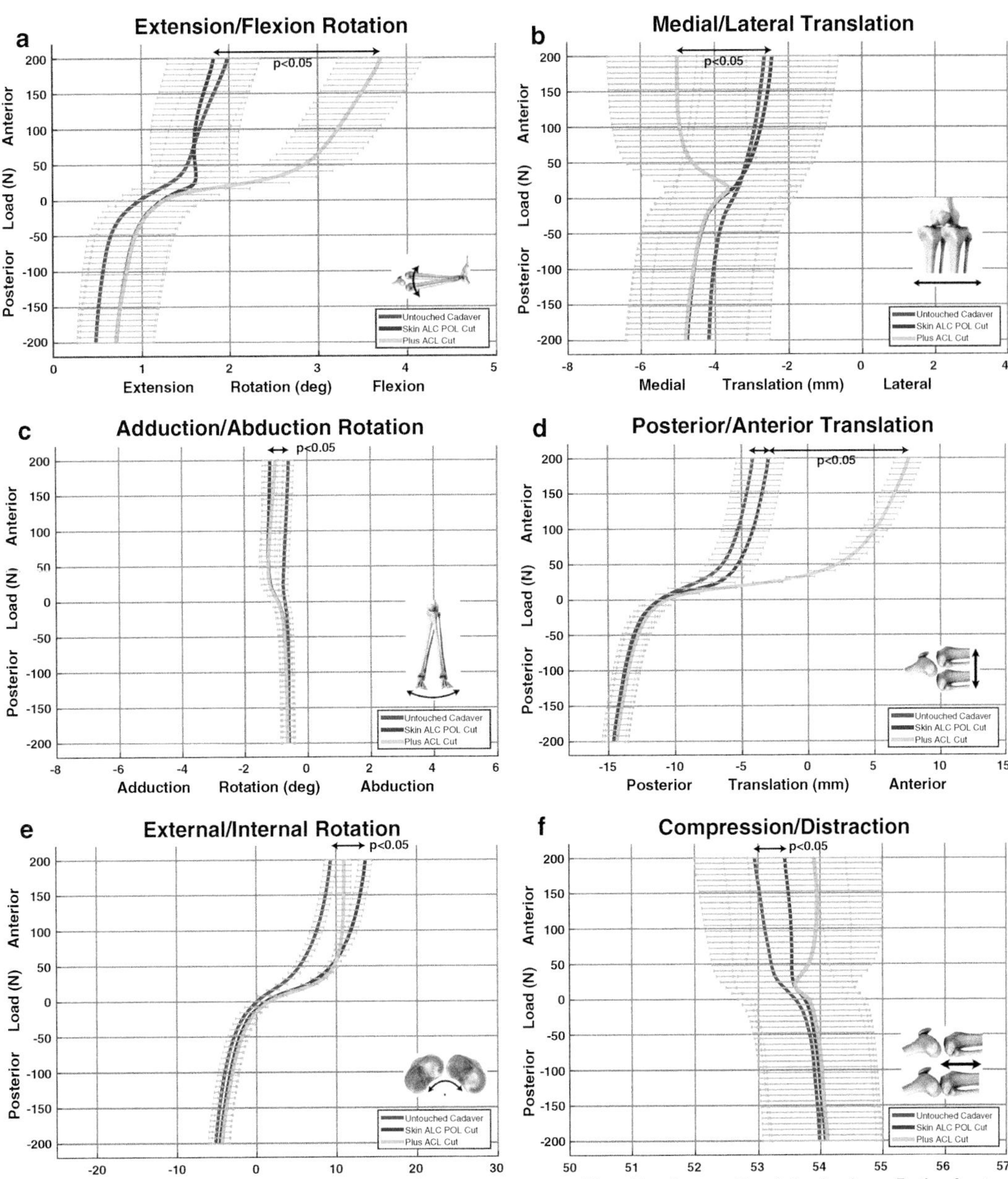

Fig. 4.6 This figure demonstrates the unimpeded motion of the tibia with respect to the femur at 30 degrees of knee flexion in all six degrees of freedom in the untouched cadaver, anterolateral corner (ALC) and posterior oblique ligament (POL) cut, and the addition of the ACL cut knees during the application of an anterior/posterior force. These are mean curves in 12 cadaver knees. All displayed motions are coupled in nature as only an anterior/posterior directed force is applied. Note that extension/flexion is not of the knee; it is extension/flexion of the tibia as the foot remains in the same location

Table 4.2 Loss of the anterior cruciate ligament (ACL) results in a loss of the coupled internal rotation with direct anterior force during the AP Lachman Test. Note that the results are similar in the STAR Robotic Test (Fig. 4.6) (modified from [47])

Mean degrees of coupled rotation during anterior translation tests for intact knees and after ligament sectioning[a]		
	Anterior test flexion angle	
	30°	90°
Intact	−8.6	−10.6
ACL	−5.4	−5.0
MCL	−11.7	−14.7
ACL & MCL	0.6	0.0

[a]Negative numbers represent internal rotation and positive numbers represent external rotation. These numbers are the change in tibial rotation from the position of the tibia after application of anterior forces or abduction moments. Intact (11 donors); ACL cut (6 donors); MCL cut (6 donors); ACL & MCL cut (6 donors).
ACL anterior cruciate ligament; MCL medial collateral ligament

Fact Box 5
Loss of all secondary stabilizers for internal rotation does not result in "valgus overlap." Only loss of the ACL allows for the potential of "valgus overlap." It represents the "unstable" state in the ACL-deficient knee.

Injury patterns within the ACL-damaged knee can be used to predict knee kinematics at the time of injury. With the MRI scan, femur and tibia contact points at the time of the injury can be seen in the form of bone contusions [21, 80, 81]. It is these anatomical points that indicate the position of the tibia under the femur at the time it breaches the "normal joint play envelope" and moves into an "unstable" or non-anatomical

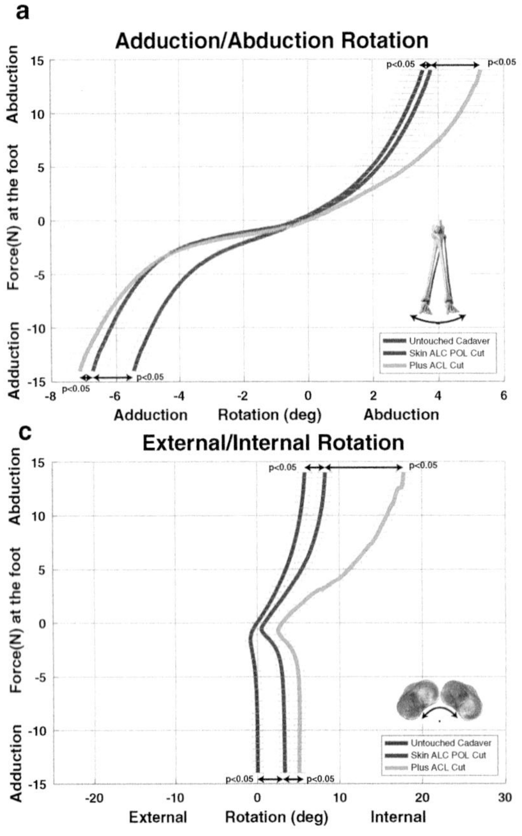

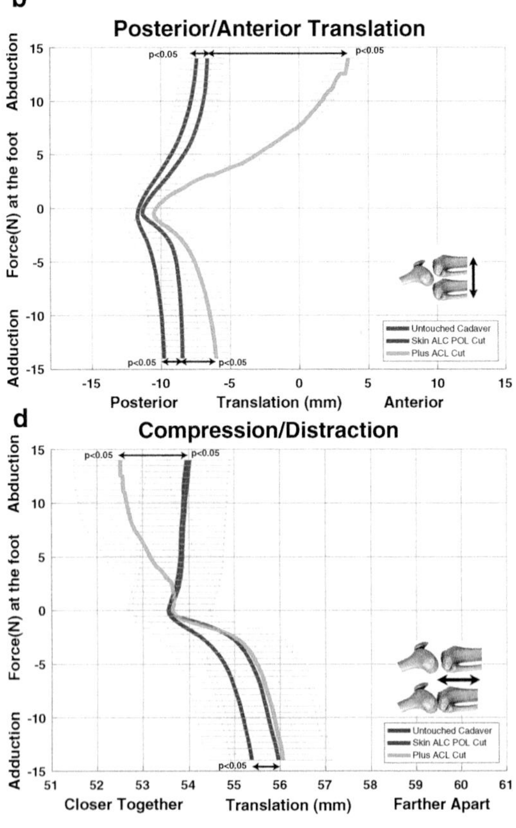

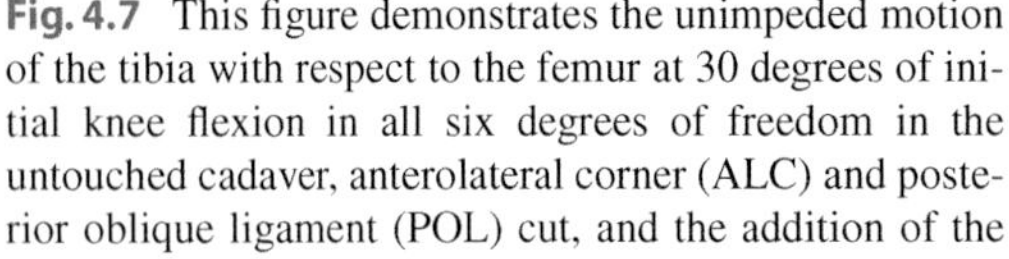

Fig. 4.7 This figure demonstrates the unimpeded motion of the tibia with respect to the femur at 30 degrees of initial knee flexion in all six degrees of freedom in the untouched cadaver, anterolateral corner (ALC) and posterior oblique ligament (POL) cut, and the addition of the ACL cut knees during the application of a knee adduction/abduction moment. These are mean curves in 12 cadaver knees. All displayed motions are coupled in nature as only the knee adduction/abduction moment is applied. Statistical significance is noted and is also in the table

state. Studying acute complete ACL tears within 45 days of injury, a pattern included bruising over the terminal sulcus of the lateral femoral condyle, and the posterolateral tibial plateau was identified. The authors suggest that this pattern may be indicative of a "pivot shift" event in which the anterior tibial translation and valgus rotation occur concurrently with an ACL tear [82]. Another study suggested that the bone bruise pattern in non-contact ACL ruptures indicated anterior tibial translation and tibial internal rotation as the major mechanisms of injury [21].

Recently, researchers used numerical optimization to determine the position of the bone necessary to maximize the overlap of a set of bone bruises to the relative positions of the femur and tibia at the time of injury (Fig. 4.8) [83]. Flexion angle, valgus orientation, internal tibial rotation, and anterior tibial translation were compared between the original positioning of the knee in the MRI and the predicted injury position. Flexion angle was near full extension, while internal tibial rotation (19 deg) and anterior tibial translation (22 mm) were increased in the predicted position of injury relative to the MRI position. Valgus angle was only slightly increased (6 deg) in the injury position as compared to the MRI position. Therefore, the results of this study would support the hypothesis that landing with an extended knee puts the ACL risk for rupture. Keep in mind that the range of "normal joint play" for valgus is 5.4 deg ± 2.1 with the application of 29 Nm of knee abduction moment [31]. These studies provide the clinician with further insight into the potential impact of postural positioning along the edge of their "joint play envelope" increasing the risk of ACL injury. The clinician must be able to identify the at-risk patient for injury to the ACL and insure that they achieve a higher level of physical training before being allowed to return to play in soccer.

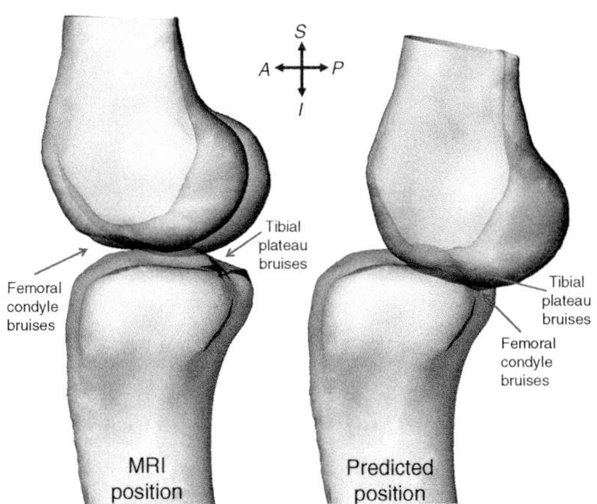

Fig. 4.8 Numerical optimization was used to maximize overlap of bone bruises on the femoral condyle (*red*) and tibial plateau (*blue*) and predict the position of injury. A sagittal view of a 3D model of one subject's knee is shown in the MRI position (*left*) and in the predicted position of injury (*right*). (*A* anterior, *P* posterior, *S* superior, *I* inferior) (Figure adapted from [29])

Fact Box 6

A knee where the tibia positions itself underneath the femur at the edge of a large joint play envelope with a femur-tibia size mismatch, a narrow notch, and an increased posterior tibial slope, combined with an "at-risk" posture, such as one that enhances abduction moments through the knee at weight-bearing impact or increases ACL strain, represents an "at-risk" knee for ACL injury.

4.7 An Algorithm for the Prediction of Knee Kinematics During ACL Injury

Setting up an algorithm for the prediction of knee kinematics during ACL injury depends on understanding stability in the biomechanical system, as well as the impact of bone morphology and normal joint play envelope on the stability of the system, and the role of posture at the time of injury. Without a clear vision of the interaction between these critical features, prediction is less reliable. The key to describing a prediction algorithm revolves around understanding the obligatory secondary motions that occur at the knee in response to outside forces as well as the position of loading at ACL injury. Before injury, a healthy knee is stable and functions within a zone that is responsive to outside forces with a predictable nature. A knee where the tibia positions itself underneath the femur at the edge of a large joint play envelope with a femur-tibia size mismatch, a narrow notch, and an increased posterior tibial slope, combined with an "at-risk" posture, such as one that enhances abduction moments through the knee at weight-bearing impact or increases ACL strain, represents an "at-risk" knee for ACL injury. While there is no absolute consensus in the literature as to high-risk knee joint motions before or during the ACL injury, there is evidence to suggest that "valgus overlap" placing the tibia under the femur in a non-anatomic position is a kinematic result, like a "pivot shift," of the post facto ACL injury itself. Furthermore, evidence exists to support the hypothesis that landing on a valgus knee in extension is a high-risk maneuver that puts the ACL at risk for injury. The clinician should develop their own algorithm with the information presented in this article to craft an athlete-specific post-injury or post-surgery physical training program for return to play, particularly in sports such as soccer.

Take-Home Message

The prediction of knee kinematics during an ACL injury takes knowledge of sports activities, population segment, posture, bone morphology, and internal biomechanics of the knee. Sports activities, such as soccer, that place a premium on jumping and landing appear to have an increased incidence of these injuries. Female athletes in these sports appear to be at a higher risk, potentially due to differences in motion patterns (i.e., increased valgus, decreased knee flexion). Bone morphology may contribute to the likelihood of ACL injury (i.e., posterior slope and relative tibial size), and the dimensions of the "joint play envelope" may help determine the amount of force necessary to cause injury. While there is no absolute consensus on the biomechanical mechanisms leading to non-contact ACL injury, there is extensive evidence to indicate that ACL injury may be the result of a combination of these factors. Clinicians should use this information to determine which athlete will require more physical training before safe return to play.

Fact Box 7

The clinician should develop their own algorithm with the information presented in this article to craft an athlete-specific post-injury or post-surgery physical training program for return to play, particularly in sports such as soccer.

Top 5 Evidence-Based References

Branch TP, Stinton SK, Browne JE, Lording TD, Hutton WC (2017) A robotic system for measuring the relative motion between the Femur and the Tibia. In: Rotatory knee instability. Springer, New York, pp 199–220

DeFrate LE, Papannagari R, Gill TJ, Moses JM, Pathare NP, Li G (2006) The 6 degrees of freedom kinematics of the knee after anterior cruciate ligament deficiency an in vivo imaging analysis. Am J Sports Med 34(8):1240–1246

Lording T, Stinton SK, Neyret P, Branch TP (2017) Diagnostic findings caused by cutting of the iliotibial tract and anterolateral ligament in an ACL intact knee using a standardized and automated clinical knee examination. Knee Surg Sports Traumatol Arthrosc 25(4):1161–1169

Li G, DeFrate LE, Rubash HE, Gill TJ (2005) In vivo kinematics of the ACL during weight-bearing knee flexion. J Orthopaedic Res 23(2): 340–344

Markolf KL, Burchfield DM, Shapiro MM, Shepard MF, Finerman GA, Slauterbeck JL (1995) Combined knee loading states that generate high anterior cruciate ligament forces. J Orthopaedic Res 13(6): 930–935

References

1. Hewett TE, Myer GD, Ford KR, Heidt RS, Colosimo AJ, McLean SG, Van den Bogert AJ, Paterno MV, Succop P (2005) Biomechanical measures of neuromuscular control and valgus loading of the knee predict anterior cruciate ligament injury risk in female athletes a prospective study. Am J Sports Med 33(4):492–501
2. Hewett TE, Roewer B, Ford K, Myer G (2015) Multicenter trial of motion analysis for injury risk prediction: lessons learned from prospective longitudinal large cohort combined biomechanical-epidemiological studies. Braz J Phys Ther 19(5):398–409
3. Myer GD, Ford KR, Khoury J, Succop P, Hewett TE (2010a) Biomechanics laboratory-based prediction algorithm to identify female athletes with high knee loads that increase risk of ACL injury. Br J Sports Med 45:245–252. bjsports 69351

4. Myer GD, Ford KR, Khoury J, Succop P, Hewett TE (2010b) Development and validation of a clinic-based prediction tool to identify female athletes at high risk for anterior cruciate ligament injury. Am J Sports Med 38(10):2025–2033
5. Collins JE, Katz JN, Donnell-Fink LA, Martin SD, Losina E (2013) Cumulative incidence of ACL reconstruction after ACL injury in adults role of age, sex, and race. Am J Sports Med 41(3):544–549
6. Griffin LY, Albohm MJ, Arendt EA, Bahr R, Beynnon BD, DeMaio M, Dick RW, Engebretsen L, Garrett WE, Hannafin JA (2006) Understanding and preventing noncontact anterior cruciate ligament injuries a review of the Hunt Valley II meeting, January 2005. Am J Sports Med 34(9):1512–1532
7. Prodromos CC, Han Y, Rogowski J, Joyce B, Shi K (2007) A meta-analysis of the incidence of anterior cruciate ligament tears as a function of gender, sport, and a knee injury–reduction regimen. Arthroscopy 23(12):1320–1325.e6
8. Quatman CE, Hewett TE (2009) The anterior cruciate ligament injury controversy: is "valgus collapse" a sex-specific mechanism? Br J Sports Med 43(5):328–335
9. Agel J, Rockwood T, Klossner D (2016) Collegiate ACL injury rates across 15 sports: National Collegiate Athletic Association Injury Surveillance System Data Update (2004-2005 through 2012-2013). Clin J Sport Med 26(6):518–523
10. Beck NA, Lawrence JTR, Nordin JD, DeFor TA, Tompkins M (2017) ACL tears in school-aged children and adolescents over 20 years. Pediatrics 139(3):e20161877
11. Kaeding CC, Léger-St-Jean B, Magnussen RA (2017) Epidemiology and diagnosis of anterior cruciate ligament injuries. Clin Sports Med 36(1):1–8
12. Sayampanathan AA, Howe BKT, Bin Abd Razak HR, Chi CH, Tan AHC (2017) Epidemiology of surgically managed anterior cruciate ligament ruptures in a sports surgery practice. J Orthop Surg (Hong Kong) 25(1):2309499016684289
13. Takahashi S, Okuwaki T (2017) Epidemiological survey of anterior cruciate ligament injury in Japanese junior high school and high school athletes: cross-sectional study. Res Sports Med 3:266–276
14. Dorf R (2001) In: Bishop RF, Modern control systems 9
15. Boden BP, Breit I, Sheehan FT (2009) Tibiofemoral alignment: contributing factors to noncontact anterior cruciate ligament injury. J Bone Joint Surg Am 91(10):2381–2389
16. LaPrade RF, Burnett QM (1994) Femoral intercondylar notch stenosis and correlation to anterior cruciate ligament injuries: a prospective study. Am J Sports Med 22(2):198–203
17. Souryal TO, Freeman TR (1993) Intercondylar notch size and anterior cruciate ligament injuries in athletes: a prospective study. Am J Sports Med 21(4):535–539
18. Souryal TO, Moore HA, Evans JP (1988) Bilaterality in anterior cruciate ligament injuries associated intercondylar notch stenosis. Am J Sports Med 16(5):449–454
19. Dienst M, Schneider G, Altmeyer K, Voelkering K, Georg T, Kramann B, Kohn D (2007) Correlation of intercondylar notch cross sections to the ACL size: a high resolution MR tomographic in vivo analysis. Arch Orthop Trauma Surg 127(4):253–260
20. Brandon ML, Haynes PT, Bonamo JR, Flynn MI, Barrett GR, Sherman MF (2006) The association between posterior-inferior tibial slope and anterior cruciate ligament insufficiency. Arthroscopy 22(8):894–899
21. Viskontas DG, Giuffre BM, Duggal N, Graham D, Parker D, Coolican M (2008) Bone bruises associated with ACL rupture correlation with injury mechanism. Am J Sports Med 36(5):927–933
22. Yu B, Lin C-F, Garrett WE (2006) Lower extremity biomechanics during the landing of a stop-jump task. Clin Biomech 21(3):297–305
23. Voos JE, Suero EM, Citak M, Petrigliano FP, Bosscher MR, Citak M, Wickiewicz TL, Pearle AD (2012) Effect of tibial slope on the stability of the anterior cruciate ligament–deficient knee. Knee Surg Sports Traumatol Arthrosc 20(8):1626–1631
24. Bojicic KM, Beaulieu ML, Imaizumi Krieger DY, Ashton-Miller JA, Wojtys EM (2017) Association between lateral posterior Tibial slope, body mass index, and ACL injury risk. Orthop J Sports Med 5(2):2325967116688664
25. Yue D, Wang B, Wang W, Guo W, Zhang Q (2013) Effects of posterior tibial slope on non-contact anterior cruciate ligament rupture and stability of anterior cruciate ligament rupture knee. Zhonghua Yi Xue Za Zhi 93(17):1309–1312
26. Branch TP, Stinton SK, Sharma A, Lavoie F, Guier C, Neyret P. The impact of bone morphology on the outcome of the pivot shift test: a cohort study. BMC Musculoskeletal Disorders DOI: 10.1186/s12891-017-1798-4
27. Musahl V, Ayeni OR, Citak M, Irrgang JJ, Pearle AD, Wickiewicz TL (2010) The influence of bony morphology on the magnitude of the pivot shift. Knee Surg Sports Traumatol Arthrosc 18(9):1232–1238
28. Edixhoven P, Huiskes R, De Graaf R (1989) Anteroposterior drawer measurements in the knee using an instrumented test device. Clin Orthop Relat Res (247):232–242
29. Edixhoven P, Huiskes R, De Graaf R, Van Rens TJ, Slooff T (1987) Accuracy and reproducibility of instrumented knee-drawer tests. J Orthop Res 5(3):378–387
30. Markolf KL, Graff-Radford A, Amstutz H (1978) In vivo knee stability. A quantitative assessment using an instrumented clinical testing apparatus. J Bone Joint Surg Am 60(5):664–674
31. Markolf KL, Mensch J, Amstutz H (1976) Stiffness and laxity of the knee--the contributions of the supporting structures. A quantitative in vitro study. J Bone Joint Surg Am 58(5):583–594
32. Shultz SJ, Shimokochi Y, Nguyen A-D, Schmitz RJ, Beynnon BD, Perrin DH (2007a) Measurement of varus-valgus and internal-external rotational knee laxities in vivo-part II: relationship with anterior-

posterior and general joint laxity in males and females. J Orthop Res 25(8):989–996
33. Shultz SJ, Shimokochi Y, Nguyen AD, Schmitz RJ, Beynnon BD, Perrin DH (2007b) Measurement of varus–valgus and internal–external rotational knee laxities in vivo—part I: assessment of measurement reliability and bilateral asymmetry. J Orthop Res 25(8):981–988
34. Bedi A, Musahl V, Lane C, Citak M, Warren RF, Pearle AD (2010a) Lateral compartment translation predicts the grade of pivot shift: a cadaveric and clinical analysis. Knee Surg Sports Traumatol Arthrosc 18(9):1269–1276
35. Bedi A, Musahl V, O'Loughlin P, Maak T, Citak M, Dixon P, Pearle AD (2010b) A comparison of the effect of central anatomical single-bundle anterior cruciate ligament reconstruction and double-bundle anterior cruciate ligament reconstruction on pivot-shift kinematics. Am J Sports Med 38(9):1788–1794
36. Citak M, Suero EM, Rozell JC, Bosscher MRF, Kuestermeyer J, Pearle AD (2011) A mechanized and standardized pivot shifter: technical description and first evaluation. Knee Surg Sports Traumatol Arthrosc 19(5):707–711
37. Hoshino Y, Araujo P, Ahlden M, Moore CG, Kuroda R, Zaffagnini S, Karlsson J, Fu FH, Musahl V (2012) Standardized pivot shift test improves measurement accuracy. Knee Surg Sports Traumatol Arthrosc 20(4):732–736
38. Lopomo N, Signorelli C, Rahnemai-Azar AA, Raggi F, Hoshino Y, Samuelsson K, Musahl V, Karlsson J, Kuroda R, Zaffagnini S (2016) Analysis of the influence of anaesthesia on the clinical and quantitative assessment of the pivot shift: a multicenter international study. Knee Surg Sports Traumatol Arthrosc:1–8
39. Muller B, Hofbauer M, Rahnemai-Azar AA, Wolf M, Araki D, Hoshino Y, Araujo P, Debski RE, Irrgang JJ, Fu FH (2016) Development of computer tablet software for clinical quantification of lateral knee compartment translation during the pivot shift test. Comput Methods Biomech Biomed Engin 19(2):217–228
40. Musahl V, Bedi A, Citak M, O'Loughlin P, Choi D, Pearle AD (2011) Effect of single-bundle and double-bundle anterior cruciate ligament reconstructions on pivot-shift kinematics in anterior cruciate ligament- and meniscus-deficient knees. Am J Sports Med 39(2):289–295
41. Musahl V, Hoshino Y, Ahlden M, Araujo P, Irrgang JJ, Zaffagnini S, Karlsson J, Fu FH (2012a) The pivot shift: a global user guide. Knee Surg Sports Traumatol Arthrosc 20(4):724–731
42. Musahl V, Hoshino Y, Becker R, Karlsson J (2012b) Rotatory knee laxity and the pivot shift. Springer
43. Petrigliano FA, Musahl V, Suero EM, Citak M, Pearle AD (2011) Effect of meniscal loss on knee stability after single-bundle anterior cruciate ligament reconstruction. Knee Surg Sports Traumatol Arthrosc 19(1):86–93
44. Suero EM, Njoku IU, Voigt MR, Lin J, Koenig D, Pearle AD (2013) The role of the iliotibial band during the pivot shift test. Knee Surg Sports Traumatol Arthrosc 21(9):2096–2100
45. Sundemo D, Alentorn-Geli E, Hoshino Y, Musahl V, Karlsson J, Samuelsson K (2016) Objective measures on knee instability: dynamic tests: a review of devices for assessment of dynamic knee laxity through utilization of the pivot shift test. Curr Rev Muscoskelet Med 9(2):148–159
46. Tanaka M, Vyas D, Moloney G, Bedi A, Pearle A, Musahl V (2012) What does it take to have a high-grade pivot shift? Knee Surg Sports Traumatol Arthrosc 20(4):737–742
47. Noyes FR (2016) Noyes' knee disorders: surgery, rehabilitation, clinical outcomes. Elsevier Health Sciences, Philadelphia, PA
48. Butler DL, Noyes F, Grood E (1980) Ligamentous restraints to anterior-posterior drawer in the human knee. A biomechanical study. JBJS 62(2):259–270
49. DeFrate LE, Nha KW, Papannagari R, Moses JM, Gill TJ, Li G (2007) The biomechanical function of the patellar tendon during in-vivo weight-bearing flexion. J Biomech 40(8):1716–1722
50. Inderhaug E, Stephen JM, Williams A, Amis AA (2017) Biomechanical comparison of anterolateral procedures combined with anterior cruciate ligament reconstruction. Am J Sports Med 45(2):347–354
51. Kittl C, El-Daou H, Athwal KK, Gupte CM, Weiler A, Williams A, Amis AA (2016) The role of the anterolateral structures and the ACL in controlling laxity of the intact and ACL-deficient knee. Am J Sports Med 44(2):345–354
52. Li G, Moses J, Papannagari R, Pathare N, Defrate L (2007a) Anterior cruciate ligament deficiency alters the in vivo motion of the tibiofemoral cartilage contact points in both the anteroposterior and mediolateral directions. J Orthop Sports Phys 37(7):421–422
53. Li G, Papannagari R, Defrate LE, Doo Yoo J, Eun Park S, J Gill T (2007b) The effects of ACL deficiency on mediolateral translation and varus–valgus rotation. Acta Orthop 78(3):355–360
54. Li G, Rudy T, Sakane M, Kanamori A, Ma C, Woo S-Y (1999) The importance of quadriceps and hamstring muscle loading on knee kinematics and in-situ forces in the ACL. J Biomech 32(4):395–400
55. Li G, Rudy TW, Allen C, Sakane M, Woo SLY (1998) Effect of combined axial compressive and anterior tibial loads on in situ forces in the anterior cruciate ligament: a porcine study. J Orthop Res 16(1):122–127
56. Li G, Zayontz S, Most E, DeFrate LE, Suggs JF, Rubash HE (2004) In situ forces of the anterior and posterior cruciate ligaments in high knee flexion: an in vitro investigation. J Orthop Res 22(2):293–297
57. Lord BR, El-Daou H, Sabnis BM, Gupte CM, Wilson AM, Amis AA (2016) Biomechanical comparison of graft structures in anterior cruciate ligament reconstruction. Knee Surg Sports Traumatol Arthrosc:1–10
58. Markolf KL, Burchfield DM, Shapiro MM, Shepard MF, Finerman GA, Slauterbeck JL (1995) Combined knee loading states that generate high anterior cruciate ligament forces. J Orthop Res 13(6):930–935
59. Chappell JD, Yu B, Kirkendall DT, Garrett WE (2002) A comparison of knee kinetics between male and

female recreational athletes in stop-jump tasks. Am J Sports Med 30(2):261–267

60. Kadaba M, Ramakrishnan H, Wootten M, Gainey J, Gorton G, Cochran G (1989) Repeatability of kinematic, kinetic, and electromyographic data in normal adult gait. J Orthop Res 7(6):849–860
61. Malinzak RA, Colby SM, Kirkendall DT, Yu B, Garrett WE (2001) A comparison of knee joint motion patterns between men and women in selected athletic tasks. Clin Biomech 16(5):438–445
62. Shultz SJ, Nguyen A-D, Leonard MD, Schmitz RJ (2009) Thigh strength and activation as predictors of knee biomechanics during a drop jump task. Med Sci Sports Exerc 41(4):857
63. Branch TP, Hunter R, Donath M (1989) Dynamic EMG analysis of anterior cruciate deficient legs with and without bracing during cutting. Am J Sports Med 17(1):35–41
64. Krosshaug T, Nakamae A, Boden BP, Engebretsen L, Smith G, Slauterbeck JR, Hewett TE, Bahr R (2007a) Mechanisms of anterior cruciate ligament injury in basketball video analysis of 39 cases. Am J Sports Med 35(3):359–367
65. Krosshaug T, Slauterbeck JR, Engebretsen L, Bahr R (2007b) Biomechanical analysis of anterior cruciate ligament injury mechanisms: three-dimensional motion reconstruction from video sequences. Scand J Med Sci Sports 17(5):508–519
66. Branch T, Lavoie F, Guier C, Branch E, Lording T, Stinton S, Neyret P (2015a) Single-bundle ACL reconstruction with and without extra-articular reconstruction: evaluation with robotic lower leg rotation testing and patient satisfaction scores. Knee Surg Sports Traumatol Arthrosc 23(10):2882–2891
67. Branch T, Stinton S, Siebold R, Freedberg H, Jacobs C, Hutton W (2017) Assessment of knee laxity using a robotic testing device: a comparison to the manual clinical knee examination. Knee Surg Sports Traumatol Arthrosc 25(8):2460–2467
68. Branch T, Stinton S, Sternberg M, Hutton W, Lavoie F, Guier C, Neyret P (2015c) Robotic axial lower leg testing: repeatability and reproducibility. Knee Surg Sports Traumatol Arthrosc 23(10):2892–2899
69. Branch TP, Stinton SK, Browne JE, Lording TD, Hutton WC (2017) A robotic system for measuring the relative motion between the femur and the tibia. In: Rotatory knee instability. Springer, New York, pp 199–220
70. Espregueira-Mendes J, Andrade R, Leal A, Pereira H, Skaf A, Rodrigues-Gomes S, Oliveira JM, Reis RL, Pereira R (2016) Global rotation has high sensitivity in ACL lesions within stress MRI. Knee Surg Sports Traumatol Arthrosc:1–11
71. Espregueira-Mendes J, Pereira H, Sevivas N, Passos C, Vasconcelos JC, Monteiro A, Oliveira JM, Reis RL (2012) Assessment of rotatory laxity in anterior cruciate ligament-deficient knees using magnetic resonance imaging with Porto-knee testing device. Knee Surg Sports Traumatol Arthrosc 20(4):671–678
72. Lording T, Stinton SK, Neyret P, Branch TP (2017) Diagnostic findings caused by cutting of the iliotibial tract and anterolateral ligament in an ACL intact knee using a standardized and automated clinical knee examination. Knee Surg Traumatol Arthrosc 25(4):1161–1169
73. Stinton S, Siebold R, Freedberg H, Jacobs C, Branch T (2016) The use of a robotic tibial rotation device and an electromagnetic tracking system to accurately reproduce the clinical dial test. Knee Surg Sports Traumatol Arthrosc 24(3):815–822
74. Li G, DeFrate LE, Rubash HE, Gill TJ (2005) In vivo kinematics of the ACL during weight-bearing knee flexion. J Orthop Res 23(2):340–344
75. Taylor K, Cutcliffe H, Queen R, Utturkar G, Spritzer C, Garrett W, DeFrate L (2013) In vivo measurement of ACL length and relative strain during walking. J Biomech 46(3):478–483
76. Taylor K, Terry M, Utturkar G, Spritzer C, Queen R, Irribarra L, Garrett W, DeFrate L (2011) Measurement of in vivo anterior cruciate ligament strain during dynamic jump landing. J Biomech 44(3):365–371
77. Utturkar G, Irribarra L, Taylor K, Spritzer C, Taylor D, Garrett W, DeFrate LE (2013) The effects of a valgus collapse knee position on in vivo ACL elongation. Ann Biomed Eng 41(1):123–130
78. DeFrate LE, Papannagari R, Gill TJ, Moses JM, Pathare NP, Li G (2006) The 6 degrees of freedom kinematics of the knee after anterior cruciate ligament deficiency an in vivo imaging analysis. Am J Sports Med 34(8):1240–1246
79. Noyes F, Grood E (1986) Classification of ligament injuries: why an anterolateral laxity or anteromedial laxity is not a diagnostic entity. Instr Course Lect 36:185–200
80. Kaplan PA, Gehl RH, Dussault RG, Anderson MW, Diduch DR (1999) Bone contusions of the posterior lip of the medial Tibial plateau (Contrecoup injury) and associated internal derangements of the knee at MR imaging 1. Radiology 211(3):747–753
81. Patel SA, Hageman J, Quatman CE, Wordeman SC, Hewett TE (2014) Prevalence and location of bone bruises associated with anterior cruciate ligament injury and implications for mechanism of injury: a systematic review. Sports Med 44(2):281–293
82. Speer KP, Spritzer CE, Bassett FH III, Feagin JRJA, Garrett JRWE (1992) Osseous injury associated with acute tears of the anterior cruciate ligament. Am J Sports Med 20(4):382–389
83. Kim SY, Spritzer CE, Utturkar GM, Toth AP, Garrett WE, DeFrate LE (2015) Knee kinematics during noncontact anterior cruciate ligament injury as determined from bone bruise location. Am J Sports Med 43(10):2515–2521

5 Match-Related Factors Influencing Injury Risk

Jaakko Ryynänen, Mats Börjesson, and Jón Karlsson

Contents

J. Ryynänen (✉)
University of Helsinki, Helsinki, Finland
e-mail: jaakko.ryynanen@helsinki.fi

M. Börjesson
University of Gothenburg, Gothenburg, Sweden

J. Karlsson
Department of Orthopaedics, Sahlgrenska University Hospital, Gothenburg University, Göteborg, Sweden

V. Musahl et al. (eds.), *Return to Play in Football*, https://doi.org/10.1007/978-3-662-55713-6_5

5.1 The Football-Playing Population, Teams' Injury Burden, and Common Types of Football Injuries

Football is likely the most popular team sport on our planet, with over 265 million FIFA-registered players worldwide [1]. Considering a popularity of this magnitude, it is easy to conclude that football players constitute a heterogeneous population. This is important to bear in mind when interpreting the results of medical research on the players' health and especially when aiming at defining treatment guidelines.

An average team of 25 male players, playing on the highest level of European football, can expect an average of 50 injuries during the course of a season [2, 3]. For the average player, this means between 1–2 injuries resulting in an average layoff time of 24–37 days from match play and training [2, 4]. In addition to being highly costly [5–7], these injuries have been shown to have adverse consequences on team performance [8] and logically on the health and career of individual players [9].

Most injuries in football affect the lower extremity, with muscle strains of the thigh, groin, and calf muscles, ligament sprains of the ankle and the knee joints, and contusions of the lower leg, the ankle, and the thigh being the most common injury types [2, 10, 11]. Also head injuries are worth mentioning, as an alarming and worldwide trend of increasing number of head injuries has been observed recently [12]. In international football tournaments, 15% of all injuries affect the head and neck, with concussion being the most common diagnosis [13].

Most football injuries are traumatic or "acute-onset" injuries, while approximately 8–28% of injuries have been reported to result from overuse [2, 3, 14]. Some traumatic injuries are contact injuries, i.e., injuries that result from player-to-player contact, as in, for example, tackle situations, while traumatic non-contact injuries occur while running or while performing other game-related actions, such as shooting the ball, jumping, and landing, or during other movements. The risk of injury is substantially, and significantly, higher during match play compared with training. A study on elite European male football with an 11-year follow-up period found an almost sevenfold injury incidence during match play compared with training [15].

A lot of epidemiological research has been conducted in order to identify risk factors for injuries. Traditionally, these factors have been divided into two broad categories: extrinsic and intrinsic risk factors [7]. Extrinsic risk factors are related to the playing conditions and environmental variables, whereas intrinsic risk factors reflect the individual players' biological and/or psychological characteristics [7]. This categorization is not always simple or even possible, as some extrinsic factors may influence intrinsic factors and vice versa.

5.2 Match Performance and Fatigue

Football is a complex sport. In addition to physical capacities, such as power, strength, and endurance, players require technical and game-specific skills, related to actions with the ball, as well as visual, perceptual, and cognitive skills [16–18]. The performance level of football players during a 90-min match is not constant. Match play is characterized by short match periods involving high-intensity activities, such as sprinting, tackling, or changing running pace, followed by low-intensity periods, necessary for the players to recover between the high-intensity periods [16]. Results of a study assessing match performance, physical fitness, and development of fatigue during professional football matches showed that 5-min match periods, during which high-intensity running peaked, were followed by 5-min periods, in which a reduction in performance below the average match level was observed [19]. Several studies have shown that the number of injuries increases toward the ends of match halves, strongly suggesting an association between the development of fatigue and an increased risk of suffering injuries [3, 4, 10, 20]. Fatigue has been found to accumulate toward the end of matches, but matches also appear to include periods of temporary fatigue [19]. Importantly, many factors, in addition to time (exposure), appear to influence the development of fatigue. These factors can be both match-related (extrinsic) factors, such as match result, match venue, and the quality of opposition, and player-related (intrinsic) factors, such as physical capacity and the age or gender of the player [21]. Future studies combining data obtained through match performance analysis with injury data could probably increase our understanding of the association between player performance and injury risk (Fig. 5.1).

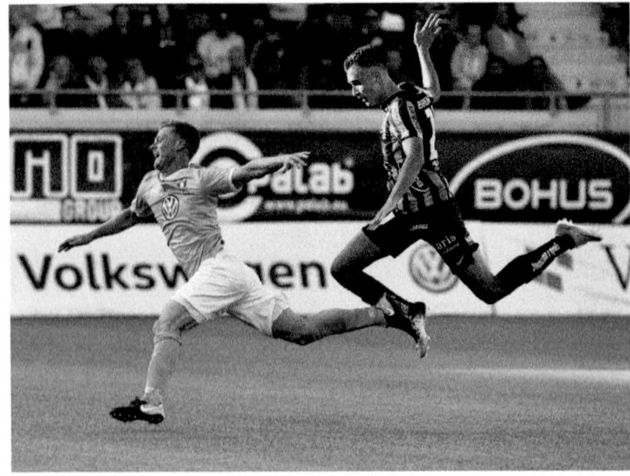

Fig. 5.1 Player involved in physical activity

The trend of an increasing injury incidence toward the end of match halves in football has been shown, specifically, for muscle injuries [20]. Muscle injuries have also been shown to increase when the recovery time between matches

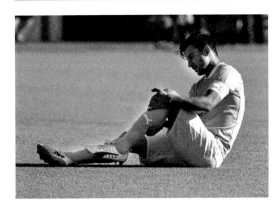

Fig. 5.2 Injured player

is short [22], further supporting the possible association between fatigue and muscle injuries. Almost all of these injuries occur by non-contact mechanisms, and they are typically muscle strains or tears of the hamstrings, the quadriceps, the groin, and the calf [20]. Muscle injuries are of a particular concern from the safe-return-to-play perspective, as they cause more than 25% of the player unavailability in professional football, and as much as 16% of muscle injuries have been shown to be re-injuries, i.e., injuries of the same type and location, that occur within 2 months of the final rehabilitation day of the previous injury [20, 23]. This suggests, alarmingly, that muscle injuries would often be inadequately rehabilitated, before the injured player returns to play. Re-injuries are a major concern in football, also because they tend to be more severe than initial injuries, i.e., they tend to result in significantly longer rehabilitation periods (layoff times) compared with initial injuries [20] (Fig. 5.2).

5.3 Fixture Congestion and Risk Taking

Fixture congestion, and its association with the risk of injuries, is a factor of particular interest from the safe-return-to-play perspective, as teams' match calendars during parts of the season can become extremely condensed, especially for teams participating in several competitions. The pressure of having a high level of player availability for squad rotation can thus be eminent. It is unfortunately not uncommon to read media reports of instances, when a conscious risk has been taken by fielding a player with a recent injury, or letting an injured player return to play after an apparent initial injury, especially when it comes to matches of great importance. This type of risk taking could potentially result in the player suffering a re-injury or worsening the initial injury. Examples of such incidents, some of which also gained widespread media coverage, occurred during the EURO 2016 and the 2014 FIFA World Cup finals. Especially a head injury of a player in the 2014 FIFA World Cup final provoked widespread discussion on how to ensure appropriate evaluations of players suffering head injuries in match conditions. Following the World Cup tournament, FIFA's Medical Committee introduced a new protocol (approved by the FIFA Executive Committee), under which the referee has the ability to interrupt the match for 3 min, whenever an incident of suspected concussion occurs, and under which the injured player will not be allowed to resume play before given authorization from the team physician [24, 25].

A male football player playing on the highest level of Europe participates on average in 254 h of football per year [15]. Most of this time (213 h) is spent in training sessions and the rest in match play [15]. Perhaps unsurprisingly, players have been shown to occasionally feel overloaded and often not completely recovered between training sessions or matches during a season, and this appears to apply for players across different age groups and skill levels [26]. Teams apply a wide range of recovery strategies for enhancing recovery between matches and between training sessions, although the efficacy of many of these methods remains to be scientifically proven. These strategies include, among others, using special nutritional intakes, cold water immersion, compression garments, massage, electrical stimulation, and different forms of active recovery [27].

Some studies have found significant associations between periods with a high fixture congestion and a higher risk of injuries [22, 28]. A UEFA injury study on top-level European football players showed that 29% players that played more than one match per week during the season and that participated in the World Cup tournament after the club season either underperformed or suffered an injury during the World Cup tournament, even though their risk of suffering injuries during the season (during the congested period) was on the same level with other players [29]. Curiously, a study on injuries in male World Cup football tournaments showed a counterintuitive, but significant, association between a longer recovery time and a higher risk of injuries [30]. Some of the differences between the results of different studies may reflect different in research methodologies, for example, regarding injury definitions, but they may also reflect differences in the populations included or the types of tournaments included in the studies. The bigger football clubs, or international teams of the highest level, may also have several top-level players for same playing positions, thus increasing their possibilities for squad rotation and consequently giving them an advantage in terms of avoiding fatigue compared with other teams. Unfortunately, data on the possible association between the level of squad rotation and injury risk are, thus far, scarce.

Players might, at least to some extent, adapt to the high physical demands posed on them by the strenuous training and match schedules during a season [19], and by appropriate planning of workloads, some injuries may be possible to prevent. Player exposure could be regarded as a value partly reflecting players' workload. Recently, an approach that differentiates between acute and chronic workloads has been encouraged and applied in research on sports injuries [31–33]. The acute workload refers to short-term workload during a specific period of the season, while chronic workload reflects the workload during a longer ("medium-term") period of time [31]. High chronic workload appears to reduce the risk of injury, whereas rapid and/or excessive increases in acute workload appear to have the opposite effect [31–33]. Results of a study on youth football players also suggest that progressive increases in chronic workload may develop physical tolerance to periods of high acute workload and potentially also reduce the risk of injuries [33]. This phenomenon could also partly explain the results of a match performance study, which suggest that professional players improve their performance level during the course of a season [19]. These results indicate that workload (or exposure) per se would not be an issue considering injury risk but that appropriate planning of match and training schedules, i.e., appropriate load management, would be beneficial from an injury-prevention point of view. This view is supported by the International Olympic Committee's (IOC) consensus statement on load in sports and the risk of injury [34]. Importantly, when monitoring load in athletes, the IOC supports a multifactorial approach, which takes into account not only factors related to physical recovery and fatigue but also factors related to non-sports-related stress, the athletes' general health and well-being, as well as vigor and motivational issues [35]. Future research applying these definitions will hopefully deepen our knowledge on the association between workload and the risk of injuries.

Fact Box 1 General extrinsic factors influencing injury risk
- Fixture congestion (match schedule)
- Workload management
- Climatic conditions and seasonal changes
- Level of play
- Gender

5.4 Foul Play, Refereeing, and Player Attitudes

In approximately a quarter of all injuries and almost half of all contact injuries in football, foul play is involved in injury causation [2, 11], and foul play has thus been regarded as the most important extrinsic risk factor for injuries [7]. Most of these "foul play injuries" are contusions and ligament sprains affecting the lower leg, ankle, knee, and thigh [2, 11, 36]. A foul is ideally awarded by the match referee every time a player breaks the rules (or the Laws of the Game), as they are outlined by FIFA. An infringement to the rules may present as use of excessive force and careless or reckless offenses on opponents by players or teams [37]. The rules, and the match referees making it sure that the rules are followed, can therefore be considered as having a role in protecting the players' health. Referees are human beings, who are, as all of us, prone to making errors and being influenced by their circumstances. Previous research suggests that referees' decisions may be influenced by several environmental factors, such as on which part of the pitch a tackle occurs, the home/away team status, the size of the crowd, and the match period [38–40], and their injury-preventive role may thus, under certain match conditions, be compromised.

Players do not always facilitate the referees' mission. A study on football players' psychological and sport-specific characteristics, across different age groups and skill levels, showed that almost all players were ready to commit a deliberate ("professional") foul, depending on the importance of the match or the match score line [26]. The same study also showed that most players thought that hidden fouls and provocation constitute a normal part of football and that more than half of the players aim at taking revenge for hidden fouls committed against them, by applying similar methods [26]. This does, of course, not mean that all fouls are deliberate. The results of a video analysis study of over 8500 tackle situations suggested that there was a high level of player error involved in tackling [41]. It is also important to remember that tackling is an essential part of football and that only 2% of all tackles result in injuries [41]. A match performance analysis study showed that an average player tackles 20 times per match [19]. The important aim is, therefore, to recognize the tackles involving a high risk of injury, in order to reduce the risk of injury by a more strict application of the rules or, in some cases, even by modifying the rules. Previous research suggests that injuries could be prevented by this kind of measures. An epidemiological study on head and neck injuries in football identified the use of the upper limb in tackles involving vertical jumping as the most common reason for severe head injuries [13]. Based on this finding, the referees were instructed to severely sanction fouls of this type, and a decrease of the number of head injuries from 25 to 13 was found between the 2002 and 2006 FIFA World Cups [42], probably at least partly due to the stricter refereeing applied (Fig. 5.3).

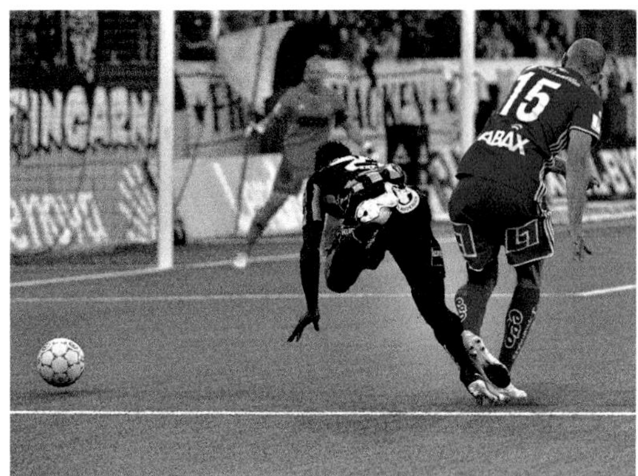

Fig. 5.3 Foul play

A study on foul play injuries in men's World Cup football showed a significant association between an increasing number of fouls in a match and an increase in injury incidence [30]. The same study showed that the variation in the risk of injuries during different match periods was similar for both injuries that involved foul play and other injuries. No differences were found between different playing positions either. This suggests that there are probably several common underlying factors for injuries that involve foul play and for other injuries. However, the association between a high number of fouls and a high risk of injury may suggest that aggressive match circumstances pose an increased risk for players to suffer injuries. Hypothetically, a player not fully recovered from a previous injury would accordingly benefit from being substituted from matches where fouls appear to accumulate.

5.5 Match Conditions and Their Influence on the Risk of Injuries

Football matches are characterized by a great number of events that have the potential to alter the course of the following match and that potentially require rapid responses from individual players, team management, and other members of team staff. Such events may include injuries to players, player substitutions, changes in the score (goals being scored), incidents in which players or sometimes even other team staff members behave aggressively, player bookings (yellow cards) or player expulsions (red cards), referees' decisions (that may or may not be erroneous), and altered weather conditions, among perhaps countless others. These events may affect player attitudes and team strategies and thus alter match conditions following the event. Players and other members of the team staff have to be able to adapt to these kinds of potential alterations in match conditions, as they characterize the sport.

As mentioned above, the fatigue developing during the course of a match is most likely a contributing factor on the trend of an increasing injury incidence toward the end of match halves. There are, however, other factors that influence the risk of injuries during the course of a game. Two studies on the influence of match events on injury risk in men's World Cup football found that the current score, referees' sanctions (yellow and red cards), and player injuries were associated with changes in the injury incidence during different match periods [43, 44]. The studies found that teams in a team currently winning ran a significantly higher risk of suffering injuries than teams currently drawing or losing, while no statistical differences were found between players in drawing and losing teams [43]. This might reflect changes in team strategies that teams apply during altered match conditions. Analysis of team tactics and ball possession strategies applied by teams has shown, for example, that losing teams aim to increase their ball possession, while winning teams tend to apply an opposite strategy [45]. This might, hypothetically, expose players of the winning team to more tackles from the losing team aiming to increase ball possession. A study on aggression in football also suggested that players of weaker teams apply more aggressive measures, as the study found that the level of injuries caused by weaker teams was greater than that of stronger teams [46]. The researchers concluded that some injuries in football were likely to be caused by deliberate aggressive behavior of certain players [46]. The studies on the influence of match events on injury risk in male World Cup football also found a higher risk of injury during 5-min match periods following goals, player injuries, and referees' sanctions (red and yellow cards) compared with other match periods [44]. Previous research has shown that players' concentration is negatively affected by social environmental settings of complexity and stress and by aroused and angry behavior [47]. Some match events may, hypothetically, contribute to this type of environmental settings. Seeing teammates being hurt by other players or seeing other athletes getting badly injured has also been found to trigger physiological responses in athletes [48]. As mentioned above, many football players also have a tendency of aiming at taking revenge when feeling being fouled and that most players find that fouls can be acceptable, depending on the match circumstances [26]. Recognizing the match periods involving a high risk of injury may be beneficial, especially for players that have undergone a recent rehabilitation period from a previous injury. A previous injury has been identified as a risk factor for a new injury [7, 49–51]. As mentioned above, the match circumstances also affect the level of the developing fatigue, providing another potential factor behind this, most likely multifactorial, association between match events and injury risk. Team personnel may, at least speculatively, be able to reduce the risk of recurrent injury by substituting the player when the risk of injury is high or at least encourage the player to play more cautiously during those match periods.

5.6 Other Match Factors and Regional Differences

One of the research questions, related to the association between injury risk and playing conditions, which has been the subject of several studies, is whether injury risk is different while playing on natural grass compared with artificial turf. Most studies have found no significant differences in the general injury risk [52–56]. Somewhat contrarily, the results of a meta-analysis comparing football injuries on natural grass and on artificial turf suggested that the injury risk could, under some match conditions, be lower while playing on artificial turf compared with natural grass [57]. However, the researchers concluded that more research was necessary in order to determine the underlying factors. A prospective study on injury risk in top-level men's football found a higher incidence of ankle sprains while playing on artificial turf compared with natural grass [56], suggesting that injury profiles may vary according to the playing surface. A speculative underlying factor for these differences may be that the playing surface affects teams' and/or players' style of play. A performance analysis study, comparing player movement patterns and technical aspects of football, while playing on natural grass versus while playing on artificial turf, found that fewer sliding tackles and more short passes were performed on artificial turf compared with natural grass [58].

Fact Box 2 Match-related factors influencing injury risk

- Fatigue
- Foul play
- Tackling
- Match events (goals, injuries, referees' sanctions)
- Pitch conditions

As becomes apparent, the match-related factors affecting injury risk are highly multifactorial, with several potential confounding factors that are sometimes impossible to assess. For example, the association between pitch conditions, or playing surface, and injury risk has been difficult to determine, as several confounding factors, such as the weather or climatic conditions and the type of footwear used, all affect the interaction between the foot and the pitch [59, 60]. The climatic conditions during a season also change with the changing seasons, as do accordingly the pitch conditions. It has been shown, for example, for hip and groin injuries, that their incidence in European male football is highest in March, October, and November, while it is lowest in May [61]. It would appear plausible to speculate, if the warmer weather in May could have a protective effect. However, teams also generally play fewer matches in the month of May, which might contribute more to the lower risk of hip and groin injuries during that period than the climate. Also hamstring injuries have been found to peak during November and January [62]. However, considering hamstring injuries that occur during training only, they have been found to peak during the warmer months of July and August [62]. An UEFA injury study showed a two- to threefold increase in hamstring injuries during the competitive season, compared with the preseason [2]. A study on ankle injuries in English professional football found a peak in the number of ankle injuries during the three first months of the season (July, August, and September) [63]. Research on the effect of climatic conditions on football injuries suggests that ankle sprains are more likely to occur in warmer weather [64]. Curiously, it has also been shown in American football that high temperatures lead to increased aggression [65]. An association between aggressive behavior and ankle injuries might also be speculated upon, as it has been shown that up to 40% of all ankle injuries in football are caused by foul play [66]. In conclusion, match-related factors influence each other, and their relative importance in causing injuries or predisposing to them is sometimes impossible to determine.

Even though, up to date, the underlying reasons remain unknown, there also appears to be some level of regional differences in injury incidence between different countries or regions. A study on regional differences in European professional football found a significantly higher injury incidence in northern European teams in comparison with geographically more southern-based teams [67]. The regional categorization applied in the study was based on a climatic classification system. The same study found that, contrarily to the overall injury incidence, non-contact anterior cruciate ligament injuries were significantly more common in southern European teams compared with northern teams. In line with this, a UEFA Champions League study found significantly higher injury incidences among English and Dutch teams, compared with teams from Spain, France, and Italy [14]. A study on injuries in Asian football tournaments found a higher injury incidence in Asian football players compared with European football players, although the injury patterns were found to be similar [68]. These findings may reflect different playing cultures, different player attitudes, different climatic conditions, and probably many other factors that could, again, potentially influence each other. A study analyzing differences in players' performances between English Premier League players and Spanish La Liga players found that the English players sprinted more during matches than their Spanish colleagues [69]. Also, South American players have been found to cover lesser total distances during matches than English players [70]. Research combining performance analysis data and injury data would probably deepen our understanding into how these regional differences affect the risk of injury or the injury patterns.

Take-Home Message

Various match factors influence the injury risk during football match play, and the risk of suffering injuries during a match is not constant. How these factors interact with each other and what their relative importance in contributing to injury risk are remain largely unknown. Players predisposed to injuries due to previous injuries should take caution, at least during periods of the playing season when the match schedule is dense and during match periods when the risk of injury is elevated. After coming back from injury, return-to-play recommendations must be followed. Avoiding playing in a state of a high level of fatigue may also be beneficial from an injury-preventive perspective.

Five Best Evidence Based References

Ekstrand J, Hägglund M, Kristenson K, Magnusson H, Waldén M (2013) Fewer ligament injuries but no preventive effect on muscle injuries and severe injuries: an 11-year follow-up of the UEFA champions league injury study. Br J Sports Med 47(12):732–737

Junge A, Dvorak J, Graf-Baumann T, Peterson L (2004) Football injuries during FIFA tournaments and the Olympic games, 1998-2001. Am J Sports Med 32(Suppl. 1):80S–89S

Junge A, Dvorak J (2013) Injury surveillance in the world football tournaments 1998–2012. Br J Sports Med 47(12):782–788

Ekstrand J, Hägglund M, Waldén M (2011) Epidemiology of muscle injuries in professional football (soccer). Am J Sports Med 39(6):1226–1232

Bengtsson H, Ekstrand J, Hägglund M (2013) Muscle injury rates in professional football increase with fixture congestion: an 11-year follow-up of the UEFA Champions League injury study. Br J Sports Med 47(12):743–747

References

1. Fédération Internationale de Football Association – Big Count. http://www.fifa.com/worldfootball/bigcount/index.html
2. Ekstrand J, Hägglund M, Waldén M (2011) Injury incidence and injury patterns in professional football: the UEFA injury study. Br J Sports Med 45(7):553–558
3. Hawkins RD, Fuller CW (1999) A prospective epidemiological study of injuries in four English professional football clubs. Br J Sports Med 33(3):196–203
4. Hawkins RD, Hulse MA, Wilkinson C, Hodson A, Gibson M (2001) The association football medical research programme: an audit of injuries in professional football. Br J Sports Med 35(1):43–47
5. Ekstrand J (2013) Keeping your top players on the pitch: the key to football medicine at a professional level. Br J Sports Med 47(12):723–724
6. Junge A, Lamprecht M, Stamm H, Hasler H, Bizzini M, Tschopp M, Reuter H, Psych D, Wyss H, Chilvers C, Dvorak J (2011) Countrywide campaign to prevent soccer injuries in Swiss amateur players. Am J Sports Med 39(1):57–63
7. Dvorak J, Junge A (2000) Football injuries and physical symptoms. A review of the literature. Am J Sports Med 28(Suppl. 5):3S–9S
8. Hägglund M, Waldén M, Magnusson H, Kristenson K, Bengtsson H, Ekstrand J (2013) Injuries affect team performance negatively in professional football: an 11-year follow-up of the UEFA champions league injury study. Br J Sports Med 47(12):738–742
9. Drawer S, Fuller C (2001) Propensity for osteoarthritis and lower limb joint pain in retired professional soccer players. Br J Sports Med 35(6):402–408
10. Junge A, Dvorak J, Graf-Baumann T, Peterson L (2004) Football injuries during FIFA tournaments and the Olympic games, 1998–2001. Am J Sports Med 32(Suppl. 1):80S–89S
11. Junge A, Dvorak J (2013) Injury surveillance in the World football tournaments 1998–2012. Br J Sports Med 47(12):782–788
12. Blennow K, Hardy J, Zetterberg H (2012) The neuropathology and neurobiology of traumatic brain injury. Neuron 76(5):886–899
13. Fuller CW, Junge A, Dvorak JA (2005) Six year prospective study of the incidence and causes of head

and neck injuries in international football. Br J Sports Med 39(Suppl. 1):i3–i9
14. Waldén M, Hägglund M, Ekstrand JUEFA (2005) Champions league study: a prospective study of injuries in professional football during the 2001–2002 season. Br J Sports Med 39(8):542–546
15. Ekstrand J, Hägglund M, Kristenson K, Magnusson H, Waldén M (2013) Fewer ligament injuries but no preventive effect on muscle injuries and severe injuries: an 11-year follow-up of the UEFA champions league injury study. Br J Sports Med 47(12):732–737
16. Stolen T, Chamari K, Castagna C, Wisløff U (2005) Physiology of soccer. Sports Med 35(6):501–536
17. Reilly T, Bangsbo J, Franks A (2000) Anthropometric and physiological predispositions for elite soccer. J Sports Sci 18(9):669–683
18. Ward P, Williams AM (2003) Perceptual and cognitive skill development in soccer : the multidimensional nature of expert performance. J Sport Exerc Psychol 25:93–111
19. Mohr M, Krustup P, Bangsbo J (2003) Match performance of high-standard soccer players with special reference to development of fatigue. J Sports Sci 21(7):519–528
20. Ekstrand J, Hägglund M, Waldén M (2011) Epidemiology of muscle injuries in professional football (soccer). Am J Sports Med 39(6):1226–1232
21. Nédélec M, McCall A, Carling C, Legall F, Berthoin S, Dupont G (2012) Recovery in soccer: part I – postmatch fatigue and time course of recovery. Sports Med 42(12):997–1015
22. Bengtsson H, Ekstrand J, Hägglund M (2013) Muscle injury rates in professional football increase with fixture congestion: an 11-year follow-up of the UEFA champions league injury study. Br J Sports Med 47(12):743–747
23. Hägglund M, Waldén M, Bahr R, Ekstrand J (2005) Methods for epidemiological study of injuries to professional football players: developing the UEFA model. Br J Sports Med 39(6):340–346
24. Fédération Internationale de Football Association 2014. http://www.fifa.com/development/news/y=2014/m=9/news=fifa-s-medical-committee-proposes-new-protocol-for-the-management-of-c-2443024.html
25. Fédération Internationale de Football Association 2014. http://www.fifa.com/about-fifa/news/y=2014/m=9/news=executive-committee-says-stop-to-third-party-ownership-of-players-econ-2444471.html
26. Junge A, Dvorak J, Rösch D, Graf-Baumann T, Chomiak J, Peterson L (2000) Psychological and sport-specific characteristics of football players. Am J Sports Med 28(Suppl. 5):22S–28S
27. Nédélec M, McCall A, Carling C, Legall F, Berthoin S, Dupont G (2013) Recovery in soccer: Part II – recovery strategies. Sports Med 43(1):9–22
28. Dupont G, Nedelec M, McCall A, McCormack D, Berthoin S, Wisløff U (2010) Effect of 2 soccer matches in a week on physical performance and injury rate. Am J Sports Med 38(9):1752–1758
29. Ekstrand J, Waldén M, Hägglund MA (2004) Congested football calendar and the wellbeing of players: correlation between match exposure of European footballers before the World Cup 2002 and their injuries and performances during that World cup. Br J Sports Med 38(4):493–497
30. Ryynänen J, Junge A, Dvorak J et al (2013) Foul play is associated with injury incidence: an epidemiological study of three FIFA World Cups (2002–2010). Br J Sports Med 47:986–991
31. Gabbett TJ The training-injury prevention paradox: should athletes be training smarter *and* harder? Br J Sports Med. https://doi.org/10.1136/bjsports-2015-095788
32. Hulin BT, Gabbett TJ, Lawson DW, Caputi P, Sampson JA The acute:chronic workload ratio predicts injury: high chronic workload may decrease injury risk in elite rugby league players. Br J Sports Med. https://doi.org/10.1136/bjsports-2015-094817
33. Bowen L, Gross AS, Gimpel M, Li F-X Accumulated workloads and the acute:chronic workload ratio relate to injury risk in elite youth football players. Br J Sports Med. https://doi.org/10.1136/bjsports-2015-095820
34. Soligard T, Schwellnus M, Alonso JM, Bahr R, Clarsen B, Dijkstra HP, Gabbett T, Gleeson M, Hägglund M, Hutchinson MR, van Rensburg CJ, Khan KM, Meeusen R, Orchard JW, Pluim B, Raftery M, Budgett R, Engebretsen L (2016) How much is too much? (Part 1) International Olympic Committee consensus statement on load in sport and risk of injury. Br J Sports Med 50:1030–1041. https://doi.org/10.1136/bjsports-2016-096581
35. Schwellnus M, Soligard T, Alonso JM, Bahr R, Clarsen B, Dijkstra HP, Gabbett T, Gleeson M, Hägglund M, Hutchinson MR, Rensburg v, Meeusen R, Orchard JW, Pluim B, Raftery M, Budgett R, Engebretsen L (2016) How much is too much? (part 2) International Olympic Committee consensus statement on load in sport and risk of illness. Br J Sports Med 50:1043–1052. https://doi.org/10.1136/bjsports-2016-096572
36. Junge A, Dvorak J, Graf-Baumann T (2004) Football injuries during the World Cup 2002. Am J Sports Med 32(Suppl. 1):23S–27S
37. Fédération Internationale de Football Association – Law 12: Fouls and misconduct. http://www.fifa.com/mm/document/afdeveloping/refereeing/law_12_fouls_misconduct_en_47379.pdf
38. Fuller CW, Junge A, Dvorak J (2004) An assessment of football referees´ decisions in incidents leading to player injuries. Am J Sports Med 32(Suppl. 1):17S–22S
39. Mallo J, Frutos PG, Juarez D, Navarro E (2012) Effect of positioning on the accuracy of decision making of association football top-class referees and assistant referees during competitive matches. J Sports Sci 30(13):1437–1445
40. Downward P, Jones M (2007) Effects of crowd size on referee decisions: analysis of the FA cup. J Sports Sci 25(14):1541–1545
41. Fuller CW, Smith GL, Junge A, Dvorak J (2004) An assessment of player error as an injury causa-

tion factor in international football. Am J Sports Med 32(Suppl. 1):28S–35S
42. Dvorak J, Junge A, Grimm K, Kirkendall D (2007) Medical report from the 2006 FIFA World Cup Germany. Br J Sports Med 41(9):578–581
43. Ryynänen J, Junge A, Dvorak J et al (2013) The effect of changes in the score on injury incidence during three FIFA World cups. Br J Sports Med 47:960–964
44. Ryynänen J, Junge A, Dvorak J et al (2013) Increased risk of injury following red and yellow cards, injuries and goals in FIFA World cups. Br J Sports Med 47:970–973
45. Lago-Peñas C, Dellal A (2010) Ball possession strategies in elite soccer according to the evolution of the match-score: the influence of situational variables. J Hum Kinet 25:93–100
46. Fuller CW (2005) An assessment of the relationship between behaviour and injury in the workplace: a case study in professional football. Saf Sci 43:213–224
47. Silva JM III (1979) Behavioral and situational factors affecting concentration and skill performance. J Sport Exerc Psychol 1(3):221–227
48. Stanger N, Kavussanu M, Willoughby A, Ring C (2012) Psychophysiological responses to sport-specific affective pictures: a study of morality and emotion in athletes. Psychol Sport Excerc 13(6):840–848
49. Hägglund M, Waldén M, Ekstrand J (2006) Previous injury as a risk factor for injury in elite football: a prospective study over two consecutive seasons. Br J Sports Med 40(9):767–772
50. Chomiak J, Junge A, Peterson L, Dvorak J (2000) Severe injuries in football players. Influencing factors. Am J Sports Med 28(Suppl. 5):58S–68S
51. Arnason A, Sigurdsson SB, Gudmunsson A, Holme I, Engebretsen L, Bahr R (2004) Risk factors for injuries in football. Am J Sports Med 32(Suppl. 1):5S–16S
52. Steffen K, Andersen TE, Bahr R (2007) Risk of injury on artificial turf and natural grass in young female football players. Br J Sports Med 41(Suppl 1):i33–i37
53. Lanzetti RM, Ciompi A, Lupariello D, Guzzini M, De Carli A, Ferretti A (2016) Safety on third-generation artificial turf in male elite professional soccer players in Italian major league. Scand J Med Sci Sports. https://doi.org/10.1111/sms.12654
54. Williams S, Hume PA, Kara SA (2011) Review of football injuries on third and fourth generation artificial turfs compared with natural turfs. Sports Med 41(11):903–923
55. Bjørneboe J, Bahr R, Andersen TE (2010) Risk of injury on third-generation artificial turf in Norwegian professional football. Br J Sports Med 44(11):794–795
56. Ekstrand J, Timpka T, Hägglund M (2006) Risk of injury in elite football played on artificial turf versus natural grass: a prospective two-cohort study. Br J Sports Med 40(12):975–980
57. Williams JH, Akogyrem E, Williams JRA (2013) Meta-analysis of soccer injuries on artificial turf and natural grass. J Sports Med. https://doi.org/10.1155/2013/380523.
58. Andersson H, Ekblom B, Krustup P (2008) Elite football on artificial turf versus natural grass: movement patterns, technical standards, and player impressions. J Sports Sci 26(2):113–122
59. Orchard JI (2002) There a relationship between ground and climatic conditions and injuries in football? Sports Med 32(7):419–432
60. Dragoo JL, Braun HJ (2010) The effect of playing surface on injury rate : a review of the current literature. Sports Med 40(10):981–990
61. Werner J, Hägglund M, Waldén M, Ekstrand JUEFA (2009) Injury study: a prospective study of hip and groin injuries in professional football over seven consecutive seasons. Br J Sports Med 43(13):1036–1040
62. Woods C, Hawkins RD, Maltby S, Hulse M, Thomas A, Hodson A (2004) The football association medical research programme: an audit of injuries in professional football – analysis of hamstring injuries. Br J Sports Med 38(1):36–41
63. Woods C, Hawkins R, Hulse M, Hodson A (2003) The football association medical research programme: an audit of injuries in professional football: an analysis of ankle sprains. Br J Sports Med 37(3):233–238
64. Orchard JW, Waldén M, Hägglund M, Orchard JJ, Chivers I, Seward H, Ekstrand J (2013) Comparison of injury incidences between football teams playing in different climatic regions. Open Access J Sports Med 4:251–260
65. Craig C, Overbeek RW, Condon MV, Rinaldo SBA (2016) Relationship between temperature and aggression in NFL football penalties. J Sports Health Science 5(2):205–210
66. Waldén M, Hägglund M, Ekstrand J (2013) Time-trends and circumstances surrounding ankle injuries in men's professional football: an 11-year follow-up of the UEFA champions league study. Br J Sports Med 47(12):748–753
67. Waldén M, Hägglund M, Orchard J, Kristenson K, Ekstrand J (2013) Regional differences in injury incidence in European professional football. Scand J Med Sci Sports 23:424–430
68. Yoon YS, Chai M, Shin DW (2004) Football injuries in Asian tournaments. Am J Sports Med 32:36S–42S
69. Dellal A, Chamari K, Wong DP, Ahmaidi S, Keller D, Barros R, Bisciotti GN, Carling C (2010) Comparison of physical and technical performance in European soccer match-play: FA premier league and la Liga. Eur J Sports Sci 11:51–59
70. Rienzi E, Drust B, Reilly T, Carter JE, Martin A (2000) Investigation of anthropometric and work-rate profiles of elite south American international soccer players. J Sports Med Phys Fitness 40(2):162–169

6 Psychological Factors Influencing Return to Sport After Anterior Cruciate Ligament Reconstruction

Kate E Webster and Julian A Feller

Contents

K.E. Webster (✉)
School of Allied Health, La Trobe University, Bundoora, Melbourne, 3086, Australia
e-mail: k.webster@latrobe.edu.au

J.A. Feller
OrthoSport Victoria, Epworth HealthCare, Richmond, Australia

6.1 Introduction

It has become clear that the return-to-sport phase following athletic injury, or surgery for an injury, is associated with a significant psychological response, which for some athletes may mean that they can never return to their sport [1]. Psychological recovery does not necessarily accord with physical recovery [2]. Some athletes are physically recovered long before they are psychologically prepared to return to sport, or conversely some may prematurely return to competition before they are physically ready. Both scenarios have negative consequences. The role that psychological factors play for a significant injury, such as an anterior cruciate ligament (ACL) rupture, may be heightened because this injury has a long rehabilitation period and a level of uncertainty about whether the athlete will be able to return to their preinjury level of sport performance [3]. It is also recognised that there is a poor correlation between objective knee function and return to sport following ACL reconstruction, suggesting that there are other factors involved [4–6]. This chapter will explore the role of psychological factors in influencing return to sport with a specific focus on ACL injury and reconstruction.

V. Musahl et al. (eds.), *Return to Play in Football*, https://doi.org/10.1007/978-3-662-55713-6_6

6.2 Psychological Impact of Athletic Injury

It is well demonstrated that athletic injuries may have profound psychological consequences. Injured athletes can experience mood disturbances, including anger and depression, and decreased self-worth [7–10]. Heightened negative emotions such as shock, frustration, tension and anger have been reported soon after an injury and also during recovery [11, 12]. The psychological response and impact of the injury may also be linked with athletic identity. For example, competitive athletes have been found to exhibit greater mood disturbances than recreational athletes [11]. Similarly, professional athletes who had severe and potentially career-ending injuries had stronger negative psychological responses compared to athletes who viewed their injury as minor [13]. Furthermore, college athletes who had their athletic careers terminated due to injury were found to report lower life satisfaction compared to athletes who did not sustain career-ending sporting injuries [14]. The athlete's psychological response may continue long after the injury has occurred, and the chain of psychological sequelae can therefore have an effect on rehabilitation and return-to-sport outcomes.

6.3 Theoretical Perspective

Returning to sport after injury is influenced both directly and indirectly by a range of physical, psychological and social/contextual factors [1, 15–17] (Fig. 6.1). Biopsychosocial models have therefore been proposed to conceptualise the myriad and complex interactions between these factors [19, 20]. In such models, psychological factors play a mediating role on physical (e.g. pain), contextual (e.g. recovery expectations) and functional performance (e.g. motor control) factors and ultimately on return to sport. Injury characteristics and sociodemographic factors (such as age and sex) have an indirect influence on return to sport via their influence on psychological, physical or social/contextual factors. An attraction of the biopsychosocial model is that there are clear pathways between psychological factors and outcome as well as the potential for psychological factors to influence return to sport via a number of different pathways [21]. The central role played by psychological factors in the biopsychosocial model highlights the importance of addressing psychological factors in the management of ACL injury.

6.4 Psychological Aspects Related to Recovery Following ACL Reconstruction

Psychological responses are prominent following ACL injury and surgery as well as during recovery and can affect the progression through rehabilitation [22, 23]. The psychological responses and emotions associated with an injury do however change over time. Whilst a negative emotional response is typically reported immediately following injury, negative emotions tend to subside during rehabilitation with studies showing improvement over time [9, 24, 25]. However, some studies show that negative emotions re-emerge once the athlete is cleared to return to sport. For example, Morrey et al. [11] described a U-shaped emotional response following ACL injury with negative peaks immediately following injury and at the time of clearance for return to sport (6 months post-reconstruction surgery).

Two psychological factors which have been shown to contribute to patient outcomes following ACL reconstruction are self-efficacy and locus of control [25–27]. Self-efficacy is the belief in one's ability to succeed in a particular situation. Self-efficacy has been found to significantly improve as athletes recover from injury. In addition, improved outcomes and patient satisfaction have been associated with higher levels of self-efficacy. Using the Knee Self-Efficacy Scale, Thomeé and colleagues [28, 29] showed that higher levels of self-efficacy were positively associated with higher levels of activity follow-

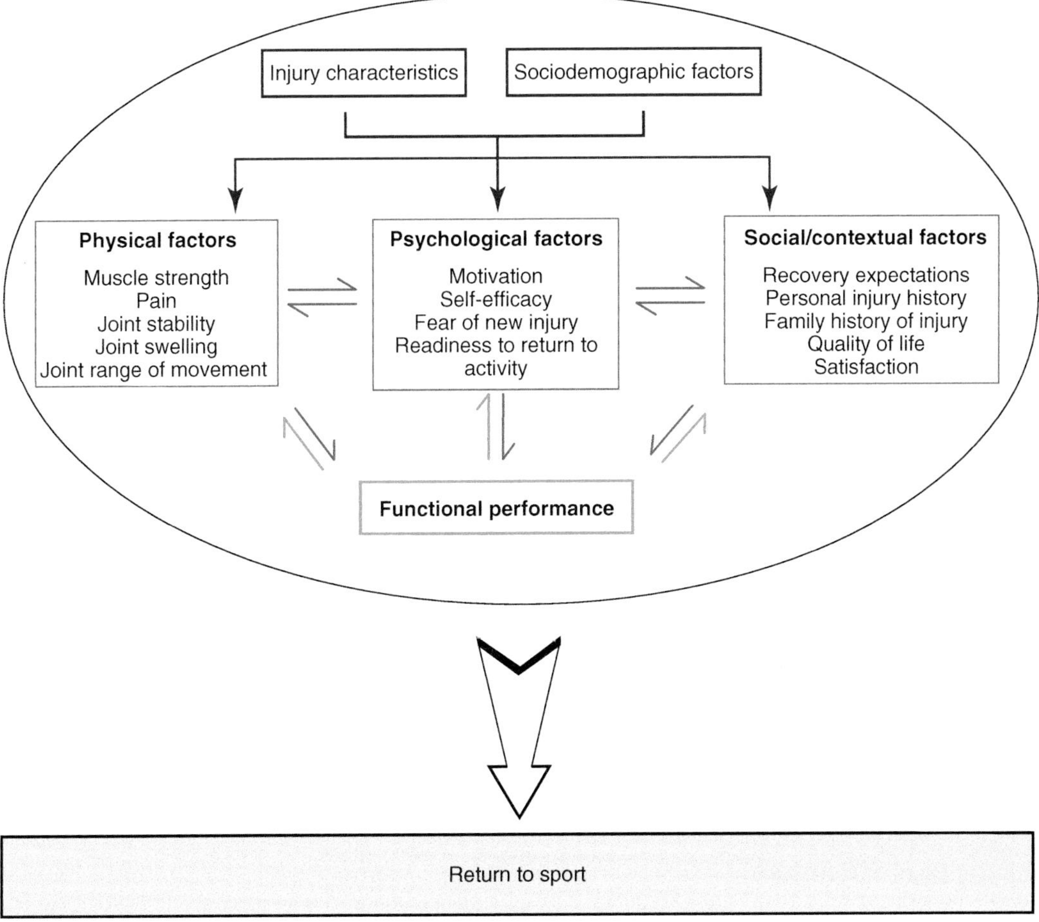

Fig. 6.1 Adapted biopsychosocial model for return to sport after injury (Reproduced from Ardern et al. [18])

ing ACL reconstruction. In a follow-up study by the same authors, preoperative self-efficacy was found to predict postoperative physical activity and return to sport [27]. Overall, there is convincing evidence that self-efficacy can play a pivotal role in successful rehabilitation and return to sport.

The second factor is locus of control, and this may contribute to an athlete's sense of self-efficacy. Locus of control refers to having the belief that there is a relationship between actions and outcomes (i.e. feeling that you have control). Athletes who have a high internal locus of control score higher on subjective outcomes following ACL reconstruction as well as reporting greater overall knee function [26]. Locus of control has also been shown to be a predictor of returning to sport at 12 months after surgery [30].

Fact Box 1

- The psychological response to injury changes over time, and negative emotions can emerge once the athlete is cleared to return to sport.
- Self-efficacy and locus of control play a pivotal role in both the success of rehabilitation and return to sport.

6.5 Psychological Factors Influencing Return to Sport from ACL Reconstruction

Athletes undergoing ACL reconstruction typically expect to be able to return to their preinjury sport. Whilst surgery addresses impairments in knee function, one in every three athletes do not make the transition back to sport after surgery, and psychological responses have been identified as a potentially modifiable factor associated with returning or not returning to the preinjury level of sport [3, 5, 16, 17]. Athletes who feel they have a greater level of control over their return to sport have greater confidence in their body, and those who feel more socially connected to their teammates are more likely to return to their previous sport [1, 18]. Higher levels of motivation during rehabilitation have also recently been shown to be associated with higher rates of return to preinjury sport following ACL reconstruction [31]. Two commonly discussed psychological factors in terms of returning to sport are 'fear of reinjury' and 'psychological readiness'.

6.5.1 Fear of Reinjury

Fear of reinjury may affect an athlete's ability to return to their previous sport and may also affect the quality of their performance. Using the Tampa Scale of Kinesiophobia, Kvist et al. [32] identified fear of reinjury as a significant factor in patients who did not return to their previous level of activity after ACL reconstruction. This finding has been supported and quantified by numerous subsequent studies with some showing that up to 50% [33] of athletes who do not return to sport cite fear of reinjury as the reason. Restriction of sporting activity due to fear of reinjury has also been reported [34].

However, exactly what constitutes fear of reinjury is unclear. It may be fear of the pain of injury itself, fear of the implications for time off work and the related loss of income, fear of not being able to return to the previous level of function or any combination of these. In a recent qualitative study, Ross et al. [35] interviewed patients who reported fear of reinjury as the sole reason for not returning to their preinjury sport to better understand factors that inform athletes' experience of fear following ACL reconstruction. Results showed that undergoing surgery with a long recovery and restricted functional capacity was one of the main factors which informed fear of reinjury. The nature of the preinjury sport also informed fear of reinjury. Specifically, once injured, many athletes reported having an increased awareness of how the movement pattern associated with the injury, such as pivoting, was common in their sport. Personality traits and social priorities (i.e. educational commitments) were also found to inform fear of reinjury.

It is interesting to consider the context in which the term fear of reinjury is used and whether it is an appropriate term. In the ACL literature specifically, fear of reinjury is most commonly used in the context of cessation of sport after ACL reconstruction. Walker et al. [36] have however suggested that 'reinjury anxiety' may be more appropriate to describe the emotional response of the athlete as fear is a biological mechanism which is stimulus specific and is associated with definite danger, whereas anxiety is associated with anticipation or uncertainty.

Ardern et al. [37] investigated whether fear of reinjury was still a consideration in athletes who made a successful return to sport after ACL reconstruction surgery. A cohort of 209 athletes answered a series of questions regarding the behavioural manifestations of fear, such as playing with hesitation and being wary of injury-provoking situations. The results showed that athletes who had successfully returned to their preinjury sport generally participated without fear of reinjury. Males who had earlier surgery (<3 months after injury) were found to participate in the preinjury sport with the least amount of fear.

6.5.2 Psychological Readiness

In a recent qualitative study, psychological readiness to return to sport was suggested to comprise three key aspects: confidence in returning to sport, realistic expectations of sporting capability and motivation to regain preinjury performance standards [38]. Confidence was specifically influenced by the athlete's belief in their rehabilitation programme and their perception that their injury was completely healed and therefore no longer at risk of being reinjured. The belief in being able to perform at the same preinjury level was also associated with increased psychological readiness to return [38, 39].

Fact Box 2

- An athlete's belief in their rehabilitation programme influences return-to-sport confidence.
- Psychological readiness to return to sport is related to an athlete's perceived ability to perform at their preinjury level of sport.

That psychological readiness is important in determining return-to-sport decisions was highlighted by Ardern et al. [30, 40]. Although multifactorial, psychological readiness is largely influenced by an athlete's emotions and confidence [18]. Confidence is thought to be derived from two elements: confidence in the injured body part and confidence in the ability to perform well [41, 42]. Developing confidence in both these aspects may provide a buffer from injury-related fear and anxiety, resulting in the athlete being in a 'psychologically ready' state to resume sport participation. In line with this, a recent systematic review concluded that an athlete's psychological readiness to return to play is a combination of the lack of fear and anxiety and confidence in performing well and remaining uninjured [43].

Fact Box 3

- *Fear of reinjury* is one of the most common reasons cited by athletes who do not return to their preinjury sport following ACL reconstruction surgery.
- *Psychological readiness* to return to sport is related to confidence, realistic expectations and motivation.
- *Psychological readiness* has been shown to have a strong association with return to sport after ACL reconstruction.

Table 6.1 Questionnaires and inventories that can be used to assess psychological readiness to return to sport

Name	Abbreviation
Injury-Psychological Readiness to Return to Sport Scale [44]	I-PRRS
Reinjury Anxiety Inventory [36]	RIAI
Knee Self-Efficacy Scale [29]	KSES
Tampa Scale of Kinesiophobia [45]	TSK
Anterior Cruciate Ligament Return to Sport After Injury scale [39]	ACL-RSI

There are several measures available to help assess psychological readiness to return to sport (Table 6.1). The Anterior Cruciate Ligament Return to Sport After Injury (ACL-RSI) scale [39] was developed as a tool to specifically measure psychological readiness to return to sport after ACL reconstruction and will thus be the focus of the following section.

6.6 The Anterior Cruciate Ligament Return to Sport After Injury (ACL-RSI) Scale

Items in the ACL-RSI scale are centred on three psychological factors associated with returning to sport: *emotions*, *confidence* and *risk appraisal* (see Table 6.2). The emotions category includes five items regarding fear of reinjury, frustration, nervousness and tension as these are commonly reported emotions experienced by athletes during rehabilitation and the commencement of sport.

In the sports setting, confidence typically refers to the amount of confidence the athlete has in their ability to perform well at their sport. However, in the case of ACL reconstruction, it also relates to the amount of confidence the athlete has in their knee function. Five items in the ACL-RSI scale therefore cover both these aspects of sport confidence. Three (items 6–8) target the athlete's confidence in their knee function, and two (items 9 and 10) measure the athlete's confidence in their overall ability to perform well at their sport. Two further items are included in the scale to investigate the cognitive risk appraisal of the athlete to reinjury.

Table 6.2 ACL-RSI items

	Scale item	Order in scale
Emotions	1. Are you nervous about playing your sport?	3
	2. Do you find it frustrating to have to consider your knee with respect to your sport?[a]	6
	3. Do you feel relaxed about playing your sport?[b]	12
	4. Are you fearful of reinjuring your knee by playing your sport?	7
	5. Are you afraid of accidentally injuring your knee by playing your sport?	9
Confidence	6. Are you confident that your knee will not give way by playing your sport?	4
	7. Are you confident that you could play your sport without concern for your knee?	5
	8. Are you confident about your knee holding up under pressure?	8
	9. Are you confident that you can perform at your previous level of sport participation?	1
	10. Are you confident about your ability to perform well at your sport?	11
Risk Appraisal	11. Do you think you are likely to reinjure your knee by participating in your sport?	2
	12. Do thoughts of having to go through surgery and rehabilitation again prevent you from playing your sport?	10

[a]Item 2 was from the Quality of Life Outcome Measure for Chronic ACL Deficiency (ACL-QOL) scale [46]
[b]Item 3 measures 'tension' with the positive antonym relaxed used to get a balance between positively and negatively worded items

In the development phase, the psychometric properties of the ACL-RSI scale were evaluated in a cohort of 220 athletes who had undergone ACL reconstruction between 8 and 22 months (mean = 12 months) prior to completing the scale [39]. The scale was found to have high internal consistency (Cronbach's alpha = 0.96), and principal component analysis confirmed the presence of one underlying factor that accounted for 67.8% of the total variance. Scores for the 12 items are therefore summed and averaged to provide a single score for the scale (from 0 to 100 with higher scores indicating a more positive psychological response). It is important to note that although the scale was designed around three constructs, these constructs were all highly related, and the scale is therefore considered unidimensional. As validation of the scale, athletes who had returned to full competition were found to score significantly higher than athletes who had given up sport and athletes who had not recommenced sport but were still planning to return [39].

6.6.1 ACL-RSI Predictive Value and Clinical Use

Given the impact of psychological factors on athletes during rehabilitation and return to sport, it is potentially useful to be able to predict which athletes may benefit from psychological counselling or intervention so that psychological recovery can occur in parallel with physical recovery. It is therefore relevant to know whether the psychological responses athletes experience during the rehabilitation period are related to sport resumption.

Two large-scale studies have been conducted which show that the ACL-RSI scale can be used to predict return-to-sport outcomes. The first enrolled 100 athletes who completed the ACL-RSI at 3, 6 and 12 months after undergoing ACL reconstruction surgery [24]. At 12 months, 51% of the athletes had returned to competitive sports. Scores on the ACL-RSI at 6 months were significantly lower in the athletes who did not return to competition sport at 12 months compared to the athletes who did. Therefore, an athlete's readiness to return to sport at 6 months post-ACL reconstruction surgery was related to whether or not they actually returned at 12 months and suggested the possibility of identifying athletes at risk of not returning to competitive sport due to psychological reasons.

Fact Box 4

- Psychological readiness to return to sport has been shown to predict subsequent return to sport.
- Psychological readiness may also identify athletes at risk of not returning to sport.

A second study of 187 patients completed a battery of psychological assessments, including the ACL-RSI scale, before ACL reconstruction surgery, as well as at 4 and 12 months after surgery [30]. At 12 months, only 56 athletes (31%) had returned to their previous level of sports participation, despite the majority (91%) having excellent physical recovery as demonstrated by an IKDC score of normal or nearly normal (category A or B) and a hop test limb symmetry index of >85%. Three variables from the psychological assessments predicted returning to sport by 12 months after surgery: readiness to return to sport, the participant's estimate of the number of months it would take to return to sport and locus of control. Psychological readiness, as assessed with the ACL-RSI scale, was the only measure that was predictive of return to sport both preoperatively and at 4 months postoperatively. The significance of this finding is that psychological readiness appears to be associated with return to sport even before the athlete undergoes surgery, and this should be taken into account during all stages of the rehabilitation. The above cohort was subsequently reviewed at 2 years to specifically see whether those who had not returned by 12 months made a later return [47]. Once again, a more positive psychological response or greater psychological readiness was associated with participation in the preinjury sport at 2 years.

The factors that contribute to an athlete's psychological readiness have not yet been clearly elucidated. Unpublished work from our group analysed a cohort of athletes who underwent ACL reconstruction, had been cleared to return to sport and completed the ACL-RSI scale at 12 months postoperatively. Results indicated that being male, having a higher frequency of preinjury sport participation, having a higher limb symmetry index on hop tests and having a higher self-rating of knee function were all associated with greater psychological readiness. It was concluded that males who participate frequently in sport before ACL injury are more likely to have a positive psychological outlook during the return-to-sport phase after ACL reconstruction surgery. Conversely, females with lower levels of function (both self-reported and on physical testing) may have a more negative outlook and therefore benefit from interventions designed to facilitate a smooth transition back to sport.

Fact Box 5

- Males who participate in sport on a frequent basis before ACL injury have a high level of psychological readiness to return to sport.
- Psychological readiness to return to sport is low in females with low levels of physical function, and, as such, this group may benefit from psychological intervention.

Work is still ongoing to determine what scores on the ACL-RSI mean clinically and what cut-off might be useful for categorising athletes as psychologically ready to return or not. A cut-off score of 56 points on the ACL-RSI was initially reported, and it had good specificity (83%) and moderate sensitivity (58%) [30]. This cut-off was based on ACL-RSI scores at 4 months and return-to-sport status at 12 months post-surgery. A further study prospectively followed 40 athletes and reported a cut-off score of 51 points based on 6-month measures, with moderate specificity (0.63) and high sensitivity (0.97) [48].

Overall, it is reasonable to suggest that athletes who score above the cut-off are highly likely to return to sport, whereas there is less certainty about those who score less than the cut-off. This is not unexpected as there will always be athletes who score low on psychological readiness and yet still return to sport for a variety of reasons, including pressure from outside sources. It is also reasonable to expect that athletes would have some level of anxiety and fear as a normal response when contemplating a return to sport. Indeed a degree of caution may be protective if it means that an athlete does not prematurely or recklessly resume sport without full consideration of the function of their knee [18]. The clinical utility of a cut-off score is that it provides clinicians with a means to identify which athlete groups may struggle to return to sport from a psychological perspective. This is important given the typically limited resources available for psychological assistance during recovery from injury. There remains a need for data which explores associations between psychological readiness and level of performance on return to sport.

Fact Box 6

- ACL-RSI scores, measured both before and after ACL reconstruction surgery, have been strongly associated with return to sport.
- Factors that contribute to higher ACL-RSI scores include being male, frequent participation in sport and higher self-rating of knee function and limb symmetry.
- Scores on the ACL-RSI scale may help clinicians identify athletes at risk of not returning to sport.

In a busy clinical environment, a short version of the ACL-RSI for rapid administration may be desirable. The ACL-RSI scale was therefore administered to 535 athletes 12 months after undergoing ACL reconstruction. The scale was found to have high internal consistency (Cronbach's alpha = 0.96) suggesting the presence of item redundancy. After a selection process, the scale was reduced to six items (items 1, 2, 4, 7, 9 and 11 in Table 6.2). Scores for the short version were found to be similar to the full version for athletes at various stages in the return to sport (Fig. 6.2), and a cut-off of 60 points was established from a 6-month data in a further sample of 250 patients (unpublished data). Interestingly, the short version ACL-RSI is less knee specific and has therefore been modified for use with shoulder, hip and Achilles tendon injuries. Copies of these scales are available from the corresponding author.

Overall the ACL-RSI scale appears to be a useful tool for assessing psychological readiness to return to sport after ACL reconstruction and may be useful for identifying athletes who may have difficulty with the resumption of sport after ACL injury due to psychological reasons. The scale had been translated from English to Swedish [49], French [50], German [51], Dutch [52] and Turkish [53] versions, with other translations currently underway.

Fact Box 7

- The ACL-RSI scale had been translated from English into many languages including Swedish, French, German, Dutch and Turkish.
- Further translations of the ACL-RSI are currently underway.

Conclusions

For many athletes, ACL rupture and subsequent reconstruction surgery have a significant psychological impact. This can occur not only at the time of injury but also throughout rehabilitation, which can in turn negatively affect recovery. From a psychological perspective, the return-to-sport phase can be particularly challenging. Negative emotions and fears can

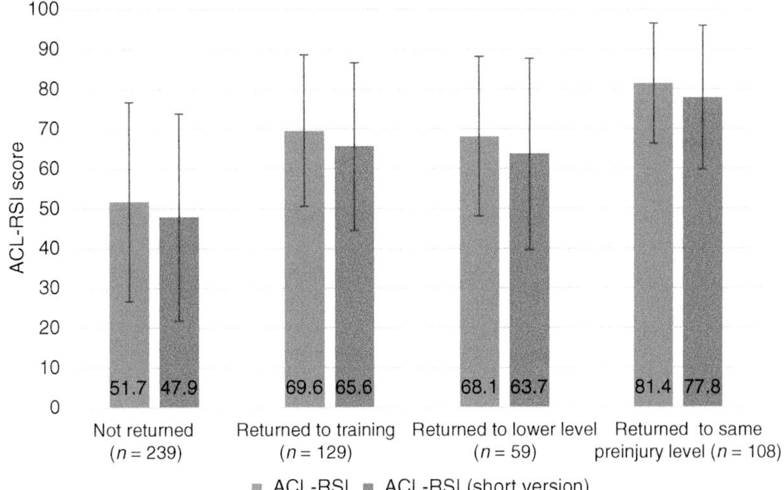

Fig 6.2 Comparative scores between the full ACL-RSI scale and a short version according to sport status

be heightened once an athlete is cleared to return to sport, and many athletes report fear of reinjury as the primary reason for not returning. Most of the psychological factors discussed in this chapter are potentially modifiable and should therefore be considered during rehabilitation in order to improve return-to-sport rates and the return-to-sport experience for athletes. This could be enabled by identifying at-risk athletes with the use of tools designed to assess psychological readiness, such as the ACL-RSI scale.

Take-Home Message

Psychological factors play a significant and continual role in the sequence of ACL injury and reconstruction, rehabilitation and return to sport. Psychological factors are potentially modifiable and should therefore be considered during the rehabilitation phase. The athlete's psychological readiness to return to sport is strongly associated with their decision whether or not to return and can be measured by tools such as the ACL-RSI scale to aid clinical decision making.

Top Five Evidence Based References

Ardern CL, Taylor NF, Feller JA, Whitehead TS, Webster KE (2013) Psychological responses matter in returning to preinjury level of sport after anterior cruciate ligament reconstruction surgery. Am J Sports Med 41:1549–1558

Ardern CL, Taylor NF, Feller JA, Whitehead TS, Webster KE (2013) Psychological responses matter in returning to preinjury level of sport after anterior cruciate ligament reconstruction surgery. Am J Sports Med 41:1549–1558

Kvist J, Ek A, Sporrstedt K, Good L (2005) Fear of re-injury: a hindrance for returning to sports after anterior cruciate ligament reconstruction. Knee Surg Sports Traumatol Arthrosc 13:393–397

Langford JL, Webster KE, Feller JA (2009) A prospective longitudinal study to assess psychological changes following anterior cruciate ligament reconstruction surgery. Br J Sports Med 43:377–381

Webster KE, Feller JA, Lambros C (2008) Development and preliminary validation of a scale to measure the psychological impact of returning to sport following anterior cruciate ligament reconstruction surgery. Phys Ther Sport 9:9–15

References

1. Ardern CL, Taylor NF, Feller JA, Webster KE (2013) A systematic review of the psychological factors associated with returning to sport following injury. Br J Sports Med 47:1120–1126
2. Podlog L, Eklund RC (2010) Returning to competition after a serious injury: the role of self-determination. J Sports Sci 28:819–831
3. te Wierike SC, van der Sluis A, van den Akker-Scheek I, Elferink-Gemser MT, Visscher C (2013) Psychosocial factors influencing the recovery of athletes with anterior cruciate ligament injury: a systematic review. Scand J Med Sci Sports 23:527–540
4. Ardern CL, Taylor NF, Feller JA, Webster KE (2012) Return-to-sport outcomes at 2 to 7 years after anterior cruciate ligament reconstruction surgery. Am J Sports Med 40:41–48

5. Ardern CL, Webster KE, Taylor NF, Feller JA (2011) Return to sport following anterior cruciate ligament reconstruction surgery: a systematic review and meta-analysis of the state of play. Br J Sports Med 45:596–606
6. Ardern CL, Webster KE, Taylor NF, Feller JA (2011) Return to the preinjury level of competitive sport after anterior cruciate ligament reconstruction surgery: two-thirds of patients have not returned by 12 months after surgery. Am J Sports Med 39:538–543
7. McLean SG, Huang X, van den Bogert AJ (2008) Investigating isolated neuromuscular control contributions to non-contact anterior cruciate ligament injury risk via computer simulation methods. Clin Biomech (Bristol, Avon) 23:926–936
8. Smith AM (1996) Psychological impact of injuries in athletes. Sports Med 22:391–405
9. Smith AM, Scott SG, O'Fallon WM, Young ML (1990) Emotional responses of athletes to injury. Mayo Clin Proc 65:38–50
10. Smith AM, Scott SG, Wiese DM (1990) The psychological effects of sports injuries coping. Sports Med 9:352–369
11. Morrey MA, Stuart MJ, Smith AM (1999 Apr) Wiese-Bjornstal DM (1999) A longitudinal examination of athletes' emotional and cognitive responses to anterior cruciate ligament injury. Clin J Sport Med 9(2):63–69
12. Walker N, Thatcher J, Lavallee D (2007) Psychological responses to injury in competitive sport: a critical review. J R Soc Promot Heal 127:174–180
13. Ruddock-Hudson M, O'Halloran P, Murphy G (2012) Exploring psychological reactions to injury in the Australian Football League (AFL). J Appl Sport Psychol 24:375–390
14. Kleiber D, Greendorfer S, Blinde E, Samdahl D (1987) Quality of exit from university sports and life satisfaction in early adulthood. Sociol Sport J 4:28–36
15. Ardern CL, Taylor NF, Feller JA, Webster KE (2014) Fifty-five per cent return to competitive sport following anterior cruciate ligament reconstruction surgery: an updated systematic review and meta-analysis including aspects of physical functioning and contextual factors. Br J Sports Med 48:1543–1552
16. Czuppon S, Racette BA, Klein SE, Harris-Hayes M (2014) Variables associated with return to sport following anterior cruciate ligament reconstruction: a systematic review. Br J Sports Med 48:356–364
17. Everhart JS, Best TM, Flanigan DC (2015) Psychological predictors of anterior cruciate ligament reconstruction outcomes: a systematic review. Knee Surg Sports Traumatol Arthrosc 23:752–762
18. Ardern CL, Kvist J, Webster KE (2015) Psychological aspects of anterior cruciate ligament injuries. Operative Tech Sports Med 24:77–83
19. Brewer B, Andersen MB, van Raalte JL (2002) Psychological aspects of sport injury rehabilitation: toward a biopsychosocial approach. In: Mostofsky D, Zaichkowsky LD (eds) Medical and psychological aspects of sport and exercise. Fitness Information Technology, Morgantown, WV, pp 41–54
20. Wiese-Bjornstal DM, Smith AM, Schaffer SM, Morrey MA (1988) An integrated model of response to sport injury: Psychological and sociological dynamics. J Appl Sport Psychol 10:46–69
21. Brewer B (2010) The role of psychological factors in sport injury rehabilitation outcomes. Rev Sport Exerc Psychol 3:40–61
22. Christino MA, Fantry AJ, Vopat BG (2015) Psychological aspects of recovery following anterior cruciate ligament reconstruction. J Am Acad Orthop Surg 23:501–509
23. Podlog L, Heil J, Schulte S (2014) Psychosocial factors in sports injury rehabilitation and return to play. Phys Med Rehabil Clin N Am 25:915–930
24. Langford JL, Webster KE, Feller JA (2009) A prospective longitudinal study to assess psychological changes following anterior cruciate ligament reconstruction surgery. Br J Sports Med 43:377–381
25. Thomeé P, Währborg P, Börjesson M, Thomeé R, Eriksson BI, Karlsson J (2007) Self-efficacy, symptoms and physical activity in patients with an anterior cruciate ligament injury: a prospective study. Scand J Med Sci Sports 17:238–245
26. Nyland J, Cottrell B, Harreld K, Caborn DN (2006) Self-reported outcomes after anterior cruciate ligament reconstruction: an internal health locus of control score comparison. Arthroscopy 22:1225–1232
27. Thomeé P, Währborg P, Börjesson M, Thomeé R, Eriksson BI, Karlsson J (2008) Self-efficacy of knee function as a pre-operative predictor of outcome 1 year after anterior cruciate ligament reconstruction. Knee Surg Sports Traumatol Arthrosc 16:118–127
28. Thomeé P, Währborg P, Börjesson M, Thomeé R, Eriksson BI, Karlsson J (2007) Determinants of self-efficacy in the rehabilitation of patients with anterior cruciate ligament injury. J Rehabil Med 39:486–492
29. Thomeé P, Währborg P, Börjesson M, Thomeé R, Eriksson BI, Karlsson J (2006) A new instrument for measuring self-efficacy in patients with an anterior cruciate ligament injury. Scand J Med Sci Sports 16:181–187
30. Ardern CL, Taylor NF, Feller JA, Whitehead TS, Webster KE (2013) Psychological responses matter in returning to preinjury level of sport after anterior cruciate ligament reconstruction surgery. Am J Sports Med 41:1549–1558
31. Sonesson S, Kvist J, Ardern C, Österberg A, Grävare Silbernagel K (2016) Psychological factors are important to return to pre-injury sport activity after anterior cruciate ligament reconstruction: expect and motivate to satisfy. Knee Surg Sports Traumatol Arthrosc. https://doi.org/10.1007/s00167-016-4294-8
32. Kvist J, Ek A, Sporrstedt K, Good L (2005) Fear of re-injury: a hindrance for returning to sports after anterior cruciate ligament reconstruction. Knee Surg Sports Traumatol Arthrosc 13:393–397
33. Flanigan DC, Everhart JS, Pedroza A, Smith T, Kaeding CC (2013) Fear of reinjury (kinesiophobia) and persistent knee symptoms are common factors for lack of return to sport after anterior cruciate ligament reconstruction. Arthroscopy 29:1322–1329

34. Mann BJ, Grana WA, Indelicato PA, O'Neill DF, George SZ (2007) A survey of sports medicine physicians regarding psychological issues in patient-athletes. Am J Sports Med 35:2140–2147
35. Ross CA, Clifford A, Louw QA (2017) Factors informing fear of reinjury after anterior cruciate ligament reconstruction. Physiother Theory Pract 33:103–114
36. Walker N, Thatcher J, Lavallee D (2010) A preliminary development of the Re-Injury Anxiety Inventory (RIAI). Phys Ther Sport 11:23–29
37. Ardern CL, Taylor NF, Feller JA, Webster KE (2012) Fear of re-injury in people who have returned to sport following anterior cruciate ligament reconstruction surgery. J Sci Med Sport 15:488–495
38. Podlog L, Banham SM, Wadey R, Hannon J (2015) Psychological readiness to return to competitive sport following injury: a qualitative study. Sport Psychologist 29:1–14
39. Webster KE, Feller JA, Lambros C (2008) Development and preliminary validation of a scale to measure the psychological impact of returning to sport following anterior cruciate ligament reconstruction surgery. Phys Ther Sport 9:9–15
40. Ardern CL, Österberg A, Tagesson S, Gauffin H, Webster KE, Kvist J (2014) The impact of psychological readiness to return to sport and recreational activities after anterior cruciate ligament reconstruction. Br J Sports Med 48:1613–1619
41. Johnston L, Carroll D (1998) The context of emotional responses to athletic injury: a qualitative analysis. J Sport Rehabil 7:206–220
42. Quinn AM, Fallon BJ (1999) The changes in psychological characteristics and reactions of elite athletes from injury onset until full recovery. J Appl Sport Psychol 11:210–229
43. Forsdyke D, Smith A, Jones M, Gledhill A (2016) Psychosocial factors associated with outcomes of sports injury rehabilitation in competitive athletes: a mixed studies systematic review. Br J Sports Med 50:537–544
44. Glazer DD (2009) Development and preliminary validation of the Injury-Psychological Readiness to Return to Sport (I-PRRS) scale. J Athl Train 44:185–189
45. French DJ, France CR, Vigneau F, French JA, Evans RT (2007) Fear of movement/(re)injury in chronic pain: a psychometric assessment of the original English version of the Tampa scale for kinesiophobia (TSK). Pain 127:42–51
46. Mohtadi N (1998) Development and validation of the quality of life outcome measure (questionnaire) for chronic anterior cruciate ligament deficiency. Am J Sports Med 26:350–359
47. Ardern CL, Taylor NF, Feller JA, Whitehead TS, Webster KE (2015) Sports participation 2 years after anterior cruciate ligament reconstruction in athletes who had not returned to sport at 1 year: a prospective follow-up of physical function and psychological factors in 122 athletes. Am J Sports Med 43:848–856
48. Müller U, Krüger-Franke M, Schmidt M, Rosemeyer B (2015) Predictive parameters for return to pre-injury level of sport 6 months following anterior cruciate ligament reconstruction surgery. Knee Surg Sports Traumatol Arthrosc 23:3623–3631
49. Kvist J, Österberg A, Gauffin H, Tagesson S, Webster K, Ardern C (2013) Translation and measurement properties of the Swedish version of ACL-Return to Sports after Injury questionnaire. Scand J Med Sci Sports 23:568–575
50. Bohu Y, Klouche S, Lefevre N, Webster K, Herman S (2015) Translation, cross-cultural adaptation and validation of the French version of the Anterior Cruciate Ligament-Return to Sport after Injury (ACL-RSI) scale. Knee Surg Sports Traumatol Arthrosc 23:1192–1196
51. Müller U, Schmidt M, Krüger-Franke M, Rosemeyer B (2014) Die ACL-Return to Sport after Injury Skala als wichtiger Parameter bei der Beurteilung Rückkehr zum Sport Level I und II nach Rekonstruktion des vorderen Kreuzbands. Ihre Übersetzung in die deutsche Sprache (ACL-Return to Sport after Injury Scale as an important Predictor for Return to Sport Level I and II after ACL Reconstruction. Translation into German Language). Sport Orthop Traumatol 30:135–144
52. Slagers AJ, Reininga IH, van den Akker-Scheek I (2017) The Dutch language anterior cruciate ligament return to sport after injury scale (ACL-RSI) - validity and reliability. J Sports Sci 35(4):393–401
53. Harput G, Tok D, Ulusoy B, Eraslan L, Yildiz TI, Turgut E et al (2016) Translation and cross-cultural adaptation of the anterior cruciate ligament-return to sport after injury (ACL-RSI) scale into Turkish. Knee Surg Sports Traumatol Arthrosc. https://doi.org/10.1007/s00167-016-4288-6

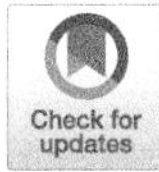

Exercise Physiology of Football: Factors Related to Performance and Health

7

Tim Meyer, Ross Julian, and Chris Thompson

Contents

7.1 Introduction

It is almost a trivial statement that football is a complex sport with a considerable number of factors affecting performance. Some of them are "physiological" ones and summarised in this chapter. However, it should be acknowledged that factors like tactics, technique, team spirit, team organisation, fan support, private circumstances, etc. do affect performance on the pitch as well. In addition, such variables may influence at least the severity of health impairments when they are present (if not act as triggers for their occurrence).

In turn, each illness, injury or other health impairment theoretically can impact on performance. This may either be due to performance-related functions being impaired or due to the sheer presence of inconvenient symptoms. This is, of course, the less important aspect when considering player eligibility with disease. Much more relevant are possible consequences from playing (or training) football when diseased. Most prominent because potentially deadly are cardiac diseases. Usually, they interfere with sufficient cardiac performance to enable playing football. However, unfortunately there are several entities which can stay undiscovered whilst being dangerous, among them chronic myocarditis, hypertrophic cardiomyopathy and anomalies of the coronary arteries or the cardiac conduction system.

7.2 Cardiorespiratory System

Due to its interval character with episodes of high-intensity activity interspersed by less intense periods, playing football typically leads to repeated activation of the sympathetic nervous system and, thus, high levels of catecholamines in the blood. Among other alterations, this leads to the well-known fluctuations

T. Meyer (✉) • R. Julian • C. Thompson
Institute of Sports and Preventive Medicine, Saarland University, Saarbrücken, Germany
e-mail: tim.meyer@mx.uni-saarland.de

V. Musahl et al. (eds.), *Return to Play in Football*, https://doi.org/10.1007/978-3-662-55713-6_7

of heart rate (HR) with considerable amounts of match time spent above 85% HRmax, and average HR is usually situated around 75–80% HRmax. These figures seem to be widely independent from age or gender of the players [1]. Of course, also blood pressure goes up due to an increased cardiac output and elevated total peripheral resistance both being a result of the increased sympathetic tone. Consequently, there is considerable volume and pressure work for the cardiac muscle during football match play.

This in turn leads to large stress on the coronary arteries because under such circumstances the myocardium has high oxygen demands which cannot be satisfied by enlarging the arteriovenous oxygen difference which is already close to maximal under low-intensity work conditions. Therefore, it is necessary to accomplish maximal dilatation of the coronary arteries to make up for the oxygen demands. It is, thus, understandable that atherosclerosis in these vessels can quickly lead to performance limitation (due to limited cardiac output) or even arrhythmias (due to suboptimal oxygen delivery to cardiomyocytes). At the same time, high concentrations of catecholamines may exert their arrhythmogenic effects which can further elevate the danger for individuals at risk—those with pre-existing cardiac diseases. This is the main reason why precompetition medical assessments (PCMAs) are considered important by most national and international football authorities and federations.

Mainly due to its endurance component, football may lead to some training-related ("chronic") adaptations of the heart, less so for the respiratory system. However, there is no "footballer's heart" or any other football-specific finding in cardiocirculatory examinations [2, 3]. Cardiac changes roughly follow the players' endurance capacity, and the relationship between cardiac size and ergometric capacity is sometimes even used to assess a possible pathological basis of heart enlargement.

Although vital capacity and lung volume of football players are slightly higher than those of the age-, gender- and anthropometry-matched population, this hardly reflects specific adaptations. Part of it may even be due to selection. Anatomical restrictions (rib cage, abdominal organs) by far prevent dimensional changes of the lungs. However, there may be tiny improvements in respiratory function due to regular football training and competition. Usually, at no time even during intense football do the lungs of a healthy player reach their functional or anatomical limits. Only pathological impairments like allergic asthma or infectious diseases may lead to the respiratory system being the limiting component for a football player. In such cases, appropriate treatment (asthma) or rest (infections) should restore full lung function.

Fact Box 1

- Independent from the league or the degree of professionalism, playing football leads to considerable activation of the sympathetic system and, consequently, to maximal cardiocirculatory responses.
- Such cardiocirculatory stress is part of the training stimulus that football delivers but at the same time constitutes an inherent risk for players with cardiac conditions. For this reason, it is advisable to ensure appropriate health when competing as a football player.
- Adaptations of the cardiovascular system are mainly elicited due to the endurance component of football. An "athlete's heart" can only be expected in the most endurant players.
- The lung is hardly a limiting factor during football play. This may happen only in players with respiratory disease and should be promptly and appropriately treated.

7.3 Hormonal System

Like for the cardiorespiratory system, there are no football-specific adaptations in the hormonal system. Acutely, the typical ensemble of hormones can be found which accompanies intense physical exercise mainly regulating metabolism and fluid balance. This means that particularly catecholamines (for the short-term maintenance of blood glucose) and cortisol (for the long-term effect) concentrations in the blood are increased with growth hormone and glucagon having a smaller effect of that kind. Physiological disturbances of the fluid balance (mainly due to losses by sweating and respiration) are usually a bit delayed compared to the immediate metabolic needs of football match play. Aldosterone and—less pronounced—antidiuretic hormone (ADH) reduce the amount of urine production and, thus, save the organism from dehydrating too quickly. All other hormones do not play major roles in the acute exercise reaction during football training or competition.

It follows that diseases of the hormonal system can, of course, affect football performance when these regulatory circuits are impaired and not treated appropriately. The most common one is diabetes mellitus which influences glucose delivery and metabolism and usually needs insulin therapy in young players. However, it is established that a well-controlled diabetes does not necessarily interfere even with participation in the highest levels of football. The main problem in football players is the adequate adaptation, i. e. lowering of insulin dosage prior to football activity. Note that insulin is a very anabolic hormone and, thus, on the list of forbidden substances ("doping list"). Therefore, application for a therapeutic use exemption (TUE, at the responsible doping control institution) is necessary when competitive football players are treated; usually there is no problem to get a TUE with normal documentation of diabetes diagnostics, of course.

Dysregulation of the catecholamines, cortisol (Cushing's and Addison's disease) or aldosterone (e.g. Conn's disease) is less frequent and typically not compatible with competitive football. Although thyroid hormones are not part of the immediate hormone response to exercise, hypo- and hyperthyroidism are to be mentioned because they are frequent and alter the basal metabolism of an affected player. Because of typical complaints like weakness/fatigue and weight changes, there is usually a need for appropriate therapy when football play is intended.

Fortunately, chronic football exposure does not lead to pathological dysregulation of hormonal circuits. However, there is some speculation that overload and overtraining syndrome can be related to an imbalance of anabolic (testosterone, insulin, growth hormone) and catabolic (particularly cortisol) hormones [4, 5]. However, so far there is no convincing evidence for this assumption. Also, trials to utilise concentrations of these hormones in the blood for diagnosing such fatigue syndromes have not been successful. Altogether, with the given low prevalence of overload syndromes under the specific circumstances of elite football, anabolic-catabolic imbalances do not seem to constitute a major problem for the medical care of players.

Effects of the menstrual cycle and sex hormones on performance in females will be discussed in the respective subchapter.

7.4 Immune System and Infectious Diseases

It has been repeatedly claimed that periods of intense exercise (or particularly strenuous competitive events like a marathon) may lead to temporary impairment of immune function and consecutive proneness to infectious diseases—particularly ones of the upper respiratory system. This theory has been named "open window" for infections [6]. Evidence, however, is mainly from laboratory measurements indicating that certain populations of lymphocytes (e.g. natural killer cells) are decreased shortly after exercise for a few hours. This downregulation may support the entry for infectious agents and—after their multiplication—finally the establishment of clinically relevant disease. Also, it has been observed that in the first days after strenuous competitions or training camps, the frequency of infections goes up in participating athletes. More convincingly, the occurrence of infection proneness has recently been linked to travel needs and circumstances and shifts between time zones in Australian and South African rugby players [7]. Therefore, under the given circumstances in competitive football, i.e. hardly more than six training sessions per week with a duration of <90 min on average, it is probably not the high physiological load that may lead to an increased incidence of infectious diseases but rather the travelling requirements (and possibly obligations for sponsors and media). Nevertheless, for infection-prone individuals, preventive (hygiene) measures should be installed to maintain their health particularly during the autumn and winter months. This includes vaccinations, regular and thorough dental care as well as hand hygiene and consequent therapy for allergies.

In turn, infectious diseases can weaken the athlete and, thus, interfere with performance. This may happen due to the simple negative effects from infection-specific complaints and also due to mediators in the blood which lead to the typical "malaise" feeling. More importantly, possible affection of organs by infectious agents is a matter of great concern. Even though there are differences between viruses, bacteria and parasites in their likelihood to cause myocarditis (the most feared complication), there should be general reluctance to let players train or compete when infected because we usually do not know what is the responsible infectious agent in the present disease. Finally, it is possible that infections may be a trigger for arrhythmia in pre-existing cardiac disease of other kind (like cardiomyopathies).

Fact Box 2

- There is no convincing evidence for an increased incidence of infections in regularly training football players—not even in the highest professional leagues.
- Of course, like in other disciplines and professions, there are certain individual football players in each team who are more prone to infections and need thorough management including hygiene and other preventive measures.
- It is rather the stress from travelling and out-of-football obligations which leads to infection proneness than the physiological load or hormonal consequences of football training and/or match play.
- Decisions about participation in training or match should be made carefully for infected football players because there is seldom sufficient information available about the responsible infectious agent and its virulence.

7.5 Musculoskeletal System and Metabolism

The acute energy requirements of football lead to not only immediate adaptations of the cardiocirculatory and respiratory system but similarly to metabolic reactions within the active tissue—the muscles. It can be assumed that about 1100–1400 kcal are expended during a football match and around 800–900 kcal per typical training session [8]. The majority of the "fuel" for energy requirements is represented by carbohydrates which may necessitate their partly substitution during the match and at halftime as well as its quick reconstitution within the first hours after cessation [9]. This also sheds light on the problematic (whilst currently frequent) habit to employ low-carb diets in competitive football players. Of course, fat metabolism also takes part in energy delivery over a whole match; however, its contribution can be considered minor. Muscle work is mainly concentric although eccentric parts can also be involved—particularly during braking movements. However, this does only mildly affect energy pathways, i.e. primarily glycolysis and citric acid cycle/respiratory chain [10]. Those metabolic diseases which affect carbohydrate turnover are hardly compatible with competitive football.

Regular training and competition of football players lead to predictable adaptations in the muscular system with hypertrophy of the calf, rectus femoris, adductor and hamstring muscles—particularly of their fast twitch fibres, of course. Also, football's endurance component usually induces mitochondrial growth and increases in metabolic enzyme concentrations as well as improved capillarization. This process can be generally considered healthy, and no resulting health impairments or associated diseases are known. An overview of musculoskeletal and metabolic training effects as related to typical training contents can be obtained from Fig. 7.1.

7.6 Mental Health

Albeit single tragic cases of suicide or at least depressive episodes have been reported in high-level football players, there is no convincing evidence that football itself leads to mental/psychiatric disorders. However, with pre-existing disease or at least a predisposition for psychiatric pathology, real existing football may create situations and constellations that serve as triggers for the initiation of such disorders or their symptoms—particularly for depressive episodes. Critical constellations may arise from a combination of external pressure and vulnerable age (like in youth academies) as well as difficult team situations and individual standing within a team. Epidemiological studies with sound methodology are completely lacking in this area. Of course, the presence of "active" psychiatric diseases is detrimental to performance. This should become evident immediately when considering the "minus symptoms" of several entities. Such a

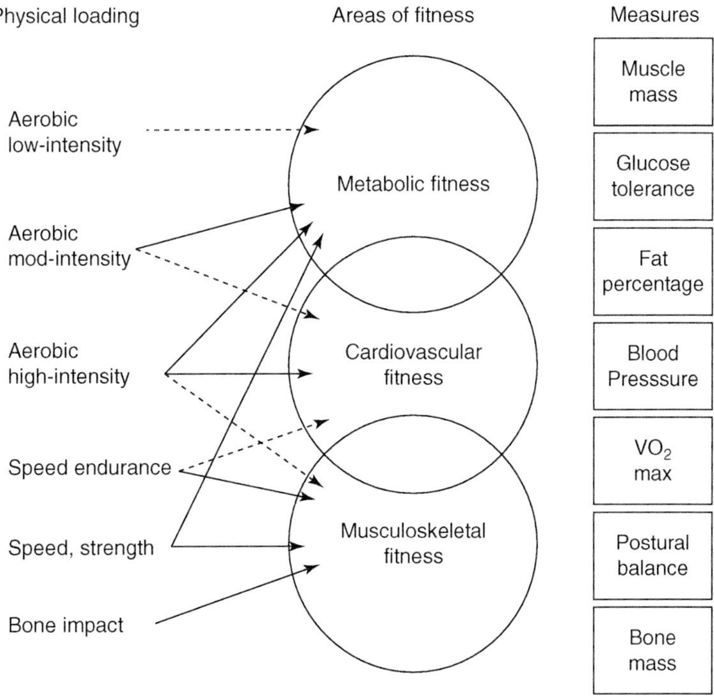

Fig. 7.1 Overview of the impact of different types of physical loading on various fitness capacities. *Full lines* denote comprehensive effects and/or well-known relationships. *Dotted lines* denote smaller yet positive effects (adapted from Krustrup et al. [11])

negative effect on performance may also lead to a selection of non-diseased individuals for football squads and, thus, an incidence of psychiatric diseases possibly slightly below the population average.

Some psychological traits do not reach the status of a disease but can nevertheless affect football performance (and possibly be triggered by events on the pitch). As an (somewhat arbitrary) example, anxiety before performing in competitive football is a common emotional trait in many players. However, it is difficult to measure the effects of anxiety on live match performance due to the multifaceted nature of the game, causing great difficulty in isolating one possible factor of performance decrement. Nevertheless, one performance parameter that has been measured is the anxiety experienced during penalty shootouts. Jordet et al. [12] found that whilst walking to the penalty spot from the halfway line, players report feelings of concentration disruption and loneliness, along with a fear and worry of goalkeeper performance.

When analysing penalties taken in elite football, it appears that a player is most likely to score when aiming at the two upper corners of the goal. Under anxiety though, players are prone to focusing on the centralised goalkeeper rather than the more likely scoring zones, which causes lower shooting accuracy [13]. Remarkably, simply adding a goalkeeper to a practice penalty shootout following previous penalty shooting practice towards an open goal resulted in a significant decline in penalty accuracy, with a greater number of centralised kicks [14]. The use of practice in focusing on the upper top corners of the goal before penalty completion resulted in greater shooting accuracy compared to a control group who received no coaching advice [15]. Confidence is a critical factor in penalty completion, as found in a study by Wood and Wilson [15], where players with higher perceptions of self-control completed a greater amount of accurate penalty kicks compared to low self-control individuals. Coaches should, thus, motivate their players and try to reduce stress and pressure before taking a penalty. Future research is required to understand the transfer of practice and coaching methods on penalty conversion in a competitive setting.

Alongside skill performance, anxiety has a negative impact on other parameters in football. In youth football, a large fear of failure is present among football players. The consequences of this fear of failure have been perceived by elite youth players to be interpersonal and intrapersonal and can have a great impact on football performance and relationships with other people [16]. These players who are not fully matured typically have poor coping strategies to these emotions and lack the necessary strategies to overcome such adversity. The stressors which cause a fear of failure/incompetence appear to differ among age categories [17]. Early adolescent (aged 12–14) players have reported greater stressors over family pressure to succeed, whilst middle adolescents (aged 15–18) face further anxiety due to physical demands of football, contractual issues and the pressure of playing at a higher level. Such experiences of anxiety must be shared with family members and/or coaching staff to allow the use of interventions (e.g. cognitive behaviour therapy) to increase mental well-being and therefore football performance.

The demands of football training and match play are well understood to be physically demanding [18]. However, the media commitments and large intake of tactical information from coaches along with the fixture congestion are just some of the factors which could induce a psychological exertion. An overload of stress to the prefrontal cortex, the brain region responsible for high-order cognitive function [19], could potentially impair both psychological and physical determinants of football performance. With this in mind, research is now being conducted to understand the effects of mental fatigue on physical performance and technical/skill performance.

Mental fatigue can be characterised as a subjective state of cognitive exertion experienced by exposure to prolonged periods of cognitive activity [20]. Feelings of tiredness and a reduction in energy are typically associated with mental fatigue [21]. Furthermore, this exertion can lead to a reduction in attention [22], task planning [23], reaction times [24], plus monitoring performance and slower adjustments in performance after errors [25]. It has been found that acutely induced mental fatigue has a detrimental effect on intermittent running [26], skill performance [27], decision making [28] and match play performance in small-sided games [29]. Although the early research in mental fatigue is promising, the methodology used (i.e. use of the Stroop test to induce subjective feelings of mental fatigue) does not accurately reflect the mental fatigue that may be experienced in reality. Future research should aim to understand the true causes of mental fatigue and whether mental fatigue is a short- and/or long-term psychological state.

7.7 Specific Aspects in Women's Football

On the surface, game characteristics and demands may appear similar across genders. Unsurprisingly, there are physical, physiological and biological differences between males and females, which cause inherent limitations that affect the pace and total work output in the women's game. Due to exercise and these biological and physiological factors, risks for health problems such as the female athlete triad (low energy availability/eating disorders, menstrual dysfunction, and low body density/osteoporosis), iron deficiency and anaemia may affect some female footballers. Furthermore, the effects of the change in hormones, due to the menstrual cycle, have the potential to alter performance and inhibit maximal activity. However, data from Scandinavia seem to indicate that the size of the problem is not that big in female football players (Table 7.1).

The hypothalamus, which regulates the levels and secretion of hormones throughout the menstrual cycle, can be affected by external stimuli, for example, high volumes of exercise. It has been well highlighted that women who encounter high training loads are exposed to a greater risk of disruptions to the normal menstrual cycle. Furthermore, it has been previously reported that menstrual dysfunction occurs in a variable percentage of women who are engaged in physical activity [30–32]. Menstrual dysfunction in athletes has been characterised by significant decreases in reproductive hormones, specifically oestrogen, and the disruption of a regularly occurring menstrual cycle. However, it is less commonly observed in the footballing population, potentially due to having less strenuous training programmes than those of other (endurance) disciplines. Also, a lower dependency on "leanness" in football may be advantageous in this regard. Therefore, a higher percentage of players with "normal" body composition and energy intake may be apparent within football compared to other sports [33] (Table 7.1). However, for those players who encounter such disturbances, health consequences can arise from the hormonal deficit. For example, supressed levels of oestrogen can heavily affect bone health through the loss of bone mineral density, as oestrogen is well-known

Table 7.1 Characteristics of the total population of athletes [33]

Mean (SD)	Football (n = 69)	Handball (n = 60)	Endurance (n = 115)	Controls (n = 607)
Age (years)	19.6 (4.1)	19.9 (3.1)	22.3 (6.3)	27.3 (7.9)
BMI (kg/m^2)	21.5 (1.6)	22.5 (2.0)	20.5 (1.8)	23.3 (4.2)
Training (h/week)	12.3 (3.7)	15.8 (4.2)	13.1 (4.5)	–
Eating disorders[a]	5.9%[b]	22.4%	25.7%	21.1%
Current use of contraceptives	35.8%	43.9%	38.2%	27.8%
Current menstrual dysfunction[c]	9.3%	18.8%	27.9%	15.2%
Stress fractures	13.6%	23.2%	13.4%	12.4%

Characteristics of the total population of athletes representing football, handball and endurance sports participating in the large screening study. *BMI* body mass index

[a]Self-reported

[b]Football significantly different from the other groups ($p < 0.05$)

[c]Oral contraceptives were excluded

to modulate bone growth and turnover. Furthermore, research has indicated a greater incidence of injuries and stress fractures among amenorrheic (absence of menstruation) and oligomenorrhoeic (infrequent menstruation) athletes compared to their eumenorrheic (normal menstrual cycle) counterparts [34]. Apart from the physical, the stresses of personal life and competition have also been associated with the disturbance of the hypothalamic-pituitary-gonadal axis which is known to regulate the menstrual cycle and hormonal secretion [35].

The fluctuating hormones of the menstrual cycle regulate many physiological processes, which are key for reproduction. However, these hormones, which rise and fall throughout this cycle, have been attributed to various alterations in common physiological processes. Adapted from Lebrun et al. [36], (Fig. 7.2) illustrates all the aspects of athletic performance, which may become affected by these fluctuations. Currently, much of the research has investigated the effects on endurance-based exercise with very limited research on the effects on team sport activity. However, recently unpublished data investigating the effects of the different phases of the menstrual cycle on football-specific performance, suggested that in a cohort of five elite teams from the two highest leagues in Germany, there was no clear relationship between cycle phase and a change in performance. The authors attributed the findings to the multifaceted and variable nature of competitive football (Julian et al., unpublished observation). There is evidence that the female footballer is more susceptible to technical errors in the pre-menses phase (~5–11 days before menses), which has been reflected in the incidence of injuries in Swedish players [37]. Finally, regarding injury, tissue qualities such as ligament laxity may be affected by oestradiol concentration (most common oestrogen type). A reduction of 17% was observed in knee stiffness at ovulation and said to be associated with knee laxity [38]. Such changes have not been observed in other tissues such as the gastrocnemius, patellar tendon or Achilles tendon, potentially contributing to the larger rates of ACL injury incidence in female footballers.

To match the physical demands of football, maintaining an energy balance that equals the energetic cost of training and match play is essential for good health. Lowered energy availability has been shown to be a contributor to the female athlete triad [39]. When energy expenditure exceeds energy intake, this increases the risk of subsequent metabolic, reproductive and bone-related health consequences. Alarmingly, previous studies indicated that energy expenditure was greater than energy intake in some female players [33]. Therefore, energy balance should be monitored and dealt with individually. Furthermore, impacts of the female athlete triad can affect bone

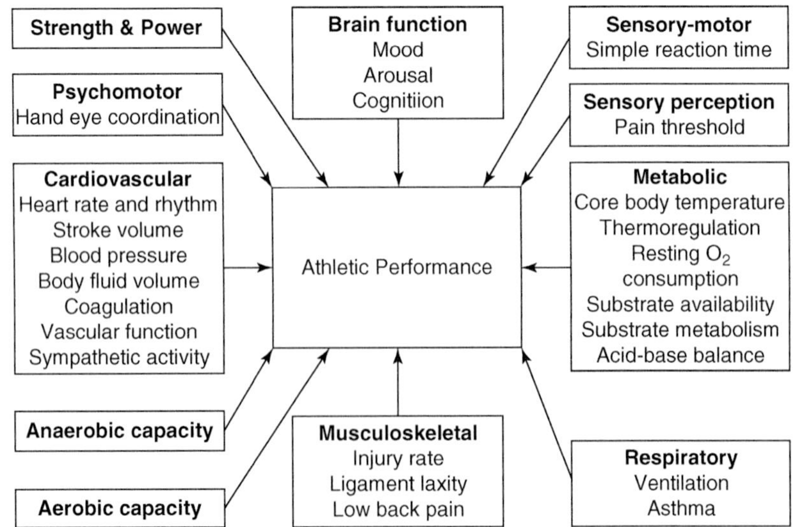

Fig. 7.2 Components of physical performance that may be affected by menstrual cycle fluctuations in endogenous hormones [36]

mineral density (BMD). If the menstrual cycle is dysfunctional, this has the potential to lead to reductions in BMD [33, 40, 41]. Reduced BMD does not inevitably have an instant physical impact. Elite footballers, if not ensuring correct nutrition or focussing on their menstrual cycles, may experience bone loss, which can lead to debilitating disorders such as osteoporosis at latter stages in life. Interestingly, it has been suggested that elite female soccer players are more susceptible to stress fractures despite having normal BMI, which could be linked to menstrual dysfunction also observed in this study [42].

Regular intense exercise is often associated with low iron stores; iron has been recognised to be particularly important in the oxygen-carrying capacity of an individual, and deficiencies may therefore compromise aerobic capacity [43]. The female athlete has been documented to be at greater risk of decreased iron status than their male counterparts; this has been heavily linked to dietary intake (lower meat intake in women) and menstrual losses as well as iron losses through sweat. Research investigating female footballers and their iron status is not highly prevalent within the scientific literature. In a recent study, of the players investigated, 57% were iron deficient and 29% had iron deficiency anaemia [44]. Continued high-level performance in football requires a myriad of attributes; however, several studies show that a better maximum aerobic capacity (VO_2max) improves soccer performance, measured as distance covered by a player during a game, as well as involvements with the ball [45]. Therefore, this high prevalence of iron deficiency may affect overall performance of the female footballer, and hence regular and continued monitoring of iron status is recommended throughout the season.

7.8 Summary

A football team physician needs thorough knowledge not only of physiological factors associated with acutely playing football but also of the expectable "normal" changes due to an ongoing typical football training process. This helps in assessing the degree of stress imposed on certain organs of football players, and it also supports in understanding the limitations caused by certain diseases as well as delineating pathological states from physiological ones.

It is necessary to identify individuals within a football squad who are more prone to suffer from certain discipline-specific factors (e.g. travelling) and are more likely to develop pathology (like infections). Some preventive measures can be confined to them. The same is true for the application of (drug) treatments, of course.

Do not underestimate the stress imposed on football players from factors besides the sheer physiological load. Obligations for sponsors and media, travel requirements as well as psychological interference from private events are relevant and worth considering for diagnostic and therapeutic decisions.

Take-Home Message

Without thorough and detailed knowledge of football-specific physiological challenges and stressors, a team physician will hardly be able to safely recognise all pathological states which may need treatment or rest. Certain subgroups of players like veterans or females may need additional attention to phenomena which are specific for them.

Top Five Evidence-Based References

Datson N, Hulton A, Andersson H, Lewis T, Weston M, Drust B, Gregson W (2014) Applied physiology of female soccer: an update. Sports Med 44(9):1225–1240

Reeves CW, Nicholls AR, McKenna J (2011) Longitudinal analysis of stressors, perceived control, coping and coping effectiveness among early and middle adolescent soccer players. Int J Sport Psychol 42(2):186–203

Schwellnus MP, Derman WE, Jordaan E, Page T, Lambert MI, Readhead C, Roberts C, Kohler R, Collins R, Kara S, Morris MI, Strauss O, Webb S (2012) Elite athletes travelling to international destinations >5 time zone differences from their home country have a 2–3-fold increased risk of illness. Br J Sports Med 46(11):816–821

Stølen T, Chamari K, Castagna C, Wisløff U (2005) Physiology of soccer: an update. Sports Med 35(6):501–536

Sundgot-Borgen J, Torstveit MK (2007) The female football player, disordered eating, menstrual function and bone health. Brit J Sport Med 41(Suppl. 1):I68–I72

References

1. Wegmann M, Steffen A, Putz K, Wurtz N, Such U, Faude O et al (2016) Cardiovascular risk and fitness in veteran football players. J Sports Sci 34:576–583
2. Bohm P, Ditzel R, Ditzel H, Urhausen A, Meyer T (2013) Resting ECG findings in elite football players. J Sports Sci 31:1475–1480
3. Bohm P, Kastner A, Meyer T (2013) Sudden cardiac death in football. J Sports Sci 31:1451–1459
4. Meister S, Faude O, Ammann T, Schnittker R, Meyer T (2013) Indicators for high physical strain and overload in elite football players. Scand J Med Sci Sports 23:156–163
5. Urhausen A, Kindermann W (2002) Diagnosis of overtraining: what tools do we have? Sports Med 32:95–102
6. Pedersen BK, Bruunsgaard H (1995) How physical exercise influences the establishment of infections. Sports Med 19:393–400
7. Schwellnus MP, Derman WE, Jordaan E, Page T, Lambert MI, Readhead C et al (2012) Elite athletes travelling to international destinations >5 time zone differences from their home country have a 2–3-fold increased risk of illness. Br J Sports Med 46:816–821
8. Ferrauti A, Giesen HT, Merheim G, Weber K (2006) Indirekte Kalorimetrie im Fußballspiel (indirect calorimetry in a soccer game). Dtsch Z Sportmed 57:142–146
9. Maughan RJ (1997) Energy and macronutrient intakes of professional football (soccer) players. Br J Sports Med 31:45–47
10. Stevens TG, De Ruiter CJ, Van Maurik D, Van Lierop CJ, Savelsbergh GJ, Beek PJ (2015) Measured and estimated energy cost of constant and shuttle running in soccer players. Med Sci Sports Exerc 47:1219–1224
11. Krustrup P, Aagaard P, Nybo L, Petersen J, Mohr M, Bangsbo J (2010) Recreational football as a health promoting activity: a topical review. Scand J Med Sci Sports 20:1–13
12. Jordet G, Elferink-Gemser MT (2012) Stress, coping, and emotions on the world stage: the experience of participating in a major soccer tournament penalty shootout. J Appl Sport Psychol 24:281–298
13. Wood G, Wilson MR (2010) A moving goalkeeper distracts penalty takers and impairs shooting accuracy. J Sports Sci 28:937–946
14. Navarro M, van der Kamp J, Ranvaud R, Savelsbergh GJ (2013) The mere presence of a goalkeeper affects the accuracy of penalty kicks. J Sports Sci 31:921–929
15. Wood G, Wilson MR (2012) Quiet-eye training, perceived control and performing under pressure. Psychol Sport and Exerc 13:721–728
16. Sagar SS, Busch BK, Jowett S (2010) Success and failure, fear of failure, and coping responses of adolescent academy football players. Int J Sport Psychol 22:213–230
17. Reeves CW, Nicholls AR, McKenna J (2011) Longitudinal analysis of stressors, perceived control, coping and coping effectiveness among early and middle adolescent soccer players. Int J Sport Psychol 42:186–203
18. Reilly T, Drust B, Clarke N (2008) Muscle fatigue during football match-play. Sports Med 38:357–367
19. Arnsten AF (2009) Stress signalling pathways that impair prefrontal cortex structure and function. Nat Rev Neurosci 10:410–422
20. Ackerman PL, Kanfer R (2009) Test length and cognitive fatigue: an empirical examination of effects on performance and test-taker reactions. J Exp Psychol Appl 15:163–181
21. Boksem MA, Tops M (2008) Mental fatigue: costs and benefits. Brain Res Rev 59:125–139
22. Chaudhuri A, Behan PO (2004) Fatigue in neurological disorders. Lancet 363:978–988
23. van der Linden D, Frese M, Meijman TF (2003) Mental fatigue and the control of cognitive processes: effects on perseveration and planning. Acta Psychol 113:45–65
24. Boksem MA, Meijman TF, Lorist MM (2005) Effects of mental fatigue on attention: an ERP study. Brain Res Cogn Brain Res 25:107–116
25. Lorist MM, Boksem MA, Ridderinkhof KR (2005) Impaired cognitive control and reduced cingulate activity during mental fatigue. Brain Res Cogn Brain Res 24:199–205
26. Smith MR, Marcora SM, Coutts AJ (2015) Mental fatigue impairs intermittent running performance. Med Sci Sports Exerc 47:1682–1690
27. Smith MR, Fransen J, Deprez D, Lenoir M, Coutts AJ (2017) Impact of mental fatigue on speed and accuracy components of soccer-specific skills. Sci Med Football 1:48–52
28. Smith MR, Zeuwts L, Lenoir M, Hens N, De Jong LM, Coutts AJ (2016) Mental fatigue impairs soccer-specific decision-making skill. J Sports Sci 34:1297–1304
29. Badin OO, Smith MR, Conte D, Coutts AJ (2016) Mental fatigue: impairment of technical performance in small-sided soccer games. Int J Sports Physiol Perform 11:1100–1105
30. Constantini NW, Warren MP (1994) Special problems of the female athlete. Baillieres Clin Rheumatol 8:199–219
31. Loucks AB, Horvath SM (1985) Athletic amenorrhea – a review. Med Sci Sports Exerc 17:56–72
32. Torstveit MK, Sundgot-Borgen J (2005) Participation in leanness sports but not training volume is associated with menstrual dysfunction: a national survey of 1276 elite athletes and controls. Brit J Sports Med 39:141–147
33. Sundgot-Borgen J, Torstveit MK (2007) The female football player, disordered eating, menstrual function and bone health. Brit J Sports Med 41:I68–I72
34. Bennell K, Matheson G, Meeuwisse W, Brukner P (1999) Risk factors for stress fractures. Sports Med 28:91–122

35. Constantini NW, Dubnov G, Lebrun CM (2005) The menstrual cycle and sport performance. Clin Sports Med 24:e51–e82. xiii-xiv
36. Lebrun C, Joyce S, Constantini NW (2013) Effects of female reproductive hormones on sports performance. In: Constantini NW, Hackney AC (eds) Endocrinology of physical activity and sport, 2nd edn. Humana Press, New York, pp 281–322. https://doi.org/10.1007/978–1–62703-314-5
37. Moller-Nielsen J, Hammar M (1989) Women's soccer injuries in relation to the menstrual cycle and oral contraceptive use. Med Sci Sports Exerc 21:126-129
38. Park SK, Stefanyshyn DJ, Ramage B, Hart DA, Ronsky JL (2009) Alterations in knee joint laxity during the menstrual cycle in healthy women leads to increases in joint loads during selected athletic movements. Am J Sports Med 37:1169–1177
39. Matzkin E, Curry EJ, Whitlock K (2015) Female athlete triad: past, present, and future. J Am Acad Orthop Surg 23:424–432
40. Dueck CA, Manore MM, Matt KS (1996) Role of energy balance in athletic menstrual dysfunction. Int J Sport Nutr 6:165–190
41. Lloyd T, Buchanan JR, Bitzer S, Waldman CJ, Myers C, Ford BG (1987) Interrelationships of diet, athletic activity, menstrual status, and bone density in collegiate women. Am J Clin Nutr 46:681–684
42. Prather H, Hunt D, McKeon K, Simpson S, Meyer EB, Yemm T et al (2016) Are elite female soccer athletes at risk for disordered eating attitudes, menstrual dysfunction, and stress fractures? PM R 8:208–213
43. Chatard JC, Mujika I, Guy C, Lacour JR (1999) Anaemia and iron deficiency in athletes – practical recommendations for treatment. Sports Med 27:229–240
44. Landahl G, Borjesson M, Rodjer S, Jacobsson S (2005) Iron deficiency and Anemia in top athletes – how to use the transferrin receptor. Med Sci Sports Exerc 37:S146–S146
45. Datson N, Hulton A, Andersson H, Lewis T, Weston M, Drust B et al (2014) Applied physiology of female soccer: an update. Sports Med 44:1225–1240

Part II

ACL: Criteria-based Return to Play

8 A Test Battery for Return to Play in Football

Felix Fischer, Christian Hoser, Elmar Herbst, Peter Gföller, and Christian Fink

Contents

F. Fischer
Research Unit of Orthopaedic Sports Medicine and Injury Prevention, ISAG/UMIT, Hall in Tirol, Austria

FIFA Medical Centre of Excellence, Innsbruck/Tirol, Austria

C. Hoser • E. Herbst • P. Gföller
FIFA Medical Centre of Excellence, Innsbruck/Tirol, Austria

Gelenkpunkt – Sport and Joint Surgery, Innsbruck, Austria

C. Fink (✉)
Research Unit of Orthopaedic Sports Medicine and Injury Prevention, ISAG/UMIT, Hall in Tirol, Austria

FIFA Medical Centre of Excellence, Innsbruck/Tirol, Austria

Gelenkpunkt – Sport and Joint Surgery, Innsbruck, Austria
e-mail: c.fink@gelenkpunkt.com

8.1 Background

Football is one of the most popular sports played by more than 260 million people all over the world [1]. Being an active player has positive effects on certain health parameters, and also untrained individuals at a recreational level benefit from improved health parameters after several weeks of training [2, 3]. However, football is also a demanding sport with high physical loads when performing sport-specific tasks such as sprinting, jumping, tackling and kicking [4]. Even higher forces act on the musculoskeletal system in the rapid deceleration of cutting, pivoting and jump-landing movements [5]. Sustained injuries in those movements are classified as non-contact injuries [6], and they account for more than 50% of the injuries [5, 7]. Injuries occur when participating in football, even if there has been a lot of effort made to implement prevention strategies [8]. A cornerstone in the investigation of injuries has been made in the consensus statement on injury definitions and data collection procedures in studies of football injuries by Fuller et al. [9]. However, football has also

V. Musahl et al. (eds.), *Return to Play in Football*, https://doi.org/10.1007/978-3-662-55713-6_8

evolved into a much faster, intensive and more competitive game, with physical and technical demands increasing substantially over the past few years [10] both at professional [11] and recreational level [12]. Despite the fact of improvements in the athlete's healthcare [13] and the implementation of injury prevention programmes [8], the risk of injury in training and gameplay and muscle and severe injury rates remains high [14].

A tear of the anterior cruciate ligament (ACL) in a football player's knee is one of the most common and devastating knee injury sustained as a result of sports participation [15]. Once the ACL is torn, it is a challenging issue, particularly in professional players [5] with around 65,000 registered professional players worldwide [1]. Considering the negative outcomes leading to reduced performance and long-term health consequences for players, there is also a financial impact [16] amounting to almost €500.000 a month for an injured player in professional football [17]. ACL reconstruction is currently the solution of choice when the ACL is torn in a football player [18], especially when the player wants to return to pre-injury level of competition [19]. In the best-case scenario, it enables the athlete to return to his pre-injury level, and the ACL reconstructed knee withstands all sporting load; in the worst outcome, it may put an athlete's career at risk. After ACL reconstruction the desired objective of an athlete is to return to sport as soon as possible, preferably performing at the same level as pre-injury without sustaining a re-rupture [20].

After a sports injury, the first question asked by most athletes (and coaches) is "When will the athlete be able to compete again?" [21]. But when is the best moment to return to training, return to play and return to competition? There is no straightforward answer to this question due to the influence of many factors [21]. The implementation of a test battery with an objective functional evaluation of the athlete's functional capacities after ACL surgery might be one piece in the puzzle when it comes to a safe return to sport [22, 23].

8.2 A Short Overview of Injuries in Football

Playing (professional) football puts the player at risk of an injury [24]. Injury rate has been estimated to be approximately 1000 times higher than the overall rate for typical high-risk industrial occupations [14]. Injury incidence of 10.2 and 35.5 injuries per 1.000 match-hours and 1.5 and 7.6 injuries per 1.000 training hours has been reported [12, 24]. Younger and less skilled players are often at higher risk for football-related injuries [25], although older age has been identified as a risk factor [26]. Approximately 60–80% of severe injuries occur in the lower extremities, most commonly at the knee or ankle [27]. In the UEFA Champions League (UCL) injury study, about 50 injuries are expected for each football team resulting in two injuries per player per season [24]. For a broader overview, please refer to the publications of the UCL study team [14, 24, 28, 29].

Fact Box 1 Injuries in football

Injuries in football	Injury risk is approximately 1000 times higher than the overall rate for typical high-risk industrial occupations [27]
	10.2 and 35.5 injuries/ 1.000 match-hours
	1.5 and 7.6 injuries/ 1.000 training hours [45, 49]
	Younger and less skilled players are often at higher risk for football-related injuries [28]
	Approximately 60–80% of severe injuries occur in the lower extremities, most commonly at the knee or ankle [22]

8.3 Severe Knee Injuries in Football and Return to Play

Knee injuries in football are common and constitute a serious problem regardless of gender or playing level [30]. One of the most common knee injuries is ACL rupture. Due to the long lay-off time from football, it is causing a threat for the athlete's career [5, 31]. With an ACL injury, the risk of a new knee injury [30] and the risk of developing osteoarthritis in the injured knee [31, 32] increases. Also high re-rupture rates within the first year of surgery have been reported [33]. The mechanism of injury often involves faulty landing technique, deceleration, pivoting or cutting with excessive anterior shear forces [27, 32]. However, the mechanism of ACL injury may differ in females and males, especially with respect to the dynamic positioning of the knee [32]. Considering a professional men's football team squad, every second year one player will suffer an ACL injury on average [30]. When an athlete suffers an ACL injury, questions such as "when will I be able to return to sports?", "will I be able to return to my preoperative level?" or "will I be able to return at all?" arise. In the last decade, research has developed variables and parameters to predict and prognosticate outcomes for ACL surgery and the following rehabilitation period to support clinicians and therapists to help and support athletes on their way back to sporting activity [20]. Each athlete is unique; therefore, the challenging path from injury back to sports should be individualized as much as possible [34]. In consequence, predictors are also classified in preoperative and postoperative values [35, 36]. Once a player suffered an ACL injury, the risk of a new knee injury is increased [31], and there are unresolved problems such as a high ACL re-rupture rate [22]. The rate of secondary ACL injury among patients who return to sports is 20%; the injury rate in younger patients (20–25 years) who return to high-risk sport is even higher meaning that nearly one out of four young athletes will sustain another major knee injury if they return to play [37, 38]. And this secondary ACL injury most likely occurs early in the return-to-play period [38]. A premature return to sports activities might be one factor that contributes to such high ACL re-rupture rates [22]. Activity modification, improved rehabilitation, return-to-play guidelines and the use of integrative neuromuscular training have been suggested to help athletes to a more safe reintegration into sport and to be beneficial in reducing a second injury [38].

Fact Box 2 Return to play after severe knee injury

Return to play	Each athlete is unique; therefore, the challenging path from injury back to sports should be individualized as much as possible [20]
	Once a player suffered an ACL injury, the risk of a new knee injury is increased, and there are unresolved problems such as a high ACL re-rupture rate [36, 46]
	A secondary ACL injury most likely occurs early in the return-to-play period [37]
	Activity modification, improved rehabilitation, return-to-play guidelines and the use of integrative neuromuscular training have been suggested [37]

8.4 Return-to-Play Criteria After Knee Injuries

Before patients are allowed to return to contact or pivoting sports, a minimum of at least 6 months between ACL reconstruction and return to sports are recommended [39, 40]; although the approach based only on time is discussed controversially [34]. Most of the athletes are pressured, or they push themselves to make their comeback as soon as possible following surgery, even if there is little firm evidence regarding the safe return to play [22]. It is desirable for the athlete to return to sport as quickly as possible; however, an accelerated return to sport may also harm the operated ACL graft [41]. Although many "return-to-play" criteria have been suggested, there are still uncertainties between time-based vs. criteria-based return-to-play decision; some are based on the time from ACL reconstruction only, while others combine time with subjective and objective criteria [20]. The decision whether an athlete can return to sporting activity in a safe and healthy way remains a major challenge. Postsurgical time as a justification for activity restriction is simply used as a surrogate for biological healing [33]. Considering only the time-based decision making, it should be noted that patients who returned to sport in <7 months were more likely to be reinjured than those who returned after 7 months [38].

Fact Box 3 Risk of re-injury in dependence of time to return to sport

Risk of re-injury	Patients who returned to sport in <7 months were more likely to be reinjured than those who returned after 7 months [37]

Thus, combining time from ACL reconstruction with subjective and objective criteria is a useful tool in evaluating an athlete's progress in the back to sport process. Most commonly described tests are isokinetic strength tests, functional tests, clinical assessment and subjective questionnaires [20]. Using various criteria is beneficial to determine an athlete's readiness to return to sport; this includes full range of motion, muscle strength and full neuromuscular function for sport-specific activities [20, 34, 35, 38].

An optimized criterion-based multifactorial return-to-sport approach based on shared decision making within a broad biopsychosocial framework [34] has been proposed in order to support clinicians in their decision making and to help athletes on their way back to sports. If athletes fulfil certain functional, physiological and psychological [42–44] requirements during and beyond the rehabilitation process, they are ready to return to sport in consideration of the postsurgical time. Assessing the functional status with test batteries has been advocated to enable the safest possible return to sport [33], and several test batteries have been developed [22, 23, 45–47]. Most test protocols include laxity measurements, subjective scores, various jump test and strength assessments [45, 47–50]. As most of these protocols require expensive equipment, are extremely time-consuming or excessively complex for implementation in daily clinical practice, the following chapter describes one possible test battery, which is evidence based and easy to use [22, 23].

Fact Box Time-based and criteria-based decision making

Time-based decision making	A minimum of at least 6 months between ACL reconstruction and return to sports are recommended [1, 47]
	Patients who returned to sport in <7 months were more likely to be reinjured than those who returned after 7 months [37]
	Time-based guidelines may lead in some instances return to play before neuromuscular function is optimized, placing the athlete at increased risk of re-injury [17]
Criteria-based decision making	Most commonly described tests are isokinetic strength tests, functional tests, clinical assessment and related subjective questionnaires [13]
	An optimized criterion-based multifactorial return-to-sport approach based on shared decision making within a broad biopsychosocial framework [20]
	Assessing the functional status with test batteries has been advocated to enable the safest possible return to sport [40]

8.5 A Test Battery for Return to Play

The back in action (BIA) test battery (CoRehab, Trento, Italy) is designed for sportive users in healthy conditions or in any phase of a recovery period after an injury. It is measuring dynamically the balance, the agility, the speed and the strength in respect to normative data from a large group of healthy individuals. As a further optional outcome, a back to sport indicator (BIA indicator) is also provided.

8.5.1 Description of the Test Battery [22]

The test battery "back in action" can be accomplished in 45 min and only needs little equipment and one room. It consisted of the following subtests: a two-legged (TL-ST) and one-legged stability test (OL-ST), a two-legged (TL-CMJ) and one-legged counter movement jump with height and power calculations (OL-CMJ), speedy jumps (OL-SY), plyometric jumps (TL-PJ) and a quick feet test (TL-QFT) [22]. The values of all the tests were categorized into five groups from "very good", "good", "normal", "weak" and "very weak" according to the age- and gender-matched normal data of 434 healthy subjects. The categorizations considered the gender, patient age and leg dominancy. For the calculation of the limb symmetry index (LSI) of the one-legged tests, the resulting absolute value of the injured leg was divided by the value of the non-affected leg and multiplied by 100. For the stability, quick feet and speedy tests, lower values were considered better than higher values, and the calculation of the LSI was different. For these tests, the LSI was calculated by dividing the measured value of the non-affected leg by the value of the injured side and multiplying by 100. The different LSI calculations were performed to achieve comparable and consistent values for all the single-legged tests. With our adaptation of the LSI formula for those tests, the LSI for the injured leg is always suspected of being inferior to the unaffected side [22].

Fact Box "Back in action" test battery

BIA test battery	Evidence based Easy to use Few equipment needed Transportable Back to sport indicator

To assess postural control, tests are performed on a disc (CoRehab, Trento, Italy) connected to a tablet PC. The disc is free to move in all directions. While balancing on the disc, the software provides instant feedback about the position of the disc. To avoid the influence of different shoe types, all trials were performed without shoes. Subjects were instructed to stand in the centre with their arms at their sides [23].

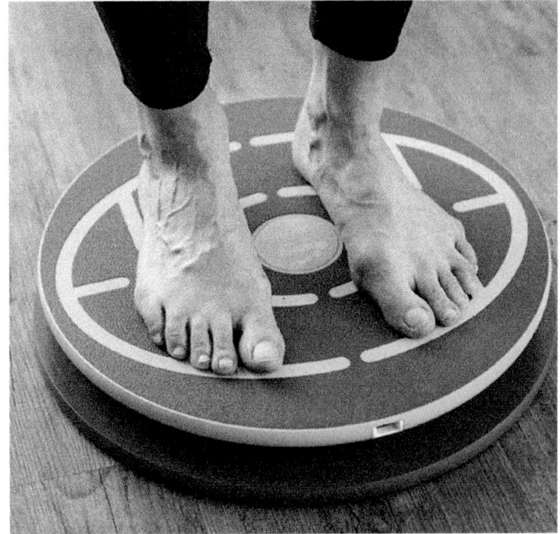

Fig. 8.1 Two-leg stability test

8.5.2 Two-Leg Stability

Subjects stand with both legs on the disc while maintaining their balance for 30 s. Three trials are conducted; the first trial is to get familiar with the testing device. Second and third trials are countable for data collection, whereby the superior trail is considered for the results. There is a 30-s break between each trial in which the subject remains with both legs on the balance board resting to one side. Data collection is immediately stopped in the case of a loss of balance (Fig. 8.1).

8.5.3 One-Leg Stability

Similar setting as the two-leg test, however, this time test is performed with only one leg. The test is performed twice, one for each leg. The subject is not allowed to stabilize the raised leg against the floor, plate or standing leg. During the break between each trial, the subject is able to put his non-testing leg on the floor, while his testing leg remains on the same position on the testing board (Fig. 8.2).

All jump tests are performed using BIA-jump sensor (CoRehab, Trento, Italy) equipment. The subjects carry a belt around their hips, and the jump sensor is placed above the greater trochanter

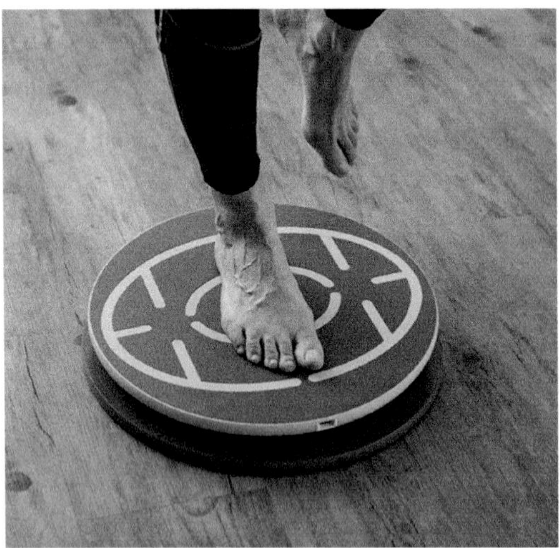

Fig. 8.2 One-leg stability test

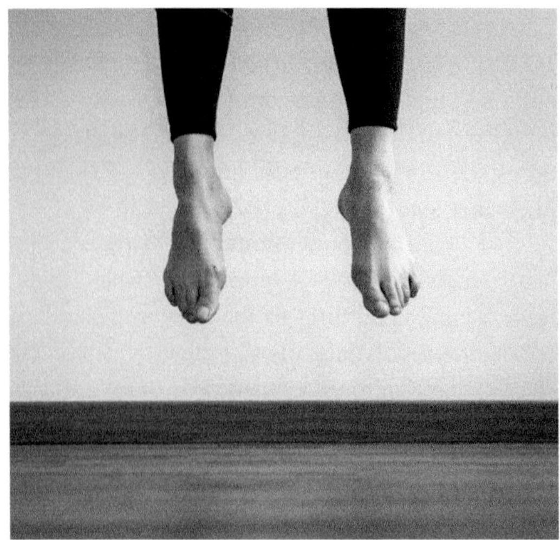

Fig. 8.3 Counter movement jump

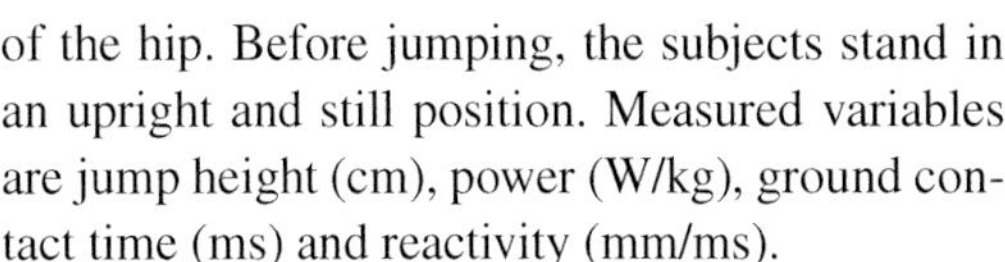

of the hip. Before jumping, the subjects stand in an upright and still position. Measured variables are jump height (cm), power (W/kg), ground contact time (ms) and reactivity (mm/ms).

8.5.4 Counter Movement Jump

A sound signal from the software announces the start of the jump. From an upright position, the subjects quickly bend their knees and then immediately jump upward, attempting to maximize their height. During this hop, arms are placed on the hips. First jump is a test trial following five jumps with 30-s pause in between each jump. Of those five jumps, the highest and lowest jump will not be considered for data collection. Mean value is calculated from the remaining three jumps (Fig. 8.3).

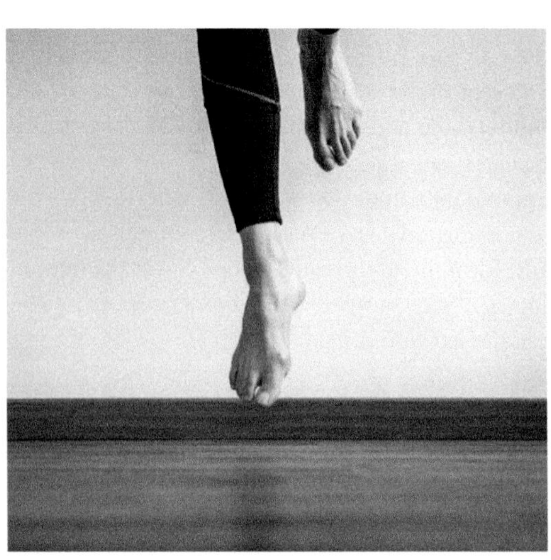

Fig. 8.4 One-leg counter movement jump

8.5.5 One-Leg Counter Movement Jump

One-leg counter movement jump is similar to the two-leg test; however, this test is performed with one leg. First jump is a test trial following three jumps with 30-s pause in between each jump. Mean value is calculated from the jumps for data collection (Fig. 8.4).

8.5.6 Plyometrics

The subjects perform three series of four consecutive two-leg jumps, focusing on a maximum jump height and a fast ground contact time. Arms could be used to assist with the jump. First jump sequence is a test trial following two jump series with 30-s pause in between each jump series (Fig. 8.5).

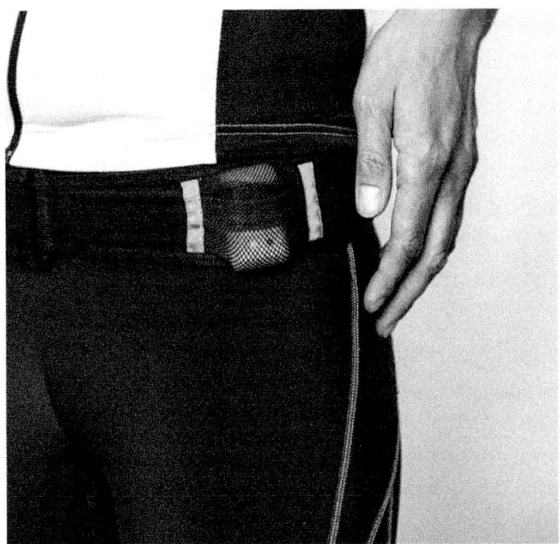

Fig. 8.5 Jump sensor placed in the belt at the position around the subjects' hip

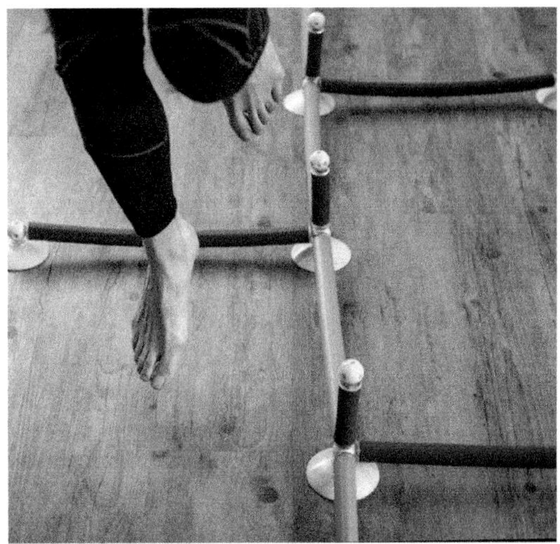

Fig. 8.6 Jump coordination path

8.5.7 Speedy Jump

The speedy basic jump set (CoRehab, Trento, Italy) is used to create the jump coordination path. The subjects perform one-footed jumps through the course of red (forward–backward–forward jumps) and blue (sideway jumps) hurdles, completing 16 jumps. The subject is advised to perform the jump coordination path as quickly as possible by jumping on one leg without a rest between the hurdles. Twisting of the hip is not allowed, and the test is immediately stopped when the raised leg touches the ground or the subject has direct contact with the speedy basic jump hurdles. Time is measured using a stopwatch included in the software. Timekeeping begins as soon as the subject starts to jump and ends when the subject reaches the finish line with one leg. The mean value is recorded for each jump. Measured variable is time (seconds) (Fig. 8.6).

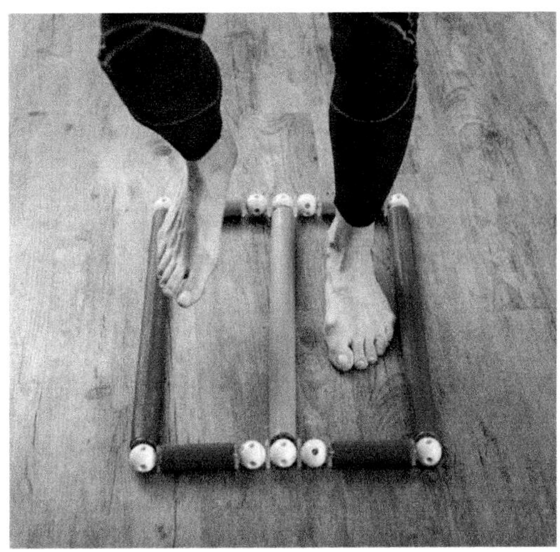

Fig. 8.7 Quick feet test

8.5.8 Quick Feet Test

Again, the speedy basic jump set (CoRehab, Trento, Italy) is used for the quick feet test as displayed in Fig. 8.7. The subject steps in and out with one foot after the other until 15 repetitions are completed. One repetition is finished when the starting leg returns to its initial position. The test is stopped if the subject reverses the order of the steps. Arms could be used to maintain balance, and stepping on the speedy pole is not allowed. Measured variable is time (seconds).

8.5.9 Clinical Experience in Using This Test Battery

In our daily practice, we use this test battery for every patient who underwent ACL reconstruction. The results ease the evaluation of one's patient functional status and detect neuromuscular and strength deficits. Our patients typically complete the first test 4–5 months after surgery. This is important to specify the next months of rehabilitation and training. In our experience all of even professional athletes have deficits in one or more parameters at this stage. On the second test, which is about 2–3 months later, we often detect some deficits. However, the return to competitive sports is then discussed individually with coaches, the athlete, the physio and the surgeon. Once athletes are cleared and ready to return to a high-risk sport, they are encouraged towards a gradual increase of training intensity and participation in competition. To compare the results of a patients status after ACL reconstruction, normative data of more than 400 healthy individuals are available. However, the test can also be conducted pre-injury to assess the individual status. Therefore, we assessed the normative data in a professional football club (see Table 8.1). Apart from semi-professional players being significantly younger than professional players, data showed only statistically significant higher values for professional players in the two-legged counter movement jump and the one-legged counter movement jump with the dominant leg (unpublished data, submitted) (Table 8.1).

Take-Home Message

Football is a very demanding sport activity with a high risk of injury. In order to return patients to athletic or demanding occupational activities as safely as possible, postoperative rehabilitation plays a critical role [51]. Participation in level I sports after ACL reconstruction within 2 years puts the athlete at a four times higher risk of re-injury; however, this rate decreases through a later return and more symmetrical quadriceps strength prior to return [33]. An athlete should therefore accomplish certain steps in the rehabilitation process, which is monitored by clinicians and other health professionals. High capabilities are seen in the combination of strict time-based and functional return-to-play criteria in order to

Table 8.1 Normative data in professional and semi-professional football players (unpublished data, submitted for publication)

	Professional players (n = 17)	Semi-professional players (n = 17)	All players (N = 34)
	Mean ± SD	Mean ± SD	Mean ± SD
Age (year)	23.8 ± 4.3	18.9 ± 1.8	21.4 ± 4.1
Height (cm)	181.3 ± 3.5	178.6 ± 5.6	179.9 ± 4.9
Weight (kg)	74.5 ± 4.9	72.7 ± 6.9	73.6 ± 6.1
BMI	22.6 ± 1.1	22.8 ± 1.4	22.7 ± 1.2
Two-leg stability	2.63 ± 0.4	2.84 ± 0.5	2.73 ± 0.5
One-leg stabilityDominant leg	2.59 ± 0.3	2.46 ± 0.5	2.53 ± 0.4
One-leg stabilityNon-dominant leg	2.47 ± 0.3	2.49 ± 0.5	2.48 ± 0.4
Counter movement jump (CMJ) (cm)	44.5 ± 5.8	39.4 ± 4	42 ± 5.6
CMJDominant leg (cm)	31.9 ± 5.6	26.6 ± 4	29.3 ± 5.4
CMJNon-dominant leg (cm)	31.1 ± 6.3	27.6 ± 4	29.4 ± 5.5
PlyometricsHeight (cm)	38.99 ± 5.1	38.98 ± 6.5	38.99 ± 5.8
PlyometricsTime (ms)	183.3 ± 28.3	188.38 ± 42.2	185.84 ± 36
Speedy testDominant leg (s)	5.45 ± 0.5	5.56 ± 0.5	5.51 ± 0.5
Speedy testNon-dominant leg (s)	5.53 ± 0.6	5.61 ± 0.4	5.57 ± 0.5
Quick feet test (s)	8.24 ± 1.2	8.31 ± 1	8.27 ± 1.1

improve long-term function and to decrease the occurrence of osteoarthritis [33]. The test battery presented in chapter 5 has shown to be safe and extremely helpful in counselling a patient with respect to further training and the timing of a return to sports [22].

Top Five Evidence-Based References

Grindem H, Snyder-Mackler L, Moksnes H, Engebretsen L, Risberg MA (2016) Simple decision rules can reduce reinjury risk by 84% after ACL reconstruction: the Delaware-Oslo ACL cohort study. Br J Sports Med 50:804–808

Herbst E, Hoser C, Hildebrandt C, Raschner C, Hepperger C, Pointner H, Fink C (2015) Functional assessments for decision-making regarding return to sports following ACL reconstruction. Part II: clinical application of a new test battery. Knee Surg Sports Traumatol Arthrosc 23:1283–1291

Hildebrandt C, Müller L, Zisch B, Huber R, Fink C, Raschner C (2015) Functional assessments for decision-making regarding return to sports following ACL reconstruction. Part I: development of a new test battery. Knee Surg Sports Traumatol Arthrosc 23:1273–1281

Kyritsis P, Bahr R, Landreau P, Miladi R, Witvrouw E (2016) Likelihood of ACL graft rupture: not meeting six clinical discharge criteria before return to sport is associated with a four times greater risk of rupture. Br J Sports Med 50:946–951

Wiggins AJ, Grandhi RK, Schneider DK, Stanfield D, Webster KE, Myer GD (2016) Risk of secondary injury in younger athletes after anterior cruciate ligament reconstruction: a systematic review and meta-analysis. Am J Sports Med 44:1861–1876

References

1. O'Brien J, Finch CF (2017) Injury prevention exercise programs for professional soccer: understanding the perceptions of the end-users. Clin J Sport Med 27:1–9
2. Krustrup P, Bangsbo J (2015) Recreational football is effective in the treatment of non-communicable diseases. Br J Sports Med 49:1426–1428
3. Randers MB, Andersen LJ, Orntoft C, Bendiksen M, Johansen L, Horton J, Hansen PR, Krustrup P (2013) Cardiovascular health profile of elite female football players compared to untrained controls before and after short-term football training. J Sports Sci 31:1421–1431
4. Arnason A, Sigurdsson SB, Gudmundsson A, Holme I, Engebretsen L, Bahr R (2004) Physical fitness, injuries, and team performance in soccer. Med Sci Sports Exerc 36:278–285
5. Waldén M, Krosshaug T, Bjørneboe J, Andersen TE, Faul O, Hägglund M (2015) Three distinct mechanisms predominate in non-contact anterior cruciate ligament injuries in male professional football players: a systematic video analysis of 39 cases. Br J Sports Med 49:1–10
6. Alentorn-Geli E, Myer GD, Silvers HJ, Samitier G, Romero D, Lázaro-Haro C, Cugat R (2009) Prevention of non-contact anterior cruciate ligament injuries in soccer players. Part 1: mechanisms of injury and underlying risk factors. Knee Surg Sports Traumatol Arthrosc 17:705–729
7. Ueblacker P, Mueller-Wohlfahrt H-W, Ekstrand J (2015) Epidemiological and clinical outcome comparison of indirect ('strain') versus direct ('contusion') anterior and posterior thigh muscle injuries in male elite football players: UEFA elite league study of 2287 thigh injuries (2001-2013). Br J Sports Med 49:1461–1465
8. Alentorn-Geli E, Myer GD, Silvers HJ, Samitier G, Romero D, Lazaro-Haro C, Cugat R (2009) Prevention of non-contact anterior cruciate ligament injuries in soccer players. Part 2: a review of prevention programs aimed to modify risk factors and to reduce injury rates. Knee Surg Sports Traumatol Arthrosc 17:859–879
9. Fuller CW, Ekstrand J, Junge A, Andersen TE, Bahr R, Dvorak J, Hägglund M, McCrory P, Meeuwisse WH (2006) Consensus statement on injury definitions and data collection procedures in studies of football (soccer) injuries. Br J Sports Med 40:193–201
10. Bowen L, Gross AS, Gimpel M, Li F-X (2016) Accumulated workloads and the acute:chronic workload ratio relate to injury risk in elite youth football players. Br J Sports Med. https://doi.org/10.1136/bjsports-2015-095820
11. Barnes C, Archer DT, Hogg B, Bush M, Bradley PS (2014) The evolution of physical and technical performance parameters in the English premier league. Int J Sports Med 35:1095–1100
12. Gatterer H, Ruedl G, Faulhaber M, Regele M, Burtscher M (2012) Effects of the performance level and the FIFA "11" injury prevention program on the injury rate in Italian male amateur soccer players. J Sports Med Phys Fitness 52:80–84
13. Fuller CW, Junge A, Dvorak J (2012) Risk management: FIFA's approach for protecting the health of football players. Br J Sports Med 46:11–17
14. Ekstrand J, Hägglund M, Kristenson K, Magnusson H, Waldén M (2013) Fewer ligament injuries but no preventive effect on muscle injuries and severe injuries: an 11-year follow-up of the UEFA champions league injury study. Br J Sports Med 47:732–737
15. Hewett TE, Di Stasi SL, Myer GD (2013) Current concepts for injury prevention in athletes after anterior cruciate ligament reconstruction. Am J Sports Med 28:374–386
16. McCall A, Davison M, Andersen TE, Beasley I, Bizzini M, Dupont G, Duffield R, Carling C, Dvorak

J (2015) Injury prevention strategies at the FIFA 2014 world cup: perceptions and practices of the physicians from the 32 participating national teams. Br J Sports Med 49:603–608

17. McCall A, Dupont G, Ekstrand J (2016) Injury prevention strategies, coach compliance and player adherence of 33 of the UEFA elite Club injury study teams: a survey of teams' head medical officers. Br J Sports Med. https://doi.org/10.1136/bjsports-2015-095259
18. Ardern CL, Taylor NF, Feller JA, Webster KE (2012) Return-to-sport outcomes at 2 to 7 years after anterior cruciate ligament reconstruction surgery. Am J Sports Med 40:41–48
19. Ardern CL, Webster KE, Taylor NF, Feller JA (2011) Return to the preinjury level of competitive sport after anterior cruciate ligament reconstruction surgery: two-thirds of patients have not returned by 12 months after surgery. Am J Sports Med 39:538–543
20. Kyritsis P, Bahr R, Landreau P, Miladi R, Witvrouw E (2016) Likelihood of ACL graft rupture: not meeting six clinical discharge criteria before return to sport is associated with a four times greater risk of rupture. Br J Sports Med 50:946–951
21. Ardern CL, Glasgow P, Schneiders A, Witvrouw E, Clarsen B, Cools A, Gojanovic B, Grif S, Khan KM, Moksnes H, Mutch SA, Phillips N, Reurink G, Sadler R, Silbernagel KG, Thorborg K, Wangensteen A, Wilk KE, Bizzini M (2016) 2016 consensus statement on return to sport from the first world congress in sports physical. Br J Sports Med 50:853–864
22. Herbst E, Hoser C, Hildebrandt C, Raschner C, Hepperger C, Pointner H, Fink C (2015) Functional assessments for decision-making regarding return to sports following ACL reconstruction. Part II: clinical application of a new test battery. Knee Surg Sports Traumatol Arthrosc 23:1283–1291
23. Hildebrandt C, Müller L, Zisch B, Huber R, Fink C, Raschner C (2015) Functional assessments for decision-making regarding return to sports following ACL reconstruction. Part I: development of a new test battery. Knee Surg Sports Traumatol Arthrosc 23:1273–1281
24. Ekstrand J, Hägglund M, Waldén M (2011) Injury incidence and injury patterns in professional football: the UEFA injury study. Br J Sports Med 45:553–558
25. Peterson L, Junge A, Chomiak J, Graf-Baumann T, Dvorak J (2000) Incidence of football injuries and complaints in different age groups and skill-level groups. Am J Sports Med 28:S51–S57
26. Arnason A, Sigurdsson SB, Gudmundsson A, Holme I, Engebretsen L, Bahr R (2004) Risk factors for injuries in football. Am J Sports Med 32:5S–16S
27. Brophy R, Silvers HJ, Gonzales T, Mandelbaum BR (2010) Gender influences: the role of leg dominance in ACL injury among soccer players. Br J Sports Med 44:694–697
28. Hägglund M, Waldén M, Ekstrand J (2009) UEFA injury study – an injury audit of European championships 2006 to 2008. Br J Sports Med 43:483–489
29. Waldén M, Hägglund M, Ekstrand J (2013) Time-trends and circumstances surrounding ankle injuries in men's professional football: an 11-year follow-up of the UEFA champions league injury study. Br J Sports Med 47:748–753
30. Waldén M, Hägglund M, Magnusson H, Ekstrand J (2011) Anterior cruciate ligament injury in elite football: a prospective three-cohort study. Knee Surg Sports Traumatol Arthrosc 19:11–19
31. Waldén M, Hägglund M, Ekstrand J (2006) High risk of new knee injury in elite footballers with previous anterior cruciate ligament injury. Br J Sports Med 40:158–162
32. Hewett TE, Myer GD, Ford KR, Paterno MV, Quatman CE (2016) Mechanisms, prediction, and prevention of ACL injuries: cut risk with three sharpened and validated tools. J Orthop Res 34:1843–1855
33. Grindem H, Snyder-Mackler L, Moksnes H, Engebretsen L, Risberg MA (2016) Simple decision rules can reduce reinjury risk by 84% after ACL reconstruction: the Delaware-Oslo ACL cohort study. Br J Sports Med 50:804–808
34. Dingenen B, Gokeler A (2017) Optimization of the return-to-sport paradigm after anterior cruciate ligament reconstruction: a critical step back to move forward. Sports Med. https://doi.org/10.1007/s40279-017-0674-6
35. Eitzen I, Holm I, Risberg MA (2009) Preoperative quadriceps strength is a significant predictor of knee function two years after anterior cruciate ligament reconstruction. Br J Sports Med 43:371–376
36. Grindem H, Risberg MA, Eitzen I (2015) Two factors that may underpin outstanding outcomes after ACL rehabilitation. Br J Sports Med 49:1425
37. McCormack RG, Hutchinson MR (2016) Time to be honest regarding outcomes of ACL reconstructions: should we be quoting 55–65% success rates for high-level athletes? Br J Sports Med 50:1167–1168
38. Wiggins AJ, Grandhi RK, Schneider DK, Stanfield D, Webster KE, Myer GD (2016) Risk of secondary injury in younger athletes after anterior cruciate ligament reconstruction: a systematic review and meta-analysis. Am J Sports Med 44:1861–1876
39. Harris JD, Abrams GD, Bach BR, Williams D, Heidloff D, C a B-J, Verma NN, Forsythe B, Cole BJ (2014) Return to sport after ACL reconstruction. Orthopedics 37:e103–e108
40. Kvist J (2004) Rehabilitation following anterior cruciate ligament injury: current recommendations for sports participation. Sports Med 34:269–280
41. Warner SJ, Smith MV, Wright RW, Matava MJ, Brophy RH (2011) Sport-specific outcomes after anterior cruciate ligament reconstruction. Arthroscopy 27:1129–1134
42. Ardern CL, Osterberg A, Tagesson S, Gauffin H, Webster KE, Kvist J (2014) The impact of psychological readiness to return to sport and recreational activities after anterior cruciate ligament reconstruction. Br J Sports Med 48:1613–1619

43. Mayer SW, Queen RM, Taylor D, Moorman CT, Toth AP, Garrett WE, Butler RJ (2015) Functional testing differences in anterior cruciate ligament reconstruction patients released versus not released to return to sport. Am J Sports Med 43:1648–1655
44. Undheim MB, Cosgrave C, King E, Strike S, Marshall B, Falvey É, Franklyn-Miller A (2015) Isokinetic muscle strength and readiness to return to sport following anterior cruciate ligament reconstruction: is there an association? A systematic review and a protocol recommendation. Br J Sports Med 49:1305–1310
45. Gustavsson A, Neeter C, Thomeé P, Silbernagel KG, Augustsson J, Thomeé R, Karlsson J (2006) A test battery for evaluating hop performance in patients with an ACL injury and patients who have undergone ACL reconstruction. Knee Surg Sports Traumatol Arthrosc 14:778–788
46. Keller M, Kurz E, Schmidtlein O, Welsch G, Anders C (2016) Interdisziplinäre Beurteilungskriterien für die Rehabilitation nach Verletzungen an der unteren Extremität : Ein funktionsbasierter Return to Activity Algorithmus. Sport Sport 30:38–49
47. Neeter C, Gustavsson A, Thomeé P, Augustsson J, Thomeé R, Karlsson J (2006) Development of a strength test battery for evaluating leg muscle power after anterior cruciate ligament injury and reconstruction. Knee Surg Sports Traumatol Arthrosc 14:571–580
48. Augustsson J, Thomeé R, Karlsson J (2004) Ability of a new hop test to determine functional deficits after anterior cruciate ligament reconstruction. Knee Surg Sports Traumatol Arthrosc 12:350–356
49. Björklund K, Sköld C, Andersson L, Dalén N (2006) Reliability of a criterion-based test of athletes with knee injuries; where the physiotherapist and the patient independently and simultaneously assess the patient's performance. Knee Surg Sports Traumatol Arthrosc 14:165–175
50. Reid A, Birmingham TB, Stratford PW, Alcock GK, Giffin JR (2007) Hop testing provides a reliable and valid outcome measure during rehabilitation after anterior cruciate ligament reconstruction. Phys Ther 87:337–349
51. Barber-Westin SD, Noyes FR (2011) Factors used to determine return to unrestricted sports activities after anterior cruciate ligament reconstruction. Arthroscopy 27:1697–1705

9 Principles and Limitations of Prehabilitation and Return to Play Strategies

Helmut Hoffmann, Werner Krutsch, and Oliver Loose

Contents

H. Hoffmann (✉)
Eden Reha, Donaustauf, Germany
e-mail: helmut.hoffmann@eden-reha.de

W. Krutsch, M.D.
Department of Trauma Surgery, University Medical Centre Regensburg, Regensburg, Germany

O. Loose, M.D.
Department of Pediatric Surgery, Hospital St. Hedwig, Regensburg, Germany

9.1 Introduction

Football is probably the most beautiful minor matter on earth - in 2006, the FIFA claimed that over 265 million people play football. On one hand, performing sports and playing football boost health and increase well-being. On the other hand, it undoubtedly involves a high risk of injury. Recent studies suggest that the injury rate among elite football players appears to be much higher than in high-risk industrial occupations.

Injury incidences in elite football vary between 4.4 and 77 per 1000 h of playing time. In

V. Musahl et al. (eds.), *Return to Play in Football*, https://doi.org/10.1007/978-3-662-55713-6_9

2015/2016, the UEFA injury study revealed 5.5 injuries per 1000 h of playing time [1–4].

Earlier, in case of severe injury such as ACL rupture, physicians, team coaches, and players intended to return to play after a defined time of rehabilitation, for instance, after 6 months. But this procedure does not comply with the individual rehabilitation process and the functional aspect of sport-specific rehabilitation and performance profiles.

Consequently, prevention is a major component of football to assure as little injury as possible. In this chapter, principles and limitations of prevention and return to play strategies are discussed.

9.2 Basic Aspects and Current Prehabilitation Strategies in Elite Football

Sport-specific characteristics and adaptions of the musculoskeletal and myofascial system.

Playing football is characterized by a high number of specific and non-varying patterns of movement: from a functional point of view, football players have to display functional power and mobility, core stability, balance, and particularly agility. Side steps, forward, and backward running, fast shifts in direction, core stability in duel, jumps and landing, and quick start and stop movements are among the requirements for a high-performing football player [5].

All these different patterns will lead to responses in specific biological structures undergoing adaptations that enable the athlete to adequately recall the movements after having trained and frequently repeated them for a long time. These transformations concern muscles, ligaments, bones, and myofascial structures and are normally not carried out in a symmetric way: in many sports, there are vast differences between the right and the left side of the athlete's body, most prominently in football with a shooting and a standing leg [6–8]. Also, the play requirements and classic movement patterns vary from one playing position to the next one. This difference is particularly striking between the goalkeeper and the field players but exists among different playing positions on the field as well.

These facts are decisive in prehabilitation and return to play settings (provided by a doctor, therapist, or trainer), as they are important to consider as to whether the adaptive changes should be prophylactically "treated" and reversed, or at least limited, with the goal of preventing future degenerative problems. There is no generally valid recommended course of action, and management decisions should be made on a case-by-case basis depending on the extent of the changes and on individual physical factors. The following factors are crucial in prehabilitation and return to play strategies.

9.3 Changes Caused by Contact of the Shooting Leg with the Ball

From a mechanical point of view, a soccer player kicking a ball is accelerating a piece of leather filled with air in a desired direction. This can be accomplished by various modes of ball contact, which impose corresponding mechanical loads on the striking area - the forehead for a header shot, the instep for an instep shot, or the inside of the foot for an inside shot. In summary, the forces of a senior ball and resulting changes for a kicking-leg through repetitive shots have to be calculated in prehabilitation and return to play strategies [9]. Besides the magnitude of the mechanical stresses associated with ball contact, the number of repetitive stereotypical loads caused by ball contact within the physiologic range can also trigger degenerative changes in the musculoskeletal system. The mechanical reaction forces generated by the ball mass have a magnitude that is within physiologic limits and generally do not exceed the stress tolerance of the biological structures. But if a large number of contacts are repeated over a long period of time, which may be measured in years, they create stimuli that act as repetitive microtrauma and will eventually evoke changes in the musculoskeletal system:

– Radiographically visible bone changes were noted only at the kicking leg side of professional soccer players who had been playing for at least 3 years [10].

- Kicking balls with a faulty, biologically unfavorable technique will quickly increase the tensile stresses on the talonavicular ligament to unphysiologically high levels that may exceed stress tolerance, resulting in an acute injury [11].

9.4 Musculoskeletal Adaptation Through Asymmetrical Muscular Changes

From a biomechanical perspective, the leg's kicking movement is an "open kinetic chain" action in which the foot is moved at maximum forward speed (moving point), while the hip is relatively stationary (fixed point). At the same time, every kicking movement will impose a "closed kinetic chain" type of load on the non-kicking side. In this case, the foot is planted on the ground (fixed point), while the overlying structures of the pelvic-leg axis and torso are in motion (moving point) and must therefore be stabilized against gravity through complex coordination. Various neuromuscular control actions, especially those that stabilize the knee joint and the entire lumbar-pelvis-hip region, initiate long-term muscular adaptations to these soccer-specific movement patterns [12]. Knebel (1988) described an increased maximum strength capacity and striking force of quadriceps muscle contraction during extension on the kicking leg side, accompanied by an increased maximum strength and striking force of the knee flexors on the support side.

These general tendencies (quadriceps stronger on the kicking side, hamstrings stronger on the support side) vary in different playing positions according to the requirements of those positions [6, 13].

9.5 Supporting Leg Changes Caused by Kicking Technique

The changes in the kicking leg described above suggest that the contralateral support leg is subjected to different loads during the kicking of a soccer ball. Interestingly, all soccer players, regardless of their performance level, tend to place their support leg in a precise position when shooting the ball (i.e., when executing an instep kick or an inside/outside kick). This causes a highly consistent pattern of stereotypical loads to act on the musculoskeletal structures (Fig. 9.1).

To permit successful ball acceleration by the kicking leg with effective momentum transfer to the ball, the support leg must be planted next to the ball on the ground. There are several observations that are significant in this regard [14] (Fact Box 1).

These side-specific changes are most clearly appreciated in the ankle joint. The greater the lateralization of the pelvic-leg axis, the greater is the lateral and shear forces acting on the joints of the foot. These forces will evoke long-term adap-

Fact Box 1

- Soccer players plant their support leg next to the ball with remarkable consistency and precision. Tests have shown that interindividual differences from one ball contact to the next are less than 1 cm!
- Soccer players plant their support leg level with the ball (relative to the frontal plane).
- As soon as the foot is planted on the ground, the body center of gravity shifts outward toward the support leg, usually moving past the left knee or even farther laterally.
- The lateral distance of the support leg from the ball can vary markedly from one player to the next. Despite these differences, however, the individual movement patterns are carried out with great precision (intraindividual consistency). But the farther the support leg is placed from the ball, the greater is the lateral shift of the body center of gravity (Fig. 9.2). The joints along the left pelvic-leg axis must stabilize and compensate for this position and adapt to it over time

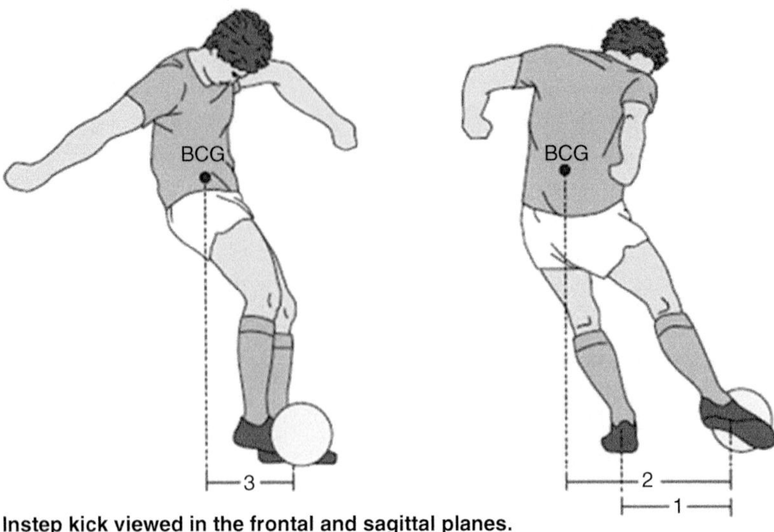

Fig. 9.1 Intraindividual differences in the position of the supporting leg for a right-side kicker during instep kick [11]

Instep kick viewed in the frontal and sagittal planes.
BCG, body's center of gravity.

1 Distance from the foot of the supporting leg to the center of the ball.

2 Distance from the BCG axis to the ball center of gravity.

3 Distance from the BCG axis to the foot of the supporting leg.

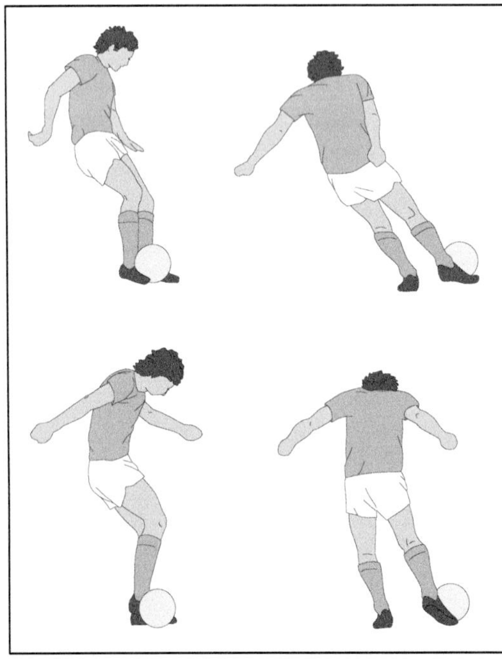

Fig. 9.2 Intraindividual differences in the position of the supporting leg for an instep kick (right-footed player) [11]

tations even in the absence of trauma or injuries. These changes are reflected not just in the stereotypical kicking actions that occur during training and play but also during ordinary walking and running.

9.6 Influence Factors and Football-Specific Prevention Strategies

Injury prevention in football is a multifactorial event, and all actors involved in the team sport can exert influence (Fig. 9.3). **Football associations**, for example, have changed the rules for an attack against the head with the elbow by punishing it with a red card. This has led to a significant reduction of head injuries in the world championship 2006. Furthermore, the adaption of the ball's size and weight according to the players' age was also a preventive procedure to reduce the risk for head injuries or degenerative changes in youth

Football player
- Age
- Gender
- Individual biomechanics and anatomy
- Technique and experience in football
- Fitness and functional stability
- Previous injury
- Behaviour on field
- Drugs and alcohol
- Medical history
- Psychological factors
Referee:
- Respecting match rules
- Fouls/penalties
- Physical performance
- Interpretations
- Behaviour on field
Medical Team
- Medical service
- Medical equipment
- Treatment of injuries
- Treatment of illness
- Doping control
- Nutrition
- Rehabilitation
- Return to play
- Prevention
- Regeneration
Sports industry
- Match equipment
- Shin guards
- Shoe equipment
- Keepers equipment
Team coach
- Physical preparation
- Mental fitness
- Rehabilitation
- Regeneration
- Return to play
- Training program
- Warm up program
- Cool down program
Football associations
- Match philosophy
- Match rules
- Match locations
- Fair play
- Environmental conditions
- Doping control
- Education

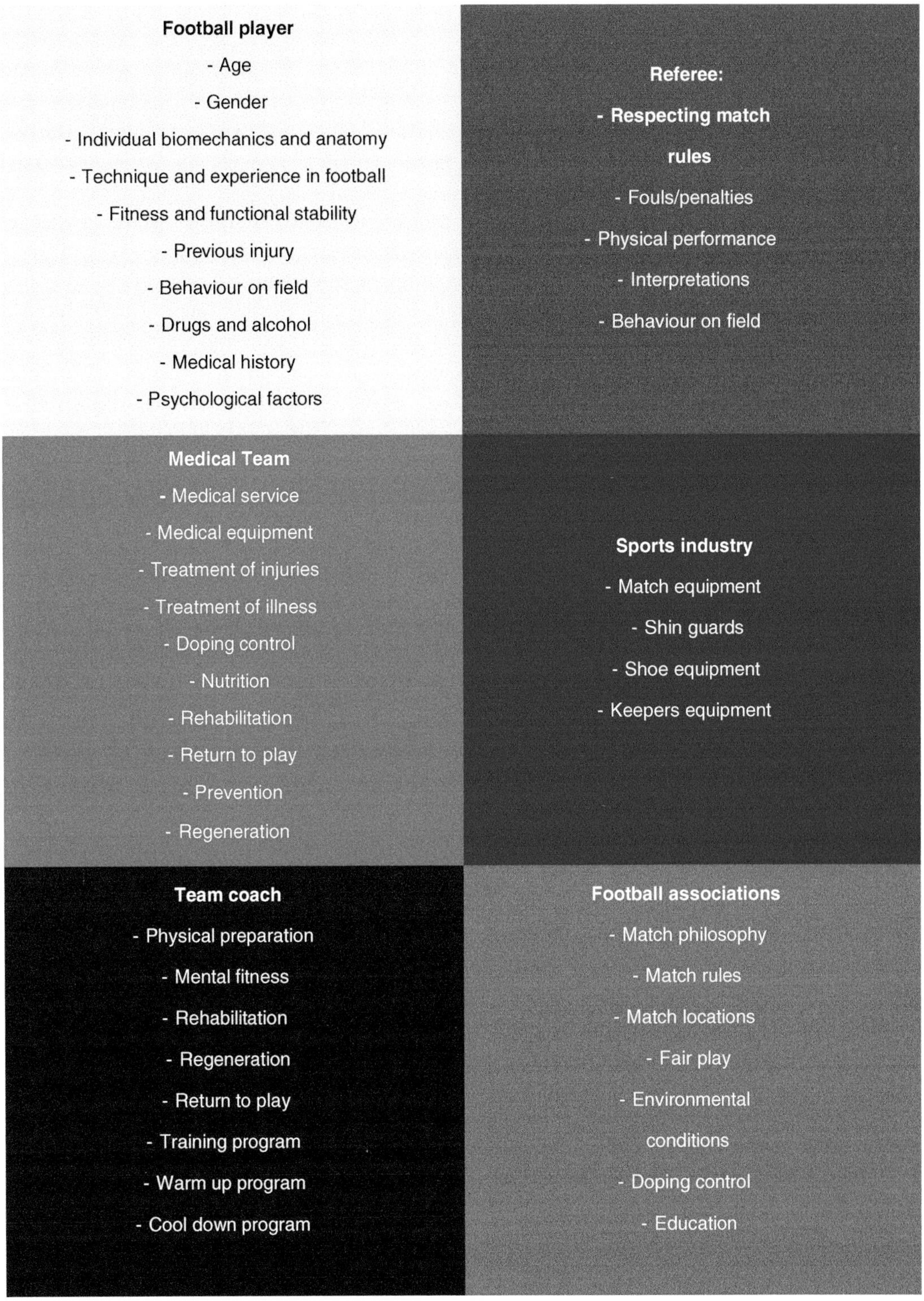

Fig. 9.3 Influence factors in prevention strategies [15]

football [8]. Other examples of the influence of associations are the prohibition of body decoration or the obligation to wear protectors in football games.

The sports industry can also contribute to strengthen prevention by adapting the football shoes to the individual requirements of players and environmental conditions: in order to compensate differences in leg dominance, an individual adaption of football shoes by means of orthopedic insoles is useful to avoid nonphysiological stress on the musculoskeletal system. It is highly recommendable to use custom-made individual shoes fitting the player's feet and anatomical predispositions. These shoes should be individualized according to biomechanical properties to select a suitable shoe model for the individual athlete. The type, number, and placement of studs on the shoe sole should be included in the analysis because they influence the value of traction potential.

One of the most important influence factors on prevention strategies are the **player** themselves: sufficient sleep and regeneration, a balanced nutrition, enough hydration, avoiding alcohol, warm-up and cooling down, and fair play have been proven in practice.

The influence of **referees** in prevention particularly refers to the surveillance of compliance with gaming rules and a good communication with players [16]. Referees must also assess the severity of injuries and decide whether to interrupt the game for medical help.

The **team coach** is another highly influential factor. He defines the training and game load; prepares the training including the warm-up phase, prevention training, and cool-down; and determines the time of regeneration. They are also responsible for the mental fitness of the players and have to interfere with all other actors in team sport.

The medical team is responsible for the treatment of injury or illness, nutrition, and anti-doping control and accompanies the players in return to play and rehabilitation process. A big part of the medical team's work is the regeneration by physiotherapy.

A survey of current prevention strategies in national teams at the FIFA 2014 World Cup showed the tests used to detect risk factors: the top five common injury risk screening tests were flexibility, physical fitness, joint mobilization/function, balance/proprioception, muscle endurance strength, and muscle peak strength. The physicians were also asked about risk factors: previous injury, accumulated fatigue, and agonist/antagonist muscle imbalance were the most frequently named intrinsic factors, whereas reduced recovery time, training load prior and during the world cup, and poor pitch quality figured among the extrinsic ones. The monitoring of the players was based on medical screen, minutes/matches played, subjective and objective wellness, and heart rate and biochemical parameters. The most important prevention exercises were flexibility, core, combined contractions, balance, and eccentric exercises [17].

9.7 Basic Aspects of Actual Return-to-Play Strategies in Elite Football

The return-to-play process after injury generally depicts the time from injury until return to the field. Earlier, the period after which to play football again after ACL rupture was defined as 6 months. But a fixed/determined date does not take into account the fact that every patient needs an individual rehabilitation process adapted on their biological healing and functional criteria (Fig. 9.4).

An optimal rehabilitation protocol starts with the **return-to-activity** period [19] after being discharged from clinical treatment to general rehabilitation training, which involves general rehabilitation training and physiotherapy. The return to sport describes the phase from the beginning of sport-specific rehabilitation training to individualized team training. Criteria for entering the **return-to-sport** phase should be:

- No stretch deficit
- Subjective knee stability (IKDC-2000 score, Lysholm score, knee outcome survey-sports activity scale)
- Objective knee stability (KT-1000 laxity testing, pivot shift test)
- Activation and innervation (functional muscle tests)

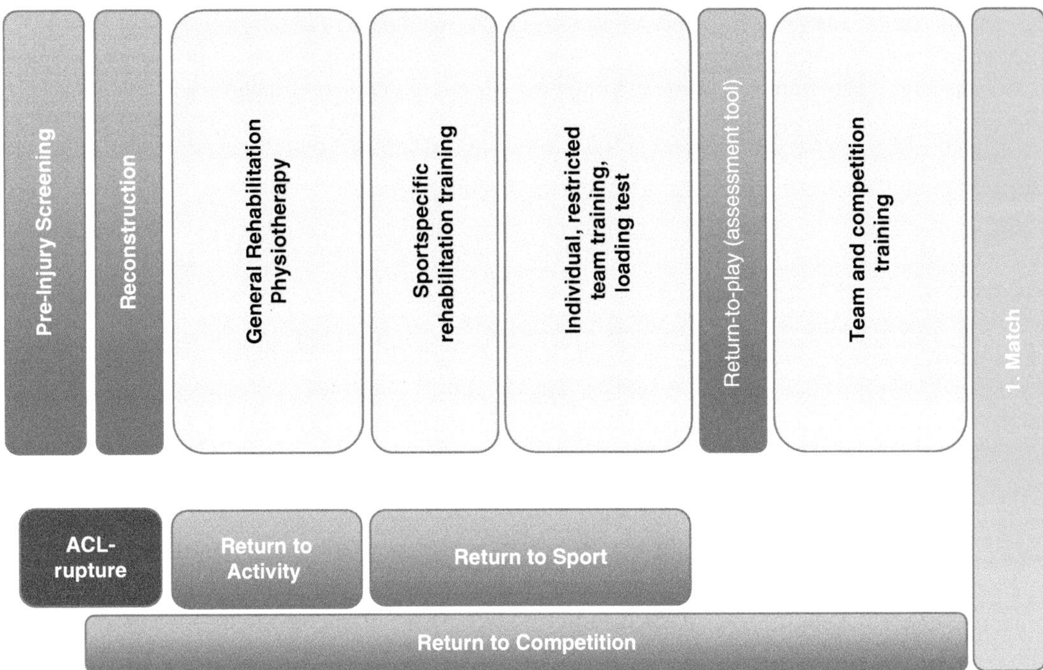

Fig. 9.4 Important steps in rehabilitation after ACL rupture [18]

- Maximal strength (minimum 85% lateral symmetry index (LSI): a comparison with **preseason screening tests** would be optimal)
- Leg axis control

The transition to the full participation in team and competition training is called the return-to-play point. The decision to transfer the player into this phase should be made by means of an interdisciplinary assessment tool (Fig. 9.5).

9.8 Time-Based Versus Criteria-Based Rehabilitation

The control of the rehabilitation process after injuries depends on the medical treatment regimen, which is usually based on the respective posttraumatic stress tolerance of the injured biological structures and their regeneration and constitutes a time-based rehabilitation concept. The focus of this information is on the current load tolerance until the restoration of the mechanical normal load (against gravitation) within the scope of ADL stereotypes. These represent the medical framework for complex rehabilitation concepts.

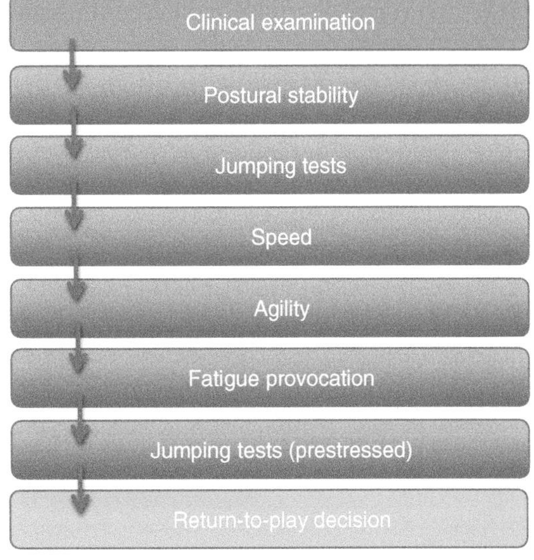

Fig. 9.5 Steps to return-to-play decision after injury [19]

The data are largely based on the findings on the respective biological wound healing processes and the associated time spans but vary considerably in practice in some cases. These time-based preconditions are certainly still relevant in the future and cannot be undershot without provoking an increased risk of re-traumatizing the affected biological tissue.

Current concepts of complex therapies control now attempt to describe each individual therapy process by means of functional criteria, taking into account the time-based minimum time spans of the wound healing processes. These represent in each case the sufficient features to initiate the next therapy step. In the ideal case, the respective individual criteria with the corresponding minimum values should be clearly defined and can be determined both qualitatively and quantitatively on the basis of evaluation methods which are as objective as possible. For example, preseason screening tests could be a possibility to define basic values in an uninjured status and could be used for a criteria-based rehabilitation.

Figure 9.6 illustrates, for example, the rehabilitation after the reconstruction of the anterior cruciate ligament, a possible time-based treatment regime according to the medical specifications of the surgeon who, in this case, provides the start of unilateral support leg phases (jogging) between the ninth and twelfth week. Experience has shown that this can also be achieved in the majority of cases. A minority of patients, however, will not be able to tolerate this burden due to a variety of reasons, which triggers corresponding reactions with delays in the rehabilitation process.

Criteria-based rehabilitation concepts allow for time-optimized progress within the therapy process, taking into account the time constraints of the wound healing processes on the basis of defined functional criteria, so that the next rehabilitation step can be initiated at the earliest possible point of time (in contrast to the time-based concept, presumably around the eighth postoperative week). Problems during rehabilitation can be avoided, and an early start, for example, in the

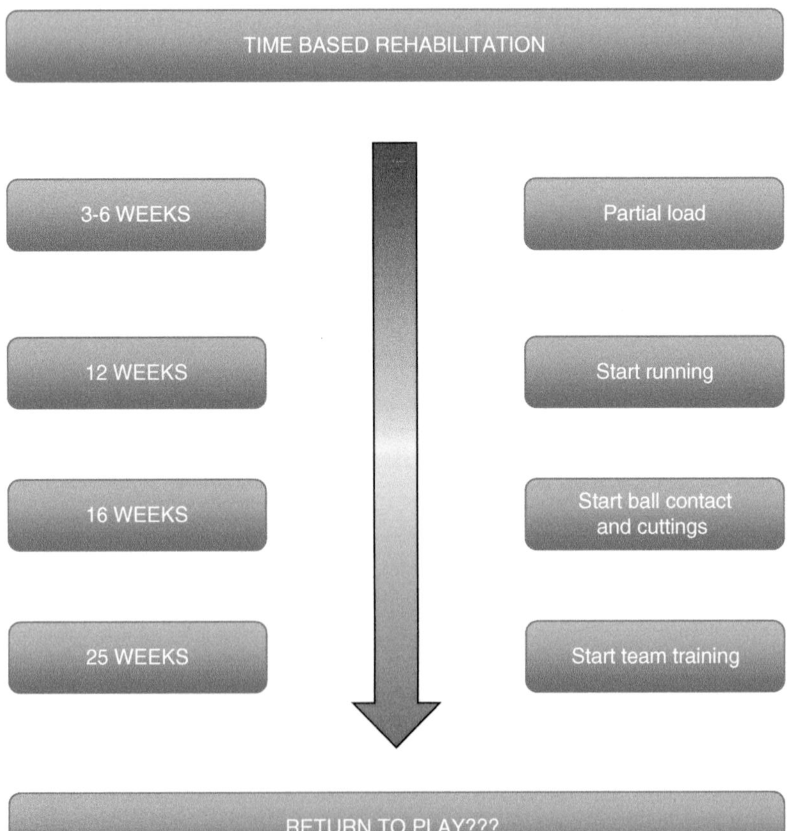

Fig. 9.6 Time-based rehabilitation

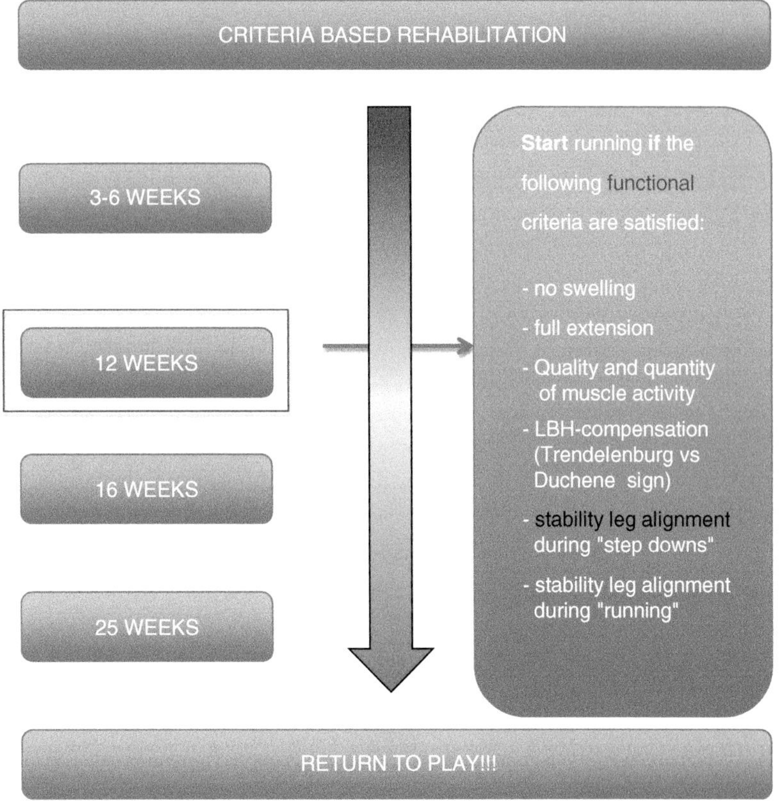

Fig. 9.7 Example of functional-based rehabilitation

20th week, might be prevented by continuing swelling problems.

For example, running loads with one-legged support phases can be determined using the methods shown in Fig. 9.7, and exemplarily illustrated parameters can be checked objectively. An appropriate test procedure should be assigned to each criterion, and the minimum quantitative expression should be defined [8].

9.9 Test Configuration for Performance Diagnostic

In general, the individual measures of physical therapy, physiotherapy, and medical training therapy within modern complex therapies following orthopedic traumatic injuries are based on biocybernetic science models. In this context, the success of training and therapy procedures in physiological structures of the musculoskeletal system must be proven. It is also important to initiate consequences in the form of reorganization or reconception in the rehabilitation process early enough if a measure has not produced the intended training or therapy success. Quantifying and/or qualifying the relevant biological parameters can be done by **performance diagnostics in the rehabilitation process**.

The individual measurement methods of rehabilitative performance diagnosis are applied several times in the course of complex therapy strategies after injuries in football:

- At the beginning of the rehabilitation period for documentation and evaluation of physical performance (quantitative and quantitative aspects)
- In the course of rehabilitation, to regulate the therapy process and to control the impulses and changes in physical function and performance that have been initiated and implied by the individual therapies (physical, therapeutic, and training therapeutic stimuli)

- For the final assessment and documentation of the rehabilitation and restored physical function and performance

A conglomerate of different methods of measurement is necessary to adequately assess the current performance after injuries in football and the football-specific determination of the earliest possible date for the reintegration of the injured player into the team training as well as the restoration of the ability to compete. These can be divided into three subcategories in a first systematization:

- Clinical criteria
- Performance criteria "indoor"
- Performance criteria "outdoor"

9.10 Clinical Return-to-Play Criteria

Clinical investigations of the injured biological structures by a physician, e.g., the reconstructed ligament structures of an ACL for the estimation of joint stability, especially the ligamentous joint stabilizers, have always been classical clinical return-to-play criteria and will continue to be in the future. Therefore, ambitious concepts are indispensable. The physician's experience in terms of the posttraumatic current stress tolerance of the affected biological structures as well as their knowledge of the necessary football-specific stress profile plays an important role in the assessment of clinical (if manually performed, semi-objective) criteria. In practice, at least to assess the functional and load-bearing capacity of ligaments, other measurement methods, such as the KT-1000 arthrometer, can also be used to quantify the tibial shift under defined pressure and the evaluation of the stability of the ACL.

9.11 Peformance Criteria "Indoor"

While the clinical criteria are predominantly aimed at functional capability and posttraumatic load-bearing capacity, the performance criteria "indoor" for football-relevant parameters are to be defined to determine the physical performance of the injured player's motions.

In general, dynamic measurement methods (such as isokinetic test systems) are preferable to static measurement methods to determine the performance of the musculoskeletal system because of the significantly higher prognosis validity. Single-joint measurements (in the so-called open kinetic system) provide information on the performance of the muscular joint stabilizers of individual joints, while multi-joint measurements (in the so-called closed kinetic system) describe the resulting performance of the entire limb. A comprehensive assessment of the performance of the musculoskeletal system always requires both measurement variants. At the moment, however, there is not yet an overarching and/or sport-specific consensus related to minimum requirements or, for example, football-specific standards of the force characteristics.

The performance and the characteristics of the test quality criteria of complex motion analysis systems also vary considerably. Kinematic parameters (location, distance, and angle-related factors in the time and their parameters such as speed and accelerations) are synchronized with dynamic parameters for the determination of the external and internal forces acting on the movement apparatus and the external forces and measured by means of measuring platforms and/or electromyography. However, the interpretation of the corresponding quantities of data and information is complex and currently lacks scientific evidence and consensus.

In addition to the criteria for assessing and evaluating the function and joint stability of individual joints, measurement methods are also used for the qualitative and quantitative assessment of the physiological stability of the lower and/or upper limb, whereas the stability of the pelvic-leg axis is used in football. There are side-specific differences and differences in the center of interest and assessment. Consensus on quantitatively justifiable limits, in order to allow training and/or competition loads again, is currently not to be recognized and derived. The performance of the pelvic axis of the pelvis, especially in the comparison of unilateral performances, can be applied by means of jump tests with good resilience and performance prediction. Both vertical jumps and horizontal jumps can be performed. In the course of these tests, side-specific differences in the sense of posttraumatic deficits appear most clearly, since these single-leg tests represent very high stresses for the neuromuscular system.

9.12 Performance Criteria "Outdoor"

In addition to the previously described clinical measurement methods and the indoor performance criteria, final return-to-play decisions also require performance criteria that closely approximate the physical requirement profile in football and should therefore be carried out under the customary football-specific external circumstances. For the assessment of the cardiorespiratory capacity, i.e., the motor endurance, a distinction is made between basic endurance and football-specific endurance. In order to evaluate the basic endurance performance, run interval tests are performed with determination of the heart rate, stress intensity, and lactate content of the venous capillary blood at the end of the respective stress intervals. According to current threshold values, the individual aerobic and anaerobic threshold (IAS) can be determined on the basis of the results. The current training intensities (by means of heart rate control or running speed control) for a regeneration training (loads up to the aerobic threshold), training for the improvement of the basic endurance (stresses in the transition area between the aerobic and anaerobic threshold), and the improvement of the anaerobic performance (football-specific endurance component) can then be targeted. A high performance predictive value demands the determination of the speed of linear stereotypes as well as the course of typical football-specific cutting movements with defined directional changes. These can be performed with or without a ball. The appropriate intermediate and total times are measured with sufficient accuracy by means of light box systems. Posttraumatically, the performance in the direction of the injured or the healthy side is of interest. A large number of sport-motor tests for the evaluation of agility, which attempt to determine the football-specific game situations and according stereotypic movements, are described in literature. Unfortunately, no binding consensus has yet emerged for a football-specific test battery, so that many institutions measure with different methods. This makes it difficult to assess the results (sufficient for training/competition loads in football?) and makes a comparison of the test results almost impossible. In addition, many test variants lack sufficient assessment of the three main test quality criteria: validity, reliability, and objectivity. In addition to the currently missing football-specific solutions, there is also the question of an adequate assessment of the various test results as well as their interpretation and formulation of the handling sequences in the assessment of the training/competition loadability. In the future, aspects of the physical claim profile as well as the football-specific adaptations must be consistently taken into account in the individual assessment criteria and parameter-specific minimum expressions. In this context, the current practice of defining side-by-side (injured vs. uninjured side) deficits below 10% as adequate performance with sufficient training/competitive resilience, while deficits of injured structures over 10% as an indicator of insufficient recovery of football-specific performance have to be rethought surely. This will lead to new decision-making and evaluation algorithms.

9.13 Basic Conception of Performance Dignostics/Evaluation Conception

For basic analysis, it is recommended to use a simple test battery which can be used on field to be independent from test centers or other institutions. In a large undergoing prevention study in elite football players, Krutsch and Loose (data collecting) integrated tests for proprioception, jumping analysis, agility, and reaction (Table 9.1):

Table 9.1 Components of VBG-prevention study of severe knee injuries

No.	Test	Category	Evaluation
1	One-leg stability test	Proprioception	Score
2	Side-hop	Jumping analysis	Lateral symmetry index (LSI) Landing error scoring system (LESS)-score Ground contact time Number of jumps (left and right)
3	Both-legged drop jump	Jumping analysis	Jumping height Ground contact time Reactivity index (Jumping height/ground contact time) LESS-score
4	Multidirectional Speedchase	Agility and reaction	Absolute time Mean turnaround time (left/right)

These tests are a part of preseason screening for performance diagnostics and are collection reference data for rehabilitation.

9.14 Limitations of Prehabilitation and Return-to-Play Activities

The following limitations of current prehabilitation and return to play strategies can therefore be viewed critically.

9.14.1 Evidence/Consensus of a Football-Specific Requirement Profile

The basis for the practical realization and implementation of the therapy strategies described above provides reliable information about the football-specific physical requirement profile. Only when it is known which physical performance is necessary for successful football games (in the partly massive different levels of achievement), it is necessary, in the context of complex therapy strategies, to work the necessary physical performance requirements out. In this area, a clear increase in scientific publications can be observed but without a current consensus of physical requirements profiles in the different performance levels.

9.14.2 Need for "Football-Specific Standard Data"

In addition to the currently insufficient number of scientific publications on the physical requirement profile of different performance levels, there is also a need for further studies on football-specific characteristics of football-related performance data as well as physiological variations of medical performance data (internal medicine, orthopedic, traumatology, and psychological studies). This leads to corresponding difficulties in the evaluation of evaluated parameters - regardless of the range of dimensions - with regard to physiological variance regions and football-specific characteristics. To this end, the authors will carry out further scientific and sport-medical research in the future, urgently needed to conceptually institutionalize adequate support as well as a targeted prevention and to systematically demonstrate and implement them with appropriate targets.

9.14.3 Interpretation of Performance-Related Data in the Context of Prehabilitation and Complex Criteria-Based Return to Play Strategies

In addition to the aspects already described, the proper interpretation of the evaluation results of the individual measurement methods of rehabilitative performance diagnostics represents a further current limitation. Present-day publications are mainly based on the comparison of the injured structure in comparison to the inviolate contralateral structure of the other side. In this case, a lateral difference of 10% is regarded and defined as the absolute limit of the lateral differences in most cases. Depending on the number of parameters evaluated, these are usually graphically as an overview of the number of "tolerable" and "non-tolerable" parameters (Figs. 9.8, 9.9, 9.10, and 9.11).

For this purpose, it must be considered whether the individual parameters represent absolute knockout criteria or whether, according to a defined algorithm, a certain number of fulfilled and unsatisfied criteria can initiate a new therapeutic milestone or can document a sufficient playability or workability of the patient. According to the authors, appropriate football-specific adaptations (if expert consensus or appropriate scientific or empirical evidence is available) should be taken into account in the evaluation and interpretation of each individual parameter/criterion, and corresponding assessment algorithms should be formulated and developed. This would demonstrate the potentially different assessments in the following example.

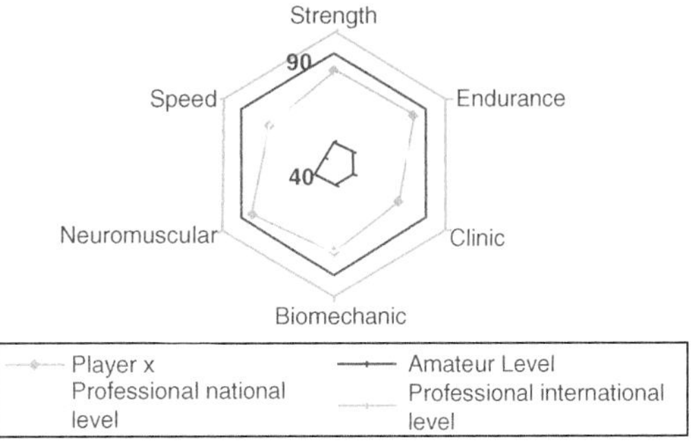

Fig. 9.8 Result presentation of rehabilitative performance diagnosis in the form of a spinning diagram

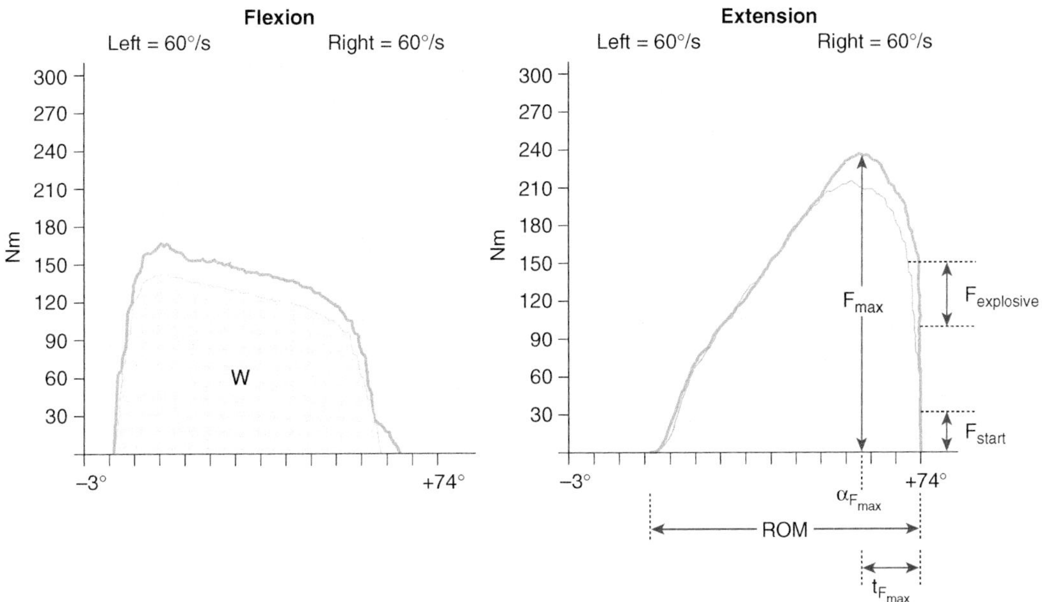

Fig. 9.9 Graphic representation of resultant joint-specific, synergistic musculoskeletal performance, illustrated for single-joint measurements with a rotatory isokinetic system. In this example, the plots for the right and left sides have been superimposed to allow side-to-side comparisons [11]. W, work; F_{max}, maximum force; α_{Fmax}, joint angle at which maximum torque is achieved; F_{start}, starting force = curve rise over a specified time interval from start of movement; $F_{explosive}$, explosive force = force increase over a specified time interval during the steepest upslope until F_{max} is reached; ROM, range of motion; t_{Fmax}, time to $_{Fmax}$

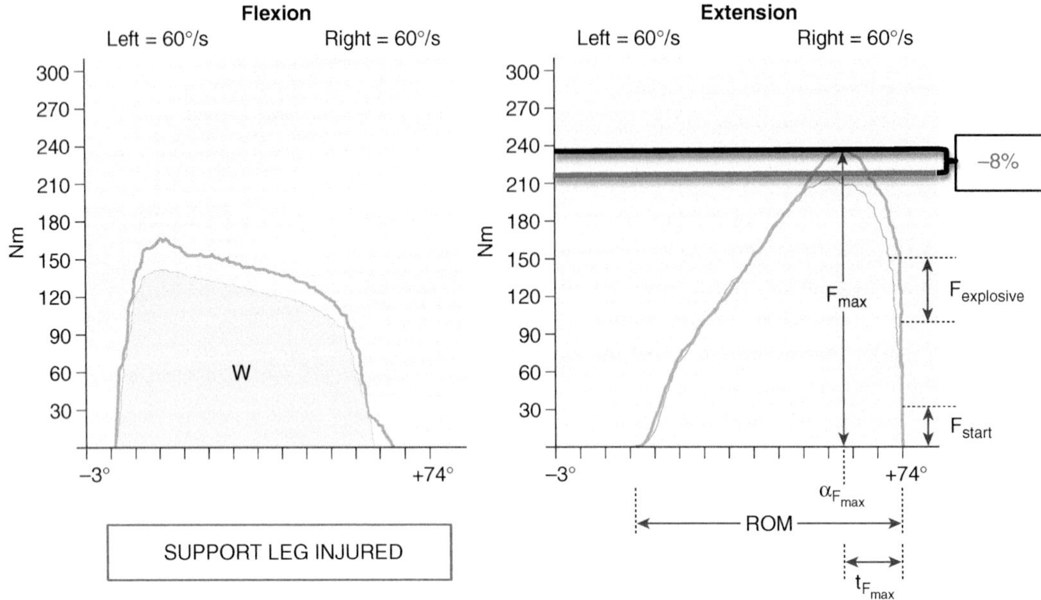

Fig. 9.10 Football-specific-related interpretation of quadriceps max. Torque: the side differences shows acceptable dimensions, when the support leg knee is injured (actual 8% injury caused deficit) [11]

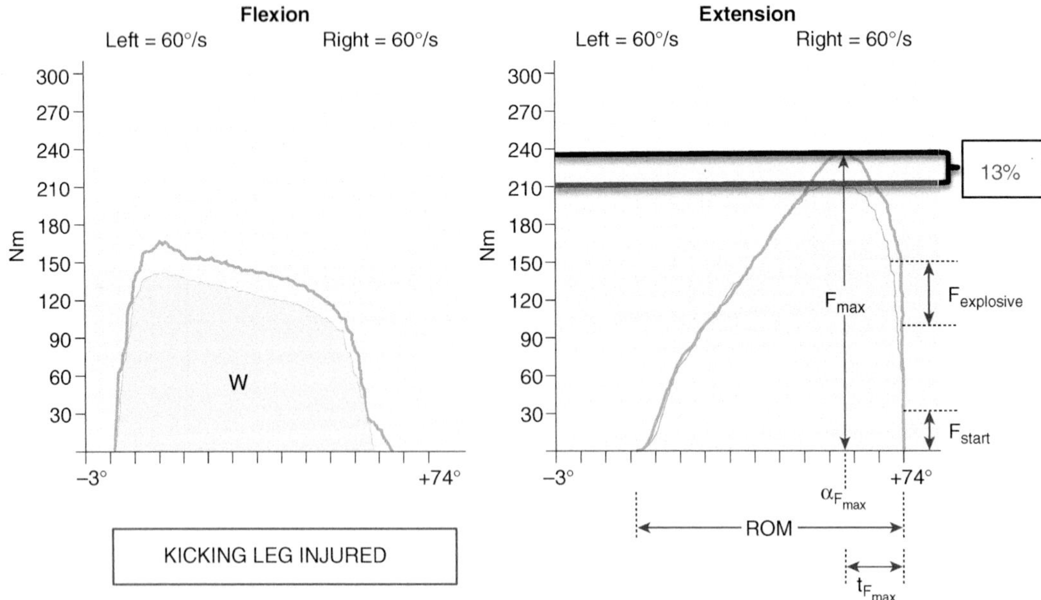

Fig. 9.11 Football-specific-related interpretation of quadriceps max. Torque: the side differences shows ongoing significant inacceptable dimensions, when the kicking leg knee is injured (actual 13% injury caused deficit) [11]

Currently, corresponding football-specific results algorithms are only rudimentary in literature and papers on future research requirements.

Take-Home Messages

1. Complex interdisciplinary return to play strategies must take into account the minimum time limits for biological wound healing processes.
2. The recovery of the physical performance of the musculoskeletal system in interdisciplinary return to play strategies should be otherwise oriented on functional criteria.
3. Functional return-to-play criteria should be evaluated objectively and validly, if possible.
4. The implementation of this return to play strategy is currently underway.
5. The absence of binding valid objective return-to-play criteria.
6. The outstanding scientific evidence with appropriate consensus-specific requirements profiles.
7. The lack of adaptation to football-specific requirements.
8. As well as through outstanding parameter-specific consensus at tolerable posttraumatic deficits (injured vs. uninjured)!

Best Evidence-Based References

Angele P, Eichhorn J, Hoffmann H, Krutsch W (2013) Prävention von vorderen Kreuzbandrupturen, SFA aktuell, Heft 26, Tuttlingen

Wohlfahrt M, Wilhelm H, Peter Ü, Lutz H (2010) Muskelverletzungen im Sport. Georg Thieme Verlag, Stuttgart New York. ISBN 978-3-13-146751-53

McCall A, Davison M, Andersen TE, Beasley I, Bizzini M, Dupont G, Duffield R, Carling C, Dvorak J (2015) Injury prevention strategies at the FIFA 2014 world cup: perceptions and practices of the physicians from the 32 participating national teams. Br J Sports Med 49(9):603–608

Dvorak J, Junge A, Grimm K (2009) F-Marc-football medicine manual, 2nd edn. RVA Druck und Medien AG, Altstätten

Eder K, Hoffmann H (2016) Verletzungen im Fußball: Vermeiden–Behandeln–Therapieren. Elsevier GmbH, München

References

1. Bollars P, Claes S, Vanlommel L, Van Crombrugge K, Corten K, Bellemans J (2014) The effectiveness of preventive programs in decreasing the risk of soccer injuries in Belgium: national trends over a decade. Am J Sports Med 42:577–582
2. Ekstrand J (2016) UEFA elite club injury report, Accessed on 29/01/2017 at http://www.uefa.org/MultimediaFiles/Download/uefaorg/Medical/02/40/27/65/2402765_DOWNLOAD.pdf
3. Ekstrand J, Hägglund M, Waldén M (2011) Injury incidence and injury patterns in professional football: the UEFA injury study. Br J Sports Med 45:553–558
4. Hawkins RD, Fuller CW (1999) A prospective epidemiological study of injuries in four English professional football clubs. Br J Sports Med 33:196–203
5. Cook G (2003) Athletic body in balance. Human Kinetics, Champaign
6. Rahnama N, Lees A, Bambaecichi E (2005) Comparison of muscle strength and flexibility between the preferred and non-preferred leg in English soccer players. Ergonomics 15:1568–1575
7. Magalhaes J, Oliveira J, Ascensao A, Soares J (2004) Concentric quadriceps and hamstrings isokinetic strength in volleyball and soccer players. J Sports Med Phys Fitness 44:119–125
8. Eder K, Hoffmann H (2006) Verletzungen im Fußball: Vermeiden–Behandeln–Therapieren. Elsevier GmbH, München
9. Hoffmann H, Brüggemann P, Ernst H (1982) Optimales Spielgerät: der Ball – biomechanische Überlegungenn zum, Einfluß der Ballmechanik auf die Belastung des Körpers, Der Übungsleiter, 1982, Heft 3. Seite:18–21
10. Brüggemann G, Hentsch P (1981) Arthrotische Veränderungen bei Fußballspielern – biomechanische Überlegungen zu ihrer Entstehung. Orthopäd Praxis 4:335–338
11. Hoffmann H, Eder K (2010) Physikalische und physiotherapeutische Maßnahmen und Rehabilitation. In: Müller-Wohlfahrt H-W, Überacker P, Hensel L (eds) Muskelverletzungen im Sport. Georg Thieme Verlag, Stuttgart/New York, pp 313–321
12. Masuda K, Kikuhara N, Demura S, Katsuta S, Yamanaka K (2005) Relationship between muscle strength in various isokinetic movements and kick performance among soccer players. J Sports Med Phys Fitness 1:44–52
13. Knebel KP, Herbeck B, Hamsen G (1988) Fußball Funktionsgymnastik. Reinbeck bei Hamburg, Rohwohlt Taschenbuch
14. Hoffmann H (1984) Biomechanik von Fußballspannstößen. Johann-Wolfgang-Goethe Universität, Unveröffentlichte Examensarbeit. Frankfurt am Main

15. Angele P, Eichhorn J, Hoffmann H, Krutsch W (2013) Prävention von vorderen Kreuzbandrupturen, SFA aktuell, Heft 26, Tuttlingen
16. Dvorak J, Junge A, Grimm K (2009) F-Marc-football medicine manual, 2nd edn. RVA Druck und Medien AG, Altstätten, Schweiz
17. McCall A et al (2016) Injury prevention strategies at the FIFA 2014 world cup: perceptions and practices of the physicians from the 32 participating national teams. Br J Sports Med 49:603–608
18. Biedert RM, Hintermann B, Hörterer H, Müller AE, Warnke K, Friederich N, Meyer S, Schmeitzky C (2006) Wissenschaftlicher Beitrag. Sports Orthopaedics and Traumatology Sport-Orthopädie – Sport-Traumatologie 22(4):249–254
19. Bloch et al (2015) Return to competition – VBG Consensus Statement, accessed on 29/901/2017on http://www.vbg.de/SharedDocs/MedienCenter/DE/Faltblatt/Pressemeldungen/ 151117_PM_Return-to-Competition.pdf?__blob=publicationFile&v=1

10 Return-to-Play Criteria: The Delaware Experience

Jacob J. Capin and Lynn Snyder-Mackler

Contents

J.J. Capin (✉)
Biomechanics and Movement Science, University of Delaware, Newark, DE, USA
e-mail: capin@udel.edu

L. Snyder-Mackler
Biomechanics and Movement Science, University of Delaware, Newark, DE, USA

Department of Physical Therapy, University of Delaware, Newark, DE, USA

10.1 Introduction

Most rehabilitation protocols and return-to-play (RTP) decisions are time-based rather than criterion-based [1]. However, time after injury or surgery alone is insufficient for determining rehabilitation progression and RTP readiness [2]. While many athletes receive RTP clearance approximately 6 months after anterior cruciate ligament (ACL) reconstruction [1], strength and functional deficits are prevalent at this time and may persist for 1 year or longer after surgery [3–8]. Therefore, evaluating functional performance and other objective criteria, in addition to appropriate healing time frames, is essential. For over two decades [9], clinician-scientists at the University of Delaware have been implementing and advocating for the use of objective criteria to guide rehabilitation progression and RTP decision-making after ACL rupture and other knee injuries [6, 9–13].

Recent, high-quality research both from our cohorts and elsewhere supports and validates the use of our objective criteria. Notably, Grindem and colleagues found that, among athletes in the Delaware-Oslo cohort, 38.2% of those who failed the objective RTP criteria we present here sustained reinjuries within 2 years of ACL reconstruction, whereas only 5.6% of those who passed these criteria sustained reinjuries within the same time frame [14]. Similarly, research from the Aspetar Orthopaedic and Sports

V. Musahl et al. (eds.), *Return to Play in Football*, https://doi.org/10.1007/978-3-662-55713-6_10

Medicine Hospital on professional athletes after ACL reconstruction found that those who returned to team training prior to meeting the objective RTP criteria we present here were at a 4.1-fold greater risk of sustaining an ACL graft rupture compared to those who met the criteria [15]. These studies [14, 15] highlight the need for using objective criteria in determining RTP clearance. This chapter will describe the Delaware approach to determining appropriate rehabilitation progression and readiness to RTP using objective criteria.

10.2 A Criterion-Based Rehabilitation Progression

Following injury or surgery and prior to considering RTP clearance, rehabilitation must occur. At the University of Delaware, clinicians adhere to a criterion-based rehabilitation that has been published previously in detail [9, 10]. To summarize briefly these publications on rehabilitation after ACL injury and reconstruction, rehabilitation progression is guided by achieving (and maintaining) clinical milestones and objective measures [9, 10, 12]. Early clinical milestones include achieving a quadriceps contraction, walking without crutches, and attaining full and symmetrical knee range of motion [10, 16]. Development of quadriceps activation and strength is essential to recovery and performance [5, 6, 10, 14, 17–19] and may be achieved through both closed- and open-kinetic-chain activities [20, 21] as well as neuromuscular electrical stimulation [19, 22]. To monitor the effectiveness of these interventions, quadriceps strength should be assessed. Clinicians should use an electromechanical dynamometer to assess strength optimally; when an electromechanical dynamometer is not available or feasible to use, however, handheld dynamometry with fixation and one-repetition maximum testing are acceptable alternatives, although they tend to overestimate the strength of the involved limb [23]. In addition to quadriceps strength testing, clinicians should monitor knee effusion and joint soreness to progress athletes through rehabilitation and also as they resume sport-specific drills and even competition.

10.2.1 Knee Effusion (Stroke Test)

Rehabilitation specialists should use the stroke test (Fig. 10.1) to assess knee joint effusion. The stroke test is a reliable measure that is used to grade the presence of effusion or intracapsular swelling within the knee [24]. Effusion indicates underlying injury or pathology [24–26] and may be responsive to changes in activity, such as when a patient returns to ambulating in school without crutches, progresses closed-chain (weight bearing) strengthening exercises too quickly, or begins running. We recommend, therefore, progression of activities only in the presence of minimal (i.e., trace) or no effusion [10, 24].

Effusion Grading Scale of the Knee Joint Based on the Stroke Test	
Grade	**Test Result**
Zero	No wave produced on downstroke
Trace	Small wave on medial side with downstroke
1+	Larger bulge on medial side with downstroke
2+	Effusion spontaneously returns to medial side after upstroke (no downstroke necessary)
3+	So much fluid that it is not possible to move the effusion out of the medial aspect of the knee

Fig. 10.1 Clinicians should monitor knee effusion throughout rehabilitation using the reliable stroke test [24]. Reproduced from Adams et al., [10]with permission from the *Journal of Orthopaedic& Sports Physical Therapy*

Soreness Rules	
Criterion	**Action**
Soreness during warm-up that continues	2 days off, drop down 1 level
Soreness during warm-up that goes away	Stay at level that led to soreness
Soreness during warm-up that goes away but redevelops during session	2 days off, drop down 1 level
Soreness the day after lifting (not muscle soreness)	1 day off, do not advance program to the next level
No soreness	Advance 1 level per week or as instructed by healthcare professional

Fig. 10.2 Clinicians should monitor and educate patients on using the soreness rules [10, 27] to appropriately progress rehabilitation and sports-related activities. Reproduced from Adams et al., [10]with permission from the *Journal of Orthopaedic& Sports Physical Therapy*

10.2.2 Soreness Rules

The soreness rules (Fig. 10.2) were originally developed by Fees et al., for weight-lifting modification after upper extremity injury [27], but have since been applied to rehabilitation after lower extremity injury, including ACL injury and reconstruction [10]. Following the soreness rules may allow for appropriate progression of activities without causing undue stress on the healing tissues. We encourage rehabilitation specialists to not only use the soreness rules to determine appropriate clinical progression but also teach their patients the soreness rules so that patients may properly progress their home exercise program, such as the running progression [10] (see below).

The soreness rules refer to joint (i.e., knee) soreness and not muscular soreness. Muscle soreness, in contrast to joint soreness, is usually acceptable and often desired as a by-product of the training necessary to promote muscular strength and hypertrophy.

10.2.3 Running Progression

We recommend that athletes begin a running progression (Fig. 10.3) [10] after they achieve both appropriate healing time frames (i.e., ≥12 weeks after ACL reconstruction) and clinical impairment resolution, operationally defined as full ROM; minimal or no effusion, pain, or joint soreness; and ≥80% quadriceps strength limb symmetry index. The running progression consists of graded exposure to running through intervals of jogging and running that progressively lengthen and intensify. We recommend that all athletes, regardless of sport, complete the running progression prior to evaluating them for readiness to RTP. We also typically do not allow athletes to begin agility drills until they have reached at least level IV of the running progression [10, 13, 28].

10.3 The University of Delaware Objective RTP Criteria

After an athlete has progressed successfully though our criterion-based rehabilitation progression, we use four broad categories of criteria to determine readiness to RTP: clinical measures (resolution of impairments), functional criteria (strength and hop testing), patient-reported outcome measures, and appropriate healing time. The following sections describe these categories and delineate the specific criteria.

10.3.1 Clinical Impairment Resolution

Achieving and maintaining resolution of clinical impairments are essential to recovery and prerequisite to initiating and progressing sport

Running Progression*		
Level	**Treadmill**	**Track**
Level 1	0.1-mi walk/0.1-mi jog, repeat 10 times	Jog straights/walk curves (2 mi)
Level 2	Alternate 0.1-mi walk/0.2-mi jog (2 mi)	Jog straights/jog 1 curve every other lap (2 mi)
Level 3	Alternate 0.1-mi walk/0.3-mi jog (2 mi)	Jog straights/jog 1 curve every lap (2 mi)
Level 4	Alternate 0.1-mi walk/0.4-mi jog (2 mi)	Jog 1.75 laps/walk curve (2 mi)
Level 5	Jog full 2 mi	Jog all laps (2 mi)
Level 6	Increase workout to 2.5 mi	Increase workout to 2.5 mi
Level 7	Increase workout to 3 mi	Increase workout to 3 mi
Level 8	Alternate between running/jogging every 0.25 mi	Increase speed on straights/jog curves
***Progress to next level when patient is able to perform activity for 2 mi without increased effusion or pain. Perform no more than 4 times in 1 week and no more frequently than every other day. Do not progress more than 2 levels in a 7-day period. Conversion: 1 mi = 1.6 km.**		

Fig. 10.3 Athletes should initiate a running progression prior to participating in higher-level activities. Reproduced from Adams et al., [10]with permission from the *Journal of Orthopaedic & Sports Physical Therapy*

activities or providing RTP testing or clearance. We do not consider evaluating athletes for RTP clearance until they can run and participate in other functional activities while maintaining minimal or no effusion, no joint soreness, and full ROM. We do, however, encourage clinicians to monitor strength, patient-reported outcome measures, and appropriate functional activities throughout rehabilitation. Examples of functional activities to monitor during rehabilitation include gait and stair climbing during the early and intermediate postoperative periods, squatting technique and running form during the late postoperative periods, and drop-jump landing and hop testing during the return-to-sport phase as well as at functional testing and follow-up. Once athletes have completed postoperative rehabilitation and maintained clinical impairment resolution, rehabilitation specialists should evaluate them on the following objective criteria to determine readiness to RTP.

10.3.2 Functional Criteria

10.3.2.1 Quadriceps Strength Index

Quadriceps strength deficits of 20% or more at 6 months and 10–15% at 1 year after ACL reconstruction are common [29]. Quadriceps weakness affects gait asymmetries [5, 30–32], functional impairments [18], and reinjury risk [14, 15]. We recommend, therefore, that athletes achieve symmetrical quadriceps strength, operationally defined as the involved limb's strength being ≥90% of the uninvolved limb's strength, prior to returning to sport. We use an electromechanical dynamometer and electrical burst superimposition technique to assess isometric quadriceps strength. This technique can also be used without the superimposed stimulation. Athletes sit securely with their knees flexed to approximately 60° (Fig. 10.4). The uninvolved limb is tested first followed by the involved limb. After warming up, such as stationary cycling followed by submaximal isometric quadriceps

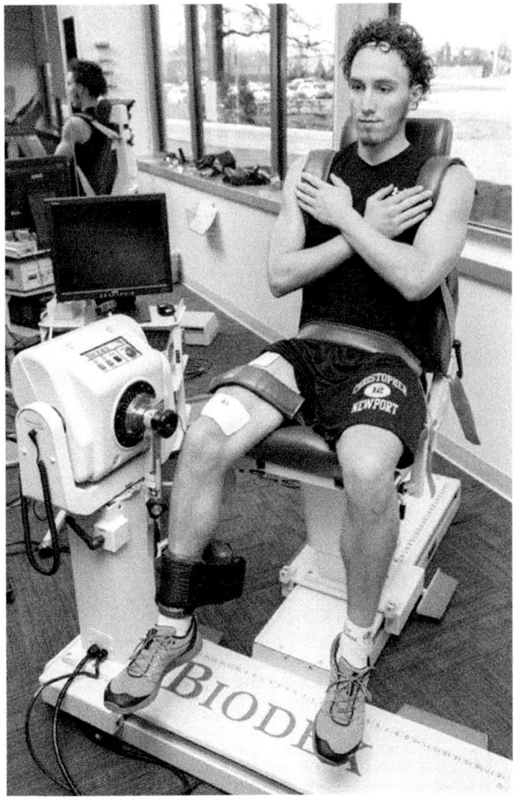

Fig. 10.4 Quadriceps strength limb symmetry index (LSI) is evaluated on an electromechanical dynamometer during a maximum volitional isometric contraction (MVIC) with an electrical burst superimposition technique [33] to assess activation of the quadriceps. Athletes must achieve ≥90% quadriceps strength LSI to meet the strength component of the Delaware RTP criteria

contractions on the dynamometer, athletes perform a maximal volitional isometric contraction (MVIC) with and without burst superimposition [33, 34]. The burst superimposition technique enables clinicians to calculate inhibition [35] and helps to ensure maximum effort by the athlete during testing, particularly of the uninvolved limb.

Isokinetic testing at angular speeds of 60°/s [14] or 60°/s, 180°/s, and 300°/s [15] using an electromechanical dynamometer is also a valid and reliable technique to measure quadriceps strength. If clinicians do not have access to an electromechanical dynamometer, the best approximation of these gold standard measures is a one-repetition maximum (1-RM) on a knee extension machine [23]. Patients should be seated in a standard leg-extension machine (with their hips and knees flexed to 90°), with the pad of the resistance arm placed just proximal to the ankle joint. The femur or pelvis need not be fixed to the knee extension machine for the 1-RM tests, but participants can use the handles for stabilization. The 1-RM method is simple and accessible but slightly underestimates strength compared to isometric testing. Instead of using a 90% threshold for symmetry with the one-repetition maximum testing method, we recommend that the RTP threshold for the athlete's involved limb strength equals or exceeds the uninvolved limb strength [23].

10.3.2.2 Single-Leg Hop Testing

Single-leg hop tests were described by Noyes et al. in 1991 [36] and have been used extensively to evaluate functional performance and limb symmetry after lower extremity injury. A 6 m by 15 cm tape affixed to a floor or flat athletic surface is used to evaluate single-leg hop performance. Athletes perform a series of four single-leg hop tests in the following order: (1) single hop for distance, (2) crossover hop for distance, (3) triple hop for distance, and (4) 6 m timed hop (Fig. 10.5). For each test, athletes per-

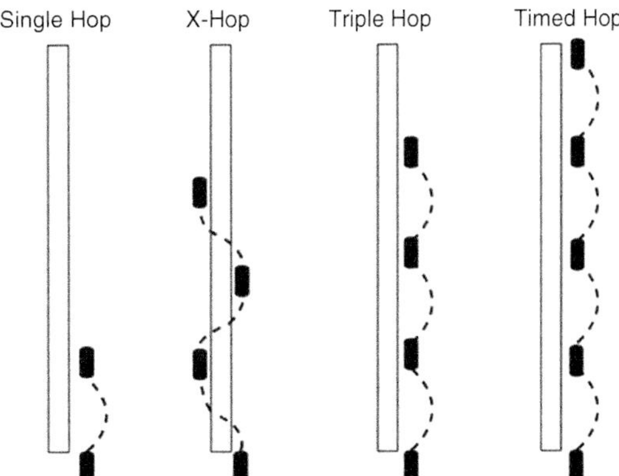

Fig. 10.5 Athletes perform a series of four single-leg hop tests [36] in the following order: 1) single hop for distance, 2) crossover hop (X-hop) for distance, 3) triple hop for distance, and 4) 6 meter timed hop. Hop tests are used to evaluate functional performance and symmetry, and athletes must achieve ≥90% LSIs on each of the four hop tests for RTP clearance. Reproduced from Adams et al., [10]with permission from the *Journal of Orthopaedic& Sports Physical Therapy*

form two practice hops followed by two recorded hops per limb, beginning with the uninvolved limb. For a trial to count for any of the three hops for distance, the athlete must "stick" the landing safely and without moving his or her landing foot, excessive body sway, or touching the contralateral lower extremity or either upper extremity to any surface or support. For the 6 m timed hop, the athlete begins behind the starting line standing on only the foot being tested; the athlete hops as quickly as safely possible across the 6 m testing strip, and the tester records the time from when the heel of the foot being tested leaves the floor until the heel of the same foot passes the 6 m mark. Interlimb comparisons are calculated using a limb symmetry index (LSI) for each test.

10.3.2.3 Limb Symmetry Indexes

Interlimb asymmetries are ubiquitous early after ACL injury and reconstruction and often persist in strength and functional activities such as walking and running for several months to even years after surgery [3, 5–8, 14, 37–39]. Therefore, to evaluate recovery of function, we contend that it is essential to compare the involved limb to the uninvolved limb. Although we typically make concurrent interlimb comparisons, comparisons to pre-injury data may be even more sensitive to detecting risk for second injury [40]. If football teams have preseason or pre-injury testing data, rehabilitation specialists should ideally compare the involved limb's post-injury or postsurgical data to the uninvolved limb's data at both the same testing session as well as pre-injury or presurgery.

We calculate limb symmetry indexes to evaluate functional performance for both quadriceps strength and each of the four single-leg hop tests. LSIs are calculated by dividing the involved limb by uninvolved limb value and multiplying by 100% for strength and the single, crossover, and triple hop tests; the LSI for the 6 m timed hop is calculated by dividing the uninvolved by involved limb value and multiplying by 100% because a faster (lower) time indicates better performance, whereas higher values for strength and distance hopped indicate better performance. Athletes must obtain at least 90% LSI for quadriceps strength and each of the four single-leg hop tests to meet the Delaware functional performance criteria for RTP clearance.

Fact Box 1 LSI calculation

Limb symmetry index = (involved limb value/uninvolved limb value) × 100%

Note that this is true for quadriceps strength index and the three single-leg hops for distance but that the 6 m timed hop LSI calculation is reversed (i.e., [uninvolved/involved] × 100%).

10.3.3 Patient-Reported Outcome Measures

10.3.3.1 Knee Outcome Survey-Activities of Daily Living Subscale

The Knee Outcome Survey-Activities of Daily Living Subscale (KOS-ADLS) is a patient-reported outcome measure used to assess knee function during activities of daily living [41]. The KOS-ADLS is reliable, valid, and responsive [41]. The KOS-ADLS allows patients to rate the effect of knee symptoms (e.g., pain, stiffness, swelling, and weakness) and functional disability on their abilities to perform activities of daily living, such as walking, stair climbing, kneeling, or rising from a chair. Scores range from 0% (minimum) to 100% (maximum) with 100% indicating no limitation in knee function during activities of daily living. Athletes must score 90% or higher on the KOS-ADLS prior to RTP clearance [6, 9–11, 13, 28, 37, 42].

10.3.3.2 Global Rating Scale of Perceived Function (GRS)

The Global Rating Scale of Perceived Function (GRS) consists of a single item, whereby patients rate their overall current knee function compared to their previous (i.e., before injury) knee function on a scale from 0 to 100% [17]. A score of zero represents a complete inability to perform pre-injury activities, while a score of 100 indicates full recovery of function. Athletes must score 90% or higher on the GRS, in conjunction with the aforementioned criteria, to receive RTP clearance [10].

10.3.4 RTP Time Frames

Clearance for returning to sport has often been granted to athletes between 4 and 9 months after ACL reconstruction [1]. Early return to sport, however, places athletes at high risk of reinjury [14, 42–45], even when they achieve objective RTP criteria [14, 42]. Recent evidence indicates that there is a 51% increase in reinjury risk for each month that an athlete returns to sport prior to 9 months after ACL reconstruction; moreover, this trend of increased risk of reinjury persisted up to 12 months after surgery, although it was no longer statistically significant beyond 9 months [14]. Given the high risk of second ACL rupture, particularly among young athletes [44–52] and those who return to level I [53, 54] sports [46, 48, 51], such as football, delaying RTP clearance until at least 9 months or longer is strongly advised—especially in these high-risk cohorts.

Fact Box 2 RTP criteria

To receive RTP clearance, athletes must meet objective criteria (i.e., ≥90% quadriceps strength index, ≥90% LSI on all four single-leg hop tests, ≥90% KOS-ADLS, and ≥90% GRS) and appropriate healing time frames (i.e., ≥9 months after primary ACL reconstruction).

10.4 Validation of the Delaware RTP Criteria

While adhering to the Delaware RTP criteria could have previously been considered level V evidence or "expert opinion," recent evidence [14, 15] validates our approach. Grindem and colleagues [14] prospectively evaluated the effect of passing or failing our seven RTP criteria prior to returning to sport on reinjury risk among 100 athletes in the Norwegian arm of the Delaware-Oslo cohort. Athletes who passed all seven of our RTP criteria prior to returning to sport were 84% less likely to sustain a reinjury within 24 months of ACL reconstruction. Returning to level I sports prior to 9 months after surgery and failing to achieve 90% quadriceps strength LSI prior to returning to level I sports, such as football, were independent risk factors for reinjury [14].

A study by Kyritsis et al. [15] also supports the use of our objective criteria for evaluating readiness to RTP after ACL reconstruction. These authors used our criteria (isokinetic quadriceps strength >90% at 60°/s and LSIs of >90% for the single, triple, and crossover single-leg hop tests) plus the graded RTP progression and an additional test, running t-test performance in <11 s. Failing to meet all six of these criteria before returning to team training placed athletes at a 4.1 times greater risk ($p \leq 0.001$) of sustaining an ACL graft rupture among 158 professional athletes, 105 of whom played football [15].

10.5 The Gradual RTP Progression

When an athlete passes all of the University of Delaware RTP criteria (Fig. 10.6), he or she does not return immediately to unrestricted sports participation and competition. Rather, the athlete begins a gradual RTP progression. During this progression, athletes begin by performing individual sport-specific drills prior to initiating unopposed team drills followed by opposed individual and then team drills, full team practice, scrimmages, and finally unrestricted competition [10, 13, 28, 55]. This progression typically occurs over a period of 2 or 3 months but may be shorter or longer depending on the time left until the competitive sport season as well as the athlete's time from surgery, age, skill level, history of injury, and other factors. Readers interested in more detailed advice on gradual RTP guidelines

Category	Criteria
Clinical Measures (Impairment Resolution)	Trace or Less Effusion: #24, (Sturgill et al., 2009) No Pain or Joint Soreness: #10 (Adams et al., 2012) and #27 (Fees et al., 1998) Hop Tests: #36 (Noyes et al., 1991) KOS-ADLS: #41 (Irrgang et al., 1998) GRS: #10 (Adams et al., 2012) and #17 (Gardinier et al., 2014) 9 Months after Primary ACL Reconstruction: #14 (Grindem et al., 2016)
Functional Measures	≥90% LSI for Quadriceps Strength ≥90% LSI for All Four Single-Leg Hop Tests [37]: Single Hop for Distance Crossover Hop for Distance Triple Hop for Distance 6 Meter Timed Hop
Patient Reported Outcomes	≥90% KOS-ADLS [21] ≥90% GRS [2, 15]
Time after Surgery	≥9 Months after Primary ACL Reconstruction [17]
Abbreviations: RTP: Return-to-Play; ROM: range of motion; LSI: limb symmetry index; KOS-ADLS: Knee Outcome Survey-Activities of Daily Living Subscale; GRS: Global Rating Scale of Perceived Function; ACL: anterior cruciate ligament	

Fig. 10.6 The Delaware RTP criteria

specific to football may consult work by Arundale and colleagues [55], who describe an interval kicking progression and RTP progression.

Fact Box 3 RTP progression
After receiving RTP clearance, athletes progress gradually through a RTP progression (individual drills, unopposed team drills, opposed individual and team drills, full practice, and scrimmages) prior to unrestricted participation in competition.

10.6 Summary

In this chapter, we present the Delaware approach to determine readiness to return to play. We discuss our criterion-based rehabilitation progression, the objective criteria we use to determine RTP clearance, and our gradual RTP progression. Athletes must first meet clinical milestones, resolve their impairments, and demonstrate an ability to maintain impairment resolution while completing a running progression and agility drills. Athletes then undergo our RTP testing battery, consisting of quadriceps strength testing, four single-leg hop tests, and two patient-reported outcome measures, the KOS-ADLS and GRS. Only when athletes achieve 90% or higher values on all RTP criteria, including LSI for quadriceps strength and all four single-leg hop tests and scores on the KOS-ADLS and GRS, as well as appropriate healing time frames or ≥9 months after primary ACL reconstruction, do they receive RTP clearance. After receiving RTP clearance, athletes progress gradually from individual and unopposed team drills to opposed drills, full practices, scrimmages, and eventually unrestricted competition. Using the Delaware approach may facilitate clinical decision-making among healthcare practitioners and reduce substantially the reinjury risk [14, 15] among the athletes they treat.

Take-Home Message
We recommend that athletes meet objective criteria, including ≥90% quadriceps strength LSI, ≥90% LSI on all four single-leg hop tests, ≥90% KOS-ADLS, and ≥90% GRS, and appropriate

time frames (i.e., ≥9 months after primary ACL reconstruction) prior to receiving RTP clearance. Athletes should then progress gradually through a RTP progression—consisting of individual drills, unopposed team drills, opposed individual and team drills, full practice, and scrimmages—prior to unrestricted participation in competition.

Top Five Evidence-Based References

Manal TJ, Snyder-Mackler L (1996) Practice guidelines for anterior cruciate ligament rehabilitation: a criterion-based rehabilitation progression. Oper Tech Orthop 6:190–196

Adams D, Logerstedt D, Hunter-Giordano A, Axe MJ, Snyder-Mackler L (2012) Current concepts for anterior cruciate ligament reconstruction: a criterion-based rehabilitation progression. J Orthop Sport Phys Ther 42:601–614

Grindem H, Snyder-Mackler L, Moksnes H, Engebretsen L, Risberg MA (2016) Simple decision rules can reduce reinjury risk by 84% after ACL reconstruction: the Delaware-Oslo ACL cohort study. Br J Sports Med 50:804–808

Kyritsis P, Bahr R, Landreau P, Miladi R, Witvrouw E (2016) Likelihood of ACL graft rupture: not meeting six clinical discharge criteria before return to sport is associated with a four times greater risk of rupture. Br J Sports Med 50:946–951

Sinacore JA, Evans AM, Lynch BN, Joreitz RE, Irrgang JJ, Lynch AD (2017) Diagnostic accuracy of handheld dynamometry and 1-repetition-maximum tests for identifying meaningful quadriceps strength asymmetries. J Orthop Sport Phys Ther 47:97–107

References

1. Barber-Westin SD, Noyes FR (2011) Factors used to determine return to unrestricted sports activities after anterior cruciate ligament reconstruction. J Arthrosc Relat Surg 27:1697–1705
2. Myer GD, Martin L, Ford KR, Paterno MV, Schmitt LC, Heidt RS, Colosimo A, Hewett TE (2012) No association of time from surgery with functional deficits in athletes after anterior cruciate ligament reconstruction: evidence for objective return-to-sport criteria. Am J Sports Med 40:2256–2263
3. Abourezk MN, Ithurburn MP, McNally MP, Thoma LM, Briggs MS, Hewett TE, Spindler KP, Kaeding CC, Schmitt LC (2017) Hamstring strength asymmetry at 3 years after anterior cruciate ligament reconstruction alters knee mechanics during gait and jogging. Am J Sports Med 45:97–105
4. Hartigan EH, Axe MJ, Snyder-Mackler L (2010) Time line for Noncopers to pass return-to-sports criteria after anterior cruciate ligament reconstruction. J Orthop Sport Phys Ther 40:141–154
5. Lewek M, Rudolph K, Axe M, Snyder-Mackler L (2002) The effect of insufficient quadriceps strength on gait after anterior cruciate ligament reconstruction. Clin Biomech 17:56–63
6. Nawasreh Z, Logerstedt D, Cummer K, Axe MJ, Risberg MA, Snyder-mackler L (2017) Do patients failing return-to-activity criteria at 6 months after anterior cruciate ligament reconstruction continue demonstrating deficits at 2 years ? Am J Sport Med 45:1037–1048
7. Roewer BD, Di Stasi SL, Snyder-Mackler L (2011) Quadriceps strength and weight acceptance strategies continue to improve two years after anterior cruciate ligament reconstruction. J Biomech 44:1948–1953
8. Schmitt LC, Paterno MV, Ford KR, Myer GD, Hewett TE (2015) Strength asymmetry and landing mechanics at return to sport after ACL reconstruction. Med Sci Sport Exerc 47:1426–1434
9. Manal TJ, Snyder-Mackler L (1996) Practice guidelines for anterior cruciate ligament rehabilitation: a criterion-based rehabilitation progression. Oper Tech Orthop 6:190–196
10. Adams D, Logerstedt D, Hunter-Giordano A, Axe MJ, Snyder-Mackler L (2012) Current concepts for anterior cruciate ligament reconstruction: a criterion-based rehabilitation progression. J Orthop Sports Phys Ther 42:601–614
11. Arundale AJH, Cummer K, Capin JJ, Zarzycki R, Snyder-Mackler L (2017) Report of the clinical and functional primary outcomes in men of the ACL-SPORTS Trial: similar outcomes in men receiving secondary prevention with and without perturbation training 1 and 2 years after ACL reconstruction. Clin Orthop Relat Res. https://doi.org/10.1007/s11999-017-5280-2. [Epub ahead of print]
12. Logerstedt D, Arundale A, Lynch A (2015) A conceptual framework for a sports knee injury performance profile (SKIPP) and return to activity criteria (RTAC). Braz J Phys Ther 19:1–20
13. White K, Di Stasi SL, Smith AH, Snyder-Mackler L (2013) Anterior cruciate ligament-specialized post-operative return-to-sports (ACL-SPORTS) training: a randomized control trial. BMC Musculoskelet Disord Mar 23:108
14. Grindem H, Snyder-Mackler L, Moksnes H, Engebretsen L, Risberg MA (2016) Simple decision rules can reduce reinjury risk by 84% after ACL reconstruction: the Delaware-Oslo ACL cohort study. Br J Sports Med 50:804–808
15. Kyritsis P, Bahr R, Landreau P, Miladi R, Witvrouw E (2016) Likelihood of ACL graft rupture: not meeting six clinical discharge criteria before return to sport is associated with a four times greater risk of rupture. Br J Sports Med 50:946–951
16. Joreitz R, Lynch A, Rabuck S, Lynch B, Davin S, Irrgang J (2016) Patient-specific and surgery-specific factors that affect return to sport after ACL reconstruction. Int J Sport Phys Ther 11:264–278

17. Gardinier ES, Manal K, Buchanan TS, Snyder-Mackler L (2014) Clinically-relevant measures associated with altered contact forces in patients with anterior cruciate ligament deficiency. Clin Biomech 29:531–536
18. Logerstedt D, Lynch A, Axe MJ, Snyder-Mackler L (2013) Pre-operative quadriceps strength predicts IKDC2000 scores 6 months after anterior cruciate ligament reconstruction. Knee 20:208–212
19. Snyder-Mackler L, Delitto A, Stralka SW, Bailey SL (1994) Use of electrical stimulation to enhance recovery of quadriceps femoris muscle force production in patients following anterior cruciate ligament reconstruction. Phys Ther 74:901–907
20. Bynum EB, Barrack RL, Alexander AH (1995) Open versus closed chain kinetic exercises after anterior cruciate ligament reconstruction. A prospective randomized study. Am J Sport Med 23:401–406
21. Mikkelsen C, Werner S, Eriksson E (2000) Closed kinetic chain alone compared to combined open and closed kinetic chain exercises for quadriceps strengthening after anterior cruciate ligament reconstruction with respect to return to sports: a prospective matched follow-up study. Knee Surg Sport Traumatol Arthrosc 8:337–342
22. Snyder-Mackler L, Ladin Z, Schepsis AA, Young JC (1991) Electrical stimulation of the thigh muscles after reconstruction of the anterior cruciate ligament. Effects of electrically elicited contraction of the quadriceps femoris and hamstring muscles on gait and on strength of the thigh muscles. J Bone Jt Surg 73:1025–1036
23. Sinacore JA, Evans AM, Lynch BN, Joreitz RE, Irrgang JJ, Lynch AD (2017) Diagnostic accuracy of handheld dynamometry and 1-repetition-maximum tests for identifying meaningful quadriceps strength asymmetries. J Orthop Sport Phys Ther 47:97–107
24. Sturgill LP, Snyder-Mackler L, Manal TJ, Axe MJ (2009) Interrater reliability of a clinical scale to assess knee joint effusion. J Orthop Sport Phys Ther 39:845–849
25. Brophy RH, Mackenzie CR, Gamradt SC, Barnes R, Rodeo S, Warren R (2008) The diagnosis and management of psoriatic arthritis in a professional football player presenting with a knee effusion: a case report. Clin J Sport Med 18:369–371
26. Johnson MW (2000) Acute knee effusions: a systematic approach to diagnosis. Am Fam Physician 61:2391–2400
27. Fees M, Decker T, Snyder-Mackler L, Axe MJ (1998) Upper extremity weight-training modifications for the injured athlete: a clinical perspective. Am J Sports Med 26:732–742
28. Capin JJ, Behrns W, Thatcher K, Arundale A, Smith AH, Snyder-mackler L (2017) On-ice return-to-hockey progression after anterior cruciate ligament reconstruction. J Orthop Sport Phys Ther 47(5):324–333
29. Palmieri-Smith RM, Thomas AC, Wojtys EM (2008) Maximizing quadriceps strength after ACL reconstruction. Clin Sports Med 27:405–424
30. DiStasi SL, Logerstedt D, Gardinier ES, Snyder-Mackler L (2013) Gait patterns differ between ACL-reconstructed athletes who pass return-to-sport criteria and those who fail. Am J Sports Med 41:1310–1318
31. Gardinier E, Manal K, Thomas B, Snyder-Mackler L (2012) Gait and neuromuscular asymmetries after acute ACL rupture. Med Sci Sport Exerc 44:1490–1496
32. Gardinier ES, Di Stasi S, Manal K, Buchanan TS, Snyder-Mackler L (2014) Knee contact force asymmetries in patients who failed return-to-sport readiness criteria 6 months after anterior cruciate ligament reconstruction. Am J Sport Med 42:2917–2925
33. Snyder-Mackler L, De Luca PF, Williams PR, Eastlack ME, Bartolozzi A (1994) Reflex inhibition of the quadriceps femoris muscle after injury of reconstuction of the anterior cruciate ligament. J Bone Jt Surg Am 76:555–560
34. Snyder-Mackler L, Delitto A, Bailey SL, Stralka SW (1995) Strength of the quadriceps femoris muscle and functional recovery after reconstruction of the anterior cruciate ligament. A prospective, randomized clinical trial of electrical stimulation. J Bone Jt Surg 77:1166–1173
35. Stackhouse SK, Dean JC, Lee SCK, Binder-MacLeod SA (2000) Measurement of central activation failure of the quadriceps femoris in healthy adults. Muscle Nerve 23:1706–1712
36. Noyes F, Barber S, Mangine R (1991) Abnormal lower limb symmetry determined by function hop tests after anterior cruciate ligament rupture. Am J Sports Med 19:513–518
37. Capin JJ, Zarzycki R, Arundale A, Cummer K, Snyder-Mackler L (2017) Report of the primary outcomes for gait mechanics in men of the ACL-SPORTS trial: secondary prevention with and without perturbation training does not restore gait symmetry in men 1 or 2 years after ACL reconstruction. Clin Orthop Relat Res. https://doi.org/10.1007/s11999-017-5279-8. [Epub ahead of print]
38. Hartigan E, Axe MJ, Snyder-Mackler L (2009) Perturbation training prior to ACL reconstruction improves gait asymmetries in non-copers. J Orthop Res 27:724–729
39. Thomeé R, Kaplan Y, Kvist J, Myklebust G, Risberg MA, Theisen D, Tsepis E, Werner S, Wondrasch B, Witvrouw E (2011) Muscle strength and hop performance criteria prior to return to sports after ACL reconstruction. Knee Surg Sport Traumatol Arthrosc 19:1798–1805
40. Wellsandt E, Failla MJ, Snyder-mackler L (2017) Limb symmetry indexes can overestimate knee function after anterior cruciate ligament injury. J Orthop Sport Phys Ther Mar 29:1–18
41. Irrgang JJ, Snyder-Mackler L, Wainner RS, FH F, Harner CD (1998) Development of a patient-reported measure of function of the knee. J Bone Jt Surg Am 80:1132–1145
42. Capin JJ, Khandha A, Zarzycki R, Manal K, Buchanan TS, Snyder-Mackler L (2016) Gait mechanics and second ACL rupture: implications for delaying

return-to-sport. J Orthop Res. https://doi.org/10.1002/jor.23476. [Epub ahead of print]

43. Laboute E, Savalli L, Puig P, Trouve P, Sabot G, Monnier G, Dubroca B (2010) Analysis of return to competition and repeat rupture for 298 anterior cruciate ligament reconstructions with patellar or hamstring tendon autograft in sportspeople. Ann Phys Rehabil Med 53:598–614
44. Paterno MV, Rauh MJ, Schmitt LC, Ford KR, Hewett TE (2012) Incidence of contralateral and ipsilateral anterior cruciate ligament (ACL) injury after primary ACL reconstruction and return to sport. Clin J Sport Med 22:116–121
45. Paterno MV, Rauh MJ, Schmitt LC, Ford KR, Hewett TE (2014) Incidence of second ACL injuries 2 years after primary ACL reconstruction and return to sport. Am J Sports Med 42:1567–1573
46. Kaeding CC, Pedroza a D, Reinke EK, Huston LJ, Spindler KP, Amendola A, Andrish JT, Brophy RH, Dunn WR, Flanigan D, Hewett TE, Jones MH, Marx RG, Matava MJ, McCarty EC, Parker RD, Wolcott M, Wolf BR, Wright RW (2015) Risk factors and predictors of subsequent ACL injury in either knee after ACL reconstruction: prospective analysis of 2488 primary ACL reconstructions from the MOON cohort. Am J Sports Med 43:1583–1590
47. Maletis GB, Chen J, Inacio MC, Funahashi TT (2016) Age-related risk factors for revision anterior cruciate ligament reconstruction: a cohort study of 21,304 patients from the Kaiser Permanente anterior cruciate ligament registry. Am J Sports Med 44:331–336
48. Mohtadi N, Chan D, Barber R, Paolucci EO (2016) Reruptures, reinjuries, and revisions at a minimum 2-year follow-up: a randomized clinical trial comparing 3 graft types for ACL reconstruction. Clin J Sport Med 26:96–107
49. Nelson IR, Chen J, Love R, Davis BR, Maletis GB, Funahashi TT (2016) A comparison of revision and rerupture rates of ACL reconstruction between autografts and allografts in the skeletally immature. Knee Surg Sport Traumatol Arthrosc 24:773–779
50. Sanders TL, Pareek A, Hewett TE, Levy BA, Dahm DL, Stuart MJ, Krych AJ (2017) Long-term rate of graft failure after ACL reconstruction: a geographic population cohort analysis. Knee Surg Sport Traumatol Arthrosc 25:222–228. https://doi.org/10.1007/s00167-016-4275-y.
51. Webster KE, Feller JA, Leigh WB, Richmond AK (2014) Younger patients are at increased risk for graft rupture and contralateral injury after anterior cruciate ligament reconstruction. Am J Sports Med 42:641–647
52. Wiggins AJ, Grandhi RK, Schneider DK, Stanfield D, Webster KE, Myer GD (2016) Risk of secondary injury in younger athletes after anterior cruciate ligament reconstruction: a systematic review and meta-analysis. Am J Sports Med 44:1861–1876
53. Daniel DM, Lou SM, Dobson BE, Fithian DC, Rossman DJ, Kaufman KR (1994) Fate of the ACL-injured patient. A prospective outcome study. Am J Sports Med 22:632–644
54. Hefti F, Muller W, Jakob RP, Staubli HU (1993) Evaluation of knee ligament injuries with the IKDC form. Knee Surg Sport Traumatol Arthrosc 1:226–234
55. Arundale A, Silvers H, Logerstedt D, Rojas J, Snyder-Mackler L (2015) An interval kicking progression for return to soccer following lower extremity injury. Int J Sports Phys Ther 10:114–127

11 Return to Play Criteria: The Norwegian Experience

Håvard Moksnes and Lars Engebretsen

Contents

11.1 Return to Play in Football: The Norwegian Model

Although the health benefits of regular physical activity are well documented, injury must be recognized as a significant "side effect" of sports. In fact, every sixth injury treated in Norwegian hospitals is caused by sports. To promote physical activity effectively, we have to deal professionally with the health problems of the active patient. This obviously means providing effective care for the injured patient but also actively promoting injury prevention measures.

In Norway, soccer and team handball account for more injuries than other sports—33% of all sports injuries occur while playing soccer, while 12% result from team handball. This does not necessarily mean that soccer and team handball are the most dangerous sports but also reflect their status as the most popular participation sports in Norway.

All injuries are not serious, but soccer and team handball—as well as alpine skiing—lead to an alarmingly high rate of serious knee injuries, especially anterior cruciate ligament (ACL) injuries. A women's elite team handball is likely to lose one player each season to an ACL injury. These injuries are a serious concern, not only since they cause a significant time loss from sport and work but above all because they lead to a significant increase in the risk of early osteoarthrosis. Unfortunately, it seems that not even modern surgical reconstruction methods can prevent future disability after an ACL injury.

Our ability to prevent injuries has been seriously hampered by our lack of understanding of the mechanisms causing injury. In particular, we have had little information on how to prevent serious knee injuries or preventive measures which can be implemented in the most popular

H. Moksnes, Ph.D. (✉)
Oslo Sport Trauma Research Center, The Norwegian School of Sport Sciences, Oslo, Norway

The Norwegian Olympic Training Center, Oslo, Norway

The Norwegian Sports Medicine Center (Idrettens Helsesenter), Oslo, Norway
e-mail: havard.moksnes@olympiatoppen.no

L. Engebretsen, M.D., Ph.D.
Oslo Sport Trauma Research Center, The Norwegian School of Sport Sciences, Oslo, Norway

Department of Orthopaedic Surgery, Oslo University Hospital, Faculty of Medicine, University of Oslo, Oslo, Norway

V. Musahl et al. (eds.), *Return to Play in Football*, https://doi.org/10.1007/978-3-662-55713-6_11

Norwegian sports. Recent years have shown progress to the extent where serious knee injuries in these sports are reduced by 50%.

Research on sports injury prevention has been scarce, and the information we have had has typically been obtained from descriptive projects outlining injury incidence, patterns and severity. However, these studies have not been designed to provide in-depth information on injury mechanisms and risk factors—information which is needed in order to propose relevant preventive measures. A concerted long-term research effort on risk factors, injury mechanisms and prevention programmes is required.

Based on this background, the Oslo Sports Trauma Research Center (OSTRC) was established at the Norwegian School of Sport Sciences in May 2000. The OSTRC is a joint venture between Oslo Orthopaedic University Clinic and The Norwegian University of Sport and Physical Education, and the centre is financed by the Royal Norwegian Ministry of Culture, the Norwegian Olympic Committee and Confederation of Sports, Norsk Tipping AS and Pfizer AS.

The main objective has been to develop a long-term research programme on injury prevention (including studies on basic epidemiology, risk factors, injury mechanisms and intervention studies). The programme focuses on the largest Norwegian sports (in terms of injuries), i.e. soccer, team handball and alpine skiing, and on the most common (e.g. ankle, hamstrings) and serious injuries (e.g. ACL). Professor Roald Bahr and Professor Lars Engebretsen chair the OSTRC, and it has produced >40 PhDs and postdoctoral students with a multidisciplinary background (medical doctors, sports scientists, physiotherapists and biomechanists). As research on prevention of injuries from our group has been published over the globe, strategies for implementation of the new knowledge have been developed. With support from IOC and industry, two new apps, Get Set (English language that will be expanded to eight languages) and Skadefri, have been developed to help athletes prevent injuries in various sports all within the Olympic framework and to help the athletes be ready for return to play (Fig. 11.1).

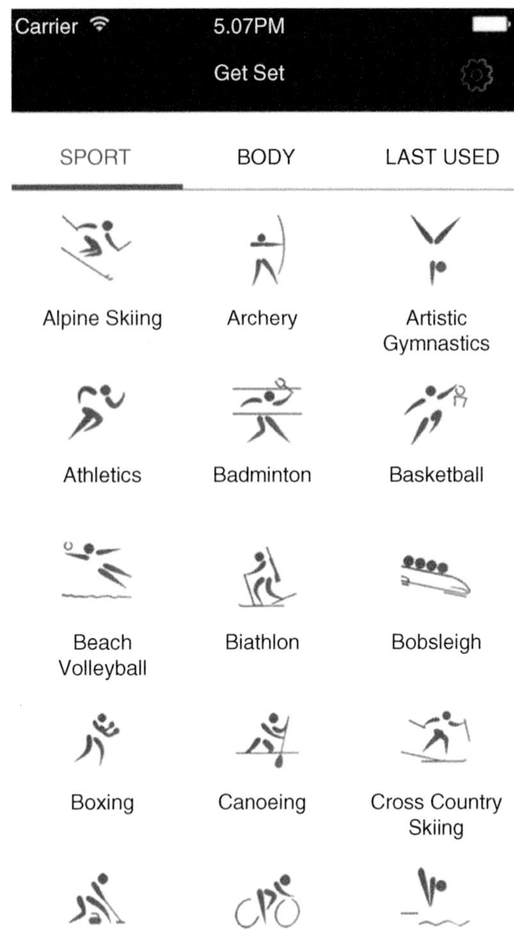

Fig. 11.1 Picture showing some of the sports represented in the Get Set app

Almost simultaneously, The Norwegian Research Center for Active Rehabilitation was started (2003) by May Arna Risberg PT, PhD, and strategic cooperation has led to many joint ventures between the two groups. The result of this has been new knowledge on prevention and rehabilitation methods based on translational and clinical research.

Returning footballers safely to full participation and matches after an injury is a challenging task for the medical support team. Recent publications highlight the importance of multi-professional collaboration and shared decision-making throughout the final stages of rehabilitation [1, 2].

Norwegian Sports Medicine clinicians and researchers have been in the forefront during the development of modern rehabilitation algorithms and functional return to play testing [3–5]. Sports injury rehabilitation is a dynamic, structured process that primarily aims to restore the injured athlete's function and performance level. Furthermore, athletes desire a quick return to sport, highlighting the second aim of the medical team, which is to return the athlete to sports participation in a safe and timely manner—with minimal risk of reinjury. Furthermore, previous injury is an important known risk factor for sports injury [6–8], and active structured rehabilitation is a critical part of returning players to play in a safe manner. Safe return to sport usually indicates that the athlete can return to their previous performance level with the lowest possible risk of a reinjury. Studies do however show that the reinjury rates are high particularly when it comes to hamstring injuries [9, 10], ACL injuries [11–13] and ankle injuries [14, 15]. Of utmost concern are the possible negative long-term health effects that have been documented following knee meniscus and ligament injuries [16, 17]. Already in 2005, Myklebust and Bahr [18] commented on the high number of athletes who never return to sport after an ACL injury and also highlighted the importance of discussing the possible long-term detrimental effects returning to sport after an ACL injury may have. The relatively low return to sport rate following ACL injury has been thoroughly documented in the latter years by Ardern et al. [19–21], although male professional football players are more frequently returning to their previous performance level [22]. Furthermore, the individual players' likelihood of returning to play is influenced by psychological factors that should be included in the return to play assessment [23, 24]. The rate of returning to sport is likely also influenced by the structure and quality of the rehabilitation, which have been shown in a Norwegian study [3]. Grindem et al. documented that a combined preoperative and post-operative rehabilitation protocol supervised by experienced sports physiotherapists led to significantly better knee function and return to sport rates compared to patients who received usual care.

The basis of sports injury rehabilitation is a gradually progressed targeted exercise programme, where the return to play decision is the natural culmination. Modern sports injury rehabilitation is progressed through phases based on sound clinical reasoning, sequenced functional achievements and the completion of functional milestones [25, 26]. Furthermore, knowledge of tissue-specific biological healing processes should be respected and will sometimes dictate parts of the progression timeline. Exercise prescription, communication and clinical reasoning are core skills for clinicians involved in rehabilitation of sports injuries [27]. Although most experienced clinicians probably are subconsciously following a progression model through rehabilitation, few theoretical models have been published [26]. Exercise therapy acts at the local tissue level and in the central nervous system. Weighted loading may be used through mechanotransduction as a direct injury treatment (mechanotherapy) [28] or to unload injured tissue via altered movement and muscle activation patterns.

In the final phases of rehabilitation, the athlete is guided towards returning to participation in sports. More traditional strength and conditioning training is usually incorporated with addition of more complexity and velocity and increasing emphasis on higher rates of force development. Physical conditioning in the gym will be similar to preseason training for the specific sport, although a majority of exercises should still be unilaterally focused to stimulate adaptation and reverse any pending impairments (Fig. 11.2).

Safe return to play is sometimes challenging due to pressure on the medical team from the athlete, coach, parents, team management and other stakeholders to return athletes to competition prematurely. Regardless of the circumstance, the medical team is obliged to ensure that the athlete's long-term health is not compromised by premature return to sport, which may have serious consequences. Over the past decade, we have experienced that the majority of pressure can be reduced if the early rehabilitation protocols include a consensus predefined sport-specific functional return to play test battery. Test

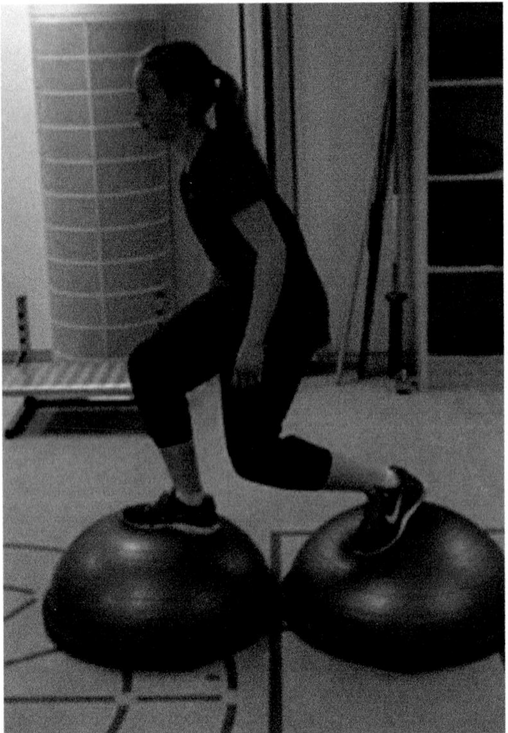

Fig. 11.2 Late-phase rehabilitation exercise with athlete following knee injury

batteries that assess the status of the athlete in different function levels are advised following most sports injuries to ensure that the athlete is fit to return to sport with minimal risk of reinjury [1, 29–34]. Unfortunately, the scientific backing regarding content and cut-off limits for these batteries are still lacking for most injuries. The evidence regarding cut-off limits has been most evaluated for return to play following ACL reconstructions. High-quality prospective studies from Qatar [35] and Norway [36] strongly indicate that returning to play after passing a battery of functional tests significantly reduces the risk of reinjury. In short, the batteries include muscle strength tests, single-legged hop tests, patient-reported outcome measures and a progressive sport-specific rehabilitation period. The sport-specific rehabilitation should include the completion of specific parts of team training sessions without symptoms during or after training. Likewise, return to match play is structured progressively with 15 min as substitute in the first match with increasing playing time in subsequent matches. Importantly, sufficient time from injury or surgery has to be provided so that the necessary biological healing can be optimal before returning to match play. Again Grindem et al. have demonstrated that the risk of a second knee injury is reduced with 51% for each month from 6 to 9 months following an ACL reconstruction [36].

Delaware–Oslo prospective cohort of 106 ACL reconstructed patients (Grindem et al. [36]):

- Patients who had passed return to sport test battery with quadriceps strength >90% of uninjured side had 5.6% secondary knee injuries compared to 32.7% in those who had not.
- Patients who returned to level I sport had 4.3 times higher risk of new knee injury compared to those who returned to a lower level.
- Patients who returned to sport earlier than 9 months after ACL reconstruction had 39.5% new knee injuries compared to 19.4% in those who returned more than 9 months after surgery.

Another important task for the clinician will be to monitor the overall load on the previously injured and healing structures, which again calls for close collaboration and clear communication with coaches and strength and conditioning professionals. Thus, a player is usually returned to matches when the specific criteria in Fig. 11.3 have been passed. Additional advice related to progression in match play is to limit availability of the player to maximum one match per week during the first 2 months with increasing playing time, i.e. 15 min → 30 min → 45 min → 60 min → 75 min → 90 min.

At the top athlete level, the Norwegian Olympic Training Center (Olympiatoppen) and the Oslo

Return to Sport criteria

Muscle strength measurements > 90%

Hop tests > 90%

With adequate strategy and quality
Performed gradual increase in sport specific training with adequate movement patterns and without pain, effusion or fear of re-injury

Fig. 11.3 Return to sport criteria following knee injury

Sports Trauma Research Center have developed and initiated a screening and monitoring programme to optimize health care for Olympic athletes [37]. The programme runs continuously with enrolment of summer and winter athletes 2 years prior to every Olympic Games since London in 2012. The programme consists of two pillars. (Pillar I) Weekly, athlete reported health monitoring by use of a smartphone app connected to an online database to which Olympic medical support teams have access. The biggest challenge in injury registration and monitoring is overuse injuries and illnesses, which have traditionally been underreported; however, new methodology ensures prospective collection of such data including the injury burden [38]. (Pillar II) Annual medical and musculoskeletal screening includes functional performance tests. The main reason for including functional performance tests is to establish baseline measurements when athletes are injury-free and healthy. These consecutive baseline measurements enable an overview and yearly assessment of physical development but also importantly serve as milestones with regard to return to play testing following subsequent injury. Thus, the test batteries in different sports are sport specific to optimize the validity related to return to sports assessments and injury patterns discovered during the continuous health monitoring. Structured performance and physical conditioning testing is already common in Norwegian male (professional) and female (semi-professional) football clubs. However, consecutive benchmarking in return to play tests and health monitoring is less frequent and may be developed, as the experiences from the Olympic programme will be shared in the future.

Sports medicine in Norway is mostly performed as a collaboration between sports medicine physicians, orthopaedic surgeons and specialized sports physiotherapists. Sports and conditioning trainers are increasingly involved particularly in professional sports. Both private and public services are used. Traditionally, the socio-democratic structure of health coverage with cost-free services for all inhabitants has been the basis throughout rehabilitation processes. As an exception, the top athletes have access to a multidisciplinary team through the designated Olympic Training Centre. However, during the past 5–10 years, public funding has been decreased. Consequently, sports insurance coverage of treatment and rehabilitation has been vastly developed and improved. Thus, all people, at all levels, who suffer a sports injury in training or competition, are guaranteed qualified treatment through the compulsory yearly participation licence. The individual cost to fund this insurance coverage is approximately 150 Euros per year.

11.2 Return to Football: Two Case Examples

The first case example is a female semi-professional football player from a top-three team in Norway. The player (born 1998) suffered an ACL injury to her left knee in August 2013. She underwent ACL reconstruction with a patellar tendon graft and returned to full participation in matches 11 months later. Subsequently she ruptured the ACL in the right knee during a training session playing with boys in December 2015. She underwent ACL reconstruction of the ligament with a patellar tendon graft in February 2016 and a concomitant partial resection of the posterior horn of the lateral meniscus. There was no indication of cartilage injury during the procedure. Post-operative rehabilitation was performed with the physiotherapist in the club with additional unsupervised sessions in the gym. From phase 2 rehabilitation, the weekly structure was periodization with six sessions per week including two muscle strength sessions, two functional stability sessions and two endurance sessions. A rehabilitation specialist was consulted every fourth week during the entire rehabilitation period. Functional tests consisting of the predefined return to play tests were performed 6, 8 and 10 months after the surgical procedure. Results are seen in Figs. 11.4, 11.5 and 11.6. Following the 6-month test, she was allowed

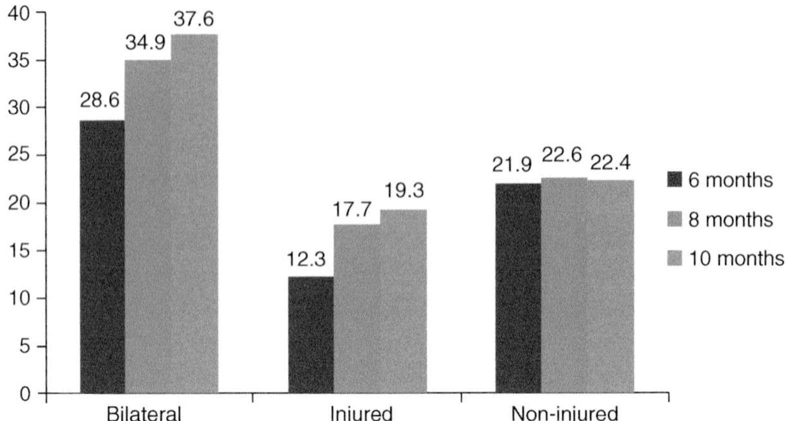

Fig. 11.4 Case 1: female soccer player with bilateral ACL. Countermovement jump bilateral and single-leg jumps (cm)

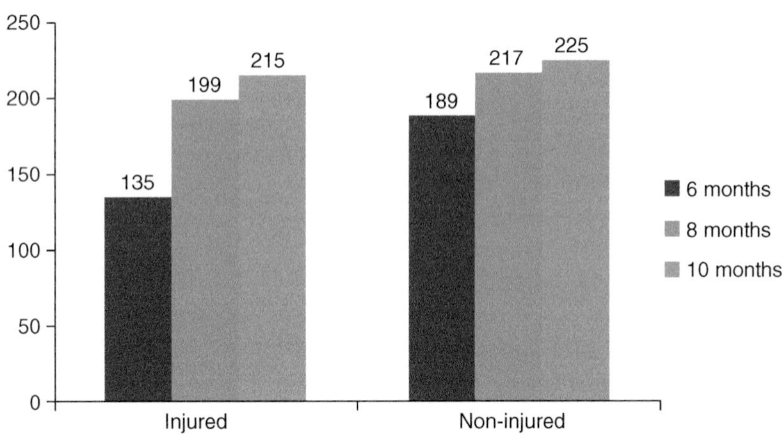

Fig. 11.5 Case 1: female soccer player with bilateral ACL. Maximum quadriceps power in leg extension exercise (watt)

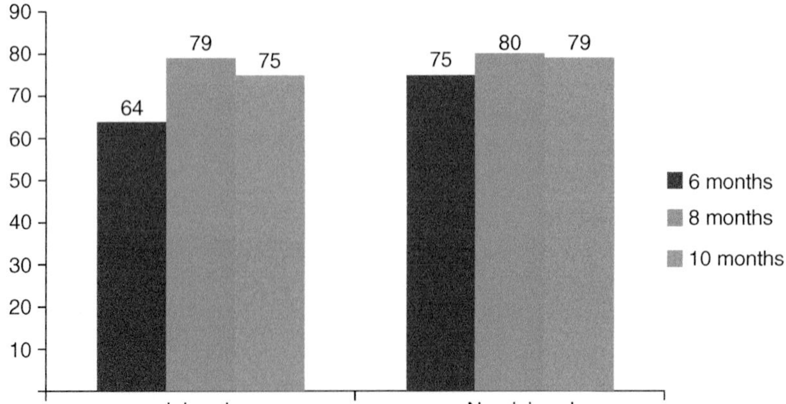

Fig. 11.6 Case 1: female soccer player with bilateral ACL. Thirty-second single-leg continuous side hop 40 cm

individual technical basic training parallel with the team every second day while still maintaining focus on strength and conditioning of the operated leg. The team physiotherapist designed the on-field rehabilitation in collaboration with the head coach. Subsequent to the 8-month test, she was permitted participation in a shielded position during parts of selected team training sessions, while continuing individual technical training and unilateral power-focused strength training. The 10-month test was performed late December 2016 after the winter break, and the current progression plan is full participation in three team sessions during January 2017. Unless symptoms of effusion, pain and insecurity appear during the next month, she will increase the number of sessions in February and is scheduled for gradual return to match play from March 2017.

The second case example is a male professional football player from a top-three team in Norway. The player (born 1992) ruptured his left Achilles tendon during a match early in March 2015. He underwent surgical repair with an open technique 3 days later in a public hospital with a specialized orthopaedic surgeon. Post-operative rehabilitation was performed in accordance with the accelerated protocol published by Olsson et al. (2013) [39]. Day-to-day rehabilitation was performed with the physiotherapist in the club, supplemented by monthly consultations with a rehabilitation specialist in Oslo. The final phases of rehabilitation were structured based on functional milestones during rehabilitation and results of validated functional tests performed 16 and 20 weeks after surgery (Figs. 11.7, 11.8 and 11.9) [31, 40].

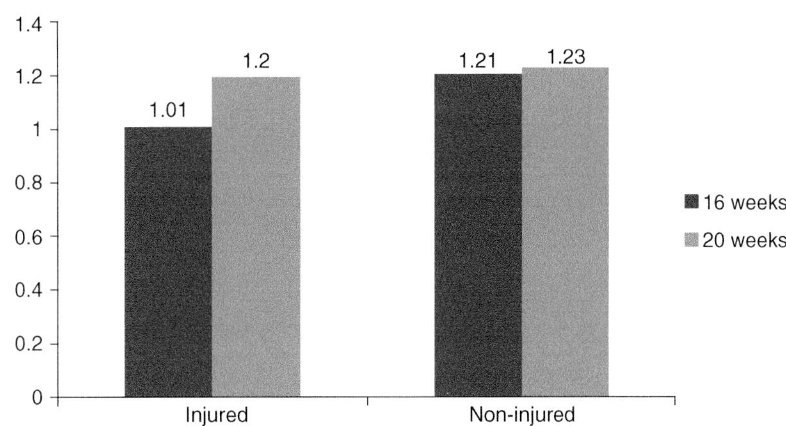

Fig. 11.7 Case 2: male soccer player with Achilles tendon rupture. Average jump coefficient (flight time/contact time) from 25 continuous maximal single-leg jumps

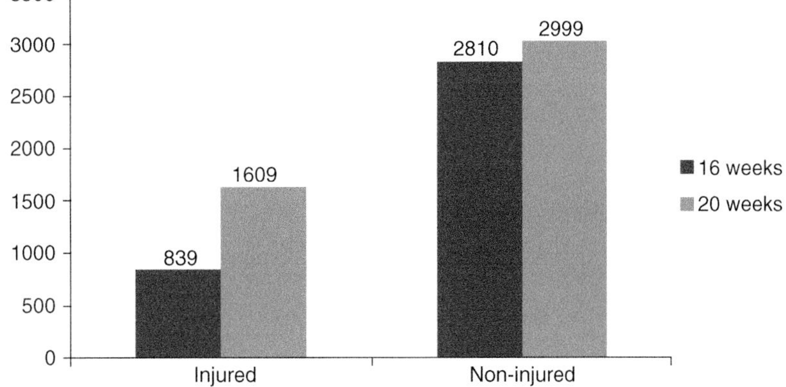

Fig. 11.8 Case 2: male soccer player with Achilles tendon rupture. Total work (Joule) performed in muscular endurance test with single-leg heel rises to failure/exhaustion

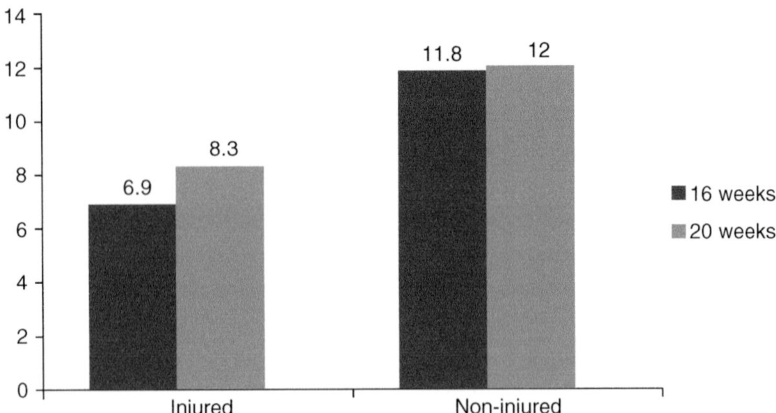

Fig. 11.9 Case 2: male soccer player with Achilles tendon rupture. Maximal heel rise height (cm) performed during muscular endurance test with single-leg heel rises to failure/exhaustion

The figures illustrate a significant improvement on the operated side during the 4 weeks of final phase rehabilitation but are also in line with the findings of Olsson et al. who describe significant deficits in functional leg symmetry indexes up to 12 months after surgical repair of Achilles tendon ruptures. The player returned to restricted football practice 13 weeks after treatment with continuous rehabilitation focused on force production and rate of force development. He participated in full unrestricted team practice in week 23 and had his first match appearance 28 weeks after surgical treatment. He played his first 90-min full match 36 weeks after surgical treatment and is still playing at the highest national level.

Take-Home Message

- The return to play decision should be made over time with a multidisciplinary approach to predefined criteria.
- Knowledge on the prevention of football injuries is growing and must be implemented better in structured training.
- Involve players in return to play decisions and provide evidence-based information on long-term consequences.
- Periodical health evaluations should include functional tests to benchmark function in probable return to play test batteries.

Top Five Evidence Based References

Grindem H, Snyder-Mackler L, Moksnes H, Engebretsen L, Risberg MA (2016) Simple decision rules can reduce reinjury risk by 84% after ACL reconstruction: the Delaware-Oslo ACL cohort study. Br J Sports Med 50(13):804–808. https://doi.org/10.1136/bjsports-2016-096031

Walden M, Hagglund M, Magnusson H, Ekstrand J (2016) ACL injuries in men's professional football: a 15-year prospective study on time trends and return-to-play rates reveals only 65% of players still play at the top level 3 years after ACL rupture. Br J Sports Med 54:744. https://doi.org/10.1136/bjsports-2015-095952

Kyritsis P, Bahr R, Landreau P, Miladi R, Witvrouw E (2016) Likelihood of ACL graft rupture: not meeting six clinical discharge criteria before return to sport is associated with a four times greater risk of rupture. Br J Sports Med 50:946. https://doi.org/10.1136/bjsports-2015-095908

Ardern CL, Osterberg A, Tagesson S, Gauffin H, Webster KE, Kvist J (2014a) The impact of psychological readiness to return to sport and recreational activities after anterior cruciate ligament reconstruction. Br J Sports Med 48(22):1613–1619. https://doi.org/10.1136/bjsports-2014-093842

Olsson N, Silbernagel KG, Eriksson BI, Sansone M, Brorsson A, Nilsson-Helander K, Karlsson J (2013) Stable surgical repair with accelerated rehabilitation versus nonsurgical treatment for acute Achilles tendon ruptures: a randomized controlled study. Am J Sports Med 41(12):2867–2876. https://doi.org/10.1177/0363546513503282

References

1. Ardern CL, Glasgow P, Schneiders A, Witvrouw E, Clarsen B, Cools A, Gojanovic B, Griffin S, Khan KM, Moksnes H, Mutch SA, Phillips N, Reurink G, Sadler R, Silbernagel KG, Thorborg K, Wangensteen A, Wilk KE, Bizzini M (2016) 2016 Consensus statement on return to sport from the First World Congress in Sports Physical Therapy, Bern. Br J Sports Med 50(14):853–864. https://doi.org/10.1136/bjsports-2016-096278
2. Shrier I (2015) Strategic Assessment of Risk and Risk Tolerance (StARRT) framework for return-to-play decision-making. Br J Sports Med 49(20):1311–1315. https://doi.org/10.1136/bjsports-2014-094569
3. Grindem H, Granan LP, Risberg MA, Engebretsen L, Snyder-Mackler L, Eitzen I (2015) How does a combined preoperative and postoperative rehabilitation programme influence the outcome of ACL reconstruction 2 years after surgery? A comparison between patients in the Delaware-Oslo ACL Cohort and the Norwegian National Knee Ligament Registry. Br J Sports Med 49(6):385–389. https://doi.org/10.1136/bjsports-2014-093891
4. Grindem H, Eitzen I, Engebretsen L, Snyder-Mackler L, Risberg MA (2014) Nonsurgical or surgical treatment of ACL injuries: knee function, sports participation, and knee reinjury: the Delaware-Oslo ACL cohort study. J Bone J Surg Am 96(15):1233–1241. https://doi.org/10.2106/JBJS.M.01054
5. Eitzen I, Moksnes H, Snyder-Mackler L, Risberg MA (2010) A progressive 5-week exercise therapy program leads to significant improvement in knee function early after anterior cruciate ligament injury. J Orthop Sports Phys Ther 40(11):705–721. https://doi.org/10.2519/jospt.2010.3345
6. Bahr R, Holme I (2003) Risk factors for sports injuries--a methodological approach. Br J Sports Med 37(5):384–392. https://doi.org/10.1136/bjsm.37.5.384
7. Kucera KL, Marshall SW, Kirkendall DT, Marchak PM, Garrett WE Jr (2005) Injury history as a risk factor for incident injury in youth soccer. Br J Sports Med 39(7):462. https://doi.org/10.1136/bjsm.2004.013672
8. van Beijsterveldt AM, van de Port IG, Vereijken AJ, Backx FJ (2013) Risk factors for hamstring injuries in male soccer players: a systematic review of prospective studies. Scand J Med Sci Sports 23(3):253–262. https://doi.org/10.1111/j.1600-0838.2012.01487.x
9. De Vos RJ, Reurink G, Goudswaard GJ, Moen MH, Weir A, Tol JL (2014) Clinical findings just after return to play predict hamstring re-injury, but baseline MRI findings do not. Br J Sports Med 48(18):1377–1384. https://doi.org/10.1136/bjsports-2014-093737
10. Freckleton G, Pizzari T (2013) Risk factors for hamstring muscle strain injury in sport: a systematic review and meta-analysis. Br J Sports Med 47(6):351–358. https://doi.org/10.1136/bjsports-2011-090664
11. Gifstad T, Foss OA, Engebretsen L, Lind M, Forssblad M, Albrektsen G, Drogset JO (2014) Lower risk of revision with patellar tendon autografts compared with hamstring autografts: a registry study based on 45,998 primary ACL reconstructions in Scandinavia. Am J Sports Med 42(10):2319–2328. https://doi.org/10.1177/0363546514548164
12. Kvist J, Kartus J, Karlsson J, Forssblad M (2014) Results from the Swedish national anterior cruciate ligament register. Arthroscopy 30(7):803–810. https://doi.org/10.1016/j.arthro.2014.02.036
13. Ageberg E, Forssblad M, Herbertsson P, Roos EM (2010) Sex differences in patient-reported outcomes after anterior cruciate ligament reconstruction: data from the Swedish knee ligament register. Am J Sports Med 38(7):1334–1342. https://doi.org/10.1177/0363546510361218
14. Janssen KW, van Mechelen W, Verhagen EA (2014) Bracing superior to neuromuscular training for the prevention of self-reported recurrent ankle sprains: a three-arm randomised controlled trial. Br J Sports Med 48(16):1235–1239. https://doi.org/10.1136/bjsports-2013-092947
15. Walden M, Hagglund M, Ekstrand J (2013) Time-trends and circumstances surrounding ankle injuries in men's professional football: an 11-year follow-up of the UEFA Champions League injury study. Br J Sports Med 47(12):748–753. https://doi.org/10.1136/bjsports-2013-092223
16. Risberg MA, Oiestad BE, Gunderson R, Aune AK, Engebretsen L, Culvenor A, Holm I (2016) Changes in knee osteoarthritis, symptoms, and function after anterior cruciate ligament reconstruction: a 20-year prospective follow-up study. Am J Sports Med 44(5):1215–1224. https://doi.org/10.1177/0363546515626539
17. Oiestad BE, Holm I, Engebretsen L, Risberg MA (2011) The association between radiographic knee osteoarthritis and knee symptoms, function and quality of life 10-15 years after anterior cruciate ligament reconstruction. Br J Sports Med 45(7):583–588. https://doi.org/10.1136/bjsm.2010.073130
18. Myklebust G, Bahr R (2005) Return to play guidelines after anterior cruciate ligament surgery. Br J Sports Med 39(3):127–131. https://doi.org/10.1136/bjsm.2004.010900
19. Ardern CL, Taylor NF, Feller JA, Webster KE (2014) Fifty-five per cent return to competitive sport following anterior cruciate ligament reconstruction surgery: an updated systematic review and meta-analysis including aspects of physical functioning and contextual factors. Br J Sports Med 48(21):1543–1552. https://doi.org/10.1136/bjsports-2013-093398
20. Ardern CL, Webster KE, Taylor NF, Feller JA (2011) Return to sport following anterior cruciate ligament reconstruction surgery: a systematic review and meta-analysis of the state of play. Br J

Sports Med 45(7):596–606. https://doi.org/10.1136/bjsm.2010.076364
21. Ardern CL, Webster KE, Taylor NF, Feller JA (2011) Return to the preinjury level of competitive sport after anterior cruciate ligament reconstruction surgery: two-thirds of patients have not returned by 12 months after surgery. Am J Sports Med 39(3):538–543. https://doi.org/10.1177/0363546510384798
22. Walden M, Hagglund M, Magnusson H, Ekstrand J (2016) ACL injuries in men's professional football: a 15-year prospective study on time trends and return-to-play rates reveals only 65% of players still play at the top level 3 years after ACL rupture. Br J Sports Med 54:744. https://doi.org/10.1136/bjsports-2015-095952
23. Ardern CL, Taylor NF, Feller JA, Whitehead TS, Webster KE (2015) Sports participation 2 years after anterior cruciate ligament reconstruction in athletes who had not returned to sport at 1 year: a prospective follow-up of physical function and psychological factors in 122 athletes. Am J Sports Med 43(4):848–856. https://doi.org/10.1177/0363546514563282
24. Ardern CL, Osterberg A, Tagesson S, Gauffin H, Webster KE, Kvist J (2014) The impact of psychological readiness to return to sport and recreational activities after anterior cruciate ligament reconstruction. Br J Sports Med 48(22):1613–1619. https://doi.org/10.1136/bjsports-2014-093842
25. Glasgow P (2015) Exercise prescription: bridging the gap to clinical practice. Br J Sports Med 49(5):277–277. https://doi.org/10.1136/bjsports-2014-094485
26. Blanchard S, Glasgow P (2014) A theoretical model to describe progressions and regressions for exercise rehabilitation. Phys Ther Sport 15(3):131–135. https://doi.org/10.1016/j.ptsp.2014.05.001
27. Gokeler A, Benjaminse A, Welling W, Alferink M, Eppinga P, Otten B (2015) The effects of attentional focus on jump performance and knee joint kinematics in patients after ACL reconstruction. Phys Ther Sport 16:114. https://doi.org/10.1016/j.ptsp.2014.06.002
28. Khan KM, Scott A (2009) Mechanotherapy: how physical therapists' prescription of exercise promotes tissue repair. Br J Sports Med 43(4):247–252. https://doi.org/10.1136/bjsm.2008.054239
29. Hagglund M, Walden M, Thomee R (2015) Should patients reach certain knee function benchmarks before anterior cruciate ligament reconstruction? Does intense 'prehabilitation' before anterior cruciate ligament reconstruction influence outcome and return to sports? Br J Sports Med 49(22):1423–1424. https://doi.org/10.1136/bjsports-2015-094791
30. Thomee R, Walden M, Hagglund M (2015) Return to sports after anterior cruciate ligament injury: neither surgery nor rehabilitation alone guarantees success-it is much more complicated. Br J Sports Med 49(22):1422. https://doi.org/10.1136/bjsports-2015-094793
31. Silbernagel KG, Gustavsson A, Thomee R, Karlsson J (2006) Evaluation of lower leg function in patients with Achilles tendinopathy. Knee Surg Sports Traumatol Arthrosc 14(11):1207–1217. https://doi.org/10.1007/s00167-006-0150-6
32. Askling CM, Nilsson J, Thorstensson A (2010) A new hamstring test to complement the common clinical examination before return to sport after injury. Knee Surg Sports Traumatol Arthrosc 18(12):1798–1803. https://doi.org/10.1007/s00167-010-1265-3
33. Griffin DR, Dickenson EJ, O'Donnell J, Agricola R, Awan T, Beck M, Clohisy JC, Dijkstra HP, Falvey E, Gimpel M, Hinman RS, Hölmich P, Kassarjian A, Martin HD, Martin R, Mather RC, Philippon MJ, Reiman MP, Takla A, Thorborg K, Walker S, Weir A, Bennell KL (2016) The Warwick Agreement on femoroacetabular impingement syndrome (FAI syndrome): an international consensus statement. Br J Sports Med 50(19):1169–1176. https://doi.org/10.1136/bjsports-2016-096743
34. Weir A, Brukner P, Delahunt E, Ekstrand J, Griffin D, Khan KM, Lovell G, Meyers WC, Muschaweck U, Orchard J, Paajanen H, Philippon M, Reboul G, Robinson P, Schache AG, Schilders E, Serner A, Silvers H, Thorborg K, Tyler T, Verrall G, de Vos RJ, Vuckovic Z, Holmich P (2015) Doha agreement meeting on terminology and definitions in groin pain in athletes. Br J Sports Med 49(12):768–774. https://doi.org/10.1136/bjsports-2015-094869
35. Kyritsis P, Bahr R, Landreau P, Miladi R, Witvrouw E (2016) Likelihood of ACL graft rupture: not meeting six clinical discharge criteria before return to sport is associated with a four times greater risk of rupture. Br J Sports Med 50:946. https://doi.org/10.1136/bjsports-2015-095908
36. Grindem H, Snyder-Mackler L, Moksnes H, Engebretsen L, Risberg MA (2016) Simple decision rules can reduce reinjury risk by 84% after ACL reconstruction: the Delaware-Oslo ACL cohort study. Br J Sports Med 50(13):804–808. https://doi.org/10.1136/bjsports-2016-096031
37. Clarsen B, Ronsen O, Myklebust G, Florenes TW, Bahr R (2014) The Oslo Sports Trauma Research Center questionnaire on health problems: a new approach to prospective monitoring of illness and injury in elite athletes. Br J Sports Med 48(9):754–760. https://doi.org/10.1136/bjsports-2012-092087
38. Clarsen B, Myklebust G, Bahr R (2013) Development and validation of a new method for the registration of overuse injuries in sports injury epidemiology: the Oslo Sports Trauma Research Centre (OSTRC) overuse injury questionnaire. Br J Sports Med 47(8):495–502. https://doi.org/10.1136/bjsports-2012-091524
39. Olsson N, Silbernagel KG, Eriksson BI, Sansone M, Brorsson A, Nilsson-Helander K, Karlsson J (2013) Stable surgical repair with accelerated rehabilitation versus nonsurgical treatment for acute Achilles tendon ruptures: a randomized controlled study. Am J Sports Med 41(12):2867–2876. https://doi.org/10.1177/0363546513503282
40. Silbernagel KG, Nilsson-Helander K, Thomee R, Eriksson BI, Karlsson J (2010) A new measurement of heel-rise endurance with the ability to detect functional deficits in patients with Achilles tendon rupture. Knee Surg Sports Traumatol Arthrosc 18(2):258–264. https://doi.org/10.1007/s00167-009-0889-7

12 Criteria-Based Return to Play After ACL Reconstruction: The Brazilian Experience

Gustavo Gonçalves Arliani, Mario Ferretti, and Moises Cohen

Contents

G.G. Arliani (✉) • M. Cohen
Centro de Traumatologia do Esporte (CETE)/Universidade Federal de São Paulo, São Paulo, Brazil
e-mail: ggarliani@hotmail.com

M. Ferretti
Hospital Israelita Albert Einstein, São Paulo, Brazil

12.1 History of Brazilian Football

Football is the most popular sport in Brazil and the world. There are over 240 million amateur football players and at least 200,000 professional players on the planet. Despite the huge growth of women's football in recent years, 80% of football players are male [1, 2].

Brazil is known as the "country of football", but the history of the sport in the South American nation is relatively recent.

There are several accounts of the arrival of football and the beginning of the sport in Brazil. However, the best-known and accepted version is that the first ball was brought from England in 1894 by Charles William Miller. Charles Miller was born in São Paulo, Brazil, in 1874. Son of a Scottish father and Brazilian mother, Miller went to study in the United Kingdom at the age of 10. When he returned to Brazil in 1894 to work with his father at the São Paulo Railway Company, Miller brought in his luggage two deflated balls, a pair of football boots, a book with the rules of football, and used uniforms.

The first organized football match in Brazil took place in the following year, 1895, between the employees of the Gas Company of São Paulo and the São Paulo Railway Company. The São Paulo Railway Company, the team of Charles Miller, won by a score of 4–2.

The São Paulo Athletic Club was the first soccer team of Brazil, formed in 1894 by Charles

V. Musahl et al. (eds.), *Return to Play in Football*, https://doi.org/10.1007/978-3-662-55713-6_12

Miller. The first club dedicated only to football was the Sport Club Internacional (São Paulo), founded in 1899 and now defunct. The Sport Club Rio Grande is considered the earliest football club founded in Brazil that remains active. In honor of that club, its founding date, July 19, has been designated "Football Day." The professionalization of sports in Brazil did not occur until the 1920s and 1930s, and football was considered a sport practiced only by members of the country's elite.

The World Cup contests began in 1930 in Uruguay. Brazil is the only nation to have participated in all World Cups and to have won five championship trophies in the most important football championship worldwide. The country has also hosted this tournament twice. Currently, Brazil has approximately 800 clubs and 30,000 professional football players. The national championship of professional football in Brazil has four divisions that play practically year-round and in most of the country's states.

12.2 Epidemiology of Injuries

The risk of injury in professional football is high. Studies have shown that the risk of injury among professional football players is 1000 times higher than that among industry workers [3]. As a sport, football has undergone many changes in recent years, mainly owing to the increasing physical demands, which force athletes to work close to their physical limits, predisposing them to injury. In Brazil we have excess games and training, which make athletes more prone to muscle, ligament, and osteoarticular injuries [4].

Fact Box 1
The risk of injury in professional football is high. Studies have shown that the risk of injury among professional football players is 1000 times higher than that among industry workers.

The incidence of soccer injuries is estimated at approximately 10–25 injuries per 1000 h of practice. Several studies have been published in recent decades describing the incidence and causes of injury in soccer. Currently the main goal of football medicine is the prevention of injuries, thus increasing the safety of athletes in the practice of sports. However, to carry out efficient preventive work, a thorough knowledge of the epidemiology of sports injuries is necessary [5].

In Brazil, the earliest epidemiological studies of soccer injuries emerged in the 1990s. Cohen et al. described the injuries that occurred in the matches of eight Brazilian soccer clubs over a period of 2 years and concluded that most injuries occurred in midfield and forward players, with muscle injuries being the most common. Most orthopedic injuries in soccer were mild and players returned to the sport within 7 days. In that study, 12% of injuries occurred in the knee, with sprains and bruises being the most common injuries in this joint [4].

Brazil is a country of continental size and tropical climate. After these first studies, we began to question whether these national differences might influence the pattern of injuries relative to soccer in European countries and other regions of the world. Thus, Arliani et al. described a national model for conducting epidemiological studies in soccer using standards previously established by FIFA. Their study presented new classifications for distances traveled to game locations and a new division in the classification of injury severity in soccer [5]. In an epidemiological study of Latin American soccer players in the 2011 Copa América, Pedrinelli et al. recorded 63 injuries in all 26 tournament matches. The incidence of injury was 70 injuries per 1000 h of play or 2.42 injuries per game. Most injuries occurred within the last 15 min of the game, with approximately 25% of injuries involving the knee [6]. Pangrazio et al. mapped the injuries that occurred during the Copa América of 2015. The authors observed that one injury occurred every 58 min of play, with an incidence of 17.25 injuries for every 1000 h of play. Anterior cruciate ligament (ACL) injuries occurred most often in the final minutes of the first half, whereas muscular injuries were more frequent in the second part of the second half of the match [7].

In a prospective study with 15 years of follow-up, it was found that a constant annual rate of ACL injuries of approximately 6% among soccer players. The ACL injury rate during games was 20 times higher than that during training [8].

Fact Box 2
A constant annual rate of ACL injuries of approximately 6% among soccer players was observed with 15 years of follow-up.

The orthopedic injuries that occurred in the first two divisions during São Paulo State Football Championship 2016 were evaluated, and it was found that 259 injuries occurred during all 361 games, an average of 0.71 injuries per game. The incidence of injury was 21.3 for every 1000 h of play for the championship overall. Most of the injuries occurred in the last 15 min of the first half, and 7.7% of the injuries required surgical treatment. Most of the surgeries (14 surgeries) were ACL reconstructions. The mean age of athletes with ACL injury was 25 years. The majority of these injuries (43%) occurred in midfielders. Regarding the timing of injury, 57% of ACL ruptures occurred in the first 30 min of the game. There was an equal division with regard to laterality (50% right side and 50% left side). Most ACL ruptures occurred without contact (65% of cases). Seventy-eight percent of ACL injuries occurred in second-division team athletes, perhaps owing to the inferior quality of the fields or poorer physical preparation of the athletes in the second division of the championship.

Fact Box 3
The majority of ACL injuries (43%) occur in midfielders, and 57% of these injuries occur in the first 30 min of the game.

12.3 Treatment

ACL injury mainly affects young, active individuals and is especially characterized by the sensation of knee distortion during movements of abrupt change of direction and running on uneven terrain. Surgical reconstruction is now the standard treatment in athletes. Football is a sport with many changes of direction, jumps, and landings, making nonsurgical treatment unlikely to be successful in professional players. Despite the almost complete consensus regarding the need for surgery after ACL rupture in professional soccer players, some aspects of the surgical procedure remain controversial, including the best options for grafting, technique, and fixation devices.

In a study of Major League Soccer (MLS), the authors reported that most US professional team surgeons performed ACL reconstruction (ACLR), preferentially within the first 4 weeks after injury. The vast majority of orthopedists (91%) performed reconstruction of the ACL with a single bundle, and 50% performed transtibial femoral tunnel drilling. The graft most often used by surgeons in ACL reconstruction in that study was a patellar tendon graft; the least commonly used was the quadriceps tendon graft [9].

In a similar study, Arliani et al. showed that most knee surgeons in Brazil opt for reconstruction of the ACL with single bundle and transtibial technique (66%). Most orthopedists participating in that study used hamstring grafts in the surgeries. Interference screws were the surgical material preferred by surgeons in graft fixation in both the tibia and femur. Regarding the time to return to the sport after surgery, orthopedists reported waiting at least 6 months for release [10].

In a systematic review, the mid- and long-term postoperative results were examined (>2 years of follow-up) of randomized and quasi-randomized clinical trials comparing patients who underwent surgery with hamstring grafts versus patellar tendon grafts. The authors concluded that there was no difference in outcomes related to graft type in ACL reconstruction. However, this study was not limited to professional soccer players, and some doubts persist for this patient group [11]. Some possible advantages of patellar tendon grafting are faster integration of the graft due to the presence of the bone plug and the possibility of a more aggressive physiotherapy protocol. Hamstring grafts cause less morbidity at the donor site and less anterior knee pain in the postoperative period. However, the hamstrings are considered secondary stabilizers of opening stress in the medial compartment of the knee, and removal of these tendons could generate discomfort in some professional players when kicking with the inner foot. Surgeons who believe this hypothesis prefer the patellar tendon graft in ACL reconstruction in professional soccer players. New high-quality studies on this subject, however, are needed to draw evidence-based conclusions.

12.4 Prevention

In a study with 11 years of follow-up of injuries occurring in some clubs participating in the UEFA Champions League, Ekstrand et al. found a 31% decrease in ligament injuries, including ACL injuries, over the 11-year period. The authors concluded that this great decrease in the incidence of ligament injuries may have resulted from the implementation in most clubs of preventive programs and proprioceptive training [12].

Yamada et al. evaluated postural stability and functional capacity in young soccer players before and after 45 min of play. The authors concluded that after 45 min of play, there was a decrease in postural stability as evaluated with the Biodex Stability System and in functional capacity as evaluated with the hop test protocol (Fig. 12.1).

This study suggested a possible association between physical fatigue, lower limb stability, and increased incidence of injury in the final 15 min of games [13].

Lundblad et al. recently investigated the possible relationship between a history of previous injuries and subsequent ACL injury in professional soccer players. The authors concluded that previous injuries do not increase the risk of ACL rupture in soccer players [14].

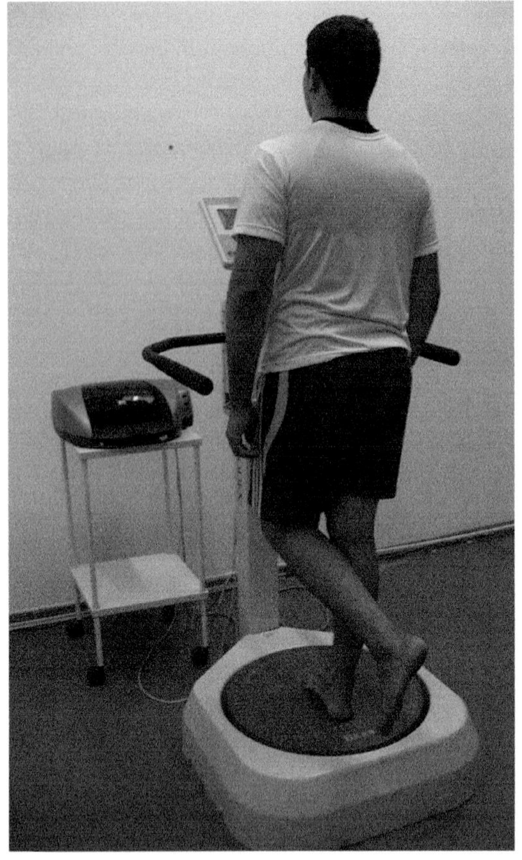

Fig. 12.1 Athlete during evaluation on Biodex Stability System platform

In the last decade, several injury prevention programs have appeared in sports generally and in football in particular. Of these programs, perhaps the most used is FIFA 11+. In 2009, FIFA created and publicized FIFA 11+, a worldwide football injury prevention program. Developed and studied by the FIFA Medical Assessment and Research Center, the program was based on a randomized clinical trial that significantly reduced injuries and health costs in football. Since the launch of FIFA 11+, major publications have confirmed the program's preventive effects and have evaluated its performance effects in professional men, professional women, and amateur soccer players alike [15]. Some studies using the FIFA 11+ program have shown a reduction of up to 40% in injuries when the program was successfully implemented [16]. Grooms et al. accompanied a male university football team with 41 athletes between 18 and 25 years of age for two consecutive seasons. In the first season, no injury prevention program was in place (control); in the second season, the FIFA 11+ program was adopted. The authors demonstrated not only a 72% reduction in the risk of lower limb injury but also a significant decrease in the severity and time to recovery of the injuries that did occur [17].

Fact Box 4

FIFA 11+ program has shown a reduction of up to 40% in injuries when the program was successfully implemented.

However, despite the excellent results in injury prevention confirmed by several quality publications, the implementation of this and other preventive programs remains a great challenge. Despite the huge publicity and promotional activities carried out by FIFA in more than 80 countries during symposia and World Cups, only 10% of FIFA's member countries have adopted the prevention program [15].

In addition to preventive programs, other approaches have emerged in recent years aimed at reducing ACL injuries as genetic research has focused on this theme. Leal et al. demonstrated that gene expression analysis is very useful in understanding the risk factors for ACL injury and failures in ACL healing. The authors concluded that at least three genes could be used as reference genes in genetic analyses [18].

12.5 Return to Football After ACL Reconstruction

Injury and consequent withdrawal from football may be the most distressing and sad occurrence in the life of a professional soccer player. After injury and surgery, the first question of athletes is how long it will take to return to the field and to play at the same level as prior to injury.

Walden et al. prospectively studied 157 ACL injuries during 15 consecutive seasons and followed these professional soccer players for a period of 3 years. The mean times from ACL reconstruction to return to training and return to games were 6.6 months and 7.4 months, respectively. The re-rupture rate before return to games was 4%. Three years after surgery, 86% of operated athletes were playing soccer; however, only 65% of players who underwent ACL reconstruction were playing professional football at the same level as prior to injury [8].

Several factors influence the return to soccer in athletes undergoing ACL reconstruction. Sandon et al. investigated these possible factors in a study of 205 players in Sweden. The authors described female gender, knee joint cartilage injuries, and pain during physical activity as independent and negative factors for return to soccer after ACL reconstruction [19].

In another study, Walden et al. investigated the risk of further knee injury in professional soccer players after ACL reconstruction. The authors found a greater risk of new knee injury, especially injuries resulting from overload, in players who previously underwent ACL reconstruction compared with players without previous surgeries [20].

Another worrying factor after ACL reconstruction in professional soccer players is the impact on health, quality of life, and knee function after retirement. Arliani et al. evaluated retired former soccer players in Brazil with a mean age of 44 years and showed that 44% of former players had been treated with infiltrated knee medications during their careers. Most of these former athletes had undergone knee surgery (ACL reconstruction and meniscectomies), and 66% of the sample showed signs of osteoarthrosis on knee radiographs. Retired players had more knee pain and poorer quality of life in the SF-36 compared with a control group [21]. In a retrospective study, Neyret et al. assessed the effect of ACL reconstruction on soccer players over a 20-year follow-up period. The authors found signs of radiographic osteoarthrosis in

77% of ex-players with a history of ACL reconstruction; 74% of these athletes were satisfied with knee function [22].

Another controversial issue is the criteria for safe return of the player to the sport. Wiggins et al. found rates of 15–20% of new ACL injury after ligament reconstruction and return to play. Determining the exact moment to release an athlete to return to football after ACL reconstruction is challenging and multifactorial [23]. In a systematic review, Barber-Westin et al. concluded that there was no consensus on the appropriate criteria and objectives for the safe return of athletes to sport. The authors showed that 40% of the studies analyzed did not have criteria for returning to sports after ACLR and 32% used only the postoperative time as a criterion for returning to sports activities [24].

In a recent prospective study involving 158 professional male soccer players, Kyritsis et al. demonstrated that players who did not meet all criteria for returning to sport after ACLR were four times more likely to have a new ACL injury, compared with players who achieved all of the proposed criteria (quadriceps and hamstring strength tests, hop tests, agility test, specific rehabilitation of sports movements in the field) (Figs. 12.2, 12.3, and 12.4). The minimum postoperative time currently suggested by most studies for return to sport after ACL reconstruction is 6 months [25]. However, recent studies have shown that returning to sports activities before 9 months after ACLR increases the risk of recurrence of ligament injury [26]. A recent review article on the subject suggested criteria for return to sport based on an analysis of several studies on the subject. The authors suggested return to sports after at least 9 months following ACL reconstruction, as well as assessments of function, symptoms, and activity scales (IKDC and Tegner), psychological assessments (ACL-RSI and K-SES), clinical evaluations, range of motion testing, KT1000 testing, muscular strength evaluation, and progressive reintegration to the sport. Despite the numerous suggested evaluations, the authors concluded that new, high-quality studies should be undertaken in the coming years to determine specific criteria with high sensitivity and sensitivity for safe return to sports after ACLR [27].

Fact Box 5
Returning to sports activities before 9 months after ACLR increases the risk of recurrence of ACL injury.

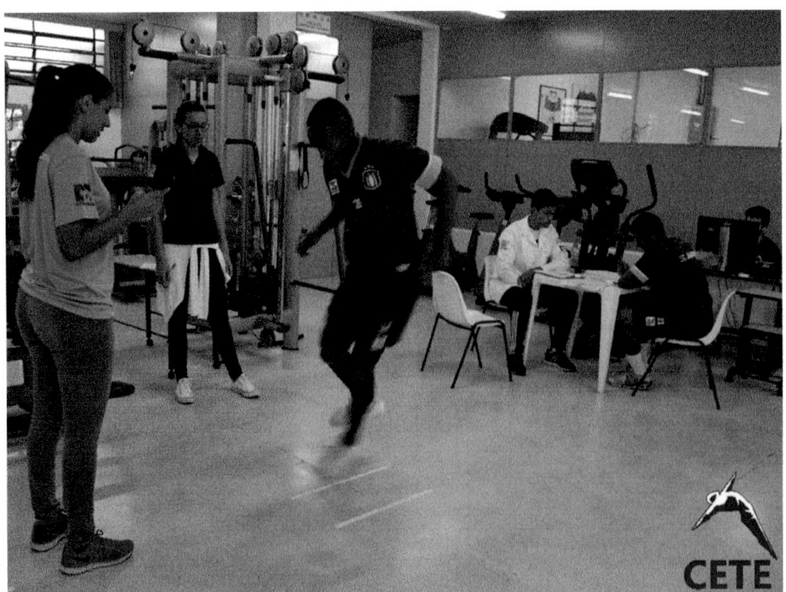

Fig. 12.2 Professional football player during a hop test evaluation

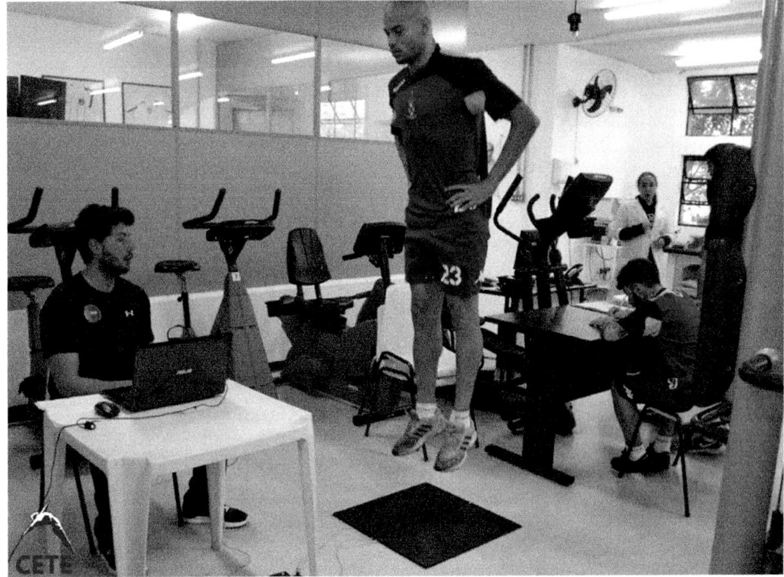

Fig. 12.3 Football player during vertical jump test evaluation

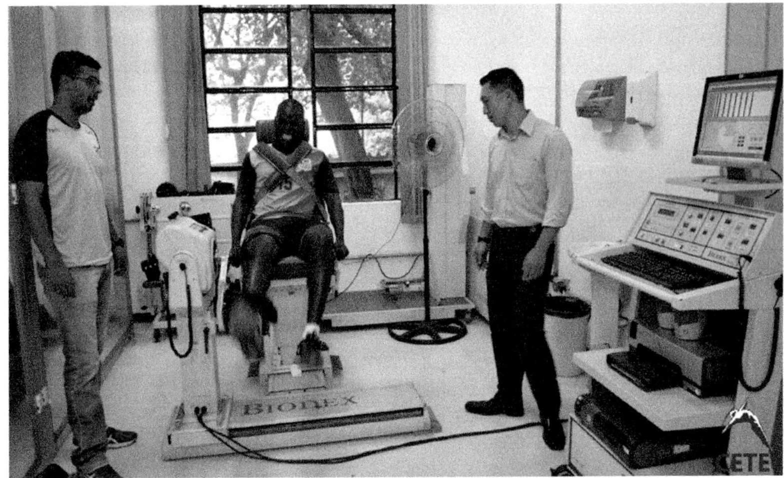

Fig. 12.4 Athlete during isokinetic muscle testing

Take-Home Message
Several factors influence the timing of return to soccer after ACL reconstruction. The surgeon should evaluate each case and each injury individually, but with the evidence available today, a later return to the sport, 8–9 months after surgery, may be preferable. In addition to the postoperative time, in Brazil, we evaluate function, symptoms, and activity with subjective questionnaires, psychological evaluation, clinical evaluations (pain, bowel movements, KT1000), and muscle-strength testing before beginning progressive reintegration of the player into sports.

Top Five Evidence-Based References

Walden M, Hagglund M, Magnusson H, Ekstrand J (2016) ACL injuries in men's professional football: a 15-year prospective study on time trends and return-to-play rates reveals only 65% of players still play at the top level 3 years after ACL rupture. Br J Sports Med 50:744–750

Ekstrand J, Hagglund M, Kristenson K, Magnusson H, Walden M (2013) Fewer ligament injuries but no preventive effect on muscle injuries and severe injuries: an 11-year follow-up of the UEFA Champions League injury study. Br J Sports Med 47:732–737

Bizzini M, Dvorak J (2015) FIFA 11+: an effective programme to prevent football injuries in various player groups worldwide-a narrative review. Br J Sports Med 49:577–579

Kyritsis P, Bahr R, Landreau P, Miladi R, Witvrouw E (2016) Likelihood of ACL graft rupture: not meeting six clinical discharge criteria before return to sport is associated with a four times greater risk of rupture. Br J Sports Med 50:946–951

Dingenen B, Gokeler A (2017) Optimization of the return-to-sport paradigm after anterior cruciate ligament reconstruction: a critical step back to move forward. Sports Med 47:1487. https://doi.org/10.1007/s40279-017-0674-6

References

1. Arliani GG, Lara PS, Astur DC, Cohen M, Goncalves JP, Ferretti M (2014) Impact of sports on health of former professional soccer players in Brazil. Acta Ortop Bras 22:188–190
2. Junge A, Dvorak J (2004) Soccer injuries: a review on incidence and prevention. Sports Med 34:929–938
3. Hawkins RD, Fuller CW (1999) A prospective epidemiological study of injuries in four English professional football clubs. Br J Sports Med 33:196–203
4. Cohen M, Abdalla RJ, Ejnisman B, Amaro JT (1997) Lesões Ortopédicas no futebol. Rev Bras Ortop 32:940–944
5. Arliani GG, Belangero PS, Runco JL, Cohen M (2011) The Brazilian Football Association (CBF) model for epidemiological studies on professional soccer player injuries. Clinics (Sao Paulo) 66:1707–1712
6. Pedrinelli A, Da Cunha GAR (2013) Estudo epidemiologico das lesoes no futebol profissional durante a Copa America de 2011. Rev Bras Ortop 48: 131–136
7. Pangrazio O, Forriol F (2016) Epidemiology of soccer players traumatic injuries during the 2015 America Cup. Muscles Ligaments Tendons J 6:124–130
8. Walden M, Hagglund M, Magnusson H, Ekstrand J (2016) ACL injuries in men's professional football: a 15-year prospective study on time trends and return-to-play rates reveals only 65% of players still play at the top level 3 years after ACL rupture. Br J Sports Med 50:744–750
9. Farber J, Harris JD, Kolstad K, McCulloch PC (2014) Treatment of anterior cruciate ligament injuries by major league soccer team physicians. Orthop J Sports Med 2:1–7
10. Arliani GG, Astur Dda C, Kanas M, Kaleka CC, Cohen M (2012) Anterior cruciate ligament injury: treatment and rehabilitation. current perspectives and trends. Rev Bras Ortop 47:191–196
11. Mohtadi NG, Chan DS, Dainty KN, Whelan DB (2011) Patellar tendon versus hamstring tendon autograft for anterior cruciate ligament rupture in adults. Cochrane Database Syst Rev:CD005960. https://doi.org/10.1002/14651858.CD005960.pub2
12. Ekstrand J, Hagglund M, Kristenson K, Magnusson H, Walden M (2013) Fewer ligament injuries but no preventive effect on muscle injuries and severe injuries: an 11-year follow-up of the UEFA Champions League injury study. Br J Sports Med 47:732–737
13. Yamada RK, Arliani GG, Almeida GP, Venturine AM, Santos CV, Astur DC et al (2012) The effects of one-half of a soccer match on the postural stability and functional capacity of the lower limbs in young soccer players. Clinics (Sao Paulo) 67:1361–1364
14. Lundblad M, Walden M, Hagglund M, Ekstrand J, Thomee C, Karlsson J (2016) No association between return to play after injury and increased rate of anterior cruciate ligament injury in men's professional soccer. Orthop J Sports Med 4:2325967116669708
15. Bizzini M, Dvorak J (2015) FIFA 11+: an effective programme to prevent football injuries in various player groups worldwide-a narrative review. Br J Sports Med 49:577–579
16. Owoeye OB, Akinbo SR, Tella BA, Olawale OA (2014) Efficacy of the FIFA 11+ warm-up programme in male youth football: a cluster randomised controlled trial. J Sports Sci Med 13:321–328
17. Grooms DR, Palmer T, Onate JA, Myer GD, Grindstaff T (2013) Soccer-specific warm-up and lower extremity injury rates in collegiate male soccer players. J Athl Train 48:782–789
18. Leal MF, Astur DC, Debieux P, Arliani GG, Silveira Franciozi CE, Loyola LC et al (2015) Identification of suitable reference genes for investigating gene expression in anterior cruciate ligament injury by using reverse transcription-quantitative PCR. PLoS One 10:e0133323
19. Sandon A, Werner S, Forssblad M (2015) Factors associated with returning to football after anterior cruciate ligament reconstruction. Knee Surg Sports Traumatol Arthrosc 23:2514–2521
20. Walden M, Hagglund M, Ekstrand J (2006) High risk of new knee injury in elite footballers with previous anterior cruciate ligament injury. Br J Sports Med 40:158–162. discussion 158-162
21. Arliani GG, Astur DC, Yamada RK, Yamada AF, Miyashita GK, Mandelbaum B et al (2014) Early osteoarthritis and reduced quality of life after retirement in former professional soccer players. Clinics (Sao Paulo) 69:589–594
22. Neyret P, Donell ST, DeJour D, DeJour H (1993) Partial meniscectomy and anterior cruciate ligament rupture in soccer players. A study with a minimum 20-year followup. Am J Sports Med 21:455–460
23. Wiggins AJ, Grandhi RK, Schneider DK, Stanfield D, Webster KE, Myer GD (2016) Risk of secondary injury in younger athletes after anterior cruciate ligament reconstruction: a systematic review and meta-analysis. Am J Sports Med 44:1861–1876
24. Barber-Westin SD, Noyes FR (2011) Factors used to determine return to unrestricted sports activities after anterior cruciate ligament reconstruction. Arthroscopy 27:1697–1705

25. Kyritsis P, Bahr R, Landreau P, Miladi R, Witvrouw E (2016) Likelihood of ACL graft rupture: not meeting six clinical discharge criteria before return to sport is associated with a four times greater risk of rupture. Br J Sports Med 50:946–951
26. Grindem H, Snyder-Mackler L, Moksnes H, Engebretsen L, Risberg MA (2016) Simple decision rules can reduce reinjury risk by 84% after ACL reconstruction: the Delaware-Oslo ACL cohort study. Br J Sports Med 50:804–808
27. Dingenen B, Gokeler A (2017) Optimization of the return-to-sport paradigm after anterior cruciate ligament reconstruction: a critical step back to move forward. Sports Med 47:1487. https://doi.org/10.1007/s40279-017-0674-6

13 Return to Sports Following Anterior Cruciate Ligament Reconstruction: Recommendations of the German Knee Society (Deutsche Kniegesellschaft, DKG)

Wolf Petersen, Christian Zantop, Andrea Achtnich, Thore Zantop, and Amelie Stöhr

Contents

W. Petersen (✉)
Martin Luther Hospital, Berlin, Germany
e-mail: wolf.petersen@pgdiakonie.de

C. Zantop
Return to Play, Straubing, Germany

A. Achtnich
Sportorthopädie, Munich, Germany

T. Zantop
Sporthopaedicum, Straubing, Germany

A. Stöhr
Orthopaedic Surgery Munich OCM, Munich, Germany

13.1 Introduction

Injury of the anterior cruciate ligament (ACL) is a frequent sports injury, which commonly leads to loss of the athletic activity level [6]. In athletes with symptomatic instability, ACL reconstruction with an autologous tendon graft is the treatment of choice [44]. Restoration of passive stability can improve the function of the joint and prevents from further injuries to meniscus and cartilage [1]. Recent systematic reviews could even confirm that ACL reconstruction can reduce the rate of osteoarthritis rates [1, 57].

Achieving the preinjury level of activity is the main goal for the ACL-reconstructed professional and recreational athlete. Especially professional athletes want to return to their preinjury activities as early as possible. However, after surgery the graft passes through a remodeling process, which weakens the graft [15, 28, 29, 31, 42, 53]. For this reason a too early return to sports can be dangerous with the risk of early re-rupture.

The discussion about the optimal time for return to sports is controversial [9, 21, 47]. A recent systematic review has shown that time

V. Musahl et al. (eds.), *Return to Play in Football*, https://doi.org/10.1007/978-3-662-55713-6_13

after surgery is the sole criterion in most studies, recommending sports clearance after 6 months [9]. Other authors report about return to sports even 3 months after surgery [52]. Recent histological biopsy studies have shown that the remodeling process of ACL grafts in humans can take up to 2 years [15, 28, 29, 31, 42]. For this reason it is to be assumed that at 6 months after surgery, the graft does not have a sufficient strength to resist functional stress during high demanding activities. However, 2-year absence of sports can mean the end of the career for a high-level athlete. Therefore, at the time of return to sports, the knee must be functionally stabilized to protect the healing graft. During the rehabilitation period, the functional stability of the joint is normally impaired because limited weight bearing and restricted range of motion lead to deficits in muscle strength, balance, and coordination. Therefore, additional functional criteria instead of postoperative time only should be used to determine if an athlete can safely return to sports.

This article summarizes a project of the ligament committee of the German Knee Society. Using objective literature research, an evidence-based return to sports algorithm was established.

13.2 Scientific Basis

13.2.1 Re-rupture Rates and Risk Factors

Re-rupture rates after ACL reconstruction and return to sports vary between 2% and 23% in current literature; the prevalence of contralateral ACL rupture is even 7–24% [18, 26, 30, 36, 49, 58]. Risk factors for re-rupture in general are age under 20 years, female gender, high activity level, and high-risk pivoting sports (e.g., soccer, basketball, handball, alpine skiing) [5, 16, 18, 66, 68, 69].

Neuromuscular deficits are likely to be a reason for the large prevalence of ACL ruptures in the nonoperated contralateral knee [24]. In female athletes a correlation between functional valgus and injury prevalence could be detected [25]. There are, however, indications that these mechanisms also apply to men.

These findings are in accordance with video analyses showing predominantly noncontact injury mechanisms in primary ACL ruptures [24]. Athletes at risk for ACL rupture often exhibit motion patterns similar to classic ACL injury mechanism: landing after a jump with a slightly flexed knee in combination with valgus alignment and the body's center of gravity behind the knee [24]. Valgus alignment here is also referred to as medial collapse or functional valgus [24].

Injury-prone valgus drift immediately following the one-legged landing or stabilization phase can be triggered by missing eccentric strength of the quadriceps muscle, missing strength of hip stabilizing muscles with consecutive pelvic tilt to the contralateral side, excess ankle eversion, as well as missing coordinative and proprioceptive properties or a combination of the abovementioned. Similar mechanisms were also identified for alpine skier and judoka.

Athletes with such motion patterns should be identified during rehabilitation after ACL reconstruction using simple functional tests. Prevention studies have shown that hazardous motion patterns can successfully be modified in special training programs with consecutive decreased reinjury rates [24, 48]. These programs comprise balance, jumping, and specific strength training for protective knee flexors, stabilizing quadriceps and hip abductors.

In conclusion, individual neuromuscular risk factors for ACL re-rupture must be taken into account during rehabilitation after ACL reconstruction. Hazardous motion patterns should be addressed by physical therapy.

13.2.2 Remodeling of ACL Grafts

The remodeling process of an ACL graft is fundamental for the return to sports decision. The duration of this healing process can barely be influenced [42, 43].

Rodeo et al. showed that osteointegration in a dog model needs 12 weeks [51]. According to the authors, the respective duration in humans is estimated to be twice as long [51]. Weiler et al.

found tendon-bone healing after 24 weeks in sheep [67]. This hypothesis is supported by an MRI study that detected substantial bone edema surrounding the bone tunnels 6 months postoperatively [3].

The remodeling process of the graft is distinguished from osteointegration [42]. The devascularized tendon graft is subject to necrosis and must be revascularized thereafter. Fibroblasts grow into the graft, new collagen is synthesized, and functional load transforms the graft into a mature ligament. According to the literature, this process can be divided into three phases [11, 42]: early healing phase, remodeling phase, and maturation phase [2, 11, 33, 42, 56].

Biopsy studies of human grafts have shown that these remodeling phases are longer than the remodeling phases observed in animal models [11, 42]. The duration of the early healing phase varies between 3 and 6 months, the remodeling phase between 3 and 12 months, and the maturation phase between 4 and 36 months [11, 42]. No difference could be shown comparing the duration of healing phases for patellar and hamstring tendon grafts. It is to be assumed that also the mechanical stability of the graft is reduced for this long period.

Many surgeons recommend a 6-month time span as sole criterion for return to sports (time-based approach) [33]. At this time grafts may be osteointegrated, but there is scientific evidence that ligamentous remodeling is not yet completed. Thus, functional stability of the knee joint must be optimal to protect the graft during this process and should be objectively assessed.

13.2.3 Joint Homeostasis After ACL Reconstruction

Injury and surgical trauma impair joint homeostasis. Typical impairments are composed of pain, swelling, reduced range of motion, and reduced passive stability. These symptoms usually normalize with rehabilitation. Persisting symptoms, however, can be hints for structural joint dysfunctions such as cyclops syndrome, arthrofibrosis, and graft failure or tunnel malpositioning.

It is obvious that an intact homeostasis of the knee joint is crucial for a safe return to sports [47].

13.2.4 Strength Deficits After ACL Reconstruction

Several systematic reviews have shown that relevant strength deficits can persist after ACL reconstruction and can often be detected even after more than 6 months postoperatively [38, 46, 70].

Weakened quadriceps muscles were seen when using patellar tendon grafts, whereas decreased knee flexion strength is accompanied with the use of hamstring tendon autografts. Both muscle groups are relevant concerning re-ruptures. Quadriceps strength coheres with hazardous motion patterns during jumps [59]. Flexors act as functional agonists to the ACL [39]. Some studies could also detect postoperative muscular deficits in the hip and foot abnormalities [46, 70]. Hip muscle deficits can negatively influence lower limb rotation and promote a functional valgus position of the knee [24, 45]. Functional valgus position can lead to a medial collapse.

In conclusion, adequate regeneration of leg muscle strength is important for return to sports and should be objectively evaluated using simple measurements and tests [62].

13.2.5 Neuromuscular Control of the Knee: Functional Stability

Athletic and activities of daily living rely on coordinated neuromuscular knee control, which can be substantially impaired after an ACL rupture [17, 54, 55]. These functional deficits seem mainly due to proprioception loss resulting in disturbed intermuscular coordination between ACL agonists (flexors) and antagonists (M. quadriceps). Subluxations and re-ruptures can probably be prevented by enhanced neuromuscular control and achievement of functional stability [17, 32, 35, 60]. Some individuals can almost completely compensate for missing passive stability using neuromuscular control mechanisms ("copers") [17, 41, 54, 55, 60].

Several studies have shown that deficits in proprioception, balance, and neuromuscular control can persist up to 12–30 months after ACL reconstruction [10, 14, 39, 40, 61, 63, 64].

In conclusion, functional knee joint stability should be considered as key point to give a safe return to sports recommendation.

Fact Box 1

- Functional or dynamic valgus is the main risk factor for ACL rupture.
- Hip muscle deficits can negatively influence lower limb rotation and promote a functional valgus position of the knee.
- Biopsy studies in humans have shown that graft remodeling can take up to 2 years.
- Knee flexors (hamstrings) act as functional agonists to the ACL and can protect the ACL.
- Several studies have shown that deficits in proprioception, balance, and neuromuscular control can persist up to 12–30 months after ACL reconstruction.
- Functional knee joint stability should be considered as one key point to give a safe return to sports recommendation.

13.3 "Return to Sports" Algorithm

These facts show that different criteria must be taken into account for an individual and safe return to sports decision. Based on this evidence, the ligament committee of the German Knee Society (DKG) has developed an algorithm for a return to sports recommendation [47]. This return to sports algorithm is shown in Fig. 13.1.

13.3.1 Temporal Aspect

It is obvious that a predetermined time period is not a sufficient stand-alone criterion since graft remodeling seems to take up to 2 years after surgery. In daily practice, most athletes however return to sporting activities between 6 and 10 months after surgery. Dedicated rehabilitation measures can normalize joint function within this time frame so that there is sufficient functional protection for further graft maturation [47].

At a time point where structural graft properties are not comparable to the normal ACL, the following prerequisites are mandatory for return to competitive sports: joint homeostasis, normal muscle strength, normal functional knee stability, and normal neuromuscular control of the lower limb.

If this is not the case, rehabilitation should be continued after ruling out structural reasons. The scope of tests to evaluate these criteria must be individually adapted to athletic ambition and available resources.

13.3.2 Joint Homeostasis

Joint homeostasis should be present for a "return to sports" decision [47]. The knee must be without effusion; range of motion and passive stability should be equivalent to the nonoperated contralateral side. These factors can be evaluated within the objective IKDC 2000 score (Fig. 13.2).

Before "returning to sports," the respective knee should be classified as "A" or "B" according to the objective IKDC score. Passive stability should be tested using Lachman and pivot shift tests. Anterior-posterior stability can be quantified by instrumented Lachman test with "KT-1000 arthrometer" or "rolimeter."

In the presence of "C" or "D" criteria according to the objective IKDC score, further diagnostics should be conducted. Graft structure, tunnel placement, cyclops lesions, and concomitant injuries can be evaluated on MRI scans. A 3D CT is helpful for further analysis of tunnel malpositioning. Laboratory results can help if there is suspicion for a joint infection. If pathologies are detected, the indication for revision surgery (arthroscopy, arthrolysis) must be considered.

A normal joint homeostasis (IKDC A or B) is prerequisite for further tests to analyze strength, functional stability, and neuromuscular function [47].

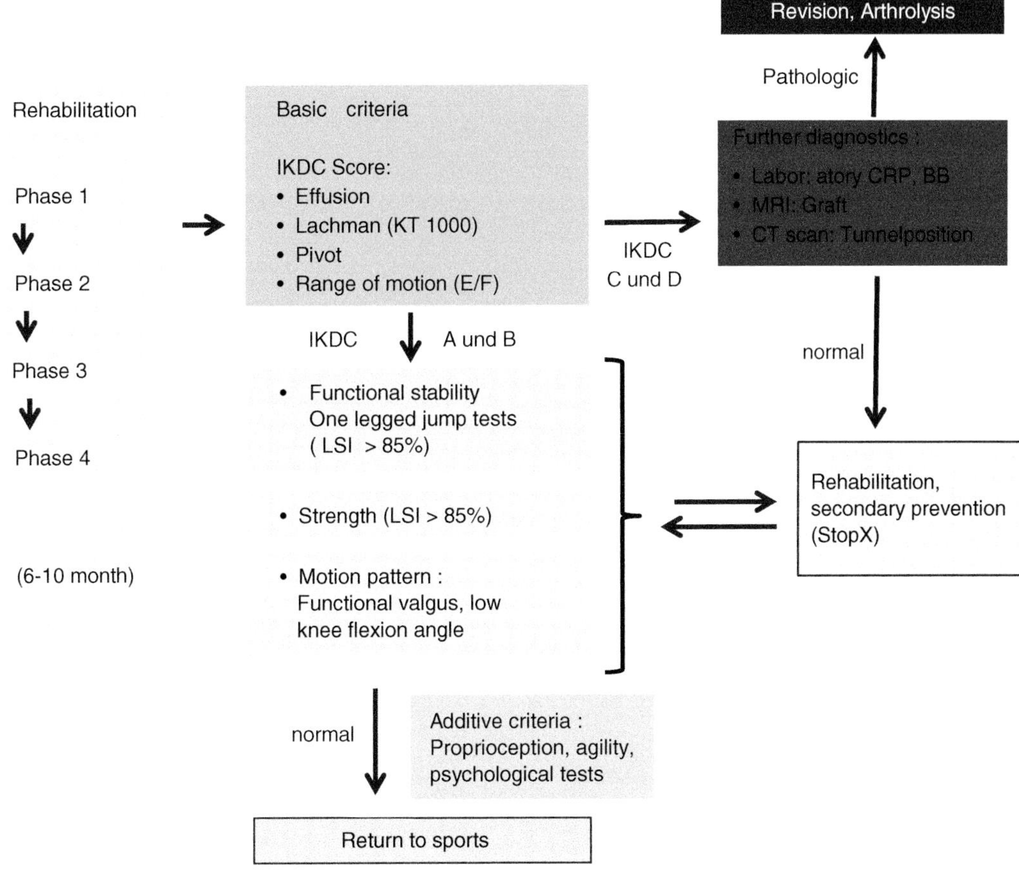

Fig. 13.1 Return to sports algorithm as recommended by the German Knee Society (Deutsche Kniegesellschaft, DKG)

	A	B	C	D
1. Effusion	None	Mild	Moderate	Severe
2. Passive range of motion				
Δ extension deficit	< 3°	3-5°	6-10°	> 10°
Δ flexion deficit	0-5°	6-15°	16-25°	> 25°
3. Ligament-examination (manual, instrumented, stress x ray)				
Δ Lachman test (mm)	1-2°	3-5°	6-10°	>10°
anterior endpoint:		☐ firm		☐ soft
Δ Pivot shift	equal	glide	gross	marked

Fig. 13.2 Objective IKDC 2000 score (https://www.sportsmed.org/AOSSMIMIS/Members/Research/IKDC_Forms/Members/Research/IKDC_Forms.aspx?hkey=4e0ca7a9-3a3c-49f9-b9b6-4e133de4ad22)

13.3.3 Muscle Strength

Muscle strength can be measured with various methods. Most common are instrumented isokinetic strength measurements of knee extensors and flexors (Fig. 13.3). The athlete has to move a lever with predetermined angular speed (e.g., 60°/s or 120°/s); different strength qualities can be measured (concentric/eccentric strength, strength endurance, etc.). Several parameters can be determined depending on the test protocol: strength (Nm), labor, power, acceleration energy, antagonist/agonist relations, muscle fatigue, and recuperation. Details concerning respective angular velocities differ in the studies [46, 70]. Angular speeds of 60–240°/s are used in practice. Maximum torque (Nm) is presented as maximum strength. The highest values for concentric strength are achieved at low angular velocities (up to 60°/s). Respective speeds are increased to evaluate springiness. Limb symmetry is the goal. Strength measurement of <90% compared to the contralateral side is a hint for rehabilitation deficits [71]. Knee flexors should receive increased attention since they can protect the ACL. Isokinetic measurements and functional stability tests should be part of the "return to sports" decision in competitive athletes.

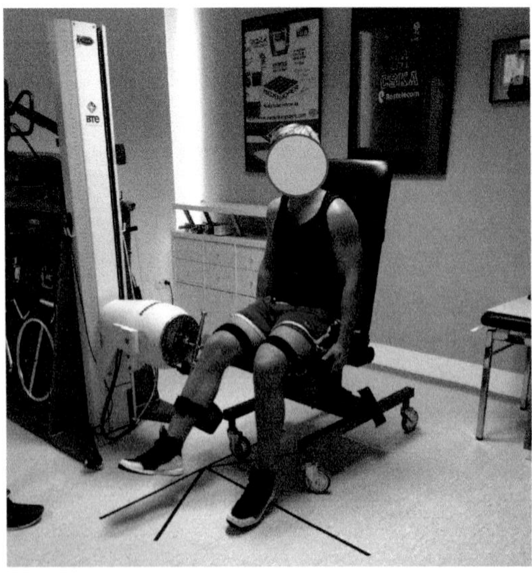

Fig. 13.3 Isokinetic strength test (Return to play, Straubing)

Due to the weakness of limb symmetry index (LSI) comparing only injured to noninjured limb, preinjury status should regularly be documented (especially in professional athletes). Thus, muscle strength should be presented as both absolute values and LSI.

More simple strength measurement methods can be used for recreational athletes. Examples are maximal strength tests with guided training devices (e.g., leg press) or circumference measurements of the lower limb (15 cm below, 10 cm and 20 cm above the medial knee joint line) as indirect method. Measurements on the operated leg should be at least 90% of the contralateral values here, too.

13.3.4 Functional Stability

Simple single-leg jump/hop tests have proven useful to evaluate functional stability [19, 20, 22, 23, 27, 37, 40, 62]. Various jump tests differing in complexity are described in literature (Table 13.1).

In practice single-leg jumps for distance tests are most feasible since they can be carried out in a large examination room (Fig. 13.4). The respective results are compared to the healthy contralateral side. These tests can easily be applied to recreational athletes and are valid predictors for good knee function. The single-leg jump test (distance) has been shown to correlate with good subjective knee function [17].

For competitive athletes, a test battery with various single-leg jump tests should be used (Table 13.1). Test-retest reliability could be shown for single-leg jump tests in several studies [20, 50]. Using them a lower limb symmetry index (LSI) can be assessed. Usually LSI is calculated with the means of three jump tests for the operated and nonoperated side. Most authors consider an LSI of >85% as a sufficient "return to sports" criterion [39, 64]. In the objective IKDC score, an LSI of more than 90% is classified as A (normal), an LSI of 89–75% as B (nearly normal), an LSI of

Table 13.1 Different jump tests which can be used for the return to sports analysis

Test	Execution
1. Distance jump test	The subject is on the test leg with arms folded on the back. He is asked to jump as far as possible with the test leg. Test is highly reliable and is the easiest to perform in clinical practice
2. Triple jump test	The subject is on the test leg with arms folded on the back. He is prompted to jump with the test leg three times as far as possible
3. Six meter jump test for time	The patient is asked to bounce on the test legs 6 m distance. The time is determined by a stopwatch
4. Vertical jump test	In the vertical jump test, the subject must jump as high as possible. The evaluation is only possible with a special measuring system (MuscleLab, Ergotest Technology) that can convert the flight time to jumping height. This test is therefore only applicable in special scientific facilities
5. Square jump test	The subject is on the test leg within a marked square. An additional 10 cm frame is marked outside this square. The subjects have to be one legged (for the right leg clockwise) for 30 s as often as they can in and outside the square. The number of jumps without affecting the frame count as a test result
6. Lateral jump test	The test person is standing on the test leg with his hands on his back. It must have side jumps between two marks (distance 40 cm). The subject must jump 30 s as often as possible between the markers. He may land only outside the markers

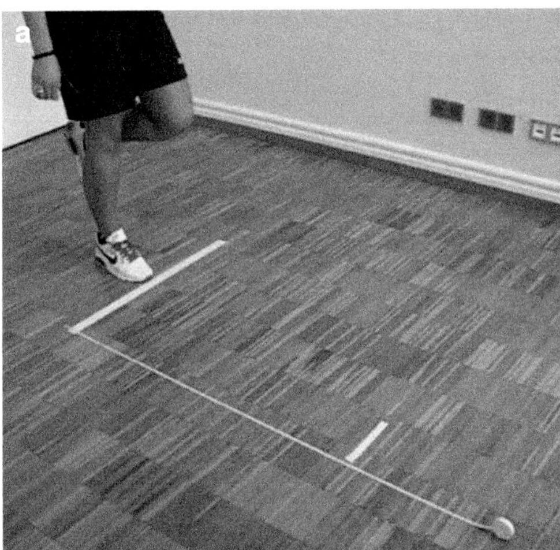
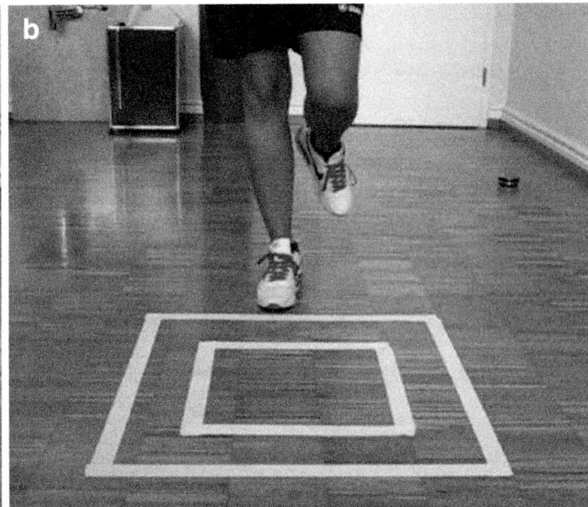

Fig. 13.4 (**a**) Distance jump test: in the one-legged jump test for distance, it is important to jump with one leg as far as possible. The jumps are repeated three times. The percentage difference between the mean values for the three jumps of the right and left leg results in the lower limb symmetry index. (**b**) Square jump test: in the square jump test, the test person should land as many jumps as possible outside the square (right and left). The lower limb symmetry index is calculated from the difference between the successful landings

75–50% as C (abnormal), and an LSI <50% as D (severely abnormal).

Jump tests are very demanding for the knee. Thus, they should only be performed under the following conditions: (1) no intra-articular effusion, (2) full ROM, (3) unrestricted straight leg lifting, (4) jumping possible without pain, and (5) patient's subjective well-being.

13.3.5 Motion Analysis: Dynamic Valgus

In recent years functional valgus of the knee has been recognized because valgus collapse is considered as a main risk factor for ACL rupture and re-rupture following ACL reconstruction [8, 24, 48]. Functional leg axis analysis has received little

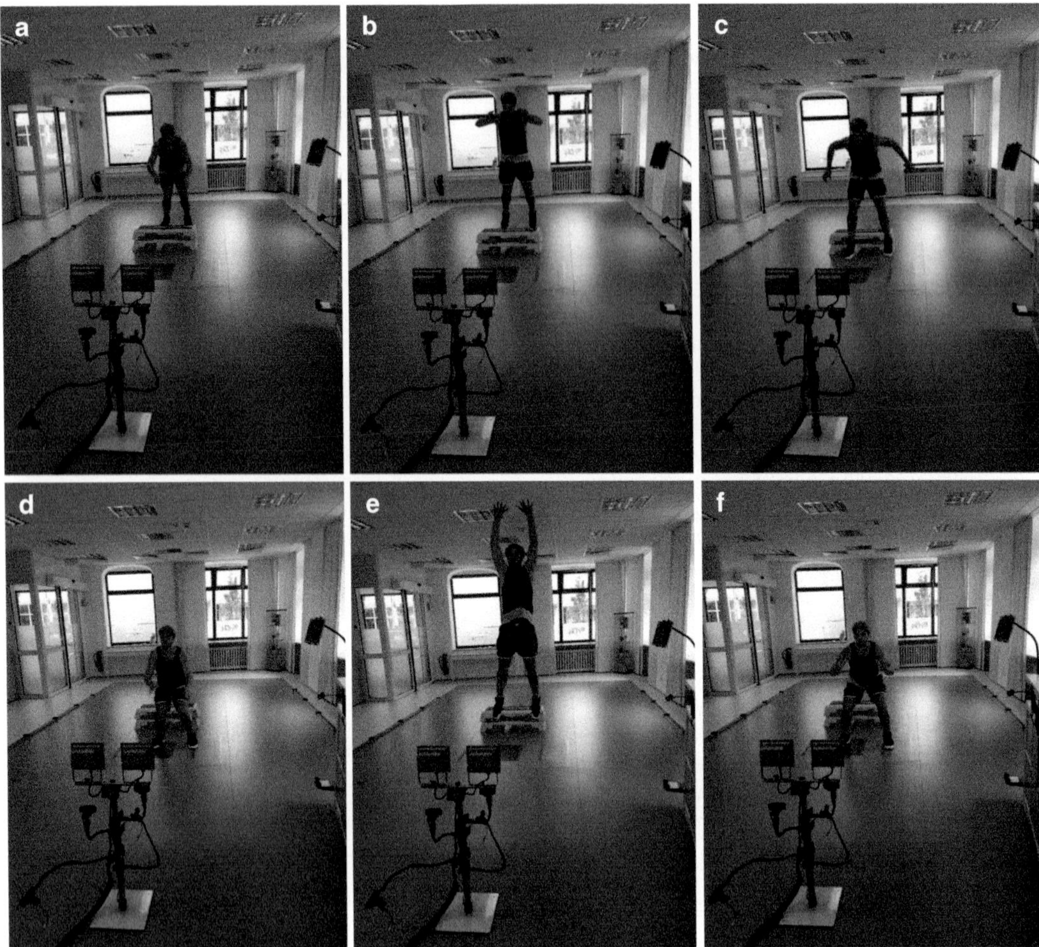

Fig. 13.5 (**a–f**) Vertical drop jump test (Return to play, Straubing)

attention in the evaluation of single-leg jump tests to date, while valgus collapse can be seen in the frontal plane during many jump tests. There are various possibilities to analyze dynamic valgus. Dichotomous classification as valgus and non-valgus is simple and clinically pragmatic. A video camera with slow motion function can be helpful for demonstration purposes; the frontal plane projection angle (FPPA) (Fig. 13.5) can be quantitatively assessed.

Today mobile phone/tablet apps can produce sufficient slow motion videos with the opportunity to measure the FFPA (e.g., "hudl" technique app).

Noyes et al. [8, 40] have described a vertical jump test from a box in which the leg axis during landing is analyzed using a video camera (more than 60% knee distance). The athletes are only instructed to jump from the box landing in a proper angle to the observer and camera and to then perform a maximal vertical hop [40]. This sequence is repeated three times, and enhanced motion analysis is possible with professional 3D imaging. However, under clinical aspects, two-dimensional methods evaluating standard camera recordings in the frontal plane have proven to be sufficient. The camera is placed 3 m from the box.

The following frames are extracted from the video recording: (1) before landing, toe-ground contact; (2) landing, lowest athlete position; and (3) takeoff, upward arm movement. The landing moment is the moment in which the knee is most out of control. Frontal plane projection angle or knee-to-ankle distance proportion can be assessed (Fig. 13.5). Minzner et al. [35] could show a correlation of two-dimensional to three-dimensional analyses for knee-to-ankle distance proportion. Qualitative evaluation of "valgus or non-valgus" can also be performed by inspection instead of recording.

Another test for dynamic valgus are single-leg squats (Fig. 13.6) [13]. Valgus collapse during this test correlates with poor hip abductor function [4, 13]. In the original version of the test, the athlete is standing on a 20 cm high box with crossed arms: he has then to perform five single-leg squats as slow as possible (each squat over 2 s) which are recorded with a video camera. According to determined criteria, the single-leg squats are classified as good, average, or poor.

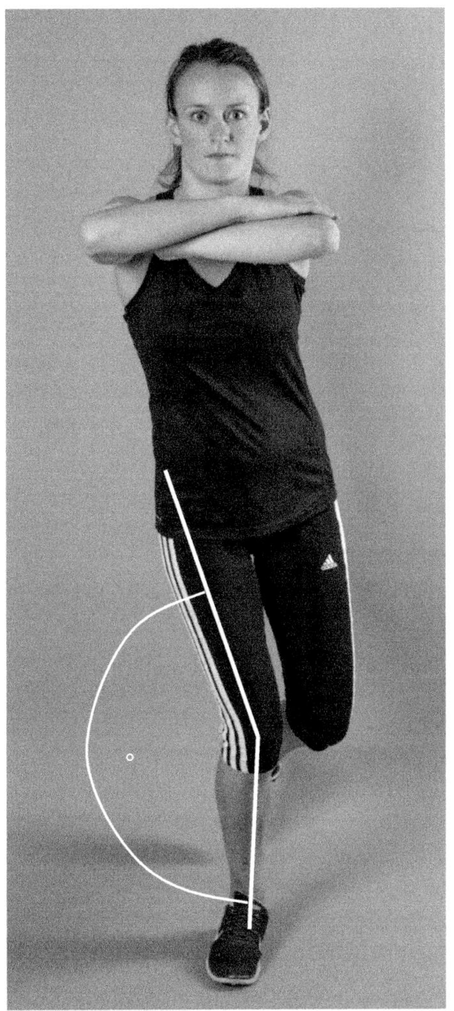

Fig. 13.6 One-legged squat for the analysis of the frontal plane projection angle (FPPA). This picture shows a low FPPA which is not desired (picture from the Stop X program, German Knee Society)

13.3.6 Additional Functional Tests

This test battery can be extended by further functional tests. This extension of the test battery involves the detection of proprioception, agility, and psychological factors and is especially recommended for professional athletes. But of course these additional tests can also be used for recreational athletes [22].

Proprioceptive or balance characteristics can be detected with the star excursion balance test (SEBT) [12]. In ACL-reconstructed patients, the SEBT reach distance was associated with lower extremity muscle strength [12].

Agility can be accessed with a speed court test [34]. Agility should be especially assessed in professional athletes (Fig. 13.7).

Psychological factors have high influence on the return to competitive sports rate [7]. Fear of new injury was the most important reason for no return to competitive sports [7]. The ACL return to sports after injury scale (ACL-RSI) is a validated questionnaire to evaluate psychological after ACL reconstruction [65].

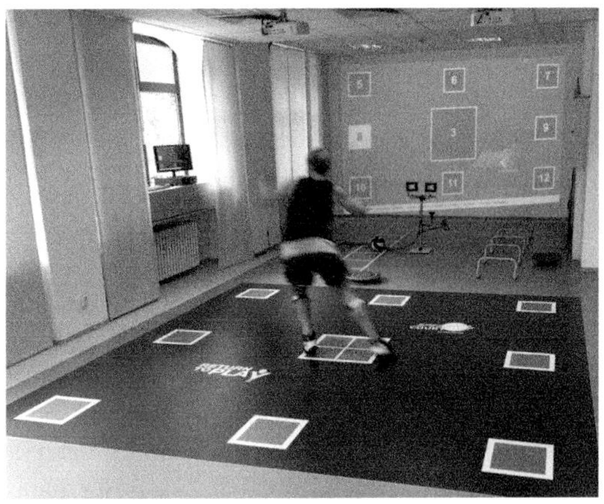

Fig. 13.7 Agility test using a speed court (Return to play, Straubing)

13.4 Secondary Prevention of ACL Ruptures: Stop X Program

Fact Box 2

- Time-based return to sports recommendations should be left in favor of functional recommendations.
- A return to sports algorithm includes basic criteria and additive criteria.
- Basic criteria are free range of motion, absence of effusion, and passive knee stability (A or B according to objective IKDC score).
- Normal basis criteria are prerequisites for further functional test such as strength test, functional stability tests, or neuromuscular function tests.
- Additive criteria include proprioception tests, agility test, and psychological tests.

If the functional analysis of the motion pattern reveals any risk factors such as dynamic valgus, the athlete should be encouraged to complete a special prevention program. For this reason the ligament committee of the German Knee Society has put together a special program for the prevention of knee injuries [48]. The name of this program is "Stop X" (Fig. 13.8). The main goal of this program is to correct the dynamic valgus [48]. More detailed information about this program can be found on these websites:

1. http://stop-x.de/
2. http://deutsche-kniegesellschaft.de/wp-content/uploads/2017/02/DKG_Stop-X_Pr%C3%A4vention-von-Sportverletzungen-am-Kniegelenk.pdf

Various studies have shown that such specific training programs can reduce the incidence of ACL injuries significantly [48]. Elements of these programs are (1) information about injury mechanism, (2) strength training with focus on hamstring and hip abductor strength, (3) jump training, (4) balance exercises, and (5) running exercises.

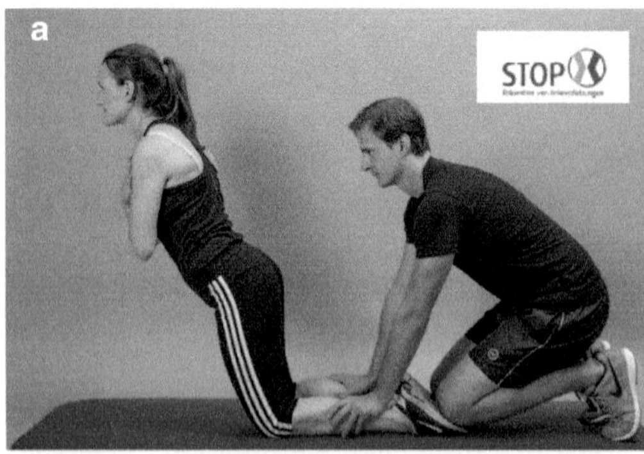

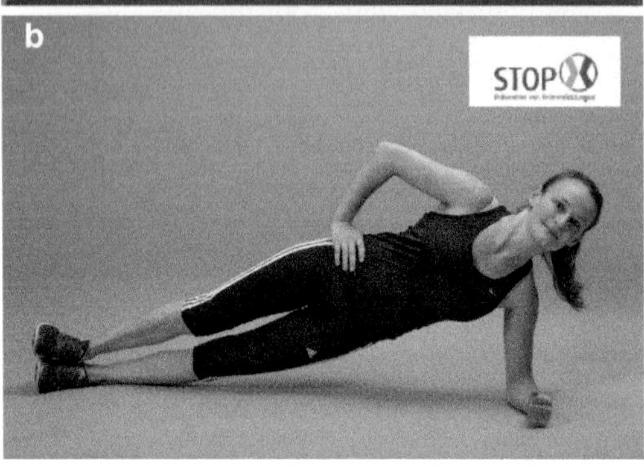

Fig. 13.8 Exercises from the German Knee Society ACL injury prevention program "Stop X." From: Petersen W, Diermeier T, Mehl J, Stöhr A, Ellermann A, Müller P, Höher J, Herbort M, Akoto R, Zantop T, Herbst E, Jung T, Patt T, Stein T, Best R, Stoffels T, Achtnich A: Prävention von Knieverletzungen und VKB-Rupturen. Empfehlungen des DKG Komitees Ligamentverletzungen. OUP 2016; 10: 542–550 DOI 10.3238/oup.2016.0542–0550. (**a**) This exercise is called "Russian hamstrings." With this exercise, the hamstring muscles can be trained. The subject should bend the upper body downward to approx. 45° and then reerect. The upper body and the thigh should be in line. The exercise is repeated up to ten times. (**b**) Static hip exercise: this exercise trains the hip abductors. The subject should hold this position as long as possible. Upper body and leg should be in line

Take-Home Message

At the time when athletes normally return to sports after ACL reconstruction (6–10 months postoperatively), graft remodeling is still not complete (duration approximately 24 months). Therefore, purely time-based return to sports recommendations should be left in favor of functional recommendations. A return to sports algorithm includes basic criteria and additive criteria. Basic criteria are free range of motion, absence of effusion, and passive knee stability (A or B according to objective IKDC score). Normal basis criteria are prerequisites for further functional test such as strength test, functional stability tests, or neuromuscular function tests. If basic criteria such as effusion, passive stability, and ROM are rated as IKDC grade A or B, functional tests (one-legged jump tests) to assess neuromuscular function and strength as well a motion analyses should be applied (vertical drop jump test, one-legged squat). Further diagnostic steps must be considered if basic criteria are rated as C or D according to IKDC classification. This algorithm can be extended by balance, agility, or psychological tests.

Additive criteria include proprioception tests, agility test, and psychological tests.

The goal of the described algorithm is to find the best possible and individual time point for a safe return to sports.

Acknowledgment All members of the ligament committee of the German Knee Society (Deutsche Kniegesellschaft, DKG) contributed to the development of the presented algorithm: Petersen W, Diermeier T, Mehl J, Stöhr A, Ellermann A, Müller P, Höher J, Herbort M, Akoto R, Zantop T, Herbst E, Jung T, Patt T, Stein T, Best R, Stoffels T, and Achtnich A.

Top Five Evidence Based References

Ajuied A, Wong F, Smith C, Norris M, Earnshaw P, Back D, Davies A (2014) Anterior cruciate ligament injury and radiologic progression of knee osteoarthritis: a systematic review and meta-analysis. Am J Sports Med 42(9):2242–2252

Andernord D, Desai N, Björnsson H, Gillén S, Karlsson J, Samuelsson K (2015) Predictors of contralateral anterior cruciate ligament reconstruction: a cohort study of 9061 patients with 5-year follow-up. Am J Sports Med 43(2):295–330

Herbst E, Hoser C, Hildebrandt C, Raschner C, Hepperger C, Pointner H, Fink C (2015) Functional assessments for decision-making regarding return to sports following ACL reconstruction. Part II: clinical application of a new test battery. Knee Surg Sports Traumatol Arthrosc 23(5):1283–1291

Pauzenberger L, Syré S, Schurz M (2013) "Ligamentization" in hamstring tendon grafts after anterior cruciate ligament reconstruction: a systematic review of the literature and a glimpse into the future. Arthroscopy 29(10):1712–1721

Petersen W, Taheri P, Forkel P, Zantop T (2014) Return to play following ACL reconstruction: a systematic review about strength deficits. Arch Orthop Trauma Surg 134(10):1417–1428

References

1. Ajuied A, Wong F, Smith C, Norris M, Earnshaw P, Back D, Davies A (2014) Anterior cruciate ligament injury and radiologic progression of knee osteoarthritis: a systematic review and meta-analysis. Am J Sports Med 42(9):2242–2225
2. Abe S, Kurosaka M, Iguchi T, Yoshiya S, Hirohata K (1993) Light and electron microscopic study of remodeling and maturation process in autogenous graft for anterior cruciate ligament reconstruction. Arthroscopy 9:394–405
3. Achtnich A, Stiepani H, Forkel P, Metzlaff S, Hänninen EL, Petersen W (2013) Tunnel widening after anatomic double-bundle and mid-position single-bundle anterior cruciate ligament reconstruction. Arthroscopy 29(9):1514–1524
4. Ageberg E, Bennell KL, Hunt MA, Simic M, Roos EM, Creaby MW (2010) Validity and inter-rater reliability of mediolateral knee motion observed during a single-limb mini squat. BMC Musculoskelet Disord 11:265
5. Andernord D, Desai N, Björnsson H, Gillén S, Karlsson J, Samuelsson K (2015) Predictors of contralateral anterior cruciate ligament reconstruction: a cohort study of 9061 patients with 5-year follow-up. Am J Sports Med 43(2):295–330
6. Ardern CL, Webster KE, Taylor NF, Feller JA (2011) Return to sport following anterior cruciate ligament reconstruction surgery: a systematic review and meta-analysis of the state of play. Br J Sports Med 45(7):596–606
7. Ardern CL, Webster KE, Taylor NF, Feller JA (2011) Return to the preinjury level of competitive sport after anterior cruciate ligament reconstruction surgery: two-thirds of patients have not returned by 12 months after surgery. Am J Sports Med 39(3):538–543
8. Barber-Westin SD, Smith ST, Campbell T, Noyes FR (2010) The drop-jump video screening test: retention of improvement in neuromuscular control in female volleyball players. J Strength Cond Res 24(11):3055–3062
9. Barber-Westin SD, Noyes FR (2011) Factors used to determine return to unrestricted sports activities after anterior cruciate ligament reconstruction. Arthroscopy 27(12):1697–1705
10. Bonfim TR, Paccola CA, Barela JA (2003) Proprioceptive and behavior impairments in individuals with anterior cruciate ligament reconstructed knees. Arch Phys Med Rehabil 84:1217–1223
11. Claes S, Verdonk P, Forsyth R, Bellemans J (2011) The "ligamentization" process in anterior cruciate ligament reconstruction: what happens to the human graft? A systematic review of the literature. Am J Sports Med 39(11):2476–2483
12. Clagg S, Paterno MV, Hewett T, Schmitt LC (2015) Performance on the modified star excursion balance test at the time of return to sports following anterior cruciate ligament reconstruction. J Orthop Sports Phys Ther 45(6):444–452

13. Crossley KM, Zhang WJ, Schache AG, Bryant A, Cowan SM (2011) Performance on the single-leg squat task indicates hip abductor muscle function. Am J Sports Med 39:866–873
14. Deneweth JM, Bey MJ, McLean SG, Lock TR, Kolowich PA, Tashman S (2010) Tibiofemoral joint kinematics of the anterior cruciate ligament-reconstructed knee during a single-legged hop landing. Am J Sports Med 38:1820–1828
15. Falconiero RP, DiStefano VJ, Cook TM (1998) Revascularization and ligamentization of autogenous anterior cruciate ligament grafts in humans. Arthroscopy 14:197–205
16. Faunø P, Rahr-Wagner L, Lind M (2014) Risk for revision after anterior cruciate ligament reconstruction is higher among adolescents: results from the danish registry of knee ligament reconstruction. Orthop J Sports Med 2(10):2325967114552405. https://doi.org/10.1177/2325967114552405
17. Fitzgerald GK, Lephart SM, Hwang JH, Wainner RS (2001) Hop tests as predictors of dynamic knee stability. J Orthop Sports Phys Ther 31(10):588–597
18. Gifstad T, Foss OA, Engebretsen L, Lind M, Forssblad M, Albrektsen G, Drogset JO (2014) Lower risk of revision with patellar tendon autografts compared with hamstring autografts: a registry study based on 45,998 primary ACL reconstructions in Scandinavia. Am J Sports Med 42(10):2319–2328
19. Gustavsson A, Neeter C, Thomeé P, Silbernagel KG, Augustsson J, Thomeé R, Karlsson J (2006) A test battery for evaluating hop performance in patients with an ACL injury and patients who have undergone ACL reconstruction. Knee Surg Sports Traumatol Arthrosc 14(8):778–788
20. Hall MP, Paik RS, Ware AJ, Mohr KJ, Limpisvasti O (2015) Neuromuscular evaluation with single-leg squat test at 6 months after anterior cruciate ligament reconstruction. Orthop J Sports Med 3(3):2325967115575900
21. Hartigan EH, Axe MJ, Snyder-Mackler L (2010) Time line for noncopers to pass return-to-sports criteria after anterior cruciate ligament reconstruction. J Orthop Sports Phys Ther 40:141–154
22. Herbst E, Hoser C, Hildebrandt C, Raschner C, Hepperger C, Pointner H, Fink C (2015) Functional assessments for decision-making regarding return to sports following ACL reconstruction. Part II: clinical application of a new test battery. Knee Surg Sports Traumatol Arthrosc 23(5):1283–1291
23. Hildebrandt C, Müller L, Zisch B, Huber R, Fink C, Raschner C (2015) Functional assessments for decision-making regarding return to sports following ACL reconstruction. Part I: development of a new test battery. Knee Surg Sports Traumatol Arthrosc 23(5):1273–1281
24. Hewett TE, Di Stasi SL, Myer GD (2013) Current concepts for injury prevention in athletes after anterior cruciate ligament reconstruction. Am J Sports Med 41(1):216–224
25. Hewett TE, Myer GD, Ford KR (2006) Preparticipation physical examination using a box drop vertical jump test in young athletes: the effects of puberty and sex. Clin J Sport Med 16:298–304
26. Hui C, Salmon LJ, Kok A, Maeno S, Linklater J, Pinczewski LA (2011) Fifteen-year outcome of endoscopic anterior cruciate ligament reconstruction with patellar tendon autograft for "isolated" anterior cruciate ligament tear. Am J Sports Med 39:89–98
27. Itoh H, Kurosaka M, Yoshiya S, Ichihashi N, Mizuno K (1998) Evaluation of functional deficits determined by four different hop tests in patients with anterior cruciate ligament deficiency. Knee Surg Sports Traumatol Arthrosc 6:241–245
28. Janssen RPA, van der Wijk J, Fiedler A (2011) Remodelling of human hamstring autografts after anterior cruciate ligament reconstruction. Knee Surg Sports Traumatol Arthrosc 19:1299–1306
29. Janssen RP, Scheffler SU (2014) Intra-articular remodelling of hamstring tendon grafts after anterior cruciate ligament reconstruction. Knee Surg Sports Traumatol Arthrosc 22(9):2102–2108
30. Keays SL, Bullock-Saxton JE, Keays AC, Newcombe PA, Bullock MI (2007) A 6-year follow-up of the effect of graft site on strength, stability, range of motion, function, and joint degeneration after anterior cruciate ligament reconstruction: patellar tendon versus semitendinosus and gracilis tendon graft. Am J Sports Med 35:729–739
31. Kondo E, Yasuda K, Katsura T et al (2012) Biomechanical and histological evaluations of the doubled semitendinosus tendon autograft after anterior cruciate ligament reconstruction in sheep. Am J Sports Med 40:315–324
32. Madhavan S, Shields RK (2011) Neuromuscular responses in individuals with anterior cruciate ligament repair. Clin Neurophysiol 122:997–1004
33. Mayr HO, Stoehr A, Dietrich M, von Eisenhart-Rothe R, Hube R, Senger S, Suedkamp NP, Bernstein A (2012) Graft-dependent differences in the ligamentization process of anterior cruciate ligament grafts in a sheep trial. Knee Surg Sports Traumatol Arthrosc 20(5):947–956
34. Mehran N, Williams PN, Keller RA, Khalil LS, Lombardo SJ, Kharrazi FD (2016) Athletic Performance at national basketball association combine after anterior cruciate ligament reconstruction. Orthop J Sports Med 25(4):2325967116648083
35. Minzner RL, Chmielewski TL, Toepke JJ, Tofte KB (2012) Comparison of 2-dimensional measurement techniques for predicting knee angle and moment during a drop vertical jump. Clin J Sport Med 22(3):221–227
36. Myklebust G, Holm I, Maehlum S, Engebretsen L, Bahr R (2003) Clinical, functional, and radiologic outcome in team handball players 6 to 11 years after anterior cruciate ligament injury: a follow-up study. Am J Sports Med 31:981–989
37. Myer GD, Paterno MV, Ford KR, Quatman CE, Hewett TE (2006) Rehabilitation after anterior cruciate ligament reconstruction: criteria-based progression through the return-to-sport phase. J Orthop Sports Phys Ther 36(6):385–402

38. Myer GD, Ford KR, Barber Foss KD, Liu C, Nick TG, Hewett TE (2009) The relationship of hamstrings and quadriceps strength to anterior cruciate ligament injury in female athletes. Clin J Sport Med 19(1):3–8
39. Noyes FR, Barber SD, Mangine RE (1991) Abnormal lower limb symmetry determined by function hop tests after anterior cruciate ligament rupture. Am J Sports Med 19:513–518
40. Noyes FR, Barber-Westin SD, Fleckenstein C, Walsh C, West J (2005) The drop-jump screening test: difference in lower limb control by gender and effect of neuromuscular training in female athletes. Am J Sports Med 33(2):197–207
41. Orishimo KF, Kremenic IJ, Mullaney MJ, McHugh MP, Nicholas SJ (2010) Adaptations in single leg hop biomechanics following anterior cruciate ligament reconstruction. Knee Surg Sports Traumatol Arthrosc 18:1587–1593
42. Pauzenberger L, Syré S, Schurz M (2013) "Ligamentization" in hamstring tendon grafts after anterior cruciate ligament reconstruction: a systematic review of the literature and a glimpse into the future. Arthroscopy 29(10):1712–1721
43. Petersen W, Laprell H (2000) Insertion of autologous tendon grafts to the bone: a histological and immunohistochemical study of hamstring and patellar tendon grafts. Knee Surg Sports Traumatol Arthrosc 8(1):26–31
44. Petersen W, Forkel P, Achtnich A, Metzlaff S, Zantop T (2013) Anatomic reconstruction of the anterior cruciate ligament in single bundle technique. Oper Orthop Traumatol 25(2):185–204
45. Petersen W, Ellermann A, Gösele-Koppenburg A, Best R, Rembitzki IV, Brüggemann GP, Liebau C (2014) Patellofemoral pain syndrome. Knee Surg Sports Traumatol Arthrosc 22(10):2264–2274
46. Petersen W, Taheri P, Forkel P, Zantop T (2014) Return to play following ACL reconstruction: a systematic review about strength deficits. Arch Orthop Trauma Surg 134(10):1417–1428
47. Petersen W, Stöhr A, Ellermann A, Achtnich A, Müller PE, Stoffels T, Patt T, Höher J, Herbort M, Akoto R, Jung T, Zantop C, Zantop T, Best R (2016) Wiederkehr zum Sport nach VKB-Rekonstruktion Empfehlungen der DKG-Expertengruppe Ligament. Deutscher Ärzte-Verlag, OUP 5(3):168
48. Petersen W, Diermeier T, Mehl J, Stöhr A, Ellermann A, Müller P, Höher J, Herbort M, Akoto R, Zantop T, Herbst E, Jung T, Patt T, Stein T, Best R, Stoffels T, Achtnich A (2016) Prävention von Knieverletzungen und VKB-Rupturen. Empfehlungen des DKG Komitees Ligamentverletzungen OUP 10:542–550. https://doi.org/10.3238/oup.2016.0542–0550
49. Pinczewski LA, Lyman J, Salmon LJ, Russell VJ, Roe J, Linklater J (2007) A 10-year comparison of anterior cruciate ligament reconstructions with hamstring tendon and patellar tendon autograft: a controlled, prospective trial. Am J Sports Med 35:564–574
50. Reid A, Birmingham TB, Stratford PW, Alcock GK, Giffin JR (2007) Hop testing provides a reliable and valid outcome measure during rehabilitation after anterior cruciate ligament reconstruction. Phys Ther 87(3):337–349
51. Rodeo SA, Arnoczky SP, Torzilli PA, Hidaka C, Warren RF (1993) Tendon-healing in a bone tunnel. A biomechanical and histological study in the dog. J Bone Joint Surg Am 75(12):1795–1803
52. Roi GS, Creta D, Nanni G et al (2005) Return to official Italian First Division soccer games within 90 days after anterior cruciate ligament reconstruction: a case report. J Orthop Sports Phys Ther 35:52–61
53. Rougraff B, Shelbourne KD, Gerth PK, Warner J (1993) Arthroscopic and histologic analysis of human patellar tendon autografts used for anterior cruciate ligament reconstruction. Am J Sports Med 21:277–284
54. Rudolph KS, Axe MJ, Snyder-Mackler L (2000) Dynamic stability after ACL injury: who can hop? Knee Surg Sports Traumatol Arthrosc 8(5):262–269
55. Rudolph KS, Axe MJ, Buchanan TS, Scholz JP, Snyder-Mackler L (2001) Dynamic stability in the anterior cruciate ligament deficient knee. Knee Surg Sports Traumatol Arthrosc 9(2):62–71
56. Sánchez M, Anitua E, Azofra J et al (2010) Ligamentization of tendon grafts treated with an endogenous preparation rich in growth factors: gross morphology and histology. Arthroscopy 26:470–448
57. Sanders TL, Kremers HM, Bryan AJ, Fruth KM, Larson DR, Pareek A, Levy BA, Stuart MJ, Dahm DL, Krych AJ (2016) Is anterior cruciate ligament reconstruction effective in preventing secondary meniscal tears and osteoarthritis? Am J Sports Med 44(7):1699–1707
58. Salmon LJ, Russell VJ, Refshauge K (2006) Long-term outcome of endoscopic anterior cruciate ligament reconstruction with patellar tendon autograft: minimum 13-year review. Am J Sports Med 34: 721–732
59. Schmitt LC, Paterno MV, Ford KR, Myer GD, Hewett TE (2015) Strength asymmetry and landing mechanics at return to sport after anterior cruciate ligament reconstruction. Med Sci Sports Exerc 47(7):1426–1434
60. Snyder-Mackler L, Fitzgerald GK, Bartolozzi AR III, Ciccotti MG (1997) The relationship between passive joint laxity and functional outcome after anterior cruciate ligament injury. Am J Sports Med 25:191–195
61. Tashman S, Kolowich P, Collon D, Anderson K, Anderst W (2007) Dynamic function of the ACL-reconstructed knee during running. Clin Orthop Relat Res 454:66–73
62. Thomeé R, Kaplan Y, Kvist J, Myklebust G, Risberg MA, Theisen D, Tsepis E, Werner S, Wondrasch B, Witvrouw E (2011) Muscle strength and hop performance criteria prior to return to sports after ACL reconstruction. Knee Surg Sports Traumatol Arthrosc 19(11):1798–1805
63. Thomeé R, Werner S (2011) Return to sport. Knee Surg Sports Traumatol Arthrosc 19(11):1795–1797
64. van Grinsven S, van Cingel RE, Holla CJ, van Loon CJ (2010) Evidence-based rehabilitation following

anterior cruciate ligament reconstruction. Knee Surg Sports Traumatol Arthrosc 18:1128–1144

65. Webster KE, Feller JA, Lambros C (2008) Development and preliminary validation of a scale to measure the psychological impact of returning to sport following anterior cruciate ligament reconstruction surgery. Phys Ther Sport 9(1):9–15
66. Webster KE, Feller JA (2016) Exploring the high reinjury rate in younger patients undergoing anterior cruciate ligament reconstruction. Am J Sports Med 44:2827. pii: 0363546516651845
67. Weiler A, Hoffmann RF, Bail HJ, Rehm O, Südkamp NP (2002) Tendon healing in a bone tunnel. Part II: Histologic analysis after biodegradable interference fit fixation in a model of anterior cruciate ligament reconstruction in sheep. Arthroscopy 18(2):124–135
68. Wiggins AJ, Grandhi RK, Schneider DK, Stanfield D, Webster KE, Myer GD (2016) Risk of secondary injury in younger athletes after anterior cruciate ligament reconstruction: a systematic review and meta-analysis. Am J Sports Med 44(7):1861–1876
69. Wright RW, Haas AK, Anderson J, Calabrese G, Cavanaugh J, Hewett TE, Lorring D, McKenzie C, Preston E, Williams G (2015) MOON Group. Anterior cruciate ligament reconstruction rehabilitation: MOON guidelines. Sports Health 7(3):239–243
70. Xergia SA, McClelland JA, Kvist J, Vasiliadis HS, Georgoulis AD (2011) The influence of graft choice on isokinetic muscle strength 4-24 months after anterior cruciate ligament reconstruction. Knee Surg Sports Traumatol Arthrosc 19(5):768–780
71. Zwolski C, Schmitt LC, Thomas S, Hewett TE, Paterno MV (2016) The utility of limb symmetry indices in return-to-sport assessment in patients with bilateral anterior cruciate ligament reconstruction. Am J Sports Med 44(8):2030–2038

14 Return to Play Criteria: The Swedish Experience

Suzanne Werner and Magnus Forssblad

Contents

S. Werner, Phys. Ed., R.P.T., Ph.D. (✉)
M. Forssblad, M.D., Ph.D.
Stockholm Sports Trauma Research Center, Karolinska Institutet, Stockholm, Sweden
e-mail: Suzanne.Werner@ki.se; Magnus@Forssblad.se

14.1 Incidence of ACL Injury in Football

The incidence of anterior cruciate ligament (ACL) injuries has been reported in a number of studies ranging between 32 and 70 injuries/100,000 inhabitants/year. In Sweden recent national data from population-based studies indicate an ACL injury incidence of about 80/100,000 inhabitants/year. Without satisfactory treatment ACL injury is a serious knee injury that often prevents young people from continuing to participate in heavy physical work or physical exercise and sport at recreational or elite level. The treatment can be either physical therapy alone or a combination of surgery (ACL reconstruction) followed by physical therapy. It is estimated that about half of all ACL injuries are not subjected to surgery for different reasons.

An injury frequency of approximately 80 per 100,000 inhabitants in Sweden would mean that some 7–8000 individuals suffer ACL injuries every year and that some 3500 would undergo surgery. Recent studies reveal that about 20% of the patients undergoing surgery require repeat surgery within a few years as a result of complications, first and foremost meniscal and/or cartilage damage, restricted mobility, or the failure of

V. Musahl et al. (eds.), *Return to Play in Football*, https://doi.org/10.1007/978-3-662-55713-6_14

the ACL reconstruction. The results after secondary surgery seem to be poorer than after primary surgery. Good results have been reported in short term after a primary operation. Only a few studies are either randomized or have a long follow-up, though (Figs. 1, 2, 3, 4, 5, 6, 7).

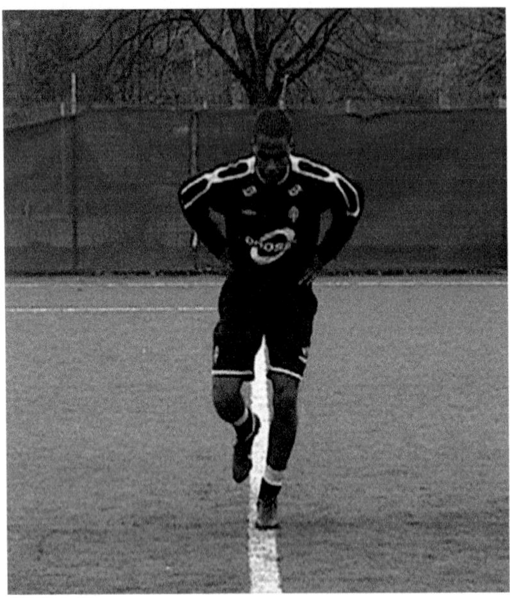

Fig. 1 One-leg hop straight forward

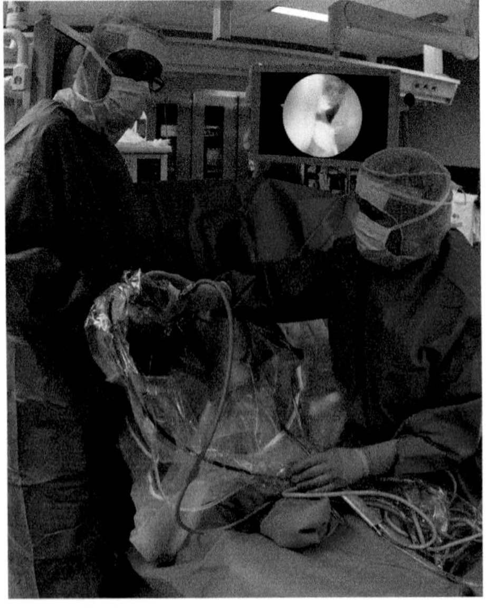

Fig. 2 Arthroscopy of the knee joint

14.2 ACL Injury Registry in Sweden

Sweden has a long tradition of orthopedic quality registries originating from the hip and knee registries in the 1970s. The Swedish ACL registry started in 2005 in cooperation with Norway and Denmark (for annual reports visit www.xbase.nu).

Fact Box 1

- Football is the leading cause of ACL injuries.
- Forty percent of all surgeons perform fewer than ten ACL reconstructions a year.
- Overall the revision rate is about 3% but increases to 10% in the younger population below 20 years of age.

The number of operations per surgeon is unevenly distributed, and about 40% of all surgeons perform fewer than 10 ACL reconstructions a year. A trend toward an increase in the number of operations per surgeon has, however, been seen since the start of the ACL registry in 2005. At the start, the ACL registry was a surgical registry, but attempts are now being made to register all patients with this knee injury, regardless of surgical or nonsurgical treatment. In Sweden we are trying to involve our physical therapists in this work and thereby make analyses of return-to-play data.

Football is still the most common activity associated with an ACL injury in male as well as female players, and this situation does not change from year to year. In 2015, football was the cause of ACL injuries in 47% of male and 34% of female players.

As football is the leading cause of ACL injuries, it is interesting that projects including prophylactic training for young people playing football are in progress in Sweden. The training is designed to create improved neuromuscular control of the lower extremities and core stability by teaching ball-playing youngsters to avoid situations in which an ACL injury could occur.

Unfortunately, only a few clinics in Sweden have collected data from physical tests per-

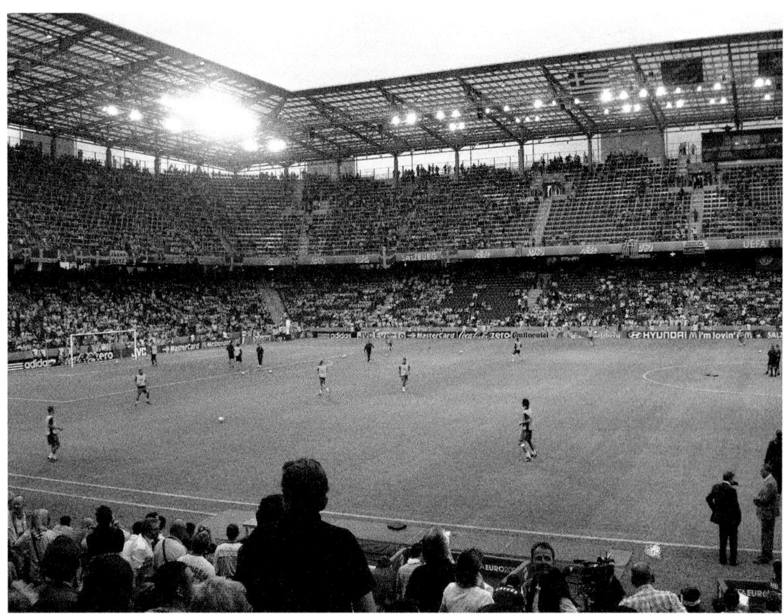

Fig. 3 Football match

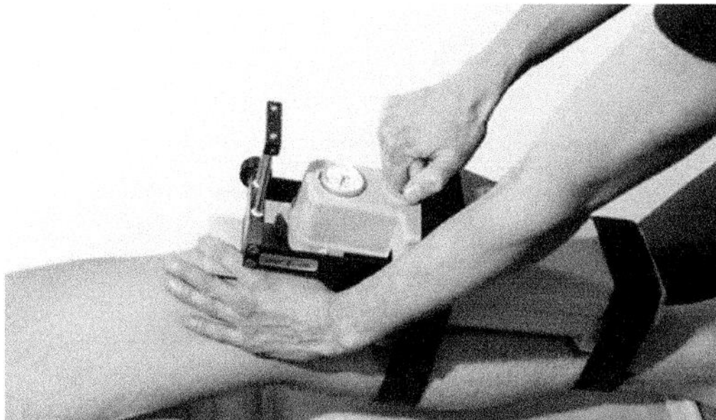

Fig. 4 KT-1000 laxity tester

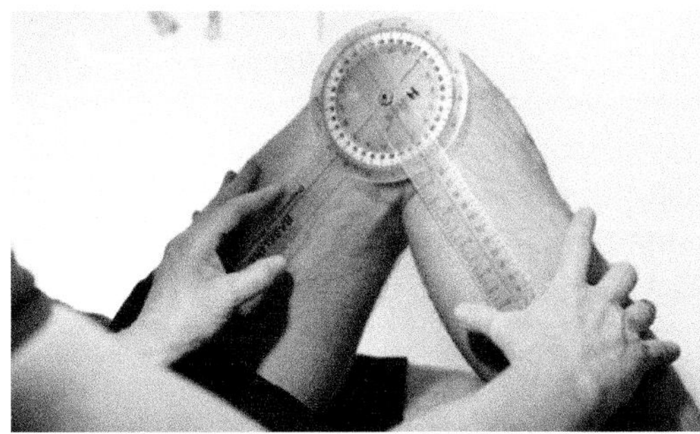

Fig. 5 Measurement of knee joint range of motion using a goniometer

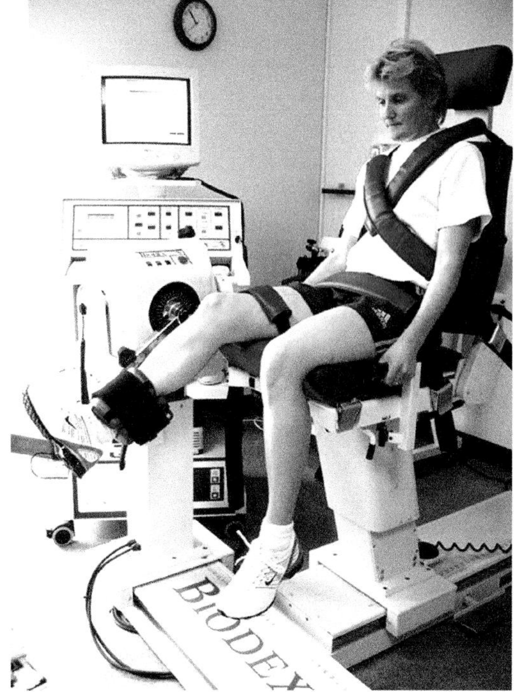

Fig. 6 Isokinetic measurement of knee extensors and knee flexors

formed 6–12 months after surgery. In the ACL registry, surgeons can follow revision surgery and data of knee function measured with Knee injury and Osteoarthritis Outcome Score (KOOS) 1, 2, 5, and 10 years postoperatively. No data are available for true re-rupture rate or about return to play except for one study presented below.

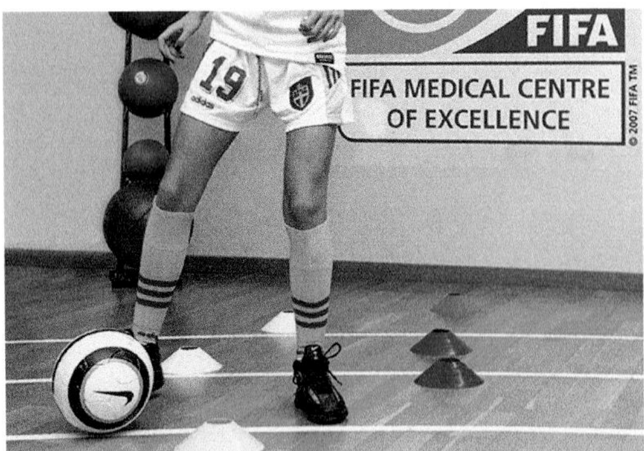

Fig. 7 Sport specific exercise for football players

14.3 ACL Injury Revision Surgery

A total of 2330 revisions were registered in the ACL registry between 2005 and 2015. If we instead choose to follow the patients who initially underwent surgery within the framework of the ACL registry and who then underwent revisions, 1290 (3.5%) new operations were registered on patients who had previously undergone surgery. In this way, the follow-up period is longest for patients who underwent surgery in 2005, while it was only possible to follow up patients who underwent surgery in 2015 during that same year. In addition, 1162 (3.2%) underwent a new ACL operation on their contralateral knee. Females underwent revisions to a larger extent than males, 3.8% compared with 3.4% for the same knee and 3.4% compared with 3.0% for the contralateral knee (www.xbase.nu).

Fact Box 2

- The overall revision rate for all patients is about 3%.
- Patients below 20 years have a revision rate of approximately 10%.
- The incidence of a new contralateral ACL injury is similar to the revision rate of the first ACL injury.

Only 63 patients, out of 33 000 procedures, underwent revisions on two occasions, and only 6 patients have undergone surgery 3 times. Based on the ACL injury registry, nobody has undergone more than three revisions.

Patients receiving hamstring tendon graft underwent revisions on the same knee in 3.6% of the cases compared with 3.0% for patients receiving patellar tendon graft. These data are difficult to assess, as the number of primary patellar tendon operations is only around 3057 compared with 31,871 for hamstring operations. As the number of patellar tendon operations was higher at the beginning of the study period, these data are probably also misleading. If the follow-up period is limited to 3 years and the period 2005–2015 is analyzed, the number of revisions using patellar tendon graft is 2.2% compared with 2.9% for hamstring tendon graft. This still indicates a larger number of revisions for hamstring tendon reconstructions than for patellar tendon reconstructions, which matches data presented from the registries in Norway and Denmark.

Patients below 20 years of age underwent revisions to a higher percentage. This is probably due to the fact that this patient group is more active and returns more frequently to sports. Six percent underwent revisions of the same knee and 6.5% of the contralateral knee.

Football players have lower revision rates compared to handball players but higher revision rates compared to alpine skiers. The reason for this is, however, unknown.

14.4 Rehabilitation After ACL Reconstruction

Tests before injury, e.g., at the start of the football season, should be mandatory in order to reveal possible physiological limitations to be used for leg comparisons at the time of the rehabilitation after an ACL injury and mainly when considering return to play. These tests should be reliable, responsive, and valid including measurements of range of motion, muscle flexibility, muscle strength, neuromuscular control (balance and coordination), as well as cardiorespiratory endurance.

A criterion-based protocol is used as a model of the rehabilitation following ACL reconstruction. There is a positive relation between goal setting and adherence, which in turn yield a positive relation with the outcome of the rehabilitation [34]. The goals of the first two postoperative weeks are based on reducing swelling, improving range of motion and the control of the quadriceps muscle group, and training to restore a normal movement and gait pattern. The rehabilitation exercises go from closed kinetic chain to open kinetic chain with gradual increasing load. Functional exercises are started approximately 12 weeks postoperatively and continue gradually toward sport-specific exercises when good muscle strength exists. During the entire rehabilitation, the muscle-strengthening exercises go from light resistance (low loads) and many repetitions to greater resistance (heavier loads) and few repetitions. At 4–6 months of conditioning exercises, agility exercises and pivoting maneuvers at different speeds are added. At approximately 6 months, the injured player is going through as well a number of physiological tests as psychological tests, mainly self-reported questionnaires, before a gradual return to play football is considered.

14.5 Project ACL: A Swedish Model of Following Up ACL-Injured Patients

The "Project ACL" is a local rehabilitation outcome registry based in Gothenburg and the western part of Sweden. This project was established in August 2014 with the primary aim to improve care and treatment of patients who sustain ACL injuries. At present, about 1200 patients between 9 and 66 years of age have been included in the project. On average ten new patients enroll to "Project ACL" each week. In addition, as of December 2016, data had been collected from approximately 3900 assessments of patient-reported outcome measures and 2400 evaluations of measurements of muscle function.

> **Fact Box 3**
>
> - The "Project ACL" is a local rehabilitation outcome registry based in Gothenburg and the western part of Sweden.
> - At present, about 1200 patients between 9 and 66 years of age have been included in the "Project ACL."
> - All patients in the "Project ACL" are carefully followed up both objectively with clinical tests and subjectively with questionnaires.

The inclusion of the "Project ACL" is voluntary. Both patients with ACL injury and their responsible orthopedic surgeon and physical therapist are asked to participate. "Project ACL" utilizes a web-based platform for regular assessment with reliable and valid patient-reported outcome measures (PROMs) and tests of muscle function for patients who have sustained an ACL injury: KOOS [26], EQ5D-3L [11], Knee Self-Efficacy Scale [29], Physical Activity Scale [14], Tegner Activity Scale [6, 28], and ACL Return to Sport Index [33]. Furthermore, the following tests for evaluating lower extremity muscle function are isokinetic muscle torque measurements of both knee extensors and knee flexors [12, 30, 31]: one-leg hop test for distance [23, 25], one-leg vertical jump [24], and one-leg side hop test [16]. This enables a thorough evaluation of the patient's physical and psychological status and recovery, which normally is difficult to perform in the standard clinical setting. With the web-based platform, the patients have the opportunity to share their results with their responsible orthopedic surgeon and physical therapist for further feedback and evaluation. This methodology has ensured a high compliance of the assessments in "Project ACL." The assessments in "Project ACL" are performed after a predefined schedule of follow-up at 10 weeks, 4 months, 8 months, 12 months, 18 months, 24 months, and every fifth year after index ACL injury or reconstructive surgery.

After every assessment, "Project ACL's" research database automatically updates. In addition, a personal report is instantly available online to the patient. Results from PROMs and tests of muscle function are reported on this patient-unique protocol after each assessment. The protocol contains the results from all assessments that the patient has performed. The scope of "Project ACL" is to be clinician friendly, and therefore, every patient has the opportunity to also make their personal report available to the responsible physician and/or physical therapist. Accordingly, a patient's participation in "Project ACL" may help the responsible orthopedic surgeon and physical therapist to evaluate the progression of recovery and rehabilitation after injury or surgery. Furthermore, the project has a unique, continuously and automatically updated, *average statistics page* available online from all assessments in "Project ACL" to support patients and clinicians in the evaluation of the rehabilitation. Additionally, there is a selection of relevant filters for stratifying the statistics to a specific subgroup, e.g., gender, age, time after injury/surgery, etc.

One concern in terms of patients with ACL injury is that previous studies have not considered the heterogeneity among patients. In addition, most studies in the literature do not have an interdisciplinary approach and may therefore be limited by confounding factors. Therefore, "Project ACL" has established collaboration with the Swedish National Knee Ligament Registry. National population-based registry studies provide a unique source of information by containing large numbers of patients that are followed over a long period of time. The collaboration comprises both orthopedic surgeons and physical therapists treating ACL-injured patients. The expectations are to utilize shared knowledge of patients with ACL injury between these medical professions to create studies covering the whole care and treatment for this patient group. In addition, together the registries include thousands of patients, enabling specific subgrouping to sport populations.

14.6 Predicting Factors for Returning to Play After ACL Reconstruction in Football Players

Football is one of the most popular sports and attracts the highest number of both male and female youngsters in Sweden today. However, it is a sport characterized by rapid changes of directions as well as cutting and pivoting movements which put heavy demands on knee joint stability. ACL rupture is a common and serious injury in football which may even lead to an end of a player's career. Therefore, most orthopedic surgeons recommend ACL reconstruction in ACL-injured football players trying to restore knee joint stability to enable return to play. Return to sports after ACL reconstruction is generally allowed after 6–12 months [7, 17].

Sandon et al. [27] tried to identify factors associated with returning to football after ACL reconstruction in a general footballing population. Two hundred five football players who had undergone ACL reconstruction were followed up 3.2 ± 1.4 years after surgery. Information about gender, age, side of injury, graft type, results of various scores, possible meniscus injury, and/or cartilage injury were collected using the Swedish ACL registry. The patients were surveyed with a questionnaire about present subjective knee function and sports participation. The results showed that 54% had returned to football, 35.5% at the same or higher level, and 18.5% to a lower level than before the ACL injury. The logistic regression analyses revealed three factors that significantly predict whether a football player will return to football after an ACL reconstruction or not. Those were gender, cartilage injury, and pain during physical activity. The regression analyses of variables illustrated no significant associations between the other types of studied variables and return to football. There was a significant gender difference with regard to returning to football. Males returned to a higher extent than females, 60% and 46%, respectively. Only 33% of those with joint cartilage injury returned to football compared to 59% of those without any joint cartilage injury. Pain was found to be the most common symptom in football players following ACL reconstruction. Almost half of the players complained of knee pain in connection with physical activities, and pain was a significant negative factor in returning to football. This finding corresponds well with the finding by Lentz et al. [20] who also reported that pain reduces the return to sports rate. In elite football players, Waldén et al. [32] reported a return-to-play rate of 94%, which is considerably higher than a rate of 54% in the present cohort and other studies [5, 27]. Ekstrand [10] argues that the access to the most experienced orthopedic surgeons and physical therapists, a rapid time to diagnosis and treatment, as well as high financial incentives in elite players could be possible reasons for these differences.

From a clinical point of view, this study [27] shows that the rehabilitation of football players after ACL reconstruction is of great importance for a successful return to sport. Another finding was that in terms of rehabilitation, extra attention should be paid to female players and knee pain.

14.7 Return to Play

Focusing on the football player's goal of returning to play should start already at the time of the ACL injury and be a continuum throughout recovery and the entire rehabilitation [22].

Including both physiological and psychological evaluation during the postoperative rehabilitation will improve the knowledge of the player's possibilities and resources for returning to play. It is most likely that this will help the physician and physical therapist to determine when the player is ready for returning to football.

Fact Box 4

Return to play should include factors like:

- Stress of returning to play
- Fear of re-injury
- Low self-efficacy
- Lack of motivation
- Pressure from outside sources, e.g., managers, trainers, and teammates

A player's safe return to football requires assessment of neuromuscular control, muscle strength, and endurance. Objective, reliable, responsive, and valid tests such as isokinetic muscle torque measurements, concentrically and eccentrically of the knee extensors and knee flexors [12, 30, 31], anterior knee laxity [9], and range of motion are recommended along with functional performance tests and football-related tests. Both muscle power tests and hop tests are recommended for evaluating knee function and thereby reveal possible functional limitations [4, 21]. However, the player's psychological readiness for football should also be taken into account when determining the appropriate time for returning to play. Psychological responses already before surgery and early recovery are associated with returning to preinjury level of sport [1], meaning that a successful return to play most likely starts already at the time of injury. There are a number of valid so-called subjective instruments, mostly questionnaires, that could reveal important personality characteristics when considering return to play such as fear of re-injury [1, 18], low self-efficacy [29], and/or lack of motivation [2, 3, 8]. The pressure that an athlete might experience from coaches, parents, and/or teammates can further complicate the ideal timing of returning to play, and the player could experience a "return-to-play stress." When it comes to ACL injuries, two evidence-based scales from a psychological point of view have been recommended, "ACL Return to Sport after Injury Scale" [19] and "Injury-Psychological Readiness to Return to Sport Scale" [13].

The criteria for returning to play are complex, and no single test can determine an athlete's readiness to return. This means that evaluation methods measuring different parameters are needed to obtain the most successful return to play (Table 1). A battery of tests measuring a variety of physiological parameters leads to higher sensitivity than a single test [15, 16, 21]. Although not always evidence based, a number of different parameters are suggested for evaluation after ACL injury and/or reconstruction. These include pain level, the player's confidence with the ACL-injured knee, range of motion, core stability, and thigh muscle strength and endurance as well as

Table 1 Suggestions for evaluating clinical status and physical performance after ACL reconstruction in football players

Clinical status	Functional performance
Anterior knee laxity	One-leg hop test for distance
Isokinetic muscle torque	Squat jump
Range of motion	Countermovement jump
Muscle flexibility	One-leg side hop test
Aerobic capacity	One-leg zigzag side hop test
	Sprint tests

patient-reported outcome scores. In addition, it is essential to determine assessments of neuromuscular control and real football-like activities that at the same time are evaluating agility, muscle strength, endurance, and core stability. The functional performance tests mirroring football should be carried out with high quality and without pain and swelling during both non-fatigued and fatigued conditions [4]. Furthermore, different types of hop tests and maneuvers requiring lateral movement as well as acceleration and deceleration should be involved in the battery of tests before considering return to play.

Take-Home Message

- In Sweden football players have the highest incidence of ACL rupture compared to athletes in other sports.
- About 50% of all ACL injuries in Sweden are treated nonsurgically. However, all athletes participating in sports with high physical demands are generally operated on 4–6 weeks after injury.
- A player's safe return to football requires assessment of neuromuscular control, muscle strength, and endurance as well as psychological factors.
- In Sweden the time to return to football usually occurs 6–9 months after the ACL injury.
- In general, only 54% of ACL-injured football players in Sweden return to play. However, most of the elite players do return.

Top Five Evidence-Based References

Ardern C, Taylor N, Feller J, Whitehead T, Webster K (2013) Psychological responses matter in returning to preinjury level of sport after anterior cruciate ligament reconstruction surgery. Am J Sports Med 41(7):1549–1558

Gustavsson A, Neeter C, Thomeé P, GrävareSilbernagel K, Augustsson J, Thomeé R, Karlsson J (2006) A test battery for evaluating hop performance in patients with an ACL injury and patients who have undergone ACL reconstruction. Knee Surg Sports Traumatol Arthrosc 14(8):778–788

Lentz TA, Zeppieri G Jr, Tillman SM, Indelicato PA, Moser MW, George SZ, Chmielewski TL (2012) Return to preinjury sports participation following anterior cruciate ligament reconstruction: contributions of demographic, knee impairment, and self-report measures. J Orthop Sports Phys Ther 42:893–901

Sandon A, Werner S, Forssblad M (2015) Factors associated with returning to football after anterior cruciate ligament reconstruction. Knee Surg Sports Traumatol Arthrosc 23(9):2514–2521

Thomeé R, Kaplan Y, Kvist J, Myklebust G, Risberg MA, Theisen D, Tsepis E, Werner S, Wondrasch B, Witvrouw E (2011) Muscle strength and hop performance criteria prior to return to sports after ACL reconstruction. Knee Surg Sports Traumatol Arthrosc 19:1798–1805

References

1. Ardern C, Taylor N, Feller J, Whitehead T, Webster K (2013) Psychological responses matter in returning to preinjury level of sport after anterior cruciate ligament reconstruction surgery. Am J Sports Med 41(7):1549–1558
2. Ardern CL, Taylor NF, Feller JA, Webster KE (2013) A systematic review of the psychological factors associated with returning to sport following injury. Br J Sports Med 47:1120–1126
3. Ardern CL (2015) Anterior cruciate ligament reconstruction–not exactly a one-way ticket back to preinjury level: a review of contextual factors affecting return to sport after surgery. Sports Health 7:224–230
4. Augustsson J, Thomeé R, Karlsson J (2004) Ability of a new hop test to determine functional deficits after anterior cruciate ligament reconstruction. Knee Surg Sports Traumatol Arthrosc 12:350–356
5. Bjordal JM, Arnły F, Hannestad B, Strand T (1997) Epidemiology of anterior cruciate ligament injuries in soccer. Am J Sports Med 25:341–345
6. Briggs KK, Lysholm J, Tegner Y, Rodkey WG, Kocher MS, Steadman JR (2009) The reliability, validity, and responsiveness of the Lysholm Score and Tegner Activity Scale for anterior cruciate ligament injuries of the knee. Am J Sports Med 37(5):890–897
7. Cascio BM, Culp L, Cosgarea AJ (2004) Return to play after anterior cruciate ligament reconstruction. Clin Sports Med 23:395–408
8. Czuppon S, Racette BA, Klein SE (2014) Variables associated with return to sport following anterior cruciate ligament reconstruction: a systematic review. Br J Sports Med 48:356–364
9. Daniel DM, Stone ML, Sachs R, Malcom L (1985) Instrumented measurements of anterior knee laxity in patients with acute anterior cruciate ligament disruption. Am J Sports Med 13:401–407
10. Ekstrand J (2011) A 94% return to elite level football after ACL surgery: a proof of possibilities with

optimal caretaking or a sign of knee abuse? Knee Surg, Sports Traumatol, Arthrosc 19(1):1–2
11. EuroQol Group (1990) EuroQol--a new facility for the measurement of health-related quality of life. Health Policy 16(3):199–208
12. Feiring DC, Christ CB, Massey BH (1990) Test-retest reliability of the Biodex isokinetic dynamometer. J Orthop Sports Phys Ther 11:298–300
13. Glazer DD (2009) Development and preliminary validation of the Injury-Psychological Readiness to Return to Sport (I-PRRS) scale. J Athl Train 44:185–189
14. Grimby G (1986) Physical activity and muscle training in the elderly. Acta Med Scand Suppl 711:233–337
15. Gustavsson A, Neeter C, Thomeé P, Grävare Silbernagel K, Augustsson J, Thomeé R, Karlsson J (2006) A test battery for evaluating hop performance in patients with an ACL injury and patients who have undergone ACL reconstruction. Knee Surg Sports Traumatol Arthrosc 14(8):778–788
16. Itoh H, Kurosaka M, Yoshiya S, Ichihashi N, Mizuno K (1998) Evaluation of functional deficits determined by four different hop tests in patients with anterior cruciate ligament deficiency. Knee Surg Sports Traumatol Arthrosc 6(4):241–245
17. Kvist J (2004) Rehabilitation following anterior cruciate ligament injury: current recommendations for sports participation. Sports Med 34:269–280
18. Kvist J, Ek A, Sporrstedt K, Good L (2005) Fear of re-injury: a hindrance for returning to sports after anterior cruciate ligament reconstruction. Knee Surg Sports Traumatol Arthrosc 13(5):393–397
19. Kvist J, Österberg A, Gauffin H, Tagesson S, Webster K, Ardern C (2011) Translation and measurement properties of the Swedish version of ACL-Return to Sports after Injury questionnaire. Scand J Med Sci Sports 23(5):568–575
20. Lentz TA, Zeppieri G Jr, Tillman SM, Indelicato PA, Moser MW, George SZ, Chmielewski TL (2012) Return to preinjury sports participation following anterior cruciate ligament reconstruction: contributions of demographic, knee impairment, and self-report measures. J Orthop Sports Phys Ther 42:893–901
21. Neeter C, Gustavsson A, Thomeé P, Augustsson J, Thomeé R, Karlsson J (2006) Development of a strength test battery for evaluating leg muscle power after anterior cruciate ligament injury and reconstruction. Knee Surg Sports Traumatol Arthrosc 14(6):571–580
22. No authors listed (2002) The team physician and return-to-play issues: a consensus statement. Med Sci Sports Exerc 34:1212–1214
23. Noyes FR, Barber SD, Mangine RE (1991) Abnormal lower limb symmetry determined by function hop tests after anterior cruciate ligament rupture. Am J Sports Med 19(5):513–518
24. Petschnig R, Baron R, Albrecht M (1998) The relationship between isokinetic quadriceps strength test and hop tests for distance and one-legged vertical jump test following anterior cruciate ligament reconstruction. J Orthop Sports Phys Ther 28(1):212–217
25. Risberg MA, Ekeland A (1994) Assessment of functional tests after anterior cruciate ligament surgery. J Orthop Sports Phys Ther 19(4):212–217
26. Roos EM, Roos HP, Ekdahl C, Lohmander LS (1998) Knee injury and osteoarthritis outcome score (KOOS)-validation of a Swedish version. Scand J Med Sci Sports 8:439–448
27. Sandon A, Werner S, Forssblad M (2015) Factors associated with returning to football after anterior cruciate ligament reconstruction. Knee Surg Sports Traumatol Arthrosc 23(9):2514–2521
28. Tegner Y, Lysholm J (1985) Rating systems in the evaluation of knee ligament injuries. Clin Orthop Relat Res 198:43–49
29. Thomeé P, Währborg P, Börjesson M, Thomeé R, Eriksson BI, Karlsson J (2006) A new instrument for measuring self-efficacy in patients with an anterior cruciate ligament injury. Scand J Med Sci Sports 16(3):181–187
30. Thomeé R, Kaplan Y, Kvist J, Myklebust G, Risberg MA, Theisen D, Tsepis E, Werner S, Wondrasch B, Witvrouw E (2011) Muscle strength and hop performance criteria prior to return to sports after ACL reconstruction. Knee Surg Sports Traumatol Arthrosc 19:1798–1805
31. Undheim MB, Cosgrave C, King E, Strike S, Marshall B, Falvey E, Franklyn-Miller A (2015) Isokinetic muscle strength and readiness to return to sport following anterior cruciate ligament reconstruction: is there an association? A systematic review and a protocol recommendation. Br J Sports Med 49(20):1305–1310
32. Waldén M, Hägglund M, Magnusson H, Ekstrand J (2011) Anterior cruciate ligament injury in elite football: a prospective three-cohort study. Knee Surg Sports Traumatol Arthrosc 19(1):11–19
33. Webster KE, Feller JA, Lambros C (2008) Development and preliminary validation of a scale to measure the psychological impact of returning to sport following anterior cruciate ligament reconstruction surgery. Phys Ther Sport 9(1):9–15
34. Wierike S, van der Sluis A, Akker-Scheek I, Elferink-Gemser M, Visscher C (2013) Psychosocial factors influencing the recovery of athletes with anterior cruciate ligament injury: a systematic review. Scand J Med Sci Sports 23(5):527–540

15 ACL: Criteria-Based Return to Play—Outcome Predictor Analysis After ACL Reconstruction

Francesco Della Villa, Jacopo Gamberini, Daniele Caminati, Margherita Ricci, and Stefano Della Villa

Contents

F. Della Villa, M.D. (✉) • J. Gamberini, M.D.
D. Caminati, P.T. • M. Ricci, M.D.
S. Della Villa, M.D.
Education and Research Department, Isokinetic Medical Group, FIFA Medical Centre of Excellence, Via Casteldebole 8/4, 40132, Bologna, Italy
e-mail: f.dellavilla@isokinetic.com

15.1 Introduction

Anterior cruciate ligament (ACL) injury and related care are critical issues in sports and moreover football medicine. Each year, worldwide, tens of thousands of patients experience such an injury. ACL injury is a serious and potentially career-threatening injury for the football player [1]. Even if a percentage of patients can deal with an ACL injury and are able to perform, the so-called copers [2], the majority of them do not.

ACL reconstruction (ACLR) remains the treatment of choice in patients willing to return to strenuous activity and pivoting sport, such as football. Given the number of procedures performed every year in the world, nearly 200,000 in the USA alone [3], the management of the ACLR athlete is a common clinical challenge for the sport physician. Normal knee function and safe return to pre-injury activity level avoiding the second ACL injury are generally the acute goals of ACLR and subsequent targeted rehabilitation. Prevention and possible mitigation of the risk of early-onset osteoarthritis are the long-term goal of ACLR.

Return to play (RTP) at the same pre-injury level is often considered as one of the main and challenging outcomes in the literature after ACLR and rehabilitation. Recent systematic reviews report RTP rates of 63–65% after primary ACLR [4, 5] which are far from the general patient's and patient's environment expectations. This low percentage of patients actually return-

V. Musahl et al. (eds.), *Return to Play in Football*, https://doi.org/10.1007/978-3-662-55713-6_15

ing to pre-injury level of sport participation underlines the fact that a lot has still to be done regarding ACLR patients.

Many variables including *patient's baseline features*, *surgery-related factors*, and finally *rehabilitation features, including functional performance* (Fig. 15.1), are believed to interact in a complex manner in determining RTP chances for the athlete.

The aim of this chapter, in which we will show original data, is to present the evidence-based state of the art in RTP predictors after ACLR.

Defining which baseline factors correlate with better or lower probability to RTP efficiently will help the clinician in targeting patient's expectations. On the other hand, underpinning which rehabilitation features, including functional test results, are associated with RTP will help the clinician to apply the best strategy to improve patient's outcomes and RTP rate.

15.2 Predicting RTP After ACLR: Literature Results

During the last years, the increased interest in registry-based research all over the world brought new insight also in the field of RTP predictors after ACLR. Many factors have been advocated to influence the RTP probability in literature.

Fact Box 1
RTP after ACLR is a complex and multifactorial outcome; a biopsychosocial model should be adopted to face the RTP decision.

15.3 Baseline Factors

Age is the first factor that may influence the RTP rate after ACLR. Lentz and Ardern [6, 7] reported that young age was positively associated with returning to pre-injury level of sport. It is shown that young patients tend also to be clinically discharged faster from rehabilitation after ACLR [8]. *Gender* appears to be a critical issue; male athletes are reported to have higher odds of RTP. A recent review shows clearly that the average pooled RTP rate for male patients is 61% vs. a 52% reported for the female counterpart [5]. Another important baseline factor is pre-injury activity level. *Elite sport athletes* have more than twice the odds of RTP if compared to nonelite athletes [5].

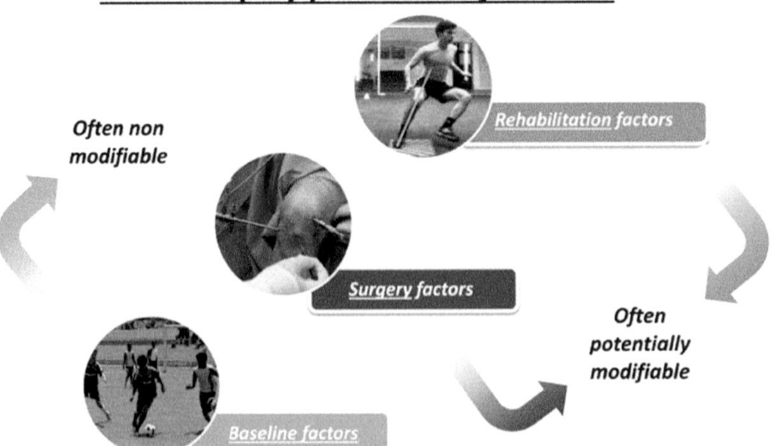

Fig. 15.1 Groups of possible predictors of RTP after ACLR. If baseline variables are often non-modifiable, surgical and especially rehabilitation factors are often potentially modifiable factors. We believe that a biopsychosocial approach should be used when considering the ACL-injured athlete. As return to play is returning to fully participate in society, we need to take into account biological, psychological and environmental factors to improve outcomes

15.4 Surgery Factors

Many surgical factors have been extensively evaluated as possible predictors of functional outcomes following ACLR, including RTP. There is still no consensus about graft choice for primary ACLR; bone patellar tendon bone (BPTB) autograft and hamstring (HT) autograft seem to have similar results in terms of RTP [5]. Also regarding surgical technique, literature is lacking of information regarding differences in RTP between different techniques. It is likely that the inner complexity of the RTP outcome is one of the reasons of this lack of differences between surgical techniques. Many athlete-related factors may influence more the decision to RTP, considering that in a high percentage of cases, this is multifactorial, and also based on psychological factors, such as fear of reinjury, inner personality traits or life's changing events [9].

On the other hand, it is clearly shown that *revision ACLR* is associated with a lower RTP rate. In a recent systematic review, we documented a 43% RTP rate for revision procedures compared to 63% for primary ACLR [4]. The *presence of a knee cartilage injury* was associated with a 70% decrease in RTP chances in a recent study on more than 200 football players [1].

15.5 Rehabilitation Factors

This wide family of possible factors correlating with RTP after ACLR has not been already studied deeply. This may be partially due to the relative predominance of surgery-based ACLR registry instead of rehabilitation based.

Associations were documented between certain physical functioning variables and RTP after ACLR. *Higher postoperative quadriceps strength, less knee effusion, lower pain* and *fewer episodes of instability* [10] correlates with higher RTP rate. On a large cohort of patients, a strong association was documented between the IKDC subjective score and the RTP rate [7], underlying the concept that a certain level of knee and physical functioning is recommended to RTP efficiently.

Psychological factors, both baseline and postoperative, had often been cited as predictors of RTP. A significant association was reported between *lower ACL-RSI scale score* (ACL Return to Sport after Injury scale) and RTP chances: patients with *lower postoperative athletic confidence* had also less chances to RTP [11]. Different types of fear are described after ACLR, fear of pain and especially *fear of reinjury*, that are negatively associated to RTP [12]. It was reported that the Tampa Scale of Kinesiophobia (TSK) score was higher (indicating more fear) in the non-RTP group and this was reflected on patient's quality of life [12]. *Higher preoperative motivation* is also considered a strong predictor. Preoperative profiling of the ACL patients was shown to be beneficial [13].

Fact Box 2

Many variables have been reported to influence patient's probability to RTP after ACLR.

Baseline and surgery factors:
- Age
- Gender
- Pre-injury activity level
- Revision ACLR
- Associated knee cartilage injury

Rehabilitation and psychological factors:
- Postoperative quadriceps strength
- Postoperative knee effusion and pain
- Fewer episodes of instability
- Athletic confidence and motivation
- Fear of reinjury

15.6 The Isokinetic Medical Group ACL Cohort

15.6.1 Study Group

From 2010 to present, we are enrolling patients after ACLR. At the time of the chapter submission, 1507 subjects were enrolled in the present study. The aim of our study was to detect possible predictors of functional outcomes after ACLR in a large "rehabilitation-based" cohort of patients. RTP, described as *return to pre-injury sport* and *activity level*, is the main outcome of our study.

Inclusion criteria were (1) *having had ACLR* and (2) *having done at least a postoperative rehabilitation medical consultation in our centres* (*Isokinetic Medical Group*). The decision of having such broad inclusion criteria is thought to include all the possible predictors of functional outcome. The patients followed the same *criterion-based RTP protocol*, as previously described in literature [14].

Baseline, *surgery factor* and *rehabilitation factor* data, including functional testing results during rehabilitation, were gathered from a systematic revision of the clinical records.

Functional testing (isokinetic test and threshold test) during rehabilitation has been performed using protocols that we have previously described [14]. 1205/1507 patients completed at least one isokinetic test. 763/1507 completed at least one threshold test.

Patients were clinically followed up annually with a dedicated form including a comprehensive return to sport assessment.

At the time of this preliminary analysis, 1279/1507 patients, corresponding to 84.8% of the cohort, completed a minimum 12-month follow-up.

15.6.2 RTP Results

Considering the whole cohort, the 94.4% of patients returned to some kind of sport or physical activity, and 76.4% returned to the same pre-injury sport, but only the 66.3% of patients returned to pre-injury sport at the same competitive level. We considered this last reported outcome (same sport at the same competitive level) as the main result of the study and our final RTP rate.

15.6.3 Isokinetic Medical Group Cohort: Baseline RTP Predictors

The baseline and surgical variables influencing the RTP rate significantly at the univariate (UV) and multivariate analysis are reported in Table 15.1, while the RTP rate for each subgroup is reported in Table 15.2 (Figs. 15.2, 15.3, 15.4 and 15.5).

Fact Box 3

Male gender, elite sport level, primary ACLR, early surgery (within 77 days) and *BMI* < 25 are positively associated with RTP rate.

Table 15.1 Predictors of RTP after ACLR. Baseline model

Baseline and surgery factor model (logistic regression analysis)						
	Univariate			Multivariate		
Factors (number of cases for each subgroup)	OR	95% C.I.	*p*	OR	95% C.I.	*p*
Male (989) vs. female (290)	**1.46**	**1.11–1.91**	**0.006**	**1.54**	**1.13–2.08**	**0.005**
Age <29 (627) vs. age >29 (652)	**1.26**	**1.00–1.59**	**0.049**	1.00	0.77–1.30	0.956
Elite (93) vs. nonelite (1177)	**2.58**	**1.48–4.48**	**0.001**	**2.00**	**1.12–3.55**	**0.017**
BMI ≥ 25 (330) vs. BMI < 25 (942)	**0.71**	**0.54–0.91**	**0.009**	**0.72**	**0.54–0.96**	**0.028**
Football (403 cases) vs. other (874 cases)	**1.44**	**1.11–1.86**	**0.005**	1.15	0.86–1.55	0.327
Revision (96 cases) vs. primary ACLR (1183)	**0.63**	**0.41–0.96**	**0.033**	**0.62**	**0.39–0.99**	**0.046**
Delayed ACLR >77 d (630) vs. early ACLR <77 d (625)	**0.58**	**0.45–0.73**	**0.000**	**0.63**	**0.49–0.82**	**0.000**

Univariate and multivariate analysis
Statistically significant result reported in bold
OR odds ratio, *CI* 95% confidence interval, *M* male, *F* female, *BMI* body mass index, *ACLR* anterior cruciate ligament reconstruction, *d* days

Table 15.2 Relationship between baseline and surgery factor and rate of RTP (1279 cases included in the analysis)

	Baseline and surgery factor affecting RTP (return to pre-injury sport at pre-injury level) after ACLR (univariate analysis)													
	Person-related factors										Surgery-related factors			
Factor (cases)	Gender		Age		Comp. level		BMI		Pre-inj. Sport		Primary or revision		Inj. to ACLR (days)	
	Men (989)	Women (290)	<29 years (627)	>29 years (652)	Elite (93)	Non-elite (1177)	<25 (942)	≥25 (330)	Football (403)	Other (875)	Primary (1183)	Revision (96)	<77 # Days (625)	>77 days (630)
RTP rate (%)	68.2*	59.5	68.9*	63.9	82.9*	65.7	68.3*	60.4	71.7*	63.7	67.0*	56.3	72.6*	60.6

RTP return to play, *ACLR* anterior cruciate ligament reconstruction, *Comp* competitive, *Inj* ACL injury, *BMI* body mass index

* = statistically significant result ($p < 0.05$) at the χ^2 test

= regarding the injury to surgery elapsed time we considered 77 days as the threshold because this is the median value of our cohort

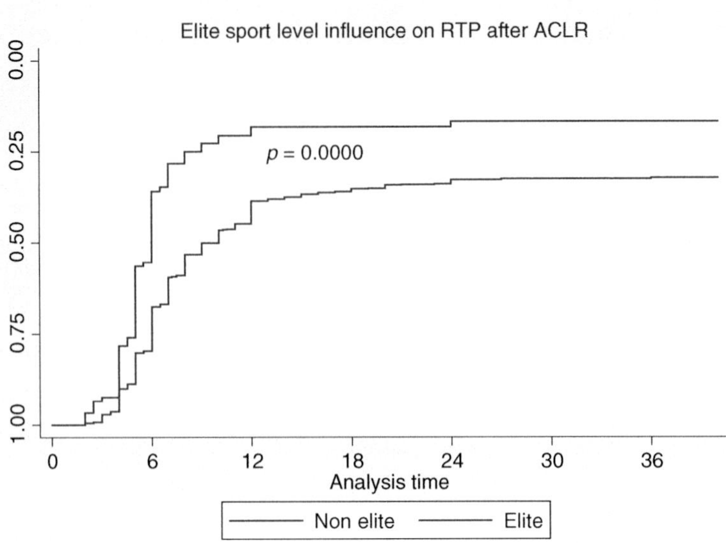

Fig. 15.2 Kaplan Meier survival estimates for RTP after ACLR. Elite sport athletes (93 cases) RTP more frequently and also faster than nonelite athletes (1177 cases). At 6 months after ACLR, over 60% of elite athletes had returned to play vs. <30% of the remaining athletes. 1270 patients included in this analysis

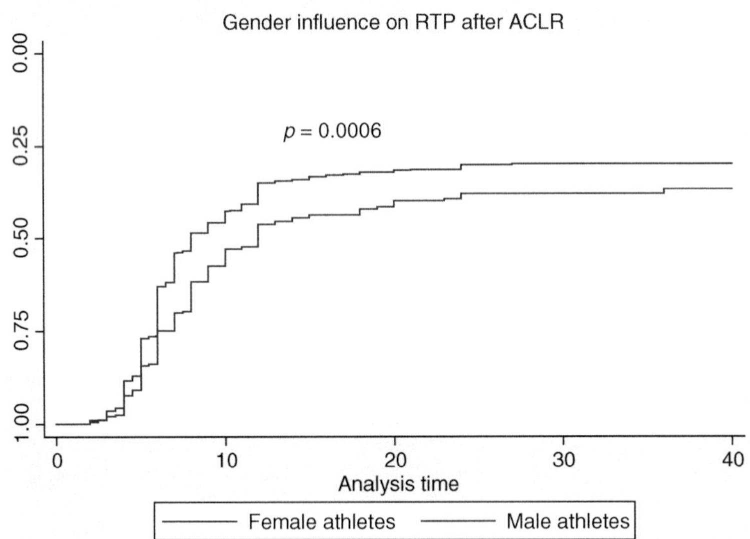

Fig. 15.3 Kaplan Meier survival estimates for RTP after ACLR. Male patients (red line) have more probability to RTP compared to the female counterpart

15.6.4 Isokinetic Medical Group Cohort: Rehabilitation RTP Predictors

Among rehabilitation factors, *quadriceps strength*, *cardiovascular fitness reconditioning* and *completing a stepwise on field rehabilitation (OFR) programme* were correlated with RTP in our cohort, as reported in Tables 15.3 and 15.4.

> **Fact Box 4**
> *Recovery of quadriceps strength*, *proper metabolic recovery* and *complete on field rehabilitation* correlate with higher rate of RTP. These factors are potentially modifiable, and the sport medicine team should focus on modifiable factors to improve the patient's outcome.

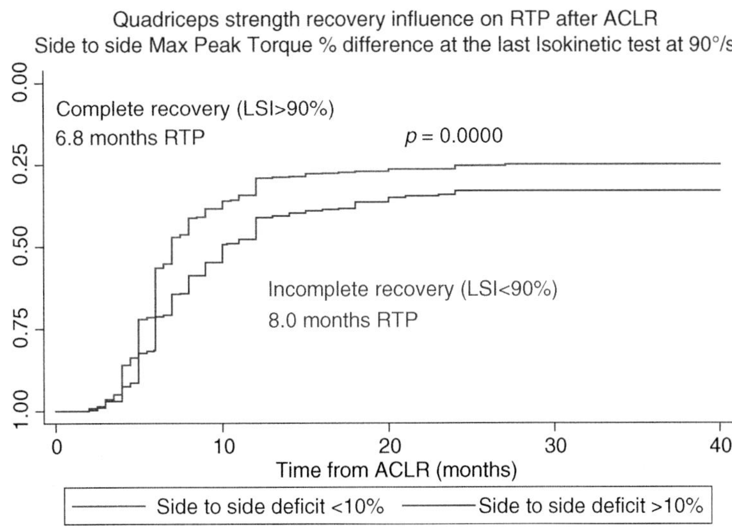

Fig. 15.4 Kaplan Meier survival estimates for RTP after ACLR. 946 included in this analysis. Patients that had achieved a complete quadriceps muscle strength recovery at the end of rehabilitation have also had constantly more probability to RTP; plus they had a faster recovery, too

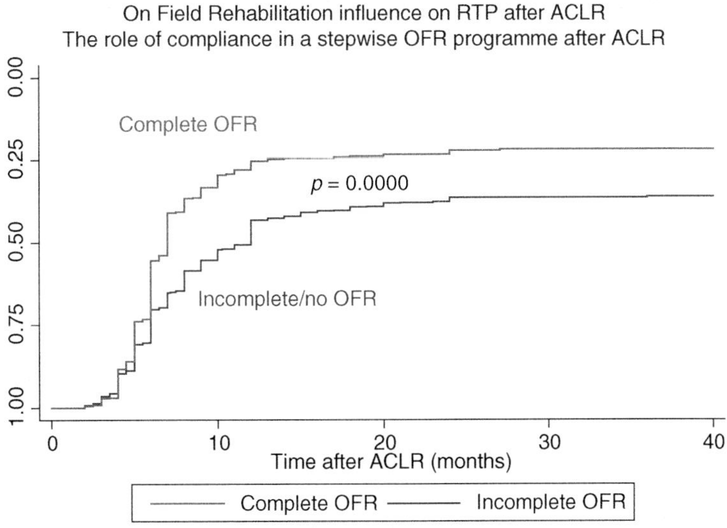

Fig. 15.5 Kaplan Meier survival estimates for RTP after ACLR. 1264 patients included in this analysis. Compliance in the OFR programme is associated constantly over time to higher RTP odds. *OFR* on field rehabilitation

Table 15.3 Relationship between rehabilitation factors and rate of RTP

	Rehabilitation factors					
Factor (cases)	Quadriceps strength recovery		On field rehabilitation		Metabolic recovery AT vel (km/h)	
	<10% (501)	>10% (445)	Complete (397)	Incomplete (867)	>8.6 (301)	<8.6 (351)
RTP rate (%)	73.4%*	64.3%	77.1%*	61.1%	72.8%*	65.4%

AT aerobic threshold velocity at the last threshold test
* = statistically significant result ($p < 0.05$)

Table 15.4 Predictors of RTP after ACLR

Rehabilitation factor model (logistic regression analysis)						
	Univariate			Multivariate		
	OR	95% C.I.	*p*	OR	95% C.I.	*p*
Quad deficit <10% vs. >10%	**1.53**	**1.16–2.02**	**0.002**	**1.45**	**1.00–2.13**	**0.049**
Complete OFR vs. incomplete	**2.14**	**1.63–2.81**	**0.000**	**1.58**	**1.06–2.35**	**0.024**
AT vel > 8.6 km/h vs. <8.6 km/h	**1.79**	**1.27–2.52**	**0.001**	**1.54**	**1.04–2.30**	**0.032**
Age (<29 vs. >29 years)				1.00	0.68–1.46	0.996
Sex (M vs. F)				1.17	0.67–1.48	0.459

Rehabilitation model
Univariate and multivariate analysis
Statistically significant result reported in bold
OR odds ratio, *CI* 95% confidence interval, *Quad* quadriceps muscle, *AT* aerobic threshold (2 mmol/l of blood lactate) velocity

15.7 Embedding Original Research into Clinical Practice

Given all the numbers, if we really want to ameliorate patient outcomes and health, original and literature research has to be translated into clinical practice (Fig. 15.6). Evidence behind functional outcomes has to be part of the clinician approach to the ACLR patient. Generating tools to share realistic numbers with patients and patient's environment is a present option in the modern sport-medicine landscape. We deeply believe that a correct implementation of study results, in an understandable way, is a crucial point to move forward.

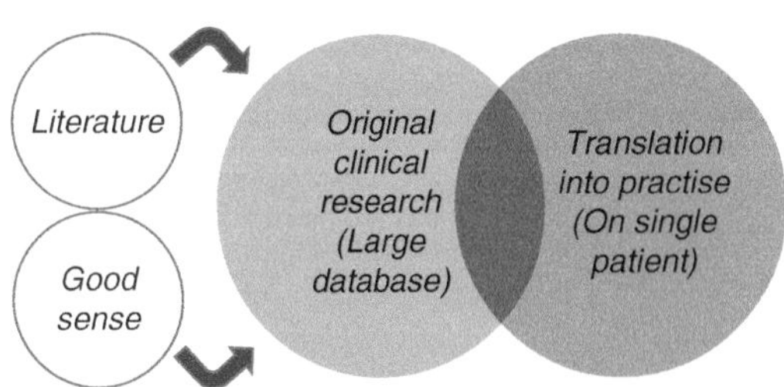

Fig. 15.6 The Blue world (original and literature research) and the Red world (clinical application) are two parts of the same "patient first" approach. Without cross talking between the worlds, we won't progress

15.8 Conclusion and RTP Recommendation

In conclusion the existing literature and the data we presented in this chapter highlight the existence of different RTP predictors after ACLR. Even if RTP decision remains a patient's choice, also based on not-knee-related factors, a number of baseline characteristics of the patient, plus a series of modifiable factors, are correlated to this decision. As physical functioning (as muscle strength and fitness reconditioning) and compliance in rehabilitation correlate with better outcomes, the importance of following (and completing) a *criteria-based rehabilitation* with full compliance should be encouraged. Following ACL injury patients need to be correctly counselled, with real numbers about RTP probabilities. Clinician should be aware about this numbers and moreover about the possibility to increase the odds of a positive outcome with a proper exercise intervention.

Although the ideal RTP test battery has not been established yet, and may never be, we purpose to base the RTP clearance decision on the criteria reported in Table 15.5. As the risk of a second ACL injury is as high as 23.5% in young active patient after RTP [15], we also need to highlight the importance of proper neuromuscular control in high-speed athletic tasks prior

Table 15.5 Isokinetic medical group RTP criteria following ACLR

Criteria to RTP after ACLR
1. No giving way episodes (<1)
2. Complete recovery of knee ROM (as the contralateral knee)
3. Complete recovery of quadriceps and hamstring strength (isokinetic test LSI 100%)
4. Hamstring/quadriceps (H/Q) ratio >0.70. Measured at isokinetic test (90°/s maximal peak torque)
5. Complete recovery of adequate qualitative movement patterns. MAT score ≥90 points/100
(a) No evidence of dynamic knee valgus
(b) Adequate pelvis and trunk stability and dynamic control
(c) Adequate shock absorption with the proficient use of knee and hip flexion
(d) The proficient use of a hip strategy, no evidence of a knee strategy
6. Cardiovascular match fitness recovery, measured at the aerobic/anaerobic threshold test. For football players aerobic threshold velocity (AT2) ≥11.5 km/h and anaerobic threshold velocity ≥13.5 km/h
7. Complete on filed rehabilitation programme

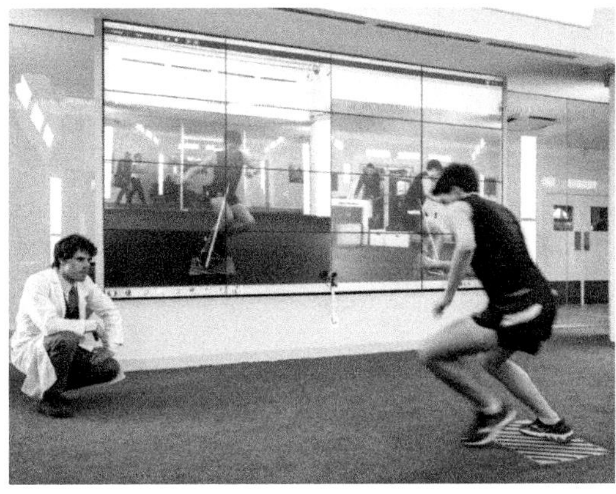

Fig. 15.7 The present and future of ACLR rehabilitation are related to the neuro-sensory-motor aspects of complex movement patterns

RTP. A *qualitative movement pattern evaluation* (Fig. 15.7) may be a critical addiction in addressing this often overlooked aspect, associated to the second injury risk in female athletes [16]. Further studies, with prospective design, are needed in order to establish the best safe RTP predictors following ACLR.

Fact Box 5

Qualitative movement pattern evaluation is at the state of the art of ACL rehabilitation and should be integrated in RTP criteria.

Take-Home Messages

- RTP following ACLR is a complex biopsychosocial outcome. In our study, the 94% of the patients returned to some kind of activity and the 76% to same sport but only the 66% RTP to same sport and same activity level.
- *Male athletes* have 50% greater probability to RTP (same sport and level) after ACLR compared to the female counterpart
- *Elite sport level* guarantees two times greater probability to RTP (same sport and level), displaying completely different results if compared to recreational level.
- *Overweight athletes* (*BMI* > *25*) had poorer results in terms of RTP in our cohort.
- *Early ACLR* (*within 2.5 months*) is associated with higher odds to RTP and maybe recommended to ACL-injured athlete, as this is a modifiable factor.
- *Revision ACLR* is associated to lower results. It seems that the second time is much more difficult to RTP efficiently.
- Achieving *complete quadriceps strength recovery* was associated to higher RTP rate and faster recovery and should be pursued in rehabilitation.
- Metabolic reconditioning should be a target of ACLR rehabilitation as *higher aerobic fitness recovery* correlated with better results.
- Attention in the last phases of rehabilitation should be high as *compliance in the OFR programme* was an important predictor of RTP in our cohort.
- Correct patient counselling on RTP rate plus a systematic addressing of the modifiable factors should be applied after ACL injury and ACLR.

Top Five Evidence Based References

Ardern CL, Taylor NF, Feller JA, Webster K (2014) Fifty-five per cent return to competitive sport following anterior cruciate ligament surgery: an updated systematic review and meta-analysis including aspects of physical functioning and contextual factors. Br J Sports Med 48(21):1543–1552

Lentz TA, Zeppieri G Jr, Tillman SM, Indelicato PA, Moser MW, George SZ, Chmielewski TL (2012) Return to preinjury sports participation following anterior cruciate ligament reconstruction: contributions of demographic, knee impairment, and self-report measures. J Orthop Sports Phys Ther 42(11):893–901

Tjong VK, Murnaghan ML, Nyhof-Young JM, Ogilvie-Harris DJ (2014) A qualitative investigation of the decision to return to sport after anterior cruciate ligament reconstruction: to play or not to play. Am J Sports Med 42(2):336–342

Fältström A, Hägglund M, Kvist J (2016) Factors associated with playing football after anterior cruciate ligament reconstruction in female football players. Scand J Med Sci Sports 26(11):1343–1352

Brophy RH, Schmitz L, Wright RW, Dunn WR, Parker RD, Andrish JT, McCarty EC, Spindler KP (2012) Return to play and future ACL injury risk after ACL reconstruction in soccer athletes from the Multicenter Orthopaedic Outcomes Network (MOON) group. Am J Sports Med 40(11):2517–2522

References

1. Sandon A, Werner S, Forssblad M (2015) Factors associated with returning to football after anterior cruciate ligament reconstruction. Knee Surg Sports Traumatol Arthrosc 23(9):2514–2521
2. Dunn WR, Spindler KP, Consortium MOON (2010) Predictors of activity level 2 years after anterior cruciate ligament reconstruction (ACLR): a Multicenter Orthopaedic Outcomes Network (MOON) ACLR cohort study. Am J Sports Med 38(10):2040–2050
3. Spindler KP, Wright RW (2008) Clinical practice. Anterior cruciate ligament tear. N Engl J Med 359(20):2135–2142
4. Andriolo L, Filardo G, Kon E, Ricci M, Della Villa F, Della Villa S, Zaffagnini S, Marcacci M (2015) Revision anterior cruciate ligament reconstruction: clinical outcome and evidence for return to sport. Knee Surg Sports Traumatol Arthrosc 23(10):2825–2845
5. Ardern CL, Taylor NF, Feller JA, Webster K (2014) Fifty-five per cent return to competitive sport following anterior cruciate ligament surgery: an updated systematic review and meta-analysis including aspects of physical functioning and contextual factors. Br J Sports Med 48(21):1543–1552
6. Ardern CL, Taylor NF, Feller JA, Whitehead TS, Webster KE (2013) Psychological responses matter in returning to preinjury level of sport after anterior cruciate ligament reconstruction surgery. Am J Sports Med 41(7):1549–1558
7. Lentz TA, Zeppieri G Jr, Tillman SM, Indelicato PA, Moser MW, George SZ, Chmielewski TL (2012) Return to preinjury sports participation following anterior cruciate ligament reconstruction: contributions of demographic, knee impairment, and self-report measures. J Orthop Sports Phys Ther 42(11):893–901
8. Della Villa F, Ricci M, Perdisa F, Filardo G, Gamberini J, Caminati D, Della Villa S (2016) Anterior cruciate ligament reconstruction and rehabilitation: predictors of functional outcome. Joints 3(4):179–185
9. Tjong VK, Murnaghan ML, Nyhof-Young JM, Ogilvie-Harris DJ (2014) A qualitative investigation of the decision to return to sport after anterior cruciate ligament reconstruction: to play or not to play. Am J Sports Med 42(2):336–342
10. Czuppon S, Racette BA, Klein SE, Harris-Hayes M (2014) Variables associated with return to sport following anterior cruciate ligament reconstruction: a systematic review. Br J Sports Med 48(5):356–364
11. Langford JL, Webster KE, Feller JA (2009) A prospective longitudinal study to assess psychological changes following anterior cruciate ligament reconstruction surgery. Br J Sports Med 43(5):377–381
12. Kvist J, Ek A, Sporrstedt K, Good L (2005) Fear of re-injury: a hindrance for returning to sports after anterior cruciate ligament reconstruction. Knee Surg Sports Traumatol Arthrosc 13(5):393–397
13. Gobbi A, Fancisco R (2006) Factors affecting return to sports after anterior cruciate ligament reconstruction with patellar tendon and hamstring graft: a prospective clinical investigation. Knee Surg Sports Traumatol Arthrosc 14(10):1021–1028
14. Della Villa S, Boldrini L, Ricci M, Danelon F, Snyder-Mackler L, Nanni G, Roi GS (2012) Clinical outcomes and return-to-sports participation of 50 soccer players after anterior cruciate ligament reconstruction through a sport-specific rehabilitation protocol. Sports Health 4(1):17–24
15. Wiggins AJ, Grandhi RK, Schneider DK, Stanfield D, Webster KE, Myer GD (2016) Risk of secondary injury in younger athletes after anterior cruciate ligament reconstruction: a systematic review and meta-analysis. Am J Sports Med 44(7):1861–1876
16. Paterno MV, Schmitt LC, Ford KR, Rauh MJ, Myer GD, Huang B, Hewett TE (2010) Biomechanical measures during landing and postural stability predict second anterior cruciate ligament injury after anterior cruciate ligament reconstruction and return to sport. Am J Sports Med 38(10):1968–1978

16 Laxity-Based Return to Play

Stefano Zaffagnini, Luca Macchiarola, Ilaria Cucurnia, Alberto Grassi, and Cecilia Signorelli

Contents

16.1 Introduction

Anterior cruciate ligament (ACL) rupture is a troublesome injury for a football player and the long-term consequences, such as early-onset osteoarthritis [1]. Interestingly, a recent study reported an increase in the number of annual ACL injuries recorded in US Major League Soccer (MLS) from 1996 to 2012: there has been at least one ACL tear per year and a greater number of ACL tears of the left versus the right knee. The ACL injury rate is 0.4 per team per season, which means that a club on average will see an ACL injury every second season [2]. In particular, injury is more frequent in female soccer players (they have almost 7 times the odds of sustaining a primary ACL tear compared with their male counterparts) [3], total rupture rate is significantly higher than the partial rupture rate, and the match ACL injury rate is 20 times higher than the training injury rate [4].

A debated risk factor in the literature is fatigue, but many of the ACL injuries actually occur early in the first half or among newly substituted players in the second half [5]. This finding suggests that if fatigue is a risk factor, it is probably more an effect of accumulated fatigue over time, for

S. Zaffagnini (✉) • L. Macchiarola • I. Cucurnia
A. Grassi
Clinica Ortopedica e Traumatologica II, Istituto Ortopedico Rizzoli, Bologna, Italy

Laboratorio di Biomeccanica e Innovazione Tecnologica, Istituto Ortopedico Rizzoli, Bologna, Italy
e-mail: stefano.zaffagnini@biomec.ior.it; luca.macchiarola@hotmail.it; ilaria.cucurnia@gmail.com

C. Signorelli
Laboratorio di Biomeccanica e Innovazione Tecnologica, Istituto Ortopedico Rizzoli, Bologna, Italy
e-mail: c.signorelli@biomec.ior.it

V. Musahl et al. (eds.), *Return to Play in Football*, https://doi.org/10.1007/978-3-662-55713-6_16

example, owing to a congested match calendar [6, 7], than energy depletion per se in the match where the ACL injury occurs.

16.2 ACL Treatment in Professional Football Players

The general opinion among football medical doctors is that football players with an ACL injury need an ACL reconstruction in order to continue playing. The rationale for surgical intervention after ACL injury is to restore the pre-injury activity level [3].

The caretaking at the elite level represents, in many ways, the optimal situation: players at this level are supported by a highly qualified medical team, the time to diagnosis for this court is as a mean 8 days, and access for a diagnostic MRI is straightforward.

Marcacci et al. compared clinical results of surgical reconstructions within 15 days, and after 3 months from the injury, they obtained better results in terms of return-to-sport and laxity testing in the early reconstruction group [8]. Early surgery can thus be another factor behind the high success rates at elite level, but it is not completely proved [9].

Another important factor is the postoperative rehabilitation. Most certainly, the rehabilitation after ACL surgery has improved markedly during the last 20 years, but the possibility of being helped by a physiotherapist also differs between elite and amateur level. In Scandinavia, for example, an amateur football player is normally helped by a physiotherapist for about 1 h 2–3 times a week following ACL surgery; on the other hand, a player at elite level normally receives help from a team physiotherapist several hours every day [10].

Even if a majority of players can return to football after ACL injury/reconstruction, some sustain further knee problems and need of surgery [11, 12].

Walden et al. [4] have previously reported that many elite football players suffer from synovitis and other overuse injuries shortly after their comeback to football, possibly indicating premature return. At the professional level, economy has to be considered as an additional factor, with monetary implications increasing the desire to return to play. The high numbers of return to play after ACL surgery might reflect a satisfactory outcome, but could also be regarded as knee abuse with a risk of further joint injury and subsequent development of osteoarthritis. Another important finding is the mean absence from full team training between 6 and 7 months after surgery. This means that, even with optimal caretaking and resources, this is the time it takes and shorter rehabilitation could create an additional problem.

> **Fact Box 1**
> Generally, all players who underwent ACL reconstruction are able to return to training, but the re-rupture rate is not negligible. Even if 89% of professional athletes play within 12 months, only 65% competes at the highest level 3 years later.

Generally, all players who underwent ACL reconstruction for a total rupture are able to return to training, but the ipsilateral re-rupture rate (4%) and the need for other ipsilateral knee surgery (3%) before return to competitive activity are not negligible. Finally, the return-to-practice (RTP) rate within a year after ACL reconstruction for a total rupture is very high within 10 months (>90%), 89% participates in elite match play within 12 months, but only 65% compete at the highest level 3 years later. ACL re-ruptures are seen especially in younger athletes who return to sports. In particular, according to Wiggins et al. [13], when they are compared to uninjured subjects, they have a 30–40 times greater risk of ACL injury higher than those for uninjured subjects. The risk for ipsilateral graft rupture seems to be greatest in the first 2 years after ACL reconstruction, and a relatively higher proportion of contralateral ACL ruptures are seen with increasing follow-up periods [14].

It is well known that release for RTP after injury/surgery is a complex process, and, trying to understand which factors could influence outcomes, it is possible to determine extrinsic and intrinsic factors.

Between extrinsic factors only the "accelerated rehabilitation" concept by Shelbourne and Gray [15] is considered a vital goal, especially for high-level athletes. Application of this principle allowed professional athletes to return to sport as soon as 6 months after ACL reconstruction. However, caution should be used, as early return to sport has been demonstrated to be related to ACL failure, especially in cases of primary reconstruction with allograft tissue [16]. There are other extrinsic factors on outcome, such as type of graft, surgical technique, or fixation technique.

Intrinsic factors are patient's anatomy, biological response, and type of lesion. Morphological knee parameters such as tibial slope, notch width, and femoral condyle shape have been correlated with increased risk of ACL injury, ACL reconstruction failure, or postoperative laxity [17]. Furthermore, with regard to knee alignment, varus deformity has been demonstrated to increase tension on the ACL [18]. Furthermore, every patient has their own specific genetic makeup and biology, and lack of incorporation of the graft and biological failure are well-recognized causes of poor outcomes after ACL reconstruction [19]. Clinicians must consider the lesion pattern and concomitant injuries: medial meniscus deficiency is responsible for increased stress on the ACL during AP tibial translation [20], while lateral meniscal deficiency is responsible for increased rotational laxity during the pivot-shift maneuver [21]. Grade II medial collateral ligament (MCL) lesions were recently recognized as a risk factor for ACL failure with an odds ratio of 13, and untreated posterolateral corner lesions have been demonstrated to increase the risk of ACL failure and to worsen outcomes [22, 23]. Finally, concomitant lesions (such as cartilage injuries) are a fundamental variable in the final return-to-sport decision, as even isolated cartilage procedures like microfractures usually need a longer recovery time compared with ACL reconstruction, about 8–12 months even in competitive athletes submitted to aggressive rehabilitation [24, 25].

16.3 The Role of Laxity Assessment

The static function of the ACL in the knee stability is to provide constraint when a force is applied (posteriorly) to the tibia, forcing it to translate forward from the femur. From a dynamic point of view, the intact ACL (especially its posterolateral bundle) limits the internal rotation and anterior subluxation of the lateral compartment of the knee, assuring its stability when complex vectors of forces are applied, such as during pivoting sports [26].

The assessment of the knee laxity represents a key factor when approaching the ACL-injured athlete in the presurgical phase, since knee laxity represents an important diagnostic tool and determinates the treatment algorithm. It was demonstrated that a high grade of pre-reconstruction knee laxity significantly increases the odds of graft failure and revision [27].

Also an intraoperative evaluation of the residual laxity might suggest the need for additional surgical procedures. In fact, although the ACL is the main ligament for static and dynamic knee stability, other anatomical structures such as menisci and the anterolateral ligament (ALL) have been demonstrated to play a minor role in knee stability [28, 29].

For this reason the authors recommend always to perform a complete assessment and reconstruction of the damaged structures, to obtain the best results in terms of return to sport.

Finally, it is useful to evaluate the knee laxity throughout the postoperative period, to verify the integration of the graft and to decide the right moment for the athlete to return to professional sport activity [30].

It was demonstrated, with a biomechanical in vivo experiment, that rotational stability of the ACL-reconstructed knees did not show much improvement at the 3-month follow-up after surgery, but at the 12-month control, they showed a rotational stability comparable to the healthy contralateral side. This suggests that the graft undergoes significant remodeling over time detectable by laxity assessment [31].

16.4 Clinical Evaluation of the Knee Laxity

In the clinical setting, the most elementary and rapid tools for the physician to evaluate the ACL function are the anterior drawer test and the Lachman test [32] for the static laxity (Fig. 16.1). The dynamic laxity is evaluated with the pivot-shift test (PS) [33] (Fig. 16.2).

These examinations were described during the 1970s and led to better accuracy in diagnosis of the ACL injuries; in particular the Lachman has been demonstrated to be the most sensitive test, while the PS is the most specific test, especially under anesthesia [34].

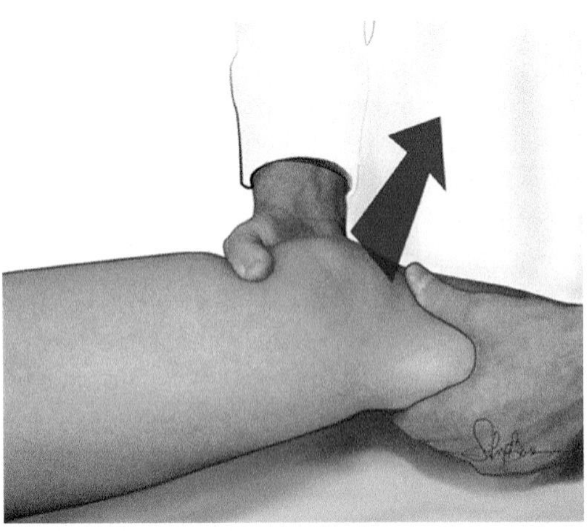

Fig. 16.1 The *arrow* shows the direction of the force applied on the tibia during the Lachman test

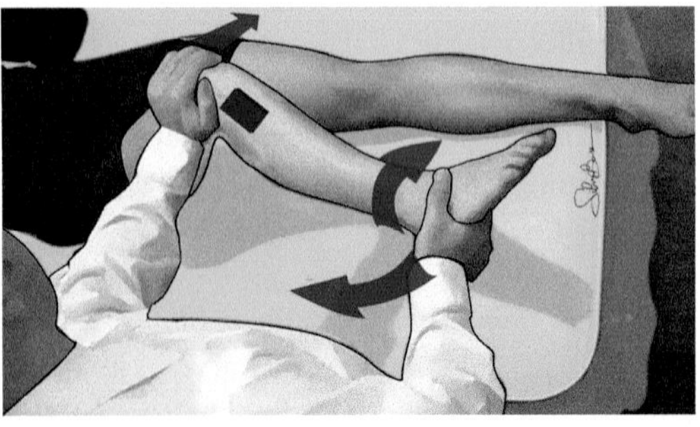

Fig. 16.2 The execution of the pivot-shift test, *arrows* show multiple vectors applied on the limb

The execution and grading of these tests are dependent on the experience of the physician and thus subjective; moreover, they involve great intra- and inter-examiner variability since applied manual loading cannot be standardized [35].

Nevertheless, a wide accepted clinical classification of the International Knee Documentation Committee (IKDC) ranks the knee laxity in four grades (from “A” to “D”) based on the millimeters of anterior tibial translation in Lachman and anterior drawer test and on the subjective feeling of tibial reduction for the PS test. In this classification the contralateral healthy side is taken as reference [36].

16.5 Instrumented Quantification of the Unidirectional Static Laxity

Among the first instruments designed for the evaluation of the ACL injuries, there are KT1000 (MEDmetric Corp, San Diego, CA, USA) and the Rolimeter (Aircast, Europe). These mechanical joint arthrometers are inexpensive and easy to use, allowing their application in an ambulatory setting. The KT1000 resembles the Lachman test in its execution and permits to calculate the force (in Newton) applied on the proximal tibia at 20° of flexion and to quantify its consequent anterior subluxation (in millimeters) [37] (Fig. 16.3).

Nowadays, this device is extensively used in the management of ACL reconstruction [38].

Rolimeter, which is normally used to quantify the anterior drawer test, is a simpler device that measures the anterior translation of the tibial tubercle, at 20° of flexion when a manual load is applied (Fig. 16.4).

Despite its simplicity, Rolimeter have been demonstrated to be as reliable and reproducible as KT1000 in the knee laxity assessment [39, 40]. Anyway, the opinion about the relation between KT1000 and Rolimeter data and clinical outcome is not unanimous, so the utility of these two instruments is not wide yet.

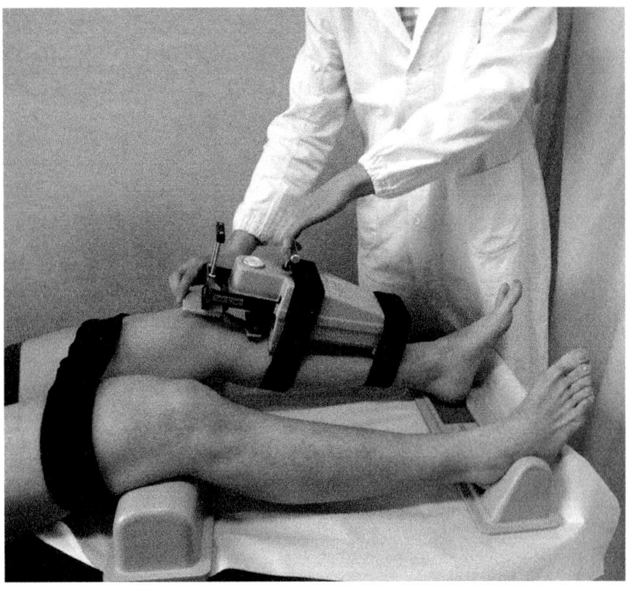

Fig. 16.3 KT1000 measures the anterior tibial translation when a standard force is applied

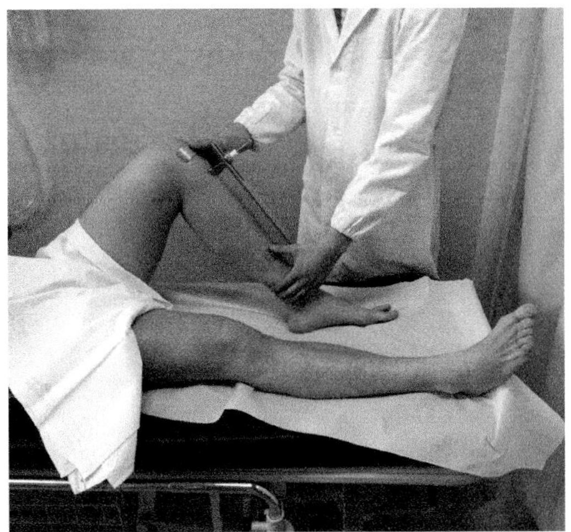

Fig. 16.4 Rolimeter measures anterior tibial translation during an anterior drawer maneuver

16.6 Assisted Assessment of the Multidirectional Dynamic Laxity with the Pivot-Shift Test

The pivot shift is a phenomenon occurring in the ACL-deficient knee when, in extension, the lateral tibial plateau is anteriorly subluxated: at a certain degree of flexion, the increased tension elicited by the iliotibial band causes a sudden reduction upon the condyles. The combined movement of the tibia during this maneuver can be divided in external rotation and posterior translation [41].

Given the complex kinematics of the PST, a number of parameters have been described in the literature for quantification. These parameter can be classified in four groups (translations, rotations, acceleration/velocity, and others), thus pointing out the lack of consensus and of standardized methodology among physicians [42].

During recent years several devices have been developed for the assessment of the knee dynamic laxity, the most promising being surgical navigation, electromagnetic sensors system, inertial sensors, and image analysis system [43].

16.6.1 Computer-Assisted Surgical Navigation

First developed during the 1990s, computer-aided surgery (CAS) has been used during ACL reconstruction to implement the tunnel drilling and the isometry of the graft and later to evaluate the knee kinematics [44].

Determination of the patient anatomy is needed for CAS, and this can be achieved with a preoperative computer tomography, intraoperatively with fluoroscopic X-rays, or more commonly with an image-free digitalization of certain anatomical structures using navigated pointers. In order to evaluate knee kinematics, either electromagnetic or optoelectronic technology is utilized to evaluate joint positions and movement. Trackers and receivers are fixed invasively to the bones under anesthesia; thus, no skin-related artifacts are present with this technology [45]. Using a navigation system (BLU-IGS, Orthokey, Lewes, Delaware, DE, USA), static and dynamic laxity measurements demonstrated that compared to single-bundle ACL-R, the double-bundle technique provides better laxity control during the PST [46].

16.6.2 Electromagnetic Sensor System

In vivo first evaluation of the knee movement during PST in 6 degree of motion (DOF) was performed by Bull et al. [41] using the electromagnetic system; they used sensors which were fixed into the femur and tibia with pins. Their measurements were accurate but the technique was invasive.

Noninvasive electromagnetic tracking devices (FASTRAK or LIBERTY, Polhemus, Colchester, VT, USA) have a sampling rate of 60 Hz and 249 Hz, respectively, and a root square accuracy of 0.03 mm and 0.15° of rotation [47].

The system is composed of three electromagnetic receivers and transmitters that produce an electromagnetic field. The first and the second receivers are fixed on the thigh and below the tibial tubercle with braces; the third is utilized to record and reconstruct the three-dimensional anatomy of the limb through seven bony landmarks. The respective movements of the tibia and femur are then visualized and analyzed on a laptop as a virtual limb [48].

Electromagnetic devices have been used for over a decade and are precise, reliable, and noninvasive. Nevertheless, metallic objects can produce signal disturbances, and wireless systems are yet to be developed to facilitate examinations.

16.6.3 Inertial Sensors

These devices have received growing attention during the last years; they exploit the fact that the lateral aspect of the tibia undergoes a sudden acceleration during reduction in the pivot-shift maneuver. This value can be calculated (in m/s^2) and visualized on a graph (Fig. 16.5).

16.6.3.1 Triaxial Accelerometer

KiRA (Orthokey, LLC, Lewes, DE, USA) is attached with a strap between the tibial tuberosity

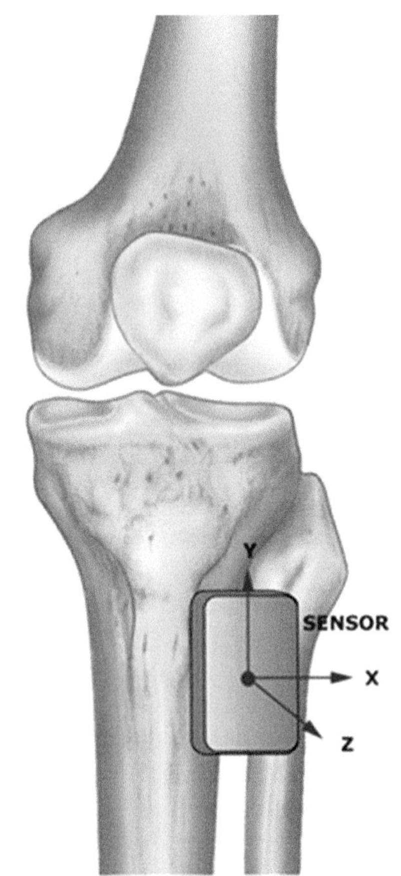

Fig. 16.5 Triaxial accelerometers are able to measure the accelerations in the three-dimensional space

and Gerdy tubercle and connected wireless with a tablet. The PST examinations can be performed before surgery and under anesthesia and is able to show statistically significant differences in acceleration between ACL injured and intact knees [49, 50].

At the 6-month follow-up, the values of acceleration normalized. However, it was shown that the specificity of the device varies from 50% to 90% depending on the experience of the tester [51].

KiRA was validated for clinical practice in the treatment of the ACL injury [52].

16.6.4 Optical Motion Capture Technique

Image analysis measures posterior translation of the tibia during pivot shift correlating with clinical grading of the PST [53, 54].

Using an iPad technology (PIVOT, Impellia Inc., USA), the recorded translation of the lateral compartment was related the IKDC clinical classification. Significant differences were found between the ACL-injured and contralateral side of the included patients; moreover, there was a significant difference in mean translation between knees graded as 1 when compared to knees graded as 2 [55]. It has been demonstrated that both inertial sensors and image analysis devices are able to differentiate between high-grade and low-grade PTS results according to the IKDC classification, making them optimal tools for diagnosis and follow-up [56].

Fact Box 2

Inertial sensors exploit the fact that the lateral aspect of the tibia undergoes a sudden acceleration during the pivot-shift maneuver: this acceleration can be on a graph. Moreover, the KiRA device has been validated for the evaluation of the anteroposterior laxity.

16.7 The Neuromuscular Factor After ACLR

There is a significant difference between PST in awake and anesthetized patients; in particular, they obtained lower values of tibial acceleration and lateral compartment translation in the awake group. This suggests that the neuromuscular component might play an important role in determining the grade of dynamic knee laxity [57]. It was also demonstrated that the local neuromuscular condition varies during the first postoperative year, influencing the stability of the knee joint as well [58].

According to the author's clinical experience and studies, KiRA device permits the evaluation when the neuromuscular response of the operated limb reaches the same level of the uninjured knee, during the rehabilitation of the athlete [59]. This can be a useful aid in the return-to-sport decision process (Fig. 16.6).

Take Home Points

- Most physicians prefer manual testing of the Lachman and PST to assess the athlete readiness to return to play [60]; in particular the PST correlates to clinical outcomes and the development of osteoarthritis [61, 62].

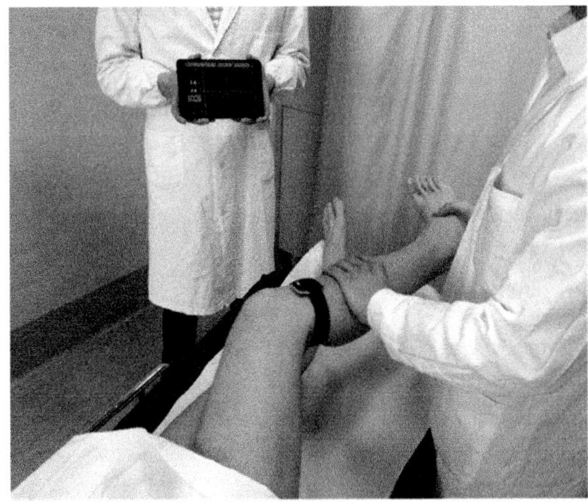

Fig. 16.6 The accelerations occurring during the pivot-shift test are measured with KiRA and visualized on a tablet

- Anterior laxity measured with KT1000 cannot predict return to football [63–65].
- Dynamic laxity 5 years postoperatively was greater in ACL-reconstructed knees than in uninjured knees, suggesting that this may affect the return to sport and risk of osteoarthritis [66].
- Currently, the timing of when an athlete returns to sport varies with rehabilitation programs, but no consensus rehabilitation program exists for athletes recovering from ACL reconstruction [67, 68].
- Actually, the return-to-sport decision is mostly based on subjective non-specific criteria [69]; on the other hand, objective criteria (like muscle strength, ROM, effusion) are used less [70].
- The vast majority of surgeons consider 6–8 months as a cut-off value for allowing sport resumption [71].
- The authors' preferred approach is using a sport-specific program to obtain more effective rehabilitation programs for athletes after surgery that allowed 95% and 62% of professional male soccer players to return to the same professional sport activity 1 and 4 years after surgery [72].
- Anyway, using a restricted test battery, the majority of patients who are 6 months after ACLR require additional rehabilitation to pass RTS criteria [73].
- It is important to create a new RTS battery with objective and restricted criteria in order to optimize the decision-making regarding RTS after ACLR with the aim to reduce incidence of second ACL injuries.

Fact Box 3

The sport resumption decision is now based on subjective non-specific criteria. Gokeler et al. demonstrated that using a more restricted test battery, the majority of patients who are 6 months after ACLR require additional rehabilitation.

Take Home Message

Despite the large number of clinical tests and accelerated rehabilitation, the improvement of diagnostic tools, and surgical technique, long-term results in professional football players are not excellent. A better pre- and postsurgical evaluation of knee laxity with new objective and restricted criteria, associated with the use in clinical practice of new devices for laxity assessment, have the potential to improve patient evaluation and to provide athletes with a safer instruction to return to sport.

Top Five Evidence Based References

Waldén M, Hägglund M, Magnusson H, Ekstrand J (2016) ACL injuries in men's professional football: a 15-year prospective study on time trends and return-to-play rates reveals only 65% of players still play at the top level 3 years after ACL rupture. Br J Sports Med 50(12):744–750

Van Eck CF, van den BekeromMP FFH, Poolman RW, Kerkhoffs GM (2013) Methods to diagnose acute anterior cruciate ligament rupture: a meta-analysis of physical examinations with and without anaesthesia. Knee Surg Sports Traumatol Arthrosc 21(8):1895–1903

Kilinc BE, Kara A, Celik H, Oc Y, Camur S (2016) Evaluation of the accuracy of Lachman and Anterior Drawer Tests with KT1000 ın the follow-up of anterior cruciate ligament surgery. J Exerc Rehabil 12(4):363–367

Zaffagnini S, Lopomo N, Signorelli C, Marcheggiani Muccioli GM, Bonanzinga T, Grassi A, Raggi F, Visani A, Marcacci M (2014) Inertial sensors to quantify the pivot shift test in the treatment of anterior cruciate ligament injury. Joints 2(3):124–129

Gokeler WW, Zaffagnini S, Seil R, Padua D (2017) Development of a test battery to enhance safe return to sports after anterior cruciate ligament reconstruction. Knee Surg Sports Traumatol Arthrosc 25:192–199

References

1. Von Porat A, Roos EM, Roos H (2004) High prevalence of osteoarthritis 14 years after an anterior cruciate ligament tear in male soccer players: a study of radiographic and 20 patient relevant outcomes. Ann Rheum Dis 63(3):269–273
2. Erickson BJ, Harris JD, Cvetanovich GL, Bach BR, Bush-Joseph CA, Abrams GD, Gupta AK, McCormick FM, Cole BJ (2014) Performance and return to sport after anterior cruciate ligament reconstruction in male

Major League Soccer players. Orthop J Sports Med 2(9):2325967114548831
3. Roos H, Ornell M, Gardsell P, Lohmander LS, Lindstrand A (1995) Soccer after anterior cruciate ligament injury, an incompatible combination? A national survey of incidence and risk factors and a 7-year follow-up of 310 players. Acta Orthop Scand 66(2):107–112
4. Waldén M, Hägglund M, Magnusson H, Ekstrand J (2016) ACL injuries in men's professional football: a 15-year prospective study on time trends and return-to-play rates reveals only 65% of players still play at the top level 3 years after ACL rupture. Br J Sports Med 50(12):744–750
5. Waldén M, Hägglund M, Magnusson H, Ekstrand J (2011) Anterior cruciate ligament injury in elite football: a prospective three-cohort study. Knee Surg Sports Traumatol Arthrosc 19:11–19
6. Dupont G, Nedelec M, McCall A, McCormack D, Berthoin S, Wisløff U (2010) Effect of 2 soccer matches in a week on physical performance and injury rate. Am J Sports Med 38:1752–1758
7. Carling C, McCall A, Le Gall F, Dupont G (2016) The impact of short periods of match congestion on injury risk and patterns in an elite football club. Br J Sports Med 50:764–768
8. Marcacci M, Zaffagnini S, Iacono F, Neri MP, Petito A (1995) Early versus late reconstruction for anterior cruciate ligament rupture. Results after 5 years of follow- up. Am J Sports Med 23(6):690–693
9. Granan LP, Bahr R, Lie SA, Engebretsen L (2009) Timing of anterior cruciate ligament reconstructive surgery and risk of cartilage lesions and meniscal tears: a cohort study based on the Norwegian National Knee Ligament Registry. Am J Sports Med 37:955–961
10. Ekstrand J (2011) A 94% return to elite level football after ACL surgery: a proof of possibilities with optimal caretaking or a sign of knee abuse? Knee Surg Sports Traumatol Arthrosc 19:1–2
11. Brophy RH, Schmitz L, Wright RW, Dunn WR, Parker RD, Andrish JT, McCarty EC, Spindler KP (2012) Return to play and future ACL injury risk after ACL reconstruction in soccer athletes from the Multicenter Orthopedic Outcomes Network (MOON) group. Am J Sports Med 40:2517–2522
12. Waldén M, Hägglund M, Ekstrand J (2006) High risk of new knee injury in elite footballers with previous anterior cruciate ligament injury. Br J Sports Med 40:158–162
13. Wiggins AJ, Grandhi RK, Schneider DK, Stanfield D, Webster KE, Myer GD (2016) Risk of secondary injury in younger athletes after anterior cruciate ligament reconstruction: a systematic review and meta-analysis. Am J Sports Med 44(7):1861–1876
14. Waldén M (2013) Return to sports after ACL reconstruction surgery: a risk for further joint injury? In: Sanchis-Alfonso V, Monllau JC (eds) The ACL-deficient knee. A problem solving approach. 1st edn. Springer, London, pp 183–188
15. Shelbourne KD, Gray T (1997) Anterior cruciate ligament reconstruction with autogenous patellar tendon graft followed by accelerated rehabilitation. A two- to nine-year follow-up. Am J Sports Med 25(6):786–795
16. van Eck CF, Schkrohowsky JG, Working ZM, Irrgang JJ, FH F (2012) Prospective analysis of failure rate and predictors of failure after anatomic anterior cruciate ligament reconstruction with allograft. Am J Sports Med 40:800–807
17. Sturnick DR, Vacek PM, DeSarno MJ, Gardner-Morse MG, Tourville TW, Slauterbeck JR, Johnson RJ, Shultz SJ, Beynnon BD (2015) Combined anatomic factors predicting risk of anterior cruciate ligament injury for males and females. Am J Sports Med 43(4):839–847
18. van de Pol GJ, Arnold MP, Verdonschot N, van Kampen A (2009) Varus alignment leads to increased forces in the anterior cruciate ligament. Am J Sports Med 37:481–487
19. Ménétrey J, Duthon VB, Laumonier T, Fritschy D (2008) "Biological failure" of the anterior cruciate ligament graft. Knee Surg Sports Traumatol Arthrosc 16:224–231
20. Spang JT, Dang AB, Mazzocca A, Rincon L, Obopilwe E, Beynnon B, Arciero RA (2010) The effect of medial meniscectomy and meniscal allograft transplantation on knee and anterior cruciate ligament biomechanics. Arthroscopy 26:192–201
21. Musahl V, Citak M, O'Loughlin PF, Choi D, Bedi A, Pearle AD (2010) The effect of medial versus lateral meniscectomy on the stability of the anterior cruciate ligament-deficient knee. Am J Sports Med 38:1591–1597
22. Ahn JH, Lee SH (2016) Risk factors for knee instability after anterior cruciate ligament reconstruction. Knee Surg Sports Traumatol Arthrosc 24(9):2936–2942
23. Bonanzinga T, Zaffagnini S, Grassi A, Marcheggiani Muccioli GM, Neri MP, Marcacci M (2013) Management of combined anterior cruciate ligament-posterolateral corner tears: a systematic review. Am J Sports Med 42:1496–1503
24. Kon E, Filardo G, Berruto M, Benazzo F, Zanon G, Della Villa S, Marcacci M (2011) Articular cartilage treatment in high- level male soccer players: a prospective comparative study of arthroscopic second-generation autologous chondrocyte implantation versus microfracture. Am J Sports Med 39:2549–2557
25. Della Villa S, Kon E, Filardo G, Ricci M, Vincentelli F, Delcogliano M, Marcacci M (2010) Does intensive rehabilitation permit early return to sport without compromising the clinical outcome after arthroscopic autologous chondrocyte implantation in highly competitive athletes? Am J Sports Med 38:68–77
26. Zantop T, Herbort M, Raschke MJ, Fu FH, Petersen W (2007) The role of the anteromedial and postero-

lateral bundles of the anterior cruciate ligament in anterior tibial translation and internal rotation. Am J Sports Med 35(2):223–227

27. Magnussen RA, Reinke EK, Huston LJ, MOON Group, Hewett TE, Spindler KP (2016) Effect of high-grade preoperative knee laxity on anterior cruciate ligament reconstruction outcomes. Am J Sports Med 44(12):3077–3082
28. Zaffagnini S, Signorelli C, Bonanzinga T, Grassi A, Galán H, Akkawi I, Bragonzoni L, Cataldi F, Marcacci M (2016) Does meniscus removal affect ACL-deficient knee laxity? An in vivo study. Knee Surg Sports Traumatol Arthrosc 24(11):3599–3604
29. Kittl C, El-Daou H, Athwal KK, Gupte CM, Weiler A, Williams A, Amis AA (2016) The role of the anterolateral structures and the ACL in controlling laxity of the intact and ACL-deficient knee. Am J Sports Med 44(2):345–354
30. Rahnemai-Azar AA, Naendrup JH, Soni A, Olsen A, Zlotnicki J, Musahl V (2016) Knee instability scores for ACL reconstruction. Curr Rev Musculoskelet Med 9(2):170–177
31. Moewis P, Duda GN, Jung T, Heller MO, Boeth H, Kaptein B, Taylor WR (2016) The restoration of passive rotational tibio-femoral laxity after anterior cruciate ligament reconstruction. PLoS One 11(7):e0159600
32. Torg JS, ConradW KV (1976) Clinical diagnosis of anterior cruciate ligament instability in the athlete. Am J Sports Med 4(2):84–93
33. Galway HR, MacIntosh DL (1980) The lateral pivot shift: a symptom and sign of anterior cruciate ligament insufficiency. Clin Orthop Relat Res (147):45–50
34. Van Eck CF, van den BekeromMP FFH, Poolman RW, Kerkhoffs GM (2013) Methods to diagnose acute anterior cruciate ligament rupture: a meta-analysis of physical examinations with and without anaesthesia. Knee Surg Sports Traumatol Arthrosc 21(8):1895–1903
35. Musahl V, Hoshino Y, Ahlden M, Araujo P, Irrgang JJ, Zaffagnini S et al (2012) The pivot shift: a global user guide. Knee Surg Sports Traumatol Arthrosc 20(4):724–731
36. Hefti F, Muller W, Jakob RP, Staubli HU (1993) Evaluation of knee ligament injuries with the IKDC form. Knee Surg Sports Traumatol Arthrosc 1(3–4):226–234
37. Daniel DM, Stone ML, Sachs R, Malcom L (1985) Instrumented measurement of anterior knee laxity in patients with acute anterior cruciate ligament disruption. Am J Sports Med 13(6):401–407
38. Kilinc BE, Kara A, Celik H, Oc Y, Camur S (2016) Evaluation of the accuracy of Lachman and Anterior Drawer Tests with KT1000 ın the follow-up of anterior cruciate ligament surgery. J Exerc Rehabil 12(4):363–367
39. Ganko A, Engebretsen L, Ozer H (2000) The rolimeter: a new arthrometer compared with the KT-1000. Knee Surg Sports Traumatol Arthrosc 8(1):36–39
40. Schuster AJ, McNicholas MJ, Wachtl SW, McGurty DW, Jakob RP (2004) A new mechanical testing device for measuring anteroposterior knee laxity. Am J Sports Med 32(7):1731–1735
41. Bull AM, Earnshaw PH, Smith A, Katchburian MV, Hassan AN, Amis AA (2002) Intraoperative measurement of knee kinematics in reconstruction of the anterior cruciate ligament. J Bone Joint Surg Br 84(7):1075–1081
42. Lopomo N, Zaffagnini S, Amis AA (2013) Quantifying the pivot shift test: a systematic review. Knee Surg Sports Traumatol Arthrosc 21(4):767–783
43. Sundemo D, Alentorn-Geli E, Hoshino Y, Musahl V, Karlsson J, Samuelsson K (2016) Objective measures on knee instability: dynamic tests: a review of devices for assessment of dynamic knee laxity through utilization of the pivot shift test. Curr Rev Musculoskelet Med 9(2):148–159
44. Zaffagnini S, Klos TV, Bignozzi S (2010) Computer-assisted anterior cruciate ligament reconstruction: an evidence-based approach of the first 15 years. Arthroscopy 26(4):546–554
45. Zaffagnini S, Bignozzi S, Martelli S, Imakiire N, Lopomo N, Marcacci M (2006) New intraoperative protocol for kinematic evaluation of ACL reconstruction: preliminary results. Knee Surg Sports Traumatol Arthrosc 14(9):811–816
46. Zaffagnini S, Signorelli C, Lopomo N, Bonanzinga T, Marcheggiani Muccioli GM, Bignozzi S, Visani A, Marcacci M (2012) Anatomic double-bundle and over-the-top single-bundle with additional extra-articular tenodesis: an in vivo quantitative assessment of knee laxity in two different ACL reconstructions. Knee Surg Sports Traumatol Arthrosc 20(1):153–159
47. Hoshino Y, Kuroda R, Nagamune K, Araki D, Kubo S, Yamaguchi M, Kurosaka M (2012) Optimal measurement of clinical rotational test for evaluating anterior cruciate ligament insufficiency. Knee Surg Sports Traumatol Arthrosc 20(7):1323–1330
48. Kuroda R, Hoshino Y (2016) Electromagnetic tracking of the pivot-shift. Curr Rev Musculoskelet Med 9(2):164–169
49. Maeyama A, Hoshino Y, Debandi A, Kato Y, Saeki K, Asai S, Goto B, Smolinski P, FH F (2011) Evaluation of rotational instability in the anterior cruciate ligament deficient knee using triaxial accelerometer: a biomechanical model in porcine knees. Knee Surg Sports Traumatol Arthrosc 19(8):1233–1238
50. Lopomo N, Zaffagnini S, Signorelli C, Bignozzi S, Giordano G, Marcheggiani Muccioli GM, Visani A (2012) An original clinical methodology for non-invasive assessment of pivot-shift test. Comput Methods Biomech Biomed Engin 15(12):1323–1328
51. Berruto M, Uboldi F, Gala L, Marelli B, Albisetti W (2013) Is triaxial accelerometer reliable in the evaluation and grading of knee pivot-shift phenomenon? Knee Surg Sports Traumatol Arthrosc 21(4):981–985
52. Zaffagnini S, Lopomo N, Signorelli C, Marcheggiani Muccioli GM, Bonanzinga T, Grassi A, Raggi F,

Visani A, Marcacci M (2014) Inertial sensors to quantify the pivot shift test in the treatment of anterior cruciate ligament injury. Joints 2(3):124–129
53. Hoshino Y, Araujo P, Irrgang JJ, FH F, Musahl V (2012) An image analysis method to quantify the lateral pivot shift test. Knee Surg Sports Traumatol Arthrosc 20(4):703–707
54. Bedi A, Musahl V, Lane C, Citak M, Warren RF, Pearle AD (2010) Lateral compartment translation predicts the grade of pivot shift: a cadaveric and clinical analysis. Knee Surg Sports Traumatol Arthrosc 18(9):1269–1276
55. Hoshino Y, Araujo P, Ahldén M, Samuelsson K, Muller B, Hofbauer M, Wolf MR, Irrgang JJ, FH F, Musahl V (2013) Quantitative evaluation of the pivot shift by image analysis using the iPad. Knee Surg Sports Traumatol Arthrosc 21(4):975–980
56. Musahl V, Griffith C, Irrgang JJ, Hoshino Y, Kuroda R, Lopomo N, Zaffagnini S, Samuelsson K, Karlsson J, PIVOT Study Group (2016) Validation of quantitative measures of rotatory knee laxity. Am J Sports Med 44(9):2393–2398
57. Lopomo N, Signorelli C, Rahnemai-Azar AA, Raggi F, Hoshino Y, Samuelsson K, Musahl V, Karlsson J, Kuroda R, Zaffagnini S, PIVOT Study Group (2016) Analysis of the influence of anaesthesia on the clinical and quantitative assessment of the pivot shift: a multicenter international study. Knee Surg Sports Traumatol Arthrosc. https://doi.org/10.1007/s00167-016-4130-1
58. Semay B, Rambaud A, Philippot R, Edouard P (2016) Evolution of the anteroposterior laxity by GnRB at 6, 9 and 12 months post-surgical anterior cruciate ligament reconstruction. Ann Phys Rehabil Med 59S:e19
59. Zaffagnini S, Signorelli C, Grassi A, Yue H, Raggi F, Urrizola F, Bonanzinga T, Marcacci M (2016) Assessment of the pivot shift using inertial sensors. Curr Rev Musculoskelet Med 9(2):160–163
60. Grassi A, Vascellari A, Combi A, Tomaello L, Canata GL, Zaffagnini S, Sports Committee SIGASCOT (2016) Return to sport after ACL reconstruction: a survey between the Italian Society of Knee, Arthroscopy, Sport, Cartilage and Orthopaedic Technologies (SIGASCOT) members. Eur J Orthop Surg Traumatol 26(5):509–516
61. Kocher MS, Steadman JR, Briggs KK, Sterett WI, Hawkins RJ (2004) Relationships between objective assessment of ligament stability and subjective assessment of symptoms and function after anterior cruciate ligament reconstruction. Am J Sports Med 32(3):629–634
62. Jonsson H, Riklund-Ahlstrom K, Lind J (2004) Positive pivot shift after ACL reconstruction predicts later osteoarthrosis: 63 patients followed 5-9 years after surgery. Acta Orthop Scand 75(5):594–599
63. Sandon A, Werner S, Forssblad M (2015) Factors associated with returning to football after anterior cruciate ligament reconstruction. Knee Surg Sports Traumatol Arthrosc 23(9):2514–2521
64. McGrath TM, Waddington G, Scarvell JM, Ball N, Creer R, Woods K, Smith D, Adams R (2016) An ecological study of anterior cruciate ligament reconstruction, Part 1: Clinical tests do not correlate with return-to-sport outcomes. Orthop J Sports Med 4(11):2325967116672208
65. Czuppon S, Racette BA, Klein SE, Harris-Hayes M (2013) Variables associated with return to sport following anterior cruciate ligament reconstruction: a systematic review. Br J Sports Med 48(5):356–364
66. Tagesson S, Öberg B, Kvist J (2015) Static and dynamic tibial translation before, 5 weeks after, and 5 years after anterior cruciate ligament reconstruction. Knee Surg Sports Traumatol Arthrosc 23(12):3691–3697
67. van Grinsven S, van Cingel RE, Holla CJ, van Loon CJ (2010) Evidence-based rehabilitation following anterior cruciate ligament reconstruction. Knee Surg Sports Traumatol Arthrosc 18:1128–1144
68. Myer GD, Paterno MV, Ford KR, Hewett TE (2008) Neuromuscular training techniques to target deficits before return to sport after anterior cruciate ligament reconstruction. J Strength Cond Res 22:987–1014
69. Barber-Westin SD, Noyes FR (2011) Factors used to determine return to unrestricted sports activities after anterior cruciate ligament reconstruction. Arthroscopy 27(12):1697–1705
70. Malinin TI, Levitt RL, Bashore C, Temple HT, Mnaymneh W (2002) A study of retrieved allografts used to replace anterior cruciate ligaments. Arthroscopy 18:163–170
71. Petersen W, Zantop T (2013) Return to play following ACL reconstruction: survey among experienced arthroscopic surgeons (AGA instructors). Arch Orthop Trauma Surg 133(7):969–977
72. Zaffagnini S, Grassi A, Marcheggiani Muccioli GM, Tsapralis K, Ricci M, Bragonzoni L, Della Villa S, Marcacci M (2014) Return to sport after anterior cruciate ligament reconstruction in professional soccer players. Knee 21:731–735
73. Gokeler W, Welling S, Zaffagnini R, Seil R, Padua D (2017) Development of a test battery to enhance safe return to sports after anterior cruciate ligament reconstruction. Knee Surg Sports Traumatol Arthrosc 25:192–199

17 MRI-Based Laxity Measurement for Return to Play

Renato Andrade, Rogério Pereira, Ricardo Bastos, Hugo Duarte, Hélder Pereira, Sérgio Rodrigues-Gomes, and João Espregueira-Mendes

Contents

17.1 Introduction

Returning to sports participation after an anterior cruciate ligament (ACL) injury has been controversial in both scientific evidence and clinical practice. In this sense, the debate between time-based and criteria-based return to play (RTP) has been extensively scrutinized by the scientific community.

R. Andrade
Clínica do Dragão, Espregueira-Mendes Sports Centre—FIFA Medical Centre of Excellence, Porto, Portugal

Dom Henrique Research Centre, Porto, Portugal

Faculty of Sports, University of Porto, Porto, Portugal

R. Pereira
Clínica do Dragão, Espregueira-Mendes Sports Centre—FIFA Medical Centre of Excellence, Porto, Portugal

Dom Henrique Research Centre, Porto, Portugal

Faculty of Sports, University of Porto, Porto, Portugal

Faculty of Health Sciences, University Fernando Pessoa, Porto, Portugal

R. Bastos
Clínica do Dragão, Espregueira-Mendes Sports Centre—FIFA Medical Centre of Excellence, Porto, Portugal

Dom Henrique Research Centre, Porto, Portugal

Fluminense Federal University, Niteroi, Brazil

H. Duarte
Hospital Riviera Chablais, Vaud-Valais, Switzerland

H. Pereira
Orthopaedic Department, Centro Hospitalar Póvoa de Varzim, Vila do Conde, Portugal

Ripoll y De Prado Sports Clinic—FIFA Medical Centre of Excellence, Madrid, Spain

3B's Research Group—Biomaterials, Biodegradables and Biomimetics, Headquarters of the European Institute of Excellence on Tissue Engineering and Regenerative Medicine, University of Minho, Guimarães, Portugal

ICVS/3B's—PT Government Associate Laboratory, Braga, Portugal

S. Rodrigues-Gomes
Clínica do Dragão, Espregueira-Mendes Sports Centre—FIFA Medical Centre of Excellence, Porto, Portugal

SMIC Serviço Médico de Imagem Computorizada, Porto, Portugal

V. Musahl et al. (eds.), *Return to Play in Football*, https://doi.org/10.1007/978-3-662-55713-6_17

J. Espregueira-Mendes (✉)
Clínica do Dragão, Espregueira-Mendes Sports Centre—FIFA Medical Centre of Excellence, Porto, Portugal

Dom Henrique Research Centre, Porto, Portugal

3B's Research Group—Biomaterials, Biodegradables and Biomimetics, Headquarters of the European Institute of Excellence on Tissue Engineering and Regenerative Medicine, University of Minho, Guimarães, Portugal

ICVS/3B's—PT Government Associate Laboratory, Braga, Portugal

Department of Orthopaedic, Minho University, Braga, Portugal
e-mail: espregueira@dhresearchcentre.com

The RTP should be a shared decision, including the healthcare professionals, the player, and the possibly other stakeholders involved (the coach, the manager, and, in some cases, the player's relatives). Still, the healthcare professional is responsible for providing objective advice on management options and possible clinical and functional outcomes, as well as the potential risks, such as reinjury and long-term health and performance deterioration [6, 19, 25, 52].

Within an average of 12 months, around 80% of elite athletes will return to their preinjury sports level, compared to 60% return to sports among nonelite athletes [45]. When focusing on football, 85% of football players return to their preinjury sports level, between 6 and 10 months [21, 37, 45, 89, 93]. Still, approximately one fourth of elite athletes may not return to sports at the same level [45], and reasons include mainly fear of reinjury [8, 44, 55] and lack of psychological readiness [7, 9].

Although having relatively high rate of RTP, the ACL graft may fail and re-rupture in around 5% of elite athletes [45]. Moreover, ACL reinjury rates may go as far as 15% (7% ipsilateral and 8% contralateral) or 23% for athletes younger than 25 years who return to sport [90]. In addition to an adequate rehabilitation process [87], objective criteria in the decision for allowing the return to high-level sports play a crucial role in decreasing the risk of ACL reinjuries [34, 85].

17.2 Residual Knee Deficits After ACL Reconstruction

Reestablishing the knee biological homeostasis (bone bruises, mechanoreceptors and sensory afferents, and graft maturation) and normal biomechanical function (mechanical stability, range of motion, neuromuscular control, quadriceps strength) plays a crucial role in RTP, as they may reduce the incidence of secondary ACL injuries [62]. These biomechanical deficits may persist for years after ACL reconstruction, or even after the player returned to competition [1, 17, 18, 31, 61, 63, 64, 71, 79, 81, 82, 92].

Residual knee laxity may be present 6–12 months after ACL reconstruction [61, 64, 69, 76]. Within this line, it has been previously shown that ACL-reconstructed knees display greater maximal anterior tibial translation during gait exercises, even after a 5-year follow-up period [79]. Furthermore, the peak ACL strain is correlated with anterior tibial translation and bipedal simulated landing, i.e., greater knee laxity produces higher levels of peak ACL strain during landing exercises. Therefore, higher peak ACL strain could place the individual at higher risk of sustaining an ACL injury [34, 48]. Additionally, increased dynamic tibial rotation that often persists after ACL-reconstruction and leads to abnormal knee motion during gait [29, 30] or running exercises [82]. These findings raise some concerns regarding RTP, particularly within those who RTP prematurely, adding further risk factors for reinjury. In addition, the increased rotatory knee laxity may, itself, decrease the player's self-efficacy and performance, as well as increase the risk of reinjury. Moreover, rotatory knee laxity deficits may contribute to associated meniscal or cartilage lesions and early development of long-term knee joint degeneration [20, 82, 88] and subsequently to a poorer associated quality of life [25, 26]. Thus, more strict criteria regarding rotatory knee laxity after ACL reconstruction should be employed in RTP battery tests.

17.3 Importance of Imaging and Laxity Measurement

Knee joint residual laxity is considered one of the major risk factors for further ACL and meniscus injury, as well as one of the reasons for ACL reconstruction failure [38, 40, 70, 73, 75, 83, 91].

Measurement of sagittal knee laxity has been extensively performed in the follow-up of ACL-reconstructed patients [2, 32, 39, 74, 86]. However, the reliability and diagnostic accuracy of KT-1000™ instrumented AP laxity testing has been questioned [27, 33]. In this regard, stress radiography, mainly through the Telos device [10, 72, 77], emerged as a potential noninvasive method to measure the tibial anterior translation.

More recently, the objective measure of rotational knee laxity has gained increasing interest from the scientific community. This has been traditionally accomplished through pivot-shift manual test. Reports concerning the lack of standardization and objective grading [3, 13, 28, 58, 59, 78] led to the development of new mechanical testing devices to assess the knee rotational laxity including arthrometers [12, 48–51, 57, 60, 65, 84], electromagnetic sensor systems [4, 35, 36, 42, 43, 54], inertial sensors [11, 41, 46, 47, 53], and stress laxity assessment within magnetic resonance imaging (MRI) evaluation [22, 23, 67, 68].

The MRI is an accurate noninvasive tool widely used in the evaluation of intra-articular knee injuries [56]. The use of MRI in the postoperative follow-up enables the clinician to assess knee effusion, graft preservation, tunnel preservation, cartilage damage, and meniscal injuries [73]. The visualization of non-healed bone bruises may also be followed by MRI and has a crucial role during the rehabilitation phases and RTP decision [15]. Moreover, graft biological integrity ("ligamentization") is an important process in the RTP decision, which MRI plays a fundamental role in the evaluation [14, 24].

The examination of partial ACL tears with MRI is important as physical examination may be unclear when assessing isolated bundle ruptures [94], and partial tears can heal on their own, which can be carefully followed using MRI [5].

Despite the MRI accuracy in evaluating and following ACL injuries, it has been highlighted that both instrumented laxity and MRI examination are needed in combination with clinical evaluation in order to obtain the greatest accuracy [16]. Thus, the ideal tool to measure the ACL laxity should be able to assess both "anatomy" and "function" on the same examination [23].

17.4 Porto-Knee Testing Device

The Porto-Knee Testing Device (PKTD) is an MRI-compatible knee laxity testing device that is capable of measuring multiplanar knee laxity, i.e., the sagittal tibiofemoral translations and tibial internal and external rotation (Fig. 17.1). The assessment of knee laxity in combination with MRI allows the correlation of both the ligament "anatomy" and "functionality" within the same exam [66].

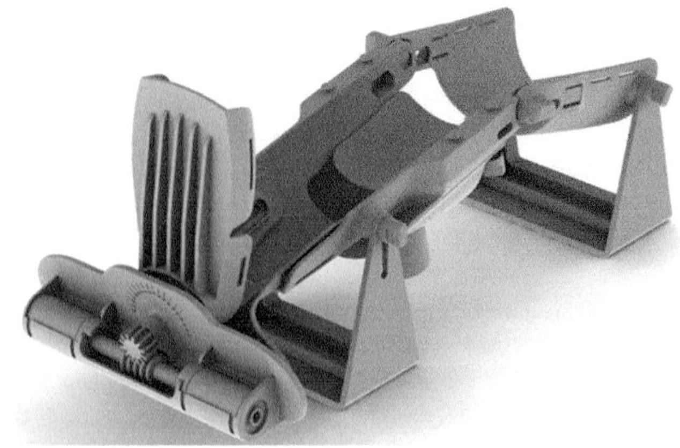

Fig. 17.1 Porto-Knee Testing Device (PKTD), developed at the Clínica do Dragão, Espregueira-Mendes Sports Centre - FIFA Medical Centre of Excellence

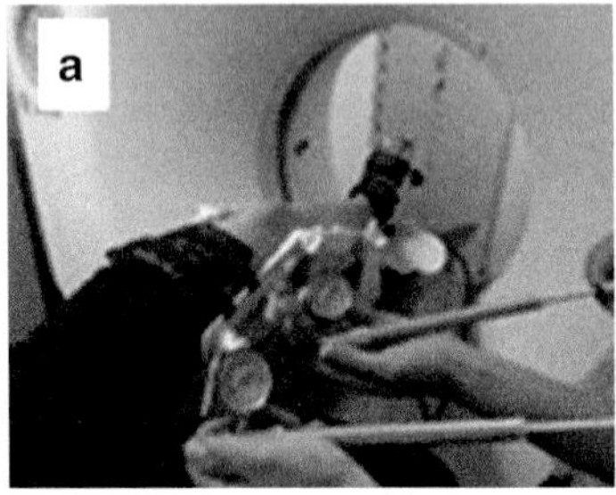

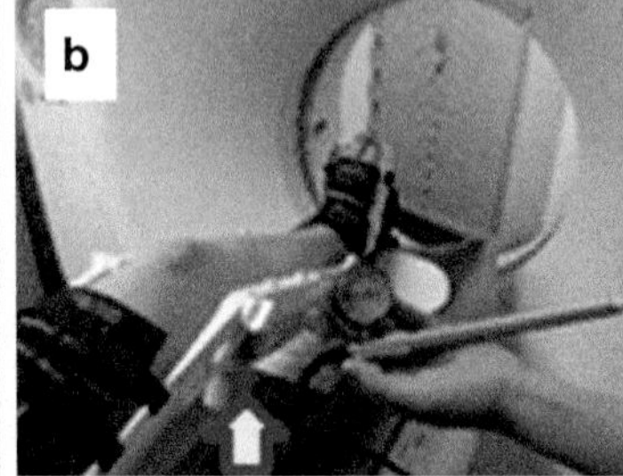

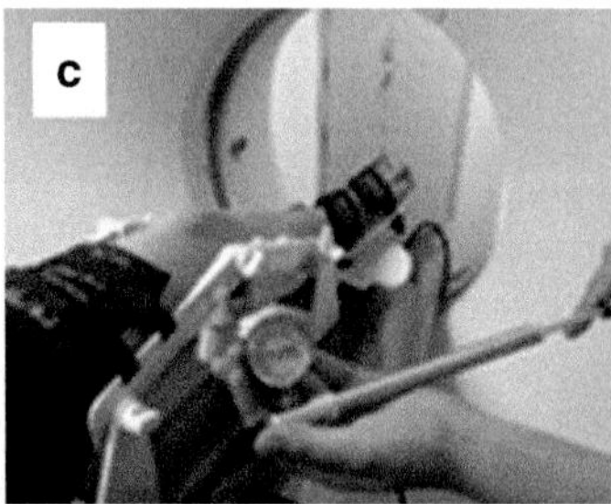

Fig. 17.2 Demonstration of PKTD sequences: without pressure (**a**), with PA pressure (**b**), and with external rotation pressure (**c**). *Arrow* indicates the tibial PA translation induced by the pressure applied in the posterior proximal calf region through the plunger pressurizing (part **b**)

The PKTD is made of polyurethane composite material, which allows to be used within the MRI and computerized tomography examination. The PKTD is capable to stress the knee at different degrees of knee flexion (from−10° to 50°) and combined with different degrees of internal/external rotation (0–90°). The tibial posteroanterior (PA) translation may be assessed alone or in combination with tibial rotation. In order to stress the ACL, a standardized pressure of 4 bar is applied to the proximal posterior calf (Fig. 17.2).

The PKTD measurements are determined through two sets of 1 mm spacing MRI slices. The first examination is made without any pressure, and a second examination is made with the application of pressure. On the obtained images, measurements (in mm) are then calculated by drawing a perpendicular line to the tibial slope, crossing the most posterior point of the tibial plateau, and a parallel line, crossing the most posterior point of the femoral condyle. This procedure is repeated for the medial and lateral tibial plateaus [80].

The laxity measurement is made by calculating the distance between the two lines, in each of the two sets of MRI slices, i.e., without and with pressure, obtaining the anterior displacement of the medial and lateral tibial plateau (Fig. 17.3). Comparison with the healthy contralateral knee can be made.

The PKTD is a reliable tool for assessment of the PA translation with a moderate-to-strong correlation with side-to-side KT-1000 measures for medial (correlation coefficient = 0.73; $p < 0.05$) and lateral (correlation coefficient = 0.5; $p < 0.05$) tibial plateaus displacement. The assessment of the rotatory knee laxity has a strong positive correlation with the pivot-shift test under anesthesia (correlation coefficient = 0.8; $p < 0.05$) and with side-to-side differences (correlation coefficient = 0.83; $p < 0.05$) [23]. More recently, two additional PKTD mea-

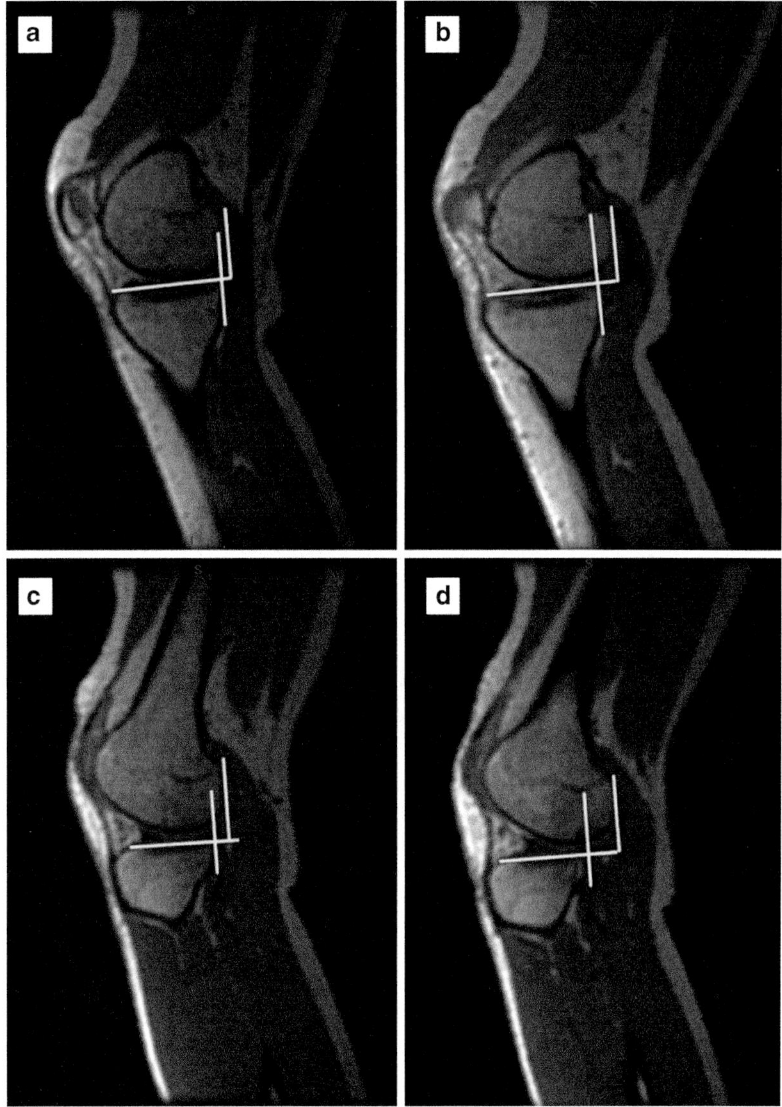

Fig. 17.3 Representation of the measurements of medial knee compartment tibial positioning without (**a**) and with pressure (**b**) and of the lateral knee compartment tibial positioning without (**c**) and with pressure (**d**), obtained from MRI slices using the PKTD

sures were investigated—the anterior global translation and the global rotation. These measurements showed high sensitivity and specificity in identifying complete ACL ruptures. The anterior global translation (PA translation of both medial and lateral tibial plateaus) has high specificity (94%), with a cutoff point of 11.1 mm. The global rotation (internal rotation at the lateral tibial plateau plus external rotation at the medial tibial plateau) is highly sensitive (93%) with a cutoff point of 15.1 mm [56].

The main purpose of the PKTD is distinguishing functional from nonfunctional ACLs or ACL grafts. Partial ACL ruptures may also be identified. By combining the sagittal and rotational laxity measurements, the PKTD is able to correlate the ligament anatomy with the functional competence of the remnant bundle

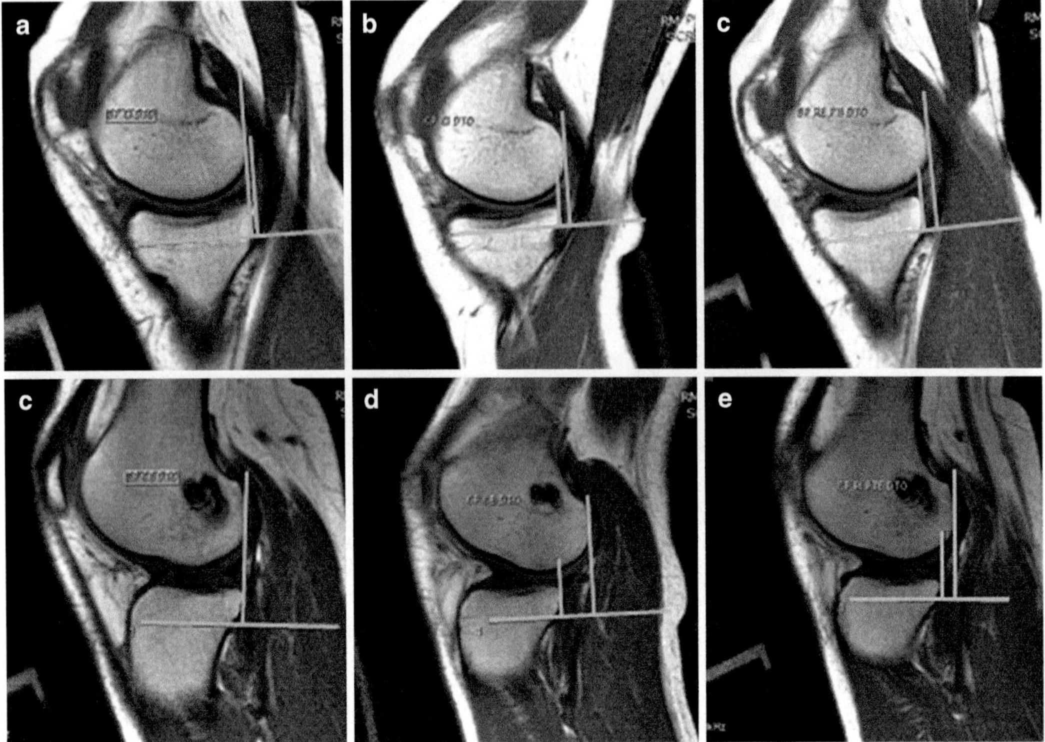

Fig. 17.4 Follow-up of PKTD-MRI; a case of an ACL-reconstructed knee with significant residual laxity in his right knee precluding return to sports. (**a**) Medial tibial plateau, no stress (−1 mm); (**b**) medial tibial plateau, posteroanterior stress (3 mm); (**c**) medial tibial plateau, external rotation stress (5 mm); (**d**) lateral tibial plateau, no stress (0 mm); (**e**) lateral tibial plateau, posteroanterior stress (13 mm); (**f**) lateral tibial plateau, internal rotation stress (4 mm)

[55]. This may play an important role in the follow-up of ACL-reconstructed patients as partial ACL graft ruptures or reconstruction failure may occur in case of surgical errors and complications, inadequate rehabilitation or anticipated RTP.

The PKTD may be used in the RTP decision by examining the functional competence of the ACL graft (Figs. 17.4 and 17.5). Residual knee laxity may indicate the need for further rehabilitation or, in case of failure, evaluate the need for new surgical intervention before allowing the player to return to competition.

Fact Box 1

The PKTD has several clinical and preventive applications within sports, including:

- Assessment of partial or total ACL ruptures
- Follow-up of ACL-reconstructed knees
- Additional objective criteria for RTP
- Planning of secondary prevention programs

Fact Box 2

Suggested additional return-to-play objective criteria based on PKTD-MRI measurements:

- Anterior global translation after PA stress <11.0 mm
- Global rotation combined measure <15.0 mm

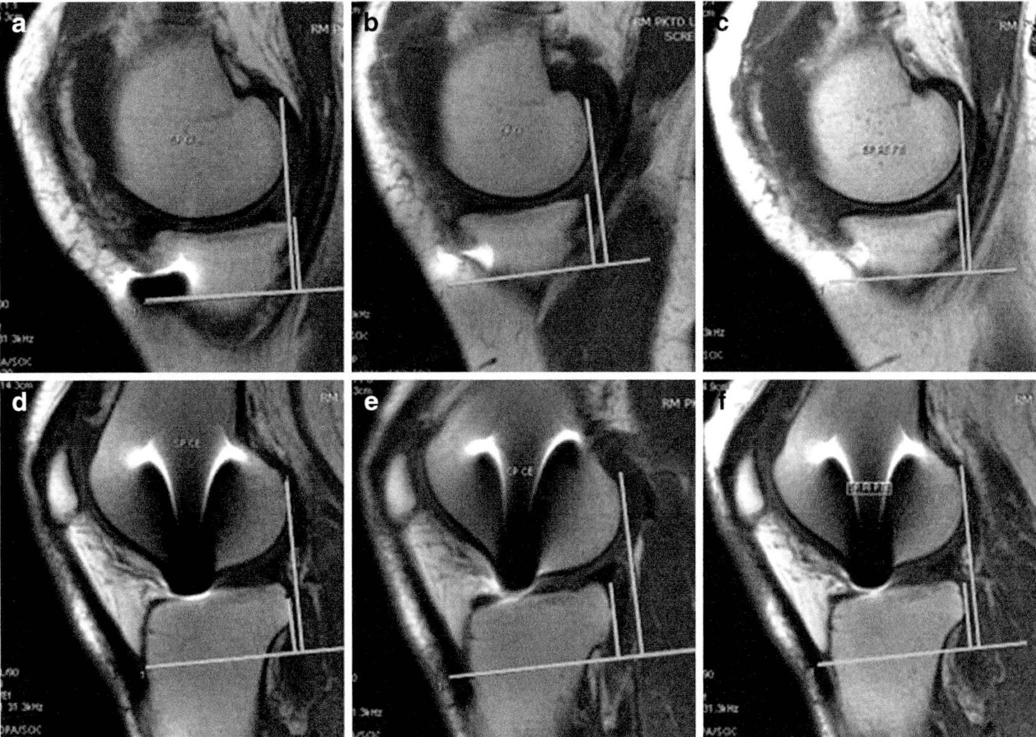

Fig. 17.5 Follow-up of PKTD-MRI; a case of an ACL-reconstructed knee with a stable joint that in presence of other achieved return-to-play criteria indicates that the player is ready to return to competition. (**a**) Medial tibial plateau, no stress (1 mm); (**b**) medial tibial plateau, posteroanterior stress (4 mm); (**c**) medial tibial plateau, external rotation stress (2 mm); (**d**) lateral tibial plateau, no stress (2 mm); (**e**) lateral tibial plateau, posteroanterior stress (6 mm); (**f**) lateral tibial plateau, internal rotation stress (3 mm)

Take Home Message

Instrumented assessment of knee laxity in combination with MRI enables the correlation of the ligament's "anatomy" and "function." In our hands, the PKTD is a helpful tool in the follow-up of football players with ACL-reconstructed knees, RTP decision-making, and planning of secondary prevention programs.

Top Five Evidence-Based References

Espregueira-Mendes J, Andrade R, Leal A, Pereira H, Skaf A, Rodrigues-Gomes S et al (2016) Global rotation has high sensitivity in ACL lesions within stress MRI. Knee Surg Sports Traumatol Arthrosc. https://doi.org/10.1007/s00167-016-4281-0

Espregueira-Mendes J, Pereira H, Sevivas N, Passos C, Vasconcelos JC, Monteiro A et al (2012) Assessment of rotatory laxity in anterior cruciate ligament-deficient knees using magnetic resonance imaging with Porto-knee testing device. Knee Surg Sports Traumatol Arthrosc 20:671–678

Musahl V, Griffith C, Irrgang JJ, Hoshino Y, Kuroda R, Lopomo N et al (2016) Validation of quantitative measures of rotatory knee laxity. Am J Sports Med 44:2393–2398

Rohman EM, Macalena JA (2016) Anterior cruciate ligament assessment using arthrometry and stress imaging. Curr Rev Musculoskelet Med 9:130–138

Sundemo D, Alentorn-Geli E, Hoshino Y, Musahl V, Karlsson J, Samuelsson K (2016) Objective measures on knee instability: dynamic tests: a review of devices for assessment of dynamic knee laxity through utilization of the pivot shift test. Curr Rev Musculoskelet Med 9:148–159

References

1. Abourezk MN, Ithurburn MP, McNally MP, Thoma LM, Briggs MS, Hewett TE et al (2017) Hamstring strength asymmetry at 3 years after anterior cruciate

ligament reconstruction alters knee mechanics during gait and jogging. Am J Sports Med 45:97–105
2. Akelman MR, Fadale PD, Hulstyn MJ, Shalvoy RM, Garcia A, Chin KE et al (2016) Effect of matching or overconstraining knee laxity during anterior cruciate ligament reconstruction on knee osteoarthritis and clinical outcomes: a randomized controlled trial with 84-month follow-up. Am J Sports Med 44: 1660–1670
3. Anderson AF, Rennirt GW, Standeffer WC Jr (1999) Clinical analysis of the pivot shift tests: description of the pivot drawer test. Am J Knee Surg 13:19–23
4. Araki D, Kuroda R, Matsushita T, Matsumoto T, Kubo S, Nagamune K et al (2013) Biomechanical analysis of the knee with partial anterior cruciate ligament disruption: quantitative evaluation using an electromagnetic measurement system. Arthroscopy 29: 1053–1062
5. Araujo P, van Eck CF, Torabi M, FH F (2013) How to optimize the use of MRI in anatomic ACL reconstruction. Knee Surg Sports Traumatol Arthrosc 21:1495–1501
6. Ardern CL, Glasgow P, Schneiders A, Witvrouw E, Clarsen B, Cools A et al (2016) 2016 Consensus statement on return to sport from the First World Congress in Sports Physical Therapy, Bern. Br J Sports Med 50:853–864
7. Ardern CL, Österberg A, Tagesson S, Gauffin H, Webster KE, Kvist J (2014) The impact of psychological readiness to return to sport and recreational activities after anterior cruciate ligament reconstruction. Br J Sports Med 48:1613–1619
8. Ardern CL, Taylor NF, Feller JA, Webster KE (2012) Fear of re-injury in people who have returned to sport following anterior cruciate ligament reconstruction surgery. J Sci Med Sport 15:488–495
9. Ardern CL, Taylor NF, Feller JA, Whitehead TS, Webster KE (2013) Psychological responses matter in returning to preinjury level of sport after anterior cruciate ligament reconstruction surgery. Am J Sports Med 41:1549–1558
10. Beldame J, Bertiaux S, Roussignol X, Lefebvre B, Adam J-M, Mouilhade F et al (2011) Laxity measurements using stress radiography to assess anterior cruciate ligament tears. Orthop Traumatol Surg Res 97:34–43
11. Berruto M, Uboldi F, Gala L, Marelli B, Albisetti W (2013) Is triaxial accelerometer reliable in the evaluation and grading of knee pivot-shift phenomenon? Knee Surg Sports Traumatol Arthrosc 21:981–985
12. Branch TP, Browne JE, Campbell JD, Siebold R, Freedberg H, Arendt EA et al (2010) Rotational laxity greater in patients with contralateral anterior cruciate ligament injury than healthy volunteers. Knee Surg Sports Traumatol Arthrosc 18:1379–1384
13. Branch TP, Mayr HO, Browne JE, Campbell JC, Stoehr A, Jacobs CA (2010) Instrumented examination of anterior cruciate ligament injuries: minimizing flaws of the manual clinical examination. Arthroscopy 26:997–1004
14. Colombet P, Graveleau N, Jambou S (2016) Incorporation of hamstring grafts within the tibial tunnel after anterior cruciate ligament reconstruction magnetic resonance imaging of suspensory fixation versus interference screws. Am J Sports Med 44:2838–2845
15. Costa-Paz M, Muscolo DL, Ayerza M, Makino A, Aponte-Tinao L (2001) Magnetic resonance imaging follow-up study of bone bruises associated with anterior cruciate ligament ruptures. Arthroscopy 17:445–449
16. Dejour D, Ntagiopoulos PG, Saggin PR, Panisset J-C (2013) The diagnostic value of clinical tests, magnetic resonance imaging, and instrumented laxity in the differentiation of complete versus partial anterior cruciate ligament tears. Arthroscopy 29:491–499
17. Di Stasi S, Hartigan EH, Snyder-Mackler L (2015) Sex-specific gait adaptations prior to and up to 6 months after anterior cruciate ligament reconstruction. J Orthop Sports Phys Ther 45:207–214
18. Di Stasi SL, Logerstedt D, Gardinier ES, Snyder-Mackler L (2013) Gait patterns differ between ACL-reconstructed athletes who pass return-to-sport criteria and those who fail. Am J Sports Med 41:1310–1318
19. Dijkstra HP, Pollock N, Chakraverty R, Ardern CL (2017) Return to play in elite sport: a shared decision-making process. Br J Sports Med 51:419–420
20. Dunn WR, Lyman S, Lincoln AE, Amoroso PJ, Wickiewicz T, Marx RG (2004) The effect of anterior cruciate ligament reconstruction on the risk of knee reinjury. Am J Sports Med 32:1906–1914
21. Erickson BJ, Harris JD, Cvetanovich GL, Bach BR, Bush-Joseph CA, Abrams GD et al (2013) Performance and return to sport after anterior cruciate ligament reconstruction in male Major League Soccer players. Orthop J Sports Med 1:2325967113497189
22. Espregueira-Mendes J, Andrade R, Leal A, Pereira H, Skaf A, Rodrigues-Gomes S et al (2016) Global rotation has high sensitivity in ACL lesions within stress MRI. Knee Surg Sports Traumatol Arthrosc. https://doi.org/10.1007/s00167-016-4281-0
23. Espregueira-Mendes J, Pereira H, Sevivas N, Passos C, Vasconcelos JC, Monteiro A et al (2012) Assessment of rotatory laxity in anterior cruciate ligament-deficient knees using magnetic resonance imaging with Porto-knee testing device. Knee Surg Sports Traumatol Arthrosc 20:671–678
24. Figueroa D, Melean P, Calvo R, Vaisman A, Zilleruelo N, Figueroa F et al (2010) Magnetic resonance imaging evaluation of the integration and maturation of semitendinosus-gracilis graft in anterior cruciate ligament reconstruction using autologous platelet concentrate. Arthroscopy 26:1318–1325
25. Filbay S, Culvenor A, Ackerman I, Russell T, Crossley K (2015) Quality of life in anterior cruciate ligament-deficient individuals: a systematic review and meta-analysis. Br J Sports Med 49:1033–1041
26. Filbay SR, Ackerman IN, Russell TG, Macri EM, Crossley KM (2014) Health-related quality of life

after anterior cruciate ligament reconstruction: a systematic review. Am J Sports Med 42:1247–1255

27. Forster I, Warren-Smith C, Tew M (1989) Is the KT1000 knee ligament arthrometer reliable? J Bone Joint Surg Br 71:843–847
28. FH F, Herbst E (2016) Editorial commentary: the pivot-shift phenomenon is multifactorial. Arthroscopy 32:1063–1064
29. Georgoulis AD, Papadonikolakis A, Papageorgiou CD, Mitsou A, Stergiou N (2003) Three-dimensional tibiofemoral kinematics of the anterior cruciate ligament-deficient and reconstructed knee during walking. Am J Sports Med 31:75–79
30. Georgoulis AD, Ristanis S, Chouliaras V, Moraiti C, Stergiou N (2007) Tibial rotation is not restored after ACL reconstruction with a hamstring graft. Clin Orthop Relat Res 454:89–94
31. Gokeler A, Benjaminse A, Van Eck C, Webster K, Schot L, Otten E (2013) Return of normal gait as an outcome measurement in acl reconstructed patients. A systematic review. Int J Sports Phys Ther 8:441–451
32. Goodwillie AD, Shah SS, McHugh MP, Nicholas SJ (2017) The effect of postoperative kt-1000 arthrometer score on long-term outcome after anterior cruciate ligament reconstruction. Am J Sports Med 45:1522. https://doi.org/10.1177/0363546517690525
33. Graham G, Johnson S, Dent C, Fairclough J (1991) Comparison of clinical tests and the KT1000 in the diagnosis of anterior cruciate ligament rupture. Br J Sports Med 25:96–97
34. Grindem H, Snyder-Mackler L, Moksnes H, Engebretsen L, Risberg MA (2016) Simple decision rules can reduce reinjury risk by 84% after ACL reconstruction: the Delaware-Oslo ACL cohort study. Br J Sports Med 50:804–808
35. Hoshino Y, Kuroda R, Nagamune K, Araki D, Kubo S, Yamaguchi M et al (2012) Optimal measurement of clinical rotational test for evaluating anterior cruciate ligament insufficiency. Knee Surg Sports Traumatol Arthrosc 20:1323–1330
36. Hoshino Y, Kuroda R, Nagamune K, Yagi M, Mizuno K, Yamaguchi M et al (2007) In vivo measurement of the pivot-shift test in the anterior cruciate ligament–deficient knee using an electromagnetic device. Am J Sports Med 35:1098–1104
37. Howard JS, Lembach ML, Metzler AV, Johnson DL (2016) Rates and determinants of return to play after anterior cruciate ligament reconstruction in National Collegiate Athletic Association Division I soccer athletes: a study of the Southeastern Conference. Am J Sports Med 44:433–439
38. Keene GC, Bickerstaff D, Rae PJ, Paterson RS (1993) The natural history of meniscal tears in anterior cruciate ligament insufficiency. Am J Sports Med 21:672–679
39. Kilinc BE, Kara A, Haluk Celik YO, Camur S (2016) Evaluation of the accuracy of Lachman and Anterior Drawer Tests with KT1000 in the follow-up of anterior cruciate ligament surgery. J Exerc Rehabil 12:363
40. Kim S-J, Kim T-E, Lee D-H, K-S O (2008) Anterior cruciate ligament reconstruction in patients who have excessive joint laxity. J Bone Joint Surg Am 90:735–741
41. Kopf S, Kauert R, Halfpaap J, Jung T, Becker R (2012) A new quantitative method for pivot shift grading. Knee Surg Sports Traumatol Arthrosc 20:718–723
42. Kuroda R, Hoshino Y (2016) Electromagnetic tracking of the pivot-shift. Curr Rev Musculoskelet Med 9:164–169
43. Kuroda R, Hoshino Y, Araki D, Nishizawa Y, Nagamune K, Matsumoto T et al (2012) Quantitative measurement of the pivot shift, reliability, and clinical applications. Knee Surg Sports Traumatol Arthrosc 20:686–691
44. Kvist J, Ek A, Sporrstedt K, Good L (2005) Fear of re-injury: a hindrance for returning to sports after anterior cruciate ligament reconstruction. Knee Surg Sports Traumatol Arthrosc 13:393–397
45. Lai CC, Ardern CL, Feller JA, Webster KE (2017) Eighty-three per cent of elite athletes return to preinjury sport after anterior cruciate ligament reconstruction: a systematic review with meta-analysis of return to sport rates, graft rupture rates and performance outcomes. Br J Sports Med. https://doi.org/10.1136/bjsports-2016-096836
46. Lopomo N, Signorelli C, Bonanzinga T, Muccioli GMM, Visani A, Zaffagnini S (2012) Quantitative assessment of pivot-shift using inertial sensors. Knee Surg Sports Traumatol Arthrosc 20:713–717
47. Lopomo N, Zaffagnini S, Signorelli C, Bignozzi S, Giordano G, Marcheggiani Muccioli GM et al (2012) An original clinical methodology for non-invasive assessment of pivot-shift test. Comput Methods Biomech Biomed Engin 15:1323–1328
48. Lorbach O, Brockmeyer M, Kieb M, Zerbe T, Pape D, Seil R (2012) Objective measurement devices to assess static rotational knee laxity: focus on the Rotameter. Knee Surg Sports Traumatol Arthrosc 20:639–644
49. Lorbach O, Kieb M, Brogard P, Maas S, Pape D, Seil R (2012) Static rotational and sagittal knee laxity measurements after reconstruction of the anterior cruciate ligament. Knee Surg Sports Traumatol Arthrosc 20:844–850
50. Lorbach O, Wilmes P, Maas S, Zerbe T, Busch L, Kohn D et al (2009) A non-invasive device to objectively measure tibial rotation: verification of the device. Knee Surg Sports Traumatol Arthrosc 17:756–762
51. Lorbach O, Wilmes P, Theisen D, Brockmeyer M, Maas S, Kohn D et al (2009) Reliability testing of a new device to measure tibial rotation. Knee Surg Sports Traumatol Arthrosc 17:920–926
52. Lynch AD, Logerstedt DS, Grindem H, Eitzen I, Hicks GE, Axe MJ et al (2015) Consensus criteria for defining 'successful outcome' after ACL injury and

reconstruction: a Delaware-Oslo ACL cohort investigation. Br J Sports Med 49:335–342

53. Maeyama A, Hoshino Y, Debandi A, Kato Y, Saeki K, Asai S et al (2011) Evaluation of rotational instability in the anterior cruciate ligament deficient knee using triaxial accelerometer: a biomechanical model in porcine knees. Knee Surg Sports Traumatol Arthrosc 19:1233–1238
54. Matsushita T, Oka S, Nagamune K, Matsumoto T, Nishizawa Y, Hoshino Y et al (2013) Differences in knee kinematics between awake and anesthetized patients during the Lachman and pivot-shift tests for anterior cruciate ligament deficiency. Orthop J Sports Med 1:2325967113487855
55. McCullough KA, Phelps KD, Spindler KP, Matava MJ, Dunn WR, Parker RD et al (2012) Return to high school–and college-level football after anterior cruciate ligament reconstruction: a Multicenter Orthopaedic Outcomes Network (MOON) cohort study. Am J Sports Med 40:2523–2529
56. Meuffels DE, Poldervaart MT, Diercks RL, Fievez AW, Patt TW, CPvd H et al (2012) Guideline on anterior cruciate ligament injury: a multidisciplinary review by the Dutch Orthopaedic Association. Acta Orthop 83:379–386
57. Mouton C, Seil R, Agostinis H, Maas S, Theisen D (2012) Influence of individual characteristics on static rotational knee laxity using the Rotameter. Knee Surg Sports Traumatol Arthrosc 20:645–651
58. Musahl V, Griffith C, Irrgang JJ, Hoshino Y, Kuroda R, Lopomo N et al (2016) Validation of quantitative measures of rotatory knee laxity. Am J Sports Med 44:2393–2398
59. Musahl V, Hoshino Y, Ahlden M, Araujo P, Irrgang JJ, Zaffagnini S et al (2012) The pivot shift: a global user guide. Knee Surg Sports Traumatol Arthrosc 20:724–731
60. Musahl V, Voos J, O'Loughlin PF, Stueber V, Kendoff D, Pearle AD (2010) Mechanized pivot shift test achieves greater accuracy than manual pivot shift test. Knee Surg Sports Traumatol Arthrosc 18:1208–1213
61. Myklebust G, Bahr R, Nilstad A, Steffen K (2017) Knee function among elite handball and football players 1-6 years after anterior cruciate ligament injury. Scand J Med Sci Sports 27:545–553
62. Nagelli CV, Hewett TE (2017) Should return to sport be delayed until 2 years after anterior cruciate ligament reconstruction? Biological and functional considerations. Sports Med 47:221–232
63. Nawasreh Z, Logerstedt D, Cummer K, Axe MJ, Risberg MA, Snyder-Mackler L (2016) Do patients failing return-to-activity criteria at 6 months after anterior cruciate ligament reconstruction continue demonstrating deficits at 2 years? Am J Sports Med 45:1037–1048
64. Noojin FK, Barrett GR, Hartzog CW, Nash CR (2000) Clinical comparison of intraarticular anterior cruciate ligament reconstruction using autogenous semitendinosus and gracilis tendons in men versus women. Am J Sports Med 28:783–789
65. Park HS, Wilson NA, Zhang LQ (2008) Gender differences in passive knee biomechanical properties in tibial rotation. J Orthop Res 26:937–944
66. Pereira H, Fernandes M, Pereira R, Jones H, Vasconcelos J, Oliveira JM et al (2015) Anterior cruciate ligament injuries identifiable for pre-participation imagiological analysis: risk factors. In: Doral MN, Karlsson J (eds) Sports injuries: prevention, diagnosis, treatment and rehabilitation. Springer, New York, NY, pp 1–15
67. Pereira H, Gomes S, Vasconcelos JC, Soares L, Pereira R, Oliveira JM et al (2017) MRI laxity assessment. In: Musahl V, Karlsson J, Kuroda R, Zaffagnini S (eds) Rotatory knee instability. Springer, New York, NY, pp 49–61
68. Pereira H, Sevivas N, Pereira R, Monteiro A, Oliveira JM, Reis R et al (2012) New tools for diagnosis, assessment of surgical outcome and follow-up. In: Hermoso JAH, Monllau JC (eds) Lesiones ligamentosas de la rodilla. Marge Medica Books, Valencia, pp 185–197
69. Rahnemai-Azar AA, Naendrup J-H, Soni A, Olsen A, Zlotnicki J, Musahl V (2016) Knee instability scores for ACL reconstruction. Curr Rev Musculoskelet Med 9:170–177
70. Ramesh R, Von Arx O, Azzopardi T, Schranz P (2005) The risk of anterior cruciate ligament rupture with generalised joint laxity. J Bone Joint Surg Br 87:800–803
71. Roewer BD, Di Stasi SL, Snyder-Mackler L (2011) Quadriceps strength and weight acceptance strategies continue to improve two years after anterior cruciate ligament reconstruction. J Biomech 44:1948–1953
72. Rohman EM, Macalena JA (2016) Anterior cruciate ligament assessment using arthrometry and stress imaging. Curr Rev Musculoskelet Med 9:130–138
73. Samitier G, Marcano AI, Alentorn-Geli E, Cugat R, Farmer KW, Moser MW (2015) Failure of anterior cruciate ligament reconstruction. Arch Bone Joint Surg 3:220
74. Sato K, Maeda A, Takano Y, Matsuse H, Ida H, Shiba N (2013) Relationship between static anterior laxity using the KT-1000 and dynamic tibial rotation during motion in patients with anatomical anterior cruciate ligament reconstruction. Kurume Med J 60:1–6
75. Scerpella TA, Stayer TJ, Makhuli BZ (2005) Ligamentous laxity and non-contact anterior cruciate ligament tears: a gender-based comparison. Orthopedics 28:656
76. Semay B, Rambaud A, Philippot R, Edouard P (2016) Evolution of the anteroposterior laxity by GnRB at 6, 9 and 12 months post-surgical anterior cruciate ligament reconstruction. Ann Phys Rehabil Med 59:e19
77. Sørensen OG, Larsen K, Jakobsen B, Kold S, Hansen T, Lind M et al (2011) The combination of radiostereometric analysis and the telos stress device results

in poor precision for knee laxity measurements after anterior cruciate ligament reconstruction. Knee Surg Sports Traumatol Arthrosc 19:355–362

78. Sundemo D, Alentorn-Geli E, Hoshino Y, Musahl V, Karlsson J, Samuelsson K (2016) Objective measures on knee instability: dynamic tests: a review of devices for assessment of dynamic knee laxity through utilization of the pivot shift test. Curr Rev Musculoskelet Med 9:148–159
79. Tagesson S, Öberg B, Kvist J (2015) Static and dynamic tibial translation before, 5 weeks after, and 5 years after anterior cruciate ligament reconstruction. Knee Surg Sports Traumatol Arthrosc 23: 3691–3697
80. Tashiro Y, Okazaki K, Miura H, Matsuda S, Yasunaga T, Hashizume M et al (2009) Quantitative assessment of rotatory instability after anterior cruciate ligament reconstruction. Am J Sports Med 37:909–916
81. Tashman S, Araki D (2013) Effects of anterior cruciate ligament reconstruction on in vivo, dynamic knee function. Clin Sports Med 32:47–59
82. Tashman S, Collon D, Anderson K, Kolowich P, Anderst W (2004) Abnormal rotational knee motion during running after anterior cruciate ligament reconstruction. Am J Sports Med 32:975–983
83. Uhorchak JM, Scoville CR, Williams GN, Arciero RA, Pierre PS, Taylor DC (2003) Risk factors associated with noncontact injury of the anterior cruciate ligament a prospective four-year evaluation of 859 west point cadets. Am J Sports Med 31:831–842
84. van Eck CF, Loopik M, van den Bekerom MP, FH F, Kerkhoffs GM (2013) Methods to diagnose acute anterior cruciate ligament rupture: a meta-analysis of instrumented knee laxity tests. Knee Surg Sports Traumatol Arthrosc 21:1989–1997
85. Van Grinsven S, Van Cingel R, Holla C, Van Loon C (2010) Evidence-based rehabilitation following anterior cruciate ligament reconstruction. Knee Surg Sports Traumatol Arthrosc 18:1128–1144
86. van Meer BL, Oei EH, Bierma-Zeinstra SM, van Arkel ER, Verhaar JA, Reijman M et al (2014) Are magnetic resonance imaging recovery and laxity improvement possible after anterior cruciate ligament rupture in nonoperative treatment? Arthroscopy 30:1092–1099
87. van Melick N, van Cingel RE, Brooijmans F, Neeter C, van Tienen T, Hullegie W et al (2016) Evidence-based clinical practice update: practice guidelines for anterior cruciate ligament rehabilitation based on a systematic review and multidisciplinary consensus. Br J Sports Med 50:1506–1515
88. Waldén M (2013) Return to sports after ACL reconstruction surgery: a risk for further joint injury? In: Sanchis-Alfonso V, Monllau JC (eds) The ACL-deficient knee. Springer, New York, NY, pp 183–188
89. Waldén M, Hägglund M, Magnusson H, Ekstrand J (2011) Anterior cruciate ligament injury in elite football: a prospective three-cohort study. Knee Surg Sports Traumatol Arthrosc 19:11–19
90. Wiggins AJ, Grandhi RK, Schneider DK, Stanfield D, Webster KE, Myer GD (2016) Risk of secondary injury in younger athletes after anterior cruciate ligament reconstruction: a systematic review and meta-analysis. Am J Sports Med 44:1861–1876
91. Wylie JD, Marchand LS, Burks RT (2017) Etiologic Factors That Lead to Failure After Primary Anterior Cruciate Ligament Surgery. Clin Sports Med 36:155–172
92. Xergia SA, Pappas E, Zampeli F, Georgiou S, Georgoulis AD (2013) Asymmetries in functional hop tests, lower extremity kinematics, and isokinetic strength persist 6 to 9 months following anterior cruciate ligament reconstruction. J Orthop Sports Phys Ther 43:154–162
93. Zaffagnini S, Grassi A, Muccioli GM, Tsapralis K, Ricci M, Bragonzoni L et al (2014) Return to sport after anterior cruciate ligament reconstruction in professional soccer players. Knee 21:731–735
94. Zantop T, Brucker PU, Vidal A, Zelle BA, FH F (2007) Intraarticular rupture pattern of the ACL. Clin Orthop Relat Res 454:48–53

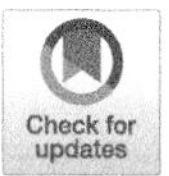

18 Development and Implementation of a Modular Return-to-Play Test Battery After ACL Reconstruction

Hendrik Bloch, Christian Klein, Patrick Luig, and Helge Riepenhof

Contents

H. Bloch (✉) • C. Klein • P. Luig
VBG, German Social Accident Insurance Institution for the Administrative Sector, Hamburg, Germany
e-mail: hendrik.bloch@vbg.de; christian.klein@vbg.de; patrick.luig@vbg.de

H. Riepenhof
BG Clinic Hamburg, Hamburg, Germany
e-mail: h.riepenhof@bgk-hamburg.de

18.1 Background

With a cumulative incidence rate of 2.5 injuries per player and season, German men's professional football in the two highest leagues demonstrates a high risk of injury. In fact, 70.7% of all injuries were lower extremity injuries, with thigh injuries (21.3%) and knee injuries (15.8%) being the most frequent. However, knee injuries alone caused 37.0% of overall short-term disability. The share of knee injuries in German football ranges between 15% and 19% accompanied with a high economic burden of approximately 50% of direct medical costs including remuneration payments (Fig. 18.1).

As the majority of knee injuries in the two highest German football leagues (58.3%) were observed during noncontact or indirect contact situations, and, additionally, 90.3% of knee injuries were completely independent of opponent's foul play, a high preventive potential may be assumed [93]. Special attention should be given to injuries of the anterior cruciate ligament (ACL), which, although represent 1.7% of all injuries, equate to almost one-third of all direct medical costs including remuneration payments (Fig. 18.2).

In addition to the high medical costs, there is a high second injury rate after sustaining an ACL tear. Returned players are at higher risk sustaining a reinjury or an ACL injury on the contralateral leg. Recent studies demonstrate that the

V. Musahl et al. (eds.), *Return to Play in Football*, https://doi.org/10.1007/978-3-662-55713-6_18

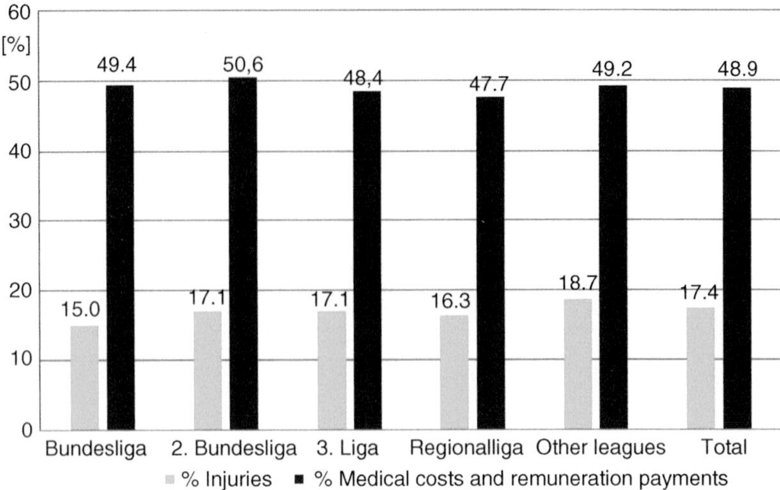

Fig. 18.1 Knee injuries in German football leagues—share of total injuries and direct medical costs

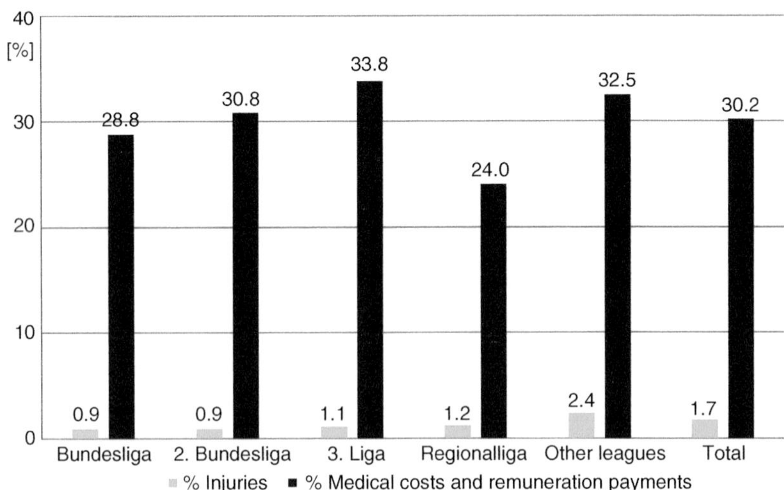

Fig. 18.2 ACL injuries in German football leagues—share of total injuries and direct medical costs

percentage sustaining a contralateral injury is even higher [98, 56]. A study in 2014 highlighted that younger athletes to the age of 25 who returned to a pivoting or cutting sport after ACL reconstruction were 15 times more likely to sustain an ACL injury in the first 12 months than a previously uninjured athlete [72]. A further study in 2017 confirmed that the risk of recurrence is greatest during the first 2 years, particularly in the first 12 months post-op [63]. It was also found that, with respect to the first 9 months post-op, a later return would reduce the risk of reinjury [41].

Moreover, reinjuries are associated with longer layoff times and a poorer medical outcome [30, 31, 49]. When a severe injury with long downtimes like the ACL tear occurs, the question arises when the athlete can resume his sport. This is not only essential for the athlete himself; it is also asked by the sporting environment, i.e., trainers, consultants, and club administrators. For team physicians and therapists, to answer this question is often the most difficult decision to make, living in a framework of conflict between the actors involved [14].

In public perception, desire and reality are widely diverging. For example, in the case of ACL injuries, a 6-month downtime is often postulated. But even at the highest international level, players return to the pitch on average 7.5 months after their ACL injury, as data from the UEFA Champions League shows [94]. Looking at the quality of this return, it is noticeable that only about 65% of the players still play on their previous level of performance 3 years after their ACL tear [94]. Across all sports, this share appears to be even lower. Only about 44–55% of athletes sustaining an ACL injury return to competition [1, 5, 6].

Although a large number of scientific publications deal with the rehabilitative treatment of injured athletes, the evidence for predictive parameters or suitable objective test methods is insufficient [8, 28, 91]. Systematic reviews showed that about 40–65% described no criteria for a return-to-play decision. Objective criteria were found in only about 13% of studies [10, 43]. A survey of 221 instructors of the German-speaking society of arthroscopy (AGA) reinforces the impression. Only three of the surgeons used a test battery as a basis for decision making. Approximately 85% of the respondents did not include a clinical score (e.g., Tegner activity score, Lysholm score, IKDC 2000 score) in their decision. This is somewhat contradictory toward the fact that a time-oriented consideration alone is not sufficient to ensure a certain decision about a safe return to play, especially as there is still disagreement as to the optimal time [74]. Investigations demonstrate that 6.5 ± 1 months after reconstruction of the ACL, only two out of 28 patients could meet all utilized test criteria. The applied test battery consisted of isokinetic force tests, four different jump tests, and two questionnaires [38]. Another investigation confirms this poor rate of return-to-play recommendations, which was received only by 17.4% of the 86 subjects, 6 months post-op [77]. A separate study found a return-to-play recommendation of 24% (n = 74) [41]. However, the tests took place in a period of 6–12 months post-op [38, 41, 77]. The low rates of recommendation confirm the necessity of objective return-to-play criteria, knowing that a hundred percent prevention of a new injury is not possible, since causes of injury are multifactorial and not all risk factors, intrinsic and extrinsic, can be influenced. Moreover, the prevalence of one or more risk factors alone does not lead to injury per se. It also requires a triggering event. However, the more risk factors that are present, or the more serious their manifestations, the lower the tolerance against occurring events. Thus, particular attention should be given to the review of risk factors prior to a return-to-play decision. In summary, there is a need to establish a consensus between the professions involved in the rehabilitation process in German football.

To implement measures, like a return-to-play test battery, it is crucial to involve important recipients at an early stage to increase the compliance of the target group [33, 46, 90]. Therefore, the VBG focuses on the transfer of existing, scientifically evaluated or expertly judged approaches into the existing sports setting of the target group.

18.2 Consensus Process

With the aim to develop a standardized test battery, the VBG, the statutory accident insurance for German professional sports, initialized a consensus conference in collaboration with the Centre for Sport and Health Research (ZfG) of the German Sport University Cologne (DSHS) in 2014. Therefore, the VBG invited relevant German research groups and a panel consisting of accredited experts from German elite team sports such as sports physicians, sports physiotherapist, rehab and athletic coaches, and sports psychologists. Thirty-five attendees followed the invitation to the conference. Five more experts were unable to participate and were consulted afterward. After an initial discussion of different return-to-play concepts within the entire expert panel, participants then selected to join smaller working groups.

The primary task of these groups was to establish a common understanding on definitions and milestones in the rehabilitation process, which, despite existing scientific approaches, was still lacking [2, 3, 89]. Within a moderated discussion, conceptual overlaps and commonalities were identified so that a first consensus on rehabilitation milestones and their definitions was achieved (Fig. 18.3 and Chap. 3).

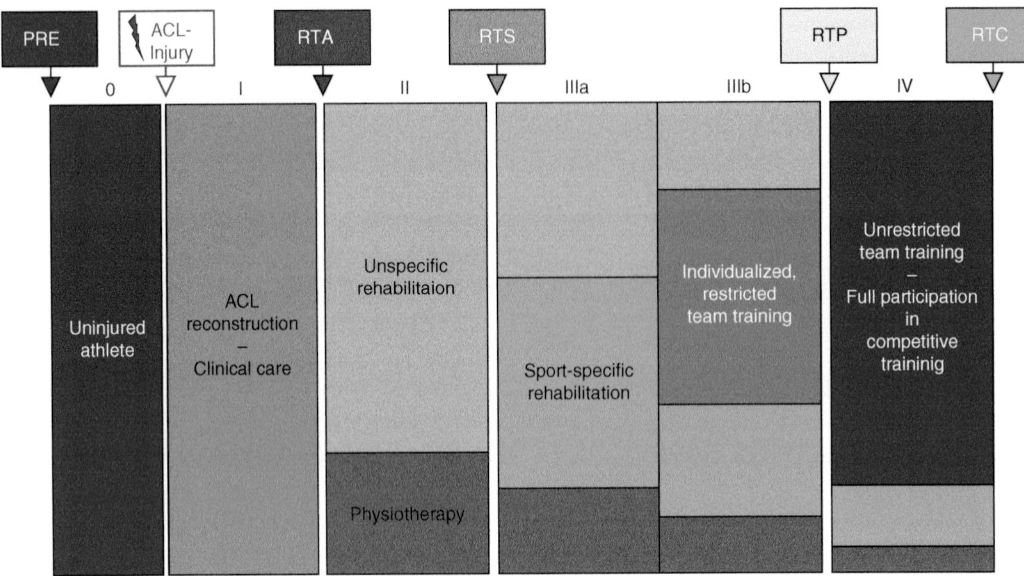

Fig. 18.3 Phases and milestones of the rehabilitation process after ACL injury. PRE = pre-injury screening, ACL = anterior cruciate ligament, RTA = return to activity, RTS = return to sport, RTP = return to play, RTC = return to competition

Recent studies have shown that comprehensive test batteries are superior to a single testing, particularly when determining the milestone of return to play [87, 91]. Therefore, as a next step, superordinate test categories and appropriate tests were debated, with focus on the return-to-play milestone.

Fact Box 1 Importance of the return-to-play milestone

The return-to-play milestone has a particular importance for the VBG, the injured athlete, and his club as it marks the athlete's end of short-term disability and herewith associated remuneration payments. Aside from the costs for medical treatment, the VBG, the statutory accident insurance for German professional sports, also bears the athlete's remuneration payments as from the 43rd day of short-term disability.

Seven test categories (i.e., clinical and psychological examination, postural control tests, hop tests, speed tests, agility tests, exhaustion test, fatigued hop tests) were determined (Fig. 18.5). Finally, based on the results of the consensus conference, a test manual was published, describing setup, execution, and interpretation of the modular test battery (Chap. 4).

18.3 Description of Phases and Milestones of the Rehabilitation Process After ACL Injury

The expert panel agreed on five distinctive milestones, i.e. (Fig. 18.4) that the injured athletes will pass during an ideal rehabilitation process.

Milestones are passages from one rehabilitation phase to the next. They are typically connected to significant gains in performance and progress in specific skills and are marked by assessments with objectively verifiable parameters. The hereby obtained findings allow the involved professions to monitor, control, and adjust the rehabilitation process and to ensure a safe progress to the next rehabilitation phase. The milestones, the expert panel agreed on, are described in the following section.

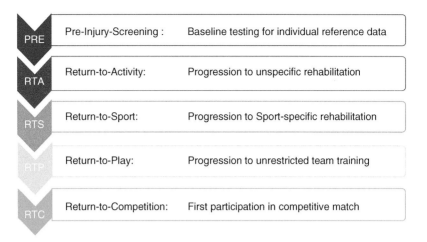

Fig. 18.4 Milestones of the rehabilitation process

18.3.1 Pre-injury Screening (PRE)

The rehabilitation after an injury always represents an individual process and depends on, i.e., the type and severity of injury, the profile of the sport of the injured athlete, and his personal goals. A pre-injury screening is a prospective data collection that provides the rehabilitation staff with important reference values for the injured athlete that can be used in the event of an injury. Moreover, individual baseline values from pre-injury screenings are superior to the frequently used limb symmetry index (LSI) or data from reference populations. Particularly in football where lower limb asymmetries due to leg dominances must be taken into consideration when interpreting test results, solely usage of the LSI seems to be questionable.

It was found that over 95% of the professional football players experienced at least one health problem that had to be treated or monitored. One-third of the athletes showed strength deficits, predominantly in the area of the hip and thigh muscles [9]. The strength of the hip abductors is again a predictor of injuries to the anterior cruciate ligament and should therefore be part of a screening in sport [53]. Besides its value in the rehabilitation process, a pre-injury screening offers the opportunity to identify individual performance deficits. This may be helpful to regulate the training process and to derive targeted individual primary prevention measures before an injury occurs.

18.3.2 Return to Activity (RTA)

Return to activity is the transition from clinical care (phase I) to general rehabilitation training (phase II) and describes the first post-traumatic milestone the injured athlete is able to achieve. After ACL surgery, the athlete passes a clinical examination by a physician who decides whether the athlete is able to start the general rehabilitation training, which then mainly focuses on regaining range of motion, stability, and movement control during basic movement patterns.

18.3.3 Return to Sport (RTS)

Return to sport marks the starting point of the crucial rehabilitation phase (phase III) from the inclusion of the sport-specific rehabilitation training (phase IIIA) to the individualized team training (phase IIIB). At the return-to-sport milestone, the athlete should already meet basic clinical and functional requirements as a result from the previous rehabilitation phase. For example, a test setting should include subjective (e.g., IKDC 2000, KOS-SAS, Lysholm score) and objective (e.g., negative pivot shift) knee stability tests, isokinetic testing, and assessments of leg axis control in the frontal plane during jumps [52, 61, 92].

After passing the RTS milestone, the rehabilitation program becomes increasingly sport specific. In later stages and with advancing athlete performance, growing parts of the rehabilitation content take place on the football field.

This phase should be developed progressively and is normally instructed through athletic coaches, rehabilitation coaches, as well as physiotherapists. It is important to consider whether the sports-specific exercises can be performed by the athlete in a coordinated manner and if they can be tolerated by the injured structure without clinical symptoms such as swelling or pain occurring. Frequently, this phase is also described as a return to restricted team training, since body contact is still deliberately omitted and the athlete participates in team training only partially or modified (i.e., by special identification of the athlete) [15, 23, 52, 92].

18.3.4 Return to Play (RTP)

Return to play refers to the successful transition from individualized and restricted team training to unrestricted participation in team and competition training. The VBG defined this milestone as the end of short-term disability for work (Fact Box 1). Thus, an interdisciplinary (i.e., sports physician, physiotherapists, athletic coaches, rehabilitation coaches, sports psychologists) decision making by means of a comprehensive test battery is essential to promote to unrestricted participation in competitive training. In the light of the collected findings, the return-to-play decision has to be ultimately made by the responsible team physician [22, 57, 92].

18.3.5 Return to Competition (RTC)

On the one hand, the return-to-competition milestone describes the first participation in a competitive match, which is finally the athlete's main goal. On the other hand, return to competition also indicates the entire reintegration process from the time of the injury to the first match play. The time span from the positive return-to-play decision and the athlete's first selection for a competitive match is the only decision that may primarily lie in the head coach's responsibility. But it is recommended that he comes to an agreement with his medical and therapeutic staff as well as the athlete himself to make a responsible decision [92].

Fact Box 2 Rehabilitation process

The rehabilitation process should be progressively structured. Criteria-based milestones help to examine interim rehabilitation goals. Despite the ultimate responsibility of team physicians (return-to-play decision) and coaches (return-to-competition decision), an interdisciplinary decision making is essential.

18.3.6 Biological Healing Process

It is important to say that the biological healing process of an ACL reconstruction is by no means accelerated through the implementation of any kind of test battery. It should be recognized that several months after the ACL reconstruction, there are still ongoing rebuilding mechanism as part of the ligamentization process [17]. Moreover, deficits in the areas of proprioception, muscular strength, and neuromuscular control (i.e., activation patterns) are common. It was noticed that athletes after ACL reconstruction do not regain or not significantly differ from baseline values until approximately 2 years post-op. Against this background, a prolonged rehabilitation and a delayed return to play of athletes under the age of 20 are currently under discussion [63]. However, the practical implementation seems questionable, especially in professional sports.

18.4 Test Manual

In the course of the consensus process, the expert panel had agreed upon seven superordinate test categories that are considered an integral part of a modular return-to-play test battery (Fig. 18.5).

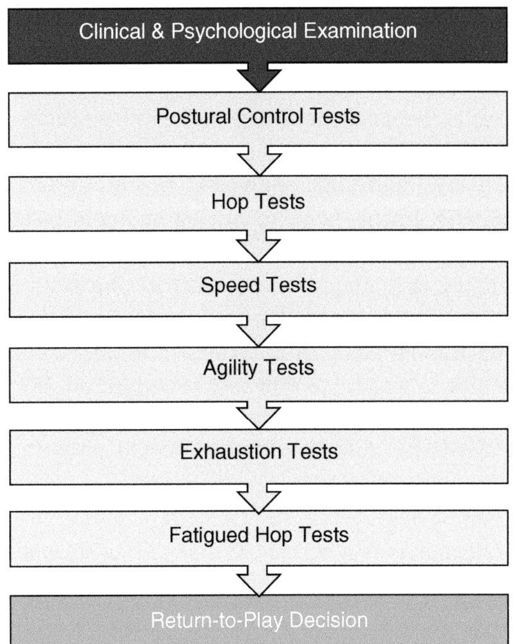

Fig. 18.5 Categories of the modular return-to-play test battery

Each category offers a choice of different tests reaching from gold standard to minimum requirements. This modular approach was chosen to reflect the heterogeneous infrastructures and capacities that are given in real-world sports rehabilitation settings, thereby facilitating the implementation and increasing adherence. Moreover, it allows a smart adjustment to different kinds of sports, if necessary.

18.4.1 Clinical and Psychological Examination

A comprehensive clinical examination is essential part of the return-to-play test battery. This examination must be conducted before the physical tests are started and should include palpation of the injured knee, knee flexion tests, the Lachman test, and isokinetic strength tests.

An isokinetic examination is elementary in ACL patients due to the frequently occurring quadriceps and hamstring strength deficits. For example, quadriceps activation failure is common in athletes after ACL reconstruction [44]. Moreover, asymmetries of the quadriceps muscles seem to be a predictor of knee injuries. It was noticed that per percentage point of improved strength, the risk of reinjury could be reduced by 3% [41].

Because of the high importance of recognizing strength asymmetries, the limb symmetry index (LSI) is commonly used to assess leg asymmetries. It is recommended to achieve a LSI of 90% for non-pivoting and noncontact sports. For pivoting, contact, and competitive sports, a LSI of 100% seems to be suitable [87]. Nevertheless, using the LSI instead of reference values from the pre-injury screening could be insufficient because of sport-specific adaptations prior sustaining an injury, e.g., strength asymmetries between the kicking and standing leg in football. Furthermore, clinical scores (i.e., KOS-SAS, IKDC2000) should complete the clinical examination.

In addition to the clinical examination, recommendations for accompanying psychological assessments were included in the test manual. In particular, motivational aspects and locus of control as well as a lack of confidence in their injured knee and the fear of injury seem to play a major role in whether athletes resume their sport or not [4, 20, 82, 92]. The ACL Return to Sport After Injury (ACL-RSI) scale, which has been developed especially for the question of a safe return after ACL injuries, is recommended as a part of the test manual [58]. Allowing a multilingual use for international players, it has been translated into various languages [16, 42, 55, 81]. The ACL-RSI should be used preoperatively or before the conservative treatment as well as in the rehabilitation process at regular intervals. In the literature, two cutoff scores, 51.3% [58] and 56% [4], were described. Athletes with conspicuous results should consult a psychological care in order to ensure a successful rehabilitation and return to play. Furthermore, other suitable instruments could be used, e.g., the Tampa Scale of Kinesiophobia or the Injury-Psychological Readiness to Return to Sports Scale [36, 45, 88].

18.4.2 Postural Control Tests

Neuromuscular and postural deficits following ACL reconstruction are common and should be assessed even in professional sports, where athletes have access to intensive rehabilitation [47]. Following an ACL injury, the accompanying reduced proprioception postural control deteriorates by approximately 25% [19, 79]. However, a decreased postural control is associated with an increased risk of injury and is considered as a predictor of recurrent ACL injuries [48, 73]. The modified Star Excursion Balance Test (SEBT) and Y Balance Test provide a minimal requirement to assess postural control [27, 40, 75]. Deficits in these tests are associated with an increased risk of injury to the lower extremity. Athletes with an anterior reach distance difference >4 cm and a composite reach distance <94% of their limb length were more likely to sustain a lower extremity injury [21, 27, 39, 40, 48, 75]. In particular, deficits in the anterior reach distance seem to have a negative effect on dynamic requirements. Athletes after ACL reconstruction who demonstrated anterior reach deficits did not tend to achieve recommended LSI values for hop tasks and isometric knee extension strength [35]. As a gold standard, computer-based posturography was determined by the expert panel.

18.4.3 Hop Tests

In the context of return-to-play decisions, uni- and bilateral hop tests are commonly used. In addition to their practicality, they have a strong proximity to the injury mechanism. In particular, unilateral landings are one of the main ACL injury mechanisms in football and other sports. Landing after heading and regaining balance after kicking are essential elements in football, which are carried out during training and competition in high repetition numbers. The landing occurs mainly on one leg only [95]. Therefore, asymmetries as well as performance deficiencies in unilateral hop tests must be taken seriously into account regarding a football-specific return-to-play decision. Moreover, ACL reconstructed athletes have altered biomechanics within their landing behavior, resulting in significant differences in the occurring hip and knee joint angles between injured and noninjured athletes [50, 65, 66, 67]. In this context, altered neuromuscular controls of the hip and knee during a dynamic landing task are essential predictors of a second ACL injury [73]. The biomechanics of unilateral hop landing tasks differ compared to double-leg landings, which are typically used [24, 60, 86]. Due to sports-related asymmetries and frequent contralateral deficits, both sides should always be tested [26, 71, 77]. To increase sensitivity, a combination of jump tests in several directions is generally recommended [51]. Within the test manual, five hop tests were described and recommended as a minimal requirement to assess demands in multiple directions and with different stretch-shortening cycles. The bilateral drop jump procedure was adopted from Padua, where the player must to jump from a box (30 cm height) with his hands on the hips to avoid additional impulses through an arm movement [70]. The unilateral drop jump should be performed from a lower height (20 cm) with a marked target at 30 cm in front of the box [59, 84]. Furthermore, the countermovement jump, the single-leg hop for distance, and the side-hop test are part of the test procedure. The athletes were permitted to make one practice trial. Afterward, each test was regularly completed twice, with the exception of the side-hop test, where only one regular trial per leg is allowed. In this test, the athlete is required to hop transversely more than 30 cm for ten repetitions as quickly as possible [51]. Quantitative measurements like the jump height, the contact time, and the reactivity index should be integral part of the hop test assessment [12, 32, 70]. Additionally, to examine the neuromuscular control and biomechanical risk factors, i.e., valgus malpositioning, an assessment of the movement quality should be realized. Risk-affected movement patterns and compensatory mechanisms in landing tasks, which are regarded as predictors of an ACL injury, can thus be detected [50, 73, 96]. The test manual recommends the 3D motion analysis and electromyography (EMG) as the gold standard. To fulfill the minimal requirements, the real-time observational screening for analyzing the frontal plane for uni- and bilateral drop jumps could be used, wherein athletes at least should show good knee control [64, 85]. Rating the movement quality from the frontal and sagittal point of view, the Landing Error Scoring System (LESS) including 17 items, is recommend with an overall assessment of good knee control. The test manual also offers a modified real-time version of the LESS as a quicker alternative consisting of ten items, wherein the athlete should show a good knee control as well [69].

18.4.4 Speed Tests

A good level of the motoric core competency speed is directly associated with a successful management of various competitive match situations and is therefore considered as an important component of sport-specific performance [13]. Speed tests also allow the identification of deficits in neuromuscular control. With the aid of the tapping test, possible frequency drops, which are associated with a faster fatigue of the neuromuscular system, and differences between the operated and nonoperated leg can be detected [11]. On a starting sign, the athlete tries to perform alternating steps on the spot with a maximum frequency. The motion amplitude should be kept as low as possible. The test is carried out once, whereby the athlete tries to achieve as many contacts as possible with his forefoot on the contact surface in 15 s. Based on the requirement profile of football with frequently recurring sprints, the repeated sprint ability test is also recommended within the test manual [15, 83, 97].

18.4.5 Agility Tests

Agility tests reflect demands of the football-specific requirement profile and confront the athlete with a test situation that is close to the injury mechanism. This includes match-related movements like accelerations, decelerations, fast changes of directions, cuttings, and unanticipated movement tasks, typically resulting from changing match situations or the behavior of teammates and opponents. It is therefore no coincidence that about 77% of the ACL injuries during competition occur in defensive actions, in which the defensive player must react to unforeseen actions of his opponent, especially in pressing situations [95]. Significant differences in the kinematics and kinetics of plant and cut maneuvers compared to hop tests make the additional examination of these risk factors indispensable [54]. As a minimal requirement, the change of direction speed should be assed, using tests like the modified agility T-test [61, 62, 80], the Illinois agility test, or the Barrow zigzag run [68, 76, 78]. Certainly, assessing agility permits an athlete to react to a stimulus which includes perceptual and decision making factors [99]. That is why usage of the mentioned tests could only assess change of direction speed, while cognitive and reactive components are missing. To achieve the gold standard, randomized multidirectional movement tasks should be assessed with the SpeedCourt or comparable systems [11, 18, 29].

18.4.6 Exhaustion Test

Training of endurance is an indispensable part in football. In addition to the development of basic endurance and sports-specific endurance, the organism's ability to regenerate and the metabolism of the operated limb are stimulated. Within the assessment tool, the exhaustion test is primarily a standardized fatigue provocation. This is due to the fact that a severe decrease in hop performance, postural control, and quality of movement as a result of ACL rupture can be observed under fatigued conditions [7, 34]. If the exhaustion test is carried out on the treadmill, it can also be combined with a gait and running analysis, since ACL patients often show altered gait patterns years after their injury [37].

18.4.7 Fatigued Hop Tests

Hop tests should be performed both under non-fatigued and fatigued test condition, because patients often displayed abnormal hop symmetry for the fatigued test condition [7]. All five recommended hop tests of the test manual (Chap. 4, Sect. 3) should be performed after the prescribed pre-exhaustion (Chap. 4, Sect. 7). If any abnormalities have already occurred in the non-fatigued test condition, patients should not carry out the corresponding hop tests under fatigued conditions in order to reduce injury risk within the test situation.

Fact Box 3 Modular return-to-play test battery

A modular test battery reflects the heterogeneous infrastructures and capacities that are given in real-world sports rehabilitation settings, thereby facilitating the implementation and increasing adherence.

A test algorithm with seven successive test categories (i.e., clinical and psychological examination, postural control tests, hop tests, speed tests, agility tests, exhaustion, and fatigued hop tests) is recommended to identify possible risk factors for recurrent injuries and to monitor the rehabilitation progress before returning to unrestricted team training.

18.5 Knowledge Transfer

The sole publication of a test manual is not sufficient to successfully implement a new test battery into real-world sports medical settings. The involvement of different professions in the return-to-play process calls for a multilateral implementation strategy to enable a widespread distribution within the target group.

Firstly, the VBG focuses on direct users of the test battery, such as team physicians, physiotherapists, athletic and rehabilitation coaches, as well as the injured players themselves. The rehabilitation manager of the VBG, who supervises the rehabilitation process, will inform the injured player about the return-to-play test and suitable test centers. This procedure is also coordinated with the attending physician. In order to raise awareness among young athletes, the VBG supports an app-based platform, which provides players from German football youth academies with information on conditioning, sports medicine, nutrition, and mental strength on their mobile phones. Using the hashtag "#ComebackStronger," specific information on the topic of return to play (i.e., added value of the return-to-play test battery) is promoted. To motivate injured players, stories about successful comebacks are illustrated and shared. Since 2015, the VBG has been conducting education modules for team physicians in the framework of the "team physician procedures," a model project that certifies team physicians in order to establish preventive sports medicine care in team sports [25]. Beside the systematic implementation of preventive standards, return-to-play guidelines should be established within the clubs. Up to now, about 200 team physicians were certified. Furthermore, the VBG, in cooperation with the *German Football Association* (*DFB*) and regional German football associations, offers free symposia on sports injury prevention. Main target groups are coaches, physiotherapist, and chairmen of elite and semi-elite football clubs. These symposia consist of keynote speeches, lectures, as well as practical workshops. The successful return-to-competition process after an ACL injury was always one of the main themes. At nine events so far, about 1500 participants were informed and trained. Through education modules in basic and advanced coach education courses of the *German Football Association* (DFB) and the *Association of German Football Coaches* (BDFL), the VBG directly reaches football coaches in theoretical and practical teaching units. In cooperation with the *Coaches Academy Cologne*, the VBG specifically addresses athletic coaches and sports physiotherapists. In summary, over 2500 coaches, athletic coaches and physiotherapists have been reached since 2014.

Fact Box 4 Multilateral implementation
The involvement of different professions in the return-to-play process calls for a multilateral implementation strategy to enable a widespread distribution within the target group of elite and semi-elite football clubs (i.e., players, coaches, athletic coaches, physiotherapists, team physicians, chairmen). Education courses of multipliers should ensure sustainable application.

18.6 Pilot Implementation

In addition to education modules, the VBG is currently implementing the modular test battery into real-world sport rehabilitation settings. Within a multicenter approach, the following key primary objectives should be reached:

- Evaluation of practicability and sensitivity of the return-to-play test battery
- Elicitation of reference values for the individual test variables as well as the final return-to-play decision
- Identification of risk factors and symptomatic deficits of the patients tested

To further the available knowledge on the etiology of ACL injuries, as well as potential risk factors, an online questionnaire, based on the German ACL registry (www.kreuzbandregister.de), was designed by the VBG. A second online questionnaire, consisting of the Knee Outcome Survey Sports Activity Scale (KOS-SAS), the 2000 IKDC subjective knee evaluation form (IKDC 2000), and the Anterior Cruciate Ligament-Return to Sport After Injury (ACL-RSI) scale, was prepared to record subjective patient parameters. Both questionnaires can thus already be answered by the patient from home. By programming mandatory responses, elementary questions cannot be skipped, which should ensure a high response rate. After answering the questions, a code word is displayed to the patients, which can be used as a control instrument for the test centers to check whether the questionnaires have already been filled out.

In addition to the primary goals, further secondary objectives should be examined:

- Analysis of the test results with regard to dependence on the rehabilitation process
- Analysis of the long-term outcomes as a function of the test results and the rehabilitation process

During pilot implementation, the focus lies on the testing of elite and semi-elite athletes with insurance coverage at the VBG from the team sports football, handball, basketball, and ice hockey with primary ruptures of the ACL. The test is carried out at the earliest 6 months' post-surgery at the time of the announced return to unrestricted team training (return to play). The recruitment is mainly carried out by the test centers' own patients as well as through the recommendation of patients by the VBG. Potentially test centers had to apply at the VBG. The application had to include information about the chosen test arrangement from the VBG test manual and the test centers recruitment process of patients. On this basis, five regionally distributed test centers were selected. The selection consciously paid attention to the fact that centers are involved that could fulfill the minimum standards or even the gold standard of the test manual (Table 18.1). Each test center should not exceed the minimum number of 40 patients. The intervention phase lasts for 14 months, and patients will be followed up after 12 and 24 months post-op. The follow-up will include information on the further course of rehabilitation, the return to competition, the current activity level, and possible injuries sustained after returning to competition (i.e., muscle injuries, second ACL injuries, other injuries).

Table 18.1 Overview of the VBG pilot implementation test centers and their modular test batteries

Category	Test center				
	I	II	III	IV	V
Clinical and psychological examination	– Palpation – Range of motion (ROM) – Lachman test – Pivot shift test – KT-1000 knee ligament arthrometer – Isokinetic (60°/s) – Hip abductor strength – Anterior Cruciate Ligament—Return to Sport after Injury (ACL-RSI) scale – International Knee Documentation Committee (IKDC) Subjective Knee Evaluation Form – Knee Outcome Survey Sports Activity Scale (KOS-SAS)	– Palpation – Range of motion (ROM) – Lachman test – Pivot shift test – KT-1000 knee ligament arthrometer – Isokinetic (60°/s) – Hip abductor strength – Anterior Cruciate Ligament—Return to Sport after Injury (ACL-RSI) scale – International Knee Documentation Committee (IKDC) Subjective Knee Evaluation Form – Knee Outcome Survey Sports Activity Scale (KOS-SAS)	– Palpation – Range of motion (ROM) – Lachman test – Pivot shift test – KT-1000 knee ligament arthrometer – Isokinetic (60°/s) – Anterior Cruciate Ligament—Return to Sport after Injury (ACL-RSI) scale – International Knee Documentation Committee (IKDC) Subjective Knee Evaluation Form – Knee Outcome Survey Sports Activity Scale (KOS-SAS)	– Palpation – Range of motion (ROM) – Lachman test – Pivot shift test – KT-1000 knee ligament arthrometer – Isokinetic (60°/s) – Hip abductor strength – Anterior Cruciate Ligament—Return to Sport after Injury (ACL-RSI) scale – International Knee Documentation Committee (IKDC) Subjective Knee Evaluation Form – Knee Outcome Survey Sports Activity Scale (KOS-SAS)	– Palpation – Range of motion (ROM) – -Lachman test – Pivot shift test – KT-1000 knee ligament arthrometer – Isokinetic (60°/s) – Anterior Cruciate Ligament—Return to Sport after Injury (ACL-RSI) scale – International Knee Documentation Committee (IKDC) Subjective Knee Evaluation Form – Knee Outcome Survey Sports Activity Scale (KOS-SAS)
Postural control tests	– Y Balance Test	– Y Balance Test	– Y Balance Test	– MFT Challenge Disc	– Y Balance Test – Interactive Balance System (IBS)
Hop tests	– Countermovement jump – Drop jump (double/single legged) – Side-hop test – Single-leg hop for distance	– Countermovement jump – Drop jump (double/single legged) – Side-hop test – Single-leg hop for distance	– Countermovement jump – Drop jump (double/single legged) – Side-hop test – Single-leg hop for distance	– Countermovement jump – Drop jump (double/single legged) – Side-hop test – Single-leg hop for distance	– Countermovement jump – Drop jump (double/single legged) – Side-hop test – Single-leg hop for distance

Category	Test center				
	I	II	III	IV	V
Motion analysis	– Landing Error Scoring System (LESS)	– Landing Error Scoring System (LESS)	– 3D motion analysis with inertial sensors – Electromyography	– 3D motion analysis with inertial sensors	– Landing Error Scoring System (LESS)
Speed tests	– Tapping test	– Tapping test	– Tapping test	– Tapping test	– Tapping test
Agility tests	– Modified agility T-test	– Modified agility T-test	– SpeedCourt®	– SpeedCourt®	– SpeedCourt®
Exhaustion tests	– Spiroergometry	– Spiroergometry	– SpeedCourt®	– SpeedCourt®	– Six-minute run on a treadmill
Fatigued hop tests	– Countermovement jump – Drop jump (double/single legged) – Side-hop test – Single-leg hop for distance	– Countermovement jump – Drop jump (double/single legged) – Side-hop test – Single-leg hop for distance	– Countermovement jump – Drop jump (double/single legged) – Side-hop test – Single-leg hop for distance	– Countermovement jump – Drop jump (double/single legged) – Side-hop test – Single-leg hop for distance	– Countermovement jump – Drop jump (double/single legged) – Side-hop test – Single-leg hop for distance

Conclusion

German elite and semi-elite football shows a high risk of injury. Mainly lower limbs are affected and lead to the biggest amount of short-term disability and medical treatment. Injuries of the ACL represent only a small share of all injuries, but they are accompanied by long downtimes, a high risk of recurrence, and high medical costs. Although test procedures for such serious injuries are required prior to the completion of the rehabilitation procedure in Germany, no standardized guidelines existed. Rather than time, which is an important factor in biological healing, objective parameters are needed to monitor, control, and optimize the rehabilitation process. Especially when it comes to the final return-to-play decision after an ACL injury, it is advisable to carry out a comprehensive test battery that considers clinical, physiological, and psychological aspects.

In the light of the ambitions to develop a standardized test battery, the VBG, the statutory accident insurance for German professional sports, conducted a consensus conference bringing together accredited experts and working groups from all professions that are typically involved in the rehabilitation process. As a result of this conference, a modular test battery was introduced to promote an accepted standard. The inclusion of the target group at an early stage in the development process of a modular test battery should contribute to an increase in the acceptance in sports practice. In the course of the consensus process, the expert panel agreed upon seven superordinate test categories (i.e., clinical and psychological examination, postural control tests, hop tests, speed tests, agility tests, exhaustion test, and fatigued hop tests), which have to be integral part of a modular return-to-play test battery. In addition to the multiplication through education of coaches, physicians, and physiotherapists, the test manual is implemented multicentrically into sports rehabilitation settings. The selected test procedures should ideally be an integral part of the pre-injury screening at the beginning of the season, so that individual reference values can be used in case of an injury. The final return-to-play and return-to-competition decision should always be an interdisciplinary agreement.

For an optimal implementation of the return-to-play test battery and a proper interpretation of the test results, a good communication between the involved actors and professions within the club is needed. Therefore, a standardized definition of the "return-to" phases in the course of the rehabilitation process is indispensable. The expert panel agreed on five distinctive milestones that the injured athletes will pass during an ideal rehabilitation process. In order to raise the awareness of responsible persons in the clubs, education of practicable screening procedures and the derivation of preventive measures are necessary, in addition to provide information about risk factors and injury patterns. During rehabilitation, as well as in training and competition, regular monitoring helps to quantify the loads of the players and to ensure optimal training control. If an injury occurs during the course of the season, systematic injury documentation could help to detect injury hot spots and context factors like injury mechanisms. In conjunction with a regular screening, this can be used to identify the causes of injury in the individual setting of the club and to identify risk factors at an early phase. Individual prevention measures derived from this help to minimize injuries, ensure high player availability, and ultimately increase the sporting success potential.

Take-Home Message

- Within an ideal rehabilitation process in team sports like football, an injured athlete must pass five essential milestones: pre-injury screening, return to activity, return to sport, return to play, and return to competition.
- Objective test procedures at these milestones are needed to monitor, control, and optimize the rehabilitation process ensuring a safe progression to the next rehabilitation phase.

- The return-to-play milestone is of utmost importance as players then progress to unrestricted training. Therefore, a comprehensive test battery is needed to determine the right moment of return-to-play.
- Seven superordinate test categories—clinical and psychological examination, postural control tests, hop tests, speed tests, agility tests, exhaustion test, and fatigued hop tests—are recommended as integral part of a modular return-to-play test battery.
- The modular setup of the test battery reflects the heterogeneous infrastructures and capacities that are given in real-world sports rehabilitation settings and will thereby increase adherence in the target population.
- To ensure successful implementation of a modular test battery, it is important that the target group (i.e., the users of the test battery) should be involved at an early stage and educated via various channels (i.e., training, consultation, and application).

Top Five Evidence-Based References

Ekstrand J, Hagglund M, Walden M (2011) Injury incidence and injury patterns in professional football: the UEFA injury study. Br J Sports Med 45:553–558

Grindem H, Snyder-Mackler L, Moksnes H, Engebretsen L, Risberg MA (2016) Simple decision rules can reduce reinjury risk by 84% after ACL reconstruction: the Delaware-Oslo ACL cohort study. Br J Sports Med 50:804–808

Harris JD, Abrams GD, Bach BR, Williams D, Heidloff D, Bush-Joseph CA et al (2014) Return to sport after ACL reconstruction. Orthopedics 37:e103–e108

Hewett TE, Myer GD, Ford KR, Heidt RS Jr, Colosimo AJ, McLean SG et al (2005) Biomechanical measures of neuromuscular control and valgus loading of the knee predict anterior cruciate ligament injury risk in female athletes: a prospective study. Am J Sports Med 33:492–501

Paterno MV, Rauh MJ, Schmitt LC, Ford KR, Hewett TE (2014) Incidence of second ACL injuries 2 years after primary ACL reconstruction and return to sport. Am J Sports Med 42:1567–1573

References

1. Ardern CL (2015) Anterior cruciate ligament reconstruction-not exactly a one-way ticket back to the preinjury level: a review of contextual factors affecting return to sport after surgery. Sports Health 7:224–230
2. Ardern CL, Bizzini M, Bahr R (2016) It is time for consensus on return to play after injury: five key questions. Br J Sports Med 50:506–508
3. Ardern CL, Glasgow P, Schneiders A, Witvrouw E, Clarsen B, Cools A et al (2016) 2016 Consensus statement on return to sport from the First World Congress in Sports Physical Therapy, Bern. Br J Sports Med 50:853–864
4. Ardern CL, Taylor NF, Feller JA, Webster KE (2014) Fifty-five per cent return to competitive sport following anterior cruciate ligament reconstruction surgery: an updated systematic review and meta-analysis including aspects of physical functioning and contextual factors. Br J Sports Med 48:1543–1552
5. Ardern CL, Taylor NF, Feller JA, Whitehead TS, Webster KE (2013) Psychological responses matter in returning to preinjury level of sport after anterior cruciate ligament reconstruction surgery. Am J Sports Med 41:1549–1558
6. Ardern CL, Webster KE, Taylor NF, Feller JA (2011) Return to the preinjury level of competitive sport after anterior cruciate ligament reconstruction surgery: two-thirds of patients have not returned by 12 months after surgery. Am J Sports Med 39:538–543
7. Augustsson J, Thomee R, Karlsson J (2004) Ability of a new hop test to determine functional deficits after anterior cruciate ligament reconstruction. Knee Surg Sports Traumatol Arthrosc 12:350–356
8. Bahr R (2016) Why screening tests to predict injury do not work-and probably never will...: a critical review. Br J Sports Med 50:776–780
9. Bakken A, Targett S, Bere T, Adamuz MC, Tol JL, Whiteley R et al (2016) Health conditions detected in a comprehensive periodic health evaluation of 558 professional football players. Br J Sports Med 50:1142–1150
10. Barber-Westin SD, Noyes FR (2011) Factors used to determine return to unrestricted sports activities after anterior cruciate ligament reconstruction. Arthroscopy 27:1697–1705
11. Bartels T, Proeger S, Brehme K, Pyschik M, Delank KS, Schulze S et al (2016) The SpeedCourt system in rehabilitation after reconstruction surgery of the anterior cruciate ligament (ACL). Arch Orthop Trauma Surg 136:957–966
12. Baumgart C, Schubert M, Hoppe MW, Gokeler A, Freiwald J (2015) Do ground reaction forces during unilateral and bilateral movements exhibit compensation strategies following ACL reconstruction? Knee Surg Sports Traumatol Arthrosc 25:1–10
13. Berschin G, Hartmann M (2011) Agility – Bedeutung, Training und Testung der Richtungswechselfähigkeit am Beispiel Fußball. Leistungssport 41:25–28
14. Best R, Bauer G, Niess A, Striegel H (2011) Return to play decisions in professional soccer: a decision algorithm from a team physician's viewpoint. Z Orthop Unfall 149:582–587

15. Bizzini M, Hancock D, Impellizzeri F (2012) Suggestions from the field for return to sports participation following anterior cruciate ligament reconstruction: soccer. J Orthop Sports Phys Ther 42:304–312
16. Bohu Y, Klouche S, Lefevre N, Webster K, Herman S (2015) Translation, cross-cultural adaptation and validation of the French version of the Anterior Cruciate Ligament-Return to Sport after Injury (ACL-RSI) scale. Knee Surg Sports Traumatol Arthrosc 23:1192–1196
17. Bonfim TR, Jansen Paccola CA, Barela JA (2003) Proprioceptive and behavior impairments in individuals with anterior cruciate ligament reconstructed knees. Arch Phys Med Rehabil 84:1217–1223
18. Born DP, Zinner C, Duking P, Sperlich B (2016) Multi-directional sprint training improves change-of-direction speed and reactive agility in young highly trained soccer players. J Sports Sci Med 15:314–319
19. Brattinger F (2012) Der Einfluss einer Ruptur des vorderen Kreuzbandes auf die posturale Kontrollfähigkeit. Universität Ulm
20. Christino MA, Fleming BC, Machan JT, Shalvoy RM (2016) Psychological factors associated with anterior cruciate ligament reconstruction recovery. Orthop J Sports Med 4:1–9
21. Clagg S, Paterno MV, Hewett TE, Schmitt LC (2015) Performance on the modified star excursion balance test at the time of return to sport following anterior cruciate ligament reconstruction. J Orthop Sports Phys Ther 45:444–452
22. Creighton DW, Shrier I, Shultz R, Meeuwisse WH, Matheson GO (2010) Return-to-play in sport: a decision-based model. Clin J Sport Med 20:379–385
23. Della Villa S, Boldrini L, Ricci M, Danelon F, Snyder-Mackler L, Nanni G et al (2012) Clinical outcomes and return-to-sports participation of 50 soccer players after anterior cruciate ligament reconstruction through a sport-specific rehabilitation protocol. Sports Health 4:17–24
24. Deneweth JM, Bey MJ, McLean SG, Lock TR, Kolowich PA, Tashman S (2010) Tibiofemoral joint kinematics of the anterior cruciate ligament-reconstructed knee during a single-legged hop landing. Am J Sports Med 38:1820–1828
25. Deters W-H, Froese E (2016) Mannschaftsarztverfahren der Verwaltungs-Berufsgenossenschaft. Trauma und Berufskrankheit 18:56–60
26. Di Stasi S, Myer GD, Hewett TE (2013) Neuromuscular training to target deficits associated with second anterior cruciate ligament injury. J Orthop Sports Phys Ther 43:777–792, A771-711
27. Dobija L, Coudeyre E, Pereira B (2016) Measurement properties of the Star Excursion Balance Test in the anterior crucial ligament-deficient subjects - preliminary analysis. Ann Phys Rehabil Med 59S:e18
28. Doyscher R, Kraus K, Hinterwimmer S, Wagner D, Wolfarth B, Haslbauer R et al (2016) Evidenz-basierte Return-to-Sport-Testung nach Gelenkeingriffen. Arthroskopie 29:38–44
29. Duking P, Born DP, Sperlich B (2016) The SpeedCourt: reliability, usefulness, and validity of a new method to determine change-of-direction speed. Int J Sports Physiol Perform 11:130–134
30. Ekstrand J (2013) Playing too many matches is negative for both performance and player availability – results from the on-going UEFA injury study. Deutsche Zeitschrift für Sportmedizin 2013:5–9
31. Ekstrand J, Hagglund M, Walden M (2011) Injury incidence and injury patterns in professional football: the UEFA injury study. Br J Sports Med 45:553–558
32. Faude OS, Andreas, Fritsche T, Treff G, Meyer T (2010) Performance diagnosis in football - methodological standards. Deutsche Zeitschrift für Sportmedizin 61:129–133
33. Finch C (2006) A new framework for research leading to sports injury prevention. J Sci Med Sport 9:3–9. discussion 10
34. Frank BS, Gilsdorf CM, Goerger BM, Prentice WE, Padua DA (2014) Neuromuscular fatigue alters postural control and sagittal plane hip biomechanics in active females with anterior cruciate ligament reconstruction. Sports Health 6:301–308
35. Garrison JC, Bothwell JM, Wolf G, Aryal S, Thigpen CA (2015) Y Balance test anterior reach symmetry at three months is related to single leg functional performance at time of return to sports following anterior cruciate ligament reconstruction. Int J Sports Phys Ther 10:602–611
36. Glazer DD (2009) Development and preliminary validation of the Injury-Psychological Readiness to Return to Sport (I-PRRS) scale. J Athl Train 44:185–189
37. Gokeler A, Benjaminse A, van Eck CF, Webster KE, Schot L, Otten E (2013) Return of normal gait as an outcome measurement in acl reconstructed patients. A systematic review. Int J Sports Phys Ther 8:441–451
38. Gokeler A, Welling W, Zaffagnini S, Seil R, Padua D (2017) Development of a test battery to enhance safe return to sports after anterior cruciate ligament reconstruction. Knee Surg Sports Traumatol Arthrosc 25:192–199
39. Gonell AC, Romero JA, Soler LM (2015) Relationship between the Y balance test scores and soft tissue injury incidence in a soccer team. Int J Sports Phys Ther 10:955–966
40. Gribble PA, Hertel J, Plisky P (2012) Using the Star Excursion Balance Test to assess dynamic postural-control deficits and outcomes in lower extremity injury: a literature and systematic review. J Athl Train 47:339–357
41. Grindem H, Snyder-Mackler L, Moksnes H, Engebretsen L, Risberg MA (2016) Simple decision rules can reduce reinjury risk by 84% after ACL reconstruction: the Delaware-Oslo ACL cohort study. Br J Sports Med 50:804–808
42. Harput G, Tok D, Ulusoy B, Eraslan L, Yildiz TI, Turgut E et al (2017) Translation and cross-cultural adaptation of the anterior cruciate ligament-return to

sport after injury (ACL-RSI) scale into Turkish. Knee Surg Sports Traumatol Arthrosc 25:159–164

43. Harris JD, Abrams GD, Bach BR, Williams D, Heidloff D, Bush-Joseph CA et al (2014) Return to sport after ACL reconstruction. Orthopedics 37:e103–e108
44. Hart JM, Pietrosimone B, Hertel J, Ingersoll CD (2010) Quadriceps activation following knee injuries: a systematic review. J Athl Train 45:87–97
45. Hartigan EH, Lynch AD, Logerstedt DS, Chmielewski TL, Snyder-Mackler L (2013) Kinesiophobia after anterior cruciate ligament rupture and reconstruction: noncopers versus potential copers. J Orthop Sports Phys Ther 43:821–832
46. Henke T, Luig P (2012) Safety in sports: general guidelines for the development and implementation of sustainable safety management schemes in high risk sports in the EU countries (D11). Universität Bochum/Fakultät für Sportwissenschaft, Bochum
47. Herbst E, Hoser C, Hildebrandt C, Raschner C, Hepperger C, Pointner H et al (2015) Functional assessments for decision-making regarding return to sports following ACL reconstruction. Part II: clinical application of a new test battery. Knee Surg Sports Traumatol Arthrosc 23:1283–1291
48. Herrington L, Hatcher J, Hatcher A, McNicholas M (2009) A comparison of Star Excursion Balance Test reach distances between ACL deficient patients and asymptomatic controls. Knee 16:149–152
49. Hewett TE, Di Stasi SL, Myer GD (2013) Current concepts for injury prevention in athletes after anterior cruciate ligament reconstruction. Am J Sports Med 41:216–224
50. Hewett TE, Myer GD, Ford KR, Heidt RS Jr, Colosimo AJ, McLean SG et al (2005) Biomechanical measures of neuromuscular control and valgus loading of the knee predict anterior cruciate ligament injury risk in female athletes: a prospective study. Am J Sports Med 33:492–501
51. Itoh H, Kurosaka M, Yoshiya S, Ichihashi N, Mizuno K (1998) Evaluation of functional deficits determined by four different hop tests in patients with anterior cruciate ligament deficiency. Knee Surg Sports Traumatol Arthrosc 6:241–245
52. Keller M, Kurz E (2016) Zurück zum Pre Injury Level nach Verletzungen der unteren Extremität – eine Einteilung funktioneller Assessments. Man Ther 20:16–18
53. Khayambashi K, Ghoddosi N, Straub RK, Powers CM (2016) Hip muscle strength predicts noncontact anterior cruciate ligament injury in male and female athletes: a prospective study. Am J Sports Med 44:355–361
54. Kristianslund E, Krosshaug T (2013) Comparison of drop jumps and sport-specific sidestep cutting: implications for anterior cruciate ligament injury risk screening. Am J Sports Med 41:684–688
55. Kvist J, Osterberg A, Gauffin H, Tagesson S, Webster K, Ardern C (2013) Translation and measurement properties of the Swedish version of ACL-Return to Sports after Injury questionnaire. Scand J Med Sci Sports 23:568–575
56. Kyritsis PWE (2014) Return to sport after anterior cruciate ligament reconstruction: a literature review. J Novel Physiother 4:1–6
57. Matheson GO, Shultz R, Bido J, Mitten MJ, Meeuwisse WH, Shrier I (2011) Return-to-play decisions: are they the team physician's responsibility? Clin J Sport Med 21:25–30
58. Müller U, Krüger-Franke M, Schmidt M, Rosemeyer B (2014) Predictive parameters for return to pre-injury level of sport 6 months following anterior cruciate ligament reconstruction surgery. Knee Surg Sports Traumatol Arthrosc 23:3623–3631
59. Munro A, Herrington L, Carolan M (2012) Reliability of 2-dimensional video assessment of frontal-plane dynamic knee valgus during common athletic screening tasks. J Sport Rehabil 21:7–11
60. Myer GD, Martin L Jr, Ford KR, Paterno MV, Schmitt LC, Heidt RS Jr et al (2012) No association of time from surgery with functional deficits in athletes after anterior cruciate ligament reconstruction: evidence for objective return-to-sport criteria. Am J Sports Med 40:2256–2263
61. Myer GD, Paterno MV, Ford KR, Quatman CE, Hewett TE (2006) Rehabilitation after anterior cruciate ligament reconstruction: criteria-based progression through the return-to-sport phase. J Orthop Sports Phys Ther 36:385–402
62. Myer GD, Schmitt LC, Brent JL, Ford KR, Barber Foss KD, Scherer BJ et al (2011) Utilization of modified NFL combine testing to identify functional deficits in athletes following ACL reconstruction. J Orthop Sports Phys Ther 41:377–387
63. Nagelli CV, Hewett TE (2017) Should return to sport be delayed until 2 years after anterior cruciate ligament reconstruction? Biological and functional considerations. Sports Med 47:221–232
64. Nilstad A, Andersen TE, Kristianslund E, Bahr R, Myklebust G, Steffen K et al (2014) Physiotherapists can identify female football players with high knee valgus angles during vertical drop jumps using real-time observational screening. J Orthop Sports Phys Ther 44:358–365
65. Oberlander KD, Bruggemann GP, Hoher J, Karamanidis K (2013) Altered landing mechanics in ACL-reconstructed patients. Med Sci Sports Exerc 45:506–513
66. Oberlander KD, Bruggemann GP, Hoher J, Karamanidis K (2014) Knee mechanics during landing in anterior cruciate ligament patients: a longitudinal study from pre- to 12 months post-reconstruction. Clin Biomech (Bristol, Avon) 29:512–517
67. Oberlander KD, Bruggemann GP, Hoher J, Karamanidis K (2012) Reduced knee joint moment in ACL deficient patients at a cost of dynamic stability during landing. J Biomech 45:1387–1392

68. Ortiz A, Olson SL, Roddey TS, Morales J (2005) Reliability of selected physical performance tests in young adult women. J Strength Cond Res 19:39–44
69. Padua DA, Boling MC, Distefano LJ, Onate JA, Beutler AI, Marshall SW (2011) Reliability of the landing error scoring system-real time, a clinical assessment tool of jump-landing biomechanics. J Sport Rehabil 20:145–156
70. Padua DA, Marshall SW, Boling MC, Thigpen CA, Garrett WE Jr, Beutler AI (2009) The Landing Error Scoring System (LESS) Is a valid and reliable clinical assessment tool of jump-landing biomechanics: the JUMP-ACL study. Am J Sports Med 37:1996–2002
71. Pairot de Fontenay B, Argaud S, Blache Y, Monteil K (2015) Contralateral limb deficit seven months after ACL-reconstruction: an analysis of single-leg hop tests. Knee 22:309–312
72. Paterno MV, Rauh MJ, Schmitt LC, Ford KR, Hewett TE (2014) Incidence of second ACL injuries 2 years after primary ACL reconstruction and return to sport. Am J Sports Med 42:1567–1573
73. Paterno MV, Schmitt LC, Ford KR, Rauh MJ, Myer GD, Huang B et al (2010) Biomechanical measures during landing and postural stability predict second anterior cruciate ligament injury after anterior cruciate ligament reconstruction and return to sport. Am J Sports Med 38:1968–1978
74. Petersen W, Zantop T (2013) Return to play following ACL reconstruction: survey among experienced arthroscopic surgeons (AGA instructors). Arch Orthop Trauma Surg 133:969–977
75. Plisky PJ, Rauh MJ, Kaminski TW, Underwood FB (2006) Star Excursion Balance Test as a predictor of lower extremity injury in high school basketball players. J Orthop Sports Phys Ther 36:911–919
76. Reiman MP, Manske RC (2009) Functional Testing in Human Performance. Tests for Sport, Fitness, Occupational Settings., p 139
77. Riepenhof H, McAleer S, Bloch H, Hennings A, Keppeler R, Holtfreter B et al (2016) Kreuzbandruptur Trauma und Berufskrankheit 18:511–514
78. Rouissi M, Chtara M, Berriri A, Owen A, Chamari K (2016) Asymmetry of the modified illinois change of direction test impacts young elite soccer players' performance. Asian J Sports Med 7:1–5
79. Rozzi SL, Lephart SM, Gear WS, FH F (1999) Knee joint laxity and neuromuscular characteristics of male and female soccer and basketball players. Am J Sports Med 27:312–319
80. Sassi RH, Dardouri W, Yahmed MH, Gmada N, Mahfoudhi ME, Gharbi Z (2009) Relative and absolute reliability of a modified agility T-test and its relationship with vertical jump and straight sprint. J Strength Cond Res 23:1644–1651
81. Slagers AJ, Reininga IH, van den Akker-Scheek I (2017) The Dutch language anterior cruciate ligament return to sport after injury scale (ACL-RSI) - validity and reliability. J Sports Sci 35:393–401
82. Sonesson S, Kvist J, Ardern C, Osterberg A, Silbernagel KG (2016) Psychological factors are important to return to pre-injury sport activity after anterior cruciate ligament reconstruction: expect and motivate to satisfy. Knee Surg Sports Traumatol Arthrosc 25:1375. https://doi.org/10.1007/s00167-016-4294-8
83. Sporis GM, Milanovic Z, Trajkovic N, Erceg M, Novak D (2013) Relationship between functional capacities and performance parameters in soccer. J Sports Med Dop Stud s2:001
84. Stalbom M, Holm DJ, Cronin J, Keogh J (2007) Reliability of kinematics and kinetics associated with horizontal single leg drop jump assessment. A brief report. J Sports Sci Med 6:261–264
85. Stensrud S, Myklebust G, Kristianslund E, Bahr R, Krosshaug T (2011) Correlation between two-dimensional video analysis and subjective assessment in evaluating knee control among elite female team handball players. Br J Sports Med 45:589–595
86. Taylor JB, Ford KR, Nguyen AD, Shultz SJ (2016) Biomechanical comparison of single- and double-leg jump landings in the sagittal and frontal plane. Orthop J Sports Med 4:1–9
87. Thomeé R, Kaplan Y, Kvist J, Myklebust G, Risberg MA, Theisen D et al (2011) Muscle strength and hop performance criteria prior to return to sports after ACL reconstruction. Knee Surg Sports Traumatol Arthrosc 19:1798–1805
88. Tichonova A, Rimdeikienė I, Petruševičienė D, Lendraitienė E (2016) The relationship between pain catastrophizing, kinesiophobia and subjective knee function during rehabilitation following anterior cruciate ligament reconstruction and meniscectomy: a pilot study. Medicina 52:229–237
89. van der Horst N, van de Hoef S, Reurink G, Huisstede B, Backx F (2016) Return to play after hamstring injuries: a qualitative systematic review of definitions and criteria. Sports Med 46:899–912
90. van Mechelen W, Hlobil H, Kemper HCG (1992) Incidence, Severity, Aetiology and Prevention of Sports Injuries. Sports Med 14:82–99
91. van Melick N, van Cingel RE, Brooijmans F, Neeter C, van Tienen T, Hullegie W et al (2016) Evidence-based clinical practice update: practice guidelines for anterior cruciate ligament rehabilitation based on a systematic review and multidisciplinary consensus. Br J Sports Med 50:1506–1515
92. VBG (2015) Return-to-competition. Testmanual zur Beurteilung der Spielfähigkeit nach Ruptur des vorderen Kreuzbands. Hamburg, Jedermann-Verlag
93. VBG (2016) VBG-Sportreport - 2016. Analyse des Unfallgeschehens in den zwei höchsten Ligen der Männer: Basketball, Eishockey, Fußball & Handball. Hamburg, Jedermann-Verlag
94. Walden M, Hagglund M, Magnusson H, Ekstrand J (2016) ACL injuries in men's professional football: a 15-year prospective study on time trends and return-

to-play rates reveals only 65% of players still play at the top level 3 years after ACL rupture. Br J Sports Med 50:744–750

95. Walden M, Krosshaug T, Bjorneboe J, Andersen TE, Faul O, Hagglund M (2015) Three distinct mechanisms predominate in non-contact anterior cruciate ligament injuries in male professional football players: a systematic video analysis of 39 cases. Br J Sports Med 49:1452–1460
96. Wojtys EM, Beaulieu ML, Ashton-Miller JA (2016) New perspectives on ACL injury: on the role of repetitive sub-maximal knee loading in causing ACL fatigue failure. J Orthop Res 34:2059–2068
97. Wragg CB, Maxwell NS, Doust JH (2000) Evaluation of the reliability and validity of a soccer-specific field test of repeated sprint ability. Eur J Appl Physiol 83:77–83
98. Wright RW, Magnussen RA, Dunn WR, Spindler KP (2011) Ipsilateral graft and contralateral ACL rupture at five years or more following ACL reconstruction: a systematic review. J Bone Joint Surg Am 93:1159–1165
99. Young W, Farrow D (2006) A review of agility. Strength Condition J 28:24–29

19 Quadriceps Strength Recovery After ACL Reconstruction Using Hamstrings Tendon Autograft and Return to Play

Yuichi Hoshino and Ryosuke Kuroda

Contents

Y. Hoshino, M.D., Ph.D.
R. Kuroda, M.D., Ph.D. (✉)
Department of Orthopaedic Surgery, Kobe University Graduate School of Medicine, 7-5-2, Kusunoki-cho, Chuo-ku, Kobe, Hyogo, Japan
e-mail: kurodar@med.kobe-u.ac.jp

19.1 Introduction

Quadriceps muscle strength is a key factor for the return to sports activity after anterior cruciate ligament (ACL) reconstruction; this is especially true in football. Quadriceps muscle weakness is a major complication of the ACL reconstruction surgery when the quadriceps tendon is used for the ACL graft [1], but quadriceps muscle weakness can be observed even when the hamstrings tendon is utilized [2, 3]. Based on the advantage of the hamstrings tendon autograft application in terms of quadriceps strength, hamstrings autograft could be selected more often than quadriceps tendon autograft for football players (Fig. 19.1). Therefore, the quadriceps muscle recovery after the ACL reconstruction using hamstrings tendon autograft should be seriously considered.

Playing football requires a variety of knee movements for running, cutting, jumping, and, of course, kicking. Given that those movements induce rotational instability in ACL-deficient knees, those who have ACL injury and reconstruction avoid those activities both intentionally and unintentionally until his/her surgeon's permission. Although some might perform pivoting sports activities as early as 3–4 months postoperatively [4, 5], such early return to sport is not generally recommended because of the weakened and healing graft (Fig. 19.2). After ACL reconstruction, patients generally go through over 6 months of rehabilitation, via a program that

V. Musahl et al. (eds.), *Return to Play in Football*, https://doi.org/10.1007/978-3-662-55713-6_19

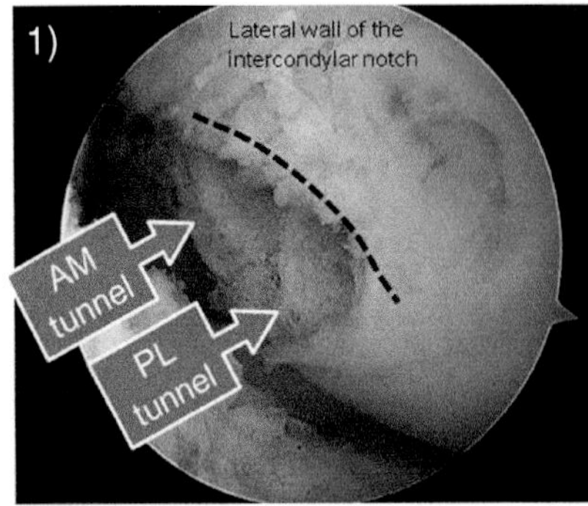

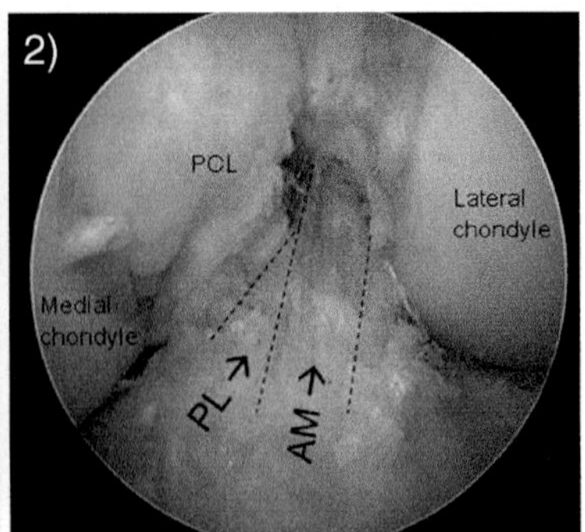

Fig. 19.1 An intraoperative arthroscopic picture during the ACL reconstruction using hamstrings. Double-bundle ACL reconstruction was performed. (**a**) Two femoral tunnels were created on the lateral wall of the intercondylar notch. Both AM and PL bundle tunnels were located posterior and proximal to the resident's ridge (marked by a *dotted line*). (**b**) Two grafts were crossed over in the middle of the joint and inserted in the tunnels separately. The edges of each bundle graft are highlighted by *dotted lines*

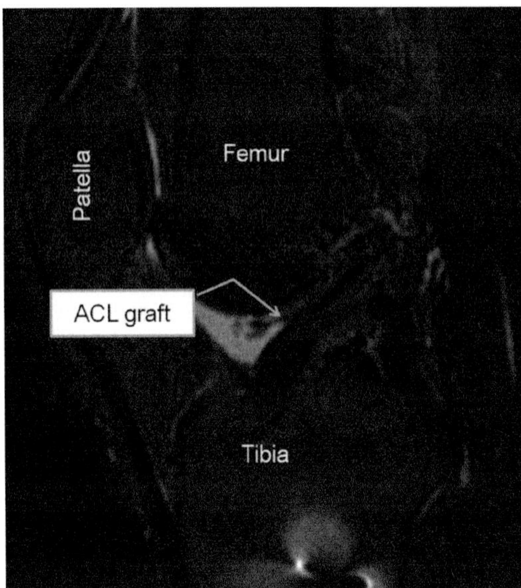

Fig. 19.2 An MRI of the knee at 6 months after the ACL reconstruction using hamstrings tendon autograft (the same knee as shown in Fig. 19.1). The reconstructed graft (indicated by an *arrow*) demonstrates taut fibers of low signal intensity in the middle but still has some high signal intensity areas which suggest incomplete maturation

aims to restore an ability to perform a high level of activities. Athletes, especially football players, are recommended to pass the return-to-sports criteria before getting back to the field. Most of those criteria include a functional movement assessment [6, 7]. Quadriceps strength has a significant impact on those functional knee movements [8]. In addition, impaired quadriceps strength has a possibility to deteriorate long-term knee joint health [9]. Wang et al. [10] reported that the increased number of patellofemoral joint chondral lesions in the patellofemoral joint could be associated with weak quadriceps strength in ACL-reconstructed patients [10]. Therefore, complete recovery of this muscle strength is needed to obtain satisfactory knee function for football players who underwent the ACL reconstruction.

The optimal or sufficient level of the quadriceps muscle strength recovery after ACL reconstruction is unknown. Side-to-side difference of the quadriceps strength in normal subjects was observed between 4 and 16%. In addition, ACL reconstructed having over 85% of the quadriceps strength in comparison to the contralateral knee would allow the performance of a one-leg jump similar to that of the contralateral knee [11]. Based on those previous studies, a deficit of within 15% of quadriceps muscle strength compared to the contralateral knee seems to be an acceptable criterion for the return to football field after ACL reconstruction.

19.2 Factors Affecting Quadriceps Muscle Recovery

It is well known that preoperative quadriceps strength is associated with postoperative quadriceps strength following an ACL reconstruction using a BPTB graft [12–14]. It was reported that patients who had preoperative quadriceps strength deficits greater than 20% had significantly lower quadriceps strength 2 years after ACL reconstruction [13]. On the other hand, patients with more than 90% preoperative quadriceps strength compared with the uninvolved leg had significantly higher quadriceps strength at 1, 2, 3, 12, and 24 months postoperatively [14]. Similar to those previous studies using a BPTB autograft, a recent study using a hamstrings tendon autograft demonstrated that preoperative quadriceps strength was associated with postoperative quadriceps strength at 6 months and 1 year [15]. Furthermore, based on a receiver operating curve analysis, more than 70% of preoperative quadriceps strength index in the ACL-involved knees in comparison to the contralateral knees could be required to achieve over 85% quadriceps strength at 6 months after the ACL reconstruction [15].

Both age and sex are also widely known to have a significant relationship with lower quadriceps in the postoperative knees of the ACL reconstruction. Iriuchishima et al. [16] found the influence of age on the residual muscle weakness 9 months after ACL reconstruction using a hamstring autograft [16], whereas a higher deficit in the peak torque of knee extension and flexion at 1 year after ACL reconstruction was demonstrated in female patients in comparison to male counterparts [17]. Ueda et al. [15] reported significant impacts of both age and sex on delayed quadriceps recovery after ACL reconstruction using a multivariate logistic regression analysis [15]. Since both age and sex seem to be highly probable to affect the postoperative quadriceps recovery, gender-specific and age-specific rehabilitation program should be considered to facilitate better muscle recovery after ACL reconstruction using a hamstrings tendon autograft.

In the postoperative knees that are painful during quadriceps strength examination, quadriceps strength is assessed to be lower than in the painless knees. Anterior knee pain can be experienced in the ACL-reconstructed knees even when a hamstrings tendon autograft is used, resulting in decreased quadriceps strength at follow-up [17, 18]. Although cartilage and meniscal injuries are widely known to induce knee pain, the direct impact of the cartilage and meniscal injuries on the postoperative quadriceps strength has not been established. It is still unknown what causes the anterior knee pain after ACL reconstruction using a hamstrings tendon autograft, and, thus, further studies are warranted.

The restriction of the range of motion occasionally happens after the ACL reconstruction due to reasons that are multifactorial; these restrictions include a cyclops lesion or arthrofibrosis [19]. Once the restriction of the range of motion occurs, the quadriceps muscle recovery could be limited [20]. One possible reason for this relationship is that reduced knee extension compromises the knee joint stability during walking or other daily activities, which prevents the patient from appropriately stimulating postoperative muscle recovery.

Some perioperative managements for the ACL reconstruction, such as tourniquet and femoral nerve block, have the potential to affect quadriceps muscle recovery. A tourniquet is often used in a wide variety of lower extremity surgeries to improve visualization during the surgical procedure, possibly leading to less operative time [21]. The ACL reconstruction can be performed without a tourniquet, but some prefer to use it to perform the operation without concern for poor arthroscopic visualization as a result of intra-articular bleeding. The effect of tourniquet use on quadriceps muscle recovery has been examined. Although the short-term influence of the tourniquet use at approximately 3 months was inconsistent between reports [22–24], it is consistently observed that the muscle recovery is similar between groups with and without tourniquet use at the time of return to sports, such as 6 months or more postoperatively. The femoral nerve block is sometimes used as an additional postoperative pain control. Better postoperative pain control after the ACL reconstruction can be obtained with the femoral nerve block, especially in the early postoperative period [25, 26]. However, the long-term detrimental effect on the muscle recovery was reported in both adult patients [27] and the younger population [28]. Therefore, femoral nerve blocks should be carefully applied in cases where strong postoperative analgesia is desired.

Surgeons should pay attention to such perioperative management for ACL reconstruction, considering their potential effect(s) on postoperative muscle recovery.

Fact Box 1

Factors affecting quadriceps muscle recovery after the ACL reconstruction using hamstrings.

1. Age	Negative correlation has been observed between age and postoperative knee extensor strength [15, 16].
2. Sex	Female patients are likely to have lower quadriceps strength in comparison to male counterparts [15, 17].
3. Preoperative quadriceps strength	Sufficient quadriceps recovery at 6 months after the ACL reconstruction, i.e., more than 85% of quadriceps strength in comparison to the contralateral side, was demonstrated in those knees which had higher preoperative quadriceps strength [15].
4. Femoral nerve block	The quadriceps recovery in the ACL-reconstructed patients with the femoral nerve block was inferior to that without it [27, 28].

19.3 Rehabilitation Strategy for Improving Quadriceps Muscle Recovery

Several rehabilitation strategies have been reported for improving recovery of quadriceps muscle strength after ACL reconstruction. Although there is no doubt about the importance of postoperative rehabilitation, preoperative rehabilitation is also vital for improving muscle recovery [14, 29, 30]. Keays et al. [30] reported that a 5-week preoperative quadriceps strength training home-based exercise program improved quadriceps recovery and further knee function [30]. Furthermore, if the exercise is controlled in a hospital-based setting, only 4 weeks of training could provide a beneficial effect on the quadriceps muscle postoperatively [31]. ACL reconstruction should be avoided if a restricted range of motion with strong inflammation is observed in the knee, especially during the acute phase after ACL injury. A significant amount of time is needed to restore the range of motion and to control inflammation in some cases. In such cases, extensive range of motion exercise and muscle training should be performed along with anti-inflammatory treatment as soon as possible after the injury.

Careful attention should be paid to the exercise scheme. The training effect would be different between concentric and eccentric contraction of muscles. The use of progressive, high-intensity, eccentric contractions has been demonstrated to have a significant effect on improving muscle size and strength [32]. Negative resistance training should be incorporated in order to maximize the effect of the muscle training after the ACL reconstruction [33, 34].

Additional muscle strengthening effect can be obtained using electrical stimulation. Transcutaneous electrical nerve stimulation (TENS) is often used in the postoperative rehabilitation after ACL reconstruction, but the main purpose of this electrical stimulation is not to stimulate the quadriceps muscle directly but to reduce the pain and joint effusion, along with cryotherapy [35]. Since the beneficial effect of postoperative usage of TENS after ACL reconstruction has been reported [36], TENS has long been widely applied. On the other hand, neuromuscular electrical stimulation (NMES) is another type of the electrical stimulation for quadriceps muscle recovery which can be used after the ACL reconstruction. Voluntary activation of quadriceps muscle is often paralyzed after the ACL injury and reconstruction; this muscle dysfunction is known as arthrogenic muscle inhibition (AMI) [37]. NMES can improve voluntary contraction of the quadriceps muscle to overcome AMI after the ACL reconstruction [38]. However, because NMES provides a higher-intensity electrical stimulation than TENS, some patients may be unable to tolerate the uncomfortable sensation and cease usage. NMES does,

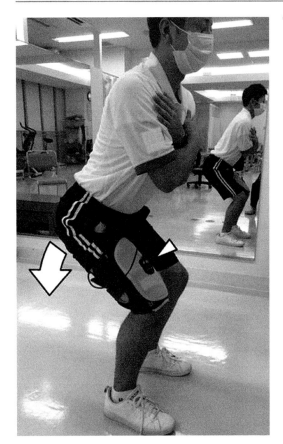

Fig. 19.3 Negative resistance training with a neuromuscular electrical stimulation (NMES). A patient is instructed to lower his hip slowly (movement direction is indicated by an *arrow*). His quadriceps muscle is voluntarily contracted with the support of NMES (NMES device's pad is indicated by an *arrowhead*)

Fact Box 2

Rehabilitation items for recovering quadriceps muscle strength after ACL reconstruction using hamstrings tendon autograft, especially against arthrogenic muscle inhibition (AMI).

1. Preoperative rehabilitation. 5 weeks of home exercise [30] and 4 weeks of controlled hospital training [31] prior to the ACL reconstruction have been proven to be effective to improve quadriceps muscle postoperatively.
2. Negative resistance training or eccentric muscle exercise. Significant improvement of muscle volume and strength has been demonstrated [32].
3. Neuromuscular electrical stimulation (NMES). Although it is too uncomfortable for some patients, NMES with eccentric exercise provides a great effect on quadriceps recovery [40].

however, have a more direct effect to induce muscle contraction than TENS, and significant improvement can be obtained in the quadriceps muscle strength and resultant knee function [39]. Moreover, the effect of the NMES on the muscle recovery can be accentuated by augmenting it with eccentric muscle training [40]. Although it is still unknown if this positive effect is sustained in the long term after the ACL reconstruction, NMES can be utilized in an supportive way to the postoperative rehabilitation, especially in the early stage after ACL reconstruction (Fig. 19.3).

Recently, blood flow restriction training has become a subject of increasing focus to stimulate muscle hypertrophy [41]. The relative anaerobic environment created by the blood flow restriction was reported to induce several localized cellular and hormonal changes that stimulate muscle hypertrophy [42]. The blood flow restriction exercise was originally used to enhance muscle training effect in athletes [43], but this technique can be more beneficial to the patients who could not perform higher-intensity training due to their own physical ability or medical restriction, with comparable training effects from low-intensity exercises [44]. This technique has been widely applied as a booster for muscle training, while there are some possible complications such as bruising on the compression site, DVT, or discomfort [45]. The clinical application of this new methodology after the ACL reconstruction has not been reported; however, some positive effect(s) on muscle recovery after ACL reconstruction would be expected.

Biological stimulation could provide a potential remedy for the postoperative quadriceps muscle atrophy and weakness after the ACL reconstruction. To date, stem cell therapy has focused more on the ligament healing [46, 47] than muscle recovery. Accelerated recovery of traumatically damaged muscle can be achieved by use of biological enhancement [48], but there was no reported biological stimulation for the muscle atrophy and weakness after the ACL reconstruction, which is mostly due to arthrogenic muscle inhibition [37]. It is still unknown what type of the biological stimulation and how much of it should be implemented to maximize the effect of muscle recovery after the ACL reconstruction, all while minimizing potential complications. Therefore, the clinical application of such biological stimulation is not widespread at the present time.

Take-Home Message

The identified factors that affect quadriceps strength after ACL reconstruction using a hamstrings tendon autograft are age, sex, knee pain, and preoperative quadriceps strength. Achieving more than 70% of quadriceps strength in the involved knees compared to the contralateral side is advisable to obtain sufficient quadriceps muscle recovery, i.e., 85% of the contralateral knees, when getting back to the football field at 6+ months postoperatively. It is generally difficult to achieve a clinically acceptable level of quadriceps muscle strength, but every effort to maximize the quadriceps recovery should be made in order to provide a safe return to the football field as soon as possible.

Acknowledgment There are no conflicts of interest to declare.

Top Five Evidence Based References

Ueda Y, Matsushita T, Araki D et al (2016) Factors affecting quadriceps strength recovery after anterior cruciate ligament reconstruction with hamstring autografts in athletes. Knee Surg Sports Traumatol Arthrosc. https://doi.org/10.1007/s00167-016-4296-6. [Epub ahead of print]

Kvist J (2004) Rehabilitation following anterior cruciate ligament injury: current recommendations for sports participation. Sports Med 34(4):269–280

Palmieri-Smith RM, Thomas AC, Wojtys EM (2008) Maximizing quadriceps strength after ACL reconstruction. Clin Sports Med 27:405–424

Lepley LK (2015) Deficits in quadriceps strength and patient-oriented outcomes at return to activity after ACL reconstruction: a review of the current literature. Sports Health 7(3):231–238

Eitzen I, Holm I, Risberg MA (2009) Preoperative quadriceps strength is a significant predictor of knee function two years after anterior cruciate ligament reconstruction. Br J Sports Med 43(5):371–376

References

1. Lepley LK (2015) Deficits in quadriceps strength and patient-oriented outcomes at return to activity after ACL reconstruction: a review of the current literature. Sports Health 7(3):231–238
2. Lautamies R, Harilainen A, Kettunen J et al (2008) Isokinetic quadriceps and hamstring muscle strength and knee function 5 years after anterior cruciate ligament reconstruction: comparison between bone-patellar tendon-bone and hamstring tendon autografts. Knee Surg Sports Traumatol Arthrosc 16(11): 1009–1016
3. Mohammadi F, Salavati M, Akhbari B et al (2013) Comparison of functional outcome measures after ACL reconstruction in competitive soccer players: a randomized trial. J Bone Joint Surg Am 95(14):1271–1277
4. Shelbourne KD, Klootwyk TE, Wilckens JH et al (1995) Ligament stability two to six years after anterior cruciate ligament reconstruction with autogenous patellar tendon graft and participation in accelerated rehabilitation program. Am J Sports Med 23(5):575–579
5. Shelbourne KD, Nitz P (1990) Accelerated rehabilitation after anterior cruciate ligament reconstruction. Am J Sports Med 18(3):292–299
6. Kvist J (2004) Rehabilitation following anterior cruciate ligament injury: current recommendations for sports participation. Sports Med 34(4):269–280
7. Myer GD, Paterno MV, Ford KR et al (2006) Rehabilitation after anterior cruciate ligament reconstruction: criteria-based progression through the return-to-sport phase. J Orthop Sports Phys Ther 36(6):385–402
8. Keays SL, Bullock-Saxton JE, Newcombe P et al (2003) The relationship between knee strength and functional stability before and after anterior cruciate ligament reconstruction. J Orthop Res 21(2):231–237
9. Slemenda C, Brandt KD, Heilman DK et al (1997) Quadriceps weakness and osteoarthritis of the knee. Ann Intern Med 127(2):97–104
10. Wang HJ, Ao YF, Jiang D et al (2015) Relationship between quadriceps strength and patellofemoral joint chondral lesions after anterior cruciate ligament reconstruction. Am J Sports Med 43(9):2286–2292
11. Ostenberg A, Roos E, Ekdahl C et al (1998) Isokinetic knee extensor strength and functional performance

in healthy female soccer players. Scand J Med Sci Sports 8(5 Pt 1):257–264
12. de Jong SN, van Caspel DR, van Haeff MJ, Saris DB (2007) Functional assessment and muscle strength before and after reconstruction of chronic anterior cruciate ligament lesions. Arthroscopy 23(1):21–28
13. Eitzen I, Holm I, Risberg MA (2009) Preoperative quadriceps strength is a significant predictor of knee function two years after anterior cruciate ligament reconstruction. Br J Sports Med 43(5):371–376
14. Shelbourne KD, Johnson BC (2004) Effects of patellar tendon width and preoperative quadriceps strength on strength return after anterior cruciate ligament reconstruction with ipsilateral bone-patellar tendon-bone autograft. Am J Sports Med 32(6):1474–1478
15. Ueda Y, Matsushita T, Araki D et al (2016) Factors affecting quadriceps strength recovery after anterior cruciate ligament reconstruction with hamstring autografts in athletes. Knee Surg Sports Traumatol Arthrosc. https://doi.org/10.1007/s00167-016-4296-6. [Epub ahead of print]
16. Iriuchishima T, Shirakura K, Horaguchi T, Wada N, Sohmiya M, Tazawa M, Fu FH (2012) Age as a predictor of residual muscle weakness after anterior cruciate ligament reconstruction. Knee Surg Sports Traumatol Arthrosc 20(1):173–178
17. Gobbi A, Domzalski M, Pascual J (2004) Comparison of anterior cruciate ligament reconstruction in male and female athletes using the patellar tendon and hamstring autografts. Knee Surg Sports Traumatol Arthrosc 12(6):534–539
18. Natri A, Jarvinen M, Latvala K, Kannus P (1996) Isokinetic muscle performance after anterior cruciate ligament surgery. Longterm results and outcome predicting factors after primary surgery and late-phase reconstruction. Int J Sports Med 17(3): 223–228
19. Mayr HO, Weig TG, Plitz W (2004) Arthrofibrosis following ACL reconstruction—reasons and outcome. Arch Orthop Trauma Surg 124(8):518–522
20. Grapar Žargi T, Drobnič M, Vauhnik R et al (2016) Factors predicting quadriceps femoris muscle atrophy during the first 12weeks following anterior cruciate ligament reconstruction. Knee 24(2):319–328. https://doi.org/10.1016/j.knee.2016.11.003. [Epub ahead of print]
21. Klenerman L (1962) The tourniquet in surgery. J Bone Joint Surg Br 44:937–943
22. Arciero RA, Scoville CR, Hayda RA et al (1996) The effect of tourniquet use in anterior cruciate ligament reconstruction. A prospective, randomized study. Am J Sports Med 24(6):758–764
23. Daniel DM, Lumkong G, Stone ML et al (1995) Effects of tourniquet use in anterior cruciate ligament reconstruction. Arthroscopy 11(3):307–311
24. Nicholas SJ, Tyler TF, McHugh MP et al (2001) The effect on leg strength of tourniquet use during anterior cruciate ligament reconstruction: a prospective randomized study. Arthroscopy 17(6):603–607
25. Iskandar H, Benard A, Ruel-Raymond J et al (2003) Femoral block provides superior analgesia compared with intra-articular ropivacaine after anterior cruciate ligament reconstruction. Reg Anesth Pain Med 28(1):29–32
26. Mulroy MF, Larkin KL, Batra MS et al (2001) Femoral nerve block with 0.25% or 0.5% bupivacaine improves postoperative analgesia following outpatient arthroscopic anterior cruciate ligament repair. Reg Anesth Pain Med 26(1):24–29
27. Krych A, Arutyunyan G, Kuzma S et al (2015) Adverse effect of femoral nerve blockade on quadriceps strength and function after ACL reconstruction. J Knee Surg 28(1):83–88
28. Luo TD, Ashraf A, Dahm DL et al (2015) Femoral nerve block is associated with persistent strength deficits at 6 months after anterior cruciate ligament reconstruction in pediatric and adolescent patients. Am J Sports Med 43(2):331–336
29. Eitzen I, Moksnes H, Snyder-Mackler L et al (2010) A progressive 5-week exercise therapy program leads to significant improvement in knee function early after anterior cruciate ligament injury. J Orthop Sports Phys Ther 40:705–721
30. Keays SL, Bullock-Saxton JE, Newcombe P et al (2006) The effectiveness of a pre-operative home-based physiotherapy programme for chronic anterior cruciate ligament deficiency. Physiother Res Int 11:204–218
31. Kim DK, Hwang JH, Park WH (2015) Effects of 4 weeks preoperative exercise on knee extensor strength after anterior cruciate ligament reconstruction. J Phys Ther Sci 27(9):2693–2696
32. LaStayo PC, Pierotti DJ, Pifer J et al (2000) Eccentric ergometry: increases in locomotor muscle size and strength at low training intensities. Am J Physiol Regul Integr Comp Physiol 278(5): R1282–R1288
33. Gerber JP, Marcus RL, Dibble LE et al (2007) Effects of early progressive eccentric exercise on muscle structure after anterior cruciate ligament reconstruction. J Bone Joint Surg Am 89(3):559–570
34. Gerber JP, Marcus RL, Dibble LE et al (2007) Safety, feasibility, and efficacy of negative work exercise via eccentric muscle activity following anterior cruciate ligament reconstruction. J Orthop Sports Phys Ther 37(1):10–18
35. Hopkins J, Ingersoll CD, Edwards J et al (2002) Cryotherapy and transcutaneous electric neuromuscular stimulation decrease Arthrogenic muscle inhibition of the Vastus Medialis after knee joint effusion. J Athl Train 37(1):25–31
36. Arvidsson I, Eriksson E (1986) Postoperative TENS pain relief after knee surgery: objective evaluation. Orthopedics 9(10):1346–1351
37. Palmieri-Smith RM, Thomas AC, Wojtys EM (2008) Maximizing quadriceps strength after ACL reconstruction. Clin Sports Med 27:405–424

38. Bremner CB, Holcomb WR, Brown CD et al (2016) The effectiveness of neuromuscular electrical stimulation in improving voluntary activation of the quadriceps: a critically appraised topic. J Sport Rehabil 11:1–21
39. Snyder-Mackler L, Delitto A, Bailey SL et al (1995) Strength of the quadriceps femoris muscle and functional recovery after reconstruction of the anterior cruciate ligament. A prospective, randomized clinical trial of electrical stimulation. J Bone Joint Surg Am 77(8):1166–1173
40. Lepley LK, Wojtys EM, Palmieri-Smith RM (2015) Combination of eccentric exercise and neuromuscular electrical stimulation to improve quadriceps function post-ACL reconstruction. Knee 22(3):270–277
41. Scott BR, Loenneke JP, Slattery KM et al (2016) Blood flow restricted exercise for athletes: a review of available evidence. J Sci Med Sport 19(5):360–367
42. Pearson SJ, Hussain SR (2015) A review on the mechanisms of blood-flow restriction resistance training-induced muscle hypertrophy. Sports Med 45(2):187–200
43. Takarada Y, Sato Y, Ishii N (2002) Effects of resistance exercise combined with vascular occlusion on muscle function in athletes. Eur J Appl Physiol 86(4):308–314
44. Loenneke JP, Wilson JM, Marín PJ et al (2012) Low intensity blood flow restriction training: a meta-analysis. Eur J Appl Physiol 112(5):1849–1859
45. Nakajima T, Kurano M, Iida H et al (2006) Use and safety of KAATSU training: results of a national survey. Int J KAATSU Train Res 2:5–13
46. Mifune Y, Matsumoto T, Ota S et al (2012) Therapeutic potential of anterior cruciate ligament-derived stem cells for anterior cruciate ligament reconstruction. Cell Transplant 21(8):1651–1665
47. Mifune Y, Matsumoto T, Takayama K et al (2013) Tendon graft revitalization using adult anterior cruciate ligament (ACL)-derived CD34+ cell sheets for ACL reconstruction. Biomaterials 34(22):5476–5487
48. Kobayashi M, Ota S et al (2016) The combined use of losartan and muscle-derived stem cells significantly improves the functional recovery of muscle in a young mouse model of contusion injuries. Am J Sports Med 44(12):3252–3261

Part III

ACL: Time-based Return to Play

20 Time-Based Return to Play: The MOON Experience

Mia Smucny and Kurt P. Spindler

Contents

M. Smucny, M.D. • K.P. Spindler, M.D. (✉)
Department of Orthopaedic Surgery, Cleveland Clinic Foundation, Garfield Heights, OH, USA
e-mail: spindlk@ccf.org

20.1 Introduction to MOON

The Multicenter Orthopaedic Outcomes Network (MOON) was established in 2001 in response to a growing need for high-quality longitudinal outcome studies on anterior cruciate ligament reconstruction (ACLR). This consortium consists of over 20 surgeons from seven institutions. With more than 3500 patients included, it is the largest prospective ACLR outcome cohort in the United States and has maintained 80% follow-up at 2, 6, and 10 years. The following chapter discusses rehabilitation guidelines used by the MOON group, the clinical evidence to support these guidelines, and the cohort's football-specific outcomes.

20.2 MOON Rehabilitation Guidelines

The ACL rehabilitation guidelines used by MOON are based on systematic reviews of level 1 and level 2 evidence [1–3]. For several aspects of ACL rehabilitation, there are no studies that qualify as "best evidence," or there are too few studies to draw confident conclusions [4]. The MOON guidelines are for primary ACLR without meniscus repair. Progression through these guidelines should be tailored by the therapist to fit the specific needs of the injured athlete. The progression through the rehabilitation guidelines is criteria-based rather than time-based, particularly after

V. Musahl et al. (eds.), *Return to Play in Football*, https://doi.org/10.1007/978-3-662-55713-6_20

12 weeks postoperatively (during the first 3 months, the guidelines are rendered more time-based as quadriceps strengthening exercises are limited, and thus injured athletes do not meet criteria to advance). It is important to respect the healing and "ligamentization" of the graft—particularly at 6–7 weeks when the graft is thought to be the weakest—and thus not accelerate patients through their rehabilitation too quickly [5, 6]. The time frames in Table 20.1 are approximate for the average patient as the fulfill criteria to move on to the next phase. Also, the guidelines in Table 20.1 refer to a primary ACL reconstruction without meniscus repair. There is no consensus among the MOON group in terms of rehabilitation for an associated meniscus repair.

AROM active range of motion, *SLR* straight-leg raises, *WBAT* weight bear as tolerated, *Quad* quadriceps, *Ham* hamstring, *TKE* terminal knee extension, *NM* neuromuscular

Table 20.1 Multicenter Orthopaedic Outcomes Network rehabilitation guidelines. These guidelines are for primary ACL reconstruction. They may be adjusted for additional procedures such as cartilage or meniscus repair or other injuries such as medial collateral ligament tear. The table continues in the following pages. Adapted from Wright RW et al. "Anterior Cruciate Ligament Reconstruction Rehabilitation: MOON Guidelines." *Sports Health* 2015; 7: Appendix

Phases	Estimated time	Goals	Exercise suggestions	Criteria for progression
0 Preoperative		• Normal gait • Minimal effusion • ROM and strength (see next column) • Patient education on postoperative exercises, crutch use, and wound care	• ROM: active 0–120° of flexion • Strength: 20 SLR without lag	• Ready for surgery when: – Minimal effusion – ROM goals met – Strength returned
1 Immediate postoperative	0–2 weeks	• Normal gait pattern – Crutches initially, WBAT • Full knee extension – No knee brace/immobilizer (if femoral nerve block, wear 24 h only) • Quad control: 20 SLR without lag • Minimize pain • Minimize swelling – Ice with compression stocking or CryoCuff® – Initially: every hour for 15 min – After acute inflammation controlled: TID for 30 min	• ROM: – Extension: low load, long duration (5 min) stretching (heel prop, prone hang, minimize co-contracture and nociceptor response) – Flexion: wall slides, heel slides, seated assisted knee flexion, bike—rocking for range – Patellar mobilization (monitor for reaction to effusion and ROM) • Strength: – Quad sets, SLR no lag, double-leg quarter squats, standing TheraBand®-resisted TKE – Ham sets, ham curls, quad/ham co-contraction supine – Side-lying hip add/abduction – Prone hip extension – Ankle pumps with TheraBand® calf press or heel raises • Other: – Cardiopulmonary: upper body erg machine – Scar massage when incision healed	• Crutches discontinued: – Normal gait pattern and can go up and down stairs without pain or instability • SLR no lag >20 • Normal gait • ROM: no greater than 5° active extension lag, 110° active flexion

Table 20.1 (continued)

Phases	Estimated time	Goals	Exercise suggestions	Criteria for progression
2 Early rehabilitation	3–6 weeks	• Full ROM • Improve muscle strength • Progress NM retraining	• ROM: – Low load, long duration – Heel slides, wall slides, heel prop, prone hang, bike with lower seat height – Flexibility stretching all major groups • Strengthening: – Quad: quad sets, mini-squats, wall squats, step-ups, knee extension, leg press, shuttle press without jump – Ham: ham curls, resistive SLR with sports cord – Hip add/abduction, multi-hip machine – Standing heel raises from double- to single-leg support, seated calf press • NM training: – Wobble board, rocker board, single-leg stance, slide board, fitter • Cardiopulmonary: – Stationary bike, elliptical, StairMaster®	Full ROM • Minimal effusion/pain • Functional strength and control in daily activities • IKDC Question #10 score of ≥7: – "How would you rate the function of your knee on a scale of 0–10 with 10 being normal, excellent function and 0 being the inability to perform any of your usual daily activities?"
3 Strengthening and control	7–12 week	• Maintain full ROM • Demonstrate ability to descent an 8" step without pain or deviation • Running without pain or swelling • Hopping without pain, swelling, or giving way	• Strengthening: – Squats, leg press, ham curl, knee extension 90°–0°, step-up/down, lunges, shuttle, sports cord, wall squats, hopping without pain (bilateral then single leg, end in 1/4 squat) • NM training: – Wobble/rocker/roller board, perturbation training, instrumented testing systems, varied surfaces • Cardiopulmonary: – Straight line running on treadmill/protected environment – Any other cardiopulmonary equipment	• Running without pain or swelling • Hopping without pain or swelling (bilateral and unilateral) • NM and strength training exercises without difficulty

(continued)

Table 20.1 (continued)

Phases	Estimated time	Goals	Exercise suggestions	Criteria for progression
4 Advanced training	13–16 weeks	• Running patterns (figure-8, pivot drills, etc.) at 75% speed without difficulty • Jumping without difficulty • Hop tests at 75% contralateral values – Cincinnati hop tests: single-leg hop for distance, triple hop for distance, crossover hop for distance, 6 m timed hop	• Aggressive strengthening: – Squats, lunges, plyometrics • Agility drills: – Shuffling, hopping, carioca, vertical jumps, running patterns at 50–75% speed (e.g., figure-8), initial sport-specific drills at 50–75% effort • NM training: – Wobble board, rocker board, roller board, perturbation training, instrumented testing systems, varied surfaces • Cardiopulmonary: – Running, other cardiopulmonary equipment	• Maximum vertical jump without pain or instability • 75% of contralateral on hop tests • Figure-8 run at 75% speed without difficulty • IKDC Question #10 score of ≥8 (see above)
5 Return to sport	17–20+ weeks	• 85% contralateral strength • 85% contralateral on hop tests • Sport-specific training without pain, swelling, or difficulty	• Aggressive strengthening: – Squats, lunges, plyometrics • Sport-specific activities: – Interval training programs, sprinting, change of direction, running patterns in football, pivot and drive in basketball, kicking in soccer, spiking in volleyball, skill/biomechanical analysis with coaches and sports medicine team • Return-to-sport evaluation recommendations: – Hop tests (see above), vertical jump, deceleration shuttle	• Return-to-sport criteria: – No functional complaints – Confidence when running, cutting, jumping at full speed – 85% contralateral values on hop tests – IKDC Question #10 score of ≥9 (see above)

20.3 Evidence Behind the MOON Guidelines

Recent systematic reviews have studied many aspects of ACL rehabilitation in depth with high-quality data [1–4]. Immediate weight-bearing following isolated ACL reconstruction was investigated by one study and found a significant decrease in patellofemoral pain from 35 to 8% [7]. Immediate range of motion has not been studied by randomized trial but is a fundamental principle. There are few studies to adequately evaluate the safety of open-chain exercises before 6 weeks postoperatively, although they appear to improve strength after 6 weeks without adversely affecting the graft.

Given the limited evidence and concern for graft strain from open-chain activities, the MOON guidelines limit these to light-load, short-arc quadriceps exercises in the first 6 weeks after surgery. Neuromuscular training such as proprioception and balance training has been found to be safe and efficacious. Other safe and effective training techniques include aquatic therapy, slide board work, stair climber, and early quadriceps strengthening with straight-leg raises. Randomized trials on accelerated rehabilitation have not found it to dramatically lessen rehabilitation to below 6 months. Scientific evidence does not support return in less than 4 months, while additional research is needed to evaluate the effect of accelerated rehabilitation on graft, menisci, and cartilage.

The use of knee immobilizers or hinged knee braces in the immediate postoperative time frame has been studied by many studies with no clinically significant improvement in safety, range of motion, or patient-reported outcome measures. Similarly, no long-term benefits or improvements in range of motion have been found with continuous massive motion. Given the cost of immediate postoperative bracing and continuous passive motion and the lack of benefit, these are not included in the MOON guidelines. There is a lack of standardization and homogeneity among studies evaluating neuromuscular electrical stimulation. The MOON group leaves the use of these devices to the therapist's discretion.

Fact Box 1

- Immediate weight-bearing should be encouraged after ACLR.
- Bracing and CPM are neither necessary nor beneficial after ACLR and add to the cost of the procedure.
- Accelerated rehabilitation after ACLR does not reduce return to play to under 6 months, and additional research is needed to evaluate its effect on the graft, menisci, and cartilage.

20.4 Rate of Return to Play in Football

In 2012, Brophy et al. used the MOON cohort to evaluate outcomes and return to play among football players after ACLR [8]. A total of 117 athletes were identified from enrollment questionnaires; 103 were contacted, and 100 were deemed eligible (3 were not actually football players), resulting in a follow-up rate of 88%. Mean age was 24, with 55 men and 45 women. The men were significantly older (27.7 vs 19.8 years, $p < 0.0001$). Sixty-nine percent received a bone-patellar tendon-bone (BTB) autograft, 28% a hamstring autograft, and 4% a BTB allograft. The dominant leg was injured in 57% of athletes.

Seventy-two percent of patients returned to football at an average of 12.2 months after surgery (76% of men and 67% of women). At long-term average follow-up of 7 ± 1 years, only 35% were still playing (38% of men and 31% of women), and only 46% of those were playing at the same or higher level of play. Both of these findings were a significant decrease from initial return to play ($p < 0.0001$). Men were more likely than women to attribute their ACL injury as the primary reason they were no longer playing football (56% versus 26%, $p = 0.02$). Leg dominance did not affect return to play (70% dominant versus 74% non-dominant), time to return (11.7 versus 12.8 months), or long-term return to play (33% dominant versus 37% non-dominant).

To determine an individual football player's ability to return to sport, multivariable analysis is required. In this study, multivariable analysis evaluated age, gender, and graft type as potential risk factors. Women were less likely than men to return to play initially (OR 0.31 [0.10–0.93], $p = 0.037$). The reasons for this are complex, as women were less likely than men to mention their ACL injury as the primary reason they were no longer playing football. Women may be more likely to limit participation due to external factors such as graduation, career, or family. Older subjects also were less likely to return (OR 0.38

[0.19–0.76], $p = 0.006$), perhaps due to loss of opportunity or interest to play. Graft type (hamstring versus BTB) did not matter.

Twelve percent of the athletes had subsequent ACL reconstruction. There were nine cases of further ACL surgery on the contralateral knee and three on the ipsilateral knee. Twenty-five percent of these athletes were still playing at final follow-up. Athletes with initial surgery on the non-dominant leg had a higher rate of contralateral ACL reconstruction than those with initial surgery on the dominant leg (16% versus 3.5%, $p = 0.03$).

Fact Box 2

- Return to play after ACLR in football players is approximately 70% after 1 year.
- Return to play after ACLR declines over time to 35% at 7 years.
- Younger athletes and men are more likely to return to play.

20.5 ACL Reconstruction Outcomes: Football Versus Other Sports

Multivariable analyses from the MOON cohort have not shown football to be a predictor of outcome after ACLR. Kaeding et al. did not find football to impact the retear rate within 2 years of ACLR (7% retear rate in football versus 8.9% in American football, 4.0% in basketball, 3.2% in "other") [9]. There was no effect of type of sport on Marx activity level 2 or 6 years after ACLR [10, 11]. Cox et al. also evaluated IKDC and KOOS scores 6 years after ACLR but did not find football to be an independent predictor [10]. Another study showed that health-related quality of life (SF-36 instrument) was not affected by type of sport at 2 or 6 years postoperatively [12]. Moreover, the type of sport also did not affect presence of a bone bruise on MRI or baseline pain (KOOS and SF-36) at the time of ACL surgery [13].

Take-Home Message

The MOON group has contributed a significant volume of high-quality evidence to the literature on ACLR. Time- and criteria-based rehabilitation guidelines for MOON were established based on systematic reviews of level 1 and 2 studies. Return to play in football in the cohort is approximately 70% at 1 year with higher rates in men and younger athletes. Compared with other sports, football is not a predictor of outcome (for revision rate, IKDC, KOOS, Marx, or SF-36 scores) after ACL reconstruction.

Top Five Evidence Based References

Brophy RH, Schmitz L, Wright RW, Dunn WR, Parker RD, Andrish JT, McCarty EC, Spindler KP (2012) Return to play and future ACL injury risk after ACL reconstruction in soccer athletes from the multicenter orthopaedic outcomes network (MOON) group. Am J Sports Med 40(11):2517–2522

Wright RW, Preston E, Fleming BC, Amendola A, Andrish JT, Bergfeld JA, Dunn WR, Kaeding C, Kuhn JE, Marx RG, McCarty EC, Parker RC, Spindler KP, Wolcott M, Wolf BR, Williams GN (2008) A systematic review of anterior cruciate ligament reconstruction rehabilitation. Part I: continuous passive motion, early weight bearing, postoperative bracing, and home-based rehabilitation. J Knee Surg 21(3):217–224

Wright RW, Preston E, Fleming BC, Amendola A, Andrish JT, Bergfeld JA, Dunn WR, Kaeding C, Kuhn JE, Marx RG, McCarty EC, Parker RC, Spindler KP, Wolcott M, Wolf BR, Williams GN (2008) A systematic review of anterior cruciate ligament reconstruction rehabilitation. Part II: open versus closed kinetic chain exercises, neuromuscular electrical stimulation, accelerated rehabilitation, and miscellaneous tips. J Knee Surg 21(3):225–234

Wright RW, Haas AK, Anderson J, Calabrese G, Cavanaugh J, Hewett TE, Lorring D, McKenzie C, Preston E, Williams G, MOON Group (2015) Anterior cruciate ligament reconstruction rehabilitation: MOON guidelines. Sports Health 7(3):239–243

Kaeding CC, Pedroza AD, Reinke EK, Huston LJ, Consortium MOON, Spindler KP (2015) Risk factors and predictors of subsequent ACL injury in either knee after ACL reconstruction: prospective analysis of 2488 primary ACL reconstructions from the MOON cohort. Am J Sports Med 43(7):1583–1590

References

1. Kruse LM, Gray B, Wright RW (2012) Rehabilitation after anterior cruciate ligament reconstruction: a systematic review. JBJS Am 94(19):1737–1748
2. Wright RW, Preston E, Fleming BC, Amendola A, Andrish JT, Bergfeld JA, Dunn WR, Kaeding C, Kuhn JE, Marx RG, McCarty EC, Parker RC, Spindler KP, Wolcott M, Wolf BR, Williams GN (2008) A systematic review of anterior cruciate ligament reconstruction rehabilitation. Part I: continuous passive motion, early weight bearing, postoperative bracing, and home-based rehabilitation. J Knee Surg 21(3):217–224
3. Wright RW, Preston E, Fleming BC, Amendola A, Andrish JT, Bergfeld JA, Dunn WR, Kaeding C, Kuhn JE, Marx RG, McCarty EC, Parker RC, Spindler KP, Wolcott M, Wolf BR, Williams GN (2008) A systematic review of anterior cruciate ligament reconstruction rehabilitation. Part II: open versus closed kinetic chain exercises, neuromuscular electrical stimulation, accelerated rehabilitation, and miscellaneous tips. J Knee Surg 21(3):225–234
4. Wright RW, Haas AK, Anderson J, Calabrese G, Cavanaugh J, Hewett TE, Lorring D, McKenzie C, Preston E, Williams G, MOON Group (2015) Anterior cruciate ligament reconstruction rehabilitation: MOON guidelines. Sports Health 7(3):239–243
5. Claes S, Verdonk P, Forsyth R, Bellemans J (2011) The "ligamentization" process in anterior cruciate ligament reconstruction: what happens to the human graft? A systematic review of the literature. Am J Sports Med 39(11):2476–2483
6. Ekdahl M, Wang JHC, Ronga M, FH F (2008) Graft healing in anterior cruciate ligament reconstruction. Knee Surg Sports Traumatol Arthrosc 16(10):935–947
7. Tyler TF, McHugh MP, Gleim GW, Nicholas SJ (1998) The effect of immediate weightbearing after anterior cruciate ligament reconstruction. Clin Orthop Relat Res 357:141–148
8. Brophy RH, Schmitz L, Wright RW, Dunn WR, Parker RD, Andrish JT, McCarty EC, Spindler KP (2012) Return to play and future ACL injury risk after ACL reconstruction in soccer athletes from the multicenter orthopaedic outcomes network (MOON) group. Am J Sports Med 40(11):2517–2522
9. Kaeding CC, Pedroza AD, Reinke EK, Huston LJ, Spindler KP, MOON Consortium (2015) Risk factors and predictors of subsequent ACL injury in either knee after ACL reconstruction: prospective analysis of 2488 primary ACL reconstructions from the MOON cohort. Am J Sports Med 43(7):1583–1590
10. Cox CL, Huston LJ, Dunn WR, Reinke EK, Nwosu SK, Parker RD, Wright RW, Kaeding CC, Marx RG, Amendola A, McCarty EC, Spindler KP (2014) Are articular cartilage lesions and meniscus tears predictive of IKDC, KOOS, and Marx activity level outcomes after anterior cruciate ligament reconstruction?: a 6-year multicenter cohort study. Am J Sports Med 42(5):1058–1067
11. Dunn WR, Spindler KP, MOON Consortium (2010) Predictors of activity level 2 years after anterior cruciate ligament reconstruction (ACLR): a multicenter orthopaedic outcomes network (MOON) ACLR cohort study. Am J Sports Med 38(10):2040–2050
12. Dunn WR, Wolf BR, Harrell FE, Reinke EK, Huston LJ, Spindler KP, MOON Knee Group (2015) Baseline predictors of health-related quality of life. J Bone Joint Surg Am 97(7):551–557
13. Dunn WR, Spindler KP, Amendola A, Andrish JT, Kaeding CC, Marx RG, McCarty EC, Parker RD, Harrell FE, An AQ, Wright RW, Brophy RH, Matava MJ, Flanigan DC, Huston LJ, Jones MH, Wolcott ML, Vidal AF, Wolf BR (2010) Which preoperative factors, including bone bruise, are associated with knee pain/symptoms at index anterior cruciate ligament reconstruction (ACLR)? A multicenter orthopaedic outcomes network (MOON) ACLR cohort study. Am J Sports Med 38(9):1778–1787

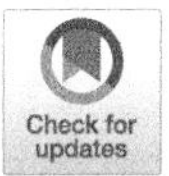

21 How Can MRI Help with Decision-Making?

Marcio Bottene Villa Albers, Jason Shin, and Freddie H. Fu

Contents

M.B.V. Albers, M.D. • J. Shin, M.D., F.R.C.S.C.
F.H. Fu, M.D., D.sc. (Hon), D.ps. (Hon) (✉)
Department of Orthopaedic Surgery, University of Pittsburgh, Pittsburgh, PA, USA
e-mail: ffu@upmc.edu

21.1 Introduction

Anterior cruciate ligament (ACL) reconstruction is the standard treatment for ACL-injured patients desiring to return to sports, particularly for athletes who play a cutting and pivoting sports, like football. Studies have shown that the knee joint undergoes biological changes that are triggered by the injury, followed by a second insult again at the time of surgery [1–3]. Such biological changes in the joint environment may affect how the graft matures over time.

Although much progress has been made in our knowledge and understanding of ACL reconstruction in the last decades, culminating in the modern individualized anatomic ACL reconstruction concept, allowing a patient to return to sport and unrestricted physical activity after surgery remains a challenging and difficult decision for the orthopedic surgeon. Psychological and physical milestones of one's rehabilitation have been shown to play a role in determining the readiness to return to play football after an ACL injury [4–6]. The individualization of the rehabilitation is a key part of this contemporary approach to patient care, aiming to optimize outcomes and avoid failures.

21.2 Diagnosing and Categorizing ACL Tear

Magnetic resonance imaging (MRI) is the gold-standard imaging modality to diagnose

V. Musahl et al. (eds.), *Return to Play in Football*, https://doi.org/10.1007/978-3-662-55713-6_21

injury to the ACL [7]. Using 3.0 Tesla (T) MRI, reported sensitivity and specificity for the diagnosis of ACL tears are 80% and 100%, respectively, while the reported accuracy of MRI in diagnosis of ACL rupture is as high as 95% [8].

In order to influence patient management and prognosis, previous studies have attempted to distinguish between clinically stable and unstable ACL tears using MRI. Relying solely on axial MRI and correlating with arthroscopic findings, studies reported that unstable ACL (unstable partial tears and complete tears) findings included cloudlike mass sign, isolated ACL bundle sign, and non-visualization of the ACL [9]. Stable ACLs were elliptical and attenuated or showed areas of increased intrasubstance signal intensity. It was reported with 100% sensitivity and 96% specificity in being able to categorize stable from unstable ACL using axial MRI.

In the latter study of 97 patients with arthroscopically confirmed ACL tears, which were surgically categorized as being stable or unstable, their knee MRIs were retrospectively reviewed [10]. Stable partial tears included mild elongation of ACL fibers and/or laxity during probing of the ligament, whereas unstable ACL included frank tearing of ligament fibers seen at arthroscopy as well as partial tears with clinical instability requiring ACL reconstruction. The study showed that MRI signs do not allow accurate distinction between clinically stable and unstable ACL injuries. Although certain signs such as anterior tibial translation, hyperbuckled PCL, and uncovering of the posterior horn of the lateral meniscus were 100% specific for unstable ACL tears, these signs had low sensitivity. The authors concluded that MRI cannot sufficiently determine which patients require ACL reconstruction. Based on these studies, determining the extent of ACL tear and the decision to treat the injured footballer should be based on their history, patient's signs and symptoms, and physical exam rather than solely on their MRI appearance.

21.2.1 MRI Recovery in Non-operatively Treated ACL Rupture

The ACL's limited healing capacity has been well documented. After ACL ruptures, a synovial tissue layer forms over the ruptured surface, hindering formation of functional scar and tissue bridging the rupture site during recovery [11]. In a recent study, 50 non-operatively treated patients were followed over 2 years to determine if ACL recovery can be shown on MRI [12]. Improvement in fiber continuity was noted in 60%, and the empty intercondylar notch resolved for 44% of patients. However, upon clinical correlation, there was no association between MRI fiber continuity improvement and Lachman test. Instead the authors demonstrated that MRI features such as decreased signal intensity, which is a MR parameter that is a function of tissue type and water content, and clear boundaries at 2 years had significant association with improvement on Lachman test [13]. Although the non-operatively treated athlete should not expect complete normalization of knee laxity, some athletes may experience partial recovery on MRI and potential clinical improvement (Fig. 21.1).

21.3 Predicting Graft Maturity Using MRI

Years ago, it was widely accepted in the orthopedic community that 6 months of rehabilitation was adequate to regain motor control and strength for returning to pre-injury levels of sport participation. There were attempts to develop accelerated recovery protocols that promised safe return to play after 3 or 4 months of surgery [14]. Recently a shift to a more conservative approach has emerged as an option to decrease the probability of early graft tear rates [15]. For successful outcome, the reconstructed graft must be adequately remodeled to be able to withstand the physiologic loads and demands that it encounters during competition.

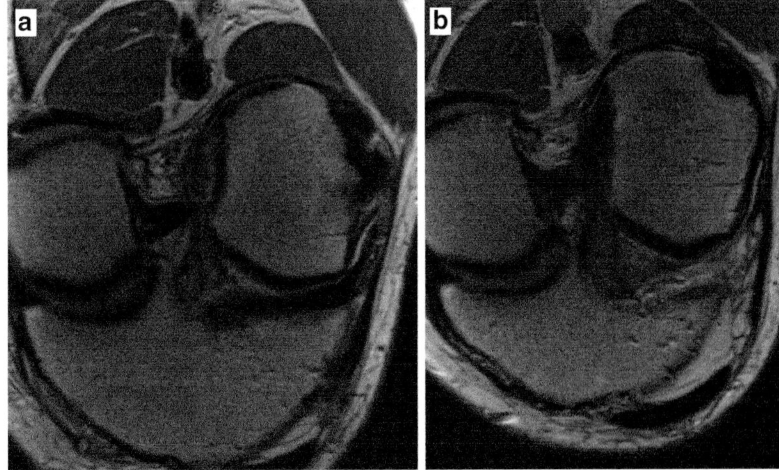

Fig. 21.1 (**a**) Coronal oblique T2 cut 2 weeks after a noncontact ACL incomplete tear; (**b**) follow-up MRI after 3 months of injury showing the healing ACL

Fact Box 1

The achievement of allograft maturation was shown to take up to 18 months after surgery.

The study of the natural history of graft maturation comes from 1988, when it was demonstrated through histologic studies that in vivo allograft maturation would take up to 18 months to fully develop [16]. Using light and electronic microscopy, it was demonstrated that the patella tendon was still immature at 12 months after surgery [17]. Although considered the gold-standard method for determining graft maturation, histological analysis, due to its invasive nature of arthroscopically acquiring a tissue sample, is impractical. Additionally, it is yet to be determined how a second invasive procedure may affect the joint, particularly newly implanted graft and cartilage [3].

Clinically, MRI offers a noninvasive tool for detecting pathologic changes in the reconstructed ACL. It can be used to evaluate ACL graft integrity and maturation following ACL reconstruction in athletes. Earlier works used magnetic resonance angiography (MRA) to demonstrate revascularization of autologous hamstring grafts and peri-ligamentous structures [18, 19]. Another study demonstrated that a branch of the medial genicular artery is responsible for revascularizing the proximal part of the graft through the posterior capsule, whereas branches of the inferior genicular arteries supply distal portion of the graft in all patients [20]. Revascularization of the graft is an important factor for the remodeling process. The same group demonstrated in 30 patients who underwent single-bundle ACL reconstruction with autogenous hamstring tendon that blood vessels from arteries reached the femoral and tibial tunnels at 2 months postoperatively, with blood flow subsequently decreasing over time [18]. Although there is near consensus in the orthopedic literature that graft healing may continue to occur for a few years after ACLR, the remodeling process is most active in the initial 6 months [21–23]. Based on these results, it is not surprising that most re-tears of the graft occur during the first 2 years after surgery [24].

In additional to revascularization studies, there have been increasing research interest to predict graft mechanical properties by MRI. Animal models have shown that MRI signal intensity of the reconstructed graft decreases with time postoperatively. There is also a negative correlation between signal and biomechanical properties including load to failure, stiffness, and tensile strength [25].

Fact Box 2

Most graft tears occur in the first 2 years after ACLR.

Using a sheep animal model, ACL reconstruction using autologous Achilles tendon graft was done to compare graft signal intensity on MRI with biomechanical and histologic parameters. After undergoing plain and gadolinium contrast-enhanced MRI, the animals were sacrificed after 6, 12, 24, 52, or 104 weeks. The author found that when signal intensity was highest at 6–12 weeks, the grafts had lowest tensile strength. Most strikingly, gadolinium-enhanced MRI signal intensity did not return to that of native ACL until 104 weeks, suggesting ongoing and late remodeling process. Although signal intensity of graft normalized at 104 weeks, the structural properties of the graft were inferior to that of healthy, uninjured ACL. Such findings suggest that normal signal intensity does not necessary reflect the graft's absolute strength but may reflect completed remodeling process which is accompanied by reduction in vascularity and water content.

In an attempt to correlate the graft mechanical properties with the T2 relaxation time signal intensity, a study using nine goats that underwent ACL reconstruction using patellar tendon autograft was conducted [26]. After 6 weeks of healing, T2 relaxation time alone did not demonstrate significant correlation to failure load or linear stiffness. However, authors found significant correlation between volume normalized by T2 relaxation time and biomechanical properties of the healing ACL. Moreover, there was a significant correlation with graft volume and anterior translation at 30° of knee flexion—when the graft volume was normalized by T2 relaxation time. The authors suggested that because T2 relaxation is not dependent on the scanner and acquisition parameters, when used in conjunction with graft volume, it is a better indicator of graft healing.

In a clinical study examining association between T2 MRI and degree of knee instability, 61 patients that previously had anatomic double-bundle ACL reconstruction were clinically and radiographically evaluated at 3, 6, and 12 months postoperatively [27]. The researchers found that at 12 months, nine of ten patients with poorly functioning grafts (anteroposterior translation ≥4 mm on side to side difference) had higher signal intensity. This study suggests that an increasing trend in T2 signal intensity may be a surrogate indicator for grafts that have more laxity.

Fact Box 3
Studies have shown that an MRI with increased T2 signal intensity indicates increased graft laxity.

21.4 Authors' Preferred Management

At the authors' institution, follow-up MRI scans are routinely ordered for those patients who are willing to return to football or other cutting and pivoting activities earlier than 9 months after ACL reconstruction (Fig. 21.2). Influenced by secondary factors and gains, this motivation for speedy return to competitive sports is especially prevalent among elite collegiate and professional athletes. We have noted that the time for graft maturation varies not only between allograft and autograft but also between different types of autografts. In our experience, the quadriceps tendon with bone block had lower signal intensity (improved maturation) than the hamstring tendons at 6 months [28]. When only one ACL bundle is torn, we encounter the ideal situation to follow-up and compare the signal intensity of the intact native ACL bundle with the reconstructed ACL graft side by side (Fig. 21.3). When following this subset of patients, the comparison between the MRI signal intensity of the remaining native ACL and the graft allows the surgeon to easily identify the different phases of the graft maturation over time.

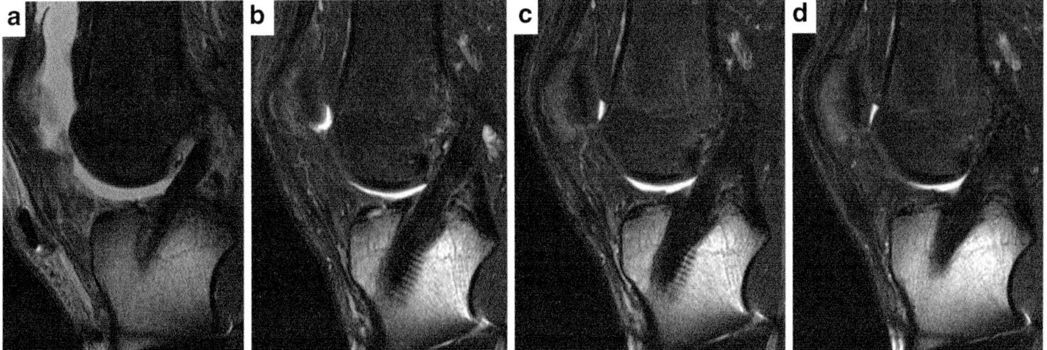

Fig. 21.2 Sagittal oblique T2 MRI showing the revascularization of the graft of a professional athlete who had an ACLR with quadriceps graft. (**a**) 1 day postoperative (PO). The graft signal intensity is comparable to the intact quadriceps tendon with no signs of revascularization; (**b**) 10 weeks PO. The graft signal intensity increased over time, as an indicative of revascularization; (**c**) 6 months PO. Although not yet mature, there is noticeable decreased graft signal intensity compared to **b**; (**d**) 10 months PO imaging showing increased maturity of the graft (lower signal intensity) when compared to the 6 months MRI

Fact Box 4

The quadriceps tendon with bone block demonstrated improved maturation compared to hamstring tendons at 6 months after ACLR.

Follow-up MRI serves as an additional tool in the decision-making process. If the patient has an immature graft on the MRI, then the athlete is advised to refrain from immediate return to competition. Conversely, if the patient has not yet achieved the adequate functional milestones in physical therapy, having a radiologically mature graft does not yield him allowance to return to play as the lack of muscle control puts the athlete at increased risk of early re-tear.

Translating the basic MRI research to the clinical setting is often not possible without some adaptations due to cost and time restrictions. For the general orthopedic surgeon, ordering a single follow-up MRI may pose a practical challenge. Acknowledging these limitations and developing a combined evaluation of the MRI signal intensity, rehabilitation milestones, psychological follow-up, and common sense are currently the best tools available to guide our footballers to safe and full functional recovery.

Take-Home Message

ACL rupture is a common injury in football resulting in significant impact on the injured athlete's quality of life as well as financial burden to society. Adequate rehabilitation is critical to safe and effective return to play. Recent studies suggest that determining the extent of ACL tear and the decision to treat the injured footballer should be based on their personal goals, history, patient's signs and symptoms, and physical exam rather than solely on their MRI appearance. Furthermore, MRI may be used to assess graft maturity and remodeling after ACL reconstruction. It is a valuable, sensitive, and noninvasive tool which can detect biomechanical changes in the graft itself and provide additional information on the athlete's readiness for return to play. An immature graft has greater risk of re-rupture and thus warrants extra time for recovery, and a better understanding of these concepts is essential to optimize the treatment of patients undergoing rehabilitation after ACL reconstruction. MRI should be used in conjunction with battery of functional and psychological tests to maximize successful, safe return to sports.

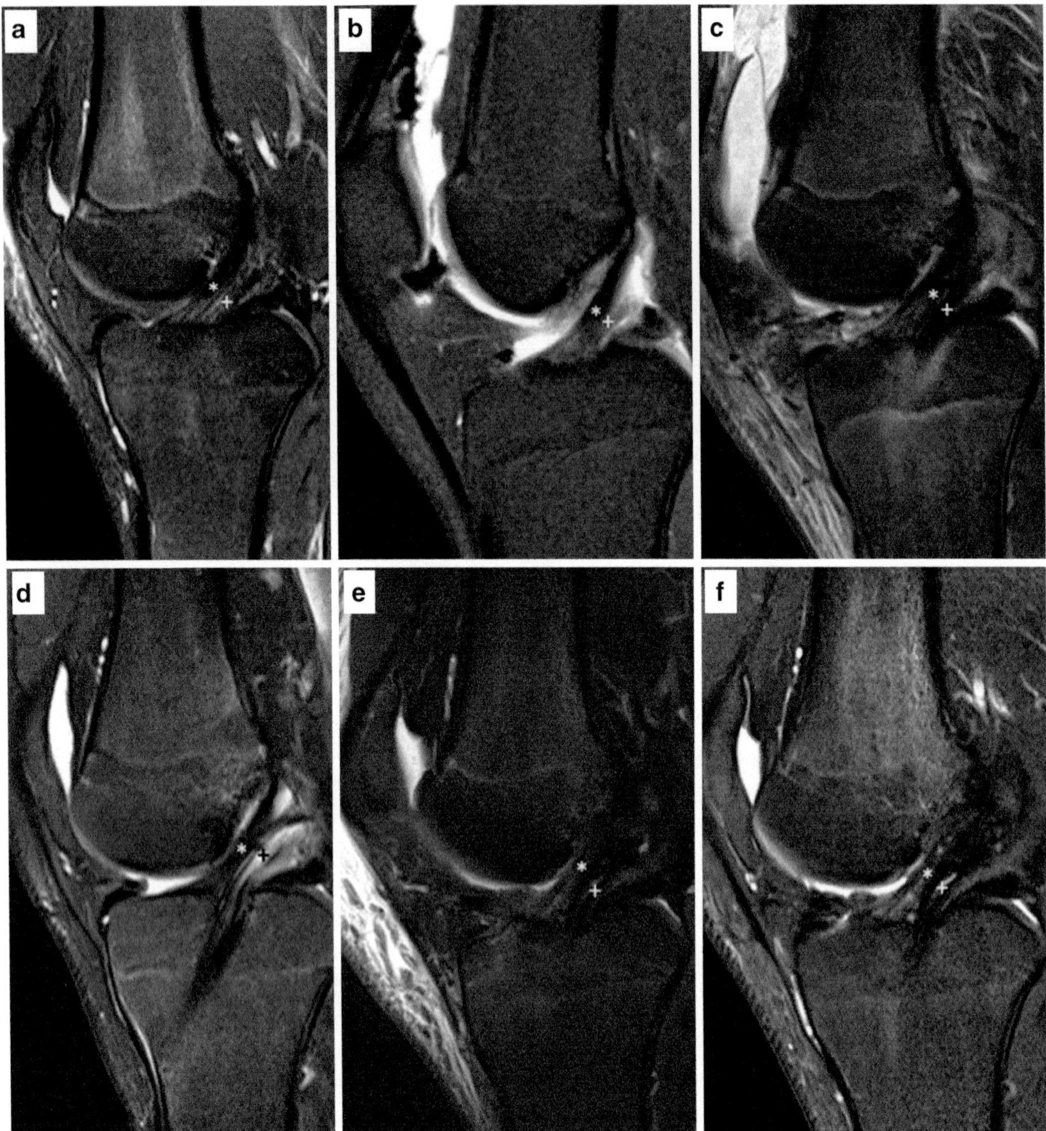

Fig. 21.3 Sagittal oblique T2 MRI of a 16-year-old athlete who had a posterolateral bundle (PL) augmentation surgery. (**a**) Intact ACL; (**b**) isolated PL tear; (**c**) immature PL graft at 2 weeks PO; (**d**) revascularization of the PL graft at 4 months PO; (**e**) and (**f**) mature graft at 1 year and 2 years PO (* indicates the intact anteromedial bundle of the native ACL; + indicates the autograft used for reconstructing the PL bundle of the ACL)

Top Five Evidence Based References

Abe S, Kurosaka M, Iguchi T, Yoshiya S, Hirohata K (1993) Light and electron microscopic study of remodeling and maturation process in autogenous graft for anterior cruciate ligament reconstruction. Arthroscopy 9(4):394–405

Howell SM, Knox KE, Farley TE, Taylor MA (1995) Revascularization of a human anterior cruciate ligament graft during the first two years of implantation. Am J Sports Med 23(1):42–49

Weiler A, Peters G, Mäurer J, Unterhauser FN, Südkamp NP (2001) Biomechanical properties and vascularity of an anterior cruciate ligament graft can be predicted by contrast-enhanced magnetic resonance imaging. Am J Sports Med 29(6):751–761

Fleming BC, Vajapeyam S, Connolly SA, Magarian EM, Murray MM (2011) The use of magnetic resonance imaging to predict ACL graft structural properties. J Biomech 44(16):2843–2846

Ma Y, Murawski CD, Rahnemai-Azar AA, Maldjian C, Lynch AD, Fu FH (2015) Graft maturity of the reconstructed anterior cruciate ligament 6 months postoperatively: a magnetic resonance imaging evaluation of quadriceps tendon with bone block and hamstring tendon autografts. Knee Surg Sports Traumatol Arthrosc 23(3):661–668

References

1. Cameron M, Buchgraber A, Passler H, Vogt M, Thonar E, Fu F, Evans CH (1997) The natural history of the anterior cruciate ligament-deficient knee. Changes in synovial fluid cytokine and keratan sulfate concentrations. Am J Sports Med 25(6):751–754
2. da Silveira Franciozi CE, Ingham SJ, Gracitelli GC, Luzo MV, FH F, Abdalla RJ (2014) Updates in biological therapies for knee injuries: anterior cruciate ligament. Curr Rev Musculoskelet Med 7(3):228–238
3. Larsson S, Struglics A, Lohmander LS, Frobell R (2017) Surgical reconstruction of ruptured anterior cruciate ligament prolongs trauma-induced increase of inflammatory cytokines in synovial fluid: an exploratory analysis in the KANON trial. Osteoarthr Cartil 25(9):1443–1451
4. Ardern CL, Osterberg A, Tagesson S, Gauffin H, Webster KE, Kvist J (2014) The impact of psychological readiness to return to sport and recreational activities after anterior cruciate ligament reconstruction. Br J Sports Med 48(22):1613–1619
5. Ardern CL, Taylor NF, Feller JA, Webster KE (2012) Fear of re-injury in people who have returned to sport following anterior cruciate ligament reconstruction surgery. J Sci Med Sport 15(6):488–495
6. Ardern CL, Taylor NF, Feller JA, Webster KE (2013) A systematic review of the psychological factors associated with returning to sport following injury. Br J Sports Med 47(17):1120–1126
7. Duc SR, Zanetti M, Kramer J, Kach KP, Zollikofer CL, Wentz KU (2005) Magnetic resonance imaging of anterior cruciate ligament tears: evaluation of standard orthogonal and tailored paracoronal images. Acta Radiol 46(7):729–733
8. Van Dyck P, Vanhoenacker FM, Lambrecht V, Wouters K, Gielen JL, Dossche L, Parizel PM (2013) Prospective comparison of 1.5 and 3.0-T MRI for evaluating the knee menisci and ACL. J Bone Joint Surg Am 95(10):916–924
9. Roychowdhury S, Fitzgerald SW, Sonin AH, Peduto AJ, Miller FH, Hoff FL (1997) Using MR imaging to diagnose partial tears of the anterior cruciate ligament: value of axial images. AJR Am J Roentgenol 168(6):1487–1491
10. Van Dyck P, Gielen JL, Vanhoenacker FM, Wouters K, Dossche L, Parizel PM (2012) Stable or unstable tear of the anterior cruciate ligament of the knee: an MR diagnosis? Skelet Radiol 41(3):273–280
11. Murray MM, Martin SD, Martin TL, Spector M (2000) Histological changes in the human anterior cruciate ligament after rupture. J Bone Joint Surg Am 82-a(10):1387–1397
12. van Meer BL, Oei EH, Bierma-Zeinstra SM, van Arkel ER, Verhaar JA, Reijman M, Meuffels DE (2014) Are magnetic resonance imaging recovery and laxity improvement possible after anterior cruciate ligament rupture in nonoperative treatment? Arthroscopy 30(9):1092–1099
13. Weiler A, Peters G, Mäurer J, Unterhauser FN, Südkamp NP (2001) Biomechanical properties and vascularity of an anterior cruciate ligament graft can be predicted by contrast-enhanced magnetic resonance imaging. Am J Sports Med 29(6):751–761
14. Shelbourne KD, Nitz P (1990) Accelerated rehabilitation after anterior cruciate ligament reconstruction. Am J Sports Med 18(3):292–299
15. Ardern CL, Webster KE, Taylor NF, Feller JA (2011) Return to the preinjury level of competitive sport after anterior cruciate ligament reconstruction surgery: two-thirds of patients have not returned by 12 months after surgery. Am J Sports Med 39(3):538–543
16. Shino K, Inoue M, Horibe S, Nagano J, Ono K (1988) Maturation of allograft tendons transplanted into the knee. An arthroscopic and histological study. J Bone Joint Surg Br 70(4):556–560
17. Abe S, Kurosaka M, Iguchi T, Yoshiya S, Hirohata K (1993) Light and electron microscopic study of remodeling and maturation process in autogenous graft for anterior cruciate ligament reconstruction. Arthroscopy 9(4):394–405
18. Arai Y, Hara K, Takahashi T, Urade H, Minami G, Takamiya H, Kubo T (2008) Evaluation of the vascular status of autogenous hamstring tendon grafts after anterior cruciate ligament reconstruction in humans using magnetic resonance angiography. Knee Surg Sports Traumatol Arthrosc 16(4):342–347
19. Howell SM, Knox KE, Farley TE, Taylor MA (1995) Revascularization of a human anterior cruciate ligament graft during the first two years of implantation. Am J Sports Med 23(1):42–49
20. Terauchi R, Arai Y, Hara K, Minami G, Nakagawa S, Takahashi T, Ikoma K, Ueshima K, Shirai T, Fujiwara H, Kubo T (2016) Magnetic resonance angiography evaluation of the bone tunnel and graft following ACL reconstruction with a hamstring tendon autograft. Knee Surg Sports Traumatol Arthrosc 24(1):169–175
21. Dong S, Xie G, Zhang Y, Shen P, Huangfu X, Zhao J (2015) Ligamentization of autogenous hamstring grafts after anterior cruciate ligament reconstruction: midterm versus long-term results. Am J Sports Med 43(8):1908–1917
22. Nagelli CV, Hewett TE (2017) Should return to sport be delayed until 2 years after anterior cruciate ligament reconstruction? Biological and functional considerations. Sports Med 47(2):221–232
23. Rougraff B, Shelbourne KD, Gerth PK, Warner J (1993) Arthroscopic and histologic analysis of

human patellar tendon autografts used for anterior cruciate ligament reconstruction. Am J Sports Med 21(2):277–284

24. Paterno MV, Rauh MJ, Schmitt LC, Ford KR, Hewett TE (2014) Incidence of second ACL injuries 2 years after primary ACL reconstruction and return to sport. Am J Sports Med 42(7):1567–1573
25. Weiler A, Peters G, Maurer J, Unterhauser FN, Sudkamp NP (2001) Biomechanical properties and vascularity of an anterior cruciate ligament graft can be predicted by contrast-enhanced magnetic resonance imaging. A two-year study in sheep. Am J Sports Med 29(6):751–761
26. Fleming BC, Vajapeyam S, Connolly SA, Magarian EM, Murray MM (2011) The use of magnetic resonance imaging to predict ACL graft structural properties. J Biomech 44(16):2843–2846
27. Hakozaki A, Niki Y, Enomoto H, Toyama Y, Suda Y (2015) Clinical significance of T2*-weighted gradient-echo MRI to monitor graft maturation over one year after anatomic double-bundle anterior cruciate ligament reconstruction: a comparative study with proton density-weighted MRI. Knee 22(1):4–10
28. Ma Y, Murawski CD, Rahnemai-Azar AA, Maldjian C, Lynch AD, FH F (2015) Graft maturity of the reconstructed anterior cruciate ligament 6 months postoperatively: a magnetic resonance imaging evaluation of quadriceps tendon with bone block and hamstring tendon autografts. Knee Surg Sports Traumatol Arthrosc 23(3):661–668

ACL: Time-Based Return to Play. "Role of Patient Reporting in Return to Play"

22

Adam J. Popchak, Mohammad A. Yabroudi, and James J. Irrgang

Contents

A.J. Popchak, P.T., Ph.D., S.C.S. (✉)
Department of Physical Therapy, University of Pittsburgh, Pittsburgh, PA, USA
e-mail: ajp64@pitt.edu

M.A. Yabroudi, P.T., M.S., Ph.D.
Department of Rehabilitation Sciences, Jordan University of Science and Technology, Irbid, Jordan

J.J. Irrgang, P.T., Ph.D., A.T.C., F.A.P.T.A.
Department of Physical Therapy, University of Pittsburgh, Pittsburgh, PA, USA

Department of Orthopaedic Surgery, University of Pittsburgh, Pittsburgh, PA, USA

22.1 Outcome Following Surgery

Increased participation in both competitive and recreational sports has led to a greater number of sports-related injuries. For the athletic population, the ultimate outcome of interest after injury is the ability to return to prior level of sports participation in terms of intensity, frequency, duration, absence of symptoms, and prevention of re-injury. Providers share the concern of returning their patients to preinjury levels of function and performance [1, 2] after a destabilizing knee injury. However, assessment of this outcome is difficult and is affected not only by physical factors but also by psychological factors [3, 4] and social behaviors. The multiple factors surrounding successful return to sports participation as well as variation in measurement methods have limited the ability to measure and improve return to sports participation. This chapter will discuss current issues with assessing return to sports participa-

V. Musahl et al. (eds.), *Return to Play in Football*, https://doi.org/10.1007/978-3-662-55713-6_22

tion in general and specifically in football, commonly used measurement scales, the success rate of surgery and rehabilitation in achieving this goal, the influence on results by the measurement method chosen, and current recommendations for assessing return to preinjury level of sports participation after ACL reconstruction.

22.2 Return to Play Overall Rates

Despite advances in surgical techniques and postoperative rehabilitation that often result in excellent recovery of knee joint stability [5] and self-report measures [5–7], many studies have shown that a substantial percentage of athletes do not return to preinjury levels of activity [8–10]. Considerable variation in return to sports participation exists in the literature, with reported rates ranging from 18% to 100% [9]. Ardern et al. [11] performed a systematic review of 7556 patients from 69 studies, where the mean age at time of surgery was 25.8 ± 3.2 years. They reported that 81% (95% CI 74–87%) returned to some form of sports, 65% (95% CI 59–72%) returned their preinjury level of play, but only 55% (95% CI 46–63%) returned to competitive sports. They [11] identified a number of non-modifiable factors that favored successful return to play such as: elite athlete status when compared to nonelite athletes, male gender, and younger age. Modifiable factors also influenced the rate of successful return, with those showing higher physical activity levels, more frequent participation, and greater psychological readiness to return to play, all favoring successful return to play following injury [11].

Return to play rates specifically in football show similar variability, ranging from approximately 50% [12, 13] to >90% [14–16]. Likewise, when assessing the rate of returning to preinjury level of participation in football, large variations are seen. Sandon et al. [13] reported that only 36% of the football players in their study returned to playing football at the same or higher level. In a cohort of female football players who were able to return to play, 59% played at the same level as before their ACL injury [12]. A retrospective study, performed by the authors, surveyed individuals 1–5 years after ACL reconstruction and compared their preinjury sports participation to their best after surgery [17]. The survey was completed by 251 individuals, 48 of which participated in football. Fifty-eight percent (58%) of football players reported returning to their preinjury level of football participation. In contrast, Walden et al. [14, 15] reported that 97% and 93% of elite level football players returned to the same level of play initially after surgery, and Zaffagnini et al. [16] reported 95% returned to the same level of football at 1 year. However, both Walden et al. [14] and Zaffagnini et al. [16] reported more modest rates of returning to preinjury levels at 3 (65%) and 4 years (62%), respectively. Factors that favored success in returning play in football included: a shorter time from injury to surgery [12], high motivation for returning to football [12], being on scholarship, [18] more years of scholastic eligibility remaining [18], and an earlier time period after surgery [14, 16]. Negative prognostic factors for returning to play in football, includes female gender, the presence of cartilage injury, and persistent knee pain with activity [13].

22.3 Reasons/Causes of Inability to Return to Sports

Some patients who fail to resume sports participation at their previous level may be physically unable to do so [19], whereas others may do so for reasons that extend beyond physical limitations [3, 20]. Fear of re-injury is the most frequently reported reason why a patient may decide to not return to their preinjury level of play [3], followed by shifting life priorities, developing a cautious personality [4], and lack of confidence. Likewise, our unpublished data examining those involved in football suggests fear of re-injury (58%), lack of confidence (42%), and work or family obligations (25%) were the reasons for not returning to participation in football. Psychological readiness to return to preinjury sports participation has also been found to be a factor, with those exhibiting greater readiness being more likely to return to preinjury levels of sports participation [3, 11]. A growing body of evidence exists suggesting factors outside of impairments in body structures may have a significant implication on returning to preinjury levels of sports participation after ACL injury [3, 4, 21, 22]. Therefore, in addition to potential ongoing limitations with physical function or performance, returning to preinjury levels of participation appears to be complex and multifactorial [3]. Secondary to the relationship between the physical and psychological components of returning to sports participation, defining what successful return to play is has been challenging and has led to considerable variation in the rates reported.

22.4 Multiple Definitions of Return to Sports

Variable definitions of return to sports likely contribute the wide range of return to sports reported. Multiple definitions of return to sports exist in the scientific literature, including returning to any sport participation, attainment of preinjury levels of activity, returning to competitive sports [11], and returning to preinjury level of competitive sports. The manner in which return to sports is assessed also varies, with some literature utilizing patient-reported outcome measures [23–26], returning to the same number of hours of sports participation per year as before the injury [27], and by using a global question of return to sports [21, 28, 29], As evidenced in the systematic review by Ardern et al. [11], the methods in which return to sports is defined can directly influence the final outcome of successful return to sports participation. The variability in the definition of return to sports participation likely contributes to the dissimilarity in return to sports rates reported in the literature and the overall estimate of the treatment effect after knee injury in athletes. Moreover, the lack of a universally accepted definition of return to sports not only limits the ability to measure return to sports, but it may also limits the ability to improve return to sports.

22.5 Measures of Activity and Participation

22.5.1 Tegner

Tegner and Lysholm [30] developed an activity scale in 1985 that graded work and sports activities numerically. This activity rating scale (Tegner activity scale) was initially constructed as a compliment to the functional score of a modified version of the Lysholm Knee Scoring Scale [31]. The Tegner activity scale [30] is presented as a single question concerning the highest level of activity possible. The activity scale covers activities of daily living and competitive and recreational sports [30]. Grading is from 10 to 0, where responses range from "competitive sports—national and international elite soccer" (10) to "sick leave or disability pension due to knee problems" (0) [30]. The initial investigation of the behavior of the Tegner activity scale [30], as it related to the Lysholm score, revealed a significantly higher Lysholm scores for those who scored 5–10 (83 ± 10) compared with those who scored a 0 (53 ± 16). Tegner and Lysholm [30] concluded the activity scale was a useful complement to the functional score derived from the Lysholm Knee Scoring Scale [31], and it provided additional information on activity level as well.

Since the initial testing of the Tegner scale was published, the scale has been widely utilized by researchers [32]. However, the Tegner scale was initially designed to be administered by a physician. In 2009, Briggs et al. [32] retested the Tegner activity scale to determine the psychometric properties when patient-administered and to determine how responsive to change the scale was in early stages of recovery post-anterior cruciate ligament reconstruction (ACLR). The Tegner scale was found to have an acceptable test-retest reliability (ICC = 0.82, 95% CI: 0.66–0.89), with a minimal detectable change of 1 [32]. Floor (8%) and ceiling (3%) effects were also considered acceptable, and the scale was significantly correlated to the IKDC subjective knee score, the Marx activity scale, and the physical component of the SF-12, which demonstrated validity of the scale [32, 33]. The Tegner scale was also found to be responsive to changes 9 months to 2 years post ACLR [32]. Overall, Briggs et al. [32] concluded the Tegner activity scale, when patient-administered, has acceptable psychometric properties and is a valid outcome measure for patients with ACL injuries and to a lesser extent patients with meniscal injuries [33]. A primary concern related to the Tegner scale is the arbitrariness of the ranking of different sports in activity level [34]. Additional concerns include the possibility that activity level for a given sport may vary among individuals and that omission of a sport may lead to misclassification [30].

22.6 Cincinnati Sports Activity Scale

Introduced by Noyes et al. [35] in 1989, the Cincinnati sports activity scale set forth to analyze the overall intensity of athletic participation by combining the type of activity and frequency of participation. The criteria for the type of activity engaged in described usual activities involved in sports and were subdivided into three levels, with an additional level for those unable to participate in sports [35]. Level I sports involved jumping, hard pivoting, and cutting. Level II sports involved running, twisting, and turning. Level III was composed of sports that did not involve running, twisting, or jumping. Finally, an activity of daily living category was established to determine severity of symptoms for those who do not participate in sports [35]. Additionally, the frequency of participation was established through 4 major categories, 4–7 times per week, 1–3 times per week, 1–3 times per month, and no sports [35]. Scores range from 100 (Level I activities, 4–7 times per week) to 0 (no sports and severe problems with ADLs). This scale is one of only a few scales that account for frequency of activity, which is an important factor to be considered [36]. Test-retest reliability has shown to be high (ICC = 0.98), and acceptable validity has been established [37]. However, some concerns have been raised in terms of its use [34]. This scale can rate subjects that do not engage in running, twisting, or jumping sports, but do so 4–7 times per week at 90 points, while subjects who do participate in jumping, hard pivoting, or cutting sports, but at 1–3 times per week at 85 [34, 37]. Marx et al. [34] raised the concern that cutting sports at a lesser frequency may place greater demands on the knee than less-demanding sports at a higher frequency, which is not be reflected in the Cincinnati sports activity scale.

22.7 International Knee Documentation Committee (IKDC)

In 1987, a group of knee surgeons from Europe and North America created the International Knee Documentation Committee Knee Ligament Evaluation Form (IKDC—KLEF) [38]. One of the main purposes of the IKDC—KLEF form was to establish an evaluation method that did not overestimate knee function by successfully satisfying parameters not important to higher level activities [38]. Additionally, the IKDC—KLEF was based only on the essential, reproducible criteria required to evaluate outcomes [39]. The full IKDC—KLEF included a documentation, qualification, and evaluation section, and was intended to be used pre- and postoperatively [38]. Widely used in the USA and Europe, the IKDC—KLEF was created with many of the factors adopted from the Cincinnati Rating System, including the sports activity scale [37]. However, in contrast to the Cincinnati Rating System, the IKDC—KLEF form was more concise and convenient, one page in length, yet still comprehensive enough to satisfy many requirements of sports [38]. Activity level, preinjury, pretreatment, and present, was defined as Level I through Level IV [38]. Level I activities included jumping, pivoting, and hard cutting, as in football or soccer. Level II activities included heavy manual work, such as skiing and tennis. Level III included light manual work, like jogging and running, and Level IV included sedentary work [38]. Symptoms were graded in terms of the highest level of activity without pain, swelling, and partial or complete giving way [38]. However, the IKDC—KLEF did not consider the frequency of activity when considering participation level.

22.8 Marx Activity Scale

Marx et al. [34] set forth to establish a rating scale to measure activity level of patients based on the principle that large variations in the frequency and intensity of sports participated in exist among patients and athletes. They claimed that activity levels are an important prognostic factor in the sports medicine population, as expectations and physical demands differ between those who are very active compared to those who are relatively sedentary [34]. The Marx activity scale was constructed to be self-administered, in an efficient and timely manner, and to allow comparisons between individuals who participate in different sports [34].

Deliberate steps were taken to avoid using specific sports as examples, as opposed to Tegner activity scale, which considers only participation in a sport [34]. Instead the focus centered on the respondent's actual activity. The scale contains four questions regarding running, cutting, decelerating, and pivoting, each rated in terms of the frequency the activity is performed. Frequencies range from less than once per month to 4 or more times per week [34]. Original test-retest reliability was shown to be excellent (ICC 0.97), and the scale correlated well with three other activity rating scales. In particular, the Marx activity scale was most highly related to the Tegner and Cincinnati sports activity scales [34]. Also noted in terms of the psychometric properties of the Marx scale was the inverse correlation with the respondent's age ($r = -0.48$). The scale presents a manner to obtain a more accurate estimation of baseline activity at the patient's highest level rather than a mere health status tool and provides an excellent goal for determining return to sports and activity after knee injury.

22.9 SPORTS Score

Initially used to assess the ability of athletes to return to sports following surgery for elbow contractures [40], the Subjective Patient Outcome for Return to Sports (SPORTS) score was developed as a simple method to evaluate an athlete's ability to return to sport [41]. The development of the 1-item SPORTS score was aimed specifically for use in evaluating athletes and their ability to return to their sport [41], regardless of being a competitive or recreational athlete. The SPORTS score consists of three main components: performing the same sport at the same level of effort, obtaining similar levels of performance, and to do so in the absence or regardless of pain [41]. The score ranges from 0 to 10, where 0 represents not returning to the same sport and 10 represents obtaining the same effort and performance as before injury without pain [41]. Test-retest reliability, criterion validity, and floor and ceiling effects have been evaluated for this instrument in a group of athletes 5–10 years after anterior cruciate ligament reconstruction [41]. Test-rest reliability of the score was found to be excellent (ICC 0.97). The instrument also showed strong correlations with the overall and sports and recreational component of the Knee Injury and Osteoarthritis Score (KOOS) and a moderate correlation with the Lysholm score [41]. Floor effects were low (9%). However, a limitation with the SPORTS scale may be in its ability to detect change at the highest levels of performance, with a reported ceiling effect of 32% [41]. Additionally, the reported psychometric properties were established via a retrospective study, which could potentially introduce recall bias. Overall, the SPORTS score does possess excellent reliability and acceptable criterion validity and may be useful in assessing return to sport, especially after ACL reconstruction.

22.10 Unidimensional Self-Report vs Multidimensional Assessments

Self-report of return to sports activity is sometimes assessed through a global question such as "Did you return to the same intensity, frequency, and duration of preinjury level of sports activity and participation?" However, it has been shown that an individual's answer and interpretation of such a question may not accurately reflect all aspects of achievement of return to preinjury levels of sports participation. Therefore when utilizing a standardized assessment, consideration should be given to a number of factors including: the type of sports engaged in, frequency of participation, duration and intensity of activity, the quality of the performance, and any symptoms that occur during or after participation. The IKDC—KLEF provides an established criteria for defining the type and level of sports criteria, with very strenuous, strenuous, moderate, and light corresponding to Levels 1 through 4 respectfully [38]. The Cincinnati sports activity scale [35] and the Marx activity scale [34] provide validated measures of the frequency of activity and how it can be assessed, typically defining frequencies as 4–7 times per week (competitive athlete), 1–3 times per week (recreational athlete), 1–3 times per month (occasional athlete), and <1 time per month. The Marx activity scale [34] provides an excellent manner to accurately estimate overall activity at the highest level and at multiple time points thereafter.

Therefore, a comprehensive manner to define return to sports can be developed by using aspects of multiple, validated patient-reported measures of the type and frequency of sports participation and activity. A multidimensional assessment [42] of return to sports that utilizes these three parameters (type of activity, frequency of participation, and Marx score) to create a comprehensive definition of return to sports is recommended. Individuals are considered to have returned to preinjury sports activity only if the type and frequency of sports participation and the Marx activity score after treatment are equal to or better than the preinjury status.

22.11 Current Recommendations

Based on the difficulty in accurately assessing return to sports, multidimensional assessment of return to sports participation and activity that considers the type and frequency of sports participation and activity and the Marx activity score is recommended. This information should be reported from the individual's perspective (i.e., self- or patient-reported measures) to minimize issues that introduce variability into the assessment. To prevent recall bias, it is important to measure preinjury level and frequency of sports participation and activity immediately after one's injury. Following the injury and during the process of recovery, it is recommended that return to activity and participation is prospectively assessed. The clinician and/or researcher should document key milestones such as return to running, cutting, jumping, agility drills, practice, competition, and full competition without restrictions as they are achieved. Additionally, the clinician and/or researcher should record symptoms and recurrent injury to the ACL-reconstructed knee as well as the contralateral knee. Comparing the frequency of running, cutting, decelerating, and pivoting with the Marx activity score before and after injury reduces the likelihood of incorrectly identifying a successful return to preinjury level of sports participation [42]. Lastly, it is important to document reasons for decreased activity and participation. Determination should be made whether reasons for reduced activity are related to the knee, lifestyle changes, or a combination of knee and lifestyle alterations [42]. Ideally, determinants of success in returning to sports should be individualized according to the goals of the patient.

22.12 Discrepancies Between Assessment Methods

There is a discrepancy between unidimensional measurements compared with comprehensive criteria that have been described to assess return to sports. It is possible that separate constructs are measured with each method of assessment. Comprehensive assessment may focus more objectively on functional abilities and participation habits, while global assessments may depend on overall patient satisfaction, which can be influenced by attitude and personality traits. There is a need for clarity and standardization in regards to what clinicians and patients are measuring when assessing successful return to sports participation. Moreover, qualitative research, including cognitive interviews, with athletes is needed to better understand the discrepancies in these definitions and to develop the most accurate definition and methods for determining return to sports.

22.13 Future Directions

Further work is needed to develop and accept a standard, universally applied definition of return to sports. The use of qualitative methods, including cognitive interviews, is needed to determine what return to sports means to the individual and how the individual interprets and constructs responses to questions about return to sports. When determining return to sports, additional work is required to determine how changes in the individual's lifestyle and interests over time should be accounted for, as well as how the quality of performance and symptoms should be incorporated. Through such future efforts, greater accuracy and generalizability can be established to assess this important outcome following knee injury in the athletic population.

22.14 Summary

Return to play rates in football show similar variability as those reported for other sports populations. When assessing return to play in the football player, it is important to define the level of return to play through not only physical abilities, but also patient-reported measures of sports activity and participation. A host of patient-reported measures of sports activity and participation exist and many have shown acceptable psychometric properties. Those patient-reported measures that assess activity level and the type and frequency of sports participation provide greater accuracy in assessing return to play over simple self-report by the athlete. Standardization of the definition of return to play and the manner in which return to play is assessed is needed to improve the generalizability and accuracy of return to play after ACL reconstruction in football.

Take Home Message

When assessing return to play in football after ACL reconstruction, assessing patient-reported function through evidence-based outcome measures is essential. Patient-reported measures that assess the type and frequency of sports participation and activity in comparison to preinjury level of sports are preferred over unidimensional scales. Comprehensive assessment of return to play limits overestimation of return and provides greater accuracy in evaluating return to play in football players.

Fact Boxes

Patient-reported outcome	Reliability	MDC or MCID	Floor effects	Ceiling effects
Tegner	ICC = 0.82	MDC = 1	8%	3%
Cincinnati sports activity scale	ICC = 0.98	NA	No	No
IKDC-SKF	ICC = 0.94	MCID = 6.3–20.5	0%	<1%
Marx activity scale	ICC = 0.97	MDC = 9.9	NA	NA

Return to sport rate	Ardern et al. [32]
Any sport	81%
Preinjury level	65%
Competitive level	55%

Factors favoring successful return to sports

- Younger age
- Male gender
- Elite athlete status
- Greater physical activity levels
- Greater frequency of participation
- Greater psychological readiness

Definitions of return to play

- Returning to any sports participation
- Attainment of preinjury levels of sports participation
- Returning to competitive play
- Returning to preinjury level of competitive play

Five Most Important References

Ardern CL, Taylor NF, Feller JA, Webster KE (2014) Fifty-five per cent return to competitive sport following anterior cruciate ligament reconstruction surgery: an updated systematic review and meta-analysis including aspects of physical functioning and contextual factors. Br J Sports Med 48:1543–1552

Walden M, Hagglund M, Magnusson H, Ekstrand J (2016) ACL injuries in men's professional football: a 15-year prospective study on time trends and return-to-play rates reveals only 65% of players still play at the top level 3 years after ACL rupture. Br J Sports Med 50:744–750

Lynch AD, Logerstedt DS, Grindem H, Eitzen I, Hicks GE, Axe MJ et al (2013) Consensus criteria for defining 'successful outcome' after ACL injury and reconstruction: a Delaware-Oslo ACL cohort investigation. Br J Sports Med 49:335–342

Marx RG, Jones EC, Allen AA, Altchek DW, O'Brien SJ, Rodeo SA et al (2001) Reliability, validity, and responsiveness of four knee outcome scales for athletic patients. J Bone Joint Surg Am 83:1459–1469

Waldén M, Hägglund M, Magnusson H, Ekstrand J (2011) Anterior cruciate ligament injury in elite football: a prospective three-cohort study. Knee Surg Sports Traumatol Arthrosc 19:11–19

References

1. Lynch AD, Logerstedt DS, Grindem H, Eitzen I, Hicks GE, Axe MJ et al (2015) Consensus criteria for defining 'successful outcome' after ACL injury and reconstruction: a Delaware-Oslo ACL cohort investigation. Br J Sports Med 49:335–342
2. Matava MJ, Howard DR, Polakof L, Brophy RH (2014) Public perception regarding anterior cruciate ligament reconstruction. J Bone Joint Surg 96:e85
3. Ardern CL (2015) Anterior cruciate ligament reconstruction—not exactly a one-way ticket back to the preinjury level: a review of contextual factors affecting return to sport after surgery. Sports Health 7:224–230
4. Tjong VK, Murnaghan ML, Nyhof-Young JM, Ogilvie-Harris DJ (2014) A qualitative investigation of the decision to return to sport after anterior cruciate ligament reconstruction to play or not to play. Am J Sports Med 42:336–342
5. Paterno MV, Weed AM, Hewett TE (2012) A between sex comparison of anterior-posterior knee laxity after anterior cruciate ligament reconstruction with patellar tendon or hamstrings autograft: a systematic review. Sports Med 42:135–152
6. Geib TM, Shelton WR, Phelps RA, Clark L (2009) Anterior cruciate ligament reconstruction using quadriceps tendon autograft: intermediate-term outcome. Arthroscopy 25:1408–1414
7. Pinczewski LA, Lyman J, Salmon LJ, Russell VJ, Roe J, Linklater J (2007) A 10-year comparison of anterior cruciate ligament reconstructions with hamstring tendon and patellar tendon autograft: a controlled, prospective trial. Am J Sports Med 35:564–574
8. Ardern CL, Taylor NF, Feller JA, Webster KE (2012) Return-to-sport outcomes at 2 to 7 years after anterior cruciate ligament reconstruction surgery. Am J Sports Med 40:41–48
9. Ardern CL, Webster KE, Taylor NF, Feller JA (2011) Return to sport following anterior cruciate ligament reconstruction surgery: a systematic review and meta-analysis of the state of play. Br J Sports Med 45:596–606
10. Ardern CL, Webster KE, Taylor NF, Feller JA (2011) Return to the preinjury level of competitive sport after anterior cruciate ligament reconstruction surgery two-thirds of patients have not returned by 12 months after surgery. Am J Sports Med 39:538–543
11. Ardern CL, Taylor NF, Feller JA, Webster KE (2014) Fifty-five percent return to competitive sport following anterior cruciate ligament reconstruction surgery: an updated systematic review and meta-analysis including aspects of physical functioning and contextual factors. Br J Sports Med 48:1543–1552
12. Faltstrom A, Hagglund M, Kvist J (2016) Factors associated with playing football after anterior cruciate ligament reconstruction in female football players. Scand J Med Sci Sports 26:1343–1352
13. Sandon A, Werner S, Forssblad M (2015) Factors associated with returning to football after anterior cruciate ligament reconstruction. Knee Surg Sports Traumatol Arthrosc 23:2514–2521
14. Walden M, Hagglund M, Magnusson H, Ekstrand J (2016) ACL injuries in men's professional football: a 15-year prospective study on time trends and

return-to-play rates reveals only 65% of players still play at the top level 3 years after ACL rupture. Br J Sports Med 50:744–750
15. Waldén M, Hägglund M, Magnusson H, Ekstrand J (2011) Anterior cruciate ligament injury in elite football: a prospective three-cohort study. Knee Surg Sports Traumatol Arthrosc 19:11–19
16. Zaffagnini S, Grassi A, Muccioli GM, Tsapralis K, Ricci M, Bragonzoni L et al (2014) Return to sport after anterior cruciate ligament reconstruction in professional soccer players. Knee 21:731–735
17. Yabroudi MA et al (2016) Predictors of revision surgery after primary anterior cruciate ligament reconstruction. Orthop J Sports Med 4(9). DOI:10.1177/2325967116666039
18. Howard JS, Lembach ML, Metzler AV, Johnson DL (2016) Rates and determinants of return to play after anterior cruciate ligament reconstruction in National Collegiate Athletic Association Division I soccer athletes: a study of the southeastern conference. Am J Sports Med 44:433–439
19. Reider B (2012) Return or retirement? Am J Sports Med 40:2437–2439
20. Ardern CL, Taylor NF, Feller JA, Whitehead TS, Webster KE (2015) Sports participation 2 years after anterior cruciate ligament reconstruction in athletes who had not returned to sport at 1 year: a prospective follow-up of physical function and psychological factors in 122 athletes. Am J Sports Med 43:848–856
21. Kvist J, Ek A, Sporrstedt K, Good L (2005) Fear of re-injury: a hindrance for returning to sports after anterior cruciate ligament reconstruction. Knee Surg Sports Traumatol Arthrosc 13:393–397
22. Langford JL, Webster KE, Feller JA (2009) A prospective longitudinal study to assess psychological changes following anterior cruciate ligament reconstruction surgery. Br J Sports Med 43:377–378
23. Fabbriciani C, Milano G, Mulas PD, Ziranu F, Severini G (2005) Anterior cruciate ligament reconstruction with doubled semitendinosus and gracilis tendon graft in rugby players. Knee Surg Sports Traumatol Arthrosc 13:2–7
24. Frobell RB, Roos HP, Roos EM, Roemer FW, Ranstam J, Lohmander LS (2013) Treatment for acute anterior cruciate ligament tear: five year outcome of randomised trial. BMJ 346:f232
25. Hasebe Y, Tanabe Y, Yasuda K (2005) Anterior-cruciate-ligament reconstruction using doubled hamstring-tendon autograft. J Sport Rehabil 14:279
26. Heijne A, Axelsson K, Werner S, Biguet G (2008) Rehabilitation and recovery after anterior cruciate ligament reconstruction: patients' experiences. Scand J Med Sci Sports 18:325–335
27. Daniel DM, Stone ML, Dobson BE, Fithian DC, Rossman DJ, Kaufman KR (1994) Fate of the ACL-injured patient a prospective outcome study. Am J Sports Med 22:632–644
28. Gobbi A, Francisco R (2006) Factors affecting return to sports after anterior cruciate ligament reconstruction with patellar tendon and hamstring graft: a prospective clinical investigation. Knee Surg Sports Traumatol Arthrosc 14:1021–1028
29. Lee DY, Karim SA, Chang HC (2008) Return to sports after anterior cruciate ligament reconstruction--a review of patients with minimum 5-year follow-up. Ann Acad Med Sinapore 37:273
30. Tegner Y, Lysholm J (1985) Rating systems in the evaluation of knee ligament injuries. Clin Orthop 198:42–49
31. Lysholm J, Gillquist J (1982) Evaluation of knee ligament surgery results with special emphasis on use of a scoring scale. Am J Sports Med 10:150–154
32. Briggs KK, Lysholm J, Tegner Y, Rodkey WG, Kocher MS, Steadman JR (2009) The reliability, validity, and responsiveness of the Lysholm score and Tegner activity scale for anterior cruciate ligament injuries of the knee: 25 years later. Am J Sports Med 37:890–897
33. Briggs KK, Kocher MS, Rodkey WG, Steadman JR (2006) Reliability, validity, and responsiveness of the Lysholm knee score and Tegner activity scale for patients with meniscal injury of the knee. J Bone Joint Surg Am 88:698–705
34. Marx RG, Stump TJ, Jones EC, Wickiewicz TL, Warren RF (2001) Development and evaluation of an activity rating scale for disorders of the knee. Am J Sports Med 29:213–218
35. Noyes FR, Barber SD, Mooar LA (1989) A rationale for assessing sports activity levels and limitations in knee disorders. Clin Orthop 246:238–249
36. Marx RG, Jones EC, Allen AA, Altchek DW, O'Brien SJ, Rodeo SA et al (2001) Reliability, validity, and responsiveness of four knee outcome scales for athletic patients. J Bone Joint Surg Am 83:1459–1469
37. Barber-Westin SD, Noyes FR, McCloskey JW (1999) Rigorous statistical reliability, validity, and responsiveness testing of the Cincinnati knee rating system in 350 subjects with uninjured, injured, or anterior cruciate ligament-reconstructed knees. Am J Sports Med 27:402–416
38. Hefti E, Müller W, Jakob R, Stäubli H-U (1993) Evaluation of knee ligament injuries with the IKDC form. Knee Surg Sports Traumatol Arthrosc 1:226–234
39. Irrgang JJ, Anderson AF, Boland AL, Harner CD, Kurosaka M, Neyret P et al (2001) Development and validation of the international knee documentation committee subjective knee form. Am J Sports Med 29:600–613
40. Blonna D, Lee G-C, O'Driscoll SW (2010) Arthroscopic restoration of terminal elbow extension in high-level athletes. Am J Sports Med 38:2509–2515
41. Blonna D, Castoldi F, Delicio D, Bruzzone M, Dettoni F, Bonasia DE et al (2012) Validity and reliability of the SPORTS score. Knee Surg Sports Traumatol Arthrosc 20:356–360
42. Joreitz R, Lynch A, Rabuck S, Lynch B, Davin S, Irrgang J (2016) Patient-specific and surgery-specific factors that affect return to sport after ACL reconstruction. Int J Sports Phys Ther 11:264–278

23 The Role of Orthobiologics in Return to Play

Graeme P. Whyte, Alberto Gobbi, and John G. Lane

Contents

G.P. Whyte, M.D., M.Sc., F.R.C.S.C.
Orthopaedic Arthroscopic Surgery International (OASI) Bioresearch Foundation, NPO, Via G.A. Amadeo, 24, 20133, Milan, Italy

Cornell University, Weill Medical College, New York Presbyterian Hospital/Queens, New York, NY, USA

A. Gobbi, M.D. (✉)
Orthopaedic Arthroscopic Surgery International (OASI) Bioresearch Foundation, NPO, Via G.A. Amadeo, 24, 20133, Milan, Italy
e-mail: gobbi@cartilagedoctor.it

J.G. Lane, M.D.
Orthopaedic Arthroscopic Surgery International (OASI) Bioresearch Foundation, NPO, Via G.A. Amadeo, 24, 20133, Milan, Italy

Musculoskeletal and Joint Research Foundation, San Diego, CA, USA

23.1 Background

Soft tissue injuries are commonly associated with disruption in sporting activities, from recreational to professional, and frequently delay or limit return to play in football. There is a wide spectrum of orthobiologic therapies that have been developed to facilitate return to play, ideally back to a pre-injury level of function. Despite advances in operative and nonoperative treatment methods, there continues to be considerable debate regarding optimal management interventions, particularly with respect to cartilage and ligamentous pathology. Biologic augmentation of healing processes is increasingly used and includes therapies that take advantage of platelet-rich plasma (PRP) and mesenchymal stem cell (MSC) preparations. These treatments are often used in an injectable form to treat an array of musculoskeletal injuries and also used in more complex procedures such as ligament repair and cartilage restoration.

The potential for the use of biologics in the treatment of functionally limiting ligament or tendon injury is encouraging [25, 27]. Regarding anterior cruciate ligament (ACL) insufficiency, reconstruction with tendon graft is considered the gold standard treatment, leading to high rates of return to play at all levels of competition. There are a number of limitations of current surgical treatments that are used to reconstruct ligaments. The incorporation of tendinous graft and restoration of ligamentous

V. Musahl et al. (eds.), *Return to Play in Football*, https://doi.org/10.1007/978-3-662-55713-6_23

stability is a slow process, particularly in case of ACL reconstruction, due to the hypocellular and hypovascular qualities of this tissue [40]. More than a year after reconstruction, the structure and mechanical characteristics of ACL repair tissue are inferior to native ligament. Additionally, following ligament reconstruction, restoration of proprioception is incomplete, joint kinematics are not normalized, and premature degenerative changes to the articular cartilage may develop [18].

Soft tissue injuries may result in substantial lifestyle modification and functional impairment, even after the injured tissue is repaired or reconstructed with contemporary surgical methods. Therapeutic approaches that utilize biologic factors, or surgical procedures that are augmented with these elements, may provide treatment alternatives with the potential to overcome some of the limitations of current management strategies.

23.2 Growth Factors and Platelet-Rich Plasma (PRP)

Growth factors have the capacity to stimulate cellular migration and proliferation, direct cellular differentiation, and to increase collagen production. There have been numerous bioactive substances shown to coordinate cellular repair processes in response to ligament and tendon injury [1]. Growth factors are upregulated following injury, playing a crucial role in orchestrating repair processes at all stages of the healing. Examples of such bioactive factors that have been shown to coordinate these processes include insulin-like growth factor-1 (IGF-1), bone morphogenetic protein (BMP), transforming growth factor beta (TGF-β), basic fibroblast growth factor (bFGF), and platelet-derived growth factor (PDGF) [14, 36, 45, 63]. Application of FGF has been demonstrated to improve vascularity and subsequent healing in an animal model, and BMP has been associated with superior healing in cases of Achilles tendon injury [2, 35]. Moreover, growth factors have been used in association with various scaffolding materials to enhance ligament repair procedures in animals [13].

Platelet-rich plasma is an increasingly used treatment containing growth factors that are released from activated platelets. Platelets contain several bioactive proteins that are capable of coordinating tissue repair processes. These factors regulate cellular differentiation, proliferation, chemotaxis, and migration, and are important in the synthesis of extracellular matrix. The potential for PRP to initiate and augment natural healing cascades is the rationale for the use of PRP in clinical practice, and so this orthobiologic is typically applied to the site of injury, where concentrated bioactive factors are released and act to stimulate healing. It is a treatment frequently used with the intention to facilitate return to play in football for a wide range of injuries, having therapeutic properties capable of reducing inflammation and optimizing formation of healthy repair tissue [26].

The initial step in isolating PRP is autologous venous blood extraction, using any one of a number of commercially available systems (Fig. 23.1). This blood subsequently undergoes a centrifugation process to isolate PRP. When injected at a site of tissue injury, platelets within the PRP are activated by endogenous thrombin and/or intra-articular collagen. To obtain a PRP gel preparation prior to clinical application, platelets are activated by calcium chloride or thrombin. A procoagulant enzyme such as batroxobin may also be used for PRP activation, which acts as a fibrinogen-cleaving enzyme, inducing rapid fibrin clot formation. Depending on the particular method of preparation, PRP can be categorized as leucocyte-poor PRP, leucocyte-rich PRP, or platelet-poor plasma [23]. Preparations of PRP vary, depending on the system used to process the autologous blood, so there continues to be difficulty in standardizing research methods and treatment protocols. Preparations of PRP that are rich in the bioactive factors IGF-1, TGF-β, and PDGF are often used, as these elements have been shown to be particularly effective at enhancing healing processes, according to in vitro studies.

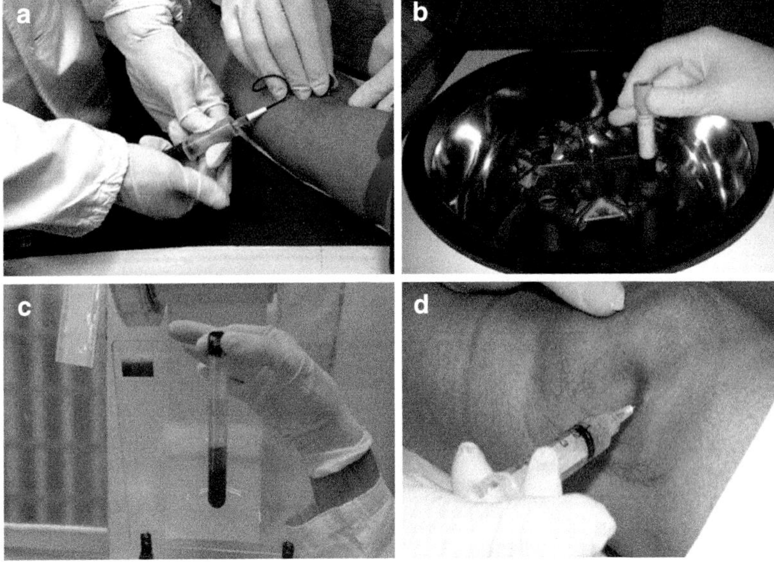

Fig. 23.1 Platelet-rich plasma (PRP) isolation and injection treatment. (**a**) Autologous venous blood extraction, (**b**) centrifugation in a commercially available system, (**c**) separation of PRP from venous blood, (**d**) intra-articular knee injection of PRP

Fact Box 1

- Bioactive growth factors coordinate and direct cellular processes that are necessary for tissue repair.
- Platelet-rich plasma (PRP) contains numerous bioactive proteins that can augment natural healing cascades after tissue injury.
- Constituents of PRP preparations vary, depending on the processing system used.

23.3 Mesenchymal Stem Cells: Cellular Biology and Healing Stimulation

There is currently an increasing interest in treatment of musculoskeletal injury with regenerative cellular therapy. Mesenchymal stem cells have factored prominently in these therapies, and have been researched extensively with in vitro models, and in protocols involving animals and human subjects. These multipotent MSCs can be isolated from a variety of tissues that include bone marrow, adipose tissue, synovium, and periosteum. A number of therapeutic protocols using MSCs sourced from bone marrow aspirate or adipose tissue have been developed, and there is optimism for wide ranging clinical applications of these therapies to treat various conditions by enhancing regenerative potential and healing processes.

Advances in cellular biology have demonstrated that MSCs are derived from pericytes, which are cells found in close association with blood vessels [10, 16, 20]. These pericytes exist in a state of quiescence within the perivascular niche [15]. Pericytes become activated and develop an MSC phenotype at times of physical injury, when damage to blood vessels initiates a process of activation and differentiation. Once activated, MSCs release a number of anti-inflammatory and trophic factors. These bioactive elements act to counter overactive immune responses and to establish a microenvironment that is favorable to regenerative processes [32]. There is stimulation of angiogenesis and proliferation of tissue-specific progenitor cells, with concurrent inhibition of apoptosis and a reduction in scar tissue formation [11, 32].

The potential for MSCs to differentiate into a variety of cell types and to repopulate cellular clus-

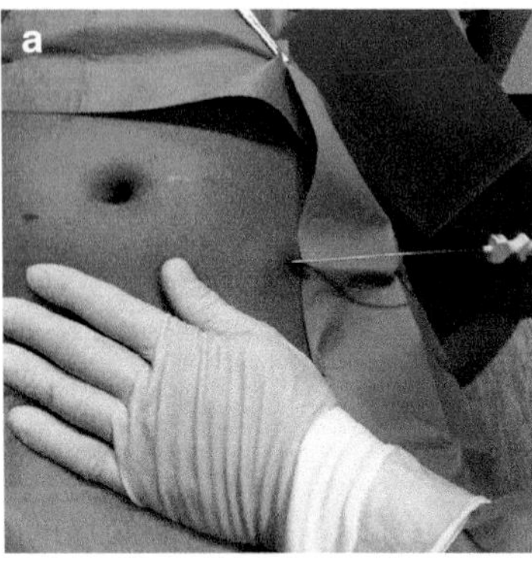
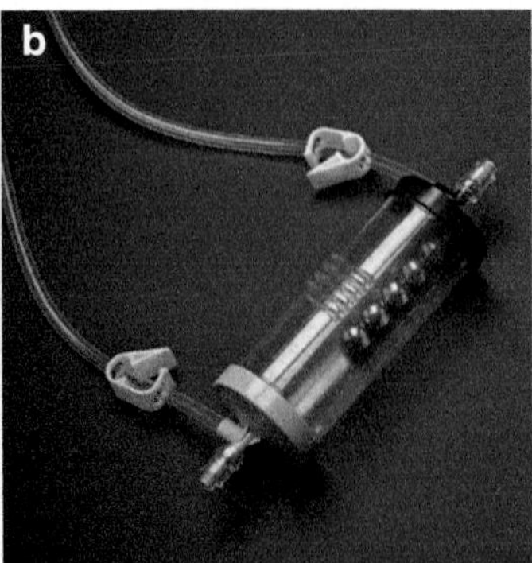
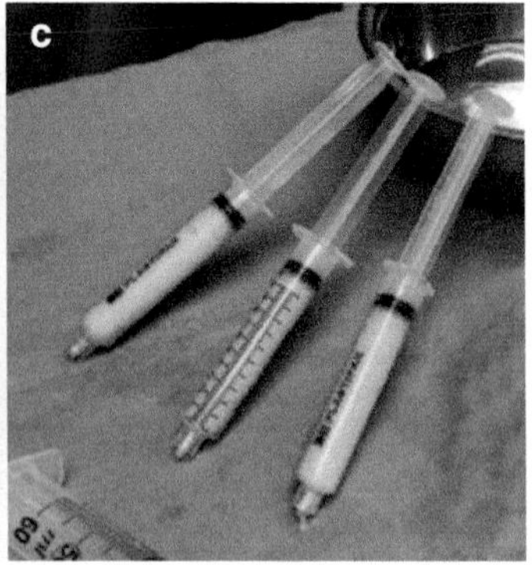

Fig. 23.2 Extraction of autologous adipose tissue and processing of lipoaspirate using the Lipogems® system (Lipogems International SpA, Milan, Italy) to isolate adipose-derived mesenchymal stem cells for intra-articular injection. (**a**) Lipoaspiration of abdominal adipose tissue, (**b**) Lipogems® processing system containing stainless steel balls for emulsification of autologous lipoaspirate, (**c**) three 10 cm^3 syringes containing micro-fragmented adipose tissue containing concentrated adipose-derived mesenchymal stem cells

ters of damaged tissue was the initial focus of clinical applications for such cells [6, 7, 24, 30, 39]. Further examination of cellular biology and physiology, based on more recent in vivo models, has highlighted the paracrine and trophic actions of these cells in the regulation of healing processes [9, 10]. MSCs have the capacity to release a plethora of cytokines and growth factors into the surrounding microenvironment of damaged tissue, with the potential to affect all biomolecular cascades responsible for tissue healing and regeneration [11, 22]. The treatment of ligamentous injury to the knee, including that of the ACL, with cellular therapies is an attractive option, given the potential to enhance the native biologic healing processes. Considering the similarities that have been identified between ACL outgrowth cells and MSCs, there is potential for these multipotent cells to augment healing of this ligament, as well as others.

In clinical practice, concentrated forms of MSCs have been primarily sourced from autologous bone marrow aspirate in recent years for use in a variety of treatments for musculoskeletal injury. Concentrations of these multipotent cells can be highly variable, depending on the tissue used to source these cells, as well as the system used to concentrate this isolate. With regard to bone marrow aspirate, 0.01–0.0001% of nucleated cells are characterized as MSCs, and the final isolate concentration of desired multipotent cells may be affected by aging [8, 12].

Mesenchymal stem cells can be isolated in abundance from autologous adipose tissue, which contains a consistently vascularized structure. Moreover, the impact of age-related variation in concentrations of the desired cellular elements may be of less concern in processed adipose tissue, as opposed to bone marrow (Fig. 23.2).

Injections of adipose-derived stem cells (ASCs) in a rabbit model have been demonstrated to have positive effects on cartilage repair processes in cases of osteoarthritic lesions [58, 59]. Furthermore, injection of ASCs resulted in a reduction in osteophyte formation and cartilage ossification. These findings are consistent with experiments in a sheep model that demonstrated chondrogenic properties of ASCs and MSCs sourced from bone marrow in cases of osteoarthritis [60]. Treatment of osteoarthritic lesions in the elbow and hip joints of dogs by injection of ASCs has also demonstrated encouraging beneficial effects [3, 4].

Studies on human subjects have demonstrated clinical improvements in cases of knee osteoarthritis treated with intra-articular ASC injection, using adipose tissue sourced from the infrapatellar fat pad [37]. Improved stability of knee articular cartilage has also been demonstrated after ASC therapy when examined by second-look arthroscopy [38]. Positive effects on human chondrocyte proliferation, organization, and cartilage matrix deposition have been demonstrated with the use of ASCs sourced from abdominal lipoaspirate [5].

23.4 Orthobiologic Augmentation of Ligamentous Healing and Ligament Repair

The progression of healing in response to injury of the ACL has been studied using a number of models [41, 42, 47, 48, 49]. After acute rupture of this ligament, there is rapid degeneration of the tissue that is associated with collagenase activity and a decrease in collagen content [41]. This is in contrast to other ligaments such as the medial collateral ligament (MCL), which has a significantly greater potential of healing through increased proliferative and migratory capacity of the reparative cells [47, 48]. The healing response of the ACL is reduced in comparison to other ligaments due to a number of factors, including a deficiency of fibrin clot formation at the site of injury, which leaves the ligamentous fibers disconnected, interfering with cellular migration and tissue reformation [50]. Circulating plasmin within the joint breaks down fibrin clot, and synovial fluid has been associated with inhibition of fibroblast proliferation and migration, further reducing healing potential of the ACL [51, 52].

Although previously attempted surgical treatments to primarily repair the injured ACL were abandoned due to poor outcomes and low rates of return to play, more recent investigations have demonstrated that primary suture repair to reappose the injured ligamentous fibers, augmented with orthobiologic factors such as PRP and bone marrow-derived MSCs, can lead to successful clinical outcomes, with high rates of return to play [31, 33, 34, 53, 54]. Advantages of primary repair with biologic augmentation may be substantial, given the greater potential to preserve native anatomy, proprioception, and joint kinematics.

Growth factors that include TGF-β, FGF2, and bFGF have been shown to regulate cellular proliferation, extracellular matrix deposition, and differentiation of precursor cells into fibroblasts in the setting of ligament injury [21, 36, 42, 46, 64]. The growth factor TGF-β1 has been shown to upregulate collagen synthesis in fibroblasts within both the ACL and MCL [43], and overexpression of FGF-2 has been associated with enhanced healing of human ACL [42]. Properly applied in the clinical setting, these growth factors are of particular interest in augmentation of healing processes that may accelerate return to play in a variety of clinical scenarios, ranging from acute ligament injury to the slowing of chronic degenerative joint changes.

Platelet-rich plasma is known to contain many of these bioactive substances that are capable of influencing all stages of the healing process after injury, by modulating inflammatory responses and directing remodeling of reparative tissue [19, 44]. Intraligamentous application of platelet-derived growth factors into the intact ACL bundle in cases of partial ACL injury has been shown to lead to a high rate of return to sport in a cohort of professional soccer players [57]. In this study by Seijas et al. [57], 18 of 19 players had returned to play at 16 weeks after treatment. Podesta et al. [55] investigated the use of PRP to treat partial ulnar collateral ligament tears of the elbow in athletes and demonstrated return to play in 88% of those treated at an average of 70 weeks after injection [55].

Prospective case series have demonstrated that partial ACL tears can be successfully treated with primary suture repair in conjunction with injection of growth factors in the form of activated PRP, leading to high rates of return to play [25, 27]. After 5 years of follow-up, this treatment effectively restored knee stability and high demand function in a group of 50 young athletes with a mean age of 28.3 years who had presented with acute partial ACL injury. This surgical technique consisted of arthroscopic suturing of the torn ligamentous fibers to approximate the proximal and distal stumps using No. 1 polydioxanone (PDS). A microfracture awl was subsequently used to release marrow elements about the anatomic femoral insertion of the ACL within the intercondylar notch. Approximately 3 cm^3 of PRP was then activated using batroxobin enzyme (Plateltex® act-S.R.O., Bratislava, SK) to create a clot of PRP gel, which was injected about the repair site. This technique has recently been modified, and the use of activated bone marrow aspirate concentrate is now preferred, which is injected about the sutured ligament repair. Second-look arthroscopy was performed in six patients in this series, consistently demonstrating

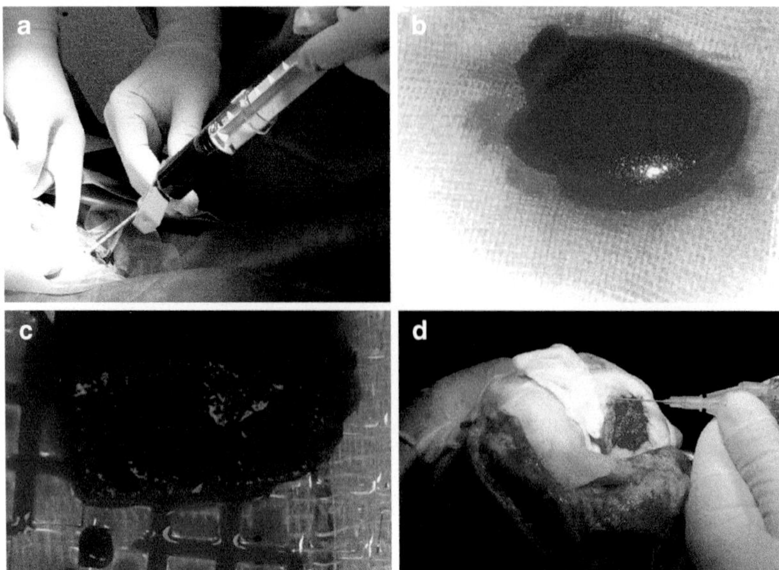

Fig. 23.3 Cartilage repair procedure of the knee using hyaluronic acid-based scaffold embedded with bone marrow aspirate concentrate (HA-BMAC). (**a**) Bone marrow aspiration from iliac crest, (**b**) clot-activated bone marrow aspirate concentrate, (**c**) activated bone marrow aspirate concentrate applied to Hyalofast scaffold (Anika Therapeutics, Italy) to create HA-BMAC graft, (**d**) application of HA-BMAC graft to cartilage lesion of medial femoral condyle of a human knee

healthy appearing, healed ACL fibers that were stable to probing.

Injury to articular cartilage of the knee may lead to significant functional limitation in sports, and orthobiologics are an important component of the treatment algorithm at our institution in order to encourage the restoration of hyaline-like cartilage, with the goal of maximizing rates of return to play. The current approach is to use a hyaluronic acid-based scaffold matrix (Hyalofast, Anika Therapeutics, Italy) embedded with activated bone marrow aspirate concentrate, to create a graft termed HA-BMAC that is used to treat cartilage lesions in the knee of wide ranging size and severity (Fig. 23.3). A prospective trial examining the outcomes of HA-BMAC cartilage repair compared to microfracture demonstrated superior clinical outcomes at 5-year follow-up after treatment with HA-BMAC and also superior rates of return to pre-injury activity levels compared to microfracture. It has also been demonstrated that this orthobiologic therapy of cartilage repair using HA-BMAC may be used successfully in patients, irrespective of age being younger or older than 45 years [28, 29]. Cartilage repair using this technique may be performed arthroscopically in appropriately indicated lesions and also in conjunction with bony inlay in cases of osteochondral injury to restore the osteochondral unit by method of biologic inlay osteochondral reconstruction (BIOR) [56, 62].

Fact Box 2

- Primary repair of partial tears of the anterior cruciate ligament augmented by platelet-rich plasma application has been shown to restore knee stability and enable return to play.
- Cell-based cartilage repair using mesenchymal stem cells sourced from bone marrow aspirate concentrate that are embedded onto hyaluronic acid-based scaffold (HA-BMAC) has been shown to provide successful clinical outcomes after medium-term follow-up of at least 5 years.

23.5 Future Advances in Orthobiologics

There are limitations of current surgical methods used to reconstruct or repair damaged tendons and ligaments, as recreation of normal pre-injury anatomy is often difficult. Engineered tissues containing a variety of scaffolds, cells, and bioactive factors continue to be developed, with the goal of improving the clinical outcomes of these procedures. Scaffolds have been the focus of much attention in the field of tissue engineering, as mechanical support for healing tissues may assist deposition of native matrix by endogenous cells. These matrices have the capacity to improve tendinous and ligamentous healing by enhancing cellular proliferation and migration, matrix deposition, and remodeling of extracellular matrix into functional tissue [61]. Scaffolds can be modified to provide an environment for improved growth factor attachment, cellular hybridization, and cellular remodeling [41]. When combined with scaffolding, biologic isolates such as PRP and MSCs have promising potential to facilitate improved healing after injury. In cases of ACL injury specifically, scaffolding can provide a sequestered microenvironment to protect the repair site from plasmin, potentiating the effects of growth factors and concentrated precursor cells. In vitro research examining collagen hydrogel in association with PRP has demonstrated enhanced ACL cell viability, metabolic activity, and collagen synthesis [17]. In a porcine model, sutured ACL repair supplemented with application of a collagen-platelet composite resulted in superior mechanical properties of the healed ACL [50]. The clinical application of these techniques using orthobiologics in combination with scaffolding or matrices has been relatively limited due to the lack thus far of data analyzed from human subjects, and much is needed in terms of randomized controlled trials to thoroughly elucidate the expected benefits of many of these newly available technologies.

Take Home Message
There is a wide variety of bioactive factors and scaffolding materials that can be used to treat an array of injuries to facilitate and accelerate return to play. Injection of orthobiologic treatments such as platelet-rich plasma and concentrated isolates of mesenchymal stem cells are becoming more widely offered as a therapeutic option for a range of conditions. These treatments contain cellular elements, bioactive proteins, and trophic growth factors that play key regulatory roles in cellular biology and tissue repair. As technology advances, composite materials of supportive scaffolds and bioactive factors will likely advance treatment options for a wide range of soft tissue injuries, enabling more precise recreation of injured anatomic structures and restoration of pre-injury musculoskeletal kinematics, leading to greater rates of return to play at all levels of competition.

Top Five Evidence Based References

Caplan AI (2016) MSCs: the sentinel and safe-guards of injury. J Cell Physiol 231(7):1413–1416

Crisan M, Yap S, Casteilla L, Chen CW, Corselli M, Park TS, Andriolo G, Sun B, Zheng B, Zhang L, Norotte C, Teng PN, Traas J, Schugar R, Deasy BM, Badylak S, Buhring HJ, Giacobino JP, Lazzari L, Huard J, Péault B (2008) A perivascular origin for mesenchymal stem cells in multiple human organs. Cell Stem Cell 3(3):301–313

Filardo G, Kon E, Roffi A, Di Matteo B, Merli ML, Marcacci M (2015) Platelet-rich plasma: why intra-articular? A systematic review of preclinical studies and clinical evidence on PRP for joint degeneration. Knee Surg Sports Traumatol Arthrosc 23(9):2459–2474

Gobbi A, Bathan L, Boldrini L (2009) Primary repair combined with bone marrow stimulation in acute anterior cruciate ligament lesions results in a group of athletes. Am J Sports Med 37(3):571–578

Gobbi A, Whyte GP (2016) One-stage cartilage repair using a hyaluronic acid-based scaffold with activated bone marrow-derived mesenchymal stem cells compared with microfracture: five-year follow-up. Am J Sports Med 44(11):2846–2854

References

1. Andia I, Sanchez M, Maffulli N (2010) Tendon healing and platelet-rich plasma therapies. Expert Opin Biol Ther 10(10):1415–1426
2. Aspenberg P, Forslund C (1999) Enhanced tendon healing with GDF 5 and 6. Acta Orthop Scand 70(1):51–54

3. Black LL, Gaynor J, Adams C, Dhupa S, Sams AE, Taylor R, Harman S, Gingerich DA, Harman R (2007) Effect of intraarticular injection of autologous adipose-derived mesenchymal stem and regenerative cells on clinical signs of chronic osteoarthritis of the elbow joint in dogs. Vet Ther 9(3):192–200
4. Black LL, Gaynor J, Gahring D, Adams C, Aron D, Harman S, Gingerich DA, Harman R (2007) Effect of adipose-derived mesenchymal stem and regenerative cells on lameness in dogs with chronic osteoarthritis of the coxofemoral joints: a randomized, double-blinded, multicenter, controlled trial. Vet Ther 8(4):272–284
5. Bosetti M, Borrone A, Follenzi A, Messaggio F, Tremolada C, Cannas M (2016) Human lipoaspirate as autologous injectable active scaffold for one-step repair of cartilage defects. Cell Transplant 25(6):1043–1056
6. Caplan AI (1991) Mesenchymal stem cells. J Orthop Res 9:641–650
7. Caplan AI (1994) The mesengenic process. Clin Plast Surg 21:429–435
8. Caplan AI (2007) Adult mesenchymal stem cells for tissue engineering versus regenerative medicine. J Cell Physiol 213(2):341–347
9. Caplan AI (2015) Adult mesenchymal stem cells: when, where, and how. Stem Cells Int 2015:628767. https://doi.org/10.1155/2015/628767
10. Caplan AI (2016) MSCs: the sentinel and safe-guards of injury. J Cell Physiol 231(7):1413–1416
11. Caplan AI, Correa D (2011) The MSC: an injury drugstore. Cell Stem Cell 9(1):11–15
12. Chamberlain G, Fox J, Ashton B, Middleton J (2007) Concise review: mesenchymal stem cells: their phenotype, differentiation capacity, immunological features, and potential for homing. Stem Cells 25(11):2739–2749
13. Chen CH (2009) Strategies to enhance tendon graft--bone healing in anterior cruciate ligament reconstruction. Chang Gung Med J 32(5):483–493
14. Chen CH, Cao Y, YF W, Bais AJ, Gao JS, Tang JB (2008) Tendon healing in vivo: gene expression and production of multiple growth factors in early tendon healing period. J Hand Surg [Am] 33(10):1834–1842
15. Chen WC, Corselli M, Péault B, Huard J (2012) Human blood-vessel-derived stem cells for tissue repair and regeneration. J Biomed Biotechnol 2012:597439. https://doi.org/10.1155/2012/597439
16. Chen WC, Péault B, Huard J (2015) Regenerative translation of human blood-vessel-derived MSC precursors. Stem Cells Int 2015:375187. https://doi.org/10.1155/2015/375187
17. Cheng M, Wang H, Yoshida R, Murray MM (2010) Platelets and plasma proteins are both required to stimulate collagen gene expression by anterior cruciate ligament cells in three-dimensional culture. Tissue Eng Part A 16(5):1479–1489
18. Cohen M, Amaro JT, Ejnisman B, Carvalho RT, Nakano KK, Peccin MS, Teixeira R, Laurino CF, Abdalla RJ (2007) Anterior cruciate ligament reconstruction after 10 to 15 years: association between meniscectomy and osteoarthrosis. Arthroscopy 23(6):629–634
19. Cole BJ, Seroyer ST, Filardo G, Bajaj S, Fortier LA (2010) Platelet-rich plasma: where are we now and where are we going? Sports Health 2(3):203–210
20. Crisan M, Yap S, Casteilla L, Chen CW, Corselli M, Park TS, Andriolo G, Sun B, Zheng B, Zhang L, Norotte C, Teng PN, Traas J, Schugar R, Deasy BM, Badylak S, Buhring HJ, Giacobino JP, Lazzari L, Huard J, Péault B (2008) A perivascular origin for mesenchymal stem cells in multiple human organs. Cell Stem Cell 3(3):301–313
21. Date H, Furumatsu T, Sakoma Y, Yoshida A, Hayashi Y, Abe N, Ozaki T (2010) GDF-5/7 and bFGF activate integrin alpha2-mediated cellular migration in rabbit ligament fibroblasts. J Orthop Res 28(2):225–231
22. de Girolamo L, Lucarelli E, Alessandri G, Avanzini MA, Bernardo ME, Biagi E, Brini AT, D'Amico G, Fagioli F, Ferrero I, Locatelli F, Maccario R, Marazzi M, Parolini O, Pessina A, Torre ML, Italian Mesenchymal Stem Cell Group (2013) Mesenchymal stem/stromal cells: a new "cells as drugs" paradigm. Efficacy and critical aspects in cell therapy. Curr Pharm Des 19(13):2459–2473
23. Dohan Ehrenfest DM, Rasmusson L, Albrektsson T (2008) Classification of platelet concentrates: from pure platelet-rich plasma (P-PRP) to leukocyte and platelet-rich fibrin (L-PRF). Trends Biotechnol 27(3):158–167
24. Gimble JM, Guilak F, Nuttall ME, Sathishkumar S, Vidal M, Bunnell BA (2008) In vitro differentiation potential of mesenchymal stem cells. Transfus Med Hemother 35(3):228–238
25. Gobbi A, Bathan L, Boldrini L (2009) Primary repair combined with bone marrow stimulation in acute anterior cruciate ligament lesions results in a group of athletes. Am J Sports Med 37(3):571–578
26. Gobbi A, Karnatzikos G, Mahajan V, Malchira S (2012) Platelet-rich plasma treatment in symptomatic patients with knee osteoarthritis: preliminary results in a group of active patients. Sports Health 4(2):162–172
27. Gobbi A, Karnatzikos G, Sankineani SR, Petrera M (2013) Biological augmentation of ACL refixation in partial lesions in a group of athletes: results at the 5-Year follow-up. Tech Orthopaed 28(2):180–184
28. Gobbi A, Scotti C, Karnatzikos G, Mudhigere A, Castro M, Peretti GM (2017) One-step surgery with multipotent stem cells and Hyaluronan-based scaffold for the treatment of full-thickness chondral defects of the knee in patients older than 45 years. Knee Surg Sports Traumatol Arthrosc 25:2494. https://doi.org/10.1007/s00167-016-3984-6
29. Gobbi A, Whyte GP (2016) One-stage cartilage repair using a hyaluronic acid-based scaffold with activated bone marrow-derived mesenchymal stem cells compared with microfracture: five-year follow-up. Am J Sports Med 44(11):2846–2854

30. Jackson L, Jones DR, Scotting P, Sottile V (2007) Adult mesenchymal stem cells: differentiation potential and therapeutic applications. J Postgrad Med 53(2):121–127
31. Kaplan N, Wickiewicz TL, Warren RF (1990) Primary surgical treatment of anterior cruciate ligament ruptures. A long-term follow-up study. Am J Sports Med 18(4):354–358
32. Kean TJ, Lin P, Caplan AI, Dennis JE (2013) MSCs: delivery routes and engraftment, cell-targeting strategies, and immune modulation. Stem Cells Int 2013:732742. https://doi.org/10.1155/2013/732742
33. Kiapour AM, Murray MM (2014) Basic science of anterior cruciate ligament injury and repair. Bone Joint Res 3(2):20–31
34. Kim S, Bosque J, Meehan JP, Jamali A, Marder R (2011) Increase in outpatient knee arthroscopy in the United States: a comparison of National Surveys of Ambulatory Surgery, 1996 and 2006. J Bone Joint Surg Am 93(11):994–1000
35. Kobayashi D, Kurosaka M, Yoshiya S, Mizuno K (1997) Effect of basic fibroblast growth factor on the healing of defects in the canine anterior cruciate ligament. Knee Surg Sports Traumatol Arthrosc 5(3):189–194
36. Kobayashi M, Itoi E, Minagawa H, Miyakoshi N, Takahashi S, Tuoheti Y, Okada K, Shimada Y (2006) Expression of growth factors in the early phase of supraspinatus tendon healing in rabbits. J Shoulder Elbow Surg 15(3):371–377
37. Koh YG, Choi YJ (2012) Infrapatellar fat pad-derived mesenchymal stem cell therapy for knee osteoarthritis. Knee 19(6):902–907
38. Koh YG, Jo SB, Kwon OR, Suh DS, Lee SW, Park SH, Choi YJ (2013) Mesenchymal stem cell injections improve symptoms of knee osteoarthritis. Arthroscopy 29(4):748–755
39. Lee AY, Lee J, Kim CL, Lee KS, Lee SH, NY G, Kim JM, Lee BC, Koo OJ, Song JY, Cha SH (2015) Comparative studies on proliferation, molecular markers and differentiation potential of mesenchymal stem cells from various tissues (adipose, bone marrow, ear skin, abdominal skin, and lung) and maintenance of multipotency during serial passages in miniature pig. Res Vet Sci 100:115–124
40. Liu CF, Aschbacher-Smith L, Barthelery NJ, Dyment N, Butler D, Wylie C (2011) What we should know before using tissue engineering techniques to repair injured tendons: a developmental biology perspective. Tissue Eng Part B Rev 17(3):165–176
41. Lohmander LS, Englund PM, Dahl LL, Roos EM (2007) The long-term consequence of anterior cruciate ligament and meniscus injuries: osteoarthritis. Am J Sports Med 35(10):1756–1769
42. Madry H, Kohn D, Cucchiarini M (2013) Direct FGF-2 gene transfer via recombinant adeno-associated virus vectors stimulates cell proliferation, collagen production, and the repair of experimental lesions in the human ACL. Am J Sports Med 41(1):194–202
43. Marui T, Niyibizi C, Georgescu HI, Cao M, Kavalkovich KW, Levine RE, Woo SL (1997) Effect of growth factors on matrix synthesis by ligament fibroblasts. J Orthop Res 15(1):18–23
44. Mishra A, Woodall J, Vieira A (2009) Treatment of tendon and muscle using platelet-rich plasma. Clin Sports Med 28(1):113–125
45. Molloy T, Wang Y, Murrell GAC (2003) The roles of growth factors in tendon and ligament healing. Sports Med 33(5):381–394
46. Muller B, Bowman KF, Bedi A (2013) ACL graft healing and biologics. Clin Sports Med 32(1):93–109
47. Murray MM, Fleming BC (2013) Biology of anterior cruciate ligament injury and repair: kappa delta ann doner vaughn award paper 2013. J Orthop Res 31(10):1501–1506
48. Murray MM, Martin SD, Martin TL, Spector M (2000) Histological changes in the human anterior cruciate ligament after rupture. J Bone Joint Surg Am 82:1387–1397
49. Murray MM, Palmer M, Abreu E, Spindler KP, Zurakowski D, Fleming BC (2009) Platelet-rich plasma alone is not sufficient to enhance suture repair of the ACL in skeletally immature animals: an in vivo study. J Orthop Res 27(5):639–645
50. Murray MM, Spindler KP, Abreu E, Muller JA, Nedder A, Kelly M, Frino J, Zurakowski D, Valenza M, Snyder BD, Conolly SA (2007) Collagen-platelet rich plasma hydrogel enhances primary repair of the porcine anterior cruciate ligament. J Orthop Res 25(1):81–91
51. Nagineni CN, Amiel D, Green MH, Berchuck M, Akeson WH (1992) Characterization of the intrinsic properties of the anterior cruciate and medial collateral ligament cells: an in vitro cell culture study. J Orthop Res 10(4):465–475
52. Nakase J, Tsuchiya H, Kitaoka K (2012) Contralateral anterior cruciate ligament injury after anterior cruciate ligament reconstruction: a case controlled study. Sports Med Arthrosc Rehabil Ther Technol 4(1):46
53. Nishimoto S, Oyama T, Matsuda K (2007) Simultaneous concentration of platelets and marrow cells: a simple and useful technique to obtain source cells and growth factors for regenerative medicine. Wound Repair Regen 15(1):156–162
54. Noyes FR, Mooar LA, Moorman CT III, McGinniss GH (1989) Partial tears of the anterior cruciate ligament. Progression to complete ligament deficiency. J Bone Joint Surg Br 71(5):825–833
55. Podesta L, Crow SA, Volkmer D, Bert T, Yocum LA (2013) Treatment of partial ulnar collateral ligament tears in the elbow with platelet-rich plasma. Am J Sports Med 41(7):1689–1694
56. Sadlik B, Gobbi A, Puszkarz M, Klon W, Whyte GP (2017) Biologic inlay osteochondral reconstruction: arthroscopic one-step osteochondral lesion repair in the knee Using morselized bone grafting and hyaluronic acid-based scaffold embedded with bone marrow aspirate concentrate. Arthrosc Tech 6:e383. https://doi.org/10.1016/j.eats.2016.10.023

57. Seijas R, Ares O, Cusco X, Alvarez P, Steinbacher G, Cugat R (2014) Partial anterior cruciate ligament tears treated with intraligamentary plasma rich in growth factors. World J Orthop 5(3):373–378
58. Toghraie FS, Chenari N, Gholipour MA, Faghih Z, Torabinejad S, Dehghani S, Ghaderi A (2011) Treatment of osteoarthritis with infrapatellar fat pad derived mesenchymal stem cells in Rabbit. Knee 18(2):71–75
59. Toghraie FS, Razmkhah M, Gholipour MA, Faghih Z, Chenari N, Torabi Nezhad S, Nazhvani Dehghani S, Ghaderi A (2012) Scaffold-free adipose-derived stem cells (ASCs) improve experimentally induced osteoarthritis in rabbits. Arch Iran Med 15(8):495–499
60. Ude CC, Sulaiman SB, Min-Hwei N, Hui-Cheng C, Ahmad J, Yahaya NM, Saim AB, Idrus RB (2014) Cartilage regeneration by chondrogenic induced adult stem cells in osteoarthritic sheep model. PLoS One 9(6):e98770
61. Vavken P, Murray MM (2009) Translational Studies in ACL repair. Tissue Eng Part B 16(1):5–11
62. Whyte GP, Gobbi A, Sadlik B (2016) Dry arthroscopic single-stage cartilage repair of the knee using a hyaluronic acid-based scaffold with activated bone marrow-derived mesenchymal stem cells (HA-BMAC). Arthrosc Tech 5(4):e913–e918
63. Wurgler-Hauri CC, Dourte LM, Baradet TC, Williams GR, Soslowsky LJ (2007) Temporal expression of 8 growth factors in tendon-to-bone healing in a rat supraspinatus model. J Shoulder Elbow Surg 16(5):198S–203S
64. Xie J, Wang C, Huang DY, Zhang Y, Xu J, Kolesnikov SS, Sung KP, Zhao H (2013) TGF-beta1 induces the different expressions of lysyl oxidases and matrix metalloproteinases in anterior cruciate ligament and medial collateral ligament fibroblasts after mechanical injury. J Biomech 46(5):890–898

Part IV

Joint Specific Return to Play Recommendations

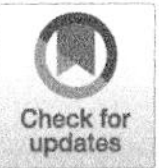

Return to Play in Football: Diagnosis, Treatment, Rehabilitation and Prevention of Spinal Injuries

24

Adad Baranto

Contents

A. Baranto
Department of Orthopaedics, Institute of Clinical Sciences at the Sahlgrenska Academy, University of Gothenburg, Gothenburg, Sweden

Sahlgrenska University Hospital, Brunastråket 11, 413 45, Gothenburg, Sweden
e-mail: adad.baranto@vgregion.se

V. Musahl et al. (eds.), *Return to Play in Football*, https://doi.org/10.1007/978-3-662-55713-6_24

Abbreviations

ACDF	Anterior cervical decompression and fusion
ALIF	Anterior lumbar interbody fusion
DDD	Degenerative disc disease
DH	Disc hernia
CDH	Cervical disc herniation
CT	Computed tomography
CTO	Cervicothoracic orthosis
FJS	Facet joint syndrome
HIZ	High intensity zones
LLIF	Lateral lumbar interbody fusion
LBP	Low back pain
LDH	Lumbar disc hernia
MRI	Magnetic resonance tomography
RTP	Return to play
ROM	Range of motion
SPECT	Single photon emission computed tomography
SCI	Spinal cord injury
SCC	Spinal cord concussion
SCN	Spinal cord neurapraxia
TDR	Total disc replacement
TLIF	Transforaminal lumbar interbody fusion

24.1 The Cervical Spine

24.1.1 Cervical Strains and Sprains

Fact Box 1

Strains and sprains cause injuries to the ligaments and muscles.

There is a lack of prevalence of soft tissue injuries of cervical spine. In case of suspicion of instability, clinical examination and radiological investigation are mandatory.

The treatment is conservative. Return to play is recommended if the athlete is pain-free and has a normal ROM.

Soft tissue injuries in the cervical spine generally include a ligamentum sprain or muscle strain in the supportive structures of the cervical spine. The injuries are often of mild character and with short duration. There is no information regarding the prevalence or incidence reported in the literature.

One critical issue is to evaluate if the athlete's cervical spine is unstable after an injury due to ligament or disc disruption. This is especially difficult in young athletes where ligament laxity is more common as a normal variant. Therefore a complete and thorough clinical examination is important. If there is a suspicion of instability, magnetic resonance tomography (MRI) is the most sensitive method to diagnose ligament injuries. Also flexion and extension plain X-ray can be a diagnostic option.

24.1.2 Treatment

The usual treatment is refraining from sports, pain killers and physiotherapy. Return to play is recommended when the athlete is pain-free and has a normal range of motion. In case of instability, confirmed by MRI or flexion/extension X-ray, the athlete should be treated with hard cervical collar during 6–10 weeks, depending on the severity of the injury and the athlete's age. After the immobilization the athlete should be treated with physiotherapy and return to play with recommendation as mentioned above, according to the described four general criteria.

Fact Box 2
The prevalence of CDH is not known.
The most affected levels are C5–C7.
Initial treatment is conservative.
ACDF is golden standard for surgical treatment of CDH.

24.2 Cervical Disc Herniation

The prevalence for cervical disc degeneration in football is not clear. A few studies have shown that the incidence of disc degeneration is increased in sports such as diving, rugby and wrestling.

Cervical disc herniation (CDH) accounts for 6% of spinal injuries and is responsible for a median of 69 days missed per incident (Fig. 24.1a).

Natural history and pathology of cervical disc herniation are well known in the general population, but however this is not well known in elite athletes. The most prevalent level of disc pathology in general population is in the lower levels, C5–C7, but in athletes with contact sports as American football, the upper cervical spine, C2–C4, is the most frequent level. The athletes are of a younger age and CDH is associated with sports-related trauma in 82% [5].

24.2.1 Treatment

Treatment of CDH is conservative with painkillers and physiotherapy. In patients who are not healed conservatively, surgery is required. Anterior cervical decompression and fusion (ACDF) has the best evidence and is "golden standard" for disc hernia surgery (Fig. 24.1b).

Fact Box 3
Recommendations for RTP are based on case series and expert opinions.
RTP is possible when the athlete meets the general recommendations.
Seventy-six percent of athletes RTP in 3–12 months.

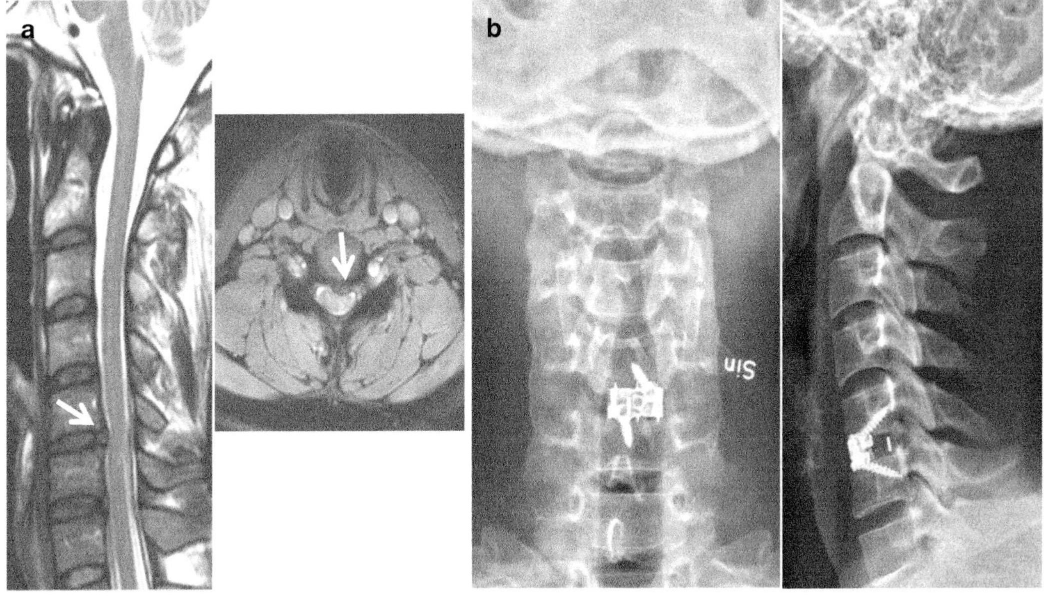

Fig. 24.1 (**a**) 31-year-old male with DH at C5–C6 level on the left side on MRI, T2 image. (**b**) 31-year-old male treated with ACDF at C5–C6 level. The disc bulging on C6–C7 is central and not symptomatic

Table 24.1 There are some recommendations in the literature regarding contraindications for returning to football play

Contraindications for returning to soccer play				
Relative	ACDF in more than 2–3 levels disc levels	ACDF on C2–C3 or C3–C4 levels	Subluxation without a safe stability of the neck	
Absolute	Myelopathy or radiculopathy	Painful stiff neck or malposition of the neck	Three or more fusioned levels	Significant central spinal stenosis

24.2.2 Return to Play

There are at present no studies on football players with cervical disc herniation who describe return to sporting activity. The recommendations are based on studies of other sports. Standard criteria for return to play after spinal surgery do not exist, especially for the football player. Therefore, the decision to clear an athlete to return to play after cervical spine surgery still remains controversial [6]. Previous studies have published guidelines for return to play after spine surgery, but their conclusions are obtained largely from case series, expert opinions and experience, rather than scientific evidence. Most authors agree that athletes who return to contact sports after spinal surgery should be asymptomatic and have stable spine with normal neurological function and range of motion. There must also be adequate space for the neural elements and adequate space for the spinal cord and nerve roots.

Return to sports requires stability of the neck, especially in collision and high-velocity sports. Success for return to competitive sports is well described after single-level ACDF due to disc herniation, but outcomes involving other cervical spinal diagnoses and surgical procedures, such as total disc replacement, still remain unclear. The time to return to the same activity level as pre-injury is not established in the literature for football players, but there are some studies on other sports that the players return to the same activity level between 3 and 12 months. Segall 2014 reported on recreational football players ($n = 14$) with cervical disc herniation that 76% of the players returned to play after approximately 3–12 months.

There are some recommendations in the literature regarding contraindications for returning to football play (Table 24.1).

Fact Box 4

Stingers or burners are common in contact sports.

Occurs due to contusion of the nerve root or brachial plexus.

The symptoms last for seconds or minutes.

The usual treatment is conservative.

24.3 Paresthesia

Paresthesia or stingers or burners are common in 30–50% of the American football players, but the incidence in football players is however not clear. They affect one arm and the injury is to the nerve root or the brachial plexus. The injury mechanism is contusion of the shoulder causing impingement of the nerve root or traction of the brachial plexus due to extension and lateral flexion of the neck. The symptoms are pain, burning and tingling down an arm and with or without transient weakness that lasts for seconds or minutes. The players are advised to return to play as soon as the symptoms have settled down. Multiple episodes require further investigation and in rare cases surgery.

24.3.1 Treatment

The nonoperative, nonsurgical treatment is symptomatic and supportive physiotherapy. Surgical treatment may be required if multiple episodes of cervical spine trauma, persistent radiculopathy signs or motor deficit. The surgical options are foraminotomy or ADCF at the affected level.

24.4 Cervical Spinal Cord Neurapraxia

Spinal cord neurapraxia or concussion (SCN/SCC) is a transient neurological deficit in more than one limb that may occur in association with sports. Tarvi et al. found in American football players an incidence of transitory paresis and paresthesias of 1.3 per 10,000 participants, and the incidence of numbness and tingling was 6.0 per 10,000 participants. The pathophysiology of SCC combines submaximal elastic stretching of the spinal cord, transient abnormality of membrane permeability and an influx of calcium without anatomic disruption that allow a complete recovery of neurological function. SCC is common in more than 80% of American football players, but athletes in other sports, such as rugby, ice hockey, basketball and soccer, are also at a risk. SCC can occur in athletes who have stenosis of the cervical spinal column, age-related degenerative changes, disc herniation or congenital abnormalities. In adults the injury is strongly related to cervical central canal stenosis (93%), while in children or in adolescents, it is related to hypermobility.

The injury mechanism is hyperextension, hyperflexion or axial load to the cervical spine. Repeated episodes of neurapraxia in adult athletes are common in 56%. The risk of recurrence is inversely related to central canal size.

The symptoms last between 15 min and 48 h and are completely reversed. The symptoms are typically burning pain, tingling, numbness and loss of sensation and may also include motor weakness and complete paralysis.

The investigation is done with the clinical examination, MRI and sometimes dynamic MRI, flexion-extension X-ray and CT if fracture is suspected [7].

24.4.1 Treatment and Returning to Sports

The treatment of SCC is conservative. However, there is still controversy whether the athlete should return to play or not. Some authors recommend that patients with SCC with central cervical stenosis can return to contact sports, where others advise from returning to sports due to the high risk of spinal cord injury [8].

If the radiological investigations do not show evidence of spinal cord injury, bony or ligament injuries—including no central spinal stenosis—then return to sports is safely advised. If the athlete has a recurrent episode of neurapraxia, further investigation is required and the recommendations may be not to engage further in athletic activity through contact or collision sports.

Fact Box 5

The symptoms are burning pain, tingling, numbness or loss of sensation, motor weakness and paralysis.

Investigation is clinically, with X-ray, CT and MRI.

Treatment is conservative.

RTP is possible when the athlete meets the general criteria.

Fact Box 6

Surgical treatment is with ACDF or posterior fixation and fusion including laminectomy. RTP is not possible in the majority of cases.

Completely recovered athletes who meet the general criteria can return to their previous sports.

24.5 Spinal Cord Injury

Spinal cord injury (SCI) is a rare but catastrophic injury for the athlete when it occurs. SCI occurs in athletes in contact sports due to central canal stenosis in adult athletes and due to hypermobility in adolescent athletes. The incidence and prevalence are not known. Athletes who develop SCI have a duration of symptoms more than 24 h [7–9].

Fact Box 7

SCI is a catastrophic injury.

In young athletes it is due to hypermobility and in adult athletes due to spinal canal stenosis.

The diagnosis is by CT and MRI.

24.5.1 Diagnosis and Treatment

Investigation of athletes with SCI is done with CT and MRI. To prevent permanent spinal cord injury, athletes with subluxation should be put in traction as soon as possible.

Treatment of SCI is early surgery with decompression and fusion. The procedure can be performed anteriorly, such as ACDF, or posteriorly due to the pathology. If MRI verifies medullar compression, surgical treatment is recommended as soon as possible. There are no specific studies on the timing of surgery, but several studies published in the past years recommend surgery as soon as possible. Van Middendorp et al. have found in a systematic review including 18 studies that early surgery was significantly associated with high motor function recovery [10].

Fact Box 8

SCC is a transient neurological deficit in more than one limb.

It's caused by hyperextension, hyperflexion or axial load to the C-spine.

The symptoms last 15 min to 48 h.

24.5.2 Returning to Football

Regarding return to sports of athletes with SCI injury, recommendations in the literature are not found. Recommendations are based on experience, such as if the athlete's neurological deficits are completely recovered and with a stable neck fixation, then the athlete can return to his/her previous sport. Nonetheless, it should be noted that this is just a recommendation without any scientific evidence.

24.6 Fractures of the Cervical Spine

24.6.1 Aetiology and Injury Mechanism

Injuries to the cervical spine, causing fractures, are usually caused by diving, road accidents and sports. The cervical spine of children, especially <10 years, is sensitive for injuries due to the ligaments' laxity. Brown et al. [11] reported in a study of cervical spine injuries in children that 27% were due to sports. American football injuries accounted for 29% of all sports-related cervical spine injuries. There are no studies reporting the specific incidence or prevalence of cervical spine injuries in athletes and especially in football players.

The classification of cervical spine fractures is according to AOSpine classification system, described by Vaccaro et al. [12]. Cervical spine fractures can be divided to the upper cervical spine (occiput to C2) and the lower cervical spine (C3–C7) due to the different injury mechanism and management.

24.6.1.1 Atlanto Occipital Luxation

Atlanto occipital luxation is rare injury. Eight percent of all of these injuries lead to mortality. These injuries account for 1–3% of all cervical fractures. The diagnosis is very difficult because it is a ligamentous injury. The treatment is posterior fixation and fusion of the occiput with C2.

24.6.1.2 Occipital Condyle Fractures

Occipital condyle fractures are also very unusual and are associated always with skull fractures. The treatment is usually with hard collar or severe cases with fracture dislocation with halo-vest.

C1 Fractures

C1 fractures are caused by axial load. The frequency in athletes is not known. The treatment is with stiff collar or cervicothoracic orthosis (CTO) or, in dislocated cases, with halo-vest. They can also be treated with transfacetal C1–C2 screw fixation.

C2 Fractures

The prevalence of dens fractures in athletes is not known. The treatment depends on the severity of the fracture. If the fracture is not dislocated, it can be treated with a stiff collar. Dislocated fractures can be treated with halo-vest, anterior screw fixation and posterior screw or hook fixation of C1–C2.

C2 Hangman Fractures

Hangman fractures of C2 are caused by hyperflexion injuries. The treatment is due to the severity of the fracture. Non-dislocated fractures can be treated with a hard collar and dislocated fractures with halo-vest and posterior screw fixation of C1–C2 or C1–C3.

C3–C7 Fractures

Fractures of the lower cervical spine are classified according AOSpine and are divided in type A (compression injuries), type B (flexion/extension and distraction injuries) and type C (rotation injuries) [12]. Luxation in the facet joints with or without fractures is very common. The injury mechanism is flexion with rotation (Fig. 24.2a, b).

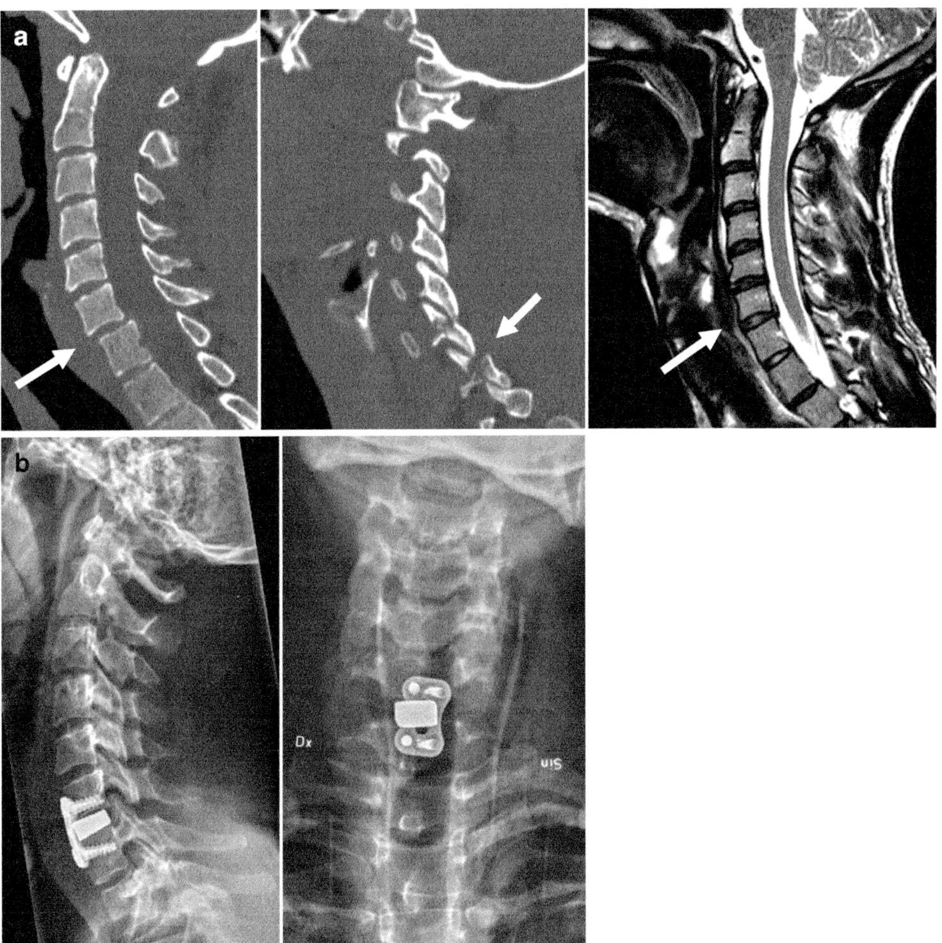

Fig. 24.2 (**a**) 32-year-old elite football player that had a head collision with another player and got fracture luxation C6–7. (*a*) CT shows slit dislocation of C6. (*b*) CT shows fracture unilateral fracture with luxation. (*c*) MRI shows disruption of the posterior annulus fibrosis on the C6–C7 disc with slit protrusion of disc material. (**b**) Postoperative pictures of the player (**a**) treated surgically with ACDF

Fact Box 9
Fractures of the C-spine are not common among football players.

Fractures of the upper cervical spine from occiput to C2 are rare.

Fractures of the lower C-spine are more common in athletes.

The treatment is with collar or surgery, due to the severity of the fracture.

RTP is allowed when the athletes meets the general criteria.

24.6.2 Treatment

Treatment of low cervical fractures depends on the severity and grade of dislocation. In case with facet joint luxation, reposition in traction is mandatory until the fracture is treated surgically either with halo-vest, ACDF or posterior fixation and fusion. Decompression is always mandatory in these cases. In athletes who are supposed to return to their sports, halo-vest is not recommended as a treatment option. In athletes who are supposed to RTP, stable fixation either with anterior or posterior fixation is mandatory. Anterior surgery is to prefer. In severe cases with luxation of the whole C-spine with spinal cord injury, anterior and posterior fixation is mandatory.

24.6.3 Return to Play

There are no specific guidelines regarding returning to play after C-fracture injuries in football players. The recommendation is the same as previously described for other cervical spinal injuries. Detailed indications and contraindications regarding RTP after cervical fractures treated with surgery are found in Table 24.1.

24.7 The Thoracolumbar Spine

24.7.1 The Thoracic Spine

There are no reported guidelines for return to play after injuries to the thoracic spine in contrast to the cervical and lumbar spine. Injuries to the thoracic spine are much less common due to its relative immobility compared to other spinal regions and the protection provided by the rib cage. Symptomatic disc hernia and spinal stenosis are less common in athletes in the thoracic spine due to the large spinal canal diameter. Athletes with pathology in the thoracic spine can return to play when they met the general criteria after conservative or surgical treatment.

24.8 The Lumbar Spine

24.8.1 Low Back Pain

The human disc is a very complex structure that undergoes extensive degenerative changes with age. The proteoglycan content of the nucleus pulposus decreases, proteoglycan aggregation decreases and proteoglycans become smaller [13]. This loss of proteoglycans in the nucleus is associated with degenerative changes in the disc [14–16]. This is assumed to lead to a reduction in the ability of the nucleus to remain hydrated. Dehydration of the disc increases and the disc becomes stiffer, less elastic and less able to accommodate a normal range of movements.

The lumbar spine of athletes usually performs demanding and extreme tasks without problems. But the poor condition puts the athlete at great risk for back injury and pain.

One of the most common reasons for missed playing time by professional athletes is pain and dysfunction of the lumbar spine. Studies have also reported that LBP in many cases was significant enough to interfere with training and competition [1].

Fact Box 10
The lifetime prevalence of LBP in athletes is 1–94%.

In football players the prevalence is 36%.

Treatment of LBP is conservative.

Fact Box 11
Injuries and pathologies in the thoracic spine are rare in athletes.

There are no guidelines for return to sports after injuries in the thoracic spine.

24.8.2 Aetiology

The epidemiology is multifactorial, and there are several risk factors such as obesity, age, previous LBP, trauma, heavy loads, depression, smoking, physical inactivity, sports with heavy loads on the spine and dissatisfaction with job [17–22]. In the past few years, heredity has been suggested to play a dominant role in explaining the variability in disc degeneration. Several of the anatomical structures in the back can cause LBP, such as the discs, the facet joints, muscles and soft tissue. In the last decades, degenerative disc disease (DDD) has been one of the main reasons for chronic LBP [22, 23]. Segmental disc degeneration or instability without olisthesis can cause chronic LBP, and the pain is thought to be discogenic due to DDD. Several studies have shown higher frequencies (up to 65%) of intervertebral disc degeneration among young athletes in sports imposing heavy demands on the back, when compared with other athletes and nonathletes [18, 24]. Baranto et al. found that disc degeneration in young divers could be related to acute spinal injuries occurring during the pubertal growth spurt early in the athletic career [25]. The results of this and previous studies suggest that degenerative changes are common among young elite athletes and that trauma to the thoracolumbar spine during the growth spurt is harmful [24, 26–28].

When the disc is degenerated, this affects the facet joints, and this initiates degeneration due to the altered loads. Arthrosis starts in the facet joints, and this changes the biomechanics and also the orientation (of facets?), known as tropism. During the last decades, there is some evidence that high intensity zones (HIZ) and inflammatory reactions in the endplates, so-called Modic changes, seen on MRI can cause chronic LBP.

24.8.3 Prevalence

Several studies have reported prevalence of LBP in athletes from 1% to 90%, which is influenced by the type of sports, gender, training intensity, frequency and technique [4, 25, 29, 30]. There are unfortunately no studies on the prevalence or incidence of LBP in football players, but there are several studies reporting in other sports. The lifetime prevalence of LBP in wrestlers has been reported to 59%, significantly higher than that of an age-matched control group (31%). A significantly higher frequency of LBP has also been reported in elite gymnasts (79%) than in controls (37%) [31]. In a prospective study of 134 former top athletes with mean age 33.2 years, it was found that wrestlers had the highest frequency of severe LBP (54%) as compared to tennis players (32%), football players (36%), gymnasts (29%) and nonathletes (32%) [21]. LBP has also been reported to be more frequent among cross-country skiers (63%) and rowers (55%) than orienteerers (49%) and a control group of nonathletes (47%) [32].

24.9 Muscle, Ligament or Tendon Injuries in the Low Back

Muscle strains and sprains are reported in the literature to be a common cause of acute LBP in athletes, but the exact prevalence is not completely known. In a study of muscle-tendon strain as a cause of LBP in young athletes and the general adult population, it was found that only 6% of the adolescent athletes were diagnosed with muscle-tendon strain compared with 27% of the adults [33, 34].

Muscle damage causes strain with the loss of fibres within the muscle belly or myotendinous junction. This is usually associated with painful muscular spasm. Sprains, on the other hand, involve damage to spinal ligaments.

24.9.1 Diagnosis

Both muscle strains and ligamentous sprains can usually not be diagnosed with radiographic examination, and the diagnosis is therefore made by anamnesis and clinical examination. Moderate and severe muscle injuries can be detected with MRI or ultrasound.

24.9.2 Treatment

The athletes with LBP complaints can resolve within a few weeks. The treatment is conservative with analgetics (anti-inflammatory medication, NSAID), absence from sports and physiotherapy. When tolerated, the player can progressively return to sporting activities. Pain should be used as a guide for advancing activity levels, and the general criteria should be met before athletes can return to competition.

24.10 Acute Low Back Pain

Acute lumbago or acute LBP is pain in the lower back with a duration of <6 weeks. Acute LBP is one of the most common reasons for patients visiting primary health care. More than 80% of the adult population will have back pain during their lifetime, but despite this the specific cause is not always completely known.

The 1-year incidence of first episode of LBP is 6.3–15.5%, while the 1-year incidence of second episode of acute LBP is between 1.5% and 36% [35]. Several studies have reported LBP prevalence of 20–30%, 1-year prevalence of 65% and lifetime prevalence of 84% the adult population [36]. The highest age for suffering of acute LBP is between 45 and 65 years of age. LBP is more common in athletes, and several studies have shown a lifetime prevalence up to 91%. The exact prevalence and incidence in football players are not completely known. LBP is the third most common injury in football, and some studies have reported a 36% prevalence, with a prevalence of 14% in young players [25, 37].

Fact Box 12
The risk factors are obesity, age, trauma, heavy loads, depression, smoking, physical activity and sports.

Heredity is a dominant risk factor.

LBP can be caused by injury or pathology to the disc, facet joints, muscles and soft tissue.

DDD is the most common reason for LBP.

24.10.1 Symptoms

Acute LBP starts in situations where the lower back is in poor muscular defence such as in lifting, coughing/sneezing or sudden movements. The most pathological movement is flexion with rotation. The patient has some stiffness, loss of motion, spasms of the paravertebral musculature and analgetic scoliosis. Sometimes the pain can radiate to the buttocks or to proximal thigs and groins.

24.10.2 Diagnosis

The diagnosis is made by clinical examination with inspection, range of motion of the spine and also complete neurological status of the lower extremities.

24.10.3 Radiology

Radiological investigation is not necessary in the first month. In athletes with a pain duration more than 3–4 weeks or if they have radiating pain, radiological investigation is mandatory. The radiological investigation should be earlier than in the general population. The athletes are at higher risks of spinal injuries, and they are also body dependent to be able to continue train and compete. Therefore, they have to be checked and also treated as soon as possible in order to safely shorten the time to return to play.

Fact Box 13
The symptoms are stiffness, loss of motion, spasm of spinal muscles and analgesic scoliosis.

Radiological examination is mandatory if the athlete's pain lasts more than 1 month.

The treatment is conservative with physiotherapy and pain killers.

Ninety percent of the athletes are pain-free within 3 months.

RTP is allowed when the athlete meets the general criteria.

24.10.4 Treatment

The treatment of LBP is conservative with pain killers and physiotherapy. It's important to rehabilitate the athletes as soon as possible to shorten the absence from training and competition. There should be no restrictions in daily living or exercise movements. In the beginning when the athletes have severe pain, they should not train or play games, but as soon as the pain has decreased, they can start to train beside the rehabilitation, and when they no longer are in pain, they can return to playing games. Surgical treatment is not indicated in players with acute LBP.

24.10.5 Prognosis

The prognosis is very good, where 60% of the patients are pain-free within 2 weeks and 90% in 3 months. There is unfortunately a lack of knowledge regarding whether football players can return to training and competition, but for the general population 60% of the patients can return to work in 1 month and 90% within 3 months. The athletes are allowed to RTP when they meet the general criteria.

24.11 Chronic Low Back Pain

Chronic LBP, non-specific LBP, segmental disc degeneration or instability or degenerative disc disease (DDD) is defined as LBP more than 3 months. Chronic LBP is very common, and the prevalence in the general population is between 5% and 10%. It usually affects individuals younger than 30 years of age, but the highest prevalence is between 40 and 50 years of age. Approximately 10% of the patients with acute LBP will develop chronic LBP.

24.11.1 Symptoms

The symptoms are stiffness and weakness of the lower back. The patients have pain, tiredness and stiffness in the back, spasms of the paravertebral musculature and sometimes radiating pain to the buttocks. The pain is of sharp or stabbing character. The pain can also radiate to the legs. The pain is aggravated by sitting, standing and walking or lifting and rotating movements. The patients have severe difficulties to rise from sitting, lying or flexion. The patients also have pain while lying in the bed for long time.

24.11.2 Diagnosis

The diagnosis of LBP is made by clinical examination of the lumbar spine and neurological examination of the lower extremities. The patient may have structural or pain-mediated scoliosis, decreased lumbar lordosis and contracted spinal muscles. The patients have difficulties with all movements of the spine, especially flexion, extension and rotation.

Fact Box 14

The prevalence of chronic LBP is 5–10%.

The most common cause is DDD.

Ten percent of athletes with acute LBP will develop a chronic LBP.

The symptoms are stiffness, weakness, pain and spasm in the lower bavck.

The diagnosis clinically and radiologically.

24.11.3 Radiology

Radiological investigation of these patients is mandatory. X-ray is the primary radiological investigation to show absence of spondylolysis, apophyseal injuries in young athletes, DDD and arthrosis in the facet joints. Sometimes CT is mandatory, if X-ray doesn't show any pathologies. MRI is mandatory to confirm early pathologies such as DDD, disc hernia and stress reaction of pars interarticularis.

24.11.4 Treatment

The initial treatment of DDD is conservative with pain killers and rehabilitation. A rehabilitation programme lasting for at least 6 months

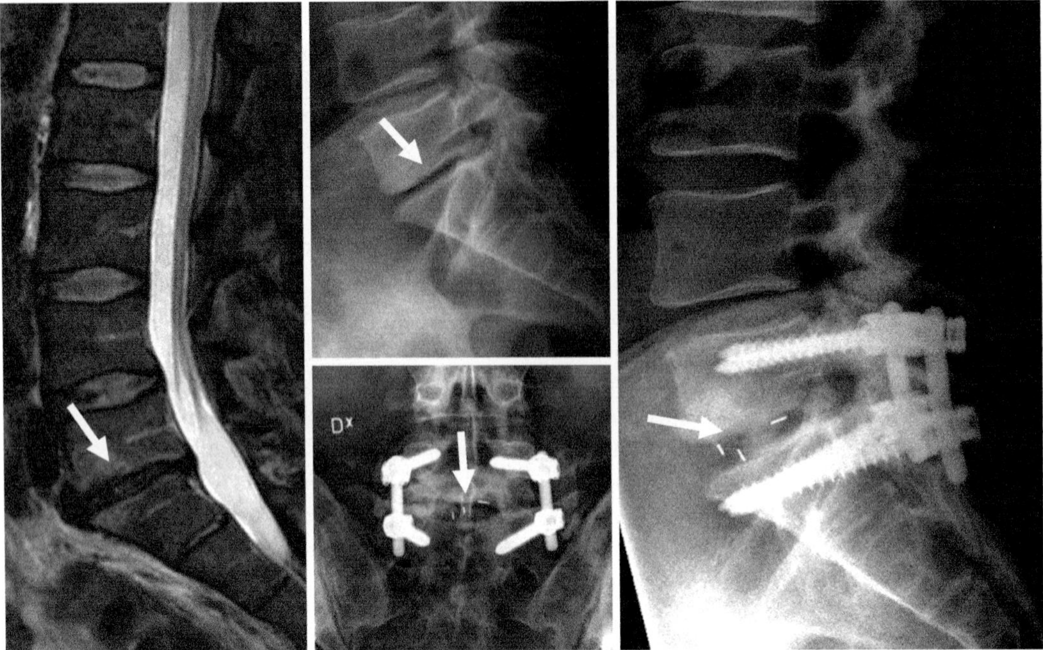

Fig. 24.3 A 35-year-old male with DDD on L5-S1 on MRI and X-ray. He is treated with TLIF. The intercorporal cage is of PEEC material, and therefore only the titanium markers are visible

is mandatory to improve the motions in the lower spine, restore the sagittal balance and also strengthen the muscles of the back. If the patient or the player doesn't get better with conservative therapy, surgical intervention can be the next step.

Fusion and fixation surgery of patients with LBP is still controversial, due to the poor scientific evidence. There are some studies showing good results of 63–70% in patients who have undergone fusion and fixation. Indication for fusion surgery of the lower spine is preserved for one or two affected disc levels. There are several randomized studies comparing fusion with conservative therapy, and there is no significant difference between these two methods, except that the surgical intervention has higher risk for complications [38].

There are several surgical techniques to perform fusion of the lower spine. Posterior fusion and fixation has during the last decades been the golden standard. The technique is fixation with pedicle screws and posterolateral fusion with bone allograft. Transforaminal lumbar interbody fusion (TLIF) has during the last decade proven to be a better fusion technique for better fusion, but it also recreates a better lumbar lordosis restauration (Fig. 24.3). During the last decade, anterior surgery has again been popular, and this can be performed with anterior lumbar interbody fusion (ALIF) or lateral lumbar interbody fusion (LLIF) (Fig. 24.4). In younger patients preservation of the range of motion of the lumbar spine is an appealing treatment option. This is done with a total disc replacement (TDR) or arthroplasty with anterior or lateral technique. The main aim is to preserve range of motion but also to reduce higher loads on the adjacent segment as is the case with fusion of segments. The theory is that TDR reduces the risk for early disc degeneration. There are some studies showing that TDR is as good as anterior fusion surgery in young individuals [39].

Fact Box 15

Surgical treatment is recommended in severe cases.

The results are good in 63–70% of patients after spinal fusion.

Anterior surgery is recommended for young athletes with ALIF or TDR.

RTP is allowed if the athlete meets the general criteria.

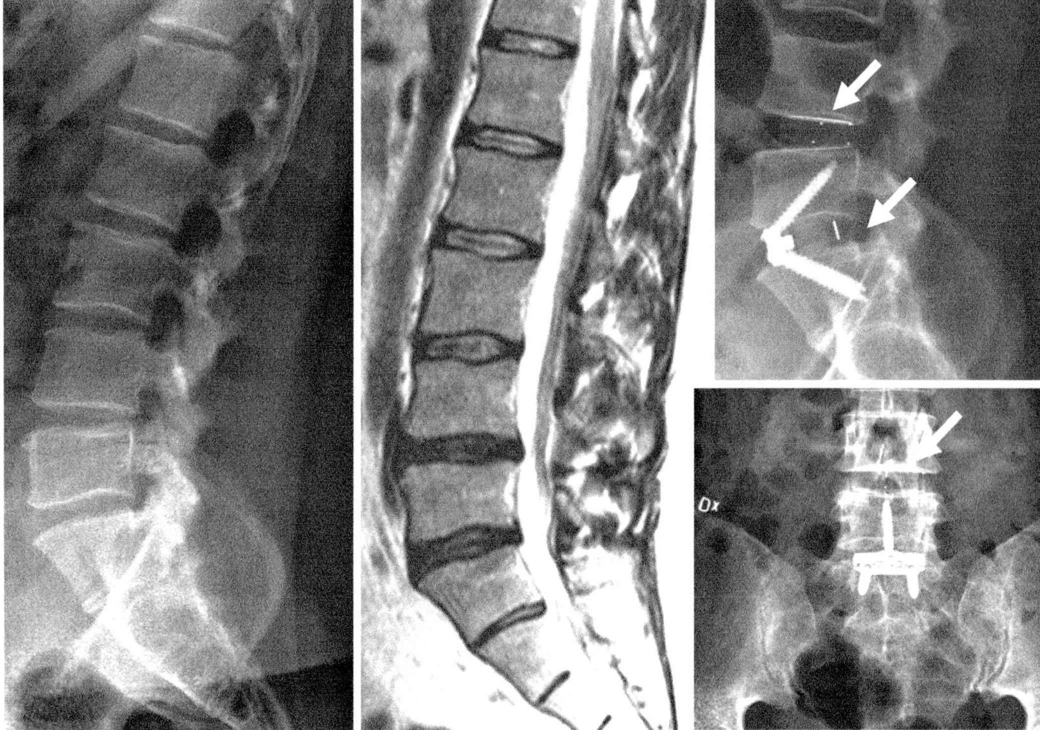

Fig. 24.4 A 35-year-old male with severe DDD (X-ray and MRI preoperatively) that is operated with anterior surgery with a hybrid technique, TDR L4-L5 and ALIF L5-S1 (X-ray postoperatively). The disc prosthesis is completely of PEEC material. The anterior part of the ALIF cage and the screws are of titanium and the rest of the cage of PEEC material

Anterior surgery is a better surgical technique for young athletes because this excludes injury to the spinal muscles. The patient has less pain and can start with rehabilitation and also return to training and competition earlier than is the case with posterior surgery. Despite the lack of studies comparing anterior and posterior surgery in young athletes, anterior surgery is a more attractive alternative surgery for young elite players. Hopefully future studies will show this difference.

24.11.5 Return to Play

There is unfortunately a lack of knowledge regarding football players that have undergone fusion surgery or TDR and returned to play and competition. The athletes are allowed to RTP if they meet the general criteria. The fusion results in the general population are still not excellent where <70 shows good results. Fusion surgery or TDR should therefore be the last treatment option for football players.

24.12 Lumbar Disc Hernia

Fact Box 16
The prevalence of LDH in athletes is up to 58%.

Athletes who have suffered from LBP and sciatica more than 2–3 weeks should be investigated with MRI.

Disc injury or degeneration is more common in elite athletes than the general population. Lumbar disc hernia (LDH) is one of the most common causing LBP in athletes. However, traumatic LDH is significantly less common in athletes. The reported prevalence of LDH in athletic population is up to 58%.

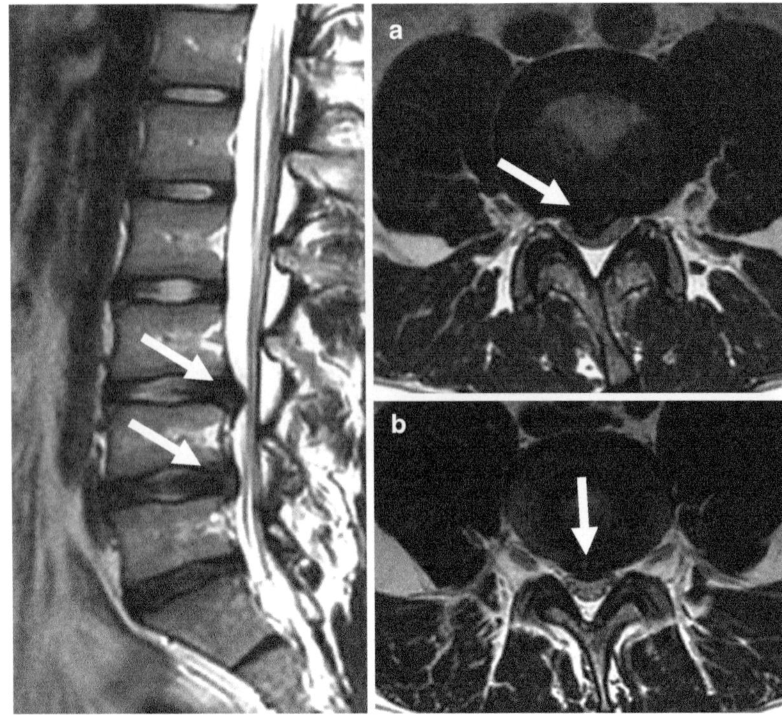

Fig. 24.5 (**a**) MRI of the spine of a 15-year-old male football player with disc hernia at L3-L4 level coursing right L4 sciatica. The athlete was treated with open mini-invasive discectomy. (**b**) The central disk hernia at L4-L5 level was asymptomatic and therefore not treated surgically

24.12.1 Diagnosis and Radiological Investigation

The athletes have LBP and radiating pain in the leg corresponding to the affected nerve root. They may also have varying forms of neurological deficits, such as numbness, loss of sensation, reflexes and muscle power, which is age dependent.

MRI is the best radiological method to diagnose LDH (Fig. 24.5). The second best is computed tomography (CT), but this method involves radiation and should therefore be avoided in young individuals.

24.12.2 Treatment

The management of LDH is a challenge in athletes, because it often forces them to a break in continuing their athletic career. Therefore the goal of the treatment is to make return to sporting activity as quickly as possible [40].

There are still no randomized controlled trials comparing conservative with surgical treatment methods in athletes with LDH in the literature. As a result, there are no scientific treatment methods or advice on the optimal strategy for the management of LDH in athletes. There is also a lack of knowledge about the time in which the athletes can return to sporting activities, which kinds of movement or load should be avoided in the rehabilitation period and special rehabilitation guidelines for different sports.

Fact Box 17

Spondylolisthesis is slippage of one vertebra in relation to another.

The main cause is spondylolysis of pars interarticularis.

LBP in athletes is in 50% caused by spondylolysis.

Persistent symptoms are due to a progressive slippage.

The diagnosis is radiologically with oblique X-ray or CT.

24.12.3 Return to Play

The long-term outcomes of conservative or surgical discectomy in athletes with lumbar disc herniation appear to be satisfactory in terms of the athletes' ability to return to their previous levels of sporting activity [40]. However, surgical intervention has more rapid rates of pain relief and recovery. It is likely that full-endoscopic discectomy is the least mini-invasive surgical intervention for the skin, paravertebral muscles and soft tissues. This technique may show better advantages in athletes when it comes to maintaining muscle function and strength in the lower back and thereby allowing an early return to participation in sporting activities [41, 42].

Several studies have shown pooled return to sporting activity within 12 months from 80% to 90% after either conservative (76%) or surgical (84%) intervention with no significant difference between the groups [40, 43–46]. The overall rate of return to sports after discectomy reported is 89% (Table 24.2). Return to play after 2–6 months is reported to be plausible for contact sports after percutaneous discectomy and microdiscectomy. The mean time reported for return to play is 5.3 months. Probably, the full-endoscopic lumbar discectomy may shorten the time for return to play due to the less invasive procedure. The pooled actual percentage of athletes returning to their previous level of sport function after discectomy is approximately 59% (range 38–65%). The differences reported in studies regarding outcomes and return to play rates are dependent on the age of the player at the time of surgery and the type of sport. The recurrence prevalence of LDH requiring secondary discectomy ranges from 9% to 31% [47].

The initial treatment is conservative.

Athletes who are not pain-free in 4 and 6 weeks are recommended surgery.

With conservative treatment the results are good in 76%.

After discectomy the results are good in 84%.

Up to 90% of athletes can RTP within 12 months.

Table 24.2 Average percentage of athletes returning to sporting activity after surgical treatment within 12 month

Returning to play				
Months	3	6	9	12
% of athletes	50%	72%	79%	84%

24.13 Spondylolisthesis

Isthmic spondylolisthesis in athletes is usually associated with spondylolysis or can on usually be congenital [48–50]. Most of the slip progression occurs during the preadolescent growth spurt [34]. Risk factors include a positive family history and sports with repetitive hyperextension, i.e. gymnastics, figure skating and dancing [51, 52].

The prevalence of spondylolisthesis in children under the age of 5 years is 1–2%, while in adults it is 6%. The prevalence in athletes with persistent LBP has been found in up to 50% [50]. It's most common at the L5-S1 disc level, because of the large forces occurring at this level, due to the fact that the lumbar spine is the link between the torso and the pelvic and lower extremities [50].

24.13.1 Diagnosis

The diagnosis is, radiologically, with a lateral lumbar view on plain radiographs. CT scans are of course more sensitive when it comes to diagnosing the spondylolysis with or without any slippage. More detailed information about spondylolisthesis and spondylolysis is in the section about traumatic thoracolumbar injuries.

24.13.2 Treatment

Fact Box 18

The majority of athletes heal conservatively.

In cases with progressive slippage and persisting pain, fusion surgery is required.

RTP is possible between 9 and 12 months, when the athlete has met the general criteria.

Spondylolisthesis may cause LBP or changes in gait and postural abnormalities, depending on the level of the slip. The first step in treatment is structured physiotherapy. To document stability and the lack of further progression, athletes should be followed with serial radiography at 6-month intervals until they have reached maturity. Athletes with slippage of >50% or with progressive slippage and those who cannot be treated conservatively may require surgery with pedicle fixation and fusion. The fusion is in most cases performed both intercorporally (PLIF/TLIF) and posterolaterally. The surgical intervention also includes some degree of repositioning of the slippage and laminectomy (so-called Gill laminectomy) [53].

24.13.3 Return to Play

There are no studies reporting return to play in football players with symptomatic spondylolisthesis. When the player is pain-free either with conservative or surgical treatment, return to play is allowed. The time to be able to return to play is still unclear but recommended when the athlete has met the general criteria. After fusion surgery it can take between 9 and 12 months for the athlete to be able to return to training and completion.

Fact Box 19
FJS is a challenging condition.
FJS cannot occur if the disc is healthy.
The prevalence of FJS may be the cause of chronic LBP in 15%.
The diagnosis is with radiology and facet joint blockades.

24.14 Facet Joint Syndrome

Facet joint syndrome (FJS) is a challenging condition for diagnosis and treatment, and there are reports that it affects up to 15% of patients with chronic LBP [54]. Despite rigorous research, there is still controversy about this diagnosis, but recent literature reports that FJS may be a primary source of LBP [55].

24.14.1 Aetiology

Facet joint pain can originate from any structure integral to both the function and configuration of the facets, including the fibrous capsule, synovial membrane, hyaline cartilage and bony articulations. The predisposing factors are spondylolisthesis, disc degeneration and old age. The conclusion from several recent studies is that disc degeneration is a more reliable indicator of ageing than facet joint osteoarthritis and that no osteoarthritis has been observed in any patient in the absence of disc degeneration [56–62]. Facet joint osteoarthritis has been found to be minimal in patients younger than 40 years [62, 63].

24.14.2 Prevalence

The prevalence rate varies widely from 5% to 90% in the literature [64–71]. However, recent studies with precise indications and methods have come to the conclusion that FJS is the cause of 15% of chronic LBP [65, 72–77].

24.14.3 Diagnosis

FJS is challenging to diagnose with the present diagnostic methods, clinical examinations, radiologically and with facet joint blocks. The main reason is that the pain from the facet joints is not always in the lower back but also usually presents as radiating or referred pain, due to the nervous distribution from the primary dorsal rami. It's therefore difficult to distinguish it from sciatica pain due to a herniated disc or foraminal stenosis.

In clinical practice, it is generally accepted that diagnostic facet joint blocks are the most reliable method of diagnosing FJS. Several guidelines and reviews have asserted that intra-articular injections and median branch blocks are equally effective [72, 73, 78–80]. However, both these methods are associated with high false-positive and false-negative rates, and their efficacy in diagnosing FJS is therefore low, and their use should be reduced.

24.14.4 Radiology

Plain radiography is not specific in diagnosing facet joint osteoarthritis (OA) in the early stages. CT scans are best at detecting degenerative facet changes. Some studies of patients with chronic LBP have reported that both the sensitivity and specificity of MRI diagnosis facet joint OA to be more than 90%, compared with CT scans [62, 65, 71, 81–83].

24.14.5 Treatment

The treatment of FJS consists of a multimodal approach comprising conservative therapy, medical management, surgical intervention and physiotherapy.

The use of intra-articular steroid injections for the treatment of FJS is still a controversial subject. When using radiofrequency denervation for FJS, studies have also produced controversial findings relating to the long-term outcome [84–86]. Studies evaluating the long-term outcomes of these two procedures have thus far provided conflicting evidence. [86] In carefully selected patients who fail to benefit from conservative treatment, such as physical and pain killers, intra-articular steroid injections and radiofrequency denervation have shown to be good treatment options [54].

Fixation and fusion of the degenerated spinal segment or arthroplasty of the facet joints are occasionally performed to treat FJS. This is despite any scientific evidence in the literature [87, 88]. Therefore, there is no convincing evidence to support any surgical intervention for FJS, except for that resulting from a traumatic dislocation or fracture.

24.14.6 Return to Play

There are no studies reporting return to play in football players that have LBP due to FJS. The management is as for athletes with LBP. When the player is pain-free either with conservative or surgical treatment, return to play is allowed. The time to be able to return to play is still unclear.

Fact Box 20

The treatment is always conservative.

In severe cases, facet joint blocks are an option.

RTP is allowed when the athlete has met the general criteria.

24.15 Fractures of the Thoracolumbar Spine

Traumatic spinal fractures in the general population account for a large percentage of musculoskeletal injuries, where approximately 75–90% occur in the thoracic and lumbar spine. Most of these fractures occur at the thoracolumbar junction (Th10-L2) and the lumbar spine, due to the rigid thoracic spine and the mobile the lumbar [89–92]. In young athletes, traumatic fractures and dislocations of the thoracolumbar spine in athletes are not as usual as in the cervical spine. There are unfortunately no statistics reporting the incidence and prevalence of fractures in the thoracic/lumbar spine in athletes. There are some case reports and series reported in American football players and basketball players. They are fortunately to a lesser rate resulting to catastrophic spinal cord injuries [93].

24.15.1 Aetiology

The mechanisms of injuries in athletes include axial compression and loading in hyperflexion or hyperextension [93]. Axial loading is usually precipitated by falls landing in a sitting position, often with combined hyperflexion of the spine.

The most common fractures in athletes are compression fractures of the vertebral endplates caused by sudden axial loading or in sports requiring jumps or high axial loads on the spine due to falls. This injury mechanism is seen in diving, skiing, snowboarding, horseback riding and gymnastics. Fractures of the thoracolumbar spine may also occur in violent collisions in contact sports, such as American football, rugby, ice hockey and soccer [93, 94].

Endplate fractures or Schmorl's nodes in paediatric athletes are common injuries [33]. These injuries represent disc extrusions through weak areas of the endplate and are more frequently seen in the thoracolumbar junction. Endplate fractures are considered to be caused by an acute axial load or by repetitive axial stresses [33]. Baranto et al. reported a higher incidence of these injuries in orienteers compared with other athletes [4].

Traumatic avulsion fractures of the posterior elements can occur during training or completion, due to a posterior direct trauma or after sudden forcible spine flexion, rotation or hyperextension. An avulsion fracture of the spinous process of the T1 vertebra, a so-called clay-shoveller fracture, can occur in weightlifters and gymnasts. Avulsion injuries are also found of the lumbar spinous and transverse processes in divers, dancers and gymnasts.

24.15.2 Classification of Thoracolumbar Fractures

The AO thoracolumbar fracture classification system is the most recent mechanistic classification system described by Magerl et al., which has globally been accepted and is used clinical pratice [95]. The AO classification system defines three major mechanisms of spinal injury: compression (type A), distraction (type B) and translation (type C). Types A and B are then divided into subgroups (i.e. A0, A1, A2, A3, A4), but not type C. The injury severity is indicated by increasing values of injury classification. This means that type A is less severe than type B, which is in turn less severe than type C (Table 24.3).

Table 24.3 Detailed description of the AO classification system (Adapted from Magerl et al. 1994 [95])

Type A	Type B	Type C
Compression injuries	Distraction injuries	Dislocation injuries
A0 Minor, non-structural	B1 Transosseous tension band disruption Chance fracture	Displacement or dislocation
A1 Wedge compression	B2 Posterior tension band disruption	
A2 Split	B3 Hyperextension	
A3 Incomplete burst		
A4 Complete burst		

Fact Box 21

75–90% of spinal fractures occur in the thoracic/lumbar spine.

The prevalence in athletes is not known.

The fractures are caused by axial compression, hyperflexion or hyperextension and loading.

The classification is according to AO.

The fractures are called types A, B and C, due to the severity.

24.15.3 Diagnosis

It's mandatory to radiologically examine athletes that are exposed to spinal trauma. If the athlete is conscious and has no neurological deficits, the first step is plain radiographs. But if the athlete is unconscious and has a neurological deficit or plain radiograph/CT scans show a fracture causing canal narrowing, MRI most be performed. Most thoracolumbar fractures can be found on plain radiographs, but CT scans are more sensitive to bony lesions. MRI is the gold standard examination for the diagnosis and evaluation of spinal cord injuries. MRI is able to detect oedema and haemorrhage in the spinal cord and is also useful for detecting compression vertebral body fractures by evidencing bony oedema. MRI should be performed in children with neurological deficits to detect eventual spinal cord injuries without radiographic fractures, so-called SCIWORA [96–99].

24.15.4 Treatment

The management of thoracolumbar fractures depends on the severity of the fracture. Type A fractures are treated conservatively with or without a brace (hyperextension brace). One exception is type A3 and A4 fractures, where the majority are instable and should therefore be treated surgically, preferably with percutaneous pedicle screw fixation. Type B and C fractures are unstable and most always be treated surgically with open pedicle fixation and fusion.

Physiotherapy is mandatory after surgery or after removal of the brace, which is approximately 2–3 months of treatment depending on the patient's age.

Fact Box 22

The diagnosis is made by CT or MRI.

The treatment is conservative, with or without brace.

Surgical treatment is required for type A3, type A4, type B and type C.

Surgical treatment is posterior pedicle fixation and fusion.

Return to play is contraindicated if the fusion is in the cervical and thoracic junction or in the thoracic and lumbar junction.

Athletes are allowed to return to play if they meet the general criteria.

The time to return to play is due to the severity of the fracture and between 3 and 24 months.

24.15.5 Return to Play

Compression fractures in the thoracic/lumbar spine are relatively rare in athletes, and therefore there is limited knowledge about the prognosis and return to play. In American football players and basketball players with compression fractures, return to play was possible after 3–24 months without any limitations.

Return to play is recommended for athletes in contact sports after healed compression fractures if the athlete meets the general criteria. For spinous process and transversal process fractures, a similar conservative treatment approach and return to play criteria have been suggested.

Traumatic fracture of the thoracic spine with instability, such as burst or Chance fractures, is reported to be a contraindication for athletic participation. However, after surgical treatment there are few proposed return to play guidelines for this condition. It is recommended that participation in contact sports after fusion treatment which include the transition zones in the cervicothoracic or thoracolumbar regions constitutes an absolute contraindication. Also, fusions which terminate at the transition zones are contraindication for return to previous play. There is a consensus that players can return to play if the fusion doesn't cross a transition zone.

24.16 Apophyseal Ring Injuries

Traumatic disc herniations are less common in young athletes. The clinical presentation in adolescents compared to adults can be less clear, where children often lack sciatica. Instead, they have mild or moderate LBP that is aggravated by activity. Disc herniation associated with avulsion fractures of the apophyseal ring is unique for the adolescent athletes [100].

24.16.1 Injury Mechanism and Incidence

Several authors have reported that apophyseal ring fractures (avulsion fracture) occur at the junction between the vertebral body and the apophysis attached to the outer annulus fibrosis [34, 101, 102]. When an avulsion fracture occurs through the growing cartilage, the ossified fragment remains attached to the annulus and posterior longitudinal ligament. Disc material always extrudes through the avulsion fracture and prevents healing of the ring to the vertebral body.

Ring apophyseal fractures occur exclusively in adolescence, before the age of full maturation around 18 years, because the cartilaginous end-plate (the attachment between the apophyseal ring and the vertebral body) is weaker than the annulus fibrosis attached by Sharpey's fibres to the apophyseal ring. Ossification of the ring begins at 13–17 years of age, and fusion to the vertebral body occurs at about 18 years, but the process is often delayed until 25 years of age.

The incidence of adolescent athletes is 5.8–28% and in all ages 5.35–8.2% [103].

Approximately 50% of these apophyseal fractures are due to acute trauma or repetitive micro-trauma [104]. Most patients are involved in sports that require repetitive hyperflexion and hyperextension of the lumbar spine, such as basketball, football, weight lifting, gymnastics and volleyball [105].

The most frequent site of ring apophyseal fractures is the inferior ring of the vertebreae in the lumbar spine, especially L4, but avulsion fractures may occurs in all the spine [33].

24.16.2 Diagnosis

Fact Box 23

The prevalence in young athletes is 6–28% and in all ages 5–8%.

Apophyseal fractures occur due to a trauma and sports are the most common cause.

The diagnosis is made by CT and MRI.

The treatment is conservative, but in patients with sciatica and neurological deficit, surgical treatment may be required.

The symptoms of apophyseal fractures are similar to a central herniated disc. The patients suffer from acute or chronic moderate or severe LBP and mild radicular pain to the buttock and posterior thigh. The symptoms are aggravated by prolonged sitting, coughing, sneezing and activities.

This avulsion fracture is difficult to find on plain radiographs. CT is most sensitive for detecting the fracture, but in most cases MRI can also diagnose the injuries with disc material in the fracture (Fig. 24.6).

24.16.3 Treatment

Treatment modalities of apophyseal fractures are conservative, with absence from sports and physiotherapy. Surgery is required if the fracture is in the posterior part of the vertebra and causes compression of the nerve root resulting in sciatica and neurological deficit. The surgical procedure is as for LDH with the addition of extirpation of the bony fragment.

24.16.4 Return to Play

There are unfortunately no reports on prognosis and recovery after apophyseal fractures, treated conservatively or surgically. The most common outcome measures are based on symptomatic relief. Most adolescent and adult cases treated surgically show good to excellent results and symptom relief.

Several clinical factors can influence the postoperative outcome such as age, type of apophyseal fracture, preoperative symptoms or associated disease, different surgical techniques and postoperative management. However the postoperative outcome is mainly dependent on the severity of the preoperative deficit. Athletes with apophyseal fracture and LDH who have undergone surgical intervention have equal clinical outcome and postoperative complications.

The exact time for return to previous or sport activity is not reported. The guidelines are the same as for LDH. Therefore the athlete shall

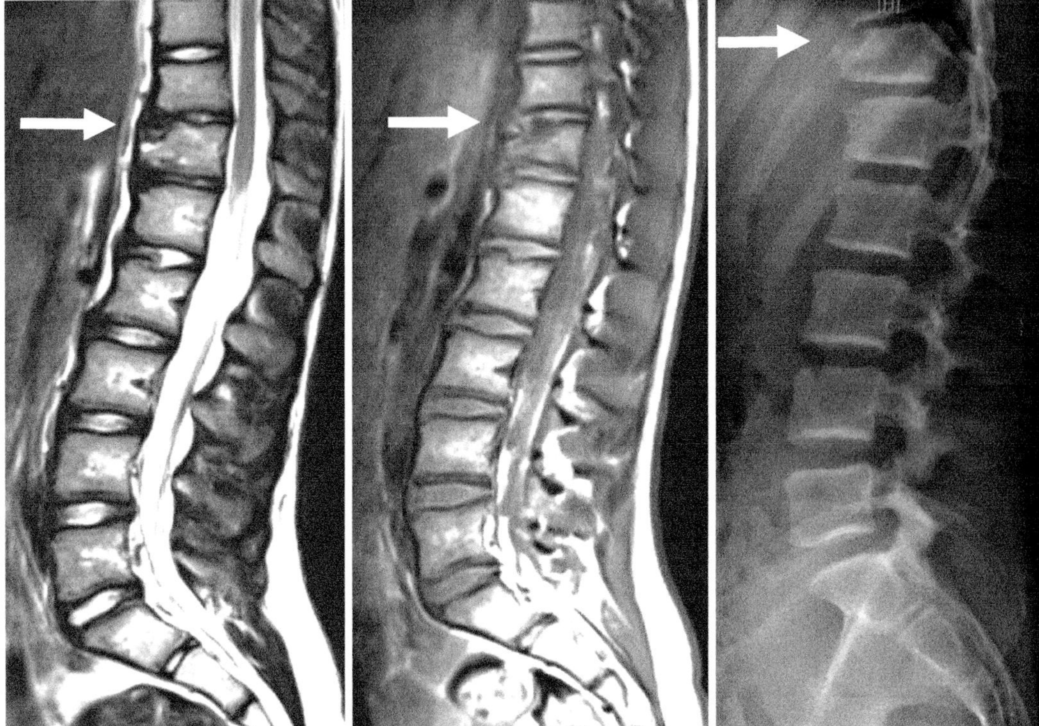

Fig. 24.6 A 13-year-old female elite gymnast with apophyseal injury at Th12 vertebra on MRI T2 and T1 waited images) and plain radiography

meet the general criteria; have no pain, muscle weakness or neurological deficit. Up to 90% of the athletes return to previous sports activities within 12 months.

24.17 Spondylolysis

Spondylolysis is a stress fracture of the pars interarticularis or the isthmus (Fig. 24.7). It's more commonly occurred in the skeletally immature young athletes due to the vulnerability of the immature pars to repeated stress loads.

The prevalence in the general population is 4–6%, and it is most common in L5 vertebrae (85–95%). However, the prevalence in athletes is much higher, especially in athletes with LBP (50%). Spondylolysis is most commonly found in children between the ages of 6 and 10 years, with a reported prevalence of 4% [106]. The prevalence in adolescent athletes is 47%, whereas 5% in the adults [52]. The prevalence in football is also very high, and there are reports of rates between 6.5% and 66.7% [107].

24.17.1 Injury Mechanism

The injury mechanism in football that puts heavy loads on the lower spine and causes spondylolysis is well described and involves three mechanisms: extension overload, unbalanced shear forces and forced rotation of the lumbar spine. This mechanism involves multiple short sprints and kicking a ball with either foot, heading the ball, occasionally throwing it with two hands above the head, collision with opponents and contact with the ground. El Rassi et al. [37] reported that 47% of the football players noticed that their pain started after a high-velocity kick. There are also anatomical abnormalities that can predispose spondylolysis such as vertical pars, long articular facet process and hyperlordotic spinal curve.

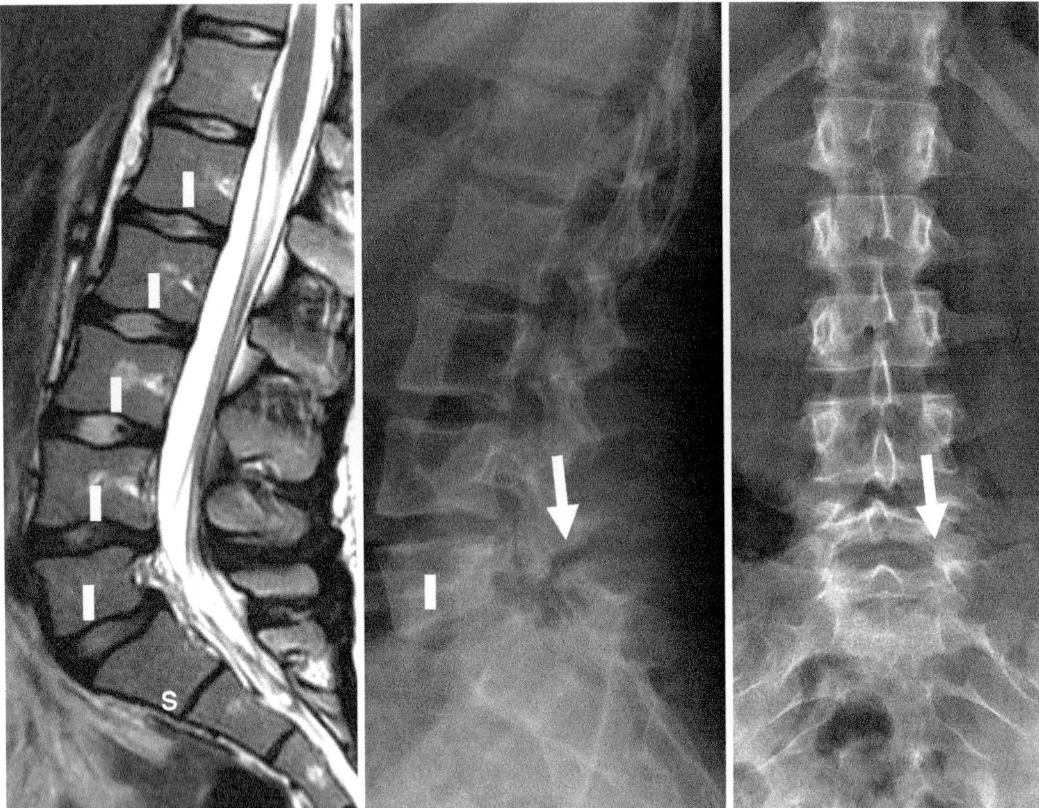

Fig. 24.7 MRI and X-ray of a 16-year-old female football player with spondylolisthesis of pars of L5 with mild retrolisthesis. The player has a lumbarized S1 vertebra. The player has had LBP since several years and cannot continue to play football

24.17.2 Diagnosis

Fact Box 24
Spondylolysis is a stress fracture of the pars interarticularis.

The prevalence in the general population is 4–6%.

The prevalence in young athletes is up to 47%.

The prevalence in football players is between 6% and 67%.

The injury mechanism is extension overload, unbalanced sheer forces and forced rotation.

The pain usually starts after a high-velocity kick.

The diagnosis is radiologically with oblique plain radiographs. The fractures are in this view called broken neck of the Scottie dog. CT scans are more sensitive when it comes to diagnosing the defect. Early stages, such as stress reactions or fractures, can be missed on plain X-rays and CT scans but are clearly seen on MRI. In paediatric athletes with back pain where plain X-rays and CT scans are negative, it is therefore recommend continuing with MRI. If all these three radiological methods are negative but there is still a high suspicion of a fracture, a single photon emission computed tomography (SPECT) can be performed. SPECT is the most sensitive method to investigate occurrence of stress reaction or fracture of the pars.

Athletes with spondylolysis or stress reaction have LBP which is aggravated by activity. They may have hyperlordosis and restricted flexion in clinical examination. Standing on one leg with the lumbar spine extended laterally may be painful. They may also have tenderness on palpation on the spinal process of the affected vertebrae.

24.17.3 Treatment

The ideal goal for treatment of spondylolysis is to achieve bone healing of the fracture at the earliest possible stage during childhood and in this way prevent spondylolisthesis with a more severe clinical condition. It is therefore mandatory to examine young athletes with LBP with radiological examinations.

The treatment is conservative with physiotherapy and absence from physical activities for at least 3 months. The athletes shall not be treated with hard or soft braces. Studies have shown that bracing delays the healing and return to play. It takes between 3 and 6 months for a pars fracture to heal with conservative treatment and absence from sports. El Rassi et al. [37] reported in a study on football player with a minimum of 2-year follow-up that 58% of the players had excellent results with no pain during sports, 35% good, 5% fair and 2% poor results with conservative treatment. They noticed also that players who ceased playing football for 3 month had better results than those who continued to play with or without a brace.

Fact Box 25

The diagnosis is with oblique X-ray, CT scans, MRI or SPECT.

The initial treatment is conservative with pain killers and physiotherapy.

In athletes with progressive slippage, inadequate healing of the fracture or neurological deficit, surgical treatment may be required.

The surgery is with posterior pedicle screw fixation and fusion.

Athletes that don't respond to conservative treatment and have continued severe LBP with progressive slippage require surgical fixation and fusion of the pars fracture. More than 70% of young athletes with bilateral spondylolysis have been reported to have forward slippage to some extent [108, 109]. Athletes that have severe slippage with radiculopathy due to nerve root stenosis at the lateral recess require also surgical treatment [110–112]. There are different surgical techniques to treat spondylolysis with or without slippage; intra-segmental pars fixation either with a laminar compression screw or using a pedicle screw, rod and a laminar hook or pedicle screw and rod construction. All these methods have shown to have good results [113].

24.17.4 Return to Play

Studies have reported good to excellent results in 80% and return to play of athletes with spondylolysis treated conservatively. Return to play is allowed once athletes have met the general criteria for contact sports, which usually takes up to 3 months. The athlete must have normal lumbar spine motion and examination without any pain, good muscular strength and stability, restored lumbar lordosis and no pain in extension provocation. Returning to previous level of sports may take between 3 and 12 months. There are still no general criteria for returning to play after surgical treatment of spondylolysis. Some surgeons do not recommend return to contact sports after fusion of spondylolysis, but others allow athletes to return to collision sports 1 year postoperatively. Therefore, fusion surgery after spondylolysis is not always a contraindication to return to contact sport activities, but the time frame for return is variable. The recommendation is, therefore, once athletes have met the general criteria, return to sports is allowed.

Fact Box 26

The results for RTP are good and up to 80%.

RTP occurs in between 3 and 12 months.

The recommendation for RTP is when the player meets the general criteria.

Take Home Message

Football is the most commonly played sports in the world, and injuries are therefore common among football players. LBP is the third most common injury in football, with a prevalence of 14% in young players and 36% in adult players.

The spine of football players is exposed both to traumatic and over-use injuries. Acute macro-trauma, repetitive micro-trauma or over-use injuries, or a combination of these two mechanisms are very common spinal injuries in football players resulting in back pain. The injury patterns are different in young athletes compared with adults, as the young athletes suffer usually form avulsion injuries of the vertebral endplates in the growth zone and the adults from vertebral body fractures or rupture of the disc.

Fractures in the spine of football players are very rare, and the specific prevalence is not known. The surgical treatment is with stabile fixation when the fracture is displaced.

Disc degeneration and other abnormalities affecting the vertebral endplates and the vertebral ring apophyses are very common among athletes in sports imposing large demands on the spine. These abnormalities appear to be relatively uncommon among top-level athletes before the adolescent growth spurt. Athletes (such as football players) with the above-mentioned radiological abnormalities have more back pain, with a frequency of up to 94%, than other athletes and nonathletes.

There are at present no specific scientific standardized consensus guidelines for return to football play after spinal injuries. Therefore, the recommendations are based on studies of other sports. Few studies have published guidelines for RTP after spine injuries, but their conclusions are obtained largely from case series, expert opinions and experience, rather than scientific evidence. However, most authors agree on four fundamental criteria that must be meeting for a player to return to playing sports:

1. The athlete must be pain-free.
2. The athlete must have full range of motion.
3. The athlete must have full strength.
4. The athlete must have no evidence of neurological deficit.

Top Five Evidence Based References

Baranto A et al (2009) Back pain and MRI changes in the thoraco-lumbar spine of top athletes in four different sports: a 15-year follow-up study. Knee Surg Sports Traumatol Arthrosc 17(9):1125–1134

Barile A et al (2007) Spinal injury in sport. Eur J Radiol 62(1):68–78

Iwamoto J et al (2010) The return to sports activity after conservative or surgical treatment in athletes with lumbar disc herniation. Am J Phys Med Rehabil 89(12):1030–1035

Nagoshi N et al (2017) Return to play in athletes with spinal cord concussion: a systematic literature review. Spine J 17(2):291–302

Swärd L et al (1991) Disc degeneration and associated abnormalities of the spine in elite gymnasts. A magnetic resonance imaging study. Spine 16(4):437–443

References

1. Jackson DW (1979) Low back pain in young athletes: evaluation of stress reaction and discogenic problems. Am J Sports Med 7(6):364–366
2. Sward L, Hellstrom M, Jacobsson B, Nyman R, Peterson L (1991) Disc degeneration and associated abnormalities of the spine in elite gymnasts. A magnetic resonance imaging study. Spine (Phila Pa 1976) 16(4):437–443
3. Baranto A, Hellstrom M, Sward L (2010) Acute injury of an intervertebral disc in an elite tennis player: a case report. Spine (Phila Pa 1976) 35:E223
4. Baranto A, Hellstrom M, Cederlund CG, Nyman R, Sward L (2009) Back pain and MRI changes in the thoraco-lumbar spine of top athletes in four different sports: a 15-year follow-up study. Knee Surg Sports Traumatol Arthrosc 17(9):1125–1134
5. Mai HT, Burgmeier RJ, Mitchell SM, Hecht AC, Maroon JC, Nuber GW, Hsu WK (2016) Does the level of cervical disc herniation surgery affect performance-based outcomes in national football league athletes? Spine (Phila Pa 1976) 41(23):1785–1789
6. Molinari RW, Pagarigan K, Dettori JR, Molinari R Jr, Dehaven KE (2016) Return to play in athletes receiving cervical surgery: a systematic review. Global Spine J 6(1):89–96
7. Torg JS, Corcoran TA, Thibault LE, Pavlov H, Sennett BJ, Naranja RJ Jr, Priano S (1997) Cervical cord neurapraxia: classification, pathomechanics, morbidity, and management guidelines. J Neurosurg 87(6):843–850
8. Nagoshi N, Tetreault L, Nakashima H, Nouri A, Fehlings MG (2017) Return to play in athletes with spinal cord concussion: a systematic literature review. Spine J 17(2):291–302
9. Torg JS, Pavlov H, Genuario SE, Sennett B, Wisneski RJ, Robie BH, Jahre C (1986) Neurapraxia of the cervical spinal cord with transient quadriplegia. J Bone Joint Surg Am 68(9):1354–1370

10. van Middendorp JJ, Hosman AJ, Doi SA (2013) The effects of the timing of spinal surgery after traumatic spinal cord injury: a systematic review and meta-analysis. J Neurotrauma 30(21):1781–1794
11. Brown RL, Brunn MA, Garcia VF (2001) Cervical spine injuries in children: a review of 103 patients treated consecutively at a level 1 pediatric trauma center. J Pediatr Surg 36(8):1107–1114
12. Vaccaro AR, Koerner JD, Radcliff KE, Oner FC, Reinhold M, Schnake KJ, Kandziora F, Fehlings MG, Dvorak MF, Aarabi B, Rajasekaran S, Schroeder GD, Kepler CK, Vialle LR (2016) AOSpine subaxial cervical spine injury classification system. Eur Spine J 25(7):2173–2184
13. Antoniou J, Steffen T, Nelson F, Winterbottom N, Hollander AP, Poole RA, Aebi M, Alini M (1996) The human lumbar intervertebral disc: evidence for changes in the biosynthesis and denaturation of the extracellular matrix with growth, maturation, ageing, and degeneration. J Clin Invest 98(4):996–1003
14. Eyre DR, Muir H (1976) Types I and II collagens in intervertebral disc. Interchanging radial distributions in annulus fibrosis. Biochem J 157(1):267–270
15. Tertti MO, Salminen JJ, Paajanen HE, Terho PH, Kormano MJ (1991) Low-back pain and disk degeneration in children: a case-control MR imaging study. Radiology 180(2):503–507
16. Kaapa E, Holm S, Inkinen R, Lammi MJ, Tammi M, Vanharanta H (1994) Proteoglycan chemistry in experimentally injured porcine intervertebral disk. J Spinal Disord 7(4):296–306
17. Holm S, Nachemson A (1988) Nutrition of the intervertebral disc: acute effects of cigarette smoking. An experimental animal study. Ups J Med Sci 93(1):91–99
18. Hellstrom M, Jacobsson B, Sward L, Peterson L (1990) Radiologic abnormalities of the thoraco-lumbar spine in athletes. Acta Radiol 31(2):127–132
19. Sward L, Hellstrom M, Jacobsson B, Peterson L (1990) Back pain and radiologic changes in the thoraco-lumbar spine of athletes. Spine (Phila Pa 1976) 15(2):124–129
20. Frymoyer JW (1992) Lumbar disk disease: epidemiology. Instr Course Lect 41:217–223
21. Lundin O, Hellstrom M, Nilsson I, Sward L (2001) Back pain and radiological changes in the thoraco-lumbar spine of athletes. A long-term follow-up. Scand J Med Sci Sports 11(2):103–109
22. Battie MC, Videman T, Parent E (2004) Lumbar disc degeneration: epidemiology and genetic influences. Spine (Phila Pa 1976) 29(23):2679–2690
23. Balague F, Troussier B, Salminen JJ (1999) Non-specific low back pain in children and adolescents: risk factors. Eur Spine J 8(6):429–438
24. Alexander CJ (1976) Effect of growth rate on the strength of the growth plate-shaft junction. Skeletal Radiol 1(2):67–76
25. Baranto A, Hellstrom M, Nyman R, Lundin O, Sward L (2006) Back pain and degenerative abnormalities in the spine of young elite divers: a 5-year follow-up magnetic resonance imaging study. Knee Surg Sports Traumatol Arthrosc 14(9):907–914
26. Arkin AM, Katz JF (1956) The effects of pressure on epiphyseal growth; the mechanism of plasticity of growing bone. J Bone Joint Surg Am 38-A(5):1056–1076
27. Goldstein JD, Berger PE, Windler GE, Jackson DW (1991) Spine injuries in gymnasts and swimmers. An epidemiologic investigation. Am J Sports Med 19(5):463–468
28. Kujala UM, Taimela S, Viljanen T, Jutila H, Viitasalo JT, Videman T, Battie MC (1996) Physical loading and performance as predictors of back pain in healthy adults. A 5-year prospective study. Eur J Appl Physiol Occup Physiol 73(5):452–458
29. Bartolozzi C, Caramella D, Zampa V, Dal Pozzo G, Tinacci E, Balducci F (1991) The incidence of disk changes in volleyball players. The magnetic resonance findings. Radiol Med (Torino) 82(6):757–760
30. Kujala UM, Taimela S, Erkintalo M, Salminen JJ, Kaprio J (1996) Low-back pain in adolescent athletes. Med Sci Sports Exerc 28(2):165–170
31. Swärd L, Hellström M, Jacobsson B, Nyman R, Peterson L (1991) Disc degeneration and associated abnormalities of the spine in elite gymnasts. A magnetic resonance imaging study. Spine 16(4):437–443
32. Bahr R, Andersen SO, Loken S, Fossan B, Hansen T, Holme I (2004) Low back pain among endurance athletes with and without specific back loading--a cross-sectional survey of cross-country skiers, rowers, orienteerers, and nonathletic controls. Spine 29(4):449–454
33. Barile A, Limbucci N, Splendiani A, Gallucci M, Masciocchi C (2007) Spinal injury in sport. Eur J Radiol 62(1):68–78
34. Sassmannshausen G, Smith BG (2002) Back pain in the young athlete. Clin Sports Med 21(1):121–132
35. Hoy D, Bain C, Williams G, March L, Brooks P, Blyth F, Woolf A, Vos T, Buchbinder R (2012) A systematic review of the global prevalence of low back pain. Arthritis Rheum 64(6):2028–2037
36. Walker BF (2000) The prevalence of low back pain: a systematic review of the literature from 1966 to 1998. J Spinal Disord 13(3):205–217
37. El Rassi G, Takemitsu M, Woratanarat P, Shah SA (2005) Lumbar spondylolysis in pediatric and adolescent soccer players. Am J Sports Med 33(11):1688–1693
38. Wilson-MacDonald J, Fairbank J, Frost H, Yu LM, Barker K, Collins R, Campbell H, Spine Stabilization Trial G (2008) The MRC spine stabilization trial: surgical methods, outcomes, costs, and complications of surgical stabilization. Spine (Phila Pa 1976) 33(21):2334–2340
39. Berg S, Tropp H (2010) Results from a randomized controlled study between total disc replacement and fusion compared with results from a spine register. SAS J 4(3):68–74
40. Iwamoto J, Sato Y, Takeda T, Matsumoto H (2010) The return to sports activity after conservative or surgical treatment in athletes with lumbar disc herniation. Am J Phys Med Rehabil 89(12):1030–1035

41. Goupille P, Mulleman D, Mammou S, Griffoul I, Valat JP (2007) Percutaneous laser disc decompression for the treatment of lumbar disc herniation: a review. Semin Arthritis Rheum 37(1):20–30
42. Watters WC III, McGirt MJ (2009) An evidence-based review of the literature on the consequences of conservative versus aggressive discectomy for the treatment of primary disc herniation with radiculopathy. Spine J 9(3):240–257
43. Watkins RG, Hanna R, Chang D, Watkins RG III (2012) Return-to-play outcomes after microscopic lumbar diskectomy in professional athletes. Am J Sports Med 40(11):2530–2535
44. Hsu WK (2011) Outcomes following nonoperative and operative treatment for cervical disc herniations in National Football League athletes. Spine (Phila Pa 1976) 36(10):800–805
45. Roberts DW, Roc GJ, Hsu WK (2011) Outcomes of cervical and lumbar disk herniations in Major League Baseball pitchers. Orthopedics 34(8):602–609
46. Iwamoto J, Takeda T, Sato Y, Wakano K (2006) Short-term outcome of conservative treatment in athletes with symptomatic lumbar disc herniation. Am J Phys Med Rehabil 85(8):667–674. quiz 675–7
47. Reiman MP, Sylvain J, Loudon JK, Goode A (2016) Return to sport after open and microdiscectomy surgery versus conservative treatment for lumbar disc herniation: a systematic review with meta-analysis. Br J Sports Med 50(4):221–230
48. Wiltse LL (1961) Spondylolisthesis in children. Clin Orthop 21:156–163
49. Ciullo JV, Jackson DW (1985) Pars interarticularis stress reaction, spondylolysis, and spondylolisthesis in gymnasts. Clin Sports Med 4(1):95–110
50. Wimberly RL, Lauerman WC (2002) Spondylolisthesis in the athlete. Clin Sports Med 21(1):133–145. vii-viii
51. Gerbino PG II, Micheli LJ (1995) Back injuries in the young athlete. Clin Sports Med 14(3):571–590
52. Micheli LJ, Wood R (1995) Back pain in young athletes. Significant differences from adults in causes and patterns. Arch Pediatr Adolesc Med 149(1):15–18
53. Gill GG (1984) Long-term follow-up evaluation of a few patients with spondylolisthesis treated by excision of the loose lamina with decompression of the nerve roots without spinal fusion. Clin Orthop Relat Res 182:215–219
54. Cohen SP, Raja SN (2007) Pathogenesis, diagnosis, and treatment of lumbar zygapophysial (facet) joint pain. Anesthesiology 106(3):591–614
55. Borenstein D (2004) Does osteoarthritis of the lumbar spine cause chronic low back pain? Curr Pain Headache Rep 8(6):512–517
56. Gotfried Y, Bradford DS, Oegema TR Jr (1986) Facet joint changes after chemonucleolysis-induced disc space narrowing. Spine (Phila Pa 1976) 11(9):944–950
57. Kirkaldy-Willis WH, Wedge JH, Yong-Hing K, Reilly J (1978) Pathology and pathogenesis of lumbar spondylosis and stenosis. Spine (Phila Pa 1976) 3(4):319–328
58. Panjabi MM, Krag MH, Chung TQ (1984) Effects of disc injury on mechanical behavior of the human spine. Spine (Phila Pa 1976) 9(7):707–713
59. Adams MA, Hutton WC (1980) The effect of posture on the role of the apophysial joints in resisting intervertebral compressive forces. J Bone Joint Surg Br 62(3):358–362
60. Haher TR, O'Brien M, Dryer JW, Nucci R, Zipnick R, Leone DJ (1994) The role of the lumbar facet joints in spinal stability. Identification of alternative paths of loading. Spine (Phila Pa 1976) 19(23):2667–2670. discussion 2671
61. Adams MA, Freeman BJ, Morrison HP, Nelson IW, Dolan P (2000) Mechanical initiation of intervertebral disc degeneration. Spine (Phila Pa 1976) 25(13):1625–1636
62. Fujiwara A, Tamai K, Yamato M, An HS, Yoshida H, Saotome K, Kurihashi A (1999) The relationship between facet joint osteoarthritis and disc degeneration of the lumbar spine: an MRI study. Eur Spine J 8(5):396–401
63. Weishaupt D, Zanetti M, Hodler J, Boos N (1998) MR imaging of the lumbar spine: prevalence of intervertebral disk extrusion and sequestration, nerve root compression, end plate abnormalities, and osteoarthritis of the facet joints in asymptomatic volunteers. Radiology 209(3):661–666
64. Long DM, BenDebba M, Torgerson WS, Boyd RJ, Dawson EG, Hardy RW, Robertson JT, Sypert GW, Watts C (1996) Persistent back pain and sciatica in the United States: patient characteristics. J Spinal Disord 9(1):40–58
65. Murtagh FR (1988) Computed tomography and fluoroscopy guided anesthesia and steroid injection in facet syndrome. Spine (Phila Pa 1976) 13(6):686–689
66. Destouet JM, Gilula LA, Murphy WA, Monsees B (1982) Lumbar facet joint injection: indication, technique, clinical correlation, and preliminary results. Radiology 145(2):321–325
67. Lau LS, Littlejohn GO, Miller MH (1985) Clinical evaluation of intra-articular injections for lumbar facet joint pain. Med J Aust 143(12-13):563–565
68. Moran R, O'Connell D, Walsh MG (1988) The diagnostic value of facet joint injections. Spine (Phila Pa 1976) 13(12):1407–1410
69. Raymond J, Dumas JM (1984) Intraarticular facet block: diagnostic test or therapeutic procedure? Radiology 151(2):333–336
70. Lewinnek GE, Warfield CA (1986) Facet joint degeneration as a cause of low back pain. Clin Orthop Relat Res 213:216–222
71. Carrera GF (1980) Lumbar facet joint injection in low back pain and sciatica: preliminary results. Radiology 137(3):665–667
72. Sowa G (2005) Facet-mediated pain. Dis Mon 51(1):18–33
73. Dreyer SJ, Dreyfuss PH (1996) Low back pain and the zygapophysial (facet) joints. Arch Phys Med Rehabil 77(3):290–300

74. Dreyfuss PH, Dreyer SJ, Nass (2003) Lumbar zygapophysial (facet) joint injections. Spine J 3(3 Suppl):50S–59S
75. Jackson RP, Jacobs RR, Montesano PX (1988) 1988 Volvo award in clinical sciences. Facet joint injection in low-back pain. A prospective statistical study. Spine (Phila Pa 1976) 13(9):966–971
76. Manchikanti L, Pampati V, Fellows B, Bakhit CE (1999) Prevalence of lumbar facet joint pain in chronic low back pain. Pain Physician 2(3):59–64
77. Newton W, Curtis P, Witt P, Hobler K (1997) Prevalence of subtypes of low back pain in a defined population. J Fam Pract 45(4):331–335
78. Dreyfuss PH, Dreyer SJ, Herring SA (1995) Lumbar zygapophysial (facet) joint injections. Spine (Phila Pa 1976) 20(18):2040–2047
79. Bogduk N (1997) International Spinal Injection Society guidelines for the performance of spinal injection procedures. Part 1: Zygapophysial joint blocks. Clin J Pain 13(4):285–302
80. Kellegren J (1939) On the distribution of pain arising from deep somatic structures with charts of segmental pain areas. Clin Sci (Lond) 4:35–46
81. Weishaupt D, Zanetti M, Boos N, Hodler J (1999) MR imaging and CT in osteoarthritis of the lumbar facet joints. Skeletal Radiol 28(4):215–219
82. Leone A, Aulisa L, Tamburrelli F, Lupparelli S, Tartaglione T (1994) The role of computed tomography and magnetic resonance in assessing degenerative arthropathy of the lumbar articular facets. Radiol Med 88(5):547–552
83. Carrera GF, Williams AL (1984) Current concepts in evaluation of the lumbar facet joints. Crit Rev Diagn Imaging 21(2):85–104
84. King JS, Lagger R (1976) Sciatica viewed as a referred pain syndrome. Surg Neurol 5(1):46–50
85. van Kleef M, Barendse GA, Kessels A, Voets HM, Weber WE, de Lange S (1999) Randomized trial of radiofrequency lumbar facet denervation for chronic low back pain. Spine (Phila Pa 1976) 24(18):1937–1942
86. Cohen SP, Hurley RW, Christo PJ, Winkley J, Mohiuddin MM, Stojanovic MP (2007) Clinical predictors of success and failure for lumbar facet radiofrequency denervation. Clin J Pain 23(1):45–52
87. Deyo RA, Nachemson A, Mirza SK (2004) Spinal-fusion surgery - the case for restraint. N Engl J Med 350(7):722–726
88. Gibson JN, Waddell G, Grant IC (2000) Surgery for degenerative lumbar spondylosis. Cochrane Database Syst Rev (3):CD001352
89. Hu R, Mustard CA, Burns C (1996) Epidemiology of incident spinal fracture in a complete population. Spine (Phila Pa 1976) 21(4):492–499
90. Wood K, Buttermann G, Mehbod A, Garvey T, Jhanjee R, Sechriest V (2003) Operative compared with non-operative treatment of a thoracolumbar burst fracture without neurological deficit. A prospective, randomized study. J Bone Joint Surg Am 85-A(5):773–781
91. Gertzbein SD (1992) Scoliosis Research Society. Multicenter spine fracture study. Spine (Phila Pa 1976) 17(5):528–540
92. Hainline B (1995) Low back injury. Clin Sports Med 14(1):241–265
93. Maxfield BA (2010) Sports-related injury of the pediatric spine. Radiol Clin North Am 48(6):1237–1248
94. Tall RL, DeVault W (1993) Spinal injury in sport: epidemiologic considerations. Clin Sports Med 12(3):441–448
95. Magerl F, Aebi M, Gertzbein SD, Harms J, Nazarian S (1994) A comprehensive classification of thoracic and lumbar injuries. Eur Spine J 3(4):184–201
96. Imhof H, Fuchsjager M (2002) Traumatic injuries: imaging of spinal injuries. Eur Radiol 12(6):1262–1272
97. Nunez DB Jr, Zuluaga A, Fuentes-Bernardo DA, Rivas LA, Becerra JL (1996) Cervical spine trauma: how much more do we learn by routinely using helical CT? Radiographics 16(6):1307–1318. discussion 1318–21
98. Takhtani D, Melhem ER (2000) MR imaging in cervical spine trauma. Magn Reson Imaging Clin N Am 8(3):615–634
99. Buldini B, Amigoni A, Faggin R, Laverda AM (2006) Spinal cord injury without radiographic abnormalities. Eur J Pediatr 165(2):108–111
100. Peh WC, Griffith JF, Yip DK, Leong JC (1998) Magnetic resonance imaging of lumbar vertebral apophyseal ring fractures. Australas Radiol 42(1):34–37
101. Sward L, Hellstrom M, Jacobsson B, Nyman R, Peterson L (1990) Acute injury of the vertebral ring apophysis and intervertebral disc in adolescent gymnasts. Spine (Phila Pa 1976) 15(2):144–148
102. Karlsson L, Lundin O, Ekstrom L, Hansson T, Sward L (1998) Injuries in adolescent spine exposed to compressive loads: an experimental cadaveric study. J Spinal Disord 11(6):501–507
103. Chang CH, Lee ZL, Chen WJ, Tan CF, Chen LH (2008) Clinical significance of ring apophysis fracture in adolescent lumbar disc herniation. Spine (Phila Pa 1976) 33(16):1750–1754
104. Stewart TD (1953) The age incidence of neural-arch defects in Alaskan natives, considered from the standpoint of etiology. J Bone Joint Surg Am 35-A(4):937–950
105. Ikata T, Morita T, Katoh S, Tachibana K, Maoka H (1995) Lesions of the lumbar posterior end plate in children and adolescents. An MRI study. J Bone Joint Surg Br 77(6):951–955
106. Trainor TJ, Trainor MA (2004) Etiology of low back pain in athletes. Curr Sports Med Rep 3(1):41–46
107. Gregory PL, Batt ME, Kerslake RW (2004) Comparing spondylolysis in cricketers and soccer players. Br J Sports Med 38(6):737–742
108. Sakai T, Sairyo K, Takao S, Nishitani H, Yasui N (2009) Incidence of lumbar spondylolysis in the general population in Japan based on multidetector computed tomography scans from two thousand subjects. Spine (Phila Pa 1976) 34(21):2346–2350

109. Seitsalo S (1990) Operative and conservative treatment of moderate spondylolisthesis in young patients. J Bone Joint Surg Br 72(5):908–913
110. Davis IS, Bailey RW (1976) Spondylolisthesis: indications for lumbar nerve root decompression and operative technique. Clin Orthop Relat Res 117:129–134
111. Edelson JG, Nathan H (1986) Nerve root compression in spondylolysis and spondylolisthesis. J Bone Joint Surg Br 68(4):596–599
112. Sairyo K, Katoh S, Sakamaki T, Komatsubara S, Yasui N (2003) A new endoscopic technique to decompress lumbar nerve roots affected by spondylolysis. Technical note. J Neurosurg 98(3 Suppl):290–293
113. Karatas AF, Dede O, Atanda AA, Holmes L Jr, Rogers K, Gabos P, Shah SA (2016) Comparison of direct pars repair techniques of spondylolysis in pediatric and adolescent patients: pars compression screw versus pedicle screw-rod-hook. Clin Spine Surg 29(7):272–280

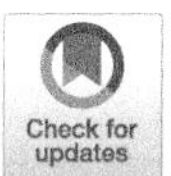

Return to Play After Rotator Cuff Surgery

25

Luca Pulici, Beatrice Zanini, Livia Carrai, Alessandra Menon, Riccardo Compagnoni, and Pietro Randelli

Contents

L. Pulici • L. Carrai • P. Randelli • A. Menon (✉)
Laboratory of Applied Biomechanics, Department of Biomedical Sciences for Health, University of Milan, Via Mangiagalli 31, 20133 Milan, Italy

U.O.C. 1° Divisione, Azienda Socio Sanitaria Territoriale Centro Specialistico Ortopedico Traumatologico Gaetano Pini-CTO, Piazza Cardinal Ferrari 1, 20122 Milan, Italy

B. Zanini • R. Compagnoni
U.O.C. 1° Divisione, Azienda Socio Sanitaria Territoriale Centro Specialistico Ortopedico Traumatologico Gaetano Pini-CTO, Piazza Cardinal Ferrari 1, 20122 Milan, Italy
e-mail: ale.menon@me.com

25.1 Introduction

The rotator cuff is a group of muscles and tendons that act as to stabilize the shoulder. The main functions of the rotator cuff are extra- and intra-rotation of the humeral head, stabilization of the humeral head into the glenoid cavity (through compressive forces), and contribution to muscular balance. The synergic work of rotator cuff muscles allows a selective movement of the humerus. Rotator cuff injury is a common cause of pain, and shoulder disability and traumatic lesions are also reported in young patients. Supraspinatus is the most frequently involved tendon, but isolated supraspinatus tears occur only in 40% of cases [1, 2]. Severe rotator cuff lesions may be caused in football players by high-energy trauma, such as macrotrauma occurred during match or training, or repeated microtrauma, which leads to weakening of soft tissues of the shoulder [3, 4]. The prognostic evaluation of rotator cuff tears must consider many factors, including the type of lesion, number of involved tendons, quality of residual tissue, and causes of the lesion.

25.2 Epidemiology

Football is one of the most popular sports worldwide; in fact, in Europe, about the 40–60% of sports-related trauma are due to football [5]. From

V. Musahl et al. (eds.), *Return to Play in Football*, https://doi.org/10.1007/978-3-662-55713-6_25

1.5 to 7.6 injuries per 1000 h of training and from 12 to 35 injuries per 1000 h of match occur in elite football players [5]. Football is a lower-limb-dominant sport, and the most common injured site is the lower limb (67.7%), followed by the upper limb (13.4%) [5]. Goalkeepers are more exposed to upper limb lesions than other football players [5]. A study regarding European professional male teams found shoulder injuries represented only 2% of all injuries during the years 2001–2008. This percentage is much lower than in other sports, where shoulder injuries are more frequently represented, respectively, 14% in rugby and 8% in volleyball and in American football [6]. In the last several years, there has been an increase in reported shoulder injuries in football players. Most likely, this change is due to the fact that modern football has been characterized by high speed, pressing and marking together with an improved overall injury detection strategy.

Fact Box 1. Epidemiology

40–60% of sports-related trauma are due to football.

An increased rate of shoulder injury has been recorded.

Isolated rotator cuff tears are rare.

A third of shoulder injuries are severe injuries (more than 28 days lost).

A previous shoulder injury is a significant risk factor for re-injury.

A study on English professional teams over 4 seasons showed that of 40,466 injury claims, 1335 (3.3%) were shoulder related, 445 serious shoulder injuries occurred each year, and the percentage increase in shoulder injuries (injuries per year/total shoulder injuries) increased from 35% in the 2006/2007 season to 89% in the 2009/2010 season [4]. A recent study reported that a third of shoulder injuries (28%) sustained by professional football players are severe and the participation in training and games is limited for at least 28 days [6].

A study of the UEFA European Championships reported 34 severe injuries, 2 of which were shoulder dislocation. A previous shoulder injury is a significant risk factor of more or repeated injuries than other football injuries in general. The majority of serious soccer shoulder injuries affect the glenoid labrum (84%), while a smaller number are labral injuries with associated rotator cuff involvement (8%), and a minority (8%) are isolated rotator cuff injuries [6].

During the Olympic Games in Athens in 2004 and UEFA EURO 2004, the percentage of shoulder damage was 3.8% and 4.4%, respectively. A recent study reported shoulder injuries between 2% and 13% during a 4-year period (from 1998 to 2001) of international tournaments. The Fédération Internationale de Football Association (FIFA) collected data during Japan/Korea World Cup (2002) and Germany World Cup (2006) reported higher percentages of upper extremity injury (4.6% and 8.2%, respectively) [5].

25.3 Etiology and Biomechanics

Many injuries in football occur as a result of a direct shoulder trauma. Consequences of these trauma are shoulder fractures (glenoid, humeral head, clavicle), glenohumeral dislocations (often with associated labral and SLAP tears), acromioclavicular dislocation, and rotator cuff lesions (full- or partial-thickness tears, tendinopathy, or contusions). Several kinds of lesions may involve rotator cuff tendons due to different injury mechanisms. Rotator cuff lesions are mainly classified in articular, bursal, and intra-tendinous, with different prognosis and treatment options. In goalkeepers, which can be considered overhead athletes, each of these types of lesions can be found. In these athletes, subacromial impingement is one of the most frequent problems affecting the shoulder. Subacromial impingement is usually classified as primary or secondary. The primary impingement is related to an unusual coracoacromial arch with a resulting lesion of the anterior surface of supraspinatus tendon. The most used classification for the acromion morphology is the one initially proposed by Bigliani et al. on outlet view radiographs that describe the acromion as flat, curved, and hooked [7]. In this report, the authors described a correlation between acromion morphology and tendon lesions. Secondary impingement is the consequence of trauma, with capsule laxity or glenohumeral ligament sprain.

Articular tears are due to intrinsic mechanism and characterized by the only degeneration of the lower portion of the tendon that leads to a progressive delamination. Intra-tendinous tears are caused by strong eccentric forces acting on the upper limb during the phase of deceleration. These lesions involve the tendon between bursal and articular sides; this kind of tear can cause much pain [8–10]. Rotator cuff tears may also be classified according to the thickness of the involved tendon (partial or complete), the etiology (degenerative or traumatic), and the number of injured tendons (isolated or massive).

The principal classification of rotator cuff tears is the Snyder classification, and its importance is due to the direct implication on the surgical treatment [11]. This classification provides the evaluation of two different features: the side involved in the lesion (articular, bursal or complete tears) and its extension.

25.4 Treatment Options and Rehabilitation Protocol

In professional athletes, it is extremely important to perform a multidimensional evaluation. In all patients, an accurate clinical evaluation is usually followed by imaging analysis, such as X-ray, ultrasonographic evaluation, and in some cases computer tomography (CT) scan or magnetic resonance imaging (MRI). In high-level athletes, some specific aspects have to be considered, including the role of the player, timing of the season, and expectations of the patient. Understanding all of these aspects is crucial for a good compliance of the patient, and more time than usual is often requested in this population [8].

Depending on these clinical, imaging, and psychological factors, the sports physician may opt for conservative or surgical treatment (Fig. 28.1).

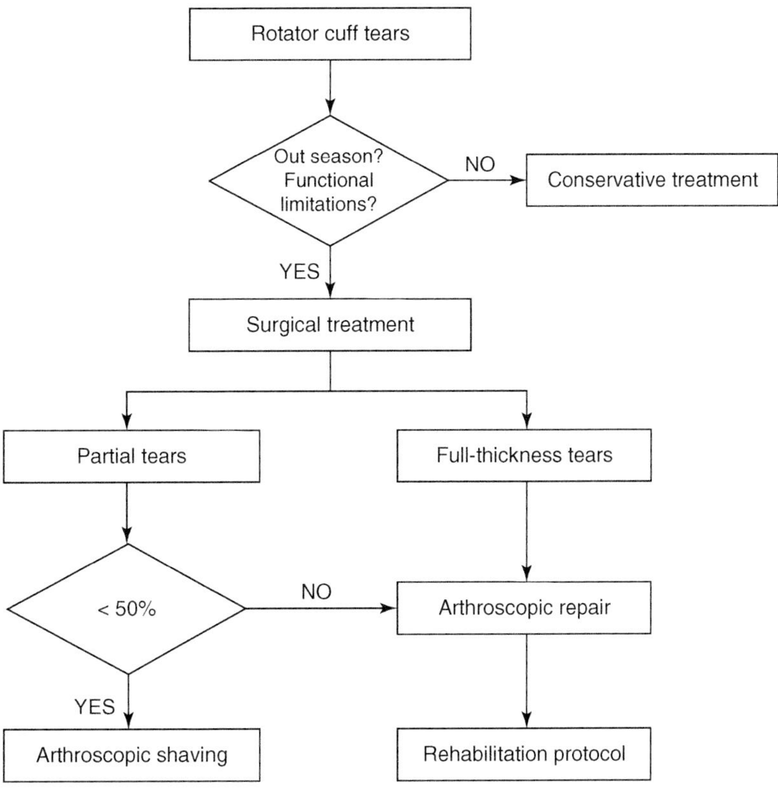

Fig. 28.1 Therapeutic approach to football players with rotator cuff tears

25.4.1 Conservative Treatment

Conservative treatment is proposed in cases of simple shoulder trauma, while relevant lesions are excluded by imaging analysis. Also, small rotator cuff tears can be initially treated in a conservative way. This approach consists of shoulder immobilization in a sling for a brief period, typically from 1 to 3 weeks. After immobilization, the treatment is focused on controlling pain and restoring full range of motion with the support of a physiotherapist, practicing neuromuscular training [12–16]. If small lesions are present and the conservative treatment have not obtained a resolution of pain along with persisting functional limitations, a surgical approach can be considered.

25.4.2 Surgical Treatment

Surgery is indicated for athletes with severe pain and/or functional limitation and when rotator cuff tears are evidenced by imaging evaluation. In these cases, the correct timing of surgery must to be planned.

Partial rotator cuff tears are usually treated with partial shaving and, according to tissue characteristics or lesion extension, may require conversion to a repair in full-thickness lesions. Repair techniques attempt to restore contact between the tendon and the humeral footprint and are performed using single-row, double-row, or transosseous equivalent techniques.

Although surgical procedures for rotator cuff repair have improved over the past decades, unsatisfying clinical results in overhead athletes are still observed. In fact, only 49.9% of professional athletes return to play at the same level after rotator cuff repair [17]. Therefore, when lesions involve <50% of tendinous thickness, arthroscopic debridement is the procedure of choice. In overhead athletes, this cutoff percentage may be increased to 75% [18].

Fact Box 2. Treatment

Treatment is based on type of lesion, symptoms, and time of sports season.

Conservative treatment: short immobilization, control pain and then restore full range of motion.

Surgical treatment might be postponed until the off-season.

Consider arthroscopy shaving in partial tear <50% and repair in other conditions.

In arthroscopic repair, the use of platelet-rich plasma at the end of the procedure has shown to be effective to reduce postoperative pain [19]. Also, better results are reported in efficacy of post-op rehabilitation. An appropriate rehabilitation protocol is necessary to reach a complete functional recovery of the shoulder.

25.4.3 Rehabilitation Protocol

Numerous postoperative rehabilitation protocols have been described. Generally, these protocols can be dichotomized as standard or accelerated. Supposed advantages of an accelerated protocol are rapid return to daily activity, less risk of articular rigidity, and faster recovery in the case of small- and medium-sized tears. Possible risks of the accelerated protocol include an increased risk of re-injury during therapy for large tears and incomplete repair; for this reason, these are usually considered as contraindications.

Fact Box 3. Rehabilitation Protocol

Choose accelerated protocol for professional football player.

Phase I: at the first and second week, patients begin passive mobilization, and from third to fourth passive motion and hydrokinesis therapy.

Phase II: active mobilization, proprioceptive, and isometric exercises for active range of motion.
Phase III: at 2 months post-op, patients start basic strengthening exercises.
Phase IV: proprioceptive and advanced strengthening exercises.
Phase V: athlete's return to sport and rehabilitation to specific athletic skills.

The rehabilitation period may be divided into the following phases (Fig. 28.2).

25.4.3.1 Phase I

Standard protocol is adopted for sedentary patients and for people presenting risk factors for accelerated protocol; it consists of immobilization for 4 weeks, removing the brace only for washing, getting dressed, and eating.

The accelerated protocol is used for young and active patients, without risk factors; during the first and second week, patient may begin passive mobilization, and then, from third and fourth week, they start pendular movements and hydrokinesitherapy with a physiotherapist.

When patient reaches almost a complete shoulder range of motion, and there is no pain at rest, they can start the phase II.

25.4.3.2 Phase II

After 4 weeks, athletes can start active mobilization, proprioceptive (in an open kinetic chain), and isometric exercises for improving muscular tropism and regaining force and complete mobility.

At the end of this phase, a complete active range of motion, compared to the contralateral side, should be observed.

25.4.3.3 Phase III

At 2 months post-op, the patient may begin the basic strengthening and proprioceptive training program. He starts to practice proprioceptive and reinforcement exercises in close kinetic chain-like push-up progression (Fig. 28.3), using exercise equipment, such as cable and pulley.

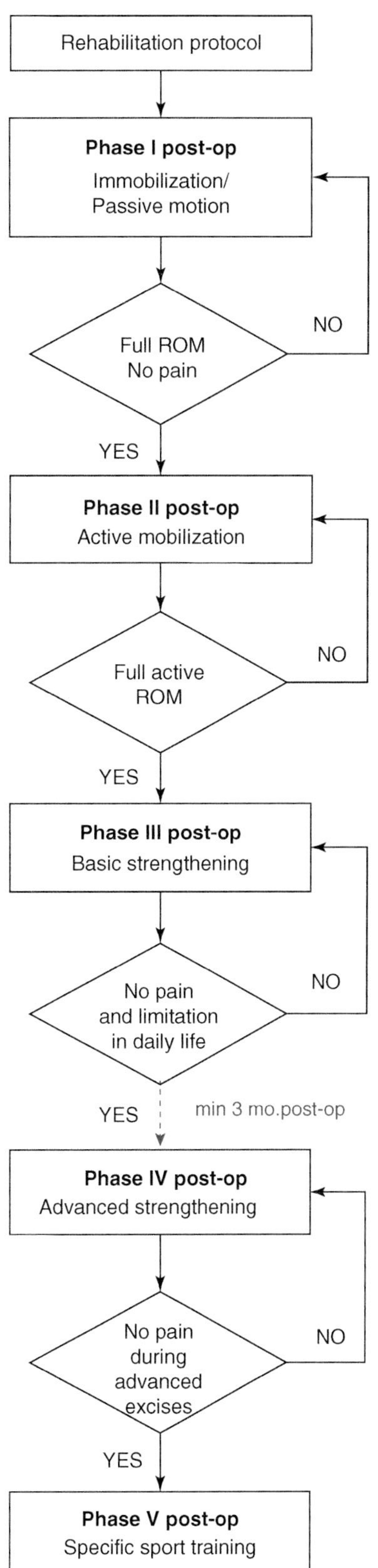

Fig. 28.2 Rehabilitation protocol after rotator cuff repair

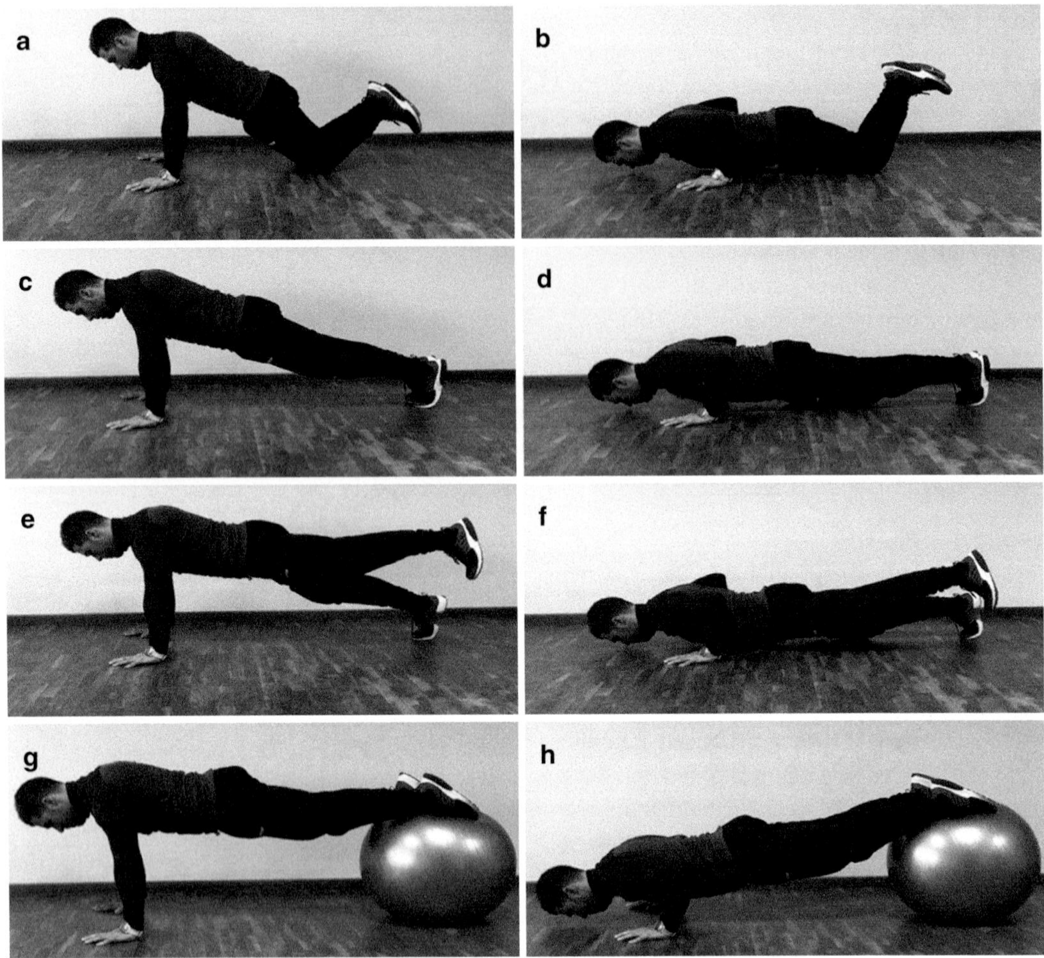

Fig. 28.3 Intensity progression of push-up exercise. Knee push-up: (**a**) starting position and (**b**) ending position. Full push-up: (**c**) starting position and (**d**) ending position. Single-leg push-up: (**e**) starting position and (**f**) ending position. Push-up with exercise ball: (**g**) starting position and (**h**) ending position

When the pain disappears at all, both at rest and practicing reinforcing exercises, patient can start the last phase of rehabilitation.

25.4.3.4 Phase IV

At minimum 3 months post-op, advanced strengthening exercises and proprioceptive exercise may be introduced (Fig. 28.4). In this period patient must carry out rehabilitation training through proprioceptive and reinforcing exercises, such as the plyometric ones, stabilization with advanced closed kinetic chain, extra rotation at 45° and 90°, and advanced push-up exercises.

25.4.3.5 Phase V

This phase is the athlete's return to sport and rehabilitation to specific athletic gestures. If there are no limitations during advanced exercises, athlete turns to practice training on field and specific sports skills training.

25.5 Return to Play

In football players may return to their athletic activity in 5–7 months, according to the type of tear, the treatment, and the role [20–23].

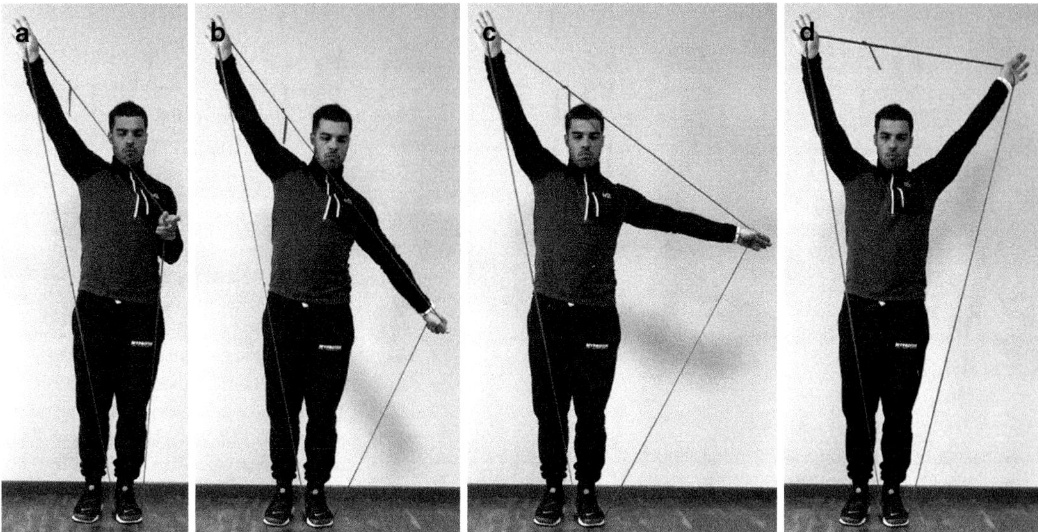

Fig. 28.4 Basic proprioceptive exercise: (**a**) starting position and (**b**–**d**) three different ending positions

Return to play is a very challenging problem, considering that limited guidelines are published and many times choices are made according to personal experience.

A good decision-based return to play model is that proposed by Creighton [24], in which there are three steps:

- Step 1: evaluation of health status
- Step 2: evaluation of participation risk (i.e., type of sport, position played, competitive level, etc.)
- Step 3: decision modification (i.e., timing and season, external pressure, conflict of interest, etc.)

For these reasons the decision to return to play should be taken by different figures [25], each one with his skills. The surgeon's instructions regarding the athlete's health status are critical for planning their return to play. Then, the sports physician should be supported by the indications of physical therapists, trainers, and coaches to evaluate steps 2 and 3.

Take-Home Message

Shoulder injuries in football players have increased over the last few years. Return to play after rotator cuff tears is challenging and few guidelines have been published.

According to the type of lesion, its symptoms, and the role of the football player, the treatment of rotator cuff tears can be surgical or conservative. Surgery consists of tendon repair, and many techniques are described in literature. Conservative treatment is based on shoulder immobilization, pain control, and restoring full range of motion with physiotherapy.

The rehabilitation protocol after surgery provides five different phases and has different duration in standard and accelerated protocols.

In football, return to play usually requires 5–7 months according to the type of tear, the treatment, and its role.

Top Five Evidence Based References

Creighton DW, Shrier I, Shultz R, Meeuwisse WH, Matheson GO (2010) Return-to-play in sport: a decision-based model. Clin J Sport Med 20(5):379–385

Ejnisman B, Barbosa G, Andreoli CV, de Castro Pochini A, Lobo T, Zogaib R, Cohen M, Bizzini M, Dvorak J (2016) Shoulder injuries in soccer goalkeepers: review and development of a FIFA 11+ shoulder injury prevention program. Open Access J Sports Med 7:75–80

Hart D, Funk L (2015) Serious shoulder injuries in professional soccer: return to participation after surgery. Knee Surg Sports Traumatol Arthrosc 23(7):2123–2129

Klouche S, Lefevre N, Herman S, Gerometta A, Bohu Y (2016) Return to sport after rotator cuff tear repair: a systematic review and meta-analysis. Am J Sports Med 44(7):1877–1887

Randelli P, Arrigoni P, Ragone V, Aliprandi A, Cabitza P (2011) Platelet rich plasma in arthroscopic rotator cuff repair: a prospective RCT study, 2-year follow-up. J Shoulder Elbow Surg 20(4):518–528

References

1. Arai R, Sugaya H, Mochizuki T et al (2008) Subscapularis tendon tear: an anatomic and clinical investigation. Arthroscopy 24:997–1004
2. Tuite MJ (2012) Magnetic resonance imaging of rotator cuff disease and external impingement. Magn Reson Imaging Clin N Am 20:187–200. ix
3. Braun S, Kokmeyer D, Millett PJ (2009) Shoulder injuries in the throwing athlete. J Bone Joint Surg Am 91:966–978
4. Dillman CJ, Fleisig GS, Andrews JR (1993) Biomechanics of pitching with emphasis upon shoulder kinematics. J Orthop Sports Phys Ther 18:402–408
5. Ejnisman B, Barbosa G, Andreoli CV et al (2016) Shoulder injuries in soccer goalkeepers: review and development of a FIFA 11+ shoulder injury prevention program. Open Access J Sports Med 7:75–80
6. Hart D, Funk L (2015) Serious shoulder injuries in professional soccer: return to participation after surgery. Knee Surg Sports Traumatol Arthrosc 23:2123–2129
7. Bigliani L, April E (1986) The morphology of the acromion and rotator cuff impingement. Orthopedic Transcription
8. Meister K, Andrews JR (1993) Classification and treatment of rotator cuff injuries in the overhand athlete. J Orthop Sports Phys Ther 18:413–421
9. Paulson MM, Watnik NF, Dines DM (2001) Coracoid impingement syndrome, rotator interval reconstruction, and biceps tenodesis in the overhead athlete. Orthop Clin North Am 32(485-493):ix
10. Walch G, Boileau P, Noel E et al (1992) Impingement of the deep surface of the supraspinatus tendon on the posterosuperior glenoid rim: an arthroscopic study. J Shoulder Elbow Surg 1:238–245
11. Snyder SJ (1994) Diagnostic arthroscopy: normal anatomy and variations. In: Shoulder arthroscopy. McGraw-Hill, Inc., New York, NY
12. Andrews JR, Broussard TS, Carson WG (1985) Arthroscopy of the shoulder in the management of partial tears of the rotator cuff: a preliminary report. Arthroscopy 1:117–122
13. Blevins FT (1997) Rotator cuff pathology in athletes. Sports Med (Auckland, NZ) 24:205–220
14. Jobe CM (1995) Posterior superior glenoid impingement: expanded spectrum. Arthroscopy 11:530–536
15. Jobe CM (1997) Superior glenoid impingement. Orthop Clin North Am 28:137–143
16. Nakagawa S, Yoneda M, Hayashida K et al (2001) Greater tuberosity notch: an important indicator of articular-side partial rotator cuff tears in the shoulders of throwing athletes. Am J Sports Med 29:762–770
17. Klouche S, Lefevre N, Herman S et al (2016) Return to sport after rotator cuff tear repair: a systematic review and meta-analysis. Am J Sports Med 44:1877–1887
18. Corpus KT, Camp CL, Dines DM et al (2016) Evaluation and treatment of internal impingement of the shoulder in overhead athletes. World J Orthoped 7:776–784
19. Randelli P, Arrigoni P, Ragone V et al (2011) Platelet rich plasma in arthroscopic rotator cuff repair: a prospective RCT study, 2-year follow-up. J Shoulder Elbow Surg 20:518–528
20. Cuff DJ, Pupello DR (2012) Prospective evaluation of postoperative compliance and outcomes after rotator cuff repair in patients with and without workers' compensation claims. J Shoulder Elbow Surg 21:1728–1733
21. Kim YS, Chung SW, Kim JY et al (2012) Is early passive motion exercise necessary after arthroscopic rotator cuff repair? Am J Sports Med 40:815–821
22. Klintberg IH, Gunnarsson AC, Svantesson U et al (2009) Early loading in physiotherapy treatment after full-thickness rotator cuff repair: a prospective randomized pilot-study with a two-year follow-up. Clin Rehabil 23:622–638
23. Koh KH, Lim TK, Shon MS et al (2014) Effect of immobilization without passive exercise after rotator cuff repair: randomized clinical trial comparing four and eight weeks of immobilization. J Bone Joint Surg Am 96:e44
24. Creighton DW, Shrier I, Shultz R et al (2010) Return-to-play in sport: a decision-based model. Clin J Sport Med 20:379–385
25. Shrier I, Safai P, Charland L (2014) Return to play following injury: whose decision should it be? Br J Sports Med 48:394–401

Return to Play After Shoulder Stabilization

26

Jason J. Shin and Bryson Lesniak

Contents

26.1 Introduction

As a lower-limb-dominant sport, most common football injuries involve the knee, ankle, and thigh musculature. Representing 2–3% of all injuries in football, far lower than the reported 28% in rugby [1] and 21% in hockey [2], shoulder injuries are less common and mostly seen in goalkeepers [3]. Nevertheless, a longitudinal epidemiologic study of English Premier League professional teams over a 4-year period revealed an increasing trend in both incidence as well as severity of shoulder injuries [4]. Although football has a relatively low incidence of shoulder injuries, with over 240 million amateur players and 200,000 professional athletes around the world, the raw number of cases as well as personal, societal, and economic impact of these injuries is tremendous.

Unlike other sports (American football, rugby) where the acromioclavicular joint often make up a large proportion of shoulder injury, majority of serious football shoulder injuries affect the glenoid labrum (84%). Although scientific literature has largely neglected research tailored toward shoulder instability in football players, more recently, there have been growing emphasis on management of such injuries within the demographic to guide the clinician on appropriate return to participation strategies.

Although glenohumeral instability is an important injury for field players, it usually does not eliminate them from return to a high level of competition. Goalkeepers represent a special subset population within football where the demands of the position subject the shoulder to injury from dives, direct falls onto shoulder, reaching and stretching for saves, as well as throwing the ball. Persistent pain and recurrent instability is considered to be more frequent in goalkeepers, and residual apprehension can negatively influence the player's ability to perform such tasks [5].

J.J. Shin, M.D., F.R.C.S.C. • B. Lesniak, M.D. (✉)
Division of Sports Medicine, University of Pittsburgh Medical Center, 3200 S Water St., Pittsburgh, PA, 15203, USA
e-mail: lesniakbp@upmc.edu

V. Musahl et al. (eds.), *Return to Play in Football*, https://doi.org/10.1007/978-3-662-55713-6_26

26.2 Biomechanics, Pathoanatomy, and Natural History

Allowing range of motion in all six degrees of freedom, the glenohumeral joint is the most mobile major joint in the human body [6]. Often described as a golf ball sitting on a tee, there is relative lack of bony congruency. While increased mobility allows for various athletic endeavors, this range of motion comes at the expense of stability and the shoulder is also the most frequently dislocated joint [7, 8]. The labrum and glenohumeral ligaments (superior, middle, and inferior) contribute to joint stability. Following a traumatic anterior dislocation, detachment of the anterior glenoid labrum and the anterior band of the inferior glenohumeral ligament (IGHL) (i.e., Bankart lesion) has been reported in 97% of young athletes.

Anterior dislocations are most common and are often result of a fall onto abducted arm, with a resultant external rotation moment applied. Other described mechanisms of dislocation include arm tugging during running, body contact to the back of the shoulder joint, as well as contact to the underside of the upper limb while in midair (heading). Although representing only a single player on a field of 11, half of shoulder injuries incurred by the team are by goalkeepers [3, 5].

Patient's age at time of initial dislocation is inversely related to recurrence rate. Although the exact number of dislocation events resulting in osteoarthritis has not been defined, the number of recurrent instability episodes is thought to correlate with development of arthritis. Moreover, repeated dislocation events likely contribute injury to cartilage, bone loss, and attenuation of the labrum and capsule.

Fact Box 1

Multiple glenohumeral dislocation events can result in to glenoid erosion and deformation of the capsule, which can lead to recurrent instability. Repeated injury and trauma to the shoulder joint can influence the surgical options as well as its outcome and prognosis.

26.3 On-Field and Early Evaluation of Shoulder Instability

After ruling out any catastrophic injuries, history can be gathered from the athlete as well as athletic trainer. Video replay, when available, may provide invaluable information regarding mechanism of injury. Anterior instability often occurs with the arm in abducted and externally rotated position. Palpable prominence of the anterior and inferior to the shoulder as well as loss of normal contour over the deltoid may be noted. The athlete will have decreased range of motion of the shoulder. After a thorough neurovascular examination of the upper limb, with special emphasis on the axillary nerve function, reduction maneuver may be attempted on the sideline. Anesthesia is often not required if reduction is performed if attempted acutely before the onset of muscle spasm. If the athlete is unable to tolerate reduction on the field or if the musculature is in spasm and reduction is difficult, he or she should be taken to the training room for an intra-articular block with local anesthetic. If there is any concern for a concomitant fracture, an acute reduction should not be attempted until radiographs are obtained. Sedation is associated with more complications and is reserved for difficult reductions. After a successful reduction, a thorough postreduction neurovascular examination as well as radiographs are performed. The authors prefer a true anteroposterior (AP) view of the glenohumeral joint as well as an axillary view to obtain orthogonal imaging to document acceptable reduction. If the athlete is unable to achieve sufficient abduction, a Velpeau view may be used instead [9]. Specific instability examinations such as apprehension test, relocation test, and load-and-shift test are rarely useful in the acute setting and reserved for the subacute situation. According to a recent meta-analysis, the surprise test, where the examiner completes the relocation test, then suddenly releases the posteriorly directed force and the patient again feels a sudden onset of instability, is the most sensitive test [10].

Magnetic resonance imaging (MRI) is essential to assess for labral-ligamentous-capsular,

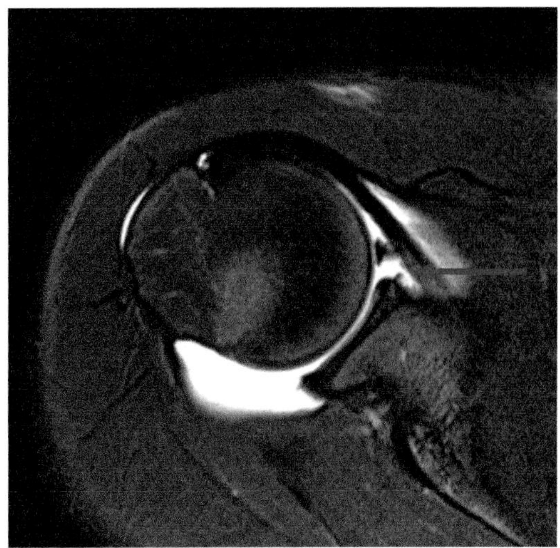

Fig. 26.1 Axial magnetic resonance arthrogram of the right shoulder. The *red arrow* is pointing to the anterior labral detachment

rotator cuff and articular cartilage abnormalities (Fig. 26.1). If the scan is obtained within a week of the dislocation, the hemarthrosis or effusion present in the joint can act as a natural contrast for arthrography [11]. In the subacute setting, intra-articular gadolinium contrast is injected into the glenohumeral space to allow for improved diagnosis of subtle injuries [12]. MRI can also be useful for quantifying glenoid bone loss. Three-dimensional (3D) computed tomography (CT) en face glenoid view has been considered to be the gold standard imaging technique to characterize glenoid morphology. Using MRI alone over CT scan has the benefit of reducing exposure to ionizing radiation in the young athlete. Recent studies suggest that 3D MRI is equivalent to 3D CT in determining glenoid bone loss [13]. In general, bone loss >20% to 25% is considered critical bone loss and dictates surgical management as well as prognosis [14, 15].

Fact Box 2
MRI with intra-articular contrast will improve diagnosis of injury to the chondral-labral junction. However, if acquired in an acute setting, hemarthrosis acts as natural contrast and a plain MRI is adequate.

26.4 Management

26.4.1 Nonoperative Management of Anterior Instability

After an athlete sustains an anterior shoulder dislocation, it is important to discuss the risks and benefits of treatment options with the athlete and/or family. The in-season athlete may elect to undergo nonoperative treatment and complete the season. Contraindications to nonoperative in-season management include failure of prior nonoperative treatment, engaging Hill-Sachs lesion, bony Bankart >20%, humeral avulsion of glenohumeral ligament lesions (HAGL), and previous failed stabilization surgery [6, 7] (Fact Box 3). Despite pressure on both the athlete and physician to return the athlete to sport as soon as possible, recognizing the relatively high rate of recurrent instability, the physician must ensure a safe and effective nonsurgical management regimen, with proper rehabilitation before clearing the athlete to return to play. Although there are no well-designed studies looking especially at timing of return to play after nonoperative management, based on lower-level evidence and expert opinion, an athlete may be authorized to return to play when he or she has minimal pain, near-normal motion, strength, functional ability, as well as sport-/position-specific skills.

Fact Box 3
Contraindications to nonoperative management of anterior shoulder instability:

In-season athlete
Failure of nonoperative treatment
Large or engaging Hill-Sachs lesion
Glenoid bone loss >20%
Humeral avulsion of glenohumeral ligament lesion
Failed previous stabilization procedure

26.4.2 Immobilization

In the last decade, there has been much debate within the orthopedic literature over the optimal position of immobilization after an instability event and its effect on recurrence. In an MRI study to assess the position of the Bankart lesion, Itoi et al. [16] described that when the shoulder was in external rotation (ER), the musculotendinous complex of the subscapularis became taut, thereby indirectly reducing the labrum back to the glenoid rim. Based on this finding, the investigators postulated that the rate of recurrence would decrease if the Bankart lesion could heal anatomically after traumatic shoulder dislocation. The MRI findings have not always translated to improved recurrence rate with ER immobilization. In a follow-up clinical study, 198 patients with first-time dislocation were randomized to either IR or ER immobilization [17]. With intention to treat analysis, the authors reported a 38.2% relative risk reduction in favor of ER immobilization. However, a recent meta-analysis of six randomized control trials (632 patients) finds no significant difference in rate of recurrence among patients treated with IR versus ER immobilization. Furthermore, the pooled Western Ontario Shoulder Instability Index scores across three studies did not demonstrate any difference between the two groups [18]. The current best available evidence does not appear to support ER immobilization after an episode of instability.

Another area of debate has been the optimal duration of immobilization. In a Swedish multicenter prospective study of primary anterior dislocation of the shoulder, 257 patients were followed for 2 years [19]. While 112 patients were immobilized for 3–4 weeks, 104 patients began to use the shoulder as early and as freely as possible. The authors found equal rate of recurrence of dislocation for both groups. Additionally, pooled data from a systematic review of six studies (five level I and one level II studies) evaluating the use of immobilization in internal rotation for varying lengths of time found no statistical difference in rate of recurrent instability in patients who had been immobilized for 1 week or less compared to patients who had been immobilized for 3 weeks or longer [20]. The current best available literature does not support prolonged immobilization after an instability event. Furthermore, this review showed that regardless of treatment period or immobilization method, age of <30 years at the time of index dislocation was significantly predictive of recurrence.

In one small study of 30 in-season athletes of various sports (wrestling, skiing, gymnastics, hockey), Buss et al. [21] were more aggressive and did not implement any period of immobilization after an instability episode. Physical therapy was initiated immediately including wand and 1 lb free weight exercises as well as periscapular strengthening. Athletes were returned to their sports when they had symmetrical strength bilaterally and a functional range of motion for full participation. Following this protocol, most athletes (26 of 30, 87%) were able to return to their sports for the complete season at an average of 10.2 days missed. Of 26 (37%) that returned to sports, 10 experienced additional instability events during the season. In total more than half (16 athletes) underwent stabilization procedure (4 in-season and 12 off-season). Despite small numbers, this study demonstrates that although more than half go onto have surgical stabilization, midseason athletes are often able to complete the season following an early rehabilitation protocol.

Braces function to prevent extreme shoulder abduction, extension, and external rotation and are associated with subjective improvement in stability. Although brace wear is advocated by many investigators, it has no proven efficiency, and no studies have demonstrated a decreased frequency of in-season instability events with bracing. Nevertheless, these braces may be utilized in outfield players where overhead and outstretched arm activities are less critical motions compared to goalkeepers.

26.4.3 Operative Management

When looking at first-time anterior dislocation, multiple studies have found 75–92% rate of recurrent instability in those treated nonoperatively, whereas those treated with surgery had 12–14% rate of recurrent instability with >30 months of follow-up [22–24]. There are no definitive markers to indicate exactly when in the season to recommend surgical stabilization. Instead based on common rationale, recurrent instability despite nonoperative measures such as maximum rehabilitative efforts, bracing, and inability of the athlete to perform sports may influence decision to pursue in-season surgery. Often for outfield players, the treatment can be performed in the off-season with minimal lost time and to facilitate adequate rehabilitation.

26.4.3.1 Arthroscopic Stabilization

With the advent of modern arthroscopic techniques, implants, and instrumentation, arthroscopic stabilization has become more popular. The arthroscopic approach has the added benefit of not disrupting the subscapularis. When performing arthroscopic soft tissue stabilization, certain principles must be adhered to such as using adequate number of suture anchors (three or more), achieving an adequate shift of capsular tissue along with plication to address the laxity, and treating of associated intra-articular disease [6, 25]. Although initial reports of recurrence rates after arthroscopic Bankart were significantly higher than open stabilization technique, more recent reviews show that no significant difference exists between the two approaches with respect to recurrence or patient-reported outcomes [26–28] (Fig. 26.2).

Terra et al. reported their outcomes after an arthroscopic capsulolabral repair in a study of 12 professional goalkeepers using suture anchors. The authors excluded athletes with glenoid bone loss >25% or engaging Hill-Sachs, humeral avulsion of glenohumeral ligament, and those with poor capsule tissue quality. The goalkeepers were allowed to resume competitive play at 6 months postoperatively. At final follow-up of 2 years, 4 of 12 (33%) reported recurrent instability and went on to have additional procedures (one Bristow coracoid transfer procedure, one open Neer's capsular shift). The authors further compared the outcomes of those who underwent stabilization following a single episode of instability to those who had surgery following multiple episodes of instability. In the acutely treated group, failure, defined as recurrence after

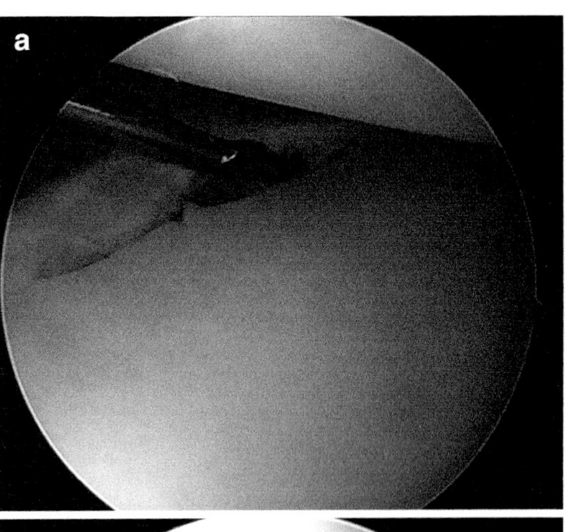

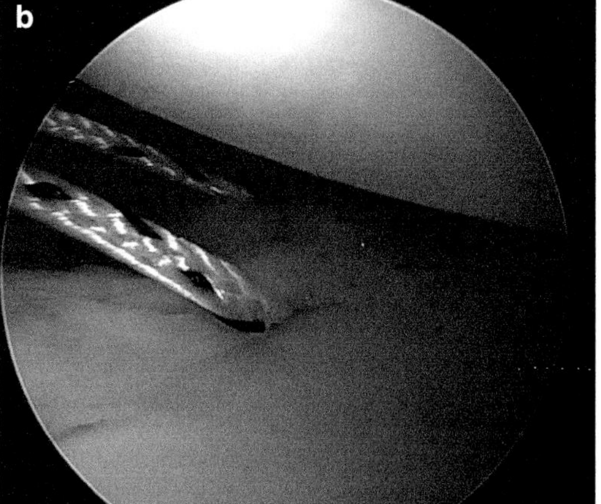

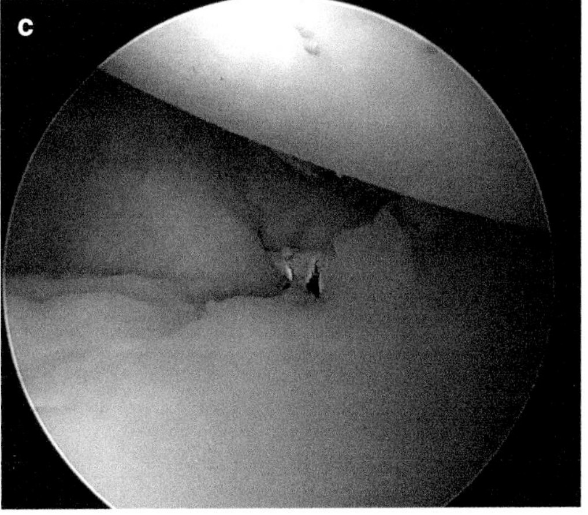

Fig. 26.2 Arthroscopic view of the right shoulder from the posterior portal demonstrating (**a**) capsulolabral detachment from the glenoid anteriorly, (**b**) passing of the labral tape around the capsule/labrum, (**c**) finished repair using a knotless suture construct

surgery, was 20%. In contrast, goalkeepers treated after multiple events had a much higher failure rate of 43%. The authors of this study concluded that even among this difficult population of professional goalkeepers, arthroscopic capsulolabral repair can be carried out with good results in those with acute dislocation without evidence of significant glenohumeral bone loss. However, this study suggests that the results arthroscopic soft tissue procedures are less predictable in goalkeepers with recurrent instability.

26.4.3.2 Bone Block

Although revision surgery by itself is not an absolute contraindication to arthroscopic approach after failed primary arthroscopic surgery, open techniques including the Latarjet procedure are often utilized. In Europe, the Latarjet procedure is often performed for primary stabilization. In a prospective case-control study of 131 consecutive patients with recurrent anterior shoulder instability, Balg and Boileau [14] developed a scoring system to identify patients who would benefit from an open procedure versus an arthroscopic Bankart procedure. Risk factors for recurrence were identified and assigned points to guide treatment (Fact Box 4). After applying this score to the study population, the authors reported if the score was six or less, the recurrence rate was 10%, but if it was more than six, the recurrence rate was significantly higher at 70%.

Fact Box 4. Balg and Boileau's Shoulder Instability Severity Index Score [14]

Age ≤20	2
Age >20	0
Competitive sports participation	2
Recreational or none	0
Contact/overhead sports	1
Noncontact sport	0
Shoulder hyperlaxity	1
Normal laxity	0
Hill-Sachs visual on AP radiograph	
Visible in ER	2
Not visible in ER	0
Glenoid loss of contour on AP radiograph	2
No lesion	0

AP anteroposterior, *ER* external rotation

Cerciello and Walch [5] reported on the outcome of Latarjet procedure in 28 shoulders of semiprofessional or professional football players with chronic anterior glenohumeral instability. Of the 28 shoulders, 8 were in goalkeepers, and patients reported an average of 7.5 dislocations before having the surgery. The surgeries were performed through a horizontal split at the superior one-third with inferior two-third junction in the subscapularis, and the coracoid was fixed with two 4.5 mm malleolar screws. One patient was unable to return to football. While 25% played football at lower level, the remainder (71.4%) were able to return to play football at the same level as they did before surgery. Only one re-dislocation was noted in a goalkeeper 6 years after the surgery. The authors concluded that Latarjet procedure is the gold standard in the treatment of chronic anterior glenohumeral instability in football players and especially in the high-risk subpopulation of goalkeepers (Fig. 26.3).

26.5 Author's Preferred Management

Nonoperative management is considered in the early season to midseason for athletes with primary instability events without significant glenohumeral bony lesions. However, for athletes who have an injury in the postseason or early preseason, depending on the athlete's goals and level of play, early operative management should be considered to allow for adequate rehabilitation for the following season. Figure 26.4 outlines the recommended algorithm for management following an instability event. They can be rehabilitated with a brief course of sling use for comfort and cryotherapy in the first week. Once past the acute phase of injury, athletes then follow a protocol of rotator cuff and periscapular strengthening exercises along with range of motion exercises. Sport- and position-specific drills are initiated prior to being cleared to play. It is especially important to achieve adequate ROM and strength through intensive rehabilitation in goalkeepers where their positional demands put them at increased risk for recurrent dislocation. After failing

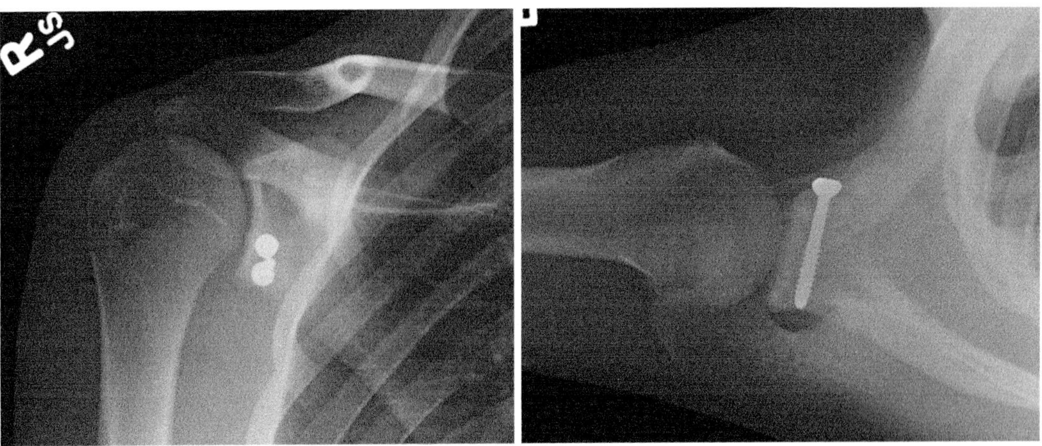

Fig. 26.3 Glenohumeral anteroposterior and axillary view of plain radiographs of the right shoulder after a Latarjet procedure

Anterior instability event

-Glenoid defect >20%
-Large Hill-Sachs
-Recurrent instability

Surgery

-Minimal or no bone loss

-Brief immobilization for comfort
-Cyrocuff

Rehabilitation
-Painless ROM
-Rotator cuff/ periscapular strengthening
-Sport/position specific drills

Return to play

Surgery

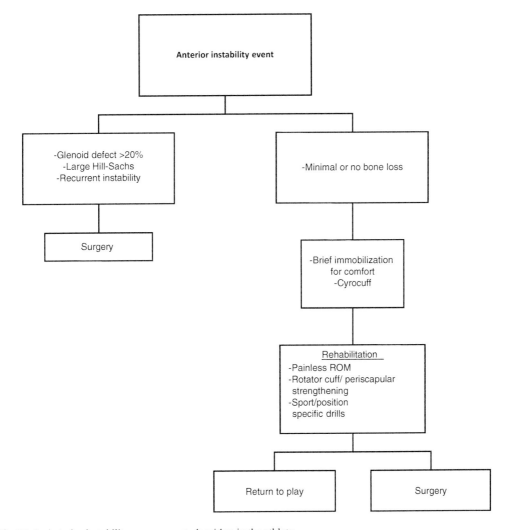

Fig. 26.4 Anterior instability management algorithm in the athlete

nonsurgical measures, athletes may undergo Bankart procedure. In the absence of significant bone loss, arthroscopic approach is the preferred approach in most primary cases. In select cases, using principles from the instability severity index score by Balg and Boileau [14], we may recommend Latarjet procedure over arthroscopic soft tissue procedure.

Anterior instability management algorithm in the athlete. ROM, range of motion.

Take-Home Message

Anterior glenohumeral dislocation and resultant chronic instability are common in young athletes. Although predominantly a lower extremity sport, epidemiologic studies have shown increasing incidence and severity of shoulder related injuries in football. As popularity of football continues to grow, team physicians and orthopedic surgeons can expect to manage increasing number of such injuries. Several factors should be considered when managing these athletes following an episode of shoulder instability. Depending on the positional demands, outfield players with predominantly soft tissue pathology may be able to quickly return to sport with dedicated rehabilitation. Although there is paucity of literature in the efficacy of using braces during competition, numerous brands are commercially available, and some athletes may find it useful. Athletes unable to perform sport-specific drills and recurrent instability are candidates for surgical stabilization. Arthroscopic approaches have become popular when treating instability with high rates of success. In setting of major bone loss and in certain revision cases, open procedures are preferred.

Top Five Evidence Based References

Arciero RA, Wheeler JH, Ryan JB, McBride JT (1994) Arthroscopic bankart repair versus nonoperative treatment for acute, initial anterior shoulder dislocations. Am J Sports Med 22:589–594

Balg F, Boileau P (2007) The instability severity index score. A simple pre-operative score to select patients for arthroscopic or open shoulder stabilisation. J Bone Joint Surg Br 89:1470–1477

Buss DD, Lynch GP, Meyer CP, Huber SM, Freehill MQ (2004) Nonoperative management for in-season athletes with anterior shoulder instability. Am J Sports Med 32:1430–1433

Hart D, Funk L (2015) Serious shoulder injuries in professional soccer: return to participation after surgery. Knee Surg Sports Traumatol Arthrosc 23:2123–2129

Hovelius L, Eriksson K, Fredin H, Hagberg G, Hussenius A, Lind B, Thorling J, Weckström J (1983) Recurrences after initial dislocation of the shoulder. Results of a prospective study of treatment. J Bone Joint Surg Am 65:343–349

References

1. Usman J, McIntosh AS (2013) Upper limb injury in rugby union football: results of a cohort study. Br J Sports Med 47:374–379
2. Matic GT, Sommerfeldt MF, Best TM, Collins CL, Comstock RD, Flanigan DC (2015) Ice hockey injuries among United States high school athletes from 2008/2009-2012/2013. Phys Sportsmed 43:119–125
3. Hart D, Funk L (2015) Serious shoulder injuries in professional soccer: return to participation after surgery. Knee Surg Sports Traumatol Arthrosc 23:2123–2129
4. Pritchard C, Mills S, Funk L, Batty P (2011) Incidence and management of shoulder injuries in premier league professional football players. Br J Sports Med 45:A15–A15
5. Cerciello S, Edwards TB, Walch G (2012) Chronic anterior glenohumeral instability in soccer players: results for a series of 28 shoulders treated with the Latarjet procedure. J Orthop Traumatol Off J Ital Soc. Orthop Traumatol 13:197–202
6. Ward JP, Bradley JP (2013) Decision making in the in-season athlete with shoulder instability. Clin Sports Med 32:685–696
7. Donohue MA, Owens BD, Dickens JF (2016) Return to play following anterior shoulder dislocation and stabilization surgery. Clin Sports Med 35:545–561
8. Owens BD, Dickens JF, Kilcoyne KG, Rue J-PH (2012) Management of mid-season traumatic anterior shoulder instability in athletes. J Am Acad Orthop Surg 20:518–526
9. Rouleau DM, Hebert-Davies J, Robinson CM (2014) Acute traumatic posterior shoulder dislocation. J Am Acad Orthop Surg 22:145–152
10. Hegedus EJ, Goode AP, Cook CE, Michener L, Myer CA, Myer DM, Wright AA (2012) Which physical examination tests provide clinicians with the most value when examining the shoulder? Update of a systematic review with meta-analysis of individual tests. Br J Sports Med 46:964–978
11. Salomonsson B, Heine A v, Dahlborn M, Abbaszadegan H, Ahlström S, Dalén N, Lillkrona U (2010) Bony Bankart is a positive predictive factor after primary shoulder dislocation. Knee Surg Sports Traumatol Arthrosc 18:1425–1431
12. Antonio GE, Griffith JF, Yu AB, Yung PSH, Chan KM, Ahuja AT (2007) First-time shoulder disloca-

tion: high prevalence of labral injury and age-related differences revealed by MR arthrography. J Magn Reson Imaging 26:983–991
13. Yanke AB, Shin JJ, Pearson I, Bach BR, Romeo AA, Cole BJ, Verma NN (2017) Three-dimensional magnetic resonance imaging quantification of glenoid bone loss is equivalent to 3-dimensional computed tomography quantification: cadaveric study. Arthroscopy 33:709
14. Balg F, Boileau P (2007) The instability severity index score. A simple pre-operative score to select patients for arthroscopic or open shoulder stabilisation. J Bone Joint Surg Br 89:1470–1477
15. Burkhart SS, De Beer JF (2000) Traumatic glenohumeral bone defects and their relationship to failure of arthroscopic Bankart repairs: significance of the inverted-pear glenoid and the humeral engaging Hill-Sachs lesion. Arthroscopy 16:677–694
16. Itoi E, Sashi R, Minagawa H, Shimizu T, Wakabayashi I, Sato K (2001) Position of immobilization after dislocation of the glenohumeral joint. A study with use of magnetic resonance imaging. J Bone Joint Surg Am 83–A:661–667
17. Itoi E, Hatakeyama Y, Sato T, Kido T, Minagawa H, Yamamoto N, Wakabayashi I, Nozaka K (2007) Immobilization in external rotation after shoulder dislocation reduces the risk of recurrence. A randomized controlled trial. J Bone Joint Surg Am 89:2124–2131
18. Whelan DB, Kletke SN, Schemitsch G, Chahal J (2015) Immobilization in external rotation versus internal rotation after primary anterior shoulder dislocation. Am J Sports Med 44:521–532
19. Hovelius L, Eriksson K, Fredin H, Hagberg G, Hussenius A, Lind B, Thorling J, Weckström J (1983) Recurrences after initial dislocation of the shoulder. Results of a prospective study of treatment. J Bone Joint Surg Am 65:343–349
20. Paterson WH, Throckmorton TW, Koester M, Azar FM, Kuhn JE (2010) Position and duration of immobilization after primary anterior shoulder dislocation: a systematic review and meta-analysis of the literature. J Bone Joint Surg Am 92:2924–2933
21. Buss DD, Lynch GP, Meyer CP, Huber SM, Freehill MQ (2004) Nonoperative Management for In-Season Athletes with Anterior Shoulder Instability. Am J Sports Med 32:1430–1433
22. Arciero RA, Wheeler JH, Ryan JB, McBride JT (1994) Arthroscopic bankart repair versus nonoperative treatment for acute, initial anterior shoulder dislocations. Am J Sports Med 22:589–594
23. Bottoni CR, Wilckens JH, DeBerardino TM, D'Alleyrand J-CG, Rooney RC, Harpstrite JK, Arciero RA (2002) A prospective, randomized evaluation of arthroscopic stabilization versus nonoperative treatment in patients with acute, traumatic, first-time shoulder dislocations. Am J Sports Med 30:576–580
24. Wheeler JH, Ryan JB, Arciero RA, Molinari RN (1989) Arthroscopic versus nonoperative treatment of acute shoulder dislocations in young athletes. Arthroscopy 5:213–217
25. Tjoumakaris FP, Bradley JP (2011) The rationale for an arthroscopic approach to shoulder stabilization. Arthroscopy 27:1422–1433
26. Cole BJ, L'Insalata J, Irrgang J, Warner JJ (2000) Comparison of arthroscopic and open anterior shoulder stabilization. A two to six-year follow-up study. J Bone Joint Surg Am 82–A:1108–1114
27. Godin J, Sekiya JK (2011) Systematic review of arthroscopic versus open repair for recurrent anterior shoulder dislocations. Sports Health 3:396–404
28. Harris JD, Gupta AK, Mall NA, Abrams GD, McCormick FM, Cole BJ, Bach BR, Romeo AA, Verma NN (2013) Long-term outcomes after Bankart shoulder stabilization. Arthroscopy 29:920–933

Joint Specific Return to Play Recommendations: "Return to Play in Non-operative Hip/Groin Pain"

27

Nolan S. Horner, Seper Ekhtiari, Allison A. Chan, Hema N. Choudur, and Olufemi R. Ayeni

Contents

27.1 Introduction

Groin pain in the athletic population presents a diagnostic and therapeutic challenge for the sports medicine physician [1]. This is due to a number of factors, including the anatomically complex nature of the hip and groin regions, as well as an extensive list of differential diagnoses that can be difficult to tease apart [2]. Furthermore, athletic groin pain is not a well-defined clinical entity and is referred to by myriad terms including "athletic pubalgia," "Gilmore's groin," "osteitis pubis," "slapshot gut," "sportsman's hernia," and many more. Hölmich et al. [1] found that the majority of causes of groin pain in a group of athletes (mostly footballers) could be categorized into three etiologies: pathology of the adductors, iliopsoas, or abdominal muscles [1].

Fact Box
Physicians must be aware of the fact that athletes presenting with groin pain may in fact have multiple pathologies causing their pain. Many etiologies for groin pain such as FAI are known to increase the incidence of other groin pain-related pathologies.

The complex anatomy of the hip and groin region leads to a strong likelihood of multiple co-occurring conditions. Biomechanically, the pubic symphysis acts as a "fulcrum for forces generated

N.S. Horner (✉) • O.R. Ayeni
Division of Orthopaedic Surgery, Department of Surgery, McMaster University, 1200 Main Street West, 4E15, Hamilton, ON, Canada, L8N 3Z5
e-mail: nolan.horner@medportal.ca; femiayeni@gmail.com

S. Ekhtiari • A.A. Chan
Michael G. DeGroote School of Medicine, McMaster University, 1280 Main St W, Hamilton, ON, Canada, L8S 4K1

H.N. Choudur
Department of Radiology, Hamilton General Hospital, 237 Barton Street East Hamilton, ON, Canada, L9L 2X2

V. Musahl et al. (eds.), *Return to Play in Football*, https://doi.org/10.1007/978-3-662-55713-6_27

at the anterior pelvis" [3]. Thus, the majority of conditions presenting with athletic groin pain are related to structures in this region, including the transversalis fascia, the distal rectus abdominis, the pubis itself, the external oblique aponeurosis, and intra-articular processes such as femoral and acetabular abnormalities. Therefore, groin injuries are common in sports that heavily engage the lower body and involve sudden changes in direction, such as football [4]. In fact, groin injuries constitute up to 13% of all football injuries [1, 5].

Within a given sport, the prevalence of groin pain depends on a number of factors, including sex and level of competition. In a study directly comparing groin pain in male and female footballers, the authors found these injuries to be much more common in males, with an odds ratio of 2.9 [2]. A 7-year prospective study conducted by the Union of European Football Associations (UEFA) found an overall groin injury prevalence of 1.1/1000 match and training hours among professional players [6], compared to a study of amateur competitive footballers which found a groin injury rate of 0.4/1000 h [7]. Interestingly, both studies reported a mean absence of 15 days due to groin injuries. However, while 76% of amateur footballers missed 8 or more days, only 53% of professionals missed the same amount of time [6, 7]. This discrepancy may be related to a number of factors, including greater availability of rehabilitation resources for professional athletes, a higher level of pre-injury of fitness, and more motivation to return to sport. In any case, with professional teams suffering a mean seven groin injuries per season, these injuries are both common and costly. In fact, over a 5-year period, a study of professional football in Australia found that groin injuries alone cost teams a total of $AUD23.2 million [8].

Not only are groin injuries costly to teams, they can also endanger the playing careers of the athletes who suffer from them. In a case series of 60 patients with chronic groin pain, only half of all patients who were treated non-operatively returned to sport after 1 year [9]. Among amateur and professional footballers, 61–73% of injuries were identified as overuse injuries as opposed to traumatic injuries [6, 7], which suggests that the prevalence of these injuries may increase with more cumulative playing time. Finally, while there was no statistically significantly difference, the UEFA injury study did find that groin injuries were more common in the dominant leg (57% vs. 43%) [6].

The following chapter will be focused on return to play in footballers following non-operative management of hip/groin pain. Return to play following operative treatment will be discussed elsewhere in this book. This chapter will be organized by etiology and begin with an overview of adductor-related hip/groin pathology before moving on to iliopsoas-related pathology including snapping hip syndrome, abdominal pathology including "sports hernia," inguinal pathologies, femoroacetabular impingement (FAI), and labral tears and, finally, a brief overview of other groin pain-related pathologies relevant to footballers. The chapter will conclude with a brief summary and takeaway points.

27.2 Adductor-Related Pathology

Hip adductor pathology represents a common source of groin pain in football players. The adductors of the hip are used when running, kicking, cutting, or pivoting, all of which are common and crucial movements while playing football [5]. Adductor injury accounted for 64% of hip/groin injuries in a 7-year prospective study of professional football players in the Union of European Football Associations (UEFA) [3].

There exist several different forms of hip adductor pathology including hip adductor strains, adductor tendinopathy, and adductor avulsions. Hip adductor strain is an injury of the hip adductor muscles at the muscle belly, the myotendinous junction, or the tendon. The adductor longus myotendinous junction is the most commonly injured site in strains [10, 11]. This is thought to be due to poor blood supply to the pubic bone at the adductor longus tendon insertion [12, 13].

In a case series following 19 football players, Schlegel et al. found approximately half of adductor avulsion injuries occurred due to eccentric overload (i.e., "cutting back" and changing directions quickly) [14]. Thorborg et al. found eccentric hip adduction strength to be lower in football players with adductor-related groin pain in the dominant leg [15]. Furthermore, disturbances to the muscular balance can increase the load on hip adductors. Examples include foot or lower leg malalignment syndromes or leg length discrepancy [5]. Ekstrand and Gillquist found that decreased preseason hip abduction range of motion correlated with future adductor injury [16]. Extrinsic risk factors for adductor injury include overuse [16]; traumatic strain when the hip is in flexion, abduction, and external rotation (FABER); as well as maximal knee extension [5].

Hip adductor strain is typically localized to the proximal groin area and acute in onset [12]. Specifically, the pain is well localized, usually to the adductor longus belly, proximal musculotendinous junction, or near the tendon origin on inferior pubic ramus [1]. On examination, there may be soft tissue swelling and bruising in the medial thigh. Symptoms worsen on hip adduction and/or flexion. Hip adductor tendinopathy may begin as a primary condition or be secondary to adductor muscle strain [12] and tends to develop with increased activity [12]. If left untreated, the groin pain can spread to the contralateral groin or suprapubic groin region. In football players, adductor tenosynovitis is a common result of overuse injury and is seen more often in preseason training [5]. Adductor longus avulsions are most commonly caused by overstretching and kicking movements [13]. An acute tear of the proximal adductor longus may also occur, though this is very rare. These tears are thought to occur as a result of eccentric overload while forcefully abducting the leg [14]. Footballers suffering from adductor pathology will often have functional limitations such as difficulty with pivoting turns, propulsion in the lateral direction, and loss of maximal sprinting speed [15]. Werner et al. found that the average absence from sport in individuals with adductor injury was 14 days [3].

The diagnosis of hip adductor pathology begins with a physical examination. The adductor tendon insertion and/or muscle belly are commonly tender to palpation. Pain on passive abduction of the hip, or pain and weakness during resisted adduction and/or flexion, is also suggestive of adductor pathology [12]. Groin pain is often reproducible with the FABER test and the adductor squeeze test [16]. To perform the squeeze test, the patient is positioned supine with both hips flexed to 45° and knees flexed to 90°. The examiner then places a fist between the knees and asks patient to squeeze their knees together which may elicit pain in patients with adductor pathology [16].

Initial investigations of adductor pathology should include plain films of the pelvis and hip. Technetium-99m bone scan, showing increased uptake, is also correlated to clinical findings of adductor-related pain in athletes, though it is not often used in practice [17]. Ultrasonography and magnetic resonance imaging (MRI) are more likely to find adductor injuries compared to clinical examination alone [3]. Ultrasonography may also be useful for dynamic evaluation of hip pathology and to compare the symptomatic extremity with its asymptomatic counterpart [18]. Hypoechoic areas and discontinuity of tendon fibers correlate with partial ruptures [13, 19]. Tendon injuries on MRI are characterized by thickening and loss of normal homogenous tendon hypointensity, with focal high signal [20]. Acute muscle strains are characterized by patterns of edema surrounding the myotendinous junction, with varying degrees of architectural distortion (retracted muscle). Specifically, the extent of anterior pubic bone enhancement and adductor longus enthesis enlargement on MRI significantly and reproducibly correlates with athletes' current symptoms in chronic adductor-related groin pain [21]. Table 27.1 summarizes differences on MRI in different adductor-related pathologies. Edema may also indicate adductor pathology but can also be present in asymptomatic athletes (Fig. 27.1).

It is generally recommended that adductor pathology be treated non-operatively at first. Initial management of an acute adductor strain is rest, ice, compression, and elevation to minimize inflammation. Nonsteroidal anti-inflammatory drugs may be used, although they have not been shown to have additive effects on healing acute

Table 27.1 Adductor-related pathology and differences on MRI

Pathology	Definition	Differences on MRI
Strain	Injury of hip adductor muscle at muscle belly, myotendinous junction, or tendon	Edema around myotendinous junction, +/– hematoma, partial disruption of junction
Tendonitis	Inflammation of adductor tendon	Thickening and loss of homogenous tendon hypointensity
Avulsions/rupture/lesion	Tear at the origin of the adductor longus muscle on the pubic bone	Complete avulsion of tendon with tendon retraction

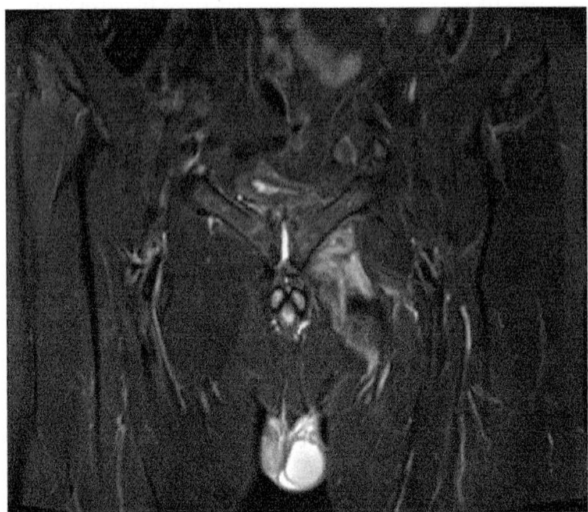

Fig. 27.1 A coronal T2 fat-saturated MR image of a high-grade adductor avulsion injury with retracted tendon ends and intervening hematoma

muscle injury [13]. The footballer should avoid painful activities and weight-bear with crutches. The athlete should then progresses to a gradual muscle strengthening program [22]. The final stage of management involves working on sports-specific skills. In an active therapy program that included muscular strengthening of the adductors, 79% of football players returned to pain-free sports activity [22].

The hip adductors should have at least 80% strength of the ipsilateral hip abductors before return to play [23]. Length of rehabilitation depends on type of pathology and severity of injury. Holmich et al. [13] found that footballers recovering from adductor strain can return to play in 4–8 weeks. Footballers with long-standing adductor-related pathology (on average 9-month injury) treated with active therapy (physiotherapy plus an emphasis on adductor muscle strengthening and improving postural stability of the pelvis) allowed 79% of athletes to return to sports in 18.5 weeks without groin pain (compared to 14% in physiotherapy only). Ueblacker et al. [24] found that the average time to return to play using non-operative management of adductor avulsion in professional football players was 13 weeks. It is essential that the patient seeks out rehabilitation guidance from an experienced therapist as there is a risk of recurrent adductor strains with improper rehabilitation or premature return to play [25]. Werner et al. found a 59% incidence of adductor reinjury in elite football players [3].

Alternative treatments include trigger point injections with lidocaine and/or corticosteroid injections if the athlete continues to be symptomatic after the above treatment options. Furthermore, there are a number of developing treatments including platelet-rich plasma injections and extracorporeal shockwave therapy; however, more research on these treatments are required to determine their effectiveness.

If non-operative therapy fails after several months, surgical options may be considered [10, 25]. Surgical options include adductor longus tenotomy, partial adductor release, and adductor reattachment with suture anchors [2]. There remains a need for more literature comparing operative and non-operative treatment. In a meta-analysis by King et al., the return-to-play rate and time to return to play after hip adductor injury were not significantly different between the surgical and non-operative treatment groups [4]. In a case series by Schlegel et al., patients with complete avulsion of the adductor tendon showed faster return to play by 6 weeks in the non-operative group compared to the operative group [14].

27.3 Iliopsoas-Related Pathology and Snapping Hip Syndrome

The iliopsoas is the primary flexor of the hip. It is also important in femoral external rotation, lateral bending, flexion, and balance of the trunk [26]. Iliopsoas pathology is the second-most common cause of athletic groin injury and is the primary cause of chronic groin pain in athletes (12–36%) [27]. In a total of 628 hip/groin injuries in European professional football players in the UEFA, 8% were due to iliopsoas injury [3]. Football players missed an average of 11 days due to iliopsoas injuries [3].

Iliopsoas pathology commonly includes iliopsoas snapping syndrome, iliopsoas tendinitis, and iliopsoas bursitis [28]. Iliopsoas snapping syndrome is also known as coxa saltans interna, or internal hip snapping syndrome. It is characterized by a snapping sound and/or sensation of the iliopsoas tendon during movement of the hip. The iliopsoas tendon may snap over a number of structures including the iliopectineal eminence of the pelvis, the lesser trochanter, the femoral head, or the iliacus [28–31].

A snapping iliopsoas tendon can lead to iliopsoas tendinitis and/or iliopsoas bursitis [32]. The iliopsoas tendon and bursa are extremely close in proximity, and inflammation of one can result in inflammation of the other [33]. As such, iliopsoas tendinitis and iliopsoas bursitis often coexist and are known together as "iliopsoas syndrome" [28].

Iliopsoas pathology is often the result of overuse. In football players, the pain is precipitated by overtraining or excessive hip hyperflexion drills [34] and aggravated by increased effort, hip flexion, running uphill, running at high speeds, and forward kicking [1, 35]. Iliopsoas pathology may also be less commonly caused by acute trauma [36].

Athletes with symptomatic snapping hip complain of painful snapping with hip flexion or repetitive twisting. It is important to distinguish internal snapping hip syndrome (iliopsoas-related) from external snapping hip syndrome (related to the iliotibial band snapping over the greater trochanter) [37]. There is generally tenderness over the area of the iliopsoas tendon [27, 38]. The examiner can also use the "active iliopsoas snapping test"[39] where the patient's hip is moved from the flexion-abduction-external rotation (FABER) position to an extended, internally rotated position while the examiner palpates the iliopsoas for snapping. The examiner may be able to block the tendon from snapping by applying pressure directly over the tendon [40]. The bicycle test is used to distinguish internal snapping hip syndrome (caused by the iliopsoas) from external snapping hip syndrome (caused by the iliotibial band snapping over the greater trochanter). To perform this test, the patient lies in lateral decubitus position with the affected side up and flexes and extends their hip while the examiner palpates the iliotibial band. If snapping is observed, this points toward external snapping hip [26].

Fact Box

Ultrasound can be useful for dynamic evaluation of snapping hip syndrome as one can range the hip while performing an ultrasound to evaluate for signs of snapping of the iliopsoas tendon.

Snapping hip syndrome is often diagnosed solely based on patient history and physical examination. Further diagnostic investigations may be used to rule out other pathologies. Plain X-rays are often normal in patients with snapping iliopsoas; however, radiographs may still be useful to rule out osseous abnormalities and evaluate for signs of femoroacetabular impingement [28, 41]. Ultrasonography is useful in diagnosing iliopsoas bursitis and tendinitis. Peritendinous fluid collection beneath and surrounding the tendon suggest bursitis, and tendon thickening and/or abnormal foci of hypoechogenicity within tendon suggest tendinitis [32, 41]. Dynamic ultrasonography allows for observation of the iliopsoas under active testing. MRI

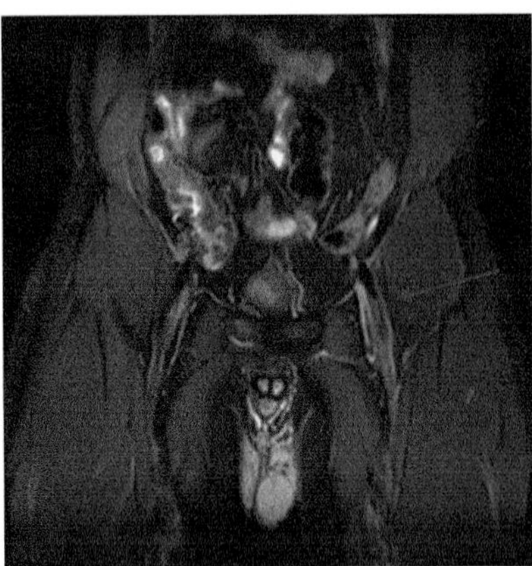
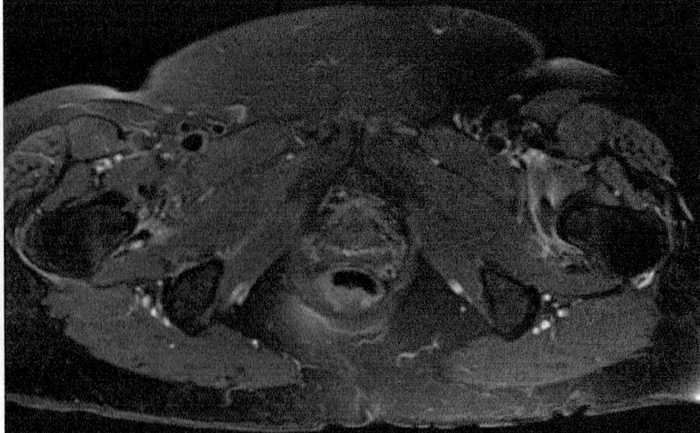

Fig. 27.2 Coronal (*left*) and axial (*right*) T2 fat-saturated MR images in a patient with bilateral iliopsoas tenosynovitis, with the *left* side being worse than the *right*

can be utilized to assess for further abnormalities, such as chondral or labral changes. MRI may also help visualize edema of the iliopsoas and bursitis [42] (Fig. 27.2).

In a pain-free snapping hip, this issue is self-limiting. Symptomatic snapping hip is initially managed conservatively [40]. The football player should avoid aggravating activities. Rest, ice, compression, elevation, and anti-inflammatory medications are initially recommended to decrease inflammation. A stretching program helps reduce the iliopsoas tension [23, 33]. Ultrasound-guided corticosteroid injection into the iliopsoas bursa temporarily reduces symptoms of iliopsoas bursitis and iliopsoas tendinitis [32, 33, 41, 43]. There remains a need for further studies to provide detailed outlines and results of conservative treatments prescribed for athletes with iliopsoas pathology, particularly football players. In a 7-year longitudinal study of UEFA football players, there was a 4% recurrence rate after 2 months in iliopsoas pathology after appropriate rehabilitation and rest [3]. Surgical intervention is indicated when patients have failed at least 3 months of a conservative management program [28]. Surgery may also be considered if the football player is unable to perform at an acceptable level [34]. Surgical procedures include releasing or lengthening of the iliopsoas tendon [2].

27.4 Abdominal Pathology and Inguinal Disruption

Fact Box

Sports hernia goes by many different terms in the literature, including but not limited to "Gilmore's groin," "sportsman's hernia," and "athletic pubalgia."

One of the etiologies of groin pain in athletes is abdominal musculature abnormalities, including "sports hernia." Sports hernia is a broad term used to describe inguinal pain in athletes [44]. Originally, it was described by Gilmore [45] in a series of 313 athletes consisting mostly of footballers [45]. It has since been referred to by various names in the literature, including sports hernia, athletic pubalgia, Gilmore's groin, and sportsman's hernia. In 2014, the British Hernia Society endorsed the term "inguinal disruption" as opposed to "sports hernia" and defined it as "pain…which occurs predominantly in the groin area…where no obvious other pathology, such as a hernia, exists to explain the symptoms"[46]. This definition and terminology will inform the focus for the following section.

The inguinal region is anatomically complex and in close proximity to the abdominal musculature. The groin triangle, as defined by Falvey et al., is a useful anatomical approach to identifying the source of groin pain in athletes [47]. The superior border of this triangle, which coincides with the location of the inguinal ligament, is the line between the anterior superior iliac spine (ASIS) and the pubic tubercle. The inguinal ligament itself is a thickening of the aponeurosis of the external oblique muscle. The structures immediately superior to this ligament, lateral to medial, include the conjoint tendon of iliopsoas passing beneath the inguinal ligament, the ilioinguinal and iliohypogastric nerves, and the genital branch of the genitofemoral nerve. Most medially, the insertions of the rectus abdominis, external oblique, internal oblique, and transversus abdominis are found close to the pubic tubercle. As well, the inguinal canal, bordered inferiorly by the inguinal ligament, runs a similar course, with its deep ring laterally and its superficial ring more medially [47]. Using the groin triangle, these superior border structures are the ones most often implicated in abdominal pathology resulting in groin pain [47].

In a study of semi-elite footballers, Hölmich et al. [1] found that lower abdominal pain was one of three major etiological categories in this group of athletes, implicated in 10% of footballers with groin pain [1]. In addition, inguinal disruption presents overwhelmingly in male athletes, with only 10% of patients being women [44]. Historically, lower rates of female athletic participation were thought to be responsible for this striking discrepancy [48]. However, given that the male-to-female ratio has not changed significantly despite increasing female participation in sports, it is likely that anatomical differences are a more important contributing factor. These differences include a lighter female pelvis and a different pattern of force distribution due to a wider subpubic angle in females [48]. It is thought that with repeated cutting, pivoting, and/or kicking motions, the rectus tendon insertion is more prone to disruption, and the posterior inguinal wall is weakened, thus predisposing footballers to inguinal disruption. The classic presentation for inguinal disruption is lower abdominal or deep groin pain, which may be of insidious or sudden onset, is worsened with activity, and improves with rest [4]. The pain may radiate into the perineal region, the suprapubic region, or the inner surface of the femur [44].

Inguinal disruption can represent a diagnostic challenge. Often, there are no findings on examination [4]. Careful palpation of the lower abdomen, adductors, and pubic tubercle and symphysis are essential [49]. In addition, a resisted sit-up while the rectus abdominis insertion is palpated may elicit the patient's symptoms [50]. On examination, it is important to rule out a true inguinal hernia (discussed in the next section), which by definition would eliminate inguinal disruption as a diagnosis. As well, while it is beyond the scope of this chapter, it is always important to consider intra-abdominopelvic etiologies for lower abdominal pain, particularly in the female athlete. Imaging can be helpful in the diagnosis of inguinal disruption. Plain radiographs are useful in ruling out bony pathology, while magnetic resonance imaging (MRI) can identify strains and tears of the abdominal muscles or the conjoint tendon, as well as bone marrow edema at the pubis. One study reported that, when compared to intraoperative findings, MRI was 68% sensitive and 100% specific for rectus abdominis pathology [51]. Finally, dynamic ultrasonography may be helpful in identifying posterior inguinal wall deficiency if it is displaced anteriorly with Valsalva, but it is difficult to identify and is quite operator-dependent [52–55] (Fig. 27.3).

The first-line treatment for inguinal disruption should be conservative management. A period of 4–8 weeks of rest (along with nonsteroidal anti-inflammatories, heat or ice, and massage) is the first step [4, 44]. This should be followed by a rehabilitation program focused on achieving better core strength and dynamic pelvic stability under the supervision of a specialized physiotherapist or sports physiologist. For athletes who are in season and wish to continue playing, a resting period of 4 weeks is recommended. As well, injections of steroids or platelet-rich plasma (PRP) may be helpful, though there is not enough evidence regarding their efficacy at this time [56]. Table 27.2 summarizes a four-phase rehabilitation protocol for athletes with inguinal disruption, which allows return to play at 10–12 weeks. Overall, there is limited evidence for long-term

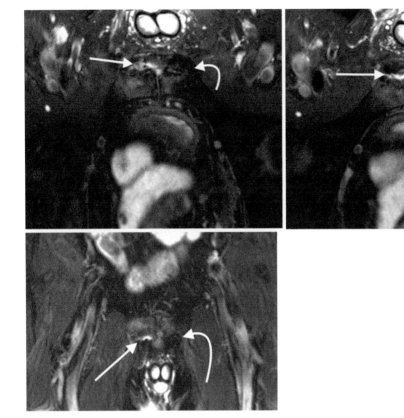

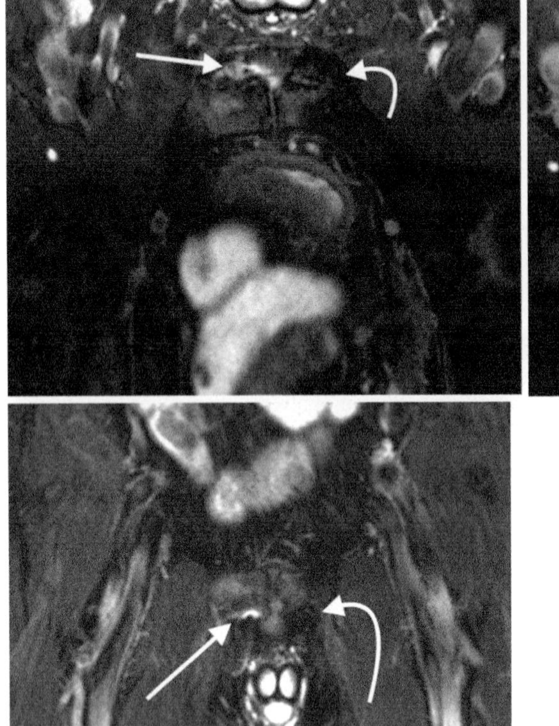

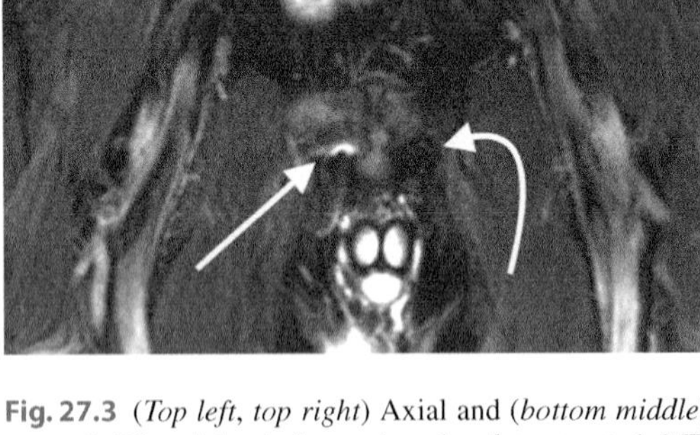

Fig. 27.3 (*Top left, top right*) Axial and (*bottom middle*) coronal T2-weighted fast spin-echo fat-saturated MR images showing disruption at the right rectus abdominis-adductor aponeurotic plate attachment at the pubis (*straight white arrows*). The *curved white arrows* show the normal-appearing aponeurotic plate attachment on the asymptomatic left side

success with conservative management of inguinal disruption, and most athletes will require surgical intervention [57–59]. Failure rates are difficult to quantify as there is a lack of literature with long-term follow-up of non-operatively treated inguinal disruption [60]. Surgical options include repair of abdominal musculature, mesh reinforcement, and pelvic floor repairs [4].

Fact Box

Abdominal Pathology and Inguinal Disruption

- Epidemiology: 90% of patients are male (likely anatomical)
- Presentation: lower abdominal or deep groin pain, insidious or sudden onset, worsened with activity, improved with rest, +/− radiating to perineal, suprapubic, or femoral regions
- Diagnosis: examination may be normal, careful palpation and resisted sit-up may elicit symptoms
- Investigations: radiographs to rule out bony pathology, MRI to investigate soft tissue pathology, dynamic ultrasonography
- Treatment
  - Non-operative: 4–8 weeks of rest, NSAIDs, ice, four-phase rehabilitation program over 10–12 weeks before return to play
  - Operative: repair of abdominal musculature, mesh reinforcement, pelvic floor repair

Table 27.2 Four-phase program for non-operative management of inguinal disruption

	Weeks post-injury	Details
Phase I	1–2	– Analgesia and anti-inflammation – Postural education – Transversus abdominis (TA) recruitment – Hip and lumbar spine ROM – Gentle active stretching – Side lying hip abduction and extension
Phase II	2–4	– Cardiovascular exercise – Gait training – Continue TA recruitment – Achieve functional to full ROM in lumbar spine, increase hip ROM – Sciatic core strengthening to maintain neutral spine – Increase recruitment of hip and pelvic stabilization – Functional strength with double leg exercises, progress to single leg – Spine and hip mobilization with addition of rotation
Criteria to be met before progression to phase III: – Decreased pain with ADLs <2/10 – Functional to full ROM in lumbar spine and hips – Ability to maintain TA contraction with single leg activity – No pain with ambulation – No Trendelenburg gait or sign		
Phase III	4–6	– Cardiovascular exercise with resistance – Good pelvic stability and TA recruitment with ambulation – Gait training and pelvic proprioceptive neuromuscular function (PNF) patterns – Functional to full ROM in lumbo-pelvic area and hips – Dynamic core training and use of unstable surfaces – Single leg functional activity and balance disturbances – Continue active stretching – Myofascial release and soft tissue work
Criteria to be met before progression to phase IV: – No pain with ADLs, ambulation, or fast-paced walking – Full function ROM in hips, pelvis, and lumbar spine – Ability to maintain neutral spine with standing, sitting, walking, single-leg activity even with unstable surfaces or perturbations – Able to recognize and correct postural dysfunction		
Phase IV	6–8	– Cardiovascular warm-up specific to sport – ROM progressed to full if previously functional – Stretching interspersed with static stretching – Strengthening in functional isotonic, isometric, and isokinetic fashion – Manual myofascial release and soft tissue mobilization – PNF training
Return to play	8–12	Progress as tolerated to full return-to-sports readiness

Adapted from Ellsworth et al. [103]

27.5 Inguinal Pathology

As discussed above, the inguinal canal is closely related to the abdominal musculature. The inguinal canal passes obliquely through the abdominal wall and is bordered inferiorly by the inguinal ligament. The anterior wall is formed by the internal oblique and external oblique muscles. The posterior wall is formed by the transversalis fascia and conjoint tendon. The posterior wall is weaker in males due to testicular descent from the abdominal cavity to the scrotal cavity.

A true inguinal hernia can be indirect or direct. Embryologically, as the testes descend from the abdomen into the scrotum, they leave behind a patent processus vaginalis. In an indirect hernia, peritoneal contents, such as mesenteric fat and/or loops of bowel, protrude into the inguinal canal. This often occurs in infants or young adults. A direct hernia occurs when there is protrusion of peritoneal content directly through a defect in the abdominal wall.

As previously discussed, the Manchester consensus definition of "inguinal disruption" must exclude a true hernia. This decision was made because true hernias were rarely found in elite and amateur athletes [55, 61]. In support of this, Falvey et al. evaluated 382 athletes with groin pain with MRI and found no true hernias [5]. Kluin et al. evaluated 14 athletes with undiagnosed groin pain under endoscopy [62]. Of the five football players who were evaluated, three presented with sportsman's hernia, one with an obturator hernia, and one with a lipoma.

Although football players are prone to inguinal disruption because of actions that weaken the posterior wall, such as kicking and twisting of the torso, they are no more prone to true inguinal hernias compared to the general public [25].

Inguinal hernias can cause a burning, aching sensation in the groin. There is a palpable abdominal bulge when the patient coughs or strains, which may disappear when patient is in prone position. Small hernias may only be painful on exertion [25].

Ultrasound and MRI can help diagnose a hernia in patients without a palpable impulse or bulge. Ultrasound is accurate in finding true inguinal hernias that correlate with clinical findings [63]. Herniography is a more invasive investigation, where radiographs are taken after iodine-based contrast medium is injected into the hernial sac. Ultrasound has been found to be more accurate than herniography [63]. In an ultrasound evaluation of the hernia, the patient must repeatedly perform Valsalva maneuvers for accuracy in diagnosis [64]. The diagnosis of a direct hernia is clear on ultrasound and is seen as abdominal contents protruding through the defect (the hernia) in Hesselbach's triangle. A positive sign for indirect inguinal hernia is internal inguinal ring dilating and abdominal contents protruding into the inguinal canal. The presence of a hernia on ultrasound will generally be more pronounced when the patient performs a Valsalva maneuver.

In the case of an asymptomatic or minimally symptomatic inguinal hernia, watchful waiting is considered first-line [61]. Surgery may be warranted if the hernia becomes symptomatic, or when acute complications occur, such as incarceration or strangulation. Surgical interventions include open or laparoscopic hernia repair [61].

27.6 Femoroacetabular Impingement

Fact Box

Cam impingement—femoral head deformity

Pincer impingement—acetabular-sided deformity

Mixed- (or combined-type) impingement—both femoral- and acetabular-sided deformities

Femoroacetabular impingement (FAI) is an intra-articular cause of groin pain that is thought be related to the development of osteoarthritis [65]. FAI occurs as a result of either abnormal femoral head and neck anatomy, termed cam impingement, or abnormal acetabular anatomy, termed pincer impingement. These deformities can occur either in isolation or in a combined-type FAI [66]. FAI is thought to occur more commonly in individuals with a high physical activity level during adolescence [67]. In particular, sports such as football that include repetitive hip flexion may cause the development of FAI and chondrolabral damage [38]. Although definitive treatment of FAI requires surgical intervention, many studies recommend a trial of non-operative management first [68].

Footballers with symptomatic FAI will typically complain of groin pain which is worsened with activity, particularly hip flexion. FAI may result in limited ROM, particularly internal rotation, either due to pain or bony impingement.

Patients will have increased groin pain with simultaneous flexion, adduction, and internal rotation of the hip, also known as an anterior impingement test. X-ray findings of cam FAI include a "pistol grip deformity," an increased alpha angle, and a decreased head-neck offset ratio. A positive crossover sign, where the posterior wall of the acetabulum crosses over the anterior wall on an anteroposterior (AP) view, is indicative of pincer impingement. A subsequent MRI of the hip joint is useful in determining the presence of other associated pathology such as labral tears. It should be noted that it is important to correlate radiographic findings with clinical symptoms and physical exam findings as many asymptomatic individuals will have radiographic findings of FAI [69].

Feeley et al. found that only 5% of all hip related injuries in National Football League players had intra-articular pathology [70]. However, football players with intra-articular pathology were found to have the highest average days missed before return to sport (94.2 days) and the highest rate of need for surgical intervention (24%). Therefore, although intra-articular pathology may be relatively uncommon as the source of groin pain in footballers, it may be the most severe.

Currently the literature reporting outcomes of patients with FAI managed non-operatively is limited. A systematic review of literature found only five primary research studies that reported outcomes after non-operative treatment of FAI [71]. Of these five primary research articles, three reported favorable outcomes. Sixty-five percent of all of the studies in this systematic review indicated that non-operative treatment as initial management was appropriate, with physical therapy and activity modification being the most common non-operative treatments recommended. It should be noted that the included studies in the review were generally of low-level evidence and included a limited number of patients [71].

The goals of physiotherapy in the management of FAI can be to increase the pain-free range of motion (ROM) of the hip, to optimize the balance between muscle strength and length, and to reduce anterior femoral glide [68, 72]. Some studies have reported positive results treating athletes with physiotherapy for FAI [70], whereas others have found it to have little to no effectiveness [73]. Despite the contradicting evidence on the utility of physiotherapy and activity modification for FAI, these modalities are generally viewed as harmless.

NSAIDs are another conservative treatment option discussed in the literature for the management of FAI [72]. NSAIDs are expected to decrease pain secondary to inflammation and increase pain-free ROM. However, many of these studies use NSAIDs in conjunction with other treatment options, making it difficult to discern the actual efficacy of these medications as the outcomes may be confounded by the other conservative treatment modalities used [72, 74].

Intra-articular corticosteroid or hyaluronic acid (HA) injections may also be useful in the treatment of FAI in football players. One case series consisting of 23 patients found significant improvement across a number of outcome measures using HA to treat patients with mild FAI [27]. A different 54-patient study found that only 37% of patients with FAI had clinically significant pain relief 2 weeks after receiving an intra-articular corticosteroid injection [75]. Intra-articular injections may also serve as a useful diagnostic tool as a negative response to an intra-articular injection with anesthetic has been shown to predict a higher likelihood of having a negative result from surgery in FAI patients [76].

To the best of the authors' knowledge, there exists no experimental data on the results obtained from osteopathic or chiropractic treatment of FAI. In fact, some authors caution the use of osteopathic methods in the treatment of FAI as strong flexing mobilization maneuvers often used by osteopaths may cause further labral injury [77].

In summary, the applicability of non-operative management in the treatment of FAI remains debatable due to limited evidence and a limited ability to address the bony deformities which cause FAI. Although there is debatable efficacy of many of these conservative treatment options, given the limited side-effect profile and the chronic nature of FAI which does not require urgent surgical treatment, a trial of conservative treatment is recommended prior to surgical management.

27.7 Other Pathologies

A number of other pathologies that may present as hip/groin pain in footballers are discussed briefly in this section. Myositis ossificans is a rare complication of traumatic muscle contusion, which is characterized by heterotopic ossification within the hematoma, most commonly in the thigh but on rare occasions presenting in the groin [78, 79]. There is limited evidence for the treatment of this condition in the athletic population; however, various case reports have successfully treated this condition both operatively and non-operatively [79–81]. Obturator nerve compression is recognized as an important cause of groin pain in athletes. It most commonly presents with radiating pain and paresthesias in the medial thigh. The definitive management for this condition is surgical neurolysis, which has shown promising results and prompt return to play in numerous studies [82–84].

Owing to its direct involvement in both sprinting and kicking motions, tears and avulsions of the rectus femoris are an important though rare injury among footballers, with incidence estimated at <1% [85]. These injuries usually present with severe, acute onset anterior thigh pain worsened with contraction of the quadriceps femoris [86]. Though there is no consensus on the appropriate management of rectus femoris avulsions, non-operative management may be attempted. This includes rest, ice, compression, elevation (RICE), nonsteroidal anti-inflammatories (NSAIDs), and a stepwise progression beginning with isometric exercises and progressing to isotonic and isokinetic exercises before return-to-sports-specific exercises. However, based on numerous reports of footballers who have sustained rectus femoris tears, surgical management was ultimately required in all cases [85, 87, 88]. Overall, hamstring injuries are among the most common injuries in football, estimated at 12–16% of all injuries [3, 16, 89, 90]. Proximal tears and avulsions of the hamstrings, however, are serious and rare injuries which can present with groin pain [91]. Due to their rarity, there is a lack of literature comparing conservative and operative management, but available data suggests better outcomes and higher rates of return to play in a variety of different sports with operative management [92–95].

Stress fractures account for 0.5% of all football injuries and occur at a rate of 0.04/1000 match and training hours at the professional level, though are much rarer in the femoral neck [3]. In the rare case that they do happen, these injuries can often be managed conservatively and prevented through reduction of training intensity and frequency [96]. Hip fractures and dislocations are uncommon in football, but need to be recognized and treated promptly with either open or closed reduction and fixation as necessary [97, 98]. Degenerative joint disease is a concern for aging and retired footballers, though it is more common in the ankle (5–7%) and knee (19–21%) than the hip (1–4%) [99]. When it does present in younger athletes, it can be a diagnostic challenge due to the higher pain tolerance, but the course of treatment is the same as in older individuals [100]. Intra-articular loose bodies, though not specific to football, can mimic other conditions such as snapping hip syndrome as they present with anterior groin pain and mechanical symptoms such as locking, clicking, and giving way [101]. In addition to traumatic causes, loose bodies can be secondary to other pathologies including Perthes disease, synovial chondromatosis, and osteoarthritis, among others [101]. Early surgical intervention and removal of loose bodies, most commonly by arthroscopy, are the gold standard of treatment [102].

Conclusions

Groin pain in football players represents a challenging clinical problem for clinicians given the fact that many different pathologies will have very similar presentations and to further complicate issues, many of the pathologies may occur simultaneously. Therefore it is critical that a thorough history and physical exam be performed in addition to appropriate imaging in order to ensure a proper diagnosis is made. Adductor pathology is the most common cause of groin pain in footballers; however, the differential diagnoses that must be considered are quite extensive as discussed in this chapter. Intra-articular sources of groin pain, although relatively uncommon, have been shown to cause footballers to miss the most time from sport. The vast majority of pathologies causing groin pain can be managed at minimum with a trial of conservative treatment. That being said, in general the literature examining the conservative management of groin pain is of low level of evidence.

Take-Home Message

- Groin pain is a common injury in footballers of all levels.
- Adductor pathology is the most common cause of groin pain in footballers, but a large differential diagnosis must be considered including abdominal, intra-articular, inguinal, and iliopsoas-related pathologies.
- Though the majority of groin pain pathologies can be treated with a trial of conservative management as first-line, the evidence for non-operative management is limited, and many ultimately require operative management.

Top Five Evidence Based References

Hölmich P (2007) Long-standing groin pain in sportspeople falls into three primary patterns, a "clinical entity" approach: a prospective study of 207 patients. Br J Sports Med 41:247–252. discussion 252

de Sa D, Hölmich P, Phillips M, Heaven S, Simunovic N, Philippon MJ, Ayeni OR (2016) Athletic groin pain: a systematic review of surgical diagnoses, investigations and treatment. Br J Sports Med 5

Werner J, Hägglund M, Waldén M, Ekstrand J (2009) UEFA injury study: a prospective study of hip and groin injuries in professional football over seven consecutive seasons. Br J Sports Med 43:1036–1040

King E, Ward J, Small L, Falvey E, Franklyn-Miller A (2015) Athletic groin pain: a systematic review and meta-analysis of surgical versus physical therapy rehabilitation outcomes. Br J Sports Med 49:1447–1451

Falvey ÉC, King E, Kinsella S, Franklyn-Miller A (2016) Athletic groin pain (part 1): a prospective anatomical diagnosis of 382 patients—clinical findings, MRI findings and patient-reported outcome measures at baseline. Br J Sports Med 50:423–430

References

1. Hölmich P (2007) Long-standing groin pain in sportspeople falls into three primary patterns, a "clinical entity" approach: a prospective study of 207 patients. Br J Sports Med 41(4):247–252
2. de Sa D, Hölmich P, Phillips M, Heaven S, Simunovic N, Philippon MJ, Ayeni OR (2016) Athletic groin pain: a systematic review of surgical diagnoses, investigations and treatment. Br J Sports Med 50(19):1181–1186
3. Werner J, Hägglund M, Waldén M, Ekstrand J (2009) UEFA injury study: a prospective study of hip and groin injuries in professional football over seven consecutive seasons. Br J Sports Med 43(13):1036–1040
4. King E, Ward J, Small L, Falvey E, Franklyn-Miller A (2015) Athletic groin pain: a systematic review and meta-analysis of surgical versus physical therapy rehabilitation outcomes. Br J Sports Med 49(22):1447–1451
5. Falvey ÉC, King E, Kinsella S, Franklyn-Miller A (2016) Athletic groin pain (part 1): a prospective anatomical diagnosis of 382 patients—clinical findings, MRI findings and patient-reported outcome measures at baseline. Br J Sports Med 50(7):423–430
6. Murar J, Birmingham PM (2015) Osteitis pubis. In: Nho S, Leunig M, Larson CM, Bedi A, Kelly BT (eds) Hip arthroscopy and hip joint preservation surgery. Springer, New York, NY, pp 737–749
7. Elattar O, Choi H-R, Dills VD, Busconi B (2016) Groin Injuries (Athletic Pubalgia) and Return to Play. Sports Health 8(4):313–323
8. Ekstrand J, Gillquist J (1983) Soccer injuries and their mechanisms: a prospective study. Med Sci Sports Exerc 15(3):267–270
9. Engström B, Johansson C, Törnkvist H (1991) Soccer injuries among elite female players. Am J Sports Med 19(4):372–375
10. Lynch SA, Renström PA (1999) Groin injuries in sport: treatment strategies. Sports Med 28(2):137–144
11. Morelli V, Weaver V (2005) Groin injuries and groin pain in athletes: part 1. Prim Care 32(1):163–183
12. Adams RJ, Chandler FA (1953) Osteitis pubis of traumatic etiology. J Bone Joint Surg Am 35-A(3):685–696
13. Hölmich P (1997) Adductor-related groin pain in athletes. Sports Med Arthrosc 5(4):285–2891
14. Schlegel TF, Bushnell BD, Godfrey J, Boublik M (2009) Success of nonoperative management of adductor longus tendon ruptures in National Football League athletes. Am J Sports Med 37(7):1394–1399
15. Thorborg K, Branci S, Nielsen MP, Tang L, Nielsen MB, Hölmich P (2014) Eccentric and isometric hip

adduction strength in male soccer players with and without adductor-related groin pain. Orthop J Sports Med 2(2):2325967114521777
16. Ekstrand J, Gillquist J (1983) The avoidability of soccer injuries. Int J Sports Med 4(2):124–128
17. Gouttebarge V, Hughes Schwab BA, Vivian A, Kerkhoffs GMMJ (2016) Injuries, matches missed and the influence of minimum medical standards in the a-league professional football: a 5-year prospective study. Asian J Sports Med 7(1):e31385
18. Weaver JS, Jacobson JA, Jamadar DA, Hayes CW (2003) Sonographic findings of adductor insertion avulsion syndrome with magnetic resonance imaging correlation. J Ultrasound Med 22(4):403–407
19. Kalebo P, Karlsson J, Sward L, Peterson L (1992) Ultrasonography of chronic tendon injuries in the groin. Am J Sports Med 20(6):634–639
20. Ansede G, English B, Healy JC (2011) Groin pain: clinical assessment and the role of MR imaging. Semin Musculoskelet Radiol 15(1):3–13
21. Robinson P, Barron DA, Parsons W, Grainger AJ, Schilders EMG, O'Connor PJ (2004) Adductor-related groin pain in athletes: correlation of MR imaging with clinical findings. Skeletal Radiol 33(8):451–457
22. Hölmich P, Uhrskou P, Ulnits L, Kanstrup IL, Bachmann Nielsen M, Bjerg AM, Krogsgaarda K (1999) Effectiveness of active physical training as treatment for long-standing adductor-related groin pain in athletes: randomised trial. Lancet 353(9151):439–443
23. Tyler TF, Nicholas SJ (2007) Rehabilitation of extra-articular sources of hip pain in athletes. N Am J Sports Phys Ther 2(4):207–216
24. Ueblacker P, English B, Mueller-Wohlfahrt H-W (2016) Nonoperative treatment and return to play after complete proximal adductor avulsion in high-performance athletes. Knee Surg Sports Traumatol Arthrosc 24(12):3927–3933
25. Bradshaw C, Holmich P (2009) Longstanding groin pain. In: Brukner P, Khan K (eds) Clinical sports medicine. McGraw-Hill, New York, NY, pp 405–426
26. Andersson E, Oddsson L, Grundstrom H, Thorstensson A (1995) The role of the psoas and iliacus muscles for stability and movement of the lumbar spine, pelvis and hip. Scand J Med Sci Sports 5(1):10–16
27. Abate M, Scuccimarra T, Vanni D, Pantalone A, Salini V (2014) Femoroacetabular impingement: is hyaluronic acid effective? Knee Surg Sports Traumatol Arthrosc 22(4):889–892
28. Anderson CN (2016) Iliopsoas: pathology, diagnosis, and treatment. Clin Sports Med 35(3):419–433
29. Deslandes M, Guillin R, Cardinal E, Hobden R, Bureau NJ (2008) The snapping iliopsoas tendon: new mechanisms using dynamic sonography. AJR Am J Roentgenol 190(3):576–581
30. Lewis CL (2010) Extra-articular snapping hip: a literature review. Sports Health 2(3):186–190
31. Schaberg JE, Harper MC, Allen WC (1984) The snapping hip syndrome. Am J Sports Med 12(5):361–365
32. Blankenbaker DG, De Smet AA, Keene JS (2006) Sonography of the iliopsoas tendon and injection of the iliopsoas Bursa for diagnosis and management of the painful snapping hip. Skeletal Radiol 35(8):565–571
33. Johnston CAM, Wiley JP, Lindsay DM, Wiseman DA (1998) Iliopsoas bursitis and tendinitis. A review. Sports Med 25(4):271–283
34. Wahl CJ, Warren RF, Adler RS, Hannafin JA, Hansen B (2009) Internal coxa saltans (snapping hip) as a result of overtraining: a report of 3 cases in professional athletes with a review of causes and the role of ultrasound in early diagnosis and management. Am J Sports Med 32(5):1302–1309
35. Mozes M, Papa MZ, Zweig A, Horoszowski H, Adar R (1985) Iliopsoas injury in soccer players. Br J Sports Med 19(3):168–170
36. Janzen DL, Partridge E, Logan PM, Connell DG, Duncan CP (1996) The snapping hip: clinical and imaging findings in transient subluxation of the iliopsoas tendon. Can Assoc Radiol J 47(3):202–208
37. Byrd JWT (2005) Snapping hip. Oper Tech Sport Med 13(1):46–54
38. Ganz R, Leunig M, Leunig-Ganz K, Harris WH (2008) The Etiology of Osteoarthritis of the Hip: an integrated mechanical concept. Clin Orthop Relat Res 466(2):264–272
39. Sammarco GJ (1984) Diagnosis and treatment in dancers. Clin Orthop Relat Res (187):176–187
40. Byrd JWT (2006) Evaluation and management of the snapping iliopsoas tendon. Instr Course Lect 55:347–355
41. Fredberg U, Hansen LB (1995) Ultrasound in the diagnosis and treatment of iliopsoas tendinitis: a case report. Scand J Med Sci Sports 5(6):369–370
42. Idjadi J, Meislin R (2004) Symptomatic snapping hip: targeted treatment for maximum pain relief. Phys Sportsmed 32(1):25–31
43. Vaccaro JP, Sauser DD, Beals RK (1995) Iliopsoas bursa imaging: efficacy in depicting abnormal iliopsoas tendon motion in patients with internal snapping hip syndrome. Radiology 197(3):853–856
44. Paksoy M, Sekmen Ü (2016) Sportsman hernia; the review of current diagnosis and treatment modalities. Ulus Cerrahi Derg 32(2):122–129
45. Gilmore OJ (1992) Gilmore's groin. Sports Med Soft Tissue Trauma 3(3):12–14
46. Sheen AJ, Stephenson BM, Lloyd DM, Robinson P, Fevre D, Paajanen H, de Beaux A, Kingsnorth A, Gilmore OJ, Bennett D, Maclennan I, O'Dwyer P, Sanders D, Kurzer M (2014) 'Treatment of the Sportsman's groin': British Hernia Society's 2014 position statement based on the Manchester Consensus Conference. Br J Sports Med 48(14):1079–1087
47. Falvey EC, Franklyn-Miller A, McCrory PR (2009) The groin triangle: a patho-anatomical approach to

the diagnosis of chronic groin pain in athletes. Br J Sports Med 43(3):213–220

48. Meyers WC, Yoo E, Devon ON, Jain N, Horner M, Lauencin C, Zoga A (2007) Understanding "sports hernia" (athletic pubalgia): the anatomic and pathophysiologic basis for abdominal and groin pain in athletes. Oper Tech Sports Med 15(4):165–177
49. Larson CM (2014) Sports Hernia/Athletic Pubalgia: evaluation and management. Sports Health 6(2):139–144
50. Hawkins RD, Hulse MA, Wilkinson C, Hodson A, Gibson M (2001) The association football medical research programme: an audit of injuries in professional football. Br J Sports Med 35(1):43–47
51. Zoga AC, Kavanagh EC, Omar IM, Morrison WB, Koulouris G, Lopez H, Chaabra A, Domesek J, Meyers WC (2008) Athletic Pubalgia and the "Sports Hernia": MR imaging findings. Radiology 247(3):797–807
52. Armfield DR, Kim DH-M, Towers JD, Bradley JP, Robertson DD (2006) Sports-related muscle injury in the lower extremity. Clin Sports Med 25(4):803–842
53. Kavanagh EC, Koulouris G, Ford S, McMahon P, Johnson C, Eustace SJ (2006) MR imaging of groin pain in the athlete. Semin Musculoskelet Radiol 10(3):197–207
54. Orchard J, Read J, Neophyton J, Garlick D (1998) Groin pain associated with ultrasound finding of inguinal canal posterior wall deficiency in Australian Rules footballers. Br J Sports Med 32(2):134–139
55. Sheen AJ, Iqbal Z (2014) Contemporary management of "Inguinal disruption" in the sportsman's groin. BMC Sports Sci Med Rehabil 6:39
56. Campbell KJ, Boykin RE, Wijdicks CA, Erik Giphart J, LaPrade RF, Philippon MJ (2013) Treatment of a hip capsular injury in a professional soccer player with platelet-rich plasma and bone marrow aspirate concentrate therapy. Knee Surg Sports Traumatol Arthrosc 21(7):1684–1688
57. Caudill P, Nyland J, Smith C, Yerasimides J, Lach J (2008) Sports hernias: a systematic literature review. Br J Sports Med 42(12):954–964
58. Farber AJ, Wilckens JH (2007) Sports hernia: diagnosis and therapeutic approach. J Am Acad Orthop Surg 15(8):507–514
59. Swan KG, Wolcott M (2007) The athletic hernia: a systematic review. Clin Orthop Relat Res 455:78–87
60. Woodward JS, Parker A, Macdonald RM (2012) Non-surgical treatment of a professional hockey player with the signs and symptoms of sports hernia: a case report. Int J Sports Phys Ther 7(1):85–100
61. Simons MP, Aufenacker T, Bay-Nielsen M, Bouillot JL, Campanelli G, Conze J, de Lange D, Fortelny R, Heikkinen T, Kingsnorth A, Kukleta J, Morales-Conde S, Nordin P, Schumpelick V, Smedberg S, Smietanski M, Weber G, Miserez M (2009) European Hernia Society guidelines on the treatment of inguinal hernia in adult patients. Hernia 13(4):343–403
62. Kluin J, den Hoed PT, van Linschoten R, IJ JC, van Steensel CJ (2004) Endoscopic evaluation and treatment of groin pain in the athlete. Am J Sports Med 32(4):944–949
63. Robinson P, Hensor E, Lansdown MJ, Ambrose NS, Chapman AH (2006) Inguinofemoral hernia: accuracy of sonography in patients with indeterminate clinical features. AJR Am J Roentgenol 187(5):1168–1178
64. Ostrom E, Joseph A (2016) The use of musculoskeletal ultrasound for the diagnosis of groin and hip pain in athletes. Curr Sports Med Rep 15(2):86–90
65. Oner A, Koksal A, Sofu H, Aykut US, Yıldırım T, Kaygusuz MA (2016) The prevalence of femoroacetabular impingement as an aetiologic factor for end-stage degenerative osteoarthritis of the hip joint: analysis of 1,000 cases. Hip Int 26(2):164–168
66. Byrd JWT (2010) Femoroacetabular impingement in athletes, Part 1: Cause and assessment. Sport Health 2(4):321–333
67. Agricola R, Bessems JHJM, Ginai AZ, Heijboer MP, van der Heijden RA, Verhaar JAN, Weinans H, Waarsing JH (2012) The development of Cam-type deformity in adolescent and young male soccer players. Am J Sports Med 40(5):1099–1106
68. Hunt D, Prather H, Harris Hayes M, Clohisy JC (2012) Clinical outcomes analysis of conservative and surgical treatment of patients with clinical indications of prearthritic, intra-articular hip disorders. PM R 4(7):479–487
69. Diesel CV, Ribeiro TA, Scheidt RB, Macedo CA de S, Galia CR (2015) The prevalence of femoroacetabular impingement in radiographs of asymptomatic subjects: a cross-sectional study. Hip Int 25(3):258–263
70. Feeley BT, Powell JW, Muller MS, Barnes RP, Warren RF, Kelly BT (2008) Hip injuries and labral tears in the national football league. Am J Sports Med 36(11):2187–2195
71. Wall PD, Fernandez M, Griffin DR, Foster NE (2013) Nonoperative treatment for femoroacetabular impingement: a systematic review of the literature. PM R 5(5):418–426
72. Emara K, Samir W, Motasem EH, El GKA (2011) Conservative treatment for mild femoroacetabular impingement. J Orthop Surg (Hong Kong) 19(1):41–45
73. Jäger M, Wild A, Westhoff B, Krauspe R (2004) Femoroacetabular impingement caused by a femoral osseous head-neck bump deformity: clinical, radiological, and experimental results. J Orthop Sci 9(3):256–263
74. Bedi A, Kelly BT (2013) Femoroacetabular impingement. J Bone Joint Surg Am 95(1):82–92
75. Krych AJ, Griffith TB, Hudgens JL, Kuzma SA, Sierra RJ, Levy BA (2014) Limited therapeutic benefits of intra-articular cortisone injection for patients with femoro-acetabular impingement and labral tear. Knee Surg Sports Traumatol Arthrosc 22(4):750–755
76. Ayeni OR, Farrokhyar F, Crouch S, Chan K, Sprague S, Bhandari M (2014) Pre-operative intra-articular

hip injection as a predictor of short-term outcome following arthroscopic management of femoroacetabular impingement. Knee Surg Sports Traumatol Arthrosc 22(4):801–805

77. Chakraverty JK, Snelling NJ (2012) Anterior hip pain – have you considered femoroacetabular impingement? Int J Osteopath Med 15(1):22–27
78. Cetin C (2004) Chronic groin pain in an amateur soccer player. Br J Sports Med 38(2):223–224
79. Mani-Babu S, Wolman R, Keen R (2014) Quadriceps traumatic myositis ossificans in a football player: management with intravenous pamidronate. Clin J Sport Med 24(5):e56–e58
80. Antao NA (1988) Myositis of the hip in a professional soccer player. A case report. Am J Sports Med 16(1):82–83
81. Marques JP, Pinheiro JP, Santos Costa J, Moura D (2015) Myositis ossificans of the quadriceps femoris in a soccer player. BMJ Case Rep. https://doi.org/10.1136/bcr-2015-210545
82. Bradshaw C, McCrory P (1997) Obturator nerve entrapment. Clin J Sport Med 7(3):217–219
83. Brukner P, Bradshaw C, McCrory P (1999) Obturator neuropathy: a cause of exercise-related groin pain. Phys Sportsmed 27(5):62–73
84. Siwiński D (2005) Neuropathy of the obturator nerve as a source of pain in soccer players. Chir Narzadow Ruchu Ortop Pol 70(3):201–204
85. García VV, Duhrkop DC, Seijas R, Ares O, Cugat R (2012) Surgical treatment of proximal ruptures of the rectus femoris in professional soccer players. Arch Orthop Trauma Surg 132(3):329–333
86. Zakaria A, Housner A (2011) Managing quadriceps strains for early return to play. J Musculoskelet Med 28(7):257–262
87. Esser S, Jantz D, Hurdle MF, Taylor W (2015) Proximal rectus femoris avulsion: ultrasonic diagnosis and nonoperative management. J Athl Train 50(7):778–780
88. Straw R, Colclough K, Geutjens G (2003) Surgical repair of a chronic rupture of the rectus femoris muscle at the proximal musculotendinous junction in a soccer player. Br J Sports Med 37(2):182–184
89. Croisier J-L (2004) Factors associated with recurrent hamstring injuries. Sports Med 34(10):681–695
90. Dauty M, Collon S (2011) Incidence of injuries in French professional soccer players. Int J Sports Med 32(12):965–969
91. Hayat Z, Konan S, Pollock R (2014) Ischiofemoral impingement resulting from a chronic avulsion injury of the hamstrings. BMJ Case Rep. https://doi.org/10.1136/bcr-2014-204017
92. Kurosawa H, Nakasita K, Nakasita H, Sasaki S, Takeda S (1996) Complete avulsion of the hamstring tendons from the ischial tuberosity. A report of two cases sustained in judo. Br J Sports Med 30(1):72–74
93. Marx RG, Fives G, Chu SK, Daluiski A, Wolfe SW (2009) Allograft reconstruction for symptomatic chronic complete proximal hamstring tendon avulsion. Knee Surg Sports Traumatol Arthrosc 17(1):19–23
94. Sallay PI, Friedman RL, Coogan PG, Garrett WE (1996) Hamstring muscle injuries among water skiers. Functional outcome and prevention. Am J Sports Med 24(2):130–136
95. Sonnery-Cottet B, Archbold P, Thaunat M, Fayard J-M, Canuto SMG, Cucurulo T (2012) Proximal hamstring avulsion in a professional soccer player. Orthop Traumatol Surg Res 98(8):928–931
96. Bettin D, Pankalla T, Böhm H, Fuchs S (2003) Hip pain related to femoral neck stress fracture in a 12-year-old boy performing intensive soccer playing activities--a case report. Int J Sports Med 24(8):593–596
97. Giza E, Mithöfer K, Matthews H, Vrahas M (2004) Hip fracture-dislocation in football: a report of two cases and review of the literature. Br J Sports Med 38(4):E17
98. Nahas RM, Netto E, Chikude T, Ikemoto R (2007) Traumatic hip fracture-dislocation in soccer: a case report. Rev Bras Med Esporte 13(4):280–282
99. Drawer S, Fuller CW (2001) Propensity for osteoarthritis and lower limb joint pain in retired professional soccer players. Br J Sports Med 35(6):402–408
100. Amoako AO, Pujalte GGA (2014) Osteoarthritis in young, active, and athletic individuals. Clin Med Insights Arthritis Musculoskelet Disord 7:27–32
101. Bare A, Guanche C (2007) Intra-articular lesions. In: Johnson DH, Pedowitz RA (eds) Practical orthopaedic sports medicine and arthroscopy. Lippincott Williams & Wilkins, Philadelphia, PA, pp 473–489
102. Keene GS, Villar RN (1994) Arthroscopic anatomy of the hip: an in vivo study. Arthroscopy 10(4):392–399
103. Ellsworth AA, Zoland MP, Tyler TF (2014) Athletic pubalgia and associated rehabilitation. Int J Sports Phys Ther 9(6):774–784

28 Return to Play Following Hip Arthroscopy for FAI and Labral Lesions

Simon Lee, Tyrrell Burrus, Pete Draovitch, and Asheesh Bedi

Contents

S. Lee, M.D., M.P.H.
University of Michigan Health System, 1500 E. Medical Center Dr., TC2912, Ann Arbor, MI 48109-5328, USA
e-mail: simlee@med.umich.edu

T. Burrus, M.D. • A. Bedi, M.D. (✉)
Domino's Farms – MedSport, University of Michigan Health System, 24 Frank Lloyd Wright Drive, Lobby A, P.O. Box 391, Ann Arbor, MI 48106, USA
e-mail: tyrrellburrus@gmail.com; abedi@med.umich.edu

28.1 Introduction

Femoroacetabular impingement (FAI) is the most common cause of pre-arthritic pain and secondary chondrolabral pathology in the non-dysplastic hip in the competitive athlete; the spectrum of complex structural variance and loading characteristics within the hip joint, potentially leading to debilitating pathology, continues to grow as an orthopedic concern [1]. Advancements in diagnostic modalities and improved practitioner awareness have resulted in significantly increased recognition and treatment of the symptomatic young, non-arthritic hip. While the concept of FAI was first described by Smith-Peterson in 1936 [2], it was Ganz and colleagues who pioneered much of the modern modalities used for the diagnosis and treatment of FAI, elucidating the pathophysiology which creates abnormal loading mechanics and results in secondary degenerative changes within the hip joint [3–5].

Mechanical impingement at terminal hip range of motion leads to regional loading of the femoral head-neck junction against the acetabular rim, precipitate tearing, or detachment of the acetabular labrum from the articular cartilage [6]. Terminal

P. Draovitch, P.T., M.S., A.T.C., C.S.C.S.
The Hip, James M. Benson Sports Rehabilitation Center, Belaire Building, Ground Floor, 525 East 71st Street, New York, NY 10021, USA
e-mail: pdraovitch@comcast.com

V. Musahl et al. (eds.), *Return to Play in Football*, https://doi.org/10.1007/978-3-662-55713-6_28

range of motion is also often restricted due to the structural pathology, often complicating intra-articular injury in football players, who often push hip range of motion to the extremes [7]. During dynamic cyclic hip motion, repetitive impaction and abnormal regional loading of the femoral head-neck junction against the acetabular rim may also cause microtrauma and chondral delamination [5, 8–12]. Football players may be particularly predisposed to injury due to the high-impact nature of the sport along with the extreme hip biomechanical movements required of the hip for participation.

Localization of these injuries is typically at the anterosuperior region of the acetabular rim with concomitant disruption at the adjacent transition zone of the articular cartilage and reflects the topography of deformity. Early diagnosis and management of these injuries are critical, as their severity often correlates with the severity of the pathomorphology and the time between symptom onset and treatment [13–17]. FAI may be particularly disabling to the high-demand football player with significant cutting and pivoting requirements; therefore, a clear understanding of the etiology, diagnosis, management, and outcomes is essential for clinicians to optimally help patients to return to play [18]. Figure 28.1 demonstrates pre- and postoperative radiographs of a

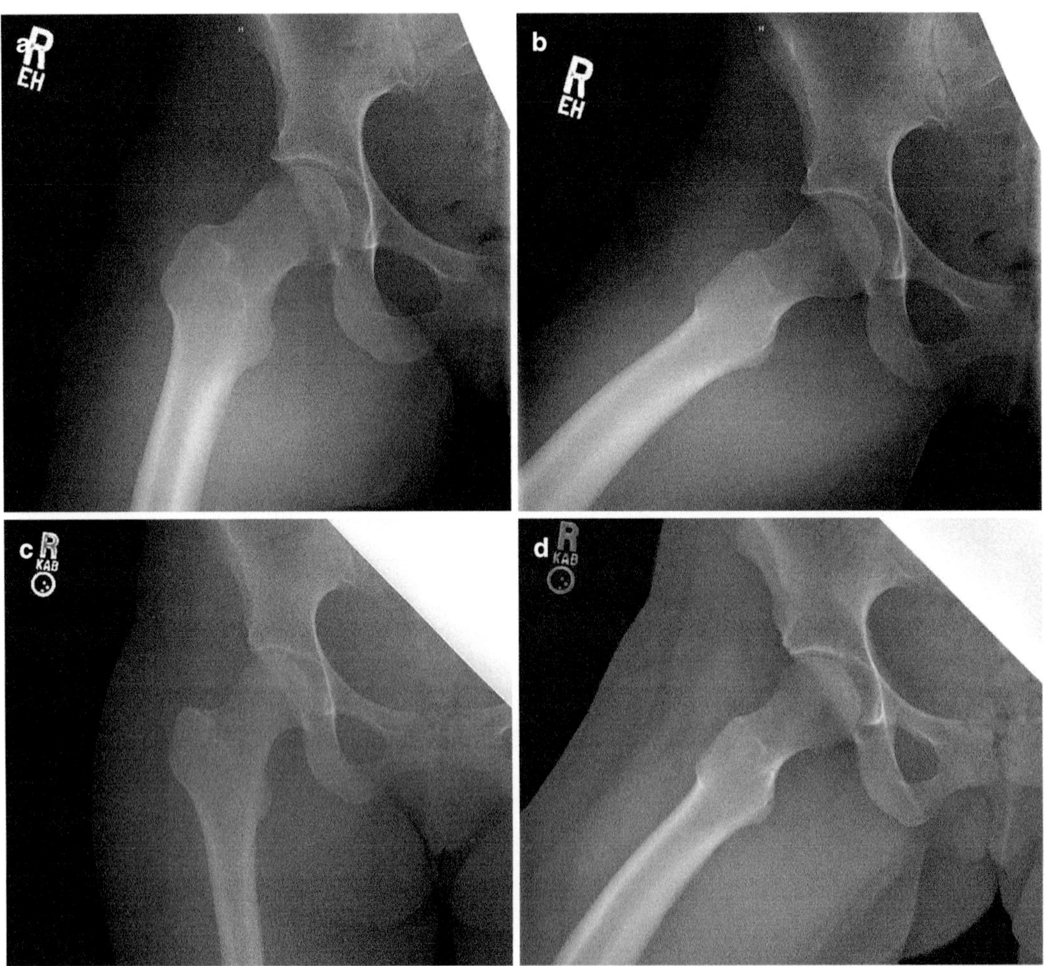

Fig. 28.1 (**a**, **b**) Anteroposterior and lateral radiographs of a right hip which demonstrates a significant femoral CAM deformity and acetabular retroversion. (**c**, **d**) Postoperative radiographs following femoral osteochondroplasty, acetabular osteochondroplasty, and labral repair, demonstrating corrected deformities

right hip which underwent hip arthroscopy for the treatment of combined-type FAI.

28.2 Femoroacetabular Impingement in Football Players

A significant number of athletes at all levels, from recreational to professional players, present with hip pain and functional disability due to FAI [19–21]. Symptomatic hip pain related to FAI is commonly diagnosed with athletic activities that may require increased ranges of motion. Examples include cutting motions and repeated changes of direction as seen in American football and soccer, increased hip flexion/abduction/internal rotation as seen in ice hockey, and supraphysiological ranges of motion as seen in dance [22]. These athletes often push their hips to extreme ranges of motion, particularly with internal rotation. Football players are subject to increased axial and rotational loads during competition, up to 12 times of their body weight. The full spectrum of competition levels is represented, from recreational weekend warriors to elite professional athletes [23, 24]. In addition, symptomatic FAI has been demonstrated to be more common in certain types of athletes as compared to the general population [25–28].

28.2.1 Hip Biomechanics in Football Players

The movement requirements of the hip and knee of elite American football athletes during dynamic, game-like athletic tasks continue to be quantified in the literature. Knowledge of the requisite hip range of motion for elite American football players is important to provide recognition of athletes with FAI who may be more susceptible to hip injury. Furthermore, this information helps to establish practical targets for restoration of motion with surgical treatment or rehabilitation. The compensatory mechanisms of injury secondary to restricted hip motion, as well as the impact of restricted hip motion on other joints in the kinetic chain such as the knee, are increasingly being recognized.

Deneweth et al. analyzed the hip and knee kinematics on 40 American National Collegiate Athletic Association (NCAA) football athletes of various position groups as they performed game-like maneuvers [29]. Average hip passive ROM across all players was measured to be 102° ± 15° of flexion, 25° ± 9° of internal rotation, and 25° ± 8° of external rotation. These ranges were not significantly different across positions. Hip internal and external rotation requirements were also similar across positions, suggesting that internal rotation ROM deficits may universally affect athletes required to perform cutting or sidestep maneuvers, independent of position. FAI has been associated with restricted hip ROM, particularly decreased terminal flexion and internal rotation, potentially causing significant loss of performance and susceptibility to injury [10].

Kapron et al. demonstrated that alpha angle and head-neck offset were significantly correlated with decreased hip internal ROM in a prospective analysis of 65 NCAA American football players [30]. Repetitive impingement and bony collisions secondary to structurally restricted hip ROM during high-intensity athletic activity may result in chondrolabral injury within the joint and subsequent progression to hip osteoarthritis [4, 5, 31]. Additional adverse compensatory musculoskeletal injuries may also be resultant from restricted hip ROM secondary to abnormal kinematic changes to the lower extremity kinetic chain [32–34]. Several recent studies have suggested a relation between radiographic indicators of hip impingement and an increased risk for anterior cruciate ligament (ACL) injury at the knee [32, 35, 36]. It has been proposed that restricted hip internal rotation results in the need to achieve a greater range of tibial internal rotation during intensive athletic motions and thereby increase the likelihood of ACL injury [32, 37].

Bedi et al. analyzed 224 American football athletes attending the 2012 NFL National Invitational Camp and found that a reduction in internal rotation of the left hip was associated with a significantly increased odds of ACL injury in the ipsilateral or contralateral knee [32]. The authors noted that that a 30-degree reduction in left hip internal rotation was associated with 4.06 and 5.29 times greater odds of ACL injury in the ipsilateral and contralateral limbs, respectively. In the same study, the authors also demonstrated that FAI systematically increased the peak ACL strain predicted during the pivot landing using an in silico biomechanical model. In addition to injuries about the hip joint, FAI may be associated with ACL injury because of the increased resistance to femoral internal axial rotation during a dynamic maneuver such as a pivot landing.

Fact Box 1

- FAI has been associated with restricted hip ROM, particularly decreased terminal flexion and internal rotation, potentially causing significant loss of performance and susceptibility to injury.
- Repetitive impingement and bony collisions secondary to structurally restricted hip ROM during high-intensity athletic activity may result in chondrolabral injury within the joint and subsequent progression to hip osteoarthritis.
- FAI may be associated with ACL injury because of the increased resistance to femoral internal axial rotation during a dynamic maneuver such as a pivot landing.

28.2.2 Demographics

Nawabi et al. recently performed a retrospective review of 622 athletes (288 high-level, 334 recreational) of various sports who underwent hip arthroscopy for FAI in an attempt to determine demographic differences in age, gender, and the need for bilateral surgery for high-level athletes as compared to recreational athletes [22]. The authors determined that high-level athletes were associated with younger age (mean age, 20.2 years vs. 33.0 years; odds ratio, 0.69; $P < 0.001$) and male gender (61.5% vs. 53.6%; odds ratio, 1.75; $P = 0.03$). The authors also found that high-level athletes received bilateral surgery more frequently (28.4% vs. 15.9%); however, the significance of this relationship was determined to be confounded by age. High-level male athletes undergoing surgery most commonly participated in ice hockey followed by American football, as compared to high-level females who most frequently participated in soccer followed by dance.

Cutting sport athletes (soccer, basketball, lacrosse, and field hockey) represented the largest group of patients by sport category, followed by athletes involved in impingement sports (ice hockey, crew/rowing, baseball catcher, water polo, equestrian polo, and breaststroke swimmer). Cutting athletes underwent surgical management at a significantly younger age (19.2 years) as compared to flexibility athletes (dance, gymnastics, yoga, cheer, figure skating, and martial arts) (20.9 years; $P = 0.03$), contact athletes (American football, rugby, and wrestling) (mean age: 21.3 years; $P = 0.005$), and impingement athletes (mean age: 21.3 years; $P < 0.001$). Athletes performing flexibility sports underwent ligamentum teres debridement significantly more frequently as compared to impingement sports ($P = 0.004$) and asymmetric sports (baseball, softball, tennis, golf, volleyball, and field events) ($P = 0.03$).

The types of sports that provoke symptomatic FAI require differing movements around the hip and the pelvis. In addition to influencing the age at which these athletes present with symptoms, the category of sport may be predictive of the pattern of intra-articular damage or compensatory pathology. For example, contact athletes may be at higher risk of impingement-induced posterior hip subluxation or dislocation because of the high-impact nature of these sports. In a case series of athletes with posterior instability and associated acetabular rim fractures, 15 of 22 patients were American football players and one was a wrestler [38].

These findings highlight that there may be important differences between athletes of different sports with corresponding implications for management and correction of deformity. In addition to age-related factors, the unique biomechanical demands on the hip applied by different categories of sport may significantly influence the development of symptomatic FAI in varying athletes. For example, the flexibility athletes are a unique group in that rehabilitation philosophy is different compared to the cutting athlete. Rehabilitation focus is on mobility in the more standard FAI patient, such as the cutting athlete, whereas undercovered patients with FAI, such as flexibility athletes, have a focus on neuromuscular stability. The category of sport may be predictive of a particular pattern of intra-articular damage or compensatory pathology. Krych et al. performed a retrospective review to analyze 22 mixed-sport athletes presenting with posterior acetabular rim fractures with subsequent posterior instability and found that 81.8% had alpha angles >45° and 77.3% had associated ligamentum teres avulsion, suggesting an association between these pathologies. Nawabi et al. also demonstrated significantly more frequent findings of ligamentum teres pathology, but these were more common in flexibility athletes. Awareness of varying demographics among different groups of athletes is important to identify the individual needs of patients when considering preventative, nonoperative, or surgical management options.

28.2.3 Increased Prevalence of FAI in American Football Players

Feeley et al. reviewed the NFL Injury Surveillance System and demonstrated a significant trend toward increased hip injuries per year among these elite athletes from 1997 to 2006 [39]. The authors noted that while intra-articular hip injuries represented only 5% of hip injuries in this cohort, they accounted for the most time lost. Fractures and dislocations resulted in the most lost time, followed by labral tears. The authors also reported on 19 NFL players who were treated at their institution for intra-articular hip injuries, 13 of which were diagnosed with labral tears. These 13 athletes also demonstrated significant evidence of femoral head and acetabular cartilage loss as well. Five of these athletes underwent surgery, while the other eight were able to return to play following a course of physical therapy. While four of the five athletes were able to return to play at an elite level by 6 months after surgery, one of the athletes demonstrated significant cartilage loss and erosive changes at the time of arthroscopy, subsequently retiring from the NFL at 35 years of age, although he was able to play one season after recovery from surgery.

The estimated prevalence of radiographic FAI is highly variable, but athletes have demonstrated an increased prevalence over the general population. In fact, radiographic evidence of FAI has been reported in up to 95% of high-level athletes [20, 27, 40]. Kapron et al. analyzed a cohort of 67 male collegiate American football players in a prospective study and showed that 95% of the 134 hips analyzed demonstrated at least one radiographic sign of cam or pincer deformity, with 21% demonstrating only cam deformity, 52% demonstrating only pincer deformity, and 77% of these hips demonstrating greater than one sign. The authors concluded that the morphologic abnormalities of FAI were common in this American football population and that its prevalence was substantially higher than seen in the general population [27].

In a sample of 123 hips with a history of hip or groin pain obtained from athletes at the National Football League Combine, Nepple et al. determined that 94.3% demonstrated radiographic evidence for FAI (cam-type, 9.8%; pincer-type, 22.8%; combined-type, 61.8%) [40]. Larson et al. corroborated these findings with another study evaluating a mixed cohort of 238 symptomatic and asymptomatic hips from the National

Football League Combine, noting that 87% exhibited at least once radiographic sign consistent with FAI. 65.3% of hips demonstrated cam deformity, 72.4% of hips demonstrated pincer deformity, and 51.9% of hips had mixed type. Additionally, 40.6% demonstrated acetabular retroversion, 2.5% demonstrated coxa profunda, 64.4% demonstrated crossover sign, and 9.2% demonstrated labral ossification. They also determined that increasing alpha angle was an independent predictor for the development of groin pain [19].

Mehran et al. analyzed all surgical procedures performed of athletes from a single NCAA Division I college American football team from the 2004–2005 season through the 2013–2014 season and found that arthroscopic hip labral repair comprised 5.9% of surgeries, and a combined femoral neck and acetabular osteoplasty was performed in 78.9% of cases [41]. Mascarenhas recently published a systematic review of imaging prevalence of FAI in patients and concluded that the majority (>90%) of American football players studied demonstrated radiographic evidence of FAI [42]. Interestingly, they noted that radiographic findings of FAI in the American football population were more consistently present as compared to soccer players, ice hockey players, and nonathletes. Domb et al. performed a retrospective analysis of 62 hip magnetic resonance imaging scans from younger retired NFL players who were evaluated in clinic for persistent hip pain which demonstrated labral tears in 89%, chondral lesions in 98%, and partial or complete ligamentum teres tears in 81% [43]. However, while radiographic evidence of FAI abnormality may be highly prevalent, symptomatology may not correlate. In a follow-up study of the previous patient cohort, Kapron et al. performed an analysis on the collegiate American football cohort and demonstrated that while 95% demonstrated radiographic evidence of FAI, only 8.5% and 2.3% of athletes were positive for pain during the impingement and FABER tests, respectively [30].

Fact Box 2

- The National Football League Injury Surveillance System demonstrated that while intra-articular hip injuries represented only 5% of hip injuries in this cohort, they accounted for the most time lost.
- 87% of hips analyzed at the National Football League Combine exhibited at least one radiographic sign consistent with FAI (65.3% of hips demonstrated cam deformity, 72.4% of hips demonstrated pincer deformity, and 51.9% of hips had mixed type).
- Radiographic signs and symptoms may not correlate, 95% of a collegiate American football cohort demonstrated radiographic evidence of FAI, and only 8.5% and 2.3% of athletes were positive for pain during the impingement and FABER tests, respectively.

28.2.4 Development of FAI During Skeletal Maturity

Increasing levels of high physical activity in adolescents have been postulated as a contributing factor in developing FAI [25, 31, 44]. Agricola et al. demonstrated in 89 elite preprofessional soccer players and 92 controls (age range: 12–19 years) that cam-type lesions on radiographs were identified significantly more often in soccer players as compared to their nonathletic peer controls (elite, 13%; controls, 0%, $P < 0.03$) [25]. The authors found cam-type lesions in athletes as young as 13 years [25].Agricola et al. subsequently reported on the radiographs of 63 preprofessional soccer players (mean age, 14.43 years; range, 12–19 years) at baseline and at a mean 2.4 years subsequent follow-up [45]. The prevalence of a head-neck prominence significantly increased from 2.1% to 17.7% ($P = 0.002$) in hips with an open growth plate at baseline, with no significant increase in the prevalence or size of the cam lesion following growth plate closure [45]. The alpha angle was also significantly increased from 59.4° at baseline to 61.3° at follow-up ($P = 0.018$). The authors concluded that cam-type lesions may gradually develop during the period of skeletal immaturity and could potentially be ameliorated through modification of athletic activity during this time [45].

In regard to American football players, Tak et al. postulated that the cam deformity is likely a reactive bony adaptation to high-impact sport practice during skeletal maturity [46]. The authors retrospectively grouped 126 hips to low-frequency versus high-frequency practice cohorts. They determined that the presence of a cam deformity was significantly lower in athletes playing American football at low frequency (≤3 times/week) from the age of 12 years or above (40.2%) as compared to athletes who started playing American football at a professional American football club before the age of 12 years (63.6%, $n = 44$, OR = 0.39, 95% CI 0.15–0.97, $p = 0.042$). When comparing the same groups, there was also a significant difference in the prevalence of a pathological cam deformity (α angle >78°) (12% vs. 30%, OR = 0.33, 95% CI 0.12–0.94, $p = 0.038$). The authors concluded there may be a probable dose-response relationship between the frequency of American football practice during skeletal maturity in the development of a cam lesion.

The currently available evidence suggests that development of FAI for the young athlete potentially starts at an early age during skeletal maturity, which for males typically occurs at about 18–22 years and for females at 14–17 years. Nepple et al. performed a systematic review analyzing the development of FAI in association with sporting activity in adolescence and demonstrated that males participating in high-level impact sports have an increased risk of cam-lesion presentation [47]. High-level male athletes were 1.9–8.0 times more likely to develop a cam lesion, with a 41% cam-lesion prevalence as compared to 17% in controls. The biomechanical stresses that the femoroacetabular joint experiences during repetitive physical activity may result in focal patterns of abnormal force on the growth plate and surrounding bone. The highly dynamic and cyclic nature of increased impact activity resulting from certain sports may generate higher mechanical joint loading with subsequent growth stimulus. These abnormal mechanical loads are produced at the extreme ranges of hip motion and therefore may be applied at areas of the joint that are relatively naïve to these types of loads. The current trend of early sport specialization may compound this effect for an even greater degree of deformity development, due to exceeding volume or intensity workload thresholds.

28.3 Return to Play in American Football Players Following Hip Arthroscopy

Rapid advances in hip arthroscopy to address symptomatic FAI have allowed for extensive visualization and management of joint pathology. The primary techniques include femoral osteochondroplasty to address the cam lesion and acetabular rim resection to address the pincer lesion. Labral injury may necessitate refixation, debridement, or reconstruction depending on the tissue quality at the time of surgery. In addition, articular cartilage damage due to abnormal joint surface forces may be addressed with microfracture techniques. Botser et al. have shown in a systematic review that hip arthroscopy provides improved return to play rates and decreased complication rates for professional athletes compared to open surgical hip dislocation, potentially due to the minimally invasive nature of the operation [48]. There have been two previous systematic reviews on the rate of return to play following surgery for FAI which demonstrate favorable outcomes [49, 50].

Improvements of in vivo hip kinematics after surgical correction of FAI have been demonstrated in the literature utilizing 3D reconstructions of CT scans [51, 52]. Kubiak-Langer et al. use a validated noninvasive 3D CT-based method for kinematic hip analysis to compare the range of motion pattern, the location of impingement, and the effect of virtual surgical reconstruction in 28 hips with anterior femoroacetabular impingement and a control group of 33 normal hips. They found that the average improvement of internal rotation was 5.4° for pincer hips, 8.5° for cam hips, and 15.7° for mixed impingement [52]. Bedi et al. analyzed ten symptomatic patients with focal cam and/or pincer impingement lesions with computer-assisted 3D modeling of high-resolution CT scans before and after surgical intervention and found that corrective femoral and rim osteoplasty resulted in significant improvements in both hip flexion 3.8° and internal rotation 9.3° [51]. Range of motion improvement, particularly internal rotation, is critical for the American football athlete to return to play and prevent future reinjury.

In a study which analyzed 45 mixed-sport professional athletes, Philippon et al. also found that 42 (93%) patients were able to return to professional competition at an average of 1.6 years (range: 6 months–5.5 years) [53]. Of the five professional American football players included in the study, one was unable to return to play and was noted to have had diffuse hip osteoarthritis present at the time of arthroscopy. A hockey player and a basketball player with extensive OA were also unable to return to play; however, a golfer with extensive OA returned to play. The authors suggested that arthroscopic treatment of FAI in the presence of OA can allow patients to return to low-impact sporting activity, however, not likely high-impact professional sports.

Nho et al. analyzed a mixed group of 47 high-level athletes (27.7% varsity high school, 53.2% college, and 19.1% professional; mean age: 22.8 ± 6.2 years) with a minimum follow-up of 1 year [54]. Four of these athletes were American football players. Of the 33 athletes who were available for follow-up, 26 (79%) returned to play at a mean of 9.4 ± 4.7 months (range: 4–26 months) postoperatively with 24 of those athletes (92.3%) returning to the same level of competition. These 24 athletes continued participating in competition at 2 years, but the level of competition at this point was not reported. The rate of return was 90% (9 of 10) in high school athletes, 59% (10 of 17) in collegiate athletes, and 83% (5 of 6) in professional athletes. Of the seven athletes who were unable to return to play, five were due to persistent hip pain. All American football players were able to return to play. Byrd and Jones performed an analysis of 200 athletic patients (28.6 years; range, 11–60 years) which included 23 professional, 56 intercollegiate, 24 high school, and 97 recreational athletes [55]. This cohort included 24 American football players (18 professional/intercollegiate and 6 high school/recreational). One hundred eighty-one athletes (90%) returned to their previous level of competition, with 95% returning at the professional level and 85% at the collegiate level and an average follow-up of 19 months (range: 12–60 months).

Malviya et al. demonstrated similar findings in a comparative analysis of 40 professional and 40 recreational athletes, 14 of which were American football players [56]. The average return-to-sport duration was 5.4 months (range: 3–10 months) for all athletes, but professional athletes required significantly less time (mean: 4.2 months) as compared to recreational athletes (mean: 6.8 months, $P = 0.03$). All athletes followed the same rehabilitation protocol, so the differential motivational or fitness aspects between professional and recreational athletes may explain this finding. Both professional and recreational groups demonstrated high rates of return to play at 6 months (78% and 65%, respectively) and 1 year (82% and 73%, respectively) without significant differences. There was a 2.6-fold improvement in the training time (from 7.8 to 20 h per week) and a 3.2-fold increase in time in competition (from 2.5 to 7.9 h per week). While professional and nonprofessional athletes both demonstrated good outcomes, the literature suggests that professional athletes may exhibit superior rate of return to play and faster return to play time. Professional athletes also returned to their previous level of activity at a higher rate. A potential explanation for this observation could be that professional athletes hold significantly greater socioeconomic investment in their sport and therefore possess elevated motivation for return to play; additionally, their unrestricted access to rehabilitation professionals and state-of-the-art physical therapy techniques and instruments may expedite their recovery. This information can be useful in setting appropriate expectations for athletes of different competition levels.

There is currently a lack of literature focusing of the analysis of return to play outcomes on American football players specifically following arthroscopic management of hip labral tears and FAI. However, outcomes of Australian Rules Football athletes following hip arthroscopy provide important insights to the potential ability to return to play of American football players. Amenbar et al. completed a retrospective review of 36 male professional Australian Football League players; 26 of 27 with at least 2 years' follow-up were available for review and found that all but one of the patients returned to play professionally for a return to play rate of 96% at an elite level [57]. At most recent follow-up, 62% were still playing professional Australian Rules Football for a mean of 52.5 months after surgery. Ten patients had retired from professional football, but they had all returned to play professionally after surgery. One player retired for causes related to hip disability. The modified Harris hip scale (MHHS) and non-arthritic hip score (NAHS) improved from 83.6 to 98 and from 85.3 to 97.1, respectively, in the players who were still playing.

Singh and O'Donnell reported on 24 consecutive Australian Rules Football players (27 hips) who underwent hip arthroscopic surgery and found that chondral lesions at the rim lesion were the most common pathology, affecting 93% of cases, followed by cam lesions in 81%. Pincer rim trimming was performed on 14%. Of note, 22% of these players underwent microfracture for significant cartilage loss. Cartilage loss was most often present at the anterosuperior acetabular rim and most often associated with a cam lesion. All players reported that they were satisfied and would have the surgery again if required. The MHHS and NAHS in all patients improved postoperatively, and they maintained their improvement from 1 year up to 4 years. One player was advised to retire from football because of the severity of the rim lesion (>40% cartilage loss) and osteoarthritis. Of 24 players, 23 returned to top-level AFL football. One player subsequently retired a year after hip surgery because of a chronic knee injury [58]. In the one patient who did not return to Australian Rules Football-level football, a >40% cartilage loss from the anterior acetabular wall was present in addition to an unstable os acetabuli and cam impingement. The player was treated with arthroscopic debridement, excision of the os, rim trimming, labral repair, microfracture of the acetabulum, and femoral osteochondroplasty. He was advised to retire from Australian Rules Football to protect his hip.

However, not all studies have demonstrated clear beneficial outcomes. Domb et al. compared the patient-reported outcomes for patients who returned to sport compared with those who did not after hip arthroscopy, a cohort which included 11 football players, and noted that football players trended toward not returning to sport [59]. However, this finding was not statistically significant as the authors noted that their study was likely not powered to detect such a difference.

Fact Box 3

- Three recent systematic reviews demonstrate favorable return to play outcomes for athletes following hip arthroscopy for FAI.
- In vivo computer modeling and CT reconstruction studies have demonstrated improvements of in vivo hip kinematics after surgical correction of FAI, particularly internal rotation, which is critical for the American football athlete to return to play and prevent future reinjury.
- Several studies demonstrate positive return to play and performance outcomes in Australian Football League athletes, a close surrogate for American football athletes.

28.3.1 Chondral Damage, Osteoarthritis, and Microfracture

Articular cartilage damage commonly occurs with the abnormal mechanical loads induced onto the joint by symptomatic FAI. Transition zone shear injuries with adjacent cartilage damage are typically caused during repetitive entry of cam lesions into the joint, subsequently resulting in chondral delamination [60]. Pincer lesions commonly result in posteroinferior articular contrecoup damage due to the levering effect of the acetabular over coverage, creating abnormal sheer forces on posterior chondral surfaces [1]. These chondral injuries may result in significant pain and functional deficit in the active athlete. As described earlier, Singh and O'Donnell analyzed 24 professional Australian Football League and found that the only athlete who was unable to return to play demonstrated >40% chondral loss on intraoperative examination, while the 23 (96%) other athletes had substantially less cartilage damage and were able to return to their previous level of professional play at a mean follow-up of 22 months [58]. Feely et al. also described an American football player who demonstrated significant cartilage loss and erosive changes at the time of arthroscopy, subsequently retiring from the NFL at 35 years of age, although he was able to play one season after recovery from surgery [39].

Microfracture at the time of hip arthroscopy has been proposed as a management option for these focal chondral injuries [61]. To evaluate the utility of hip arthroscopy in the management of chondral lesions in elite athletes, McDonald et al. recently performed a comparative study between 39 male hips who underwent microfracture for discrete Outerbridge grade IV chondral lesions and 94 male control hips without microfracture [62]. The two groups did not significantly differ in terms of return to play, as 30 athletes (77%) undergoing microfracture were able to return to competition at some point as compared to 79 control athletes (84%). Interestingly, 22 athletes (70%) undergoing microfracture continued professional play at an average of three seasons postoperatively (range: 1–11 seasons), while only 43 control athletes (54%) continued professional play at an average of 2.8 seasons (range: 1–11 seasons). However, there was no statistically significant difference detected. In the cohort of 200 mixed-level athletes reported by Byrd et al., 88% had Outerbridge grade III or grade IV articular damage [55]. Forty-nine of those athletes underwent microfracture surgery with a resultant 92% return to play rate postoperatively, similar to athletes undergoing hip arthroscopy without the additional microfracture procedure.

While the natural history of these chondral lesions is unclear, the current literature suggests that these injuries may continue to progress in severity and ultimately result in early-onset hip osteoarthritis if left unmanaged [63]. Byrd and Jones followed 15 athletes (mean age, 31.7 years; range, 14–70 years) who underwent hip arthroscopy and analyzed their return to play at minimum follow-up of 10 years [64]. While 13 (87%) athletes were initially able to return to play, five of these patients did not have sustained symptomatic relief from the procedure and progressed to failure. The authors found that all five of these athletes presented with arthritis at the time of surgery, all of whom progressed to total hip arthroplasty at an average of 73 months (range: 4–119 months) and demonstrated significantly inferior outcomes ($P < 0.006$). Additionally, the retrospective analysis of 45 mixed-sport professional athletes reviewed earlier by Philippon et al. concluded that the presence of diffuse osteoarthritis was a predictor for worse postoperative outcomes as all five patients with this finding were unable to ultimately return to play [53].

When management is initiated in the athlete prior to radiographic signs of significant osteoarthritis, athletes are generally able to return to competition. For microfracture to be effective, it is important that the athletes commit to follow a consistent postoperative and rehabilitation protocol [61]. Taken together, athletes undergoing additional microfracture procedures for focal chondral defects secondary to FAI exhibit high rates of return to play, with competition-level durability similar to other athletes without chondral defects. However, the athlete receiving microfracture must have a high level of commitment to the rehabilitation process if they are to have a good outcome. Platelet-rich plasma is an evolving technique as a conjunction to hip arthroscopy in the setting of articular damage and early osteoarthritis. While some studies have demonstrated some improved tissue healing, the body of literature is lacking, and higher levels of evidence are required to infer any clinical utility for athletes [65].

28.3.2 Labral Reconstruction

Disruption of the longitudinal fibers may functionally cripple the labrum and provide minimal viable tissue to primary repair, necessitating a reconstruction technique with tissue grafting [66]. Clinical and functional outcomes have demonstrated positive results in the general population; however, specific literature focusing on athletes is sparse [67]. The restoration of a competent labrum is especially important in the athletic population as the return of physiologic hip biomechanics is critical to achieve the mobility necessary to these patients. Boykin et al. performed a retrospective review of 21 elite athletes (23 hips; mean age, 28.0 years; range, 19–41 years) who underwent arthroscopic labral reconstruction with iliotibial band graft with an average follow-up of 41.4 months (range: 20–74 months). Four professional American football players were included in the analysis. The authors determined that the athletes achieved a high rate of return to play (17 of 18 athletes, 85.7%), 17 (81%) of which returned to a similar level of competition [68]. The authors also found significant improvements in the MHHS (67–84, $P = 0.026$) and hip outcome score sport subscale (HOS SS) (56–77, $P = 0.009$) [68]. Of the 23 hips, two required joint replacement: one at 24 months and one at 23 months after reconstruction. Both players were older (37 years and 31 years, respectively) than the average age of the remaining athletes, and both had evidence of osteoarthritis on preoperative imaging with <2 mm of joint space on at least one point of measurement. Their preoperative MHHS values were 65 and 59.4. One was a professional baseball player, and one was a professional American football player. The American football player was able to return to the practice field with his National Football League team but never returned to game action; he retired from professional American football 16 months after reconstruction. Four athletes were professional American football players: one linebacker, one free safety, one cornerback, and one placekicker. The linebacker progressed to arthroplasty within the follow-up period. All the rest returned to play at the professional level and have thus far had good return to play outcomes, similar to their pre-injury performance.

In a systematic review evaluating outcomes following labral reconstruction, Ayeni et al. concluded that the ideal candidates for the technique were young, active patients with >2 mm of joint space preservation [67]. Philippon et al. found that patient age was an independent predictor for patient satisfaction for a general population undergoing labral reconstruction with iliotibial band [66]. The average age of the 9% progressing to total hip arthroplasty in this cohort was significantly older as compared to those who did not require replacement (49 years vs. 36 years, $P = 0.027$). The two athletes who progressed to arthroplasty in the study by Boykin et al. were older (37 and 31 years) compared to the other patients and exhibited evidence of osteoarthritis and <2 mm joint space preservation on radiographs. Both of these factors have been shown to be independent predictors of hip arthroscopy failure [69]. The available evidence is limited, but labral reconstruction appears to provide improved short-term outcomes and good return to play rates in the younger athletic population who do not have evidence of osteoarthritis. Longer-term prospective studies will be required to evaluate the durability of these grafts to preserve high-level functioning and to mitigate early-onset osteoarthritis.

28.4 Rehabilitation

Postoperative rehabilitation protocols should include activities that can accurately evaluate an athlete's physical status and determine appropriate progressions for safe return to play. Phillipon et al. have previously published a rehabilitation protocol in a professional American football athlete following arthroscopic repair of intra-articular disorders which focus on a four-phase progression [70]. Phase 1 consists of mobility and protection, protecting the repaired tissue while initiating early but restricted passive range of motion. This initial phase emphasized hip circumduction, flexion, and internal rotation PROM to avoid potential adhesion formation within the joint capsule, as well as focusing on isometric exercises which were implemented to mitigate muscle inhibition and atrophy. Phase 2 focuses on stabilization of the hip joint with core stabilization exercises and progressive resistive exercise in addition to continue PROM and gait training. Balance training and neuromuscular reeducation were initiated to promote proper gait mechanics. Phase 3 marks the initiation of strengthening with focus on muscle endurance strength and cardiovascular conditioning. Advanced cord-resisted agility and single-leg-bend activities were started to prepare the patient for the functional return-to-sport test. Phase 4 was the return-to-sport aspect in which the athlete was integrated into team practice in preparation for competitive return to high-level sport. Table 28.1 demonstrates our preferred progression of rehabilitation with specific activity examples which mirrors many of these core principles. Figures 28.1, 28.2, 28.3, 28.4, 28.5, 28.6, and 28.7 illustrate the detailed maneuvers within the rehabilitation protocol.

Table 28.1 Hip arthroscopy rehabilitation—labral repair with or without FAI component

Postoperative time period	Rehabilitation activities and progressions
Weeks 0–2	• Focus on decreasing soft tissue swelling and restoring gliding of adjacent tissues • Stationary bicycle for 20 min/day (up to twice a day) • ROM progression—Stool rotations (AAROM hip IR), pelvic tilts, supine hip log rolling, limit external rotation to <20° (Fig. 28.2) • Hip isometrics (no flexion)—Prone leg curls, prone abdominal/gluteal/quad-hamstring/dorsiflexion isometric holds, quadruped hand heel rocks with stable core, supine bridges • Neuromuscular electrical stimulation to quadriceps with short-arc quadriceps if indicated or appropriate • Sustained stretching for psoas with cryotherapy (two pillows under hips) • Gait training every session to prevent the development of poor motion
Weeks 2–4	• Progress weight bearing—Wean off crutches at weeks 3–4 • Progress hip ROM as tolerated—Bent knee fall outs (week 4), stool rotations for ER (week 3–4), hip hiking (week 4) • Gluteal/piriformis stretching • Progress core and hip strengthening (avoid hip flexor tendonitis)—Bilateral cable column rotations (weeks 3–4) (Fig. 28.3), isotonic exercises (no flexion), clam shells→isometric side lying hip abduction (Fig. 28.4) • Step ups and downs starting with 4″ box building to 8″ box • Begin proprioception/balance training—Balance boards, single-leg stance (Fig. 28.5) • Aquatic therapy in low end of water
Weeks 4–8	• Progress strengthening—Introduce hip flexion prone isometrics to AAROM, multi-hip machine (open and closed chain), leg press (bilateral→unilateral), single-leg wall push, windmills, lawn mowers, resistive hip hikes (begin with doing all exercises as the stance leg first to insure muscular strength, endurance, and neuromuscular control prior to the moving leg) (Fig. 28.6) • Progress core strengthening—Prone/side planks • Progress proprioception/balance—Standing rotations with rocker bottom boards • Treadmill side stepping (week 6) • Elliptical (weeks 4–6) • Hip flexor, gluteus/piriformis, and IT band stretching—Seated eccentric hip flexor stretch (Fig. 28.7) • Three-point step with TheraBand progressing to side stepping with TheraBand (Fig. 28.8)

Table 28.1 (continued)

Postoperative time period	Rehabilitation activities and progressions
Weeks 8–12	• Progressive hip ROM • Progressive extremity and core strengthening using challenging surfaces or perturbations • Endurance activities around the hip • Dynamic balance activities
Weeks 12–16	• Progressive extremity and core strengthening • Plyometrics—Begin with in-place double-leg progressing to single-leg jumps, hops, and bounds being sure to monitor sets, foot contacts, and rest between sets • Begin treadmill or field running program • Sport-specific agility drills • Return to supervised modified weight room program • Begin developing a time-based plan for return to activity and sport

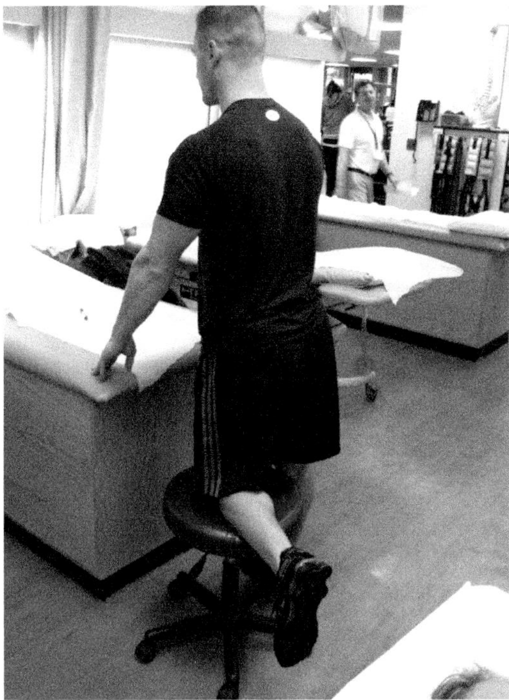

Fig. 28.2 Stool rotations to participate in active assisted range of motion exercises, particularly hip internal/external rotation

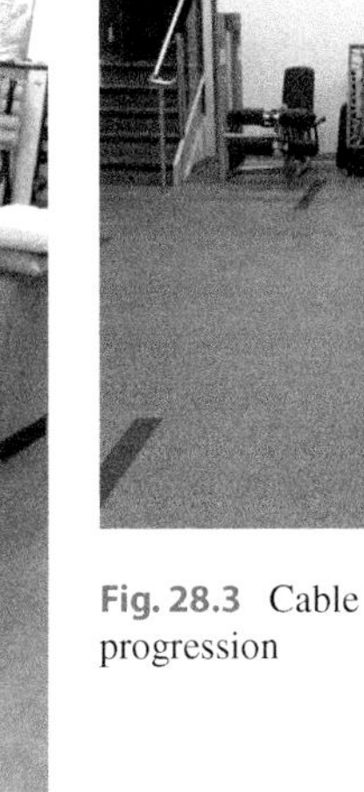

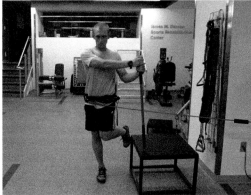

Fig. 28.3 Cable column rotations for core strengthening progression

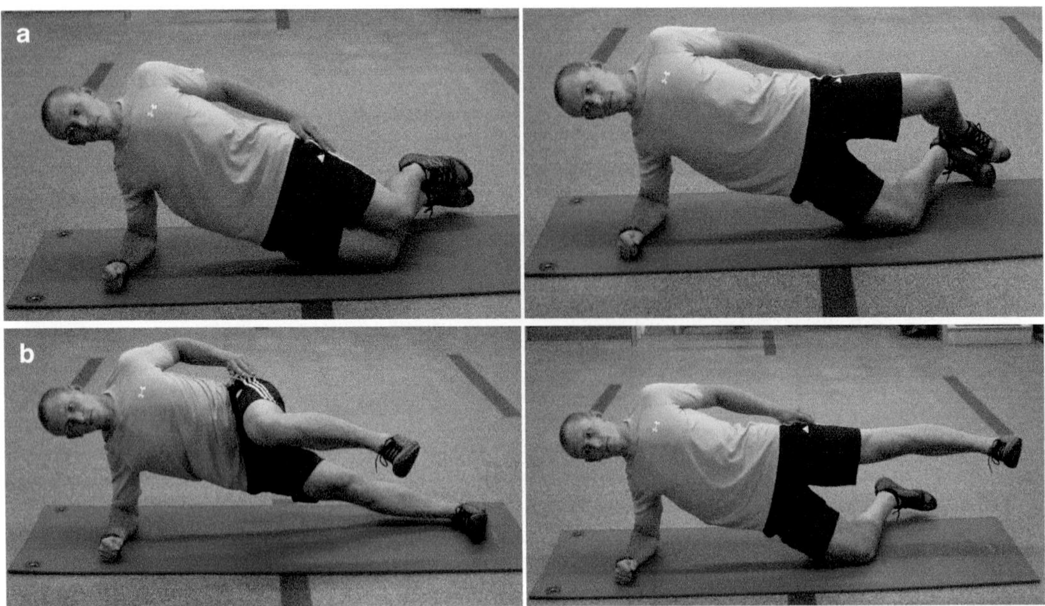

Fig. 28.4 (**a**) Clam shell exercise for hip external rotation and abduction, (**b**) progression to isometric side lying hip abduction

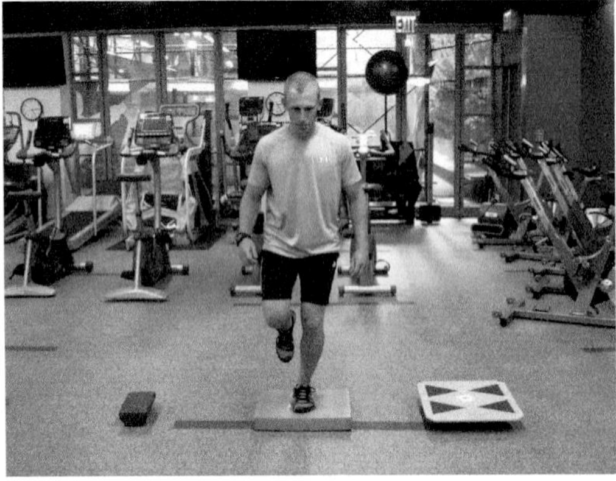

Fig. 28.5 Proprioception and balance training utilizing a variety of devices

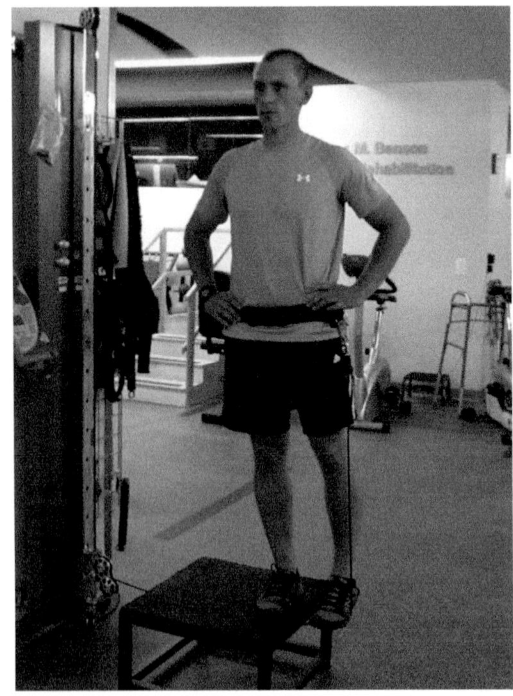

Fig. 28.6 Resistive hip hikes

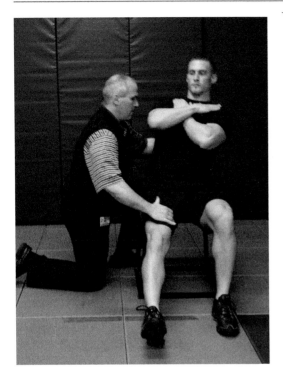

Fig. 28.7 Seated eccentric hip flexor stretch

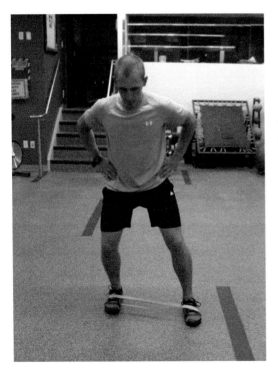

Fig. 28.8 Progressing to side stepping with resistance band

Conclusion

Intra-articular pathology leading to symptomatic hip pain results in significant morbidity and functional deficits in the athlete. Symptomatic FAI is the most common cause of pre-arthritic hip pain in the non-dysplastic hip. If nonoperative treatment fails to adequately alleviate symptoms or sufficiently restore function in the American football player, hip arthroscopy can lead to improved pain, improved range of motion, and high rates of return to play with proper postoperative rehabilitation. Important considerations include the ability to achieve the diagnosis in a timely manner and to exercise caution in older athletes with the presence of pre-existing osteoarthritis or diminished joint space. American football athletes who did not return to play in the literature tended to also demonstrate more severe chondral damage at the time of arthroscopy. Expectations should be managed in these patients as the literature demonstrates suboptimal outcomes in these populations. Higher quality of evidence with long-term prospective studies is required to determine the effectiveness of this technique to durably maintain athletes in athletic activity and alter the natural history of disease progression.

Take-Home Message

- Femoroacetabular impingement (FAI) may be particularly disabling to the high-demand athlete, especially those with significant cutting and pivoting requirements such as American football players.
- Awareness of varying requirements among different groups of athletes, particularly American football players, is important to identify the individual needs of patients when considering preventative, nonoperative, or surgical management options.
- Important considerations in the management of American football players with FAI include the importance of achieving the diagnosis in a timely manner and exercising caution in older athletes with the presence of pre-existing

osteoarthritis or diminished joint space, as the literature demonstrates suboptimal outcomes in this population.

Top Five Evidence Based References

Alradwan H, Philippon MJ, Farrokhyar F, Chu R, Whelan D, Bhandari M, Ayeni OR (2012) Return to preinjury activity levels after surgical management of femoroacetabular impingement in athletes. Arthroscopy 28:1567–1576

Casartelli NC, Leunig M, Maffiuletti NA, Bizzini M (2015) Return to sport after hip surgery for femoroacetabular impingement: a systematic review. Br J Sports Med 49:819–824

Bedi A, Chen N, Robertson W, Kelly BT (2008) The management of labral tears and femoroacetabular impingement of the hip in the young, active patient. Arthroscopy 24:1135–1145

Feeley BT, Powell JW, Muller MS, Barnes RP, Warren RF, Kelly BT (2008) Hip injuries and labral tears in the national football league. Am J Sports Med 36:2187–2195

Philippon MJ, Christensen JC, Wahoff MS (2009) Rehabilitation after arthroscopic repair of intra-articular disorders of the hip in a professional football athlete. J Sport Rehabil 18:118–134

References

1. Bedi A, Dolan M, Leunig M, Kelly BT (2011) Static and dynamic mechanical causes of hip pain. Arthroscopy 27:235–251
2. Smith-Petersen MN (2009) The classic: treatment of malum coxae senilis, old slipped upper femoral epiphysis, intrapelvic protrusion of the acetabulum, and coxa plana by means of acetabuloplasty. Clin Orthop Relat Res 467:608–615
3. Ganz R, Gill TJ, Gautier E, Ganz K, Krügel N, Berlemann U (2001) Surgical dislocation of the adult hip: a technique with full access to the femoral head and acetabulum without the risk of avascular necrosis. J Bone Joint Surg Br 83–B:1119–1124
4. Ganz R, Leunig M, Leunig-Ganz K, Harris WH (2008) The Etiology of Osteoarthritis of the Hip. Clin Orthop Relat Res 466:264–272
5. Ganz R, Parvizi J, Beck M, Leunig M, Nötzli H, Siebenrock KA (2003) Femoroacetabular impingement: a cause for osteoarthritis of the hip. Clin Orthop Relat Res:112–120
6. Wenger DE, Kendell KR, Miner MR, Trousdale RT (2004) Acetabular labral tears rarely occur in the absence of bony abnormalities. Clin Orthop Relat Res:145–150
7. Beck M, Kalhor M, Leunig M, Ganz R (2005) Hip morphology influences the pattern of damage to the acetabular cartilage: femoroacetabular impingement as a cause of early osteoarthritis of the hip. J Bone Joint Surg Br 87:1012–1018
8. Allen D, Beaulé PE, Ramadan O, Doucette S (2009) Prevalence of associated deformities and hip pain in patients with cam-type femoroacetabular impingement. J Bone Joint Surg Br 91–B:589–594
9. Anderson LA, Peters CL, Park BB, Stoddard GJ, Erickson JA, Crim JR (2009) Acetabular cartilage delamination in femoroacetabular impingement risk factors and magnetic resonance imaging diagnosis. J Bone Joint Surg Am 91:305–313
10. Bedi A, Chen N, Robertson W, Kelly BT (2008) The management of labral tears and femoroacetabular impingement of the hip in the young, active patient. Arthroscopy 24:1135–1145
11. Crawford JR, Villar RN (2005) Current concepts in the management of femoroacetabular impingement. J Bone Joint Surg Br 87–B:1459–1462
12. Khanduja V, Villar RN (2006) Arthroscopic surgery of the hip: current concepts and recent advances. J Bone Joint Surg Br 88–B:1557–1566
13. Burnett RSJ, Della Rocca GJ, Prather H, Curry M, Maloney WJ, Clohisy JC (2006) Clinical presentation of patients with tears of the acetabular labrum. J Bone Joint Surg Am 88:1448–1457
14. Dolan MM, Heyworth BE, Bedi A, Duke G, Kelly BT (2011) CT reveals a high incidence of osseous abnormalities in hips with labral tears. Clin Orthop Relat Res 469:831–838
15. Johnston TL, Schenker ML, Briggs KK, Philippon MJ (2008) Relationship between offset angle alpha and hip chondral injury in femoroacetabular impingement. Arthroscopy 24:669–675
16. Kelly BT, Weiland DE, Schenker ML, Philippon MJ (2005) Arthroscopic labral repair in the hip: surgical technique and review of the literature. Arthroscopy 21:1496–1504
17. Nepple JJ, Zebala LP, Clohisy JC (2009) Labral disease associated with femoroacetabular impingement: do we need to correct the structural deformity? J Arthroplasty 24:114–119
18. Bennell K, Hunter DJ, Vicenzino B (2012) Long-term effects of sport: preventing and managing OA in the athlete. Nat Rev Rheumatol 8:747–752
19. Larson CM, Sikka RS, Sardelli MC, Byrd JWT, Kelly BT, Jain RK, Giveans MR (2013) Increasing alpha angle is predictive of athletic-related "hip" and "groin" pain in collegiate National Football League prospects. Arthroscopy 29:405–410
20. Weir A, de Vos RJ, Moen M, Hölmich P, Tol JL (2011) Prevalence of radiological signs of femoroacetabular impingement in patients presenting with long-standing adductor-related groin pain. Br J Sports Med 45:6–9
21. Yuan BJ, Bartelt RB, Levy BA, Bond JR, Trousdale RT, Sierra RJ (2013) Decreased range of motion is associated with structural hip deformity in asymptomatic adolescent athletes. Am J Sports Med 41:1519–1525

22. Nawabi DH, Bedi A, Tibor LM, Magennis E, Kelly BT (2014) The demographic characteristics of high-level and recreational athletes undergoing hip arthroscopy for femoroacetabular impingement: a sports-specific analysis. Arthroscopy 30:398–405
23. Hammoud S, Bedi A, Magennis E, Meyers WC, Kelly BT (2012) High incidence of athletic pubalgia symptoms in professional athletes with symptomatic femoroacetabular impingement. Arthroscopy 28:1388–1395
24. Siebenrock KA, Kaschka I, Frauchiger L, Werlen S, Schwab JM (2013) Prevalence of cam-type deformity and hip pain in elite ice hockey players before and after the end of growth. Am J Sports Med 41:2308–2313
25. Agricola R, Bessems JHJM, Ginai AZ, Heijboer MP, van der Heijden RA, Verhaar JAN, Weinans H, Waarsing JH (2012) The development of Cam-type deformity in adolescent and young male soccer players. Am J Sports Med 40:1099–1106
26. Gerhardt MB, Romero AA, Silvers HJ, Harris DJ, Watanabe D, Mandelbaum BR (2012) The Prevalence of Radiographic Hip Abnormalities in Elite Soccer Players. Am J Sports Med 40:584–588
27. Kapron AL, Anderson AE, Aoki SK, Phillips LG, Petron DJ, Toth R, Peters CL (2011) Radiographic prevalence of femoroacetabular impingement in collegiate football players: AAOS exhibit selection. J Bone Joint Surg Am 93:e111(1-10)
28. Silvis ML, Mosher TJ, Smetana BS, Chinchilli VM, Flemming DJ, Walker EA, Black KP (2011) High prevalence of pelvic and hip magnetic resonance imaging findings in asymptomatic collegiate and professional hockey players. Am J Sports Med 39:715–721
29. Deneweth JM, Pomeroy SM, Russell JR, McLean SG, Zernicke RF, Bedi A, Goulet GC (2014) Position-specific hip and knee kinematics in NCAA football athletes. Orthop J Sports Med 2:2325967114534591
30. Kapron AL, Anderson AE, Peters CL, Phillips LG, Stoddard GJ, Petron DJ, Toth R, Aoki SK (2012) Hip internal rotation is correlated to radiographic findings of cam femoroacetabular impingement in collegiate football players. Arthroscopy 28:1661–1670
31. Bedi A, Lynch EB, Sibilsky Enselman ER, Davis ME, Dewolf PD, Makki TA, Kelly BT, Larson CM, Henning PT, Mendias CL (2013) Elevation in circulating biomarkers of cartilage damage and inflammation in athletes with femoroacetabular impingement. Am J Sports Med 41:2585–2590
32. Bedi A, Warren RF, Wojtys EM, YK O, Ashton-Miller JA, Oltean H, Kelly BT (2016) Restriction in hip internal rotation is associated with an increased risk of ACL injury. Knee Surg Sports Traumatol Arthrosc 24:2024–2031
33. Powers CM (2010) The influence of abnormal hip mechanics on knee injury: a biomechanical perspective. J Orthop Sports Phys Ther 40:42–51
34. Scher S, Anderson K, Weber N, Bajorek J, Rand K, Bey MJ (2010) Associations among hip and shoulder range of motion and shoulder injury in professional baseball players. J Athl Train 45:191–197
35. Ellera Gomes JL, Palma HM, Becker R (2010) Radiographic findings in restrained hip joints associated with ACL rupture. Knee Surg Sports Traumatol Arthrosc 18:1562–1567
36. Gomes JLE, de Castro JV, Becker R (2008) Decreased hip range of motion and noncontact injuries of the anterior cruciate ligament. Arthroscopy 24:1034–1037
37. Kelly BT, Bedi A, Robertson CM, Dela Torre K, Giveans MR, Larson CM (2012) Alterations in internal rotation and alpha angles are associated with arthroscopic cam decompression in the hip. Am J Sports Med 40:1107–1112
38. Krych AJ, Thompson M, Larson CM, Byrd JWT, Kelly BT (2012) Is posterior hip instability associated with cam and pincer deformity? Clin Orthop Relat Res 470:3390
39. Feeley BT, Powell JW, Muller MS, Barnes RP, Warren RF, Kelly BT (2008) Hip injuries and labral tears in the national football league. Am J Sports Med 36:2187–2195
40. Nepple JJ, Brophy RH, Matava MJ, Wright RW, Clohisy JC (2012) Radiographic findings of femoroacetabular impingement in National Football League Combine athletes undergoing radiographs for previous hip or groin pain. Arthroscopy 28:1396–1403
41. Mehran N, Photopoulos CD, Narvy SJ, Romano R, Gamradt SC, Tibone JE (2016) Epidemiology of operative procedures in an NCAA Division I Football Team over 10 seasons. Orthop J Sports Med 4:2325967116657530
42. Mascarenhas VV, Rego P, Dantas P, Morais F, McWilliams J, Collado D, Marques H, Gaspar A, Soldado F, Consciência JG (2016) Imaging prevalence of femoroacetabular impingement in symptomatic patients, athletes, and asymptomatic individuals: a systematic review. Eur J Radiol 85:73–95
43. Domb BG, Jackson TJ, Carter CC, Jester JR, Finch NA, Stake CE (2014) Magnetic resonance imaging findings in the symptomatic hips of younger retired national football league players. Am J Sports Med 42:1704–1709
44. Philippon MJ, Stubbs AJ, Schenker ML, Maxwell RB, Ganz R, Leunig M (2007) Arthroscopic management of femoroacetabular impingement - osteoplasty technique and literature review. Am J Sports Med 35:1571–1580
45. Agricola R, Heijboer MP, Ginai AZ, Roels P, Zadpoor AA, Verhaar JAN, Weinans H, Waarsing JH (2014) A cam deformity is gradually acquired during skeletal maturation in adolescent and young male soccer players: a prospective study with minimum 2-year follow-up. Am J Sports Med 42:798–806
46. Tak I, Weir A, Langhout R, Waarsing JH, Stubbe J, Kerkhoffs G, Agricola R (2015) The relationship between the frequency of football practice during skeletal growth and the presence of a cam defor-

mity in adult elite football players. Br J Sports Med 49:630–634
47. Nepple JJ, Vigdorchik JM, Clohisy JC (2015) What is the association between sports participation and the development of proximal femoral cam deformity? A systematic review and meta-analysis. Am J Sports Med 43:2833–2840
48. Botser IB, Smith TW, Nasser R, Domb BG (2011) Open surgical dislocation versus arthroscopy for femoroacetabular impingement: a comparison of clinical outcomes. Arthroscopy 27:270–278
49. Alradwan H, Philippon MJ, Farrokhyar F, Chu R, Whelan D, Bhandari M, Ayeni OR (2012) Return to preinjury activity levels after surgical management of femoroacetabular impingement in athletes. Arthroscopy 28:1567–1576
50. Casartelli NC, Leunig M, Maffiuletti NA, Bizzini M (2015) Return to sport after hip surgery for femoroacetabular impingement: a systematic review. Br J Sports Med 49:819–824
51. Bedi A, Dolan M, Hetsroni I, Magennis E, Lipman J, Buly R, Kelly BT (2011) Surgical treatment of femoroacetabular impingement improves hip kinematics: a computer-assisted model. Am J Sports Med 39(Suppl):43S–49S
52. Kubiak-Langer M, Tannast M, Murphy SB, Siebenrock KA, Langlotz F (2007) Range of motion in anterior femoroacetabular impingement. Clin Orthop Relat Res 458:117–124
53. Philippon M, Schenker M, Briggs K, Kuppersmith D (2007) Femoroacetabular impingement in 45 professional athletes: associated pathologies and return to sport following arthroscopic decompression. Knee Surg Sports Traumatol Arthrosc 15:908–914
54. Nho SJ, Magennis EM, Singh CK, Kelly BT (2011) Outcomes after the arthroscopic treatment of femoroacetabular impingement in a mixed group of high-level athletes. Am J Sports Med 39(Suppl): 14S–19S
55. Byrd JWT, Jones KS (2011) Arthroscopic management of femoroacetabular impingement in athletes. Am J Sports Med 39(Suppl):7S–13S
56. Malviya A, Paliobeis CP, Villar RN (2013) Do professional athletes perform better than recreational athletes after arthroscopy for femoroacetabular impingement? Clin Orthop Relat Res 471:2477–2483
57. Amenabar T, O'Donnell J (2013) Return to sport in Australian football league footballers after hip arthroscopy and midterm outcome. Arthroscopy 29:1188–1194
58. Singh PJ, O'Donnell JM (2010) The outcome of hip arthroscopy in Australian football league players: a review of 27 hips. Arthroscopy 26:743–749
59. Domb BG, Dunne KF, Martin TJ, Gui C, Finch NA, Vemula SP, Redmond JM (2016) Patient reported outcomes for patients who returned to sport compared with those who did not after hip arthroscopy: minimum 2-year follow-up. J Hip Preserv Surg 3:124–131
60. Leunig M, Beck M, Kalhor M, Kim Y-J, Werlen S, Ganz R (2005) Fibrocystic changes at anterosuperior femoral neck: prevalence in hips with femoroacetabular impingement. Radiology 236:237–246
61. Crawford K, Philippon MJ, Sekiya JK, Rodkey WG, Steadman JR (2006) Microfracture of the hip in athletes. Clin Sports Med 25:327–335. x
62. McDonald JE, Herzog MM, Philippon MJ (2013) Return to play after hip arthroscopy with microfracture in elite athletes. Arthroscopy 29:330–335
63. Ellis HB, Briggs KK, Philippon MJ (2011) Innovation in hip arthroscopy: is hip arthritis preventable in the athlete? Br J Sports Med 45:253–258
64. Byrd JWT, Jones KS (2009) Hip arthroscopy in athletes 10-year follow-up. Am J Sports Med 37:2140–2143
65. Engebretsen L, Steffen K, Alsousou J, Anitua E, Bachl N, Devilee R, Everts P, Hamilton B, Huard J, Jenoure P, Kelberine F, Kon E, Maffulli N, Matheson G, Mei-Dan O, Menetrey J, Philippon M, Randelli P, Schamasch P, Schwellnus M, Vernec A, Verrall G (2010) IOC consensus paper on the use of platelet-rich plasma in sports medicine. Br J Sports Med 44:1072–1081
66. Philippon MJ, Briggs KK, Hay CJ, Kuppersmith DA, Dewing CB, Huang MJ (2010) Arthroscopic labral reconstruction in the hip using iliotibial band autograft: technique and early outcomes. Arthroscopy 26:750–756
67. Ayeni OR, Alradwan H, de Sa D, Philippon MJ (2014) The hip labrum reconstruction: indications and outcomes--a systematic review. Knee Surg Sports Traumatol Arthrosc 22:737–743
68. Boykin RE, Patterson D, Briggs KK, Dee A, Philippon MJ (2013) Results of arthroscopic labral reconstruction of the hip in elite athletes. Am J Sports Med 41:2296–2301
69. Philippon M, Briggs K, Yen Y-M, Kuppersmith D (2009) Outcomes following hip arthroscopy for femoroacetabular impingement with associated chondrolabral dysfunction: minimum two-year follow-up. [miscellaneous article]. J Bone Joint Surg Br 91:16–23
70. Philippon MJ, Christensen JC, Wahoff MS (2009) Rehabilitation after arthroscopic repair of intra-articular disorders of the hip in a professional football athlete. J Sport Rehabil 18:118–134

Return to Play After Ankle Injuries

29

Frank G.J. Loeffen, Yoshiharu Shimozono, Gino M.M.J. Kerkhoffs, and John G. Kennedy

Contents

29.1 Introduction

Football is associated with high injury rates. Due to repetitive kicking and frequent changing in direction, the ankle is particularly vulnerable to injury. Historically, the ankle used to be the most common location of injury in professional football (around 30% of total injuries). However, more recent studies suggest a lower ankle injury rate, accounting for 10–15% of all

Frank G. J. Loeffen and Yoshiharu Shimozono contributed equally to this work.

F.G.J. Loeffen, M.D. (✉)
Gino M.M.J. Kerkhoffs, M.D., Ph.D.
Department of Orthopaedic Surgery, Academic Medical Center, Amsterdam, The Netherlands

Academic Center for Evidence-based Sports Medicine (ACES), Amsterdam, The Netherlands

Amsterdam Collaboration for Health and Safety in Sports (ACHSS), AMC/VUmc IOC Research Center, Amsterdam, The Netherlands
e-mail: fgjloeffen@gmail.com; g.m.kerkhoffs@amc.uva.nl

Y. Shimozono, M.D. • J.G. Kennedy, M.D., M.Ch., M.M.Sc., F.R.C.S.
Hospital for Special Surgery, 523 East 72nd Street, Suite 507, New York, NY, USA
e-mail: yshimozono13@gmail.com; kennedyj@hss.edu

V. Musahl et al. (eds.), *Return to Play in Football*, https://doi.org/10.1007/978-3-662-55713-6_29

injuries [25, 118]. Possible explanations of this declining trend include successful implantation of prevention strategies, stricter enforcement of existing rules or new rules and, possibly, different injury definitions [140]. As a recent long-term study in professional football reported an ankle injury rate of 1/1000 h [140], a professional 25-player squad will suffer around seven ankle injuries in each season. Increased ankle injury rates have been found in older players, dominant leg, during competition and later in each half of a match time [18]. The overall ankle reinjury rate in football is between 4% and 29% [18, 55, 140]. In terms of time loss, an average of 16–24 calendar days was missed per ankle injury [17, 18, 140, 145]. Severe injuries, i.e. more than 28 days absence, represent 10–17% of all ankle injuries in professional football [25, 140, 145].

29.2 Lateral Ligament Lesions

29.2.1 Introduction

Ankle sprains account for 67–72% of all football-related ankle injuries [18, 70, 97, 140, 145]. Most ankle sprains in football are caused by player contact, mainly tackling (54%) [145]. Foul play is involved in 40% of the match-related ankle sprains [140]. Football players with a previous ankle sprain are two to five times more likely to sustain a recurrent ankle sprain than players without previous ankle sprains [3, 70, 136]. Mean lay-off per ankle sprain in football is between 7 and 18 days [70, 140, 145]. A total of 83–89% of the ankle sprains required football players to miss 1 month or less [25, 140, 145], suggesting that it is the incidence rather than severity of ankle sprains that makes them problematic [145]. However, up to 40% of the patients in the general population report residual symptoms after standard treatment for an acute ankle sprain [28, 134], including chronic pain, recurrent instability and muscular weakness.

Injury to the lateral ligamentous complex represents 70–91% of all ankle sprains in football [24, 42, 70, 145]. This is partly explained by the natural tendency for the ankle to go into inversion and the relative weakness of the lateral ligaments. The ankle joint is stabilized laterally by three ligaments: the anterior talofibular ligament (ATFL), the calcaneofibular ligament (CFL) and the posterior talofibular ligament (PTFL). The most common mechanism of injury is inversion of the plantar-flexed foot. A video analysis of ankle sprains in football revealed two mechanisms that put the ankle in this vulnerable position: (1) impact by opponent on the medial aspect of the leg just before or at foot strike, resulting in a laterally directed force causing the player to land with the ankle in a vulnerable inverted position, and (2) forced plantar flexion when the injured player hits the opponent's foot when attempting to shoot or clear the ball [2]. As the ATFL is maximally stretched with inversion of the plantar-flexed foot and has the lowest tolerance to loads (approximately 150 N [71, 116]), it is the first and often only ligament to sustain injury. As a result, the ATFL is the most frequently injured ligament of the ankle (90–95% [70, 145]). When the mechanism of injury continues around the lateral aspect of the ankle, rupture of the ATFL is followed by damage to the CFL and finally to the PTFL. An MRI study showed that 41% of the patients with an ankle inversion trauma injured both the ATFL and CFL, whereas only 5% had damaged the PTFL [69]. Associated injuries include fractures, osteochondral lesions and damage to both the peroneus tendon and nerve.

29.2.2 Clinical Presentation

History taking and video footage are particularly useful in identifying the injured ligaments. It is important to distinguish a simple distortion from a (lateral) ligament rupture, since adequate treatment is associated with a better prognosis and time to return to play (RTP) [128, 130]. Ask for the ability to bear weight and the location of pain and swelling. Patients with lateral ligamentous rupture report more immediate swelling and are more frequently compelled to stop their activities, than those without a rupture [124].

All ligamentous and bony structures should be palpated for tenderness, including the whole length of the fibula and the base of the fifth metatarsal. If there is no pain on palpation of the ATFL, there is no lateral ligament rupture [128, 130]. The anterior drawer test evaluates ATFL laxity, whereas the talar tilt test aids in identifying CFL instability. If a haematoma is present, accompanied by pressure pain at palpation or a positive stress test or both, it is most likely that a (partial) lateral ligamentous rupture exists [128, 130]. However, manual stress test is less reliable in the acute phase, because of pain and swelling. Therefore, delayed physical examination (4–5 days) gives better diagnostic results and is considered the gold standard in the diagnosis of acute lateral ligament injury. The sensitivity to correctly diagnose an acute lateral ligament rupture during a delayed physical examination is 96 %, with a specificity of 84% [128, 130].

29.2.3 Diagnosis

The Ottawa ankle rules are an accurate instrument to rule out fractures of the injured ankle, with a sensitivity of almost 100% [5]. Stress radiographs are generally not indicated in the routine diagnosis of lateral ligament injury, as they are difficult to perform and will not change the treatment protocol.

Ultrasonography has been demonstrated to be an accurate investigation for ligamentous injury, but images may be difficult to interpret on retrospective review by other physicians. The sensitivity and specificity of ultrasonography for a lateral ligament rupture are 92% and 64%, respectively [130]. If ultrasonography is performed after an inconclusive delayed physical examination, sensitivity increases to 100% and specificity to 72% [130].

MRI is reliable in the diagnosis of lateral ligamentous ruptures and other associated injuries, including tendinous and syndesmotic tears, occult fractures and osteochondral lesions. The sensitivity and specificity of MRI for ATFL injuries are 92–100% and 100%, respectively [58, 90]. In comparison with arthroscopy, MR images correctly located the injured portion of the ATFL in 93%, whereas ultrasonography was able to identify 63% [90]. Overall, MRI is our imaging modality of choice for lateral ligament injury in the professional football player. There are no known studies on the value of MRI in monitoring recovery and RTP decisions of athletes with lateral ligament lesions, let alone football players.

29.2.4 Treatment and Rehabilitation

A grading system has been devised to aid in guiding the treatment of lateral ligament injuries [38, 59]. It incorporates anatomical damage with patient's symptoms and is only reliable with delayed physical examination. Grade I (mild) injuries include stretching of the ligaments. There is minor swelling and tenderness, little to no functional loss and no increased laxity. Grade II (moderate) injuries include partial tearing of the ligaments, with moderate pain, swelling and tenderness. There is a mild to moderate increase in laxity, some loss of motion and moderate functional disability. In grade III (severe) injuries, a complete rupture of the ligaments and the joint capsule is present with severe bruising, swelling and pain. There is major loss of function and an increased laxity. The patient is most frequently unable to bear weight. In clinical practice, only the difference between a simple sprain (grade I) and real instability (grade II or III) is relevant. The majority of acute grades I–III lateral ligament injuries can be managed by non-operative measures [94].

Treatment of lateral ligament injury is based upon the three stages of ligament healing: the inflammatory phase, the proliferation phase (up to 6 weeks to 3 months after trauma) and the remodelling or maturation phase (until 1 year post-injury). The initial treatment is directed towards avoiding or diminishing excess swelling and ongoing injury. This involves the RICE principle for the first days: rest, ice (cryotherapy), compression and elevation. The use of oral or topical nonsteroidal anti-inflammatory drugs (NSAID) leads to less pain without an increase in adverse events [126]. Manual mobilization of the ankle has limited added value and must be discouraged [67]. No effect was found for ultrasound therapy, laser therapy and electrotherapy [67]. Long-term immobilization (>2 weeks) leads to poorer outcomes than functional treatment [64, 94]. However, a short period of immobilization (max 10 days) in a below-knee cast or removable boot can be advantageous for severe lateral ligamentous injury, i.e. faster recovery when compared to compression bandage [73, 94].

During the proliferation phase, controlled stress on the injured ligament will promote proper collagen fibre orientation, whereas protection of inversion is important to prevent excess formation of weaker type III collagen. The use of an external ankle support is advocated (for longer than 8 weeks [52]). Elastic bandage is associated with a slower RTP and more instability than an ankle brace [65]. Although a recent study found no differences in outcome between tape, semi-rigid brace and a lace-up brace 6 months after treatment [127], most studies report superior results for protection with a brace [61, 94]. Since it is also more cost-effective and gives less skin irritation, the use of a (semi-rigid) brace in the proliferation phase is preferable. Exercise therapy combined with progressive weight bearing is an essential element of the functional treatment of lateral ligament injury [62]. Early active range of motion (ROM) exercises are essential, both passive and active. Strength deficits for the ankle evertors, invertors and plantar flexors have been reported following ankle injury [60]. Rehabilitation programmes should emphasize strengthening of all muscle groups using both eccentric and concentric exercises, followed by proprioceptive training and functional exercises. Activities in the last phase should progressively simulate the physical demands of football, including running and cutting drills. More detailed rehabilitation for acute lateral ligamentous injury can be found in several best evidence-based schedules [60, 102, 150], although none are specifically designed for football players.

The treatment of grade III lateral ligament injury remains controversial. Most reviews comparing surgical versus conservative treatment failed to demonstrate a superior approach [62, 94]. Therefore, functional treatment is preferred in most cases [62, 94]. However, surgical treatment may be beneficial on an individual basis in professional athletes [66]. The advantage of surgical repair is significantly less objective instability when compared to non-operative treatment [62]. Since increased objective instability is predictive for future ankle sprains [137] and RTP is not delayed after surgical treatment [66], acute repair should be considered in professional football players [66, 94, 124] (Fig. 29.1). The time of the season, athletes' expectations, sports-specific ankle load, individual history, stage of his or her career, time from trauma to diagnosis, collateral ankle joint damage and access to an expert orthopaedic surgeon are all features to take into account when considering an operative treatment in the professional football player [124]. When performing repair, a direct anatomical reconstruction of the ruptured lateral ligaments in a high-volume centre by an experienced surgeon is recommended [66, 124]. The rehabilitation regime after direct anatomic reconstruction is a lower-leg cast for 1–2 weeks, followed by 2–4 weeks in a walking boot. Then an active rehabilitation protocol with the use of an ankle support is advised, as recently described in an evidence-based guideline [93].

29.2.5 Return to Play and Prevention

After a lateral ligamentous injury, it is difficult to determine when a football player can RTP. Furthermore, residual disability of ankle sprains is often caused by inadequate rehabilitation and a potentially overly hurried RTP [102]. When assessing a player's ability to return, all functional limitations as a result of the injury must be restored, cardiovascular fitness should be equal to or greater than pre-injury status, and there should be no apprehension from the player or other members of the rehabilitation team about the player's safety. The RTP process itself will often be progressive as well. In determining a player's ability to progress to the next phase or RTP, objective data are required. Although self-

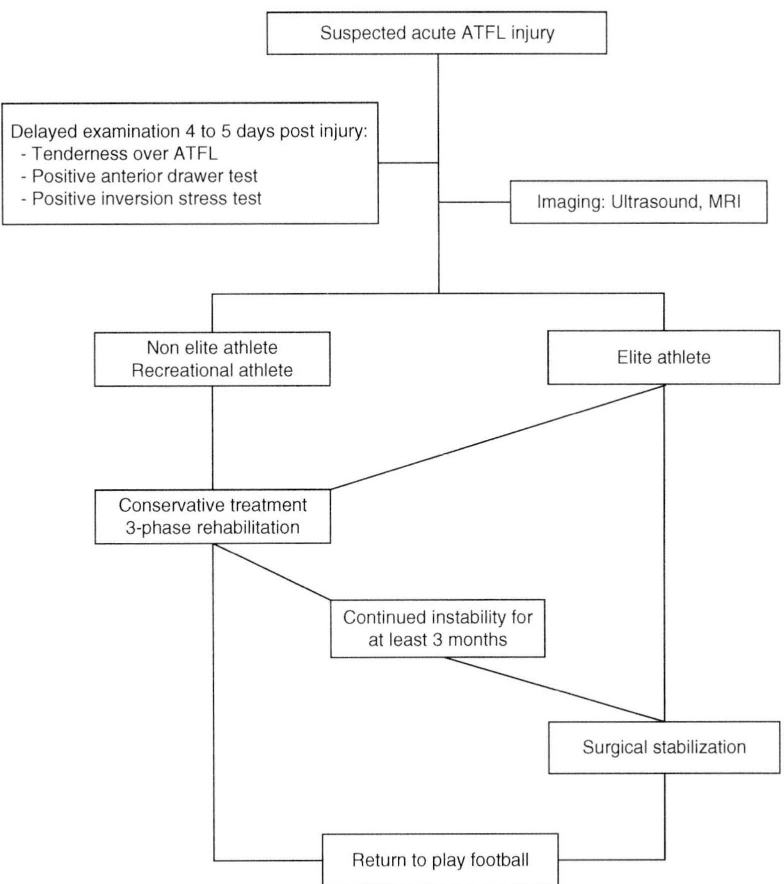

Fig. 29.1 Treatment algorithm for suspected injury of the ATFL (*Adapted from Ballal et al., 2016* [6])

reported ankle scoring systems are not validated for RTP decisions, they can be useful to evaluate the effectiveness of the rehabilitation protocol. For instance, the Foot and Ankle Disability Index (FADI) includes an optional 8-item sports subscale that is geared towards individuals returning to athletic activities [81]. Furthermore, the use of functional performance tests to assess the footballer's ability to perform sports-specific skills is considered helpful [60]. Tests can progress from relatively simple tasks such as the single-legged balance test [31] to more complex tests in different domains, such as the (modified) Star Excursion Balance Test (Fig. 29.2) [45], the Y Balance Test [95] and the agility *T*-test [92]. Dynamic balance tests are considered more accurate in assessing lower extremity function than static tests [103]. The outcomes of these tests should be evaluated throughout the rehabilitation process, thereby quantifying progress, and compared to pre-injury and contralateral scores. As several functional tests have been found to be predictive of ankle injuries in uninjured athletes [37, 83, 92, 96], the use of these tests in the RTP decision of football players with lateral ligamentous injury should be validated. A minimal score on functional test for RTP, e.g. 90% of pre-injury or contralateral ankle, has been advised [54] but warrants further research [60]. Baseline values of these functional tests should preferably be established before the start of the football season.

In summary, minimal criteria for a safe RTP following a lateral ligament injury should include full ROM, 90% of pre-injury score on both strength and functional performance tests and a normal and pain-free gait pattern when performing football-specific tasks, including cutting and running. The rehabilitation process should never abruptly be stopped after RTP, as deficits can erroneously be overlooked during the RTP

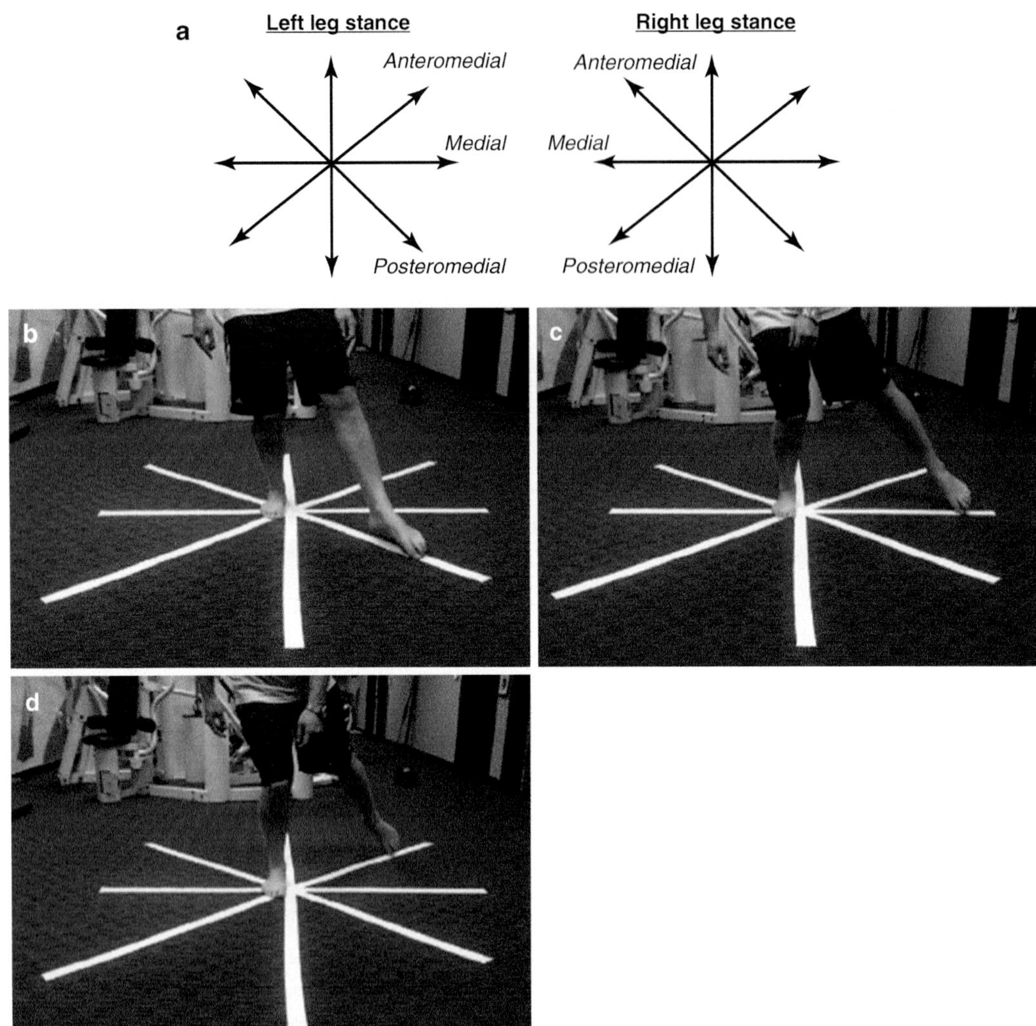

Fig. 29.2 (**a–d**) Modified Star Excursion Balance Test. The test has been simplified to include only three reach directions: anteromedial, medial and posteromedial (*Reprinted with permission from Richie et al., 2015* [103])

evaluation. Moreover, certain deficits may only be present after the player has been thoroughly fatigued. Continuing sports-specific rehabilitation will help to minimize this risk.

The time needed to RTP in lateral ligamentous injury depends on several factors, including severity of the injury, patient's ability and rehabilitation facilities available. Reported RTP in amateur and professional football players has been 7 days and 15 ± 19 days, respectively [70, 140]. There was no documentation on the severity of injuries. A case series of professional athletes who underwent surgical repair reported a median RTP of 77 days for isolated lateral ligamentous injuries and 105 days for those with concomitant injuries [93].

The most important risk factor for an ankle sprain is a previous ankle sprain. This is due to reduced proprioceptive function and reduced mechanical stability. There is good evidence from high-level studies that neuromuscular training, especially balance training (e.g. wobble board), is effective for the prevention of recurrent ankle sprains. It is controversial if neuromuscular training is beneficial in normal healthy ankles in preventing sprains [124], although the recently introduced FIFA 11 injury prevention programme decreased lower extremity injury risk in footballers by 24% [1].

There is consensus that external ankle support reduces the risk of recurrent ankle injury in previously injured athletes [65] (by approximately 70% [22]). These results were reproduced in football players [113, 118]. As ruptured ankle ligaments need at least 6 months to achieve full strength, prophylactic ankle brace should be worn for a minimum of 6 months after RTP [103]. It is unclear whether a brace is more effective than a tape [66]. Both have their advantages and disadvantages. Tape can lead to skin irritation and loses 40–50% of its effect after 15 min of vigorous exercise [29]. However, some football players tend to dislike braces because they do not seem to fit in the typical football shoes. Braces are reusable and readjustable, and minimal expertise is required for correct application. Contrary to popular belief, an external ankle support does not impede speed, agility and kicking accuracy in football players [91, 99]. A combination of both treatment modalities could be considered, especially in professional football players with recurrent ankle sprains.

Fact Box

- Delayed physical examination of the lateral ankle ligaments (4–5 days) gives better results than within 48 h.
- The majority of acute lateral ligament injuries can be treated conservatively with adequate rehabilitation.
- Surgery is considered in professional athletes with acute grade III injuries, as surgery provides lower incidence of chronic ankle instability than conservative treatment.
- RTP criteria should include strength and functional performance tests (e.g. 90% pre-injury score)

29.3 Medial Ligament Lesions

29.3.1 Introduction

The ankle joint is stabilized medially by the medial ligament complex (MLC), also known as the deltoid ligament. It consists of six adjacent bands [12, 85], either belonging to a superficial or deep layer. The superficial component is weaker than the deep part. The primary mechanism of isolated MLC injury is pronation or external rotation of the ankle. Such injuries commonly occur during an off-balanced landing on an uneven surface [46] or due to a lateral contact to the weight-bearing ankle [36]. Furthermore, MLC injury may be caused by severe supination and external rotation (SER) injuries. As the deltoid ligaments have a higher load to failure than the lateral ligaments [4], considerable forces are required to injure the MLC. Isolated MLC injury is rare, usually involves the superficial layer and has a good prognosis. Complete disruption of both the deep and superficial parts is almost always associated with other injury patterns, including syndesmotic injury, rotational ankle fractures and lateral ligament injury.

Injury to the MLC represents 10–16% of all ankle sprains in football [70, 140, 145]. The average lay-off per isolated MLC injury in professional football is 13.6 ± 15.4 days, with a reinjury rate of 11% [140]. However, medial ankle injuries tend to be more severe in nature than the more common lateral ankle sprains (because of associated injuries). Therefore, the recovery time is generally much longer [20].

29.3.2 Clinical Presentation

Signs of a MLC injury include medial soft-tissue swelling, often ecchymosis and tenderness over the course of the ligament. In contrast to lateral ligament injury, one or a combination of these findings has a relatively low predictive value for MLC rupture [125]. If MLC injury is suspected, it is important to evaluate the ankle for associated injuries, including the entire fibula and the tibiofibular joint. Several stress tests have been described to evaluate the integrity of the MLC [7], e.g. valgus stress test and external rotation stress test, but these tests generally lack external validity. Since swelling and pain hinder stress tests, delayed examination might be beneficial.

29.3.3 Diagnosis

The Ottawa ankle rules also apply to medial sprains. In the case of a disrupted syndesmosis and MLC, the distance between the medial talus and the medial malleolus on the mortise view will be widened. A medial clear space (MCS) of 4 and 5 mm on the mortise view has a false-positive rate for MLC rupture of 53.6% and 26.9%, respectively [110]. However, isolated MLC rupture does not cause widening of the MCS on static radiographs, because the lateral malleolus holds the talus in position. Furthermore, SER fractures of the ankle (80% of all ankle injuries) may present with a MLC rupture that is not apparent on the initial radiographs. In other words, an isolated lateral malleolar fracture with an intact ankle mortise on the static radiographs does not exclude MLC injury. Historically, external rotation stress radiographs were used to detect occult MLC injuries. However, patients generally experience pain during these examinations, leading to possible suboptimal radiographs. As an alternative, the gravity stress test was developed, showing at least equivalent results [35, 109]. A MCS of ≥5 mm on the gravity stress radiographs is accepted to represent a deep MLC rupture [119]. More recently, the use of delayed weight-bearing radiographs has been advocated [142]. Patients with an isolated lateral malleolar fracture and an intact mortise on the initial radiographs (with medial sided symptoms and/or signs) underwent weight-bearing radiographs 1 week after the injury. Compared to both rotation and gravity stress test, it resulted in a decreased false-positive rate and good clinical outcome [41, 48, 50, 142].

MRI has a high sensitivity and specificity for confirmation of injury to both the superficial and deep layers of the MLC [82]. It may especially be helpful for individual cases in which doubt about joint stability and soft-tissue integrity exists [47, 119]. Furthermore, it provides information about possible concomitant pathology [106] and is, therefore, the authors' imaging technique of choice in the (professional) football player.

Ultrasonography might represent an alternative to MRI for assessing MLC injury, although data are scarce. When used in SER ankle fractures, both a 100% sensitivity and specificity for MLC rupture were reported [15, 43]. A recent study also found 100% sensitivity for complete MLC rupture, but only 50% of the partial rupture were correctly identified by ultrasonography [75].

29.3.4 Treatment and Rehabilitation

There is little evidence to guide the management of deltoid injuries without a fracture, let alone in football. Isolated superficial or partial MLC injuries with no instability are mostly treated conservatively. The first step of treatment is the RICE principle. Further treatment consists of 4–6 weeks in a cast or brace, sometimes preceded by a non-weight-bearing (NWB) period of 5–7 days [80, 82]. It should be combined with a progressive functional rehabilitation programme.

The treatment of complete rupture of both the deep and superficial components of the MLC remains controversial [82]. These are almost always associated with other injuries that may require surgical intervention, especially fractures. It is beyond the scope of this book to provide a detailed discussion on these surgical indications, but inaccurate assessment of MLC injury could predispose to early posttraumatic osteoarthritis [119]. In general, the decision between surgically and conservatively treating the acute MLC injury in a combination injury will depend on the severity of the combined lateral ligament, syndesmotic and osseous injuries and resultant instability. The authors' preference for ankle fractures with additional MLC injury in professional football players involves arthroscopic inspection (and treat additional osteochondral pathology if present), open reduction internal fixation and, if necessary after inspection or stress exams, open MLC repair and syndesmotic fixation [80, 82]. The postoperative protocol varies, depending on the severity of the associated injuries, but generally implies a minimum of 6 weeks NWB in a cast or boot. A removable cast or boot allows for early ROM exercises.

29.3.5 Return to Play and Prevention

RTP for MLC injury generally takes longer as would be predicted were the injury on the lateral side. In the case of an isolated superficial MLC injury, return to full weight bearing (FWB) and light training is expected after 6–8 weeks [82]. However, faster RTP is described in professional football: 2–4 weeks [140]. Potential explanations for this discrepancy include supervision by a multidisciplinary sports medicine team, availability of rehabilitation facilities (e.g. aquatic therapy or antigravity treadmills) and, possibly, milder injury in professional athletes due to prophylactic bracing or neuromuscular training. The time to RTP in MLC injury with additional fracture varies, depending on the severity of associated injuries [21]. In the case of a bimalleolar equivalent fracture with deltoid repair, RTP can be expected as early as 8–10 weeks after stabilization [57]. Predictors of RTP after operative fixation of an unstable ankle fracture at 1 year include younger age, male gender, no or mild systemic disease and a less severe ankle fracture [19].

The ability to RTP in medial ligamentous injury requires a pain-free full ROM with no swelling and symptoms on stress testing. Furthermore, functional performance tests (Sect. 29.2.5) can guide the rehabilitation process and help in making the final RTP decision.

All preventive studies on ankle sprains only involve lateral ankle sprains. As ankle support significantly reduces ROM for both inversion and eversion [117], the use of a brace or tape in the prevention of MLC reinjury is presumably beneficial as well. Neuromuscular training in the prevention of recurrent MLC injury is also potentially helpful but warrants further research.

Fact Box

- Isolated MLC injuries are rare.
- Arthroscopy to identify MLC injury and treat additional osteochondral pathology is advocated for high-level athletes suffering a complete deep and superficial MLC injury.
- RTP in isolated MLC injuries is expected after 6–8 weeks.

29.4 Syndesmotic Ligament Lesions

29.4.1 Introduction

Although the syndesmosis is technically a joint, the term syndesmotic injury is used to describe injury of the syndesmotic ligaments. It is often referred to as a high ankle sprain. The syndesmotic ligament complex consists of the anterior inferior tibiofibular ligament (AITFL), the posterior inferior tibiofibular ligament (PITFL) and the interosseous ligament (IOL). It ensures the stability between distal tibia and fibula, and it resists the axial, rotational and translation forces which tend to distend the distal tibia and fibula.

The most accepted mechanism of injury for syndesmotic ankle sprains is a forceful external rotation of the foot and ankle with the ankle in dorsiflexion and the foot pronated [148]. As the talus rotates in the mortise, the fibula rotates externally and moves posteriorly and laterally, separating the distal tibia and fibula, sequentially tearing the AITFL (weakest ligament) and deep MLC or causing a malleolar fracture, the IOL and finally the PITFL [9, 147]. Ruptures of the syndesmosis are therefore rarely isolated injuries but generally occur in association with fractures of either the fibula or the posterior and medial malleoli. Combined deltoid and syndesmosis injury critically disrupts talar stability [148]. The amount of force and how long it is applied will determine how proximal the syndesmotic and interosseous injury extends, sometimes resulting in a proximal fibula fracture (Maisonneuve fracture) [144]. Another injury mechanism for syndesmotic ankle sprains is hyperdorsiflexion. Forced dorsiflexion of the ankle causes the wider anterior talus to act as a wedge that can cause injury to the syndesmotic ligaments.

Injury to the syndesmotic ligaments occurs in 3–6% of footballers with an ankle sprain [70, 145]. It is likely that this is an underestimate, since 20% of athletes suffering an acute ankle sprain had evidence of syndesmotic injury on MRI [104]. Football has a relatively high incidence rate of syndesmotic ankle sprains (31 per 100,000 athletic exposures) [141]. Male sex, higher level of competition and a planovalgus foot alignment are risk factors for syndesmotic injury in athletes [141, 144]. Syndesmotic involvement following lateral ligamentous injury was the most predictive factor of chronic ankle dysfunction at 6 months post-injury [33]. Missed and chronically unstable syndesmotic injuries may to lead to early osteoarthritis [144].

29.4.2 Clinical Presentation

Patients with syndesmotic injury may complain of the inability to bear weight, swelling, pain during the push-off phase of gait and pain anteriorly between distal tibia and fibula, as well as posteromedially at the level of the ankle joint [49]. Inspection may reveal oedema and ecchymoses around the lateral aspect of the ankle. ROM is often limited with an empty or painful end feel at terminal dorsiflexion [87]. Anterior tenderness between tibia and fibula should be evaluated; there is a significant correlation between how far this tenderness extends up the leg and injury severity and time to RTP [89]. Local tenderness is, however, not specific in the acute setting, as 40% of the patients with an ATFL disruption reported pain in the area of the AITFL, while arthroscopy showed no syndesmotic injury [130].

Numerous special tests are used to detect syndesmotic injury. The external rotation test and the squeeze test are the most commonly described tests, but the Cotton test and the fibular translation test are also widely used. A systematic review on eight different tests reported a low diagnostic accuracy of all tests [115]. As no single test was sufficient to identify ankle syndesmosis injury with certainty, the authors speculated that a combination of tests and inclusion of other elements, such as symptoms and the patient's history, might further assist in the diagnosis [115]. The recommended clinical tests in the most recent consensus statement on isolated syndesmotic injuries include tenderness on palpation over the AITFL and PITFL, the fibular translation test and the Cotton test [129]. If clinical tests raise suspicion of a syndesmotic injury, additional imaging should be performed. One study examined the ability of syndesmotic tests to predict recovery time; athletes with a positive test on either the external rotation test or the dorsiflexion-compression test were significantly more likely to have a delayed RTP.

29.4.3 Diagnosis

Initial radiographs are recommended to assess bony integrity and stability of the ankle mortise. If there is a clinical or radiographical suspicion of a Maisonneuve fracture, radiographs with full-length views of the lower leg are needed. The tibiofibular clear space, defined as the distance between the medial border of the fibula and the lateral border of the posterior tibia, provides the most reliable radiographic parameter of diastasis (e.g. syndesmotic injury) [40]. It should not exceed 6 mm in both the AP and mortise views [40]. Biomechanical studies suggest that stress radiographs probably offer little advantage over plain views in assessing syndesmotic stability [10, 129]. Recently, bilateral standing CT is emerging as an alternative diagnostic stress view, although prospective comparatively controlled data is lacking [139].

MRI effectively displays the structures of the syndesmosis and possible associated injuries and is the authors' investigation of choice for suspected syndesmotic ligament injury [129]. MRI showed a sensitivity of 100% and a specificity of 93% for AITFL injuries and sensitivity and specificity of 100% for PITFL tears [120]. However, there is no association between the extent of syndesmotic injury on MRI and the time to RTP [51]. A high prevalence of associated injuries was found in a retrospective MRI study, including osteochondral lesions (28%), bone contusions (24%) and osteoarthritis (10%) [13].

Dynamic ultrasound examination showed a 66–100% sensitivity and 91–100% specificity for AITFL rupture [84, 86]. It has the disadvantage that it lacks the ability to detect associated injuries and it is investigator dependent [129]. The use of ultrasonography for diagnosing isolated syndesmotic injury is not recommended in the latest consensus statement [129].

29.4.4 Treatment and Rehabilitation

Treatment is based on the severity of the syndesmotic injury: grade I represents a mild sprain to the AITFL without instability; grade II involves a tear of the AITFL and a partial tear of the IOL with some instability; and grade III represents definite instability with complete rupturing of all the syndesmotic ligaments [33].

Grade I injuries without instability and only partial disruption of the AITFL are treated with non-surgical management [82]. A three-phase approach is recommended: an acute phase, a subacute phase and an advanced training phase. In the acute phase, management entails immediate RICE. If the patient has significant pain, immobilization in a NWB cast or boot using crutches for 2–3 weeks can be considered [129]. Partial weight bearing (PWB) commences when pain complaints have subsided or approximately 3 weeks post-injury as tolerated. Elite athletes, however, might show quicker recovery: 3–5 days NWB in a boot, followed by 7–10 days of weight bearing [53]. ROM and light proprioception exercises are started early, although end-range dorsiflexion should be limited in the early stage of rehabilitation to prevent excess stress on the injured distal tibiofibular joint, for instance, by the use of tape or altered exercise positions [87]. Patients are progressed to the subacute phase of treatment when pain and oedema are controlled and the patient can walk with a minimally antalgic gait on various surfaces. It consists of progressive mobilization, strengthening in the pain-free ROM and FWB. Progression to the advanced training phase is based on the ability to jog and hop repetitively without pain [143]. In this last phase, the athlete is prepared for a safe RTP. This includes more advanced neuromuscular, agility drills and sports-specific tasks, such as dribbling in football [144]. Exercises begin slow, with movement in a single direction, and progressively become more quick, intense and dynamic. A (stirrup) brace or tape is frequently used to support the ankle joint.

Treatment of grade II injuries depends on stability [129]. Recreational football players with a competent PITFL and MLC without diastasis can be treated nonoperatively with good results [53]. Conservative treatment consists of a NWB cast for 6–8 weeks. The athlete is then transitioned to progressive weight bearing in a walking cast and then eventually to a soft ankle brace. A recent study in athletes with a clinically stable syndesmosis, however, showed good results with only 10 days of NWB and a minimum of 3 weeks weight bearing in a walking boot [14]. This study also found that a positive squeeze test and injury to the ATFL and MLC are important factors in differentiating stable (grade IIa) from dynamically unstable grade II injuries (grade IIb). Rehabilitation of grade IIa injuries is commenced as described above. For a high-level football player with a grade II injury and clinical or radiological suspicion of dynamic instability (type IIb) (Fig. 29.3), an examination under anaesthesia and arthroscopic visualization of the syndesmosis is recommended [53, 68]. Dynamic diastasis of 2 mm or more warrants fixation [82]. Early anatomic reduction and fixation lead to a potential quicker RTP in comparison with non-surgical treatment [57].

Grade III injuries are uncommon in (professional) football, inherently unstable and often associated with other injuries. Operative fixation is necessary to maintain anatomic reduction of the mortise. Screws or suture buttons (Fig. 29.4)

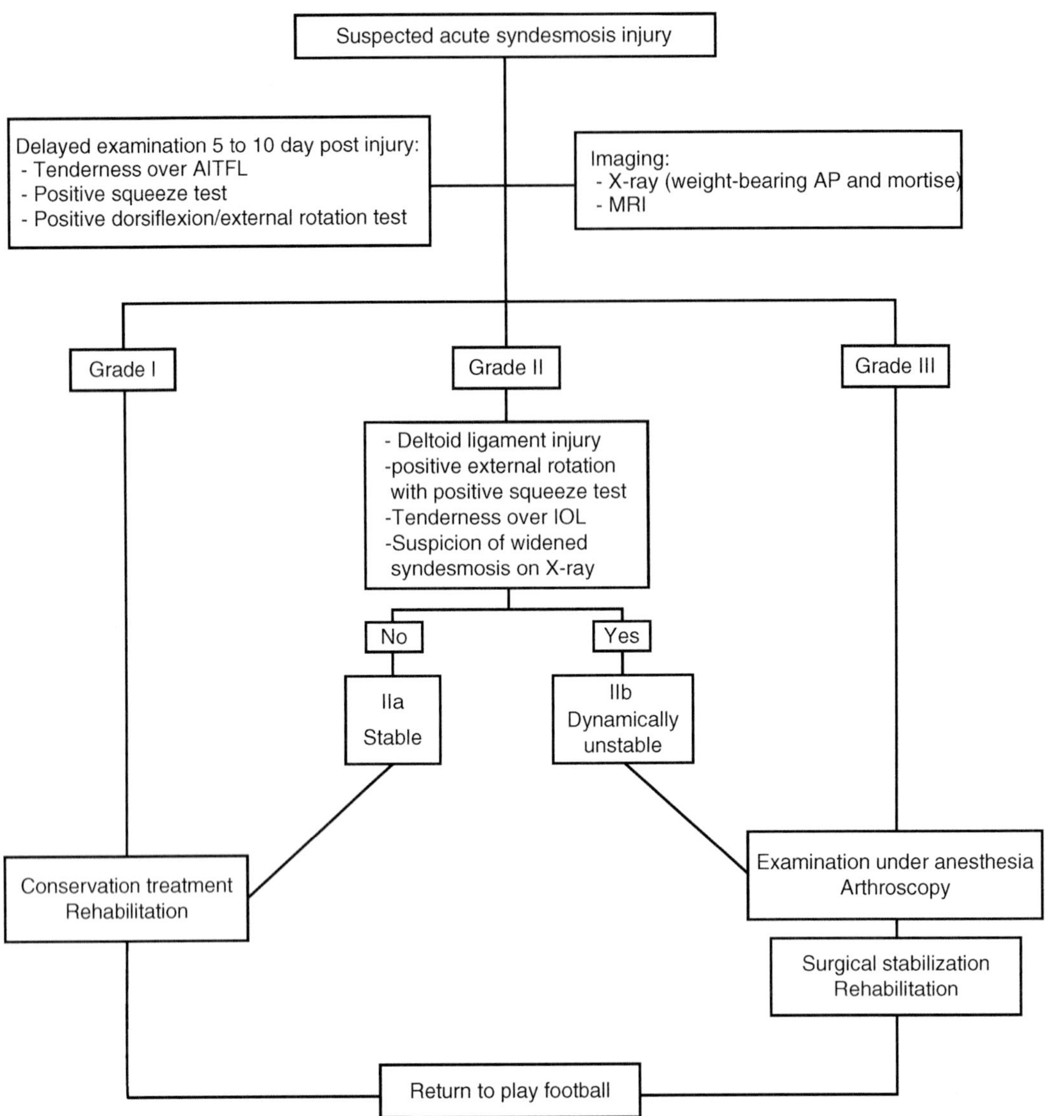

Fig. 29.3 Treatment algorithm for suspected injury of the syndesmosis (*Adapted from Ballal et al., 2016* [6])

are used to stabilize the syndesmosis. Outcomes are similar, but the use of suture button devices might lead to a quicker RTP and a lower rate of implant removal [108, 129]. Arthroscopic visualization can identify and address any additional intra-articular pathology. Postoperatively, the ankle is treated in a NWB splint for 10–14 days, followed by early ROM exercises with PWB at 3–4 weeks postoperative. FWB is commenced at 4 weeks as tolerated with continuation of strength and proprioception training.

Syndesmotic ruptures are commonly associated with ankle fractures. After reduction and fixation of the malleolar fractures and/or associated ligaments, intraoperative testing of the syndesmotic stability should be performed. The Hook or Cotton test is regarded as the most reliable intraoperative stress tests [123]. Arthroscopy can aid in the diagnosis of syndesmotic injury and possibly help in determining the stability of the syndesmosis [14], although a ruptured AITFL does not automatically mean instability.

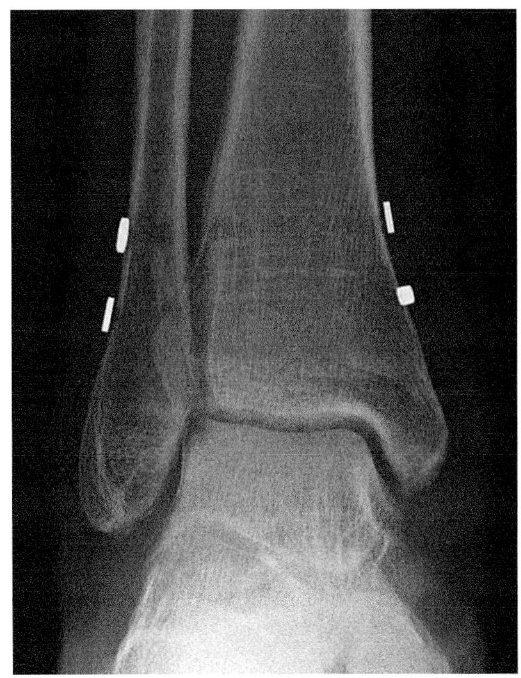

Fig. 29.4 Postoperative radiograph of ankle following two TightRopes® fixation

Whenever in doubt about syndesmotic instability, stabilization should be performed, because of the problems caused by chronic syndesmotic instability [123].

29.4.5 Return to Play and Prevention

Athletes who sustain an associated syndesmotic injury take twice as long to RTP compared to those who sustain an isolated lateral ligament injury [146]. This finding was reconfirmed in professional football players: mean lay-off of 43 ± 33 days for syndesmotic injury versus 15 ± 19 days for lateral ligament injury [140].

RTP in grade I injuries is usually at 6–8 weeks post-injury. A RTP prediction formula with a 95% confidence interval for athletes with syndesmotic injury, without a fracture or frank diastasis, was developed: time to RTP equals 5 + (0.93 × [tenderness length in centimetres]) ± 3.72 days [89].

Professional athletes with stable isolated grade II syndesmotic injuries are reported to RTP at a mean of 45 days, compared with 64 days for those with unstable grade II injuries [14]. All athletes returned to the same level of professional sports. Furthermore, athletes with injury to both the AITFL and deltoid ligament took longer to RTP than those with an AITFL injury alone, and IOL injury on MRI and PITFL injury on MRI were both independently associated with a delay in RTP [14].

RTP in surgically treated grade III injuries is between 10 and 14 weeks post-injury [53, 144], although RTP as early as 6 weeks has been described [122]. When comparing surgically treated grade III syndesmotic injuries with conservative treatment, there is little long-term difference in symptoms and athletic performance. However, RTP in the surgically treated athletes was on average 3 weeks quicker. As RTP for professional football players is critical, a more aggressive surgical treatment is recommended. To enhance the outcomes in non-operative syndesmotic injury, two studies evaluated the use of ultrasound-guided platelet-rich plasma (PRP) injection in the AITFL in athletes suffering a grade III syndesmotic injury [74, 105]. Athletes receiving PRP injections returned to play significantly sooner (21 days and 19 days, respectively) and also had less pain than controls. However, further study is warranted for this potential treatment before it can be recommended as part of routine management options [139].

RTP in syndesmotic injury is permitted when able to single-leg hop for 30 s without significant pain [82]. Furthermore, patients should be able to perform football-specific tasks at game speed with good movement quality and little to no pain or instability [143]. Another study defined RTP criteria for syndesmotic injury as follows: comfort with push-off and cutting manoeuvres, 80–90% symmetry in single-leg broad jumps and normal FADI scores. To our knowledge, there are no specific studies on prevention of syndesmotic reinjury. Although it might be assumed that neuromuscular bracing and/or taping is beneficial, injury mechanisms differ, and further investigation is required to increase our understanding of syndesmotic injuries and improve treatment and prevention of this significant injury [144].

Fact Box

- Syndesmotic injury generally occurs in association with other osteoligamentous injuries, especially fractures.
- Stable syndesmotic injuries (grades I and IIa) should be treated conservatively, whereas unstable injuries (grades IIb and III) warrant surgical fixation.
- RTP is generally prolonged in syndesmotic injury and allowed when able to single-leg hop for 30 s.

29.5 Osteochondral Defects

29.5.1 Introduction

An osteochondral defect (OCD) is a lesion involving the articular cartilage and its subchondral bone. An OCD is mostly caused by a single or repetitive trauma. Non-traumatic aetiologic factors have been described as well ("osteochondritis dissecans") [101]. OCDs can either heal and remain asymptomatic, stabilize or progress to subchondral bone cysts.

Ankle sprains are considered the most common cause of ankle OCDs. During an ankle sprain, the talus twists inside the ankle mortise, and the cartilage linings of distal tibia and talar dome are forcefully pushed upon each other. The degree of injury depends on the force exerted and on the range of abnormal motion. The impact may lead to subchondral bruising and subsequent softening of the cartilage, to a crack and subsequent cyst formation or to the shearing off of a chondral or osteochondral fragment. Most OCDs are located on the talar dome, especially on the anterolateral and posteromedial side [101]. Medial talar lesions are caused by an inversion of the foot and a plantar-flexed ankle, whereas lateral talar lesions are caused by eversion of the foot with the ankle in dorsal flexion. Medial talar OCDs are not only more common (62% vs. 34%) but are larger and deeper than lateral lesions [26].

The reported incidence of OCDs varies widely, both in acute ankle sprains (5–73% [76, 77, 121]) and chronic ankle instability (7–41% [11, 121]). There are no studies on the incidence and severity of OCDs in football. Early and accurate diagnosis of OCDs of the talus is important because optimal ankle joint function requires talar integrity. However, both clinical and radiological recognitions of an OCD can be difficult, potentially leading to suboptimal treatment.

29.5.2 Clinical Presentation

Symptoms of an acute OCD are often unrecognized, as the swelling and pain from the ligament injury prevail. If these symptoms persist 4–6 weeks post-injury, the possibility of an OCD should be considered [101]. Patients generally present with deep ankle pain on weight bearing. Lateral OCDs in general cause more symptoms than medial ones [131]. Reactive swelling and stiffness can be present, but the absence of swelling does not rule out an OCD. Locking and catching are symptoms of a displaced fragment, although this is less common [78]. Most patients demonstrate a normal ROM. Recognizable tenderness is typically not present, as most OCDs are not reachable by palpation, but can be present in the case of synovitis.

29.5.3 Diagnosis

If an OCD is suspected, plain radiographs should be taken. A heel-rise view with the ankle in a plantar-flexed position may be helpful in detecting a posteromedial or posterolateral defect [138]. Displaced or large OCDs are likely to be detected on initial radiographs. More often, no abnormalities are found on the primary radiographs. By repeating the radiographs in a later stage, the defect sometimes becomes visible [149]. A combination of medical history, physical examination and radiographs results in a sensitivity of 59% and a specificity of 91% [138].

CT scans provide a more detailed visualization of the lesion. It is useful in determining the size, location, shape and degree of displacement of osteochondral fragments. Furthermore, a CT provides information about possible associated cysts. CT is often invaluable in preoperative planning and is our imaging modality of choice in OCDs. The sensitivity and specificity of CT to detect an OCD are 81% and 99%, respectively [138].

MRI offers the advantage of visualizing the articular cartilage and subchondral bone, as well as oedema and other associated soft-tissue injuries. Nevertheless, CT has proven to be as valuable as MRI in diagnosing an OCD [138]. Moreover, the true extent of the OCD may be obscured by concomitant bone marrow oedema [72].

29.5.4 Treatment and Rehabilitation

Several classification systems for ankle OCDs exist. Historically, a staging system based on plain radiographs was used [8]. In grade I, there is local compression of the cartilage and subchondral bone, and usually there are no radiographic findings. In grade II, there is avulsion or partial detachment of the osteochondral fragment, but the main part is still attached to the talus. In grade III, there is complete avulsion of an osteochondral fragment without any displacement. In grade IV, the osteochondral fragment is completely detached and displaced inside the ankle joint. Later, grade V was added, which included subchondral cysts [78]. More recent classifications systems are based on CT, MRI and arthroscopic findings [16, 27, 44, 98]. The use of these classification systems is questionable, since none of the systems are sufficient to direct the choice of treatment [138].

Conservative treatment should be considered for nondisplaced OCDs, as well as for asymptomatic or mild symptomatic lesions [79, 101]. It consists of rest and/or limited (athletic) activities, sometimes by cast immobilization for 3 weeks up to 4 months [138], NSAIDs and protected weight bearing [39]. The aim is to unload the damaged cartilage, so oedema can be resolved and necrosis is prevented [101]. Systematic reviews on conservative treatment of talar OCDs showed a success rate of only 45–56% [138, 149]. These low overall success rates are mostly due to the avascular nature of the hyaline cartilage, which limit the healing potential of the articular surface [79].

Operative treatment is indicated in the acute setting when the lesion is displaced and in the more chronic setting when conservative treatment fails to improve patient symptoms. A wide variety of surgical techniques has been described [39]. It generally involves repair or replacement of the damaged OCD. The specific operative techniques utilized vary based on symptomatology, size and location of the defect and whether a primary or secondary OCD. Current literature suggests that arthroscopic bone marrow stimulation (BMS) via drilling or microfracture is the preferred treatment for primary talar lesions up to 15 mm in diameter [39]. However, a recent systematic review suggested that BMS may be best reserved for lesions of <107 mm^2 in area or 10 mm in diameter [100]. Overall, short- and midterm results of BMS of small isolated talar OCDs are generally good [23, 79]. Recent studies have attempted to augment OCD healing by injecting PRP or hyaluronic acid as an adjunct to arthroscopic microfracture [56, 112]. Although functional improvement has been reported following injection, further double-blinded evaluations in greater numbers are necessary [79].

For larger or secondary OCDs, autologous osteochondral transplantation (AOT) techniques are used [39]. Autologous osteochondral grafts are most commonly harvested from the ipsilateral knee and implanted as single or multiple plugs (mosaicplasty). The primary concern with osteochondral autografts is donor-site morbidity, which is seen in up to 12% of the cases [79, 149]. This is especially relevant for professional football players, since knee pain may prevent the patient from returning to play [32]. AOT provides good functional outcomes in the short- and medium term [34]. Some larger primary fragments are best treated with reduction and fixation [63]. Osteochondral allograft transplantation and, more recently, cell-based techniques, such as autologous chondrocyte implantation, have been used for the treatment of large OCDs. Well-designed clinical trials of high methodological quality are, however, lacking, and these techniques should only be used in carefully considered patients in whom other primary techniques have failed previously [63]. The course of rehabilitation in larger or secondary lesions depends on the specific surgical technique but generally involves longer periods of PWB. In the case of fixation or procedures involving malleolar osteotomy, at least 4–6 weeks of NWB is advised [88]. Prolonged periods of immobilization lead to muscle atrophy and joint stiffness, so training for ROM and strength is especially important in the early phase of rehabilitation. Further training of proprioception and later sports-specific skills is then commenced.

29.5.5 Return to Play and Prevention

For arthroscopic BMS, a four-level activity rehabilitation scheme has been proposed (Fig. 29.5) [132], derived from rehabilitation after Achilles tendon rupture. The first level of activity phase is a gradual return to normal walking. Early training for ROM is important in this phase. Allowing FWB depends on the size and location of the defect; a lesion up to 1 cm is allowed to progress to FWB within 2–4 weeks, whereas larger and anteriorly located lesions require up to 6 weeks of PWB [132]. The second level of activity phase involves progression from walking to running on even ground. This is usually permitted between 12 and 16 weeks postoperatively. Proprioception should be optimized, whereas lower-leg left/right strength differences should be <12%. After increased activity, pain and swelling should have ceased after 24 h. The third level of activity phase is a return to noncontact activities. This is usually possible between 20 and 24 weeks. Further training of sports-specific skills is then commenced. Some pain may occur after increased activity but should be absent after 24 h. The fourth and final level activity phase involves return to contact sports, which is permitted from 24 weeks and up. Final training for speed, muscle strength and endurance should enable running on uneven ground, generating explosive force, changing direction and other sports-specific movements.

An average RTP of 15 ± 4 weeks in athletes treated with BMS has, however, been reported [107]. With regard to football players after BMS, a 94% RTP is described [111], although studies in a mixed population generally report lower rates (63–79%) [63, 133]. Prognostic factors for early RTP have been established as younger age, lower body mass index, smaller OCD size and coordinated physical therapy [114].

The RTP in athletes treated with autologous bone grafts is significantly longer than that of the BMS group (19.6 ± 5.9 weeks) [107]. Ninety percent of professional athletes and 87% of recreational athletes were able to return to pre-injury activity levels [30]. Additional medial malleolar osteotomy only resulted in 2 weeks extra RTP delay. Medial malleolar osteotomy is, however,

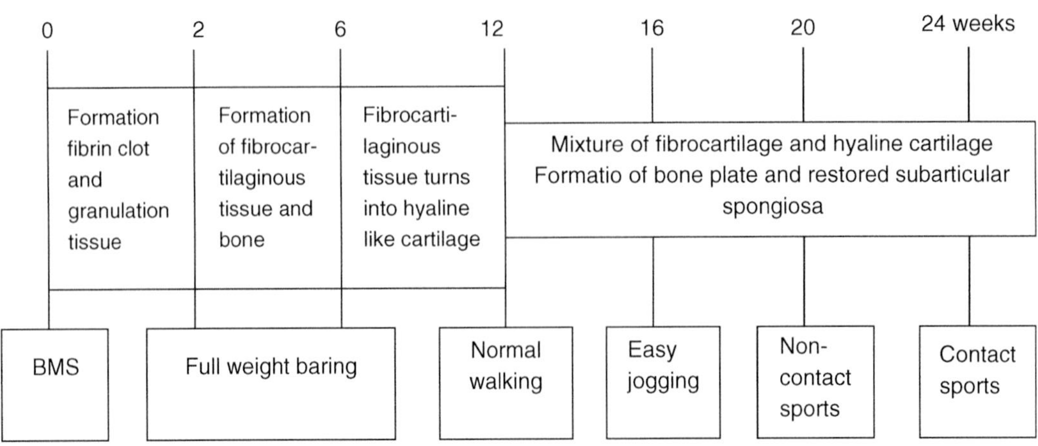

Fig. 29.5 Timetable recovery after BMS (*Reprinted with permission from Gerards R et al., 2014* [32])

not recommended in professional football players, since it could lead to persisting ankle stiffness, malunion, non-union and degenerative changes due to the osteotomy [32]. In a case series of athletes who underwent autologous bone grafting, 90% of the athletes were still competing at a mean follow-up of 6 years [30]. A recently introduced arthroscopic "one-step" bone marrow-derived cell transplantation technique showed a RTP of 6.6 ± 4.8 months post-injury. All patients were able to return to activity, and 73% were able to resume sports at pre-injury level [135].

As sprains are the major cause of OCDs, ankle injury prevention should be stressed. Multiple ankle sprains should especially be avoided, since repetitive micro damage can accumulate in macroscopic failure. Various modes of prevention have been discussed in the preceding chapters, including neuromuscular training and the use of tape or braces.

Fact Box

- Ankle sprains are considered the most common cause of OCDs.
- Displaced or chronic symptomatic OCDs should be treated surgically: <10–15 mm with BMS and larger or secondary OCDs with autologous grafts or fixation.
- Approximately 90% of professional football players can RTP in both BMS and autologous graft procedures.

Take-Home Message

Ankle injuries are common in modern football. Adequate examination and appropriate imaging are necessary to identify ankle injuries, including potential associated pathology. Most (ligamentous) ankle injuries in football can be treated conservatively. However, early surgical fixation is sometimes indicated and could lead to an earlier RTP. Rehabilitation should be performed according to the biological phases of healing. Full ROM, normal running pattern without pain and 90% pre-injury score on both strength and functional performance tests are minimal requirements for RTP.

Top Five Evidence Based References

Calder JD, Bamford R, Petrie A, McCollum GA (2016) Stable versus unstable grade ii high ankle sprains: a prospective study predicting the need for surgical stabilization and time to return to sports. Arthroscopy 32(4):634–642

Hannon CP, Smyth NA, Murawski CD, Savage-Elliott I, Deyer TW, Calder JD et al (2014) Osteochondral lesions of the talus: aspects of current management. Bone Joint J 96(2):164–171

McCollum GA, van den Bekerom MP, Kerkhoffs GM, Calder JD, van Dijk CN (2013) Syndesmosis and deltoid ligament injuries in the athlete. Knee Surg Sports Traumatol Arthrosc 21(6):1328–1337

van den Bekerom MP, Kerkhoffs GM, McCollum GA, Calder JD, van Dijk CN (2013) Management of acute lateral ankle ligament injury in the athlete. Knee Surg Sports Traumatol Arthrosc 21(6):1390–1395

Waldén M, Hägglund M, Ekstrand J (2013) Time-trends and circumstances surrounding ankle injuries in men's professional football: an 11-year follow-up of the UEFA Champions League injury study. Br J Sports Med 47(12):748–753

References

1. Al Attar WS, Soomro N, Pappas E, Sinclair PJ, Sanders RH (2016) How effective are F-MARC injury prevention programs for soccer players? A systematic review and meta-analysis. Sports Med 46(2):205–217
2. Andersen TE, Floerenes TW, Arnason A, Bahr R (2004) Video analysis of the mechanisms for ankle injuries in football. Am J Sports Med 32(1 Suppl):69S–79S
3. Arnason A, Sigurdsson SB, Gudmundsson A, Holme I, Engebretsen L, Bahr R (2000) Risk factors for injuries in football. Am J Sports Med 32(1 Suppl):5S–16S
4. Attarian DE, McCrackin HJ, DeVito DP, McElhaney JH, Garrett WE Jr (1985) Biomechanical characteristics of human ankle ligaments. Foot Ankle 6(2):54–58
5. Bachmann LM, Kolb E, Koller MT, Steurer J, ter Riet G (2003) Accuracy of Ottawa ankle rules to exclude fractures of the ankle and mid-foot: systematic review. BMJ 326(7386):417
6. Ballal MS, Pearce CJ, Calder JD (2016) Management of sports injuries of the foot and ankle: an update. Bone Joint J 98-B(7):874–883

7. Beals TC, Crim J, Nickisch F (2010) Deltoid ligament injuries in athletes: techniques of repair and reconstruction. Oper Tech Sports Med 18(1):11–17
8. Berndt AL, Harty M (1959) Transchondral fractures (osteochondritis dissecans) of the talus. J Bone Joint Surg Am 41(6):988–1020
9. Beumer A, Valstar ER, Garling EH, Niesing R, Ginai AZ, Ranstam J et al (2006) Effects of ligament sectioning on the kinematics of the distal tibiofibular syndesmosis. Acta Orthop 77(3):531–540
10. Beumer A, Valstar ER, Garling EH, van Leeuwen WJ, Sikma W, Niesing R et al (2003) External rotation stress imaging in syndesmotic injuries of the ankle: comparison of lateral radiography and radiostereometry in a cadaveric model. Acta Orthop Scand 74(2):201–205
11. Bosien WR, Staples OS, Russell SW (1955) Residual disability following acute ankle sprains. J Bone Joint Surg Am 37(6):1237–1243
12. Boss AP, Hintermann B (2002) Anatomical study of the medial ankle ligament complex. Foot Ankle Int 23(6):547–553
13. Brown KW, Morrison WB, Schweitzer ME, Parellada JA, Nothnagel H (2004) MRI findings associated with distal tibiofibular syndesmosis injury. AJR Am J Roentgenol 182(1):131–136
14. Calder JD, Bamford R, Petrie A, McCollum GA (2016) Stable versus unstable grade ii high ankle sprains: a prospective study predicting the need for surgical stabilization and time to return to sports. Arthroscopy 32(4):634–642
15. Chen PY, Wang TG, Wang CL (2008) Ultrasonographic examination of the deltoid ligament in bimalleolar equivalent fractures. Foot Ankle Int 29(9):883–886
16. Cheng MS, Ferkel RD, Applegate GR (1995) Osteochondral lesions of the talus: a radiologic and surgical comparison. In: Presented at the annual meeting of the American Academy of Orthopedic Surgeons, New Orleans, 16–21 Feb 1995. American Academy of Orthopedic Surgeons, New Orleans
17. Cloke DJ, Ansell P, Avery P, Deehan D (2011) Ankle injuries in football academies: a three-centre prospective study. Br J Sports Med 45(9):702–708
18. Cloke DJ, Spencer S, Hodson A, Deehan D (2009) The epidemiology of ankle injuries occurring in English Football Association academies. Br J Sports Med 43(14):1119–1125
19. Colvin AC, Walsh M, Koval KJ, MLCaurin T, Tejwani N, Egol K (2009) Return to sports following operatively treated ankle fractures. Foot Ankle Int 30(4):292–296
20. Cox JS (1985) Surgical and nonsurgical treatment of acute ankle sprains. Clin Orthop Relat Res (198):118–126
21. Del Buono A, Smith R, Coco M, Woolley L, Denaro V, Maffulli N (2013) Return to sports after ankle fractures: a systematic review. Br Med Bull 106:179–191
22. Dizon JM, Reyes JJ (2010) A systematic review on the effectiveness of external ankle supports in the prevention of inversion ankle sprains among elite and recreational players. J Sci Med Sport 13(3):309–317
23. Donnenwerth MP, Roukis TS (2012) Outcome of arthroscopic debridement and microfracture as the primary treatment for osteochondral lesions of the talar dome. Arthroscopy 28(12):1902–1907
24. Ekstrand J, Gillquist J (1983) Soccer injuries and their mechanisms: a prospective study. Med Sci Sports Exerc 15(3):267–270
25. Ekstrand J, Hägglund M, Waldén M (2011) Injury incidence and injury patterns in professional football: the UEFA injury study. Br J Sports 45(7):553–558
26. Elias I, Zoga AC, Morrison WB, Besser MP, Schweitzer ME, Raikin SM (2007) Osteochondral lesions of the talus: localization and morphologic data from 424 patients using a novel anatomical grid scheme. Foot Ankle Int 28(2):154–161
27. Ferkel RD, Sgaglione NA, Del Pizzo W (1990) Arthroscopic treatment of osteochondral lesions of the talus: technique and results. Orthop Trans 14:172–173
28. Ferran NA, Maffulli N (2006) Epidemiology of sprains of the lateral ankle ligament complex. Foot Ankle Clin 11(3):659–662
29. Frankeny JR, Jewett DL, Hanks GA, Sebastianelli WJ (1993) A comparison of ankle-taping methods. Clin J Sport Med 3(1):20–25
30. Fraser EJ, Harris MC, Prado MP, Kennedy JG (2016) Autologous osteochondral transplantation for osteochondral lesions of the talus in an athletic population. Knee Surg Sports Traumatol Arthrosc 24(4):1272–1279
31. Freeman MA, Dean MR, Hanham IW (1965) The etiology and prevention of functional instability of the foot. J Bone Joint Surg Br 47(4):678–685
32. Gerards R, Zengerink M, van Dijk CN (2014) Osteochondral defects in the ankle joint. In: The ankle in football. Springer, Paris, pp 101–117
33. Gerber JP, Williams GN, Scoville CR, Arciero RA, Taylor DC (1998) Persistent disability associated with ankle sprains: a prospective examination of an athletic population. Foot Ankle 19(10): 653–660
34. Gianakos AL, Yasui Y, Hannon CP, Kennedy JG (2017) Current management of talar osteochondral lesions. World J Orthop 8(1):12–20
35. Gill JB, Risko T, Raducan V, Grimes JS, Schutt RC Jr (2007) Comparison of manual and gravity stress radiographs for the evaluation of supination-external rotation fibular fractures. J Bone Joint Surg Am 89(5):994–999
36. Giza E, Fuller C, Junge A, Dvorak J (2003) Mechanisms of foot and ankle injuries in soccer. Am J Sports Med 31(4):550–554
37. Gonell AC, Romero JA, Soler LM (2015) Relationship between the Y-balance test scores and

soft tissue injury incidence in a soccer team. Int J Sports Phys Ther 10(7):955–966
38. Hamilton WG (1982) Sprained ankles in ballet dancers. Foot Ankle 3(2):99–102
39. Hannon CP, Smyth NA, Murawski CD, Savage-Elliott I, Deyer TW, Calder JD et al (2014) Osteochondral lesions of the talus: aspects of current management. Bone Joint J 96(2):164–171
40. Harper MC (1993) An anatomic and radiographic investigation of the tibiofibular clear space. Foot Ankle 14(8):455–458
41. Hastie GR, Akhtar S, Butt U, Baumann A, Barrie JL (2015) Weightbearing radiographs facilitate functional treatment of ankle fractures of uncertain stability. J Foot Ankle Surg 54(6):1042–1046
42. Hawkins RD, Hulse MA, Wilkinson C, Hodson A, Gibson M (2001) The association football medical research programme: an audit of injuries in professional football. Br J Sports Med 35(1):43–47
43. Henari S, Banks LN, Radovanovic I, Queally J, Morris S (2011) Ultrasonography as a diagnostic tool in assessing deltoid ligament injury in supination external rotation fractures of the ankle. Orthopedics 34(10):e639–e643
44. Hepple S, Winson IG, Glew D (1999) Osteochondral lesions of the talus: a revised classification. Foot Ankle Int 20(12):789–793
45. Hertel J, Miller SJ, Denegar CR (2000) Intratester and intertester reliability during the star excursion balance tests. J Sport Rehabil 9(2):104–116
46. Hintermann B (2003) Medial ankle instability. Foot Ankle Clin 8(4):723–738
47. Hintermann B (2005) What the orthopaedic foot and ankle surgeon wants to know from MR Imaging. Semin Musculoskelet Radiol 9(3):260–271
48. Holmes JR, Acker WB II, Murphy JM, McKinney A, Kadakia AR, Irwin TA (2016) A novel algorithm for isolated weber b ankle fractures: a retrospective review of 51 nonsurgically treated patients. J Am Acad Orthop Surg 24(9):645–652
49. Hopkinson WJ, St Pierre P, Ryan JB, Wheeler JH (1990) Syndesmosis sprains of the ankle. Foot Ankle 10(6):325–330
50. Hoshino CM, Nomoto EK, Norheim EP, Harris TG (2012) Correlation of weightbearing radiographs and stability of stress positive ankle fractures. Foot Ankle Int 33(2):92–98
51. Howard DR, Rubin DA, Hillen TJ, Nissman DB, Lomax J, Williams T et al (2012) Magnetic resonance imaging as a predictor of return to play following syndesmosis (high) ankle sprains in professional football players. Sports Health 4(6):535–543
52. Hubbard TJ, Cordova M (2009) Mechanical instability after an acute lateral ankle sprain. Arch Phys Med Rehabil 90(7):1142–1146
53. Hunt KJ, Phisitkul P, Pirolo J, Amendola A (2015) High ankle sprains and syndesmotic injuries in athletes. J Am Acad Orthop Surg 23(11):661–673
54. Hupperets MD, Verhagen EA, van Mechelen W (2009) Effect of unsupervised home based proprioceptive training on recurrences of ankle sprain: randomised controlled trial. BMJ 339:b2684
55. Jain N, Murray D, Kemp S, Calder J (2014) Frequency and trends in foot and ankle injuries within an English Premier League Football Club using a new impact factor of injury to identify a focus for injury prevention. Foot Ankle Surg 20(4):237–240
56. Jazzo SF, Scribner D, Shay S, Kim KM (2016) Patient-reported outcomes following platelet-rich plasma injections in treating osteochondral lesions of the talus: a critically appraised topic. J Sport Rehabil 19:1–23
57. Jelinek JA, Porter DA (2009) Management of unstable ankle fractures and syndesmosis injuries in athletes. Foot Ankle Clin 14(2):277–298
58. Joshy S, Abdulkadir U, Chaganti S, Sullivan B, Hariharan K (2010) Accuracy of MRI scan in the diagnosis of ligamentous and chondral pathology in the ankle. Foot Ankle Surg 16(2):78–80
59. Kaikkonen A, Kannus P, Järvinen M (1994) A performance test protocol and scoring scale for the evaluation of ankle injuries. Am J Sports Med 22(4):462–469
60. Kaminski TW, Hertel J, Amendola N, Docherty CL, Dolan MG, Hopkins JT et al (2013) National Athletic Trainers' Association position statement: conservative management and prevention of ankle sprains in athletes. J Athl Train 48(4):528–545
61. Kemler E, van de Port I, Backx F, van Dijk CN (2011) A systematic review on the treatment of acute ankle sprain: brace versus other functional treatment types. Sports Med 41(3):185–197
62. Kerkhoffs GM, Handoll HH, de Bie R, Rowe BH, Struijs PA (2007) Surgical versus conservative treatment for acute injuries of the lateral ligament complex of the ankle in adults. Cochrane Database Syst Rev 2:CD000380
63. Kerkhoffs GM, Reilingh ML, Gerards RM, de Leeuw PA (2016) Lift, drill, fill and fix (LDFF): a new arthroscopic treatment for talar osteochondral defects. Knee Surg Sports Traumatol Arthrosc 24(4):1265–1271
64. Kerkhoffs GM, Rowe BH, Assendelft WJ, Kelly K, Struijs PA, van Dijk CN (2002) Immobilisation and functional treatment for acute lateral ankle ligament injuries in adults. Cochrane Database Syst Rev 3:CD003762
65. Kerkhoffs GM, Struijs PA, Marti RK, Assendelft WJ, Blankevoort L, van Dijk CN (2002) Different functional treatment strategies for acute lateral ankle ligament injuries in adults. Cochrane Database Syst Rev 3:CD002938
66. Kerkhoffs GM, Tol JL (2012) A twist on the athlete's ankle twist: some ankles are more equal than others. Br J Sports Med 46(12):835–836

67. Kerkhoffs GM, van den Bekerom M, Elders LA, van Beek PA, Hullegie WA, Bloemers GM et al (2012) Diagnosis, treatment and prevention of ankle sprains: an evidence-based clinical guideline. Br J Sports Med 46(12):854–860
68. Kerkhoffs GMMJ, de Leeuw PAJ, Tennant JN, Amendola A (2014) Ankle ligament lesions. In: The ankle in football. Springer, Paris, pp 81–96
69. Khor YP, Tan KJ (2013) The anatomic pattern of injuries in acute inversion ankle sprains: a magnetic resonance imaging study. Orthop J Sports Med 1(7):2325967113517078
70. Kofotolis ND, Kellis E, Vlachopoulos SP (2007) Ankle sprain injuries and risk factors in amateur soccer players during a 2-year period. Am J Sports Med 35(3):458–466
71. Krips R, de Vries J, van Dijk CN (2006) Ankle instability. Foot Ankle Clin 11(2):311–329
72. Lahm A, Erggelet C, Steinwachs M, Reichelt A (2000) Arthroscopic management of osteochondral lesions of the talus: results of drilling and usefulness of magnetic resonance imaging before and after treatment. Arthroscopy 16(3):299–304
73. Lamb SE, Marsh JL, Hutton JL, Nakash R, Cooke MW, Collaborative Ankle Support Trial (CAST Group) (2009) Mechanical supports for acute, severe ankle sprain: a pragmatic, multicentre, randomised controlled trial. Lancet 373(9663):575–581
74. Laver L, Carmont MR, McConkey MO, Palmanovich E, Yaacobi E, Mann G et al (2015) Plasma rich in growth factors (PRGF) as a treatment for high ankle sprain in elite athletes: a randomized control trial. Knee Surg Sports Traumatol Arthrosc 23(11):3383–3392
75. Lechner R, Richter H, Friemert B, Palm HG, Gottschalk A (2015) The value of ultrasonography compared with magnetic resonance imaging in the diagnosis of deltoid ligament injuries--is there a difference? Z Orthop Unfall 153(4):408–414
76. Leontaritis N, Hinojosa L, Panchbhavi VK (2009) Arthroscopically detected intra-articular lesions associated with acute ankle fractures. J Bone Joint Surg Am 91(2):333–339
77. Lippert MJ, Hawe W, Bernett P (1989) Surgical therapy of fibular capsule-ligament rupture. Sportverletz Sportschaden 3(1):6–13
78. Loomer R, Fisher C, Lloyd-Smith R, Sisler J, Cooney T (1993) Osteochondral lesions of the talus. Am J Sports Med 21(1):13–19
79. Looze CA, Capo J, Ryan MK, Begly JP, Chapman C, Swanson D et al (2017) Evaluation and management of osteochondral lesions of the talus. Cartilage 8(1):19–30
80. Lötscher P, Lang TH, Zwicky L, Hintermann B, Knupp M (2015) Osteoligamentous injuries of the medial ankle joint. Eur J Trauma Emerg Surg 41(6):615–621
81. Martin RL, Burdett RG, Irrgang JJ (1999) Development of the foot and ankle disability index (FADI) [abstract]. J Orthop Sports Phys Ther 29:A32–A33
82. McCollum GA, van den Bekerom MP, Kerkhoffs GM, Calder JD, van Dijk CN (2013) Syndesmosis and deltoid ligament injuries in the athlete. Knee Surg Sports Traumatol Arthrosc 21(6):1328–1337
83. McGuine TA, Greene JJ, Best T, Leverson G (2000) Balance as a predictor of ankle injuries in high school basketball players. Clin J Sport Med 10(4):239–244
84. Mei-Dan O, Kots E, Barchilon V, Massarwe S, Nyska M, Mann G (2009) A dynamic ultrasound examination for the diagnosis of ankle syndesmotic injury in professional athletes: a preliminary study. Am J Sports Med 37(5):1009–1016
85. Milner CE, Soames RW (1998) Anatomy of the collateral ligaments of the human ankle joint. Foot Ankle Int 19(11):757–760
86. Milz P, Milz S, Steinborn M, Mittlmeier T, Putz R, Reiser M (1998) Lateral ankle ligaments and tibiofibular syndesmosis. 13-MHz high-frequency sonography and MRI compared in 20 patients. Acta Orthop Scand 69(1):51–55
87. Mulligan EP (2011) Evaluation and management of ankle syndesmosis injuries. Phys Ther Sport 12(2):57–69
88. Murawski CD, Kennedy JG (2013) Operative treatment of osteochondral lesions of the talus. J Bone Joint Surg Am 95(11):1045–1054
89. Nussbaum ED, Hosea TM, Sieler SD, Incremona BR, Kessler DE (2001) Prospective evaluation of syndesmotic ankle sprains without diastasis. Am J Sports Med 29(1):31–35
90. Oae K, Takao M, Uchio Y, Ochi M (2010) Evaluation of anterior talofibular ligament injury with stress radiography, ultrasonography and MR imaging. Skeletal Radiol 39(1):41–47
91. Paris DL (1992) The effects of the Swede-O, New Cross, and McDavid ankle braces and adhesive ankle taping on speed, balance, agility, and vertical jump. J Athl Train 27(3):253
92. Pauole K, Madole K, Garhammer J, Lacourse M, Rozenek R (2000) Reliability and validity of the T-Test as a measure of agility, leg power, and leg speed in college aged men and women. J Strength Cond Res 14(4):443–450
93. Pearce CJ, Tourné Y, Zellers J et al (2016) Rehabilitation after anatomical ankle ligament repair or reconstruction. Knee Surg Sports Traumatol Arthrosc 24(4):1130–1139
94. Petersen W, Rembitzki IV, Koppenburg AG, Ellermann A, Liebau C, Brüggemann GP, Best R (2013) Treatment of acute ankle ligament injuries: a systematic review. Arch Orthop Trauma Surg 133(8):1129–1141
95. Plisky PJ, Gorman PP, Butler RJ, Kiesel KB, Underwood FB, Elkins B (2009) The reliability of an instrumented device for measuring components

of the star excursion balance test. N Am J Sports Phys Ther 4(2):92–99
96. Plisky PJ, Rauh MJ, Kaminski TW, Underwood FB (2006) Star Excursion Balance Test as a predictor of lower extremity injury in high school basketball players. J Orthop Sports Phys Ther 36(12):911–919
97. Price RJ, Hawkins RD, Hulse MA, Hodson A (2004) The Football Association medical research programme: an audit of injuries in academy youth football. Br J Sports Med 38(4):466–471
98. Pritsch M, Horoshovski H, Farine I (1986) Arthroscopic treatment of osteochondral lesions of the talus. J Bone Joint Surg Am 68(6):862–865
99. Putnam AR, Bandolin SN, Krabak BJ (2012) Impact of ankle bracing on skill performance in recreational soccer players. PM R 4(8):574–579
100. Ramponi L, Yasui Y, Murawski CD, Ferkel RD, DiGiovanni CW, Kerkhoffs GM et al (2017) Lesion size is a predictor of clinical outcomes after bone marrow stimulation for osteochondral lesions of the talus: a systematic review. Am J Sports Med 45:1698. https://doi.org/10.1177/0363546516668292
101. Reilingh ML, van Bergen CJA, van Dijk CN (2009) Diagnosis and treatment of osteochondral defects in the ankle. South Afr Orthop 8(2):44–55
102. Renström PA, Konradsen L (1997) Ankle ligament injuries. Br J Sports Med 31(1):11–20
103. Richie DH, Izadi FE (2015) Return to play after an ankle sprain: guidelines for the podiatric physician. Clin Podiatr Med Surg 32(2):195–215
104. Roemer FW, Jomaah N, Niu J, Almusa E, Roger B, D'Hooghe P, Geertsema C, Tol JL, Khan K, Guermazi A (2014) Ligamentous injuries and the risk of associated tissue damage in acute ankle sprains in athletes: a cross-sectional MRI study. Am J Sports Med 42(7):1549–1557
105. Samra DJ, Sman AD, Rae K, Linklater J, Refshauge KM, Hiller CE (2015) Effectiveness of a single platelet-rich plasma injection to promote recovery in rugby players with ankle syndesmosis injury. BMJ Open Sport Exerc Med 1(1):e000033
106. Savage-Elliott I, Murawski CD, Smyth NA, Golano P, Kennedy JG (2013) The deltoid ligament: an in-depth review of anatomy, function, and treatment strategies. Knee Surg Sports Traumatol Arthrosc 21(6):1316–1327
107. Saxena A, Eakin C (2007) Articular talar injuries in athletes: results of microfracture and autogenous bone graft. Am J Sports Med 35(10):1680–1687
108. Schepers T (2012) Acute distal tibiofibular syndesmosis injury: a systematic review of suture-button versus syndesmotic screw repair. Int Orthop 36(6):1199–1206
109. Schock HJ, Pinzur M, Manion L, Stover M (2007) The use of gravity or manual-stress radiographs in the assessment of supination-external rotation fractures of the ankle. J Bone Joint Surg Br 89(8):1055–1059
110. Schuberth JM, Collman DR, Rush SM, Ford LA (2004) Deltoid ligament integrity in lateral malleolar fractures: a comparative analysis of arthroscopic and radiographic assessments. J Foot Ankle Surg 43(1):20–29
111. Seijas R, Alvarez P, Ares O, Steinbacher G, Cuscó X, Cugat R (2010) Osteocartilaginous lesions of the talus in soccer players. Arch Orthop Trauma Surg 130(3):329–333
112. Shang XL, Tao HY, Chen SY, Li YX, Hua YH (2016) Clinical and MRI outcomes of HA injection following arthroscopic microfracture for osteochondral lesions of the talus. Knee Surg Sports Traumatol Arthrosc 24(4):1243–1249
113. Sharpe SR, Knapik J, Jones B (1997) Ankle braces effectively reduce recurrence of ankle sprains in female soccer players. J Athl Train 32(1):21–24
114. Shimozono Y, Yasui Y, Ross AW, Kennedy JG (2017) Osteochondral lesions of the talus in the athlete: up to date review. Curr Rev Musculoskelet Med 10(1):131–140
115. Sman AD, Hiller CE, Refshauge KM (2013) Diagnostic accuracy of clinical tests for diagnosis of ankle syndesmosis injury: a systematic review. Br J Sports Med 47(10):620–628
116. St Pierre RK, Rosen J, Whitesides TE, Szczukowski M, Fleming LL, Hutton WC (1983) The tensile strength of the anterior talofibular ligament. Foot Ankle 4(2):83–85
117. Stryker SM, Di Trani AM, Swanik CB, Glutting JJ, Kaminski TW (2016) Assessing performance, stability, and cleat comfort/support in collegiate club soccer players using prophylactic ankle taping and bracing. Res Sports Med 24(1):39–53
118. Stubbe JH, van Beijsterveldt AM, van der Knaap S, Stege J, Verhagen EA, van Mechelen W, Backx FJ (2015) Injuries in professional male soccer players in the Netherlands: a prospective cohort study. J Athl Train 50(2):211–216
119. Stufkens SA, van den Bekerom MP, Knupp M, Hintermann B, van Dijk CN (2012) The diagnosis and treatment of deltoid ligament lesions in supination-external rotation ankle fractures: a review. Strategies Trauma Limb Reconstr 7(2):73–85
120. Takao M, Ochi M, Oae K (2003) Diagnosis of a tear of the distal tibiofibular syndesmosis. The role of arthroscopy of the ankle. J Bone Joint Surg Br 85(3):324–329
121. Takao M, Ochi M, Uchio Y, Naito K, Kono T, Oae K (2003) Osteochondral lesions of the talar dome associated with trauma. Arthrosc J Arthrosc Relat Surg 19(10):1061–1067
122. Taylor DC, Tenuta JJ, Uhorchak JM, Arciero RA (2007) Aggressive surgical treatment and early return to sports in athletes with grade III syndesmosis sprains. Am J Sports Med 35(11):1833–1838
123. Van den Bekerom MP (2011) Diagnosing syndesmotic instability in ankle fractures. World J Orthop 2(7):51–56
124. Van den Bekerom MP, Kerkhoffs GM, McCollum GA, Calder JD, van Dijk CN (2013) Management of

acute lateral ankle ligament injury in the athlete. Knee Surg Sports Traumatol Arthrosc 21(6):1390–1395
125. Van den Bekerom MP, Mutsaerts EL, van Dijk CN (2009) Evaluation of the integrity of the deltoid ligament in supination external rotation ankle fractures: a systematic review of the literature. Arch Orthop Trauma Surg 129(2):227–235
126. Van den Bekerom MP, Sjer A, Somford MP, Bulstra GH, Struijs PA, Kerkhoffs GM (2015) Non-steroidal anti-inflammatory drugs (NSAIDs) for treating acute ankle sprains in adults: benefits outweigh adverse events. Knee Surg Sports Traumatol Arthrosc 23(8):2390–2399
127. Van den Bekerom MP, van Kimmenade R, Sierevelt IN, Eggink K, Kerkhoffs GM, van Dijk CN et al (2016) Randomized comparison of tape versus semi-rigid and versus lace-up ankle support in the treatment of acute lateral ankle ligament injury. Knee Surg Sports Traumatol Arthrosc 24(4):978–984
128. Van Dijk CN, Lim LS, Bossuyt PM, Marti RK (1996) Physical examination is sufficient for the diagnosis of sprained ankles. J Bone Joint Surg Br 78(6):958–962
129. Van Dijk CN, Longo UG, Loppini M, Florio P, Maltese L, Ciuffreda M et al (2016) Classification and diagnosis of acute isolated syndesmotic injuries: ESSKA-AFAS consensus and guidelines. Knee Surg Sports Traumatol Arthrosc 24(4):1200–1216
130. Van Dijk CN, Mol BW, Lim LS, Marti RK, Bossuyt PM (1996) Diagnosis of ligament rupture of the ankle joint. Physical examination, arthrography, stress radiography and sonography compared in 160 patients after inversion trauma. Acta Orthop Scand 67(6):566–570
131. Van Dijk CN, Reilingh ML, Zengerink M, van Bergen CJ (2010) Osteochondral defects in the ankle: why painful? Knee Surg Sports Traumatol Arthrosc 18(5):570–580
132. Van Eekeren IC, Reilingh ML, van Dijk CN (2012) Rehabilitation and return-to-sports activity after debridement and bone marrow stimulation of osteochondral talar defects. Sports Med 42(10):857–870
133. Van Eekeren IC, van Bergen CJ, Sierevelt IN, Reilingh ML, van Dijk CN (2016) Return to sports after arthroscopic debridement and bone marrow stimulation of osteochondral talar defects: a 5- to 24-year follow-up study. Knee Surg Sports Traumatol Arthrosc 24(4):1311–1315
134. Van Rijn RM, van Os AG, Bernsen RMD, Luijsterburg PA, Koes BW, Bierma-Zeinstra SMA (2008) What is the clinical course of acute ankle sprains? A systematic literature review. Am J Med 121:324–331
135. Vannini F, Cavallo M, Ramponi L, Castagnini F, Massimi S, Giannini S, Buda RE (2017) Return to sports after bone marrow-derived cell transplantation for osteochondral lesions of the talus. Cartilage 8(1):80–87
136. Vereijken AJ (2012) Risk factors for ankle sprain injury in male amateur soccer players: a prospective cohort study. http://dspace.library.uu.nl/handle/1874/252485. Accessed 4 Jan 2017.
137. Verhagen EA, Van der Beek AJ, Bouter LM, Bahr RM, Van Mechelen W (2004) A one season prospective cohort study of volleyball injuries. Br J Sports Med 38(4):477–481
138. Verhagen RA, Maas M, Dijkgraaf MG, Tol JL, Krips R, van Dijk CN (2005) Prospective study on diagnostic strategies in osteochondral lesions of the talus. Is MRI superior to helical CT? J Bone Joint Surg Br 87(1):41–46
139. Vopat ML, Vopat BG, Lubberts B, DiGiovanni CW (2017) Current trends in the diagnosis and management of syndesmotic injury. Curr Rev Musculoskelet Med 10:94. https://doi.org/10.1007/s12178-017-9389-4
140. Waldén M, Hägglund M, Ekstrand J (2013) Time-trends and circumstances surrounding ankle injuries in men's professional football: an 11-year follow-up of the UEFA Champions League injury study. Br J Sports Med 47(12):748–753
141. Waterman BR, Belmont PJ Jr, Cameron KL, Svoboda SJ, Alitz CJ, Owens BD (2011) Risk factors for syndesmotic and medial ankle sprain: role of sex, sport, and level of competition. Am J Sports Med 39(5):992–998
142. Weber M, Burmeister H, Flueckiger G, Krause FG (2010) The use of weightbearing radiographs to assess the stability of supination-external rotation fractures of the ankle. Arch Orthop Trauma Surg 130(5):693–698
143. Williams GN, Allen EJ (2010) Rehabilitation of syndesmotic (high) ankle sprains. Sports Health 2(6):460–470
144. Williams GN, Jones MH, Amendola A (2007) Syndesmotic ankle sprains in athletes. Am J Sports Med 35(7):1197–1207
145. Woods C, Hawkins R, Hulse M, Hodson A (2003) The Football Association Medical Research Programme: an audit of injuries in professional football: an analysis of ankle sprains. Br J Sports Med 37(3):233–2388
146. Wright RW, Barlie J, Suprent DA, Matave MJ (2004) Ankle syndesmosis sprains in national hockey league players. Am J Sports Med 32(8):1941–1945
147. Xenos JS, Hopkinson WJ, Mulligan ME, Olson EJ, Popovic NA (1995) The tibiofibular syndesmosis: evaluation of the ligamentous structures, methods of fixation, and radiographic assessment. J Bone Joint Surg Am 77(6):847–856
148. Zalavras C, Thordarson D (2007) Ankle syndesmosis injury. J Am Acad Orthop Surg 15(6):330–339
149. Zengerink M, Struijs PA, Tol JL, van Dijk CN (2010) Treatment of osteochondral lesions of the talus: a systematic review. Knee Surg Sports Traumatol Arthrosc 18(2):238–246
150. Zöch C, Fialka-Moser V, Quittan M (2003) Rehabilitation of ligamentous ankle injuries: a review of recent studies. Br J Sports Med 37(4):291–295

30 Return to Play in Stress Fractures of the Foot

Pieter d'Hooghe and Athol Thomson

Contents

P. d'Hooghe (✉)
Department of Orthopaedic Surgery, Aspetar Orthopaedic and Sports medical Hospital, Aspire Zone, Sports city street 1, P.O. Box 29222, Doha, Qatar
e-mail: pieter.dhooghe@aspetar.com

A. Thomson
Department of Sports Podiatry, Aspetar Orthopaedic and Sports medical Hospital, Aspire Zone, Sports city street 1, P.O. Box 29222, Doha, Qatar
e-mail: athol.thomson@aspetar.com

30.1 Introduction

A football-induced stress fracture in the foot occurs when the bone is unable to withstand the recurrent stresses of training or game. There is scarce literature in male football (see five best evidence-based citations box), but we know that every team can expect a lower extremity stress fracture every third season [1]. It also shows that the most common stress fracture site is the fifth

V. Musahl et al. (eds.), *Return to Play in Football*, https://doi.org/10.1007/978-3-662-55713-6_30

Table 30.1 Important risk factors for stress fractures

Intrinsic risk factors	Extrinsic risk factors
1. Age – *Male*: incidence decreases after 17 years of age – *Female*: incidence increases after menarche	1. Long-distance running
2. Low body mass index (BMI)	2. Hard-surface running
3. Decreased muscle strength	3. Training schedule changes
4. Anatomical factors – *Low cross-sectional area* – *Leg length discrepancy*	4. Alcohol/smoking
5. Lack of physical activity	5. Vitamin D low levels
6. Female athlete triad (menstrual dysfunction, low bone mineral density, eating disorders)	

metatarsal (78%), that younger players are more prone to suffer from one and that 29% are reinjuries. In female football the overall reported incidence of stress fractures is 13.6%, and the specific importance of the pathogenesis in the female athlete has been highlighted in recent reports [2]. Risk factors can be identified (Table 30.1) in an attempt to target the "high-risk" groups in order to prevent stress fractures in the football players' feet. A high index of suspicion is required since many players that complain will present with normal plain radiographs that can underestimate the incidence.

30.2 Stress Fracture of the Navicular

30.2.1 Functional Anatomy

The area available for blood supply is limited because the navicular bone is extensively covered by articular cartilage. The blood supply to the navicular bone is received via the dorsalis pedis and the posterior tibial arteries. The blood supply enters the bone mainly via the dorsal and plantar surfaces at the insertion of the tibialis posterior tendon. The vascular network branches out medially and laterally, but the central third is relatively avascular. This area has been described as "a watershed area" and is the site most vulnerable to stress fractures and non-union [3, 4].

30.2.2 Biomechanics

The navicular bone functions biomechanically as the link between the midfoot and the hindfoot and couples the movement between the talo-navicular and the subtalar joint. It serves as a keystone of the medial longitudinal column, and it relates anatomically to the head of the talus as well as the anterior process of the calcaneus. The talo-navicular joint needs to be mobile if it wants the subtalar joint to function properly. In case a navicular stress fracture occurs, the medial longitudinal arch can collapse and result in a combined loss of supination [3, 5, 6].

During football foot strike, the navicular bone is maximally compressed between the proximally located talar head and the distally located first and second metatarso-cuneiform (MTC) joints. When sprinting for a ball, the navicular bone experiences maximum compressive forces during the end of the stance phase when the forefoot becomes loaded. Maximum compressive and shear stresses are seen at the central third of the navicular at the junction between the first and the second MTC joints (nutcracker effect) [7]. Knowing that this area is also the watershed area of blood supply, it makes it the most vulnerable area to stress fractures. Therefore, football players who engage in forceful push-offs, sprints, deceleration twists and jumps (e.g. wingers) are more prone to navicular stress fractures.

30.2.3 Risk Factors

Pes cavus, limited ankle dorsiflexion, restricted subtalar motion, short first MT, long second MT and metatarsus adductus have all been labelled as predisposing factors for navicular stress fracture ([7], Table 30.1). Football players have frequently some grade of reduced ankle dorsiflexion (anterior impingement) that is accumulated by these potential predisposing factors. This makes the midfoot to compensate with a larger excursion and increases motion, resulting in navicular impingement during dorsiflexion.

30.2.4 Clinical Assessment

Football-induced stress fractures of the foot require a high clinical index of suspicion since the clinical signs can be very limited. Due to the initial non-specific and mild symptoms, delay in diagnosis is common in most of the reported series [4]. Players typically present with activity-related dorsal (or occasionally non-specific) foot pain that abates at rest. No obvious swelling or bruising is commonly seen, but the pain may be aggravated while standing on tiptoes. At a later stage, the symptoms can affect activities of daily living, and the pain will present over the dorsum of the navicular between the tendons of tibialis anterior and extensor hallucis longus. This area corresponds to the central third of the navicular and has been termed *the N spot* [3]. Frequently, players present with a cavo-varus alignment, normal ankle ROM and normal strength. Cavo-varus alignment is related to reduced midfoot motion that can absorb less the required loads during football activity. Once identified, this can be addressed by adequate orthotic support. Other risk factors like aberrant technique, equipment issues and training/match overuse should also be addressed and carefully ruled out.

Fact Box 1

Always suspect a stress fracture in an athlete who presents with dull foot pain, localized to the bone, that increases on activity and is relieved on rest.

30.2.5 Investigations

30.2.5.1 Plain Radiograph

A standard first-line imaging tool is the weight-bearing anteroposterior, lateral and oblique view on the plain radiograph of the foot. However, there is a low sensitivity of plain radiographs in the diagnosis of a navicular stress fracture. The main reason is that navicular stress fractures occur in the sagittal plane and involve the central third. That makes it difficult to get the X-ray beam truly perpendicular to the fracture plane. Another reason is that most of these fractures are incomplete and do not involve the plantar cortex which makes them invisible on plain radiographs until osteoclastic resorption has taken place [4]. Additional imaging such as 3D bone scintigraphy (bone scan), computed tomography (CT) or magnetic resonance imaging (MRI) are very helpful in case of clinical suspicion towards definitive diagnosis. There is no superiority of one investigation over the other, and each has its specific diagnostic advantages (Tables 30.2 and 30.3) as described below:

Table 30.2 Typical features of imaging modalities in lower extremity stress fractures

Imaging modality	Sensitivity (%)	Specificity (%)
Plain radiograph	12–56	88–96
Ultrasound	43–99	13–79
CT scan	32–38	88–98
MRI scan	68–99	4–97
Bone scan (scintigraphy)	50–97	33–98

Table 30.3 Kaeding and Miller classification system (a validated stress fracture classification system)

Grade	Pain	Imaging
1	No	No fracture line (CT, sclerosis; MRI, oedema; bone scan, increased uptake)
2	Yes	No fracture line (CT, sclerosis; MRI, oedema; bone scan, increased uptake)
3	Yes	Undisplaced fracture
4	Yes	Displaced fracture
5	Yes	Non-union

Fact Box 2

Do not rely on plain radiographs only for the diagnosis of foot stress fractures. MRI and/or bone scan is often needed to make the correct diagnosis.

30.2.5.2 Bone Scan

Bone scan has a high sensitivity but low specificity and s-hould not be used as a first-line

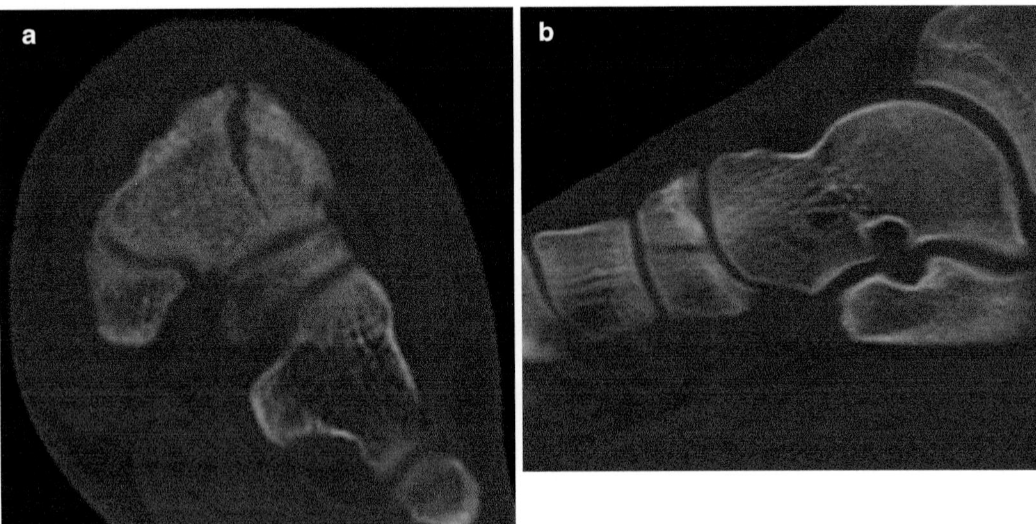

Fig. 30.1 28-year-old elite football player with a navicular stress fracture. (**a**) Axial CT view, (**b**) sagittal CT view

investigation. However, it can be helpful when CT and/or MRI fail to demonstrate a clear diagnosis [3].

30.2.5.3 CT Scan

CT scan can delineate fracture lines accurately and is a reliable modality in the stress fracture spectrum (Fig. 30.1). It is recommended to ask for thin coronal slices (0.625 mm) through the plane of the talo-navicular joint. A CT-based classification system based on the fracture pattern was introduced by Saxena et al. ([8], Box 1).

Although clinical union often precedes signs of radiological union, CT scan can also be used to monitor healing. As early as 6 weeks after injury, dorsal cortical proliferation can be seen as the first radiologic sign of healing. Fracture consolidation can be expected between 3 and 4 months, but a persistent medullary cyst or cortical notching can remain even after complete fracture healing [9].

30.2.5.4 MRI Scan

MRI scan is superior to detect pre-fracture stage bone oedema and stress reaction but is inferior to CT scan in identifying the stress fracture itself. When a stress fracture is suspected, the initial imaging modality should be CT to visualize the fracture line. If the CT does not demonstrate a fracture, an MRI is the next appropriate imaging modality to determine whether a stress reaction is occurring ([3], Fig. 30.2).

30.2.6 Differential Diagnosis

- Navicular stress reaction (NSR): This represents a stress reaction with identical clinical fracture-like symptoms and changes on bone scan and MRI but no obvious fracture line seen on CT scan. The observed bony changes can be considered as a precursor to a frank stress fracture and a bone remodelling attempt in response to stress/load [7]. In case of early NSR identification, a conservative protocol with gradual return to football is advised.
- Osteochondritis dissecans (OCD): This entity should not be confused with a stress fracture or a stress reaction. It usually has a traumatic aetiology and affects the central third of the navicular just like a stress injury. Most football players are affected around the age of late teens to 20s, although occasionally it can be seen at a later age. In this condition, a cartilage injury occurs usually at the junction of the

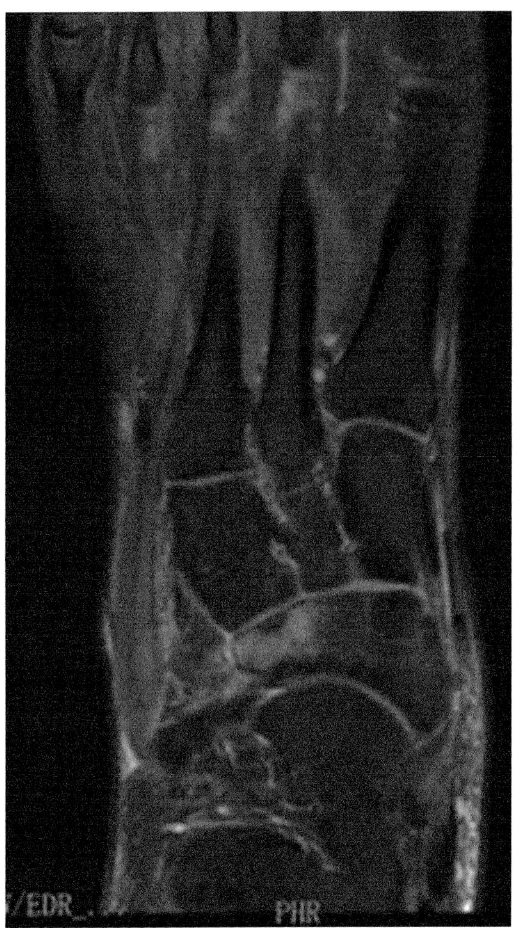

Fig. 30.2 Axial T2 MRI view of navicular stress reaction over the typical "nutcracker effect" area (23-year-old football player)

middle and medial third of the navicular. Frequently, fragmentation and cyst formation can be seen on CT just below the articular surface, and on the MRI a "halo" of increased signal denotes a more active lesion. This condition starts dorsally and proximally and heads distally but does not extend to the plantar area of the navicular bone and does not progress to a stress fracture. Since OCD is often self-limiting, a conservative treatment with activity modification, orthotic support, injection and relative rest is indicated. In case of significant articular damage, the prognosis for return to play is poor, and surgery can be indicated.

30.2.7 Therapeutical Options and/or Surgical Technique

There are no clear guidelines supported by solid literature regarding the best treatment options. In order to guide management, stress fractures of the lower extremities have been divided into "high-risk" and "low-risk" groups that can assist in making the proper treatment choice ([1], Table 30.4).

Most literature that compares surgery versus conservative therapy is retrospective, not representing equal groups and struggles with underpowered sample sizes. Incomplete reporting, lack of validated outcome tools and inconsistent follow-up make it impossible to rely on the presented guidelines. Recent meta-analyses present a 6–8 week non-weight-bearing cast as the treatment of choice for incomplete fractures and non-displaced complete fractures [10–12]. Gradual return to football training is then genuinely started 8 weeks post trauma. The three-fracture type classification by Saxena et al. ([8], Box 1) can also guide the treatment of navicular stress fractures.

Box 1 Classification of navicular stress fractures (Saxena et al.)

Type 1: fracture involves dorsal cortex only

Type 2: fracture extends from dorsum into the navicular body

Type 3: complete bicortical disruption

From Saxena A, Fullem B, Hannaford D. Results of treatment of 22 navicular stress fractures and a new proposed radiographic classification system. J Foot Ankle Surg 2000:39(2);98

Table 30.4 Foot/ankle "high-risk" stress fractures with surgical indication and "low-risk" stress fractures

High-risk stress fractures	*Low-risk* stress fractures
Medial malleolar fractures	Calcaneus
Talar neck fractures	Cuboid
Central-dorsal navicular fractures	Cuneiform
Hallux sesamoidal fractures	Lateral malleolus
Fifth metatarsal fractures	

A conservative non-invasive treatment is advised in type 1 fractures and surgery for type 2 and 3 fractures. In selected elite football cases, however, surgery can be indicated even in a type 1 fracture to assist in early return to play and reduce the refracture rate. This is supported by recent literature [13] stating that there is a low threshold for surgery in the elite athlete, even in type 1 fractures. Further research is needed to define and fine-tune the treatment guidelines in these three-type fracture patterns.

Open or percutaneous surgery is indicated in displaced fractures, delayed union or non-union [4, 14]. A longitudinal incision between the tibialis anterior and tibialis posterior tendons is used just medial to the neurovascular bundle [15]. After identifying the fracture, any sclerotic bone must be removed, and a bone graft (autologous iliac crest) can be impacted in the remaining gap while stabilizing the fracture with (preferably) two compressive screws. Commonly, two partial-threaded cannulated screws, placed lateral to medial, are used in a parallel fashion, but also cross-screw configurations have been described. It is recommended to place the first screw from proximal and dorsal, while the second screw should be more distal and plantar. Due to the helicoidal shape of the navicular bone, caution must be taken not to enter the joint. Therefore, it is mandatory to use intraoperative fluoroscopy, even in an open procedure. Sometimes it can be challenging to achieve an anatomical reduction, and in difficult cases, the use of assisted intraoperative CT scan can be very helpful. CT can also be helpful postoperatively to confirm bony healing and allow a return to football training.

30.2.8 Clinical Outcomes

Clinical outcome is positively correlated with the severity of the fracture, and (since this is a gradual progressive condition) early diagnosis/treatment is key ([16], Box 2). Up to 50% of players remain symptomatic over the *N spot* despite bony consolidation and appear to not return to their previous level [17]. On average, it takes 4 months for a fracture to heal and 5 months before players return to sports [12]. Complications of navicular stress fractures include delayed union (25%), non-union (rare), refracture, persistent pain and degenerative arthritis.

Box 2 Recommended non-weight-bearing regimen for navicular stress fractures (de Clercq et al.)

0–6 weeks: non-weight bearing

6–8 weeks: weight bearing as able in removable cast

8–10 weeks: weight bearing out of cast, resistive strengthening exercise, light jogging

10–12 weeks: full running, sport-specific training

>12 weeks: full return to sports; patients progress to the next stage only if they remain asymptomatic

From de Clercq PFG, Bevernage BD, Leemrijse T. Stress fracture of the navicular bone. Acta OrthopBelg 2008;74(6):725–34

30.3 Metatarsal (MT) Stress Fractures

The metatarsal area is a common site for stress fractures in football players [1]. Stress fractures of the second or the fifth MT are more common than the rest. Because of its unique anatomy and differing function, it is conventional to group MT fractures into fractures of the medial column (first MT), central column (second–third MT) and the lateral column (fourth–fifth MT).

30.3.1 Anatomy

Shape is not uniform across the five metatarsal bones. The first MT is the stoutest and bears maximum load, which is approximately one-third of the total body weight. Therefore, any displacement of the first MT is poorly tolerated and results in a loss of normal weight-bearing function. The second MT is the longest of all five and absorbs the greatest stresses during normal weight bearing. The second tarsometatarsal joint

(TMT) is a stable joint and is consequently the least mobile of all MTs.

The MT bones are supported by strong ligamentous attachments, proximally to the tarsal and phalangeal bones as well as distally. The MT heads are supported by deep-binding transverse MT ligaments, and therefore isolated fractures usually do not displace significantly.

In case of a MT fracture, the flexor digitorum longus and the intrinsic muscles can pull the distal fragment to plantar flexion, which then displaces the MT head plantar and proximal. This deformation results in metatarsalgia and plantar keratosis due to the increased localized loading there. Most stress fractures however present normally undisplaced. The fourth and the fifth MTs are attached firmly to the cuboid bone. This makes them more prone to delayed union because of the traction stresses that they need to absorb.

The proximal diaphysis of the fifth MT is supplied by a short recurrent single nutrient artery. The tuberosity of the fifth MT is supplied by numerous metaphyseal arteries. A watershed area exists between these two sources of blood supply and is located at the proximal metadiaphyseal junction distal to the tuberosity. This area is prone to delayed healing after a stress fracture [3].

30.3.2 Biomechanics

The MT length is considered an important factor in distributing the forefoot load during weight bearing. There is no clear evidence, however, of any relation between MT length and stress fracture. Recent studies found that the MT length does not correlate with peak plantar loading pressure [3, 18, 19] and that maximum stress on the MT 5 occurs 3–4 cm from the proximal end. This area responds with the typical location of the MT 5 stress fracture [20]. The most typical area of fracture is proximally at the first MT and midshaft or more distally at the second to fourth MTs. The second MT is most prone to stress fractures because it needs to take on the highest bending stresses. This is especially true in women because they have a higher middle forefoot loading than men.

The plantar aponeurosis supports the longitudinal arch of the foot that is higher medial than lateral. It elevates and depresses the arch by the "windlass" and the "reverse windlass" mechanism, respectively. By doing so, it can modulate forefoot stress. Injury or surgery on this plantar aponeurosis therefore increases the MT strain on weight bearing.

30.3.3 Risk Factors

Risk factors for MT stress fractures generally are divided into several categories (Table 30.1).

Fact Box 3
Always enquire about changes in the training schedule ("spikes" in load) and playing surface since changes are important risk factors in football.

30.3.4 Clinical Assessment

The injured football player presents with a sudden physical activity-induced aggravation of chronic (prodromal) pain and inability to weight bear. Depending on the time of presentation swelling, ecchymosis and palpable callus may also be present.

To elicit any possible risk factors, a thorough history should be taken, and the threshold for investigation is to be low. The focus of clinical examination should be systematic and specifically assess gait, hindfoot alignment, flexibility, deformity, Achilles tendon tightness, ankle range of motion and callosity at the lateral border.

30.3.5 Return to Play

Stress fractures potentially result in prolonged absence from football. For stress fractures of the fifth MT, the mean absence from football is 3 months [1, 2].

30.3.5.1 First Metatarsal Stress Fracture

Stress fractures at the first MT are rare, and most reports of proximal base stress fracture show healing with conservative management [21].

30.3.5.2 Second to Third Metatarsal Stress Fracture

Football players predominantly present with a fracture just proximal to the MT neck, but they can also occur even more proximal at the base [22]. Proximal fractures are at high risk for non-union, while the distal stress fractures have a good prognosis and faster recovery through conservative management. In football, extreme plantar flexion (e.g. while jumping for a header) increases the risk for proximal fractures. Potential risk factors for proximal fractures are having a short first toe, tibialis anterior tightness, low bone mass and multiple fractures [23].

30.3.5.3 Fourth to Fifth Metatarsal Stress Fracture

The proximally localized stress fractures are also the problematic ones at the fourth and fifth MT. Stress fractures occur typically at the metadiaphyseal junction and are prone to delayed union [24]. More distal fractures are known to be more amenable to conservative management [25].

Players with cavus feet are especially at risk for sustaining a stress fracture at the fifth MT. Associations between restriction in hip rotation and elevated calcaneal pitch have been found in football.

The so-called *Jones fracture* is an eponymous term that has given rise to widespread confusion in the literature between an acute fracture and a stress fracture. Stress fractures of the fifth MT have a typical presentation and occur at a specific site in the bone (Fig. 30.3). Anatomic site is the best way to describe these fractures. Although

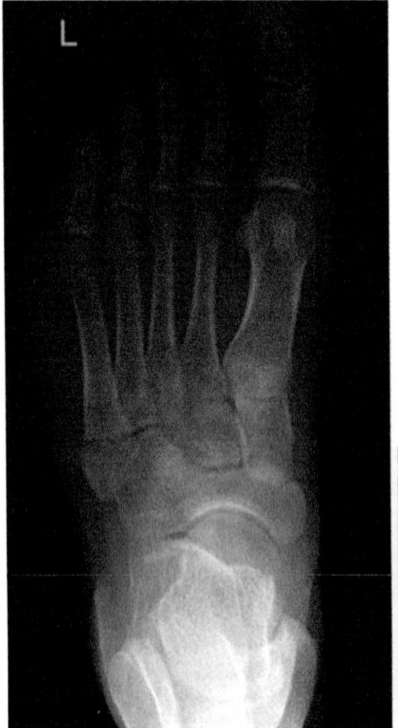

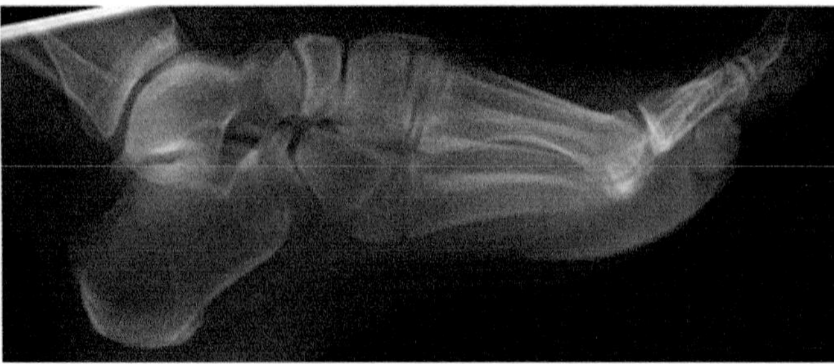

Fig. 30.3 Anteroposterior and lateral radiograph view of a "Jones fracture"

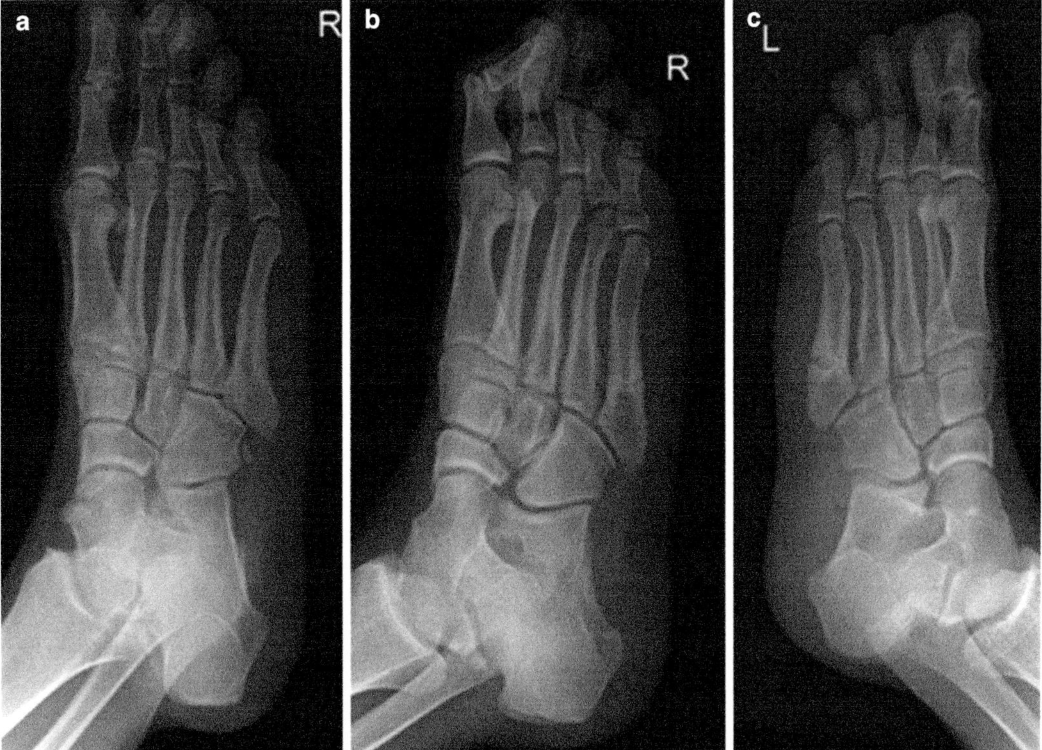

Fig. 30.4 Anteroposterior plain radiograph view of the three Torg types of MT 5 stress fractures in elite football players (**a** Torg 1, **b** Torg 2, **c** Torg 3)

there might be some overlap in the anatomical site of the injury, the site of a Jones fracture is typically more proximal than the classic fifth MT stress fracture. Delayed and non-union can also occur in type 3 fractures according to this classification, but these type 3 fractures are not typically stress fractures.

The differentiation between these two fracture types can be made by clinical examination and radiographs. Most stress fractures have prodromal signs, risk factors and a typical radiograph that differs from the clear radiolucent line in an acute fracture.

Fifth MT stress fractures have been classified by Torg in three types (Fig. 30.4) of which type 2 and 3 require surgical treatment ([26], Box 3). Several classifications have been introduced to cover all aspects of this MT 5 stress fracture type, location, imaging signs and amount of diastasis (Boxes 3–6).

Box 3 Classification for fifth metatarsal stress fractures (Torg et al.)

Type 1: periosteal reaction, early stress fracture (acute fracture lacking sclerosis)

Type 2: widened fracture line and intramedullary sclerosis, delayed union

Type 3: complete obliteration on intramedullary canal with sclerotic bone, established non-union

From Torg JS, Balduini FC, Zelko RR, et al. Fractures of the base of the fifth metatarsal distal to the tuberosity. Classification and guidelines for non-surgical and surgical management. J Bone Joint Surg Am 1984;66(2):209–14

Box 4 Classification for fifth metatarsal stress fractures (Logan et al.)

Type I: at the junction of extra- and intra-articular parts of the tuberosity
Type II: at the proximal fourth–fifth intermetatarsal joints
Type III: at the distal fourth–fifth intermetatarsal joints
Type IV: more distally in the diaphysis

From Logan AJ, Dabke H, Finlay D, et al. Fifth metatarsal base fractures: a simple classification. Foot Ankle Surg 2007;13(1):30–4

Box 5 Classification for fifth metatarsal stress fractures (Steward et al.)

Zone I: fracture involving the styloid process
Zone II: fracture involving the base (Jones' fracture)
Zone III: fracture involving the metaphysiodiaphyseal junction (stress fracture)

From Steward IM. Jones' fracture: fracture of base of fifth metatarsal. ClinOrthop 1960;16:190–8

Box 6 Classification for fifth metatarsal stress fractures (Lee et al.)

Type A: complete fracture
- A1: acute complete stress fracture
- A2: acute on chronic complete stress fracture

Type B: incomplete fracture
- B1: plantar gap <10 mm as measured on oblique radiograph
- B2: plantar gap >10 mm

From Lee KT, Kim KC, Park YU. Radiographic evaluation of foot structure following fifth metatarsal stress fracture. Foot Ankle Int 2011;32:796–801

30.3.6 Investigation

30.3.6.1 Vitamin D

In football, there is a growing awareness of the importance of the role of vitamin D levels, particularly in Northern Europe (even the elite players), with several studies showing hypovitaminosis (some among the lowest levels) especially in winter [27].

Fact Box 4
In female football players, enquire about specific risk factors such as menstrual disorders, eating disturbances and weight loss.

30.3.6.2 Radiograph

Weight-bearing AP, lateral and oblique views of the foot need to be included in the radiological request. The initial stage may not show any changes on radiograph, but at later stages, periosteal reaction and callus formation appear (Fig. 30.5). In the first MT, *periosteal reaction* is

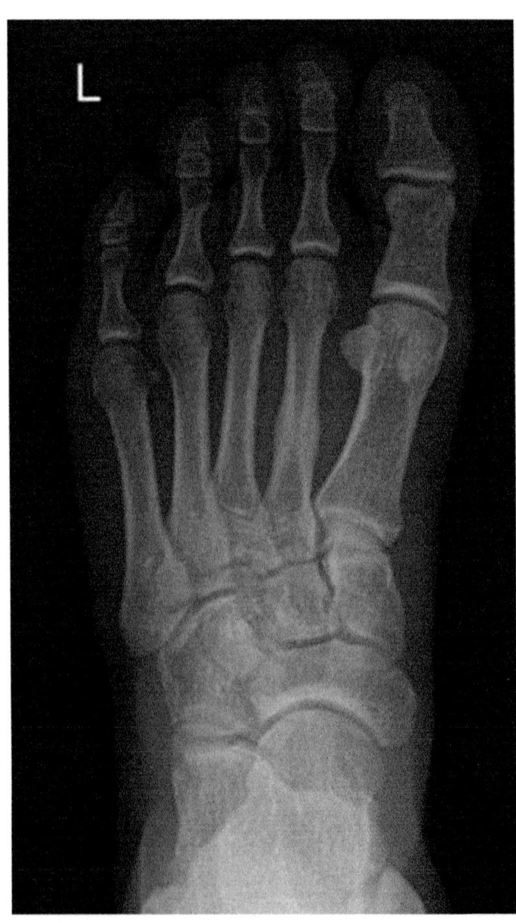

Fig. 30.5 Anteroposterior plain radiograph view of an MT 2 stress fracture in a national team football player. Note the periosteal reaction on the MT 2 shaft

uncommon but usually presents as *linear sclerosis*. About half of the MT stress fractures are unrecognized on plain radiographs, and (in case of clinical suspicion) it is advised to repeat radiographs after 2 weeks.

30.3.6.3 Ultrasound

Most professional football teams have direct access to ultrasound examination. Ultrasound is sensitive, is easily accessible and can identify early stress reaction. In case of a normal radiograph, it is advised to ask for an ultrasound to identify periosteal reaction and oedema since the bony stress reaction generally commences dorsally.

30.3.6.4 MRI

MRI is helpful especially in early cases in managing football players at risk. It allows early recognition of bony oedema before a fracture becomes evident and allows measures to be taken to prevent development of a frank stress fracture.

30.3.6.5 Bone Scan

When radiographs are negative and the clinical suspicion remains, a bone scan can be helpful to show changes in early phase of injury. In case of a stress fracture, it can be positive in all three phases, in contrast to soft tissue injury where it hypercaptates only in the first phase.

30.3.7 Treatment

Most MT stress fractures can be treated by conservative treatment. A detailed three-phase rehabilitation programme (that takes into account the physiology of stress fracture repair) allows the player to progress with gradual activity modification until symptoms subside [28].

Phase I (weeks 1–3): The emphasis of this phase is to remove stress, control pain and allow bone to commence healing with angiogenesis and periosteal and osteocyte maturation. Limited weight bearing with crutches is recommended. Patients can be provided with a hard-sole shoe, off-the-shelf walker boot or a short-leg walking cast. Ice massage may help improve swelling. Patients should be allowed to gradually increase weight bearing from partial to full weight bearing as tolerated. Lower extremity conditioning exercises are also recommended at this stage. These include towel toe curl, ankle isometrics, etc. This phase is taken to be completed when normal activities become pain-free.

Phase II (lasts for 2–3 weeks after resolution of pain): The focus of this stage is general conditioning and strengthening specific to the injured extremity. Ice compression is continued, pool training should progress from walking to jogging, and wobble board exercise can also include weight bearing. The aim of this phase is to be able to fully weight bear without pain for at least 30 min three times a week.

Phase III: Activities at this stage aim to allow gradual remodelling of the bone. This phase alternates with 2 weeks of gradually increasing stress followed by a week of rest. It is thought that alternating between stress and rest helps the osteocytes and periosteum to mature quicker at this stage. Patients are allowed for running and functional activities and progress to plyometrics [3, 28].

30.3.8 Surgery

Although surgery is mainly recommended in delayed union or non-union cases, surgery will be recommended for elite football players in selected cases to allow earlier return to play. Percutaneous, mini-open and open reduction and internal fixation techniques are available and used upon surgical preference. The combined use of a bone graft is generally recommended for management of delayed union and non-union and revision cases. Some reports promote immediate use of a bone graft in a primary case with good results and earlier return to play [3].

For the fifth MT Torg types II and III fractures and for stress fractures displaced more than 2 mm, surgery is recommended [26, 29]. The use of augmented autologous bone graft with intramedullary screw fixation may give better results compared to fixation without. A partially threaded

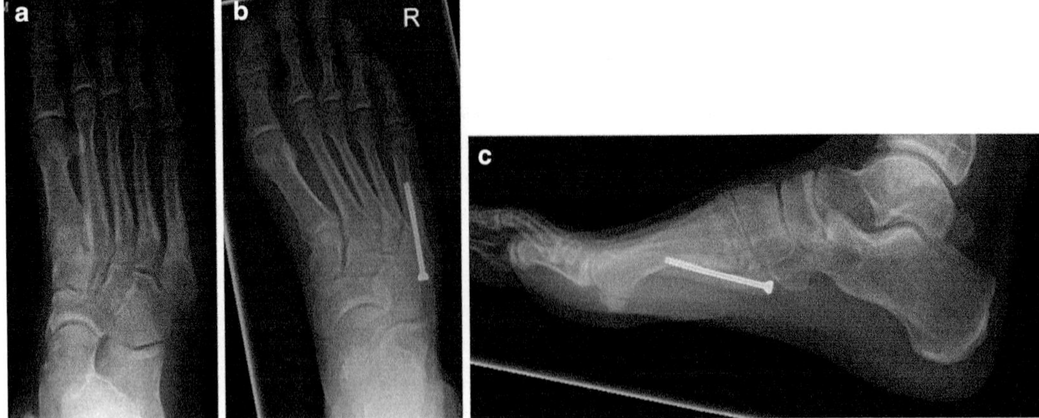

Fig. 30.6 Anteroposterior and lateral plain radiograph view of an MT 5 stress fractures in a national team football winger who was treated with a mini-open fixation technique using a 5 mm cannulated screw (**a** double stress fracture line, **b**, **c** 2.5 months postoperative)

cannulated screw is the gold standard although good results are reported with headless compression screws [30]. It is recommended to use the largest diameter cannulated screw that fits the width of the intramedullary canal with a minimum diameter of 4 mm, and the screw should be at least 50 mm in length ([31, 32], Fig. 30.6).

Proximally, the screw should avoid irritation to the cuboid or the fourth/fifth intermetatarsal joint. Due to the dorsal curvature of the proximal fifth MT, care must be taken that the screw tip aligns as closely as possible to the bone axis [31]. Postoperatively a non-weight-bearing cast or controlled ankle movement walker boot can be used to off-load the fifth MT in the initial recovery phase [33].

30.3.9 Complications

Delayed union and non-union are a specific point of concern in MT stress fractures in conservative treatment as well as surgery. The use of adjuvant bone grafting at the time of surgical fixation in acute stress fractures is therefore recommended in the football player ([30], Fig. 30.7). Early return to sports, increased body mass index and a protruding fifth MT [34] are known risk factors for recurrent fracture, and the role of podiatry is key to reduce this risk. The so-called plantar gap functions as a prognostic factor for time to union after surgical treatment of a fifth MT stress fracture. This "plantar gap" is the distance between the fracture margins on the plantar lateral side of the fifth MT bone and is best viewed on an oblique radiograph of the foot.

30.4 Player Load and Shoe-Surface Interaction in Fifth MT Stress Fractures

Among the modifiable risk factors for sustaining a fifth MT stress fracture, management of player load is of vital importance. Attention must be paid to prodromal "warning" signs (such as pain at lateral forefoot) following training or matches and subsequent modification of load prescribed to avoid stress fracture [1]. Monitoring player load (increasingly by GPS/accelerometer systems) is therefore important to identify relative "spikes" in workload.

Examination of the loading that occurs between the player and the surface at the shoe-surface interface can shed light on how fifth MT stress fractures may develop. The fifth MT bone experiences compressive, torsional and tension forces from the ground reaction forces and muscle/ligament/joint attachments. These forces incur bending moments on the bone during

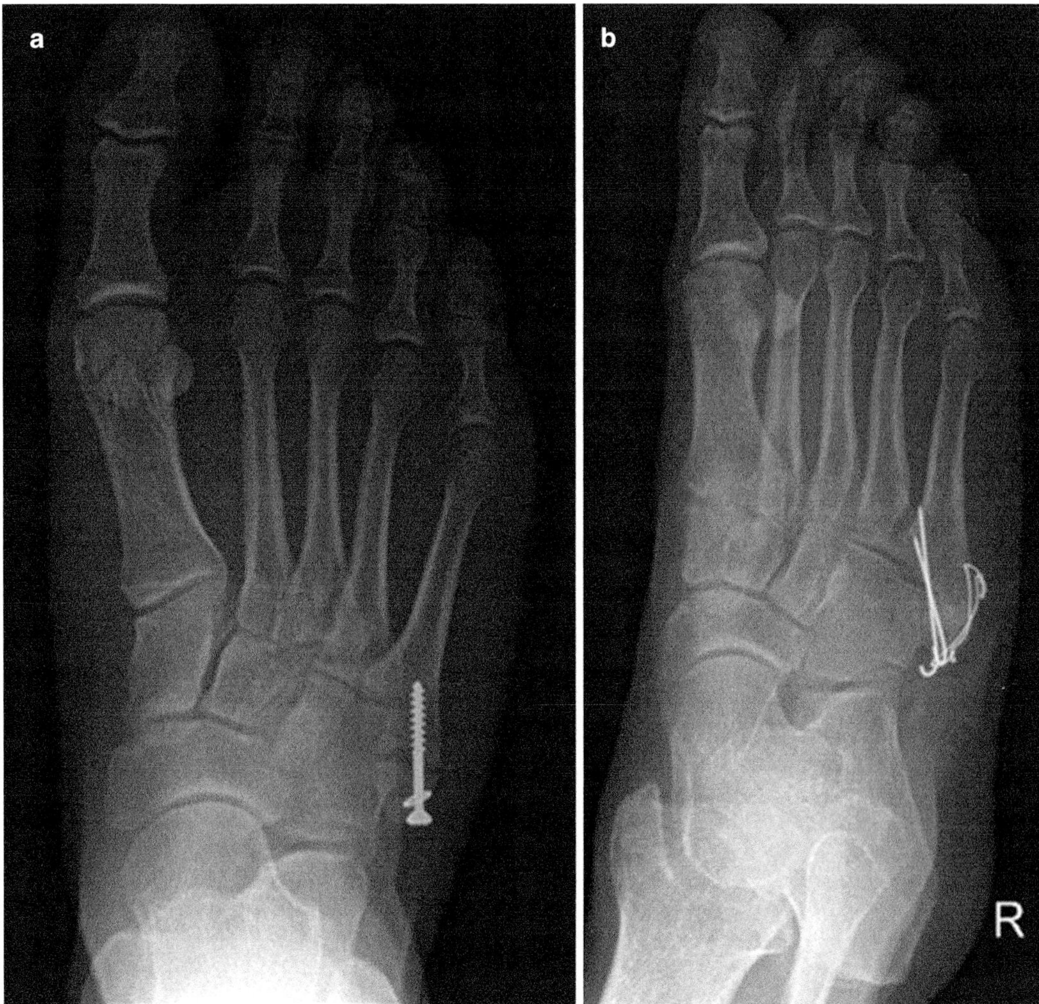

Fig. 30.7 Anteroposterior plain radiograph view of an MT 5 stress fracture in an elite football player who suffered from a non-union after fixation (**a**). He was treated with an iliac autologous bone graft interpositioning and tension band wire fixation and healed 3.5 months postoperatively (**b**)

football-specific movements. Studying the magnitude and timing of such forces will give insight to clinicians about the mechanical contributions to fifth MT stress fracture.

Certain football-specific movements have been studied using in-shoe pressure analysis, while the player performs a task on the field of play (Fig. 30.8a). Of the movements studied, plantar load is highest at the lateral forefoot during acceleration into a curved run, cross cutting task [35] and when performing a set-piece "corner" kick (at the stance leg) [36] (Fig. 30.8b). Conversely, straight-line running at a moderate to fast pace increases loading at the medial forefoot as does cutting [37]. Gender differences are apparent in some football-specific movements with an increase in plantar loading at the lateral foot in males when compared to females [38].

Fifth MT stress fractures are more common in the non-dominant or stance leg [39]. Plantar loading data may help explain why that is the case. Significantly higher force, pressure and relative loads occur at the lateral forefoot while performing a full-effort set-piece kick when compared to sprinting or cutting [36, 37]. Prodromal symptoms at the lateral foot should lead to a

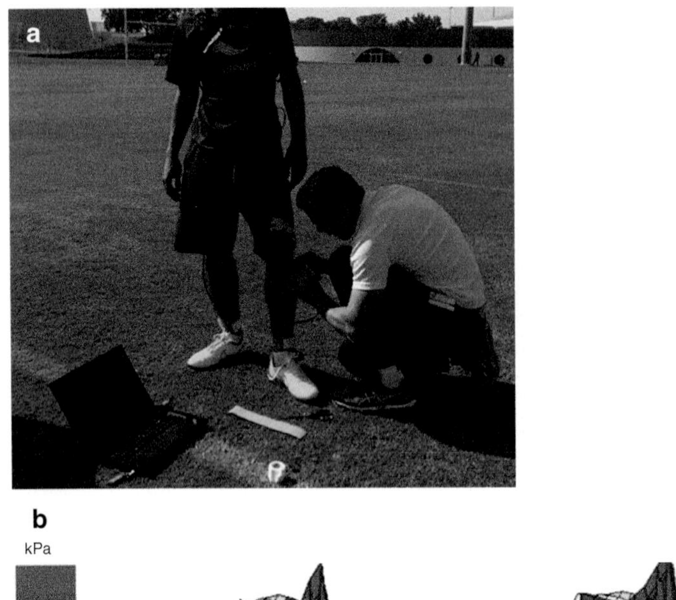

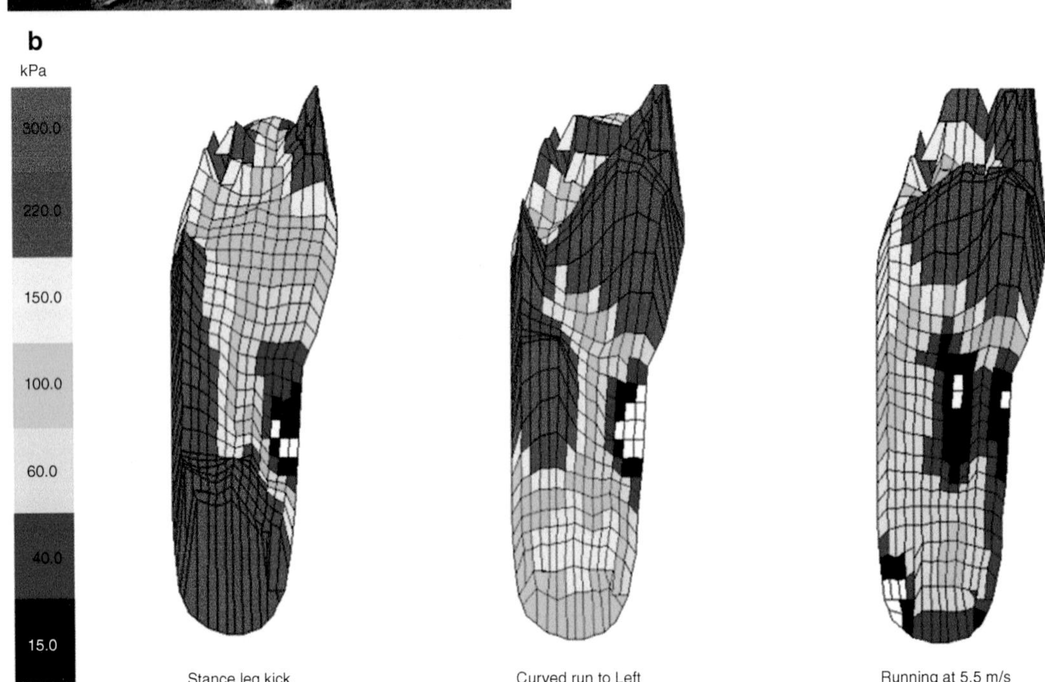

Fig. 30.8 (**a**) In-shoe plantar loading on the field of play (Novel PedarX). (**b**) Plantar loading in common football movements

reduction of tasks such as accelerated curved runs, crosses, corner and penalty kicks during training to decrease load at the fifth MT. Plantar loading data suggests that straight-line running (using running or turf shoes) may be continued at this time of "load modification" for fitness levels, as the medial aspect of the foot is under greater demand (Fig. 30.8b, [36, 37]). Further studies are required to assess if loading intervention at the prodromal sign stage is effective in preventing progression to stress fracture.

30.4.1 Surface

Recent advances in the preparation and maintenance of natural grass playing surfaces are changing the way the game is played. New hybrid pitches used in elite football allow for more consistent mechanical properties for player-surface interaction (traction and shock absorption) and ball-surface interaction (ball bounce and roll) and are less affected by weather conditions. However, due to the sand-based construction and reinforcement with artificial fibres, they may be harder than natural grass pitches of the past [40]. Surface hardness affects penetration of the studs or cleats on the outsole of football shoes. To avoid areas of high pressure under the fifth metatarsal, it is recommended that shoes be selected that allow adequate stud penetration for the given playing surface (Fig. 30.9).

30.4.2 Footwear

Greater impact forces, plantar pressure and loading rates occur when running in football shoes compared to training or turf shoes for a given surface [35, 41]. Turf shoes with forefoot cushioning and many multiple studs on the outsole are advised for players returning to training following fifth MT stress fracture.

Subjective comfort and fit of the shoe are important parameters especially the width of the stud plate on the outsole, the material properties of the outsole and the stud placement or configuration (Fig. 30.10).

In-shoe pressure analysis can be used to assess plantar pressures at the metatarsals for

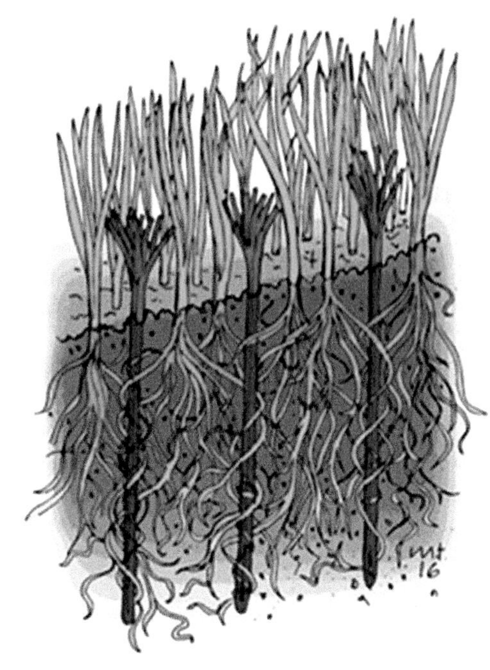

Fig. 30.9 Example of a hybrid playing surface. Sand-based root-zone with long artificial fibres (*dark green*) to reinforce the natural grass surface (Figure credit Mr. Mike Todd (Brisbane, Australia))

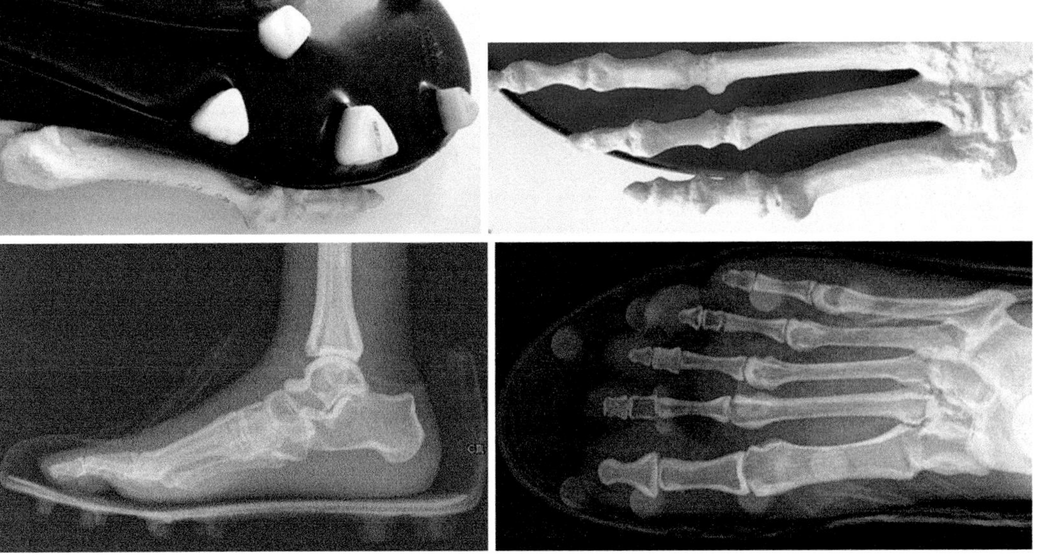

Fig. 30.10 The sole plate should be wide enough to accommodate the fifth MT and constructed from a material of adequate stiffness to prevent studs pushing through and causing high-localized pressure areas

individual player shoe-surface combinations to avoid stud placement that may be detrimental. In the absence of such technology, use of subjective comfort ratings from the player after running a functional traction course on the playing surface is advised [42].

Much debate remains over the effect blade-style cleats have on plantar loading and subsequent fifth MT stress fracture. Medical staff and football managers have expressed fears over blade-style cleats with a higher incidence of fifth metatarsal stress fractures being among the chief concerns [43, 44]. However, the findings are conflicting and unclear when comparing plantar loading and different stud or cleat types. With the natural anatomic variation seen in football players' feet, it is suggested footwear should be tailored to the individual in respect to shape, fit and stud placement. Player wellness monitoring should be utilized post training and matches to pick up on any prodromal signs after using new footwear.

30.4.3 Insoles, Orthoses and Rigid Carbon Inserts

Generic off-the-shelf foot orthoses with medial arch support increase the plantar forces and pressures at the fifth MT in basketball players [45]. It is unclear if these findings extend to football. Monitoring for prodromal symptoms at the fifth MT is recommended for any new orthotic or insole use to assess for changes in load.

Rigid carbon fibre inserts are ineffective at decreasing the plantar loading during side or cross-over cutting manoeuvres. Queen et al. [46] reported increased plantar loading at the lateral forefoot with carbon fibre inserts and as such advised caution with their use for rehabilitation following fifth MT stress fracture. It is possible that the rigid plates alter the bending moments at the fifth MT bone; however, this has not been measured to date. Raikin et al. [47] reported 0% refracture rate when using a rigid custom-made orthotic with lateral wedging that extends along the lateral forefoot in 20 patients post-surgery fixation for Jones fracture. It is recommended that any orthoses used in football shoes following fifth MT stress fracture be custom-made to the specific anatomical and biomechanical requirements of each player.

In summary, specific football shoe and insole combinations do alter plantar pressure at the fifth MT, and as such a tailored footwear/insole evaluation in which subjective and dynamic biomechanical data are combined may lead to optimal shoe/insole combinations that are both surface and subject specific [48].

Fact Box 5

Monitor for prodromal or "warning" signs at the fifth metatarsal following changes in training load, footwear, orthotic insoles or playing surface. Load modification is essential at this stage as certain football movements cause very high plantar loading at the lateral forefoot (Fig. 30.8b). The aim is to prevent progression to stress fracture.

30.5 Other Stress Fractures

- *Cuboid*: Most of the cuboid stress fractures occur in the *female* football player (Fig. 30.11). A potential predisposing factor to this entity is the cavus foot alignment and the hypermobile foot. The role of podiatry and tailored orthotics is key in treatment and prevention.
- *Talus*: A primarily undisplaced stress fracture of the talus is rare, but it is important for the clinician to be alerted on the possible secondary displacement (Fig. 30.12). Plain radiographs have a typically low diagnostic accuracy, and a high index of suspicion is necessary. Although treatment guidelines are not well defined, a 6 weeks NWB immobilization can be indicated. In case of secondary displacement signs, early surgical intervention is recommended to avoid the risk of increased morbidity (*Hawkins sign*) and delayed return to play [49].

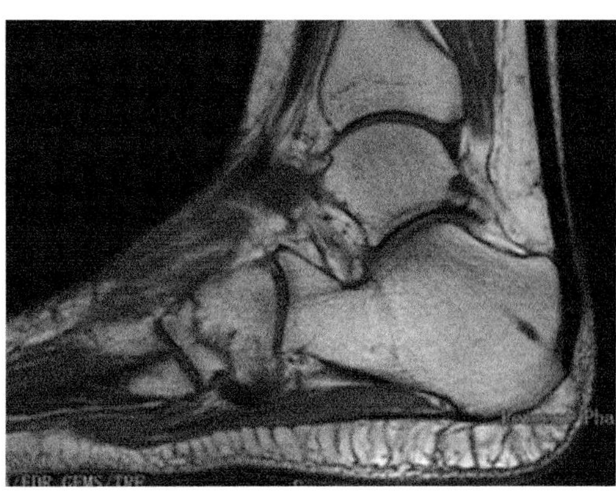

Fig. 30.11 Sagittal T1 MRI view of a cuboid stress fracture in a national league female football player

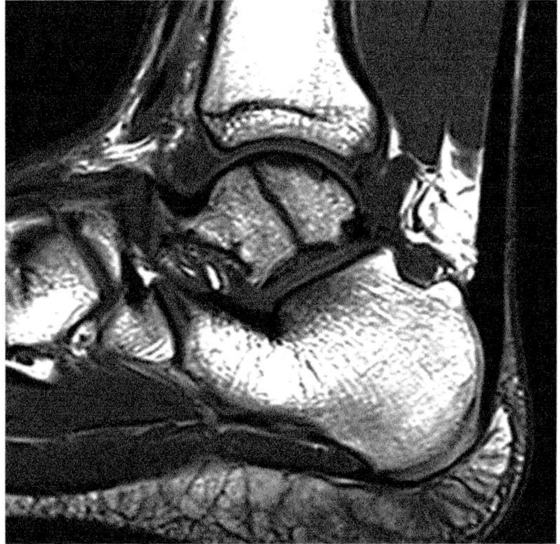

Fig. 30.12 Sagittal T1 MRI view of a talar body stress fracture in a 16-year-old youth national team football player

- *Calcaneal*: These stress fractures are infrequent and occur mainly preseason and during long-distance running in training. They present with pain, and 2–3 weeks after the onset of symptoms, a sclerotic or radiolucent line often appears on the radiograph. MRI is the best tool to identify early oedema and visualize the fracture line. The differential diagnosis includes plantar fasciitis, Achilles tendinopathy, Baxter nerve entrapment and retrocalcaneal bursitis. Calcaneal stress fractures can be managed with activity modification alone (no cast or surgery required).
- *Sesamoid*: Typically, the *medial* sesamoid is affected by stress fractures. Plain radiographs can be difficult to interpret, and the use of a CT scan is advised in case of clinical suspicion. Normally, conservative management with rest, boot, orthotics, injection and progressive loading is standard. In the salvage case where surgery is required, a partial sesamoidectomy is the treatment of choice. Prediction towards return to play is difficult to predict, and the player must be informed [1].

Fact Box 6

The major pitfalls in the diagnosis and management of stress fractures are:

1. Inadequate clinical workup: failure to identify the prodromal symptoms of stress fractures and failure to localize the site of bony tenderness upon palpation
2. Reliance on plain radiographs alone for the diagnosis of foot stress fractures
3. Failure to identify the "high-risk" stress fractures from the "low-risk" stress fractures (Table 30.3)
4. Failure to identify and rectify the extrinsic risk factors which may predispose to stress fractures (Table 30.1)

30.6 General Principles in the Treatment of Foot Stress Fractures That Are Commonly Extrapolated to Football

A football-induced stress fracture occurs when the mechanical forces during training or gameplay outweigh the biological abilities of the bone. Since the foot is key for performance in football, it is therefore essential to ensure that the forces are minimized and the biology is optimized.

30.6.1 Biomechanical Therapy for Stress Fractures

The major components in the treatment of any stress fracture are "rest" and "activity modification". Especially during in-season in football, a team approach (medical staff, coach, agent, director) is key in the management of setting up treatment goals and return to play criteria. Although this sometimes means to temporarily unload and immobilize a player, cycling, rowing, swimming and even specific running (to maintain cardiovascular fitness and lower limb strength) can be continued. The focus should be on altering the nature of the training, individualizing the programme and type of surface and shoe. Hydrotherapy and antigravity treadmill are useful in this stage to keep the player's fitness while allowing the stress fracture to heal. Careful evaluation of malalignment, muscular imbalance and abnormal loading patterns needs to be assessed and corrected meanwhile.

30.6.2 Biological Therapy in the Management of Stress Fractures

Several adjuvant treatment strategies, such as bone morphogenetic protein (BMP), shock wave therapy (ESWT), low-intensity pulsed ultrasound therapy (LIPUS), teriparatide, electromagnetic stimulation and hyperbaric oxygen, have been recommended in the literature to enhance stress fracture healing. Controversy remains due to the heterogeneity of patient populations, the interventions offered as well as the different outcome measures considered. In addition, most of the published reports are case series instead of controlled trials.

30.6.3 Shock Wave Therapy (ESWT)

ESWT can have a role in the upregulation of local angiogenesis and concentration of growth factors. Although quality research is lacking, ESWT has shown improved healing potential and earlier return to play in chronic and non-union cases [50, 51].

30.6.4 Low-Intensity Pulsed Ultrasound Therapy (LIPUS)

LIPUS has been introduced in the world of football as a promising alternative to treat non-union or delayed union. A recent systematic review however concluded that LIPUS does not reduce the time to return to activity for conservatively treated stress fractures [52].

30.6.5 Electrical Stimulation (ES)

There is laboratory evidence that endochondral bone formation and growth factor expression may be appropriately stimulated by the application of an electromagnetic field. Electrical stimulation (ES) therapy can be provided via several modes: direct current, capacitive coupling, inductive coupling and pulsed electromagnetic field. Although in football the pressure can be high to try out these "new tools", there is little evidence for the use of ES in the management of stress fractures [53].

30.6.6 Bone Morphogenetic Protein

BMPs belong to "transforming growth factor b superfamily proteins" and act as osteoinductive agents to enhance fracture healing. Several BMPs have been isolated like BMP2 and BMP7 that are subjected to clinical trials. In stress fractures, there is no evidence to support the use of BMP's [53].

30.6.7 Teriparatide

Teriparatide is a bone anabolic agent (recombinant human parathyroid hormone analogue) used in the treatment of osteoporosis by stimulating osteoblasts. A recent RCT showed that it can shorten the time to fracture healing compared to placebo but no credible data in *stress fractures* is available yet [3, 54].

Take-Home Message

- Stress fractures are common in athletes and have specific characteristics in football.
- A high index of suspicion is appropriate, and early investigation may prevent progression to frank fractures and delayed return to play in football.
- Both navicular and fifth metatarsal (MT) stress fractures are considered high-risk fractures where early surgery may be indicated in the early phase.
- There is limited evidence at present for biological treatment of stress fractures, but biological agents may be useful adjuncts.
- Identification and alleviation of risk factors are essential parts of management of stress fractures.

Top Five Evidence Based References

D'Hooghe P, Wiegerinck JI, Tol JL, Landreau PA (2015) 22-year-old professional soccer player with atraumatic ankle pain. Br J Sports Med 49(24):1589–1590

Ekstrand J, van Dijk CN (2013) Fifth metatarsal fractures among male professional footballers: a potential career-ending disease. Br J Sports Med 47(12):754–758

Saxena A, Fullem B, Hannaford D (2000) Results of treatment of 22 navicular stress fractures and a new proposed radiographic classification system. J Foot Ankle Surg 39(2):96–103

Torg JS, Balduini FC, Zelko RR et al (1984) Fractures of the base of the fifth metatarsal distal to the tuberosity. Classification and guidelines for non-surgical and surgical management. J Bone Joint Surg Am 66(2):209–214

Torstveit M, Sundgot-Borgen J (2005) The elite female athlete triad: are elite athletes at increased risk? Med Sci Sports Exerc 37:184–193

References

1. Ekstrand J, van Dijk CN (2013) Fifth metatarsal fractures among male professional footballers: a potential career-ending disease. Br J Sports Med 47(12):754–758
2. Torstveit M, Sundgot-Borgen J (2005) The elite female athlete triad: are elite athletes at increased risk? Med Sci Sports Exerc 37:184–193
3. Hossain M, Clutton J, Ridgewell M, Lyons K, Perera A (2015) Stress fractures of the foot. Clin Sports Med 34:769–790
4. Mann JA, Pedowitz DI (2009) Evaluation and treatment of navicular stress fractures, including nonunions, revision surgery, and persistent pain after treatment. Foot Ankle Clin 14(2):187–204
5. Kapandji IA (1970) The physiology of the joints: annotated diagrams of the mechanics of the human joints, 2nd edn. Churchill Livingstone, London
6. vanLangelaan EJ (1983) A kinematical analysis of the tarsal joints. An X-ray photogram- metric study. Acta Orthop Scand Suppl 204:1–269
7. Lee S, Anderson RB (2004) Stress fractures of the tarsal navicular. Foot Ankle Clin 9(1):85–104
8. Saxena A, Fullem B, Hannaford D (2000) Results of treatment of 22 navicular stress fractures and a new proposed radiographic classification system. J Foot Ankle Surg 39(2):96–103
9. Tuthill HL, Finkelstein ER, Sanchez AM et al (2014) Imaging of tarsal navicular disorders: a pictorial review. Foot Ankle Spec 7(3):211–225
10. Fowler JR, Gaughan JP, Boden BP et al (2011) The non-surgical and surgical treatment of tarsal navicular stress fractures. Sports Med 41(8):613–619
11. Khan KM, Fuller PJ, Brukner PD et al (1992) Outcome of conservative and surgical management of navicular stress fracture in athletes. Eighty-six cases proven with computerized tomography. Am J Sports Med 20(6):657–666
12. Torg JS, Moyer J, Gaughan JP et al (2010) Management of tarsal navicular stress fractures: conservative versus surgical treatment: a meta-analysis. Am J Sports Med 38(5):1048–1053
13. Jacob KM, Paterson RS (2013) Navicular stress fractures treated with minimally invasive fixation. Indian J Orthop 47(6):598–601
14. Fitch KD, Blackwell JB, Gilmour WN (1989) Operation for non-union of stress fracture of the tarsal navicular. J Bone Joint Surg Br 71(1):105–110
15. Choi LE, Chou LB (2006) Surgical treatment of tarsal navicular stress fractures. Oper Tech Sports Med 14(4):248–251
16. Saxena A, Fullem B (2006) Navicular stress fractures: a prospective study on athletes. Foot Ankle Int 27(11):917–921
17. Burne SG, Mahoney CM, Forster BB et al (2005) Tarsal navicular stress injury: long- term outcome and clinicoradiological correlation using both computed tomography and magnetic resonance imaging. Am J Sports Med 33(12):1875–1881
18. Davidson G, Pizzari T, Mayes S (2007) The influence of second toe and metatarsal length on stress fractures at the base of the second metatarsal in classical dancers. Foot Ankle Int 28(10):1082–1086
19. Kaipel M, Krapf D, Wyss C (2011) Metatarsal length does not correlate with maximal peak pres-

sure and maximal force. Clin Orthop Relat Res 469(4):1161–1166
20. Arangio GA, Beam H, Kowalczyk G et al (1998) Analysis of stress in the metatarsals. Foot Ankle Surg 4:123–128
21. Harato K, Ozaki M, Sakurai A et al (2014) Stress fracture of the first metatarsal after total knee arthroplasty: two case reports using gait analysis. Knee 21(1):328–331
22. Watson HI, O'Donnell B, Hopper GP et al (2013) Proximal base stress fracture of the second metatarsal in a Highland dancer. BMJ Case Rep 2013
23. Chuckpaiwong B, Cook C, Pietrobon R et al (2007) Second metatarsal stress fracture in sport: comparative risk factors between proximal and non-proximal locations. Br J Sports Med 41(8):510–514
24. Saxena A, Krisdakumtorn T, Erickson S (2001) Proximal fourth metatarsal injuries in athletes: similarity to proximal fifth metatarsal injury. Foot Ankle Int 22(7):603–608
25. Rongstad KM, Tueting J, Rongstad M et al (2013) Fourth metatarsal base stress fractures in athletes: a case series. Foot Ankle Int 34(7):962–968
26. Torg JS, Balduini FC, Zelko RR et al (1984) Fractures of the base of the fifth metatarsal distal to the tuberosity. Classification and guidelines for non-surgical and surgical management. J Bone Joint Surg Am 66(2):209–214
27. Clutton J, Perera A (2016) Insufficiency and deficiency of vitamin D in patients with fractures of the fifth metatarsal. Foot (Edinb) 27:50–52
28. Romani WA, Gieck JH, Perrin DH et al (2002) Mechanisms and management of stress fractures in physically active persons. J Athl Train 37(3):306–314
29. Logan AJ, Dabke H, Finlay D et al (2007) Fifth metatarsal base fractures: a simple classification. Foot Ankle Surg 13(1):30–34
30. Nagao M, Saita Y, Kameda S et al (2012) Headless compression screw fixation of jones fractures: an outcomes study in Japanese athletes. Am J Sports Med 40(11):2578–2582
31. Tsukada S, Ikeda H, Seki Y et al (2012) Intramedullary screw fixation with bone autografting to treat proximal fifth metatarsal metaphyseal-diaphyseal fracture in athletes: a case series. Sports Med Arthrosc Rehabil Ther Technol 4(1):25
32. Ochenjele G, Ho B, Switaj PJ et al (2015) Radiographic study of the fifth metatarsal for optimal intramedullary screw fixation of Jones fracture. Foot Ankle Int 36(3):293–301
33. Hunt KJ, Goeb Y, Esparza R et al (2014) Site-specific loading at the fifth metatarsal base in rehabilitative devices: implications for Jones fracture treatment. PM R 6(11):1022–1029
34. Lee KT, Park YU, Jegal H et al (2013) Factors associated with recurrent fifth metatarsal stress fracture. Foot Ankle Int 34(12):1645–1653
35. Queen RM, Charnock BL, Garrett WE et al (2008) A comparison of cleat types during two football-specific tasks on fieldturf. Br J Sports Med 42(4):278–84; discussion 284
36. Thomson A, Akenhead R, D'hooghe P, et al (2017) Plantar loading in elite male football players with 5th metatarsal fracture. (In review) .
37. Eils E, Streyl M, Linnenbecker S et al (2004) Characteristic plantar pressure distribution patterns during soccer-specific movements. Am J Sports Med 32(1):140–145
38. Sims EL, Hardaker WM, Queen RM (2008) Gender differences in plantar loading during three soccer-specific tasks. Br J Sports Med 42(4):272–277
39. Fujitaka K, Taniguchi A, Isomoto S et al (2015) Pathogenesis of fifth metatarsal fractures in college soccer players. Orthop J Sports Med 3(9):2325967115603654
40. Thomson A, Rennie D (2016) Evolution of natural grass playing surfaces for elite football. Aspetar J 5(2)
41. Smith N, Dyson R, Janaway L (2004) Ground reaction force measures when running in soccer boots and soccer training shoes on a natural turf surface. Sports Eng 73:159–167
42. Sterzing T, Müller C, Hennig EM et al (2009) Actual and perceived running performance in soccer shoes: a series of eight studies. Footwear Sci 1(1):5–17
43. Bentley JA, Ramanathan AK, Arnold GP, Wang W, Abboud RJ (2011) Harmful cleats of football boots: a biomechanical evaluation. Foot Ankle Surg 17(3):140–144
44. Jain N, Murray D, Kemp S et al (2012) Foot & ankle injuries in elite professional footballers: the findings of one English Premier League team. J Bone Joint Surg Br 94:249–249
45. Yu B, Preston JJ, Queen RM, Byram IR, Hardaker WM, Gross MT et al (2007) Effects of wearing foot orthosis with medial arch support on the fifth metatarsal loading and ankle inversion angle in selected basketball tasks. J Orthopaed Sports Phys Ther 37(12):186–191
46. Queen RM, Abbey AN, Verma R et al (2014) Plantar loading during cutting while wearing a rigid carbon fiber insert. J Athl Train 49(3):297–303
47. Raikin SM, Slenker N, Ratigan B (2008) The association of a varushindfoot and fracture of the fifth metatarsal metaphyseal-diaphyseal junction: the jones fracture. Am J Sports Med 36(7):1367–1372
48. Nunns MP, Dixon SJ, Clarke J, Carré M (2015) Boot-insole effects on comfort and plantar loading at the heel and fifth metatarsal during running and turning in soccer. J Sports Sci 22:1–8
49. D'Hooghe P, Wiegerinck JI, Tol JL, Landreau PA (2015) 22-year-old professional soccer player with atraumatic ankle pain. Br J Sports Med 49(24):1589–1590. (Free Article)
50. Moretti B, Notarnicola A, Garofalo R et al (2009) Shock waves in the treatment of stress fractures. Ultrasound Med Biol 35(6):1042–1049
51. Furia JP, Rompe JD, Cacchio A et al (2010) Shock wave therapy as a treatment of non-unions, avascular

necrosis, and delayed healing of stress fractures. Foot Ankle Clin 15(4):651–662
52. Busse JW, Kaur J, Mollon B et al (2009) Low intensity pulsed ultrasonography for fractures: systematic review of randomised controlled trials. BMJ 338:b351
53. Beck BR, Matheson GO, Bergman G et al (2008) Do capacitively coupled electric fields accelerate tibial stress fracture healing? A randomized controlled trial. Am J Sports Med 36(3):545–553
54. Raghavan P, Christofides E (2012) Role of teriparatide in accelerating metatarsal stress fracture healing: a case series and review of literature. Clin Med Insights Endocrinol Diabetes 5(5):39–45

Return to Play in Stress Fractures of the Hip, Thigh, Knee, and Leg

31

Hélder Pereira, Duarte Sousa, Pieter d'Hooghe, Sérgio Gomes, Joaquim Miguel Oliveira, Rui L. Reis, João Espregueira-Mendes, Pedro L. Ripoll, and Kenneth Hunt

Contents

H. Pereira (✉) • J.M. Oliveira
3B's Research Group–Biomaterials, Biodegradables and Biomimetics, University of Minho, Headquarters of the European Institute of Excellence on Tissue Engineering and Regenerative Medicine, AvePark, Parque de Ciência e Tecnologia, Zona Industrial da Gandra, 4805-017 Barco, Guimarães, Portugal

ICVS/3B's–PT Government Associate Laboratory, Braga, Guimarães, Portugal

Orthopedic Department, Centro Hospitalar Póvoa de Varzim, Vila do Conde, Portugal

Ripoll y De Prado Sports Clinic—FIFA Medical Centre of Excellence, Murcia, Madrid, Spain

International Sports Traumatology Centre of Ave, Taipas Termal, Caldas das Taipas, Portugal

Dom Henrique Research Centre, Porto, Portugal
e-mail: helderduartepereira@gmail.com

V. Musahl et al. (eds.), *Return to Play in Football*, https://doi.org/10.1007/978-3-662-55713-6_31

D. Sousa
Orthopedic Department, Centro Hospitalar Póvoa de Varzim, Vila do Conde, Portugal

P. d'Hooghe
Department of Orthopaedic Surgery, ASPETAR Orthopaedic and Sports Medicine Hospital, Aspire Zone, Doha, Qatar

S. Gomes
International Sports Traumatology Centre of Ave, Taipas Termal, Caldas das Taipas, Portugal

Clínica do Dragão, Espregueira-Mendes Sports Centre—FIFA Medical Centre of Excellence, Porto, Portugal

R.L. Reis
3B's Research Group–Biomaterials, Biodegradables and Biomimetics, University of Minho, Headquarters of the European Institute of Excellence on Tissue Engineering and Regenerative Medicine, AvePark, Parque de Ciência e Tecnologia, Zona Industrial da Gandra, 4805-017 Barco, Guimarães, Portugal

ICVS/3B's–PT Government Associate Laboratory, Guimarães, Braga, Portugal

J. Espregueira-Mendes

Clínica do Dragão, Espregueira-Mendes Sports Centre—FIFA Medical Centre of Excellence, Porto, Portugal

Dom Henrique Research Centre, Porto, Portugal

3B's Research Group–Biomaterials, Biodegradables and Biomimetics, Headquarters of the European Institute of Excellence on Tissue Engineering and Regenerative Medicine, University of Minho, AvePark, Parque de Ciência e Tecnologia, Zona Industrial da Gandra, Barco, 4805-017 Guimarães, Portugal

ICVS/3B's–PT Government Associate Laboratory, Guimarães, Braga, Portugal

Department of Orthopaedic, Minho University, Braga, Portugal

P.L. Ripoll
Ripoll y De Prado Sports Clinic—FIFA Medical Centre of Excellence, Murcia, Madrid, Spain

K. Hunt
Department of Orthopaedic Surgery, University of Colorado School of Medicine, Aurora, CO, USA

31.1 Introduction

31.1.1 Epidemiology and Clinical Presentation

In brief, "stress fractures" occur when a normal (or pathologic) bone is incapable of recovery from repeated strains that occur during physical activity [1]. Typically, such fractures have been linked to specific groups like military personnel or athletes from running and jumping sports, but in fact they can occur in anybody from general population [2].

The relationship between these fractures and military has historical origins. The first description of such injuries comes from the nineteenth century and was described as the "swollen feet syndrome" found after long marches in Prussian soldiers. Such swelling was demonstrated to be due to metatarsal stress fractures [3].

The incidence among military recruits varies from 5% to 30% per year, and it has been shown to be significantly higher among women [2, 4, 5].

Among athletes (nonmilitary), the incidence ranges from 1.1% to 31% per year and is highest among long-distance runners [2, 6–8]. Such fractures represent 10–20% of sports injuries due to overtraining [9–11]. They can affect any bone; however, it has been recognized that 90% of these are lower extremity stress fractures (Fact Box 1) [12]. The most affected bone in footballers is the fifth metatarsal, and the second most affected is the tibia [10, 13–15].

Regardless of competitive level, football is one of the most frequent sports worldwide [16]. Thus, football-related injuries have a high socioeconomic impact [17, 18]. Moreover, concerning high-level athletes, injuries lead to absence from competition (with all related consequences), costs related to treatment, and potential endangerment of an athlete's career [17].

Despite the former, there remains limited data and research in this topic related to footballers [1, 19–24]. In a recent study on elite male football players, stress fractures accounted for 0.5% of all injuries, and the incidence was 0.04/1000 h [19]. Thus, one might conclude that a team with 25–28 players could expect a stress fracture every third season [19]. Another study reinforces the influence of gender as risk factor, finding a 13.6% incidence of stress fractures among female football players [22].

Fact Box 1

Distribution of lower extremity stress fractures in male footballers [19]	
Stress fracture site	Frequency (%)
Fifth metatarsal	78.4
Tibia	11.7
Pelvis	5.8
Tarsal bones	1.9
Fibula	1.9

31.1.1.1 Clinical Presentation

The early diagnosis of a stress fracture relies on a careful clinical history and physical examination. The team physician must be aware of prodromal symptoms before the onset of more serious injuries. Typically, patients with stress fractures present with insidious onset of localized pain. The athlete's complaints often correlate with, or are aggravated by, physical activity and are relieved by rest, reappearing after repeated effort. The absence of rest pain helps on differential diagnosis of stress fractures with a variety of conditions, including inflammatory processes, acute fractures, and tumors.

Many times, there is a history of change/increase in vigor of training/physical activity, change in pattern or effort, change in footwear, or a different training field (e.g., harder surfaces) [1, 25]. Athletes with stress fractures might experience pain on palpation or strain on the involved bone—the athlete typically recognizes the pain he/she feels after the activity when the examiner presses over [26]. Swelling, redness, or warmth may or may not be present.

31.1.2 Mechanism of Injury, Risk Factors, High- Versus Low-Risk Injuries

The skeleton is subjected to several types of forces during motion and activity. The human bone follows *Wolff's law*, which describes the way this tissue will adapt to mechanical stress [27]. As the force acting on bone rises, it will deform accordingly, given the inherent elasticity of the tissue. If loading on a particular bone increases, the bone will remodel itself over time in order to become stronger and to be capable to resist that kind of stress. The internal architecture of the tissue suffers adaptive modifications (e.g., temporary elastic deformation), followed by secondary changes to the external cortical portion of the bone, which can become thicker as a result. The inverse is also true: if the loading on a bone decreases, the bone will become less dense and weaker due to the lack of the stimulus required for continued remodeling. Thus, balance is required to promote a healthy bone [28].

When the bone is exposed to forces within its capacity to support them, it undergoes elastic deformation, recovering its histological configuration as soon as the load discontinues. However, when these strains exceed bone's resistance, the elastic deformation is superseded by plastic deformation: there is no return to the previous situation, and, in case the repetitive forces remain, microfractures can occur. In such cases, bone reabsorption will occur.

Once this balance is disrupted (e.g., consecutive microtrauma without permitting the bone to recover completely from the initial stress) and microtrauma accumulates, a "stress fracture" can occur [28].

According to the described mechanism, stress fractures occur in three phases: microfracture, propagation of the microfracture, and complete fracture [28, 29]. Such fractures typically occur in places submitted to high tension [25, 27, 29, 30]. This is different from the mechanism involved on a normal acute fracture. In this case, a single load exceeds the bony resistance and crates a failure of the tissue. Opposing, stress fractures typically derive from repeated microtauma. In these cases, not only the strain intensity but also its frequency and duration, among other physical conditions, are determinant [31–33].

There are still a number of questions to be answered concerning the precise conditions, which might lead to these injuries, thus enabling improved prevention strategies and early diagnosis. However, several risk factors (intrinsic and extrinsic) have been identified, for example, gender and a predilection for young people and athletes [34]. Fact Box 2 summarizes the risk factors which gather higher level of scientific support [1].

Fact Box 2 (Based on [1])

Important risk factors for "stress fractures"	
Intrinsic factors	Extrinsic factors
Diminished physical activity	Changes in training program
Low "body mass index" and low bone mineral density	Running on hard surfaces
Age: In men, the incidence lowers above the age of 17 In women, the incidence increases after the menarche	Long-distance runners
Diminished muscle strength	Alcohol
Anatomical factors: e.g., leg-length discrepancy, low cross-sectional area	Smoking
Eating disorders	Low vitamin D levels
Menstrual dysfunction	

31.1.2.1 Risk Factors

Several intrinsic and extrinsic risk factors have been proposed [1]. Extrinsic factors include change in training program, sports on hard surfaces, and type of sports (e.g., long-distance runners) [35–37]. The influence of shoewear has been proposed but remains somewhat controversial with some discrepancies in literature [1]. In a recent study, it was proposed that a sports shoe with more than 6 months of regular use and training in hard surfaces increases the risk of stress injuries by diminishing the capacity to dissipate energy when the foot strikes the pitch [38]. Caffeine, alcohol, and tobacco can also increase the risk for bone stress injury [39].

Intrinsic factors that have been proposed include gender (female with higher risk), age (higher in young ages), physical condition, anatomic features, and history of previous stress fractures [34, 40–42]. Most studies suggest that females have higher risk of stress fractures, in part related to the "female athlete triad" [43]. In addition, differences among genders also include lower cross-sectional bone area and neuromuscular response [44, 45].

Other intrinsic factors include leg-length discrepancy, history of previous surgeries or trauma, hyperlaxity, instability, and muscle weakness [10, 46, 47]. Muscle weakness has been considered an important risk factor once muscles help to dissipate the energy thus lowering strain transmitted to bone during running or jumping [48]. This theory has been described as the "neuromuscular hypothesis" [28, 37]. Training overload with short recovery times might lead to overtraining [49]. This condition increases risk of bone stress injury and leads to paradoxical lowering of performance [50].

Finally, some stress fractures have been linked to specific anatomic features. For example, tibial stress fractures have been linked to anatomic conditions such as *cavus* foot, smaller tibial bone, and foot overpronation [51, 52].

31.1.2.2 High-Risk and Low-Risk Stress Fractures

High-risk injuries occur on the side of maximal tension (e.g., tension-sided femoral neck fractures, anterior tibial diaphyseal fractures, tension-sided patellar fractures) and hypovascular zones [53, 54]. High-risk lesions have higher probability for longer recovery; are more prone to progression to complete fracture, delayed union, and chronic pain [53, 54]; and more often require surgical treatment [1].

31.2 Imaging of Lower Extremity Stress Fractures

31.2.1 Radiographies

Given the low cost and availability, plain radiographs are usually the first imaging exam to be performed. Plain radiographs provide important anatomic information and can identify cortical thickening, impingement lesions, and displaced fractures. However, they have very low sensitivity for stress fractures, particularly in the first 3–4 weeks, particularly in the presence of osteopenia [25, 55, 56]. Stress fractures can sometimes be seen as a subtle linear sclerosis, focal endosteal or periosteal reaction, or a fracture overlapped and hidden by a periosteal reaction [25]. So, a negative X-ray cannot exclude a stress fracture. Sometimes the X-ray will be positive later in the course (typically weeks to months) showing bone callus and remodeling in the later phase of this condition (possibly much latter than the full clinical recovery) [57]. If there is the clinical suspicion and a negative X-ray, another imaging exam should be obtained (e.g., MRI, bone scan, or CT) [58].

31.2.2 Bone Scan

Three-phase bone scintigraphy used to be the gold standard given its high sensitivity in detecting the early phases of stress fractures (detects the increased metabolic activity around the injury site) [59]. However, bone scintigraphy is accompanied by a high level of inherent radiation and very low specificity with up to 40% of false positives [60]. It cannot distinguish from inflammatory processes, infection, or tumor diseases [58]. Moreover, it can show increased uptake in the injury site up to 2 years after an injury is clinically resolved [60].

31.2.3 CT Scan

Computed tomography (CT) scans can be highly valuable for assessment of bone stress injuries, despite exposing patients to radiation. In the scope of stress fractures, CT scans remain useful in sacral fractures and spondylolysis and in differentiating tumors, infection, or bone stress reaction from stress fractures [58].

31.2.4 MRI

MRI is currently the most used imaging exam given its high sensitivity and specificity (ranging from 85% to 100%) [9, 61, 62]. Under the clinical suspicion of bone stress injury, negative plain radiography, and pain without defined etiology, MRI is the first-line exam [63]. It is possible to identify fracture lines hypointense in T1 and T2 sequences, usually combined with bone marrow edema, and hyperintensity in surrounding soft tissue on SatFat or STIR sequences [33]. The presence of bone edema is not specific but is highly sensitive for stress reaction [33]. MRI assessment besides confirming the diagnosis is usually helpful in determining the severity of the condition. In this way, it also helps in the decision for choice of treatment and can be useful in deciding the timing to return to play (by assessing the severity of the lesion). One of the most used classifications for tibial stress fractures characteristics in MRI has been described by Fredericson and others [33, 64–68]. Table 31.1 represents the Fredericson classification as one example of how MRI can be used to assess the most common type of stress fracture herein described (tibial). Table 31.2 summarizes another classification method based on MRI and used as guideline for treatment [64].

Table 31.1 MRI Fredericson classification for tibial stress fractures

Grade	Periosteal edema	Marrow STIR SI	Marrow T1 SI	Intracortical sign
0	No	Normal	Normal	Normal
1	Yes	Normal	Normal	Normal
2	Yes	High	Normal	Normal
3	Yes	High	Low	Normal
4°	Yes	High	Low	Focal abnormality
4b	Yes	High	Low	Linear fracture

STIR short-TI inversion recovery; *SI* signal intensity [65]

Table 31.2 Stages/grades of Arendt and Griffiths [64] for stress fracture, based on magnetic resonance imaging (MRI) findings and correlation with period of rest required

Classification of Arendt and Griffiths		
Grade of injury	MRI findings	Required period of rest (weeks)
I	STIR-positive	3
II	STIR and T2-weighted positive images	3–6
III	T1- and T2-positive without definition of cortical rupture	12–16
IV	T1- and T2-positive with definition of cortical rupture and visible fracture line	>16

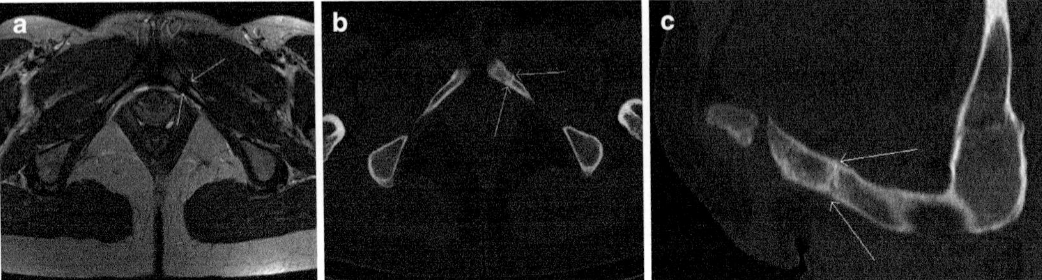

Fig. 31.1 Inferior pubic ramus stress fracture (*white arrows*) on MRI (**a**) and CT views (**b**, **c**)

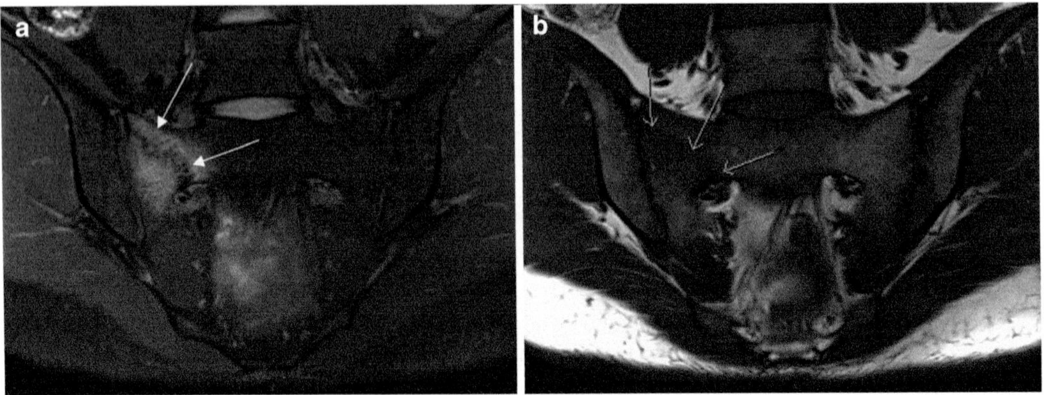

Fig. 31.2 MRI views of sacral stress fracture (*white arrows*) on STIR (**a**) and T1 (**b**)

31.3 Pelvic Stress Fractures

Pelvic stress fractures can occur in a wide spectrum of structures, such as the pubic rami (Fig. 31.1), the sacrum (Fig. 31.2), and the apophyses (e.g., anterior superior iliac spine or the ischial tuberosity). Stress fractures around the pelvis represent the third most common type of stress fractures encountered in football [19]. Stress fractures of the pubic rami are rare and usually occur in the medial portion or at the junction between the inferior pubic ramus and the symphysis pubis [69].

The occurrence of sacral stress fractures (Fig. 31.2) is probably underreported, given the general lack of awareness of this condition and the nonspecificity of symptoms. Stress fractures of the sacrum have been described primarily in long-distance runners, especially females and military [70–72]. They are described as fatigue and insufficiency fractures. The diagnosis is often delayed or inaccurate due to limited overall awareness of this condition and the lack of specific symptoms [71].

The clinical presentation of athletes with pelvic stress fractures consists of insidious onset of pain in the hip or lower back. Despite its low sensitivity, radiographs can identify pubic ramus stress fractures, which might be visible as nondisplaced fracture lines. However, it can be difficult to identify sacral stress fractures on plain radiography, which is particularly difficult given the overlying bowel gas. CT scan or MRI is necessary for accurate diagnosis. Treatment consists of a period of rest and medication. It has been stated that most fractures heal well within 6–10 weeks [51, 73].

31.4 Femoral Stress Fractures

Femoral stress fractures (Fig. 31.3) represent 4.2–48% of all stress fractures in athletes [1, 51, 73]. Femoral stress fractures are less common than pelvic stress fractures and are more common among female runners [74]. Femoral stress fractures (Fig. 31.3) can occur in the femoral neck or the femoral shaft [74].

Plain radiographies often fail to detect femur stress fractures. A high index of suspicion is required in order to achieve early diagnosis in an initial phase of this condition and avoid more severe consequences, such as displacement of a fracture. MRI is an important imaging tool since it enables detection of bone edema and hypointense lines representing fractures on early stages (Fig. 31.3) [74]. Kiuru et al. have described a helpful system for MRI grading of pelvic bones and proximal femur [75].

31.4.1 Femur Neck Stress Fractures

Considering the same biomechanical principles, the superolateral section of the femoral neck corresponds to its tensile site opposing to the inferomedial part (compression). The morphology of the proximal femur probably plays a role in the susceptibility of the patient to develop a stress fracture. *Coxa vara* predisposes to femoral neck stress fracture [76]. *Coxa vara* substantially modifies the biomechanical conditions of the femoral neck, increasing the effect of direct muscle pull and leading to fatigue of opposing muscle groups favoring stress fractures [76]. Femoral neck stress fractures have been linked to female

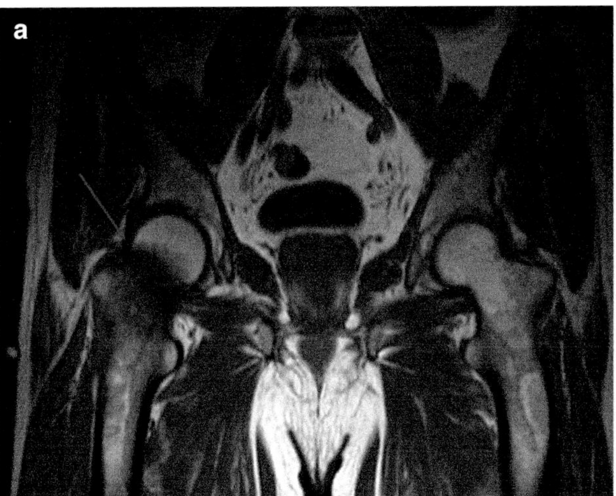

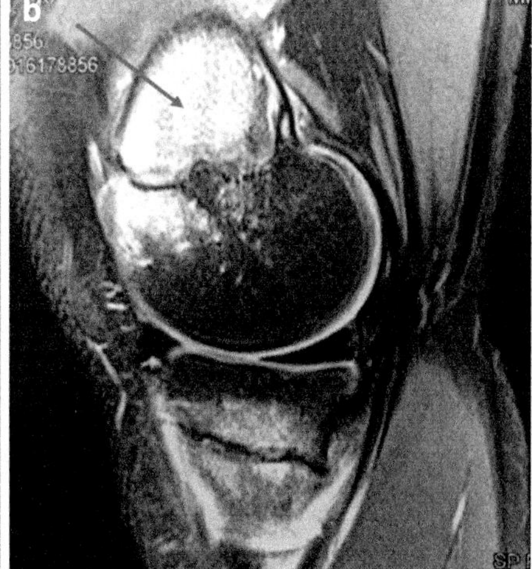

Fig. 31.3 MRI views of femoral neck stress fracture (*red arrow*) (**a**) and stress reaction (*blue arrow*) of the distal femur of an immature footballer (**b**)

athlete triad and might occur in either tension or compression sites [7, 77].

The tension-sided femoral neck fractures are higher-risk injuries with a worse prognosis (i.e., higher risk for displacement) [74]. The presence of displacement increases the risk of a worse clinical outcome (higher morbidity and lower functional results) and increases the risk of complications (osteonecrosis, refracture, or pseudarthrosis) [77]. Considering the potential consequences of complete fracture, tension-sided femoral neck fractures are surgically treated even in early stages (most often by osteosynthesis with three screws) [1]. Considering the biomechanical risk factors in the femoral neck, fractures in the compression side might be managed conservatively, but refractory cases typically require surgical repair.

31.4.2 Femoral Shaft Stress Fractures

Considering human anatomy, the femoral diaphysis has slight anterolateral bowing. Bearing this in mind, the anterolateral surface corresponds to the tension site, while the posteromedial surface corresponds to the compression site. In this case, most stress fractures occur as a consequence of repetitive microtrauma on the compression side, at the junction of its proximal and middle thirds. The pathophysiological explanation is that this is the area of origin of the *vastus medialis* muscle and the insertion of the *adductor brevis muscle*, both of which may be implicated in repeated stresses [78, 79].

Most athletes with femoral shaft stress fractures are managed nonoperatively with good results [80, 81]. This option requires a variable period of rest with return to full sports activity between 12 and 18 weeks [74, 82]. One of the most frequently cited protocols for nonoperative management has been proposed by Arendt and Griffiths (Table 31.2), in which treatment is adapted according to the MRI grading of the injury [64, 81, 83]. Nonoperative treatment must consider the possible complication of displacement dictating the need for surgery.

Currently, when surgical treatment is required, the first option is intramedullary nail fixation [83]. There is no study assessing return to sports after surgical treatment of femoral stress fracture. On a cohort of military recruits, a mean of 3.5 months was required for bone union [84].

31.5 Tibia, Fibula, and Patella Stress Fractures

31.5.1 Shin Splint and Tibia Stress Fracture

The tibia is the second most frequent site for stress fractures among football players (Fig. 31.4) [19]. Stress fractures may occur at any location of the tibia. However, the tibial diaphysis is most commonly affected [1]. Tibial diaphyseal stress fractures may be divided in anterolateral (tension sided) and posteromedial (compression sided). Stress-sided anterior or anterolateral diaphyseal tibial stress fractures are considered high-risk fractures [85]. From an anatomical and biomechanical perspective, the tibia is a component of both the knee and the ankle joints. Therefore, changes in the knee or ankle joint biomechanics play a key role in loading of the tibia during activity. The tibia is bowed anterolaterally due to the powerful tensile stress of the gastrocnemius-soleus complex. In addition, the anterior surface of the tibia is poorly vascularized, increasing the risk for stress fracture [85].

Stress fractures of the tibia must be distinguished from medial tibial stress syndrome (MTSS), also known as "shin splints." "Shin splints" refers to periostitis of the posteromedial tibia that occurs due to the pulling stress of the gastrocnemius-soleus complex [86–88]. It has been proposed that "shin splints" might be an early stage of tibia stress fracture and that both entities are the same in different stages. However, there is no consensus on this statement, and both continue to be considered with their clinical and imaging differences [1].

The most important symptom of tibial stress fracture is pain. For both entities, pain develops insidiously and is aggravated by activity and

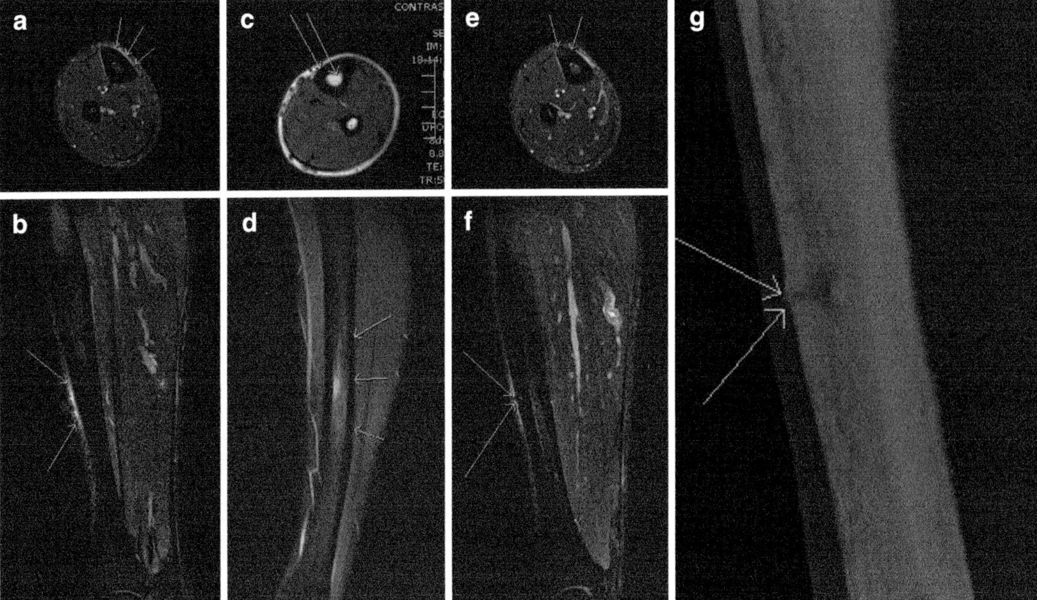

Fig. 31.4 **Fredericson grade I lesion**—Axial (**a**) and lateral (**b**) MRI views of the tibia with visible periosteal edema (*white arrows*), without bone marrow or cortical changes. **Fredericson grade 2 lesion**—without signal changes in T1 (two *white arrows*) (**c**) but bone marrow edema in STIR (three *white arrows*) without cortical changes (**d**). **Fredericson grade 4b lesion**—Axial (**e**) and sagittal views (**f**) with periosteal, bone marrow, and cortical changes (*white arrows*) including linear fracture which is also visible in CT image (*white arrows*) (**g**)

relieved by rest [25]. For tibial stress fracture, pain is located at the site of the stress fracture, and clinical examination reveals focal tenderness localized to the site of injury. Conversely, "shin splint" patients present with diffuse pain and tenderness along the posteromedial surface of the tibia [1]. One must emphasize that changes in training schedule or program as well as return to sports by people with physical deconditioning predispose to the onset of complaints.

A thorough search is required to identify any risk factors. *Pes planus* and *cavus*, tarsal coalition, muscle imbalance, or joint stiffness may alter the biomechanics of the ankle and predispose to "shin splint" and stress fractures [86–88]. Edema and palpable periosteal thickening are often observed in patients with tibial stress fractures while being usually absent from patients with "shin splint" [87]. The vibrating tuning fork test has been nearly abandoned since it is not reliable [89]. The single-leg hop test has also been commonly used in the evaluation of all lower extremity stress fractures; however, its sensitivity and specificity are very low [26]. It is critical to distinguish low-risk from high-risk fractures given their implication on the choice of treatment (surgical versus conservative) but also for prognosis and possible complications.

Stress-sided anterior or anterolateral diaphyseal tibial stress fractures are considered as high-risk fractures [85, 90]. These have higher risk for prolonged recovery, complete fracture, delayed union, nonunion, or chronic pain [53, 54].

However, most tibial stress fractures are posteromedial (compression sided), thus representing low-risk lesions that can be successfully treated nonoperatively [8]. Nonoperative management requires discontinuation of sports activities and avoidance of any activity that may load the tibia significantly until the patient can walk without pain. Non-weight bearing and rarely immobilization in a cast or brace may be needed if the athlete shows no improvement after 3–4 weeks [81]. Most rehabilitation protocols are divided into two stages [91–93]. The first stage is focused on rest and pain management. During this stage, athletes might use deep water running and/or antigravity treadmill in order to keep cardiovascular conditioning while treating the bone in a protected environment. Some data suggest that this approach might lead to an earlier return to play [91–93].

The second stage is focused on the return to previous activity and competition [9]. The second stage includes correction of risk factors, muscle conditioning, and balance and proprioception training [46].

Resistance training incorporating repetitions with no loading or lower magnitude loading is used to improve muscle performance and bone recovery [46, 94]. The American College of Sports Medicine usually recommends resistance training 2–3 times per week [95]. There is general consensus that athletes should only return to sports after a minimum of 2 weeks free of symptoms [31]. On the other hand, the need for imaging control prior to return to play does not have consensus [96, 97]. For anterior tibial stress fractures, non-weight bearing for a period of 4–8 weeks is recommended, while for posteromedial fractures, a period up to 3 weeks is required [46, 96].

Using Fredericson's scale, it has been proposed that Grade 1 lesions might require 2–3 weeks before return to play, Grade 2 to Grade 4a injuries will take 6–7 weeks, and Grade 4b injuries will require a minimum of 9–10 weeks prior to return to sports [62, 98]. Low-risk fractures not responding to nonoperative treatment might require surgical treatment.

High-risk anterior fractures often require surgical treatment [99]. Intramedullary nailing is the preferred surgical method and is associated with high union rates, low rates of complications, and high return to sport [51, 96, 100, 101]. Approximately 10–12 weeks are required to return to sports activity after surgical treatment of tibial stress fractures [51, 96, 100, 101].

31.5.2 Fibula Stress Fractures

Fibula stress fractures are quite rare and can therefore be overlooked by the team physician (Fig. 31.5). From a biomechanical perspective, the load transmission to the fibula, with the ankle in neutral rotation, is only 6–7% of body weight [102]. The proportion of fibular stress fractures among runners on a recent systematic review was reported as 7–12% of all stress fractures [38]. However, in female and male long-distance runners, this proportion may be as high as 33% and 20% of stress fractures, respectively [103].

Most fibular stress fractures represent a simple injury that can be successfully treated with rest and activity modification in 6–12 weeks [104]. Stress fractures of the fibula are most common in its distal third and cause pain in the lateral distal third of the lower leg [38, 105]. Differential diagnosis of conditions that may cause pain in this location include *fibularis* muscle strain or tendinopathy particularly *fibularis brevis* and lateral ankle ligament sprain [105]. MRI or bone scan is usually required for diagnosis on an early stage. On rare occasions, dysfunction of the ankle syndesmosis may contribute to the development of a distal fibular stress fracture. This fact should be considered in the global assessment of pain along the fibula [104].

Proximal fibula stress fractures are very rare. The mechanism might be repetitive pressure of the proximal fibula, a consequence of repeated jumping with both knees completely flexed in a squatting position, causing a repeated strong pull of the muscles attached to the fibula (e.g., *soleus*, *peroneus longus*, *tibialis posterior*, and flexor *hallucis longus*) [104]. In long-distance runners, *biceps femoris* contraction forces have been implicated [38]. Among football players, its description has been associated with running and jumping [106]. Cessation of activity results in complete healing and strengthening, and flexibility exercises of ankle dorsiflexors, ankle plantar flexors, peroneals, and hamstrings are helpful in recovery and avoid recurrence [104].

31.5.3 Patella Stress Fractures

Although patella stress fractures have been increasingly recognized, the patella remains a

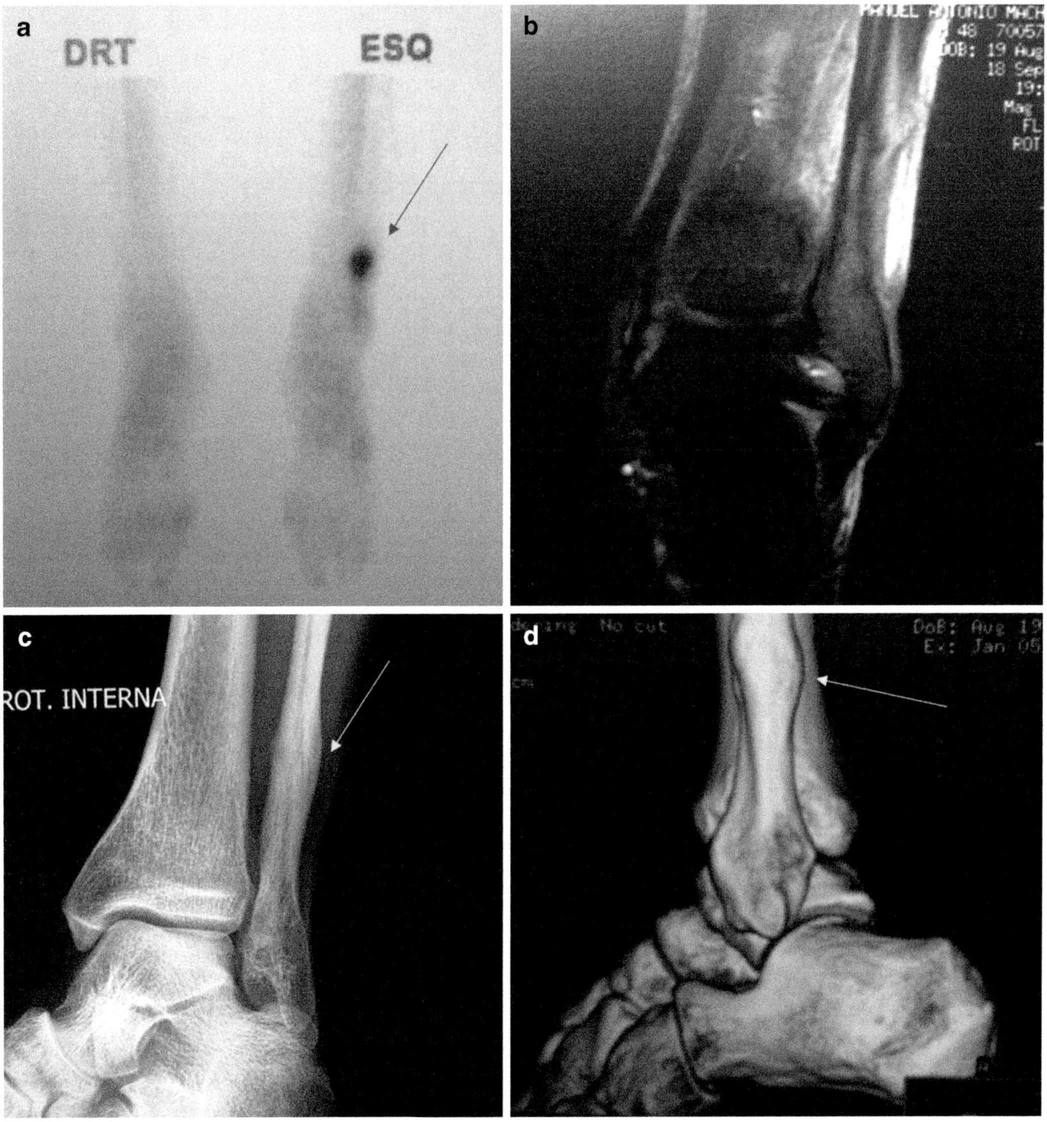

Fig. 31.5 Bone scan showing increased activity in the painful fibula site (*red arrow*) on the early stage of the condition (**a**); MRI view confirming periosteal edema, cortical and bone marrow changes (*red arrow*) (**b**); X-ray after 3 months confirming fracture healing and callus formation (*yellow arrow*) (**c**) which is also visible on CT (**d**) with exuberant bone callus (*yellow arrow*)

rare site for stress fractures [107]. The published data are comprised of individual case reports and small case series. The patella is a sesamoid bone lying within the extensor mechanism of the patellar tendon, linking the quadriceps to the tibia and functions under a quite demanding biomechanical environment of the patellofemoral joint. The force knee vector acting in it reaches more than three times the body weight going up and down the stairs and up to eight times the body weight during deep knee flexion [108].

In order to identify and differentiate a patella stress fracture from the numerous causes of anterior knee pain, a high index of suspicion is necessary. The anterior (tension side) stress fracture of the patella is considered a high-risk lesion and might require surgical treatment, while compression side fractures will respond better to rest and nonoperative treatment [1].

Patients will present with an atypical history of anterior knee pain. Often, there will have been a recent change inactivity levels or a change in training program or training load, applying higher stresses or shorter periods of rest between exercises. Most cases describe a sudden onset of pain during activity, often associated with a pop or crack, but this is typically preceded by weeks or months of anterior knee pain. Transverse fractures are more frequent considering the axial loading applied, although longitudinal fractures may also occur. The most common injury site is at the junction of the middle and distal thirds of the patella where distal quadriceps and proximal patellar tendon fibers merge and insert.

Plain radiographs may demonstrate an obvious fracture, either non-displaced or displaced, although the features of chronic stress, such as sclerotic fracture margins (Fig. 31.6) or cystic changes, may be noticed. Bone scan and MRI will help to detect the early stages of this condition, and CT scan can help better define it once identified.

Concerning treatment, most often when there is a positive bone scan but X-rays are normal, patients can be managed conservatively by a period of rest. If X-rays show a non-displaced fracture, it is possible to choose conservative treatment by immobilization in extension (cast or brace) 4–6 weeks with partial weight bearing followed by passive range of motion exercises, quadriceps strengthening, and progressive return to activity within a period of 3 months. If a displaced fracture is present, surgical treatment is required by tension band wiring or compression screws. It is important, if sclerotic fracture margins are present, to debride and curettage these margins to create healthy, vascularized surfaces for bone healing. The postoperative protocol will depend on the achieved fixation and bone quality.

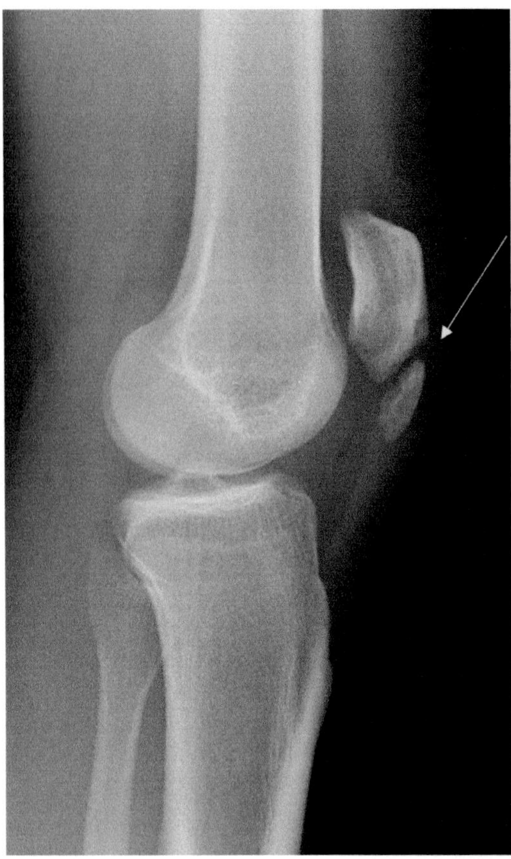

Fig. 31.6 Radiography of lateral view of late stage patella stress fracture (*yellow arrow*). Notice the sclerotic border of fracture line confirming the slowly developing process

31.6 Recent Therapeutic Options

With recent therapeutic biotechnical advances, several new modalities (both biological and physical agents based) are being developed in order to accelerate the healing process and return to play. These are used in combination with general fracture management principles but aim to achieve the maximal benefits of biological and physical stimulation methods [109]. However, many of these options remain experimental and lack evidence-based support.

31.6.1 Hyperbaric Oxygen Therapy (HBOT)

This method consists of intermittently administering 100% oxygen at pressures greater than one atmosphere absolute (ATA) in a pressure vessel. It has been attempted as therapy for several conditions. However, despite some basic-science support as an effective way to stimulate the osteoblasts [110], there is still no clinical evidence on its effectiveness in promoting bone healing [111]. Its use remains controversial and somewhat experimental.

31.6.2 Bisphosphonates

Bisphosphonates suppress bone reabsorption by osteoclasts. By this mechanism, bisphosphonates might prevent bone loss during the initial remodeling phase following high bone stresses and facilitate bone recovery. A small series in collegiate athletes suggested a positive effect of intravenous pamidronate [112]. There is no further evidence of its benefit. Considering the costs and potential adverse effects of bisphosphonates, its use cannot be widely indicated for the treatment of stress fractures in athletes, and prudency is advised [113, 114]. Moreover, their prophylactic effect has also not been demonstrated for bone stress injuries [113, 114].

31.6.3 Growth Factors

The use of growth factors and preparations rich in growth factors (PRGF) has become increasingly popular, particularly in the sports population [115, 116]. These include the growth factors that are produced by platelets in a number of forms of application. Besides remaining controversial in different tissues, with contradictory results found in literature, there is even less evidence concerning its use in stress fractures given the paucity of studies. It has been stated that autologous preparations rich in growth factors might enhance the healing of hypertrophic nonunions when applied during internal fixation surgery and also enhance healing by injection application on stable nonunions [117]. However, more definitive knowledge is required before supporting its widespread use to treat these conditions.

31.6.4 Bone Morphogenetic Proteins (BMPs)

These proteins belong to a family of growth factors (TGF-beta superfamily) that are known to have osteoinductive properties and have been used to promote bone healing [118]. These have been demonstrated to be useful during surgical approaches of fractures and cases of nonunion [119]. Ongoing work is aiming for its clinical percutaneous application, which might be helpful in some stress fracture conditions [118, 119]. Cost-effectiveness must also be taken into account, but this is a promising approach.

31.6.5 Recombinant Parathyroid Hormone

Parathyroid hormone (PTH) increases serum calcium levels by enhancing gastrointestinal calcium absorption, increases renal calcium and phosphate absorption, and releases calcium from the skeleton when required. Although with regular administration of PTH promotes osteoclast activity, intermittent exposure to PTH can also stimulate osteoblasts and results in increased bone formation.

Some studies have shown positive effect in bone healing [120]. Systemic intermittent PTH treatment can enhance either endochondral or intramembranous bone repair [121]. Once more, there is limited knowledge specifically in stress fractures, but this is also a promising and interesting area for future developments.

31.6.6 Low-Intensity Pulsatile Ultrasound Therapy

High-frequency sound waves that are above the audible capacity of humans can influence the bone and the surrounding soft tissues by creating microstress and tension that are capable of stimulate healing. Despite the method being effective in accelerating acute fracture consolidation [122], the exact mechanism remains unclear but is ostensibly related to increased synthesis of extracellular matrix proteins [123]. There remains a paucity of available data concerning ultrasound and stress fractures. A meta-analysis of the effect of low-intensity pulsed ultrasound on the healing of all types of fractures found conflicting results and concluded that most studies had relevant methodological limitations [124].

31.6.7 Magnetic Field Application

Electric fields are recognized to promote bone healing in vitro given the fact they induce cellular stimulation and protein synthesis [123]. There are two main methods to consider: capacity-coupled electrical field (CCEF) devices or pulsed electromagnetic field (PEMF) stimulation [123]. CCEF requires operative placement of an electrode in the fracture site. PEMF promotes release of calcium stored inside the cells, while CCEF uses the calcium ions present in the extracellular fluid. CCEF has been shown to result in higher DNA increase in bone tissue [123]. From a clinical perspective, there are few studies evaluating these methods [125–127]. Further research is needed.

31.7 Return to Sports After Stress Fractures

Fact Box 3

1. A stress fracture should always be considered in an athlete who presents insidious pain, referred to a bony structure, which typically increases after effort and diminishes on rest.
2. Radiographies alone are not feasible (very low sensitivity) for the diagnosis of stress fractures; diagnosis often requires MRI and/or a bone scan.
3. It is mandatory to investigate changes in the training schedule and/or playing surface in footballers.
4. Concerning women athletes, always search history of menstrual disorders, eating disturbances, and weight loss.
5. General rule: return to play (training) is allowed after 2–3 weeks free of symptoms.
6. There is currently no consensus on imaging criteria prior to return to play.

Stress fractures can result in prolonged absence from football, particularly the high-risk variety. The time taken from diagnosis to full recovery and return to play depends on multiple factors: the injury site, sports activity, injury type, and severity and possibility of correcting intrinsic and extrinsic risk factors [1, 81, 83].

Low-risk stress fractures and those manageable by conservative treatment usually make possible for the patient to return to their previous activities 4–17 weeks after the injury [128]. Ekstrand and Torstveit reported that the mean absence from football was 3 months for stress fractures of the tibia and 4–5 months for pelvic stress fractures [19]. However, tibial stress fractures, according to its classification, might range from 2 to 12 weeks prior to return to play [62, 98]. If surgery is required to treat stress fractures, it will typically take at least 3 months after surgery to resume sports activity [51, 96, 100, 101]. Femoral stress fractures usually require 12–18 weeks before full return to sports [74, 82].

The criteria that might be used to allow an athlete to return to play include absence of pain at the affected site during sports activity, absence of symptoms during provocative tests, and absence of abnormalities in imaging examinations. It is of paramount relevance that the athlete, the coach, the manager, and the technical team understand the risk factors and conditions that led to the injury. This way, necessary steps can take place in order to mitigate these risk factors and prevent recurrence and reappearance of injuries [1, 83]. The gradual return to sports activity should be started after the patient has been free from pain for 10–14 days, with 10% increases in training intensity per week [81]. Imaging information confirming complete healing might also be considered as previously discussed.

Fact Box 4

General criteria for athlete's return to play after "stress fractures":

No pain at the injured site during sports activity

No symptoms during provocative tests

Progressive return to sports activity after the athlete is without complaints for 10–14 days, with 10% increases in training intensity per week

No evidence of imaging abnormalities

Take-Home Message

Despite being infrequent conditions, a stress fracture should always be considered in an athlete who presents with insidious pain, referred to a bony structure, which typically increases after effort and diminishes on rest. The tibia is the second most frequent bone affected by stress fracture in football, followed by the pelvis. Understanding the biomechanical feature of tension and compression sites helps establishing higher-risk lesions.

Radiographies have very low sensitivity for the diagnosis of stress fractures; thus, MRI and/or a bone scan is often required for early detection.

In the athletic population, it is mandatory to investigate changes in the training schedule and/or playing surface. Female athletes have specific risk factors that need to be considered. Identifying biologic contributing factors, such as nutritional or hormonal deficiencies, is an important part of management.

During the healing phase, the athlete should focus on conventional methods of relative rest, analgesia, and rehabilitation. Although surgical stabilization involves iatrogenic trauma to the area, the pain related to surgery may well force the athlete to rest, thus promoting healing and recovery.

As a general rule, return to play (training) should be allowed only after the athlete remains 2–3 weeks free of symptoms. There is currently no consensus on imaging criteria prior to return to play; however, some classifications have proven useful and the team physician must be aware of this to assure safe return to play for footballers.

Top Five Evidence Based References

Dhillon MS et al (2016) Stress fractures in football. J ISAKOS Joint Disord Orthopaedic Sports Med **1**(4):229–238

Ekstrand J, Torstveit MK (2012) Stress fractures in elite male football players. Scand J Med Sci Sports 22:341–346

Sundgot-Borgen J, Torstveit MK (2007) The female football player, disordered eating, menstrual function and bone health. Br J Sports Med 41(Suppl 1):i68–i72

Wright AA et al (2016) Diagnostic accuracy of various imaging modalities for suspected lower extremity stress fractures: a systematic review with evidence-based recommendations for clinical practice. Am J Sports Med 44(1):255–263

Changstrom BG et al (2015) Epidemiology of stress fracture injuries among US high school athletes, 2005-2006 through 2012-2013. Am J Sports Med 43(1):26–33

References

1. Dhillon MS, Ekstrand J, Mann G, Sharma S (2016) Stress fractures in football. J ISAKOS Joint Disord Orthopaed Sports Med 1:229–238
2. Mann G, Constantini N, Nyska M, Dolev E, Barchilon V, Shabat S et al (2012) Stress fractures: overview. In: Doral MN, Tandoğan RN, Mann G, Verdonk R (eds) Sports injuries. Springer, Berlin, pp 787–813
3. Stechow AW (1897) Fussödem und Röntgenstrahlen. Deutsche Militärärztliche Zeitschrift 26:465
4. Milgrom C, Giladi M, Stein M, Kashtan H, Margulies JY, Chisin R et al (1985) Stress fractures in military recruits. A prospective study showing an unusually high incidence. J Bone Joint Surg Br 67:732–735
5. Valimaki VV, Alfthan H, Lehmuskallio E, Loyttyniemi E, Sahi T, Suominen H et al (2005) Risk factors for clinical stress fractures in male military recruits: a prospective cohort study. Bone 37:267–273
6. Changstrom BG, Brou L, Khodaee M, Braund C, Comstock RD (2015) Epidemiology of stress fracture injuries among US high school athletes,

2005-2006 through 2012-2013. Am J Sports Med 43:26–33
7. Chen YT, Tenforde AS, Fredericson M (2013) Update on stress fractures in female athletes: epidemiology, treatment, and prevention. Curr Rev Musculoskelet Med 6:173–181
8. Matheson GO, Clement DB, McKenzie DC, Taunton JE, Lloyd-Smith DR, MacIntyre JG (1987) Stress fractures in athletes. A study of 320 cases. Am J Sports Med 15:46–58
9. Fredericson M, Jennings F, Beaulieu C, Matheson GO (2006) Stress fractures in athletes. Top Magn Reson Imaging 17:309–325
10. Fredericson M, Jennings F, Beaulieu C, Matheson GO (2006) Stress fractures in athletes. Top Magn Reson Imaging 17:309–325
11. Pegrum J, Crisp T, Padhiar N (2012) Diagnosis and management of bone stress injuries of the lower limb in athletes. BMJ 344:e2511
12. Berger FH, de Jonge MC, Maas M (2007) Stress fractures in the lower extremity. The importance of increasing awareness amongst radiologists. Eur J Radiol 62:16–26
13. Csizy M, Babst R, Fridrich KS (2000) Fehldiagnose "Knochentumor" bei Stressfraktur am medialen Tibiaplateau. Unfallchirurg 103:993–995
14. Edwards PH Jr, Wright ML, Hartman JF (2005) A practical approach for the differential diagnosis of chronic leg pain in the athlete. Am J Sports Med 33:1241–1249
15. Wall J, Feller JF (2006) Imaging of stress fractures in runners. Clin Sports Med 25:781–802
16. Lee BJ, Kim TY (2016) A study on the birth and globalization of sports originated from each continent. J Exerc Rehabil 12:2–9
17. Ekstrand J, Hagglund M, Walden M (2011) Injury incidence and injury patterns in professional football: the UEFA injury study. Br J Sports Med 45:553–558
18. Timpka T, Ekstrand J, Svanstrom L (2006) From sports injury prevention to safety promotion in sports. Sports Med 36:733–745
19. Ekstrand J, Torstveit MK (2012) Stress fractures in elite male football players. Scand J Med Sci Sports 22:341–346
20. Ekstrand J, van Dijk CN (2013) Fifth metatarsal fractures among male professional footballers: a potential career-ending disease. Br J Sports Med 47:754–758
21. Sundgot-Borgen J, Torstveit MK (2007) The female football player, disordered eating, menstrual function and bone health. Br J Sports Med 41(Suppl 1):i68–i72
22. Torstveit MK, Sundgot-Borgen J (2005) The female athlete triad: are elite athletes at increased risk? Med Sci Sports Exerc 37:184–193
23. Walden M, Hagglund M, Ekstrand J (2005) UEFA Champions League study: a prospective study of injuries in professional football during the 2001-2002 season. Br J Sports Med 39:542–546
24. Warden SJ, Creaby MW, Bryant AL, Crossley KM (2007) Stress fracture risk factors in female football players and their clinical implications. Br J Sports Med 41(Suppl 1):i38–i43
25. Daffner RH, Pavlov H (1992) Stress fractures: current concepts. AJR Am J Roentgenol 159:245–252
26. Lesho EP (1997) Can tuning forks replace bone scans for identification of tibial stress fractures? Mil Med 162:802–803
27. Chamay A, Tschantz P (1972) Mechanical influences in bone remodeling. Experimental research on Wolff's law. J Biomech 5:173–180
28. Kaeding CC, Miller T (2013) The comprehensive description of stress fractures: a new classification system. J Bone Joint Surg Am 95:1214–1220
29. Bennell KL, Malcolm SA, Wark JD, Brukner PD (1996) Models for the pathogenesis of stress fractures in athletes. Br J Sports Med 30:200–204
30. Krestan C, Hojreh A (2009) Imaging of insufficiency fractures. Eur J Radiol 71:398–405
31. Harrast MA, Colonno D (2010) Stress fractures in runners. Clin Sports Med 29:399–416
32. Kaeding CC, Spindler KP, Amendola A (2004) Management of troublesome stress fractures. Instr Course Lect 53:455–469
33. Matcuk GR Jr, Mahanty SR, Skalski MR, Patel DB, White EA, Gottsegen CJ (2016) Stress fractures: pathophysiology, clinical presentation, imaging features, and treatment options. Emerg Radiol 23:365–375
34. Pepper M, Akuthota V, McCarty EC (2006) The pathophysiology of stress fractures. Clin Sports Med 25(1-16):vii
35. Gilchrist J, Jones BH, Sleet DA, Kimsey CD (2000) Exercise-related injuries among women: strategies for prevention from civilian and military studies. MMWR Recom Rep 49:15–33
36. Kaeding CC, Najarian RG (2010) Stress fractures: classification and management. Phys Sportsmed 38:45–54
37. Miller TL, Kaeding CC (2012) Upper-extremity stress fractures: distribution and causative activities in 70 patients. Orthopedics 35:789–793
38. Kahanov L, Eberman LE, Games KE, Wasik M (2015) Diagnosis, treatment, and rehabilitation of stress fractures in the lower extremity in runners. Open Access J Sports Med 6:87–95
39. Gardner L Jr, Dziados JE, Jones BH, Brundage JF, Harris JM, Sullivan R et al (1988) Prevention of lower extremity stress fractures: a controlled trial of a shock absorbent insole. Am J Public Health 78:1563–1567
40. Korpelainen R, Orava S, Karpakka J, Siira P, Hulkko A (2001) Risk factors for recurrent stress fractures in athletes. Am J Sports Med 29:304–310
41. Tenforde AS, Sayres LC, McCurdy ML, Sainani KL, Fredericson M (2013) Identifying sex-specific risk factors for stress fractures in adolescent runners. Med Sci Sports Exerc 45:1843–1851
42. Warden SJ, Burr DB, Brukner PD (2006) Stress fractures: pathophysiology, epidemiology, and risk factors. Curr Osteoporos Rep 4:103–109

43. Bennell KL, Malcolm SA, Thomas SA, Wark JD, Brukner PD (1996) The incidence and distribution of stress fractures in competitive track and field athletes. A twelve-month prospective study. Am J Sports Med 24:211–217
44. Bell DG, Jacobs I (1986) Electro-mechanical response times and rate of force development in males and females. Med Sci Sports Exerc 18:31–36
45. Miller GJ, Purkey WW Jr (1980) The geometric properties of paired human tibiae. J Biomech 13:1–8
46. Liem BC, Truswell HJ, Harrast MA (2013) Rehabilitation and return to running after lower limb stress fractures. Curr Sports Med Rep 12:200–207
47. Muthukumar T, Butt SH, Cassar-Pullicino VN (2005) Stress fractures and related disorders in foot and ankle: plain films, scintigraphy, CT, and MR Imaging. Semin Musculoskelet Radiol 9:210–226
48. Hoffman JR et al (1999) The effect of leg strength on the incidence of lower extremity overuse injuries during military training. Mil Med 164(2): p. 153–156
49. Meeusen R, Duclos M, Foster C, Fry A, Gleeson M, Nieman D et al (2013) Prevention, diagnosis, and treatment of the overtraining syndrome: joint consensus statement of the European College of Sport Science and the American College of Sports Medicine. Med Sci Sports Exerc 45:186–205
50. Madigan DJ, Stoeber J, Passfield L (2017) Perfectionism and training distress in junior athletes: a longitudinal investigation. J Sports Sci 35(5): p. 470–475
51. Behrens SB, Deren ME, Matson A, Fadale PD, Monchik KO (2013) Stress fractures of the pelvis and legs in athletes: a review. Sports Health 5:165–174
52. Bennell K, Crossley K, Jayarajan J, Walton E, Warden S, Kiss ZS et al (2004) Ground reaction forces and bone parameters in females with tibial stress fracture. Med Sci Sports Exerc 36:397–404
53. Boden BP, Osbahr DC (2000) High-risk stress fractures: evaluation and treatment. J Am Acad Orthop Surg 8:344–353
54. McInnis KC, Ramey LN (2016) High-risk stress fractures: diagnosis and management. PM R 8:S113–S124
55. Browne GJ, Barnett P (2016) Common sports-related musculoskeletal injuries presenting to the emergency department. J Paediatr Child Health 52:231–236
56. Kiuru MJ, Pihlajamaki HK, Ahovuo JA (2004) Bone stress injuries. Acta Radiol 45:317–326
57. Boden BP, Osbahr DC, Jimenez C (2001) Low-risk stress fractures. Am J Sports Med 29:100–111
58. Wright AA, Hegedus EJ, Lenchik L, Kuhn KJ, Santiago L, Smoliga JM (2016) Diagnostic accuracy of various imaging modalities for suspected lower extremity stress fractures: a systematic review with evidence-based recommendations for clinical practice. Am J Sports Med 44:255–263
59. Roub LW, Gumerman LW, Hanley EN Jr, Clark MW, Goodman M, Herbert DL (1979) Bone stress: a radionuclide imaging perspective. Radiology 132:431–438
60. Bryant LR, Song WS, Banks KP, Bui-Mansfield LT, Bradley YC (2008) Comparison of planar scintigraphy alone and with SPECT for the initial evaluation of femoral neck stress fracture. AJR Am J Roentgenol 191:1010–1015
61. Nachtrab O, Cassar-Pullicino VN, Lalam R, Tins B, Tyrrell PN, Singh J (2012) Role of MRI in hip fractures, including stress fractures, occult fractures, avulsion fractures. Eur J Radiol 81:3813–3823
62. Swischuk LE, Jadhav SP (2014) Tibial stress phenomena and fractures: imaging evaluation. Emerg Radiol 21:173–177
63. Gaeta M, Minutoli F, Scribano E, Ascenti G, Vinci S, Bruschetta D et al (2005) CT and MR imaging findings in athletes with early tibial stress injuries: comparison with bone scintigraphy findings and emphasis on cortical abnormalities. Radiology 235:553–561
64. Arendt EA, Griffiths HJ (1997) The use of MR imaging in the assessment and clinical management of stress reactions of bone in high-performance athletes. Clin Sports Med 16:291–306
65. Fredericson M, Bergman AG, Hoffman KL, Dillingham MS (1995) Tibial stress reaction in runners. Correlation of clinical symptoms and scintigraphy with a new magnetic resonance imaging grading system. Am J Sports Med 23:472–481
66. Fredericson M, Bergman AG, Hoffman KL, Dillingham MS (1995) Tibial stress reaction in runners: correlation of clinical symptoms and scintigraphy with a new magnetic resonance imaging grading system. Am J Sports Med 23:472–481
67. Saxena A, Fullem B, Hannaford D (2000) Results of treatment of 22 navicular stress fractures and a new proposed radiographic classification system. J Foot Ankle Surg 39:96–103
68. Torg JS, Balduini FC, Zelko RR, Pavlov H, Peff TC, Das M (1984) Fractures of the base of the fifth metatarsal distal to the tuberosity. Classification and guidelines for non-surgical and surgical management. J Bone Joint Surg Am 66:209–214
69. Bertolini FM, Vieira RB, Oliveira LH, Lasmar RP, Junior Ode O (2011) Pubis stress fracture in a 15-year-old soccer player. Rev Bras Ortop 46:464–467
70. Johnson AW, Weiss CB Jr, Stento K, Wheeler DL (2001) Stress fractures of the sacrum. An atypical cause of low back pain in the female athlete. Am J Sports Med 29:498–508
71. Longhino V, Bonora C, Sansone V (2011) The management of sacral stress fractures: current concepts. Clin Cases Miner Bone Metab 8:19–23
72. Shah MK, Stewart GW (2002) Sacral stress fractures: an unusual cause of low back pain in an athlete. Spine (Phila Pa 1976) 27:E104–E108
73. Liong SY, Whitehouse RW (2012) Lower extremity and pelvic stress fractures in athletes. Br J Radiol 85:1148–1156
74. Niva MH, Kiuru MJ, Haataja R, Pihlajamaki HK (2005) Fatigue injuries of the femur. J Bone Joint Surg Br 87:1385–1390

75. Kiuru MJ, Pihlajamaki HK, Ahovuo JA (2003) Fatigue stress injuries of the pelvic bones and proximal femur: evaluation with MR imaging. Eur Radiol 13:605–611
76. Carpintero P, Leon F, Zafra M, Serrano-Trenas JA, Roman M (2003) Stress fractures of the femoral neck and coxa vara. Arch Orthop Trauma Surg 123:273–277
77. Goolsby MA, Barrack MT, Nattiv A (2012) A displaced femoral neck stress fracture in an amenorrheic adolescent female runner. Sports Health 4:352–356
78. DeFranco MJ, Recht M, Schils J, Parker RD (2006) Stress fractures of the femur in athletes. Clin Sports Med 25:89–103. ix
79. Koenig SJ, Toth AP, Bosco JA (2008) Stress fractures and stress reactions of the diaphyseal femur in collegiate athletes: an analysis of 25 cases. Am J Orthop (Belle Mead NJ) 37:476–480
80. Ivkovic A, Bojanic I, Pecina M (2006) Stress fractures of the femoral shaft in athletes: a new treatment algorithm. Br J Sports Med 40:518–520. discussion 520
81. Raasch WG, Hergan DJ (2006) Treatment of stress fractures: the fundamentals. Clin Sports Med 25:29–36. vii
82. Johnson AW, Weiss CB Jr, Wheeler DL (1994) Stress fractures of the femoral shaft in athletes--more common than expected. A new clinical test. Am J Sports Med 22:248–256
83. Royer M, Thomas T, Cesini J, Legrand E (2012) Stress fractures in 2011: practical approach. Joint Bone Spine 79(Suppl 2):S86–S90
84. Salminen ST, Pihlajamaki HK, Visuri TI, Bostman OM (2003) Displaced fatigue fractures of the femoral shaft. Clin Orthop Relat Res:250–259. https://doi.org/10.1097/01.blo.0000058883.03274.17
85. Caesar BC, McCollum GA, Elliot R, Williams A, Calder JD (2013) Stress fractures of the tibia and medial malleolus. Foot Ankle Clin 18:339–355
86. Craig DI (2009) Current developments concerning medial tibial stress syndrome. Phys Sportsmed 37:39–44
87. Moen MH, Tol JL, Weir A, Steunebrink M, De Winter TC (2009) Medial tibial stress syndrome: a critical review. Sports Med 39:523–546
88. Tweed JL, Avil SJ, Campbell JA, Barnes MR (2008) Etiologic factors in the development of medial tibial stress syndrome: a review of the literature. J Am Podiatr Med Assoc 98:107–111
89. Toney CM, Games KE, Winkelmann ZK, Eberman LE (2016) Using tuning-fork tests in diagnosing fractures. J Athl Train 51:498–499
90. Liimatainen E, Sarimo J, Hulkko A, Ranne J, Heikkila J, Orava S (2009) Anterior mid-tibial stress fractures. Results of surgical treatment. Scand J Surg 98:244–249
91. Knobloch K, Schreibmueller L, Jagodzinski M, Zeichen J, Krettek C (2007) Rapid rehabilitation programme following sacral stress fracture in a long-distance running female athlete. Arch Orthop Trauma Surg 127:809–813
92. Saxena A, Granot A (2011) Use of an anti-gravity treadmill in the rehabilitation of the operated achilles tendon: a pilot study. J Foot Ankle Surg 50:558–561
93. Tenforde AS, Watanabe LM, Moreno TJ, Fredericson M (2012) Use of an antigravity treadmill for rehabilitation of a pelvic stress injury. PM R 4:629–631
94. Westcott WL (2012) Resistance training is medicine: effects of strength training on health. Curr Sports Med Rep 11:209–216
95. Ratamess NA, Alvar BA, Evetoch TK, Housh TJ, Kibler WB, Kraemer WJ et al (2009) American College of Sports Medicine position stand. Progression models in resistance training for healthy adults. Med Sci Sports Exerc 41:687–708
96. Feldman JJ, Bowman EN, Phillips BB, Weinlein JC (2016) Tibial Stress Fractures in Athletes. Orthop Clin North Am 47:733–741
97. Tenforde AS, Kraus E, Fredericson M (2016) Bone Stress Injuries in Runners. Phys Med Rehabil Clin N Am 27:139–149
98. Kijowski R, Choi J, Shinki K, Del Rio AM, De Smet A (2012) Validation of MRI classification system for tibial stress injuries. AJR Am J Roentgenol 198:878–884
99. McCormick F, Nwachukwu BU, Provencher MT (2012) Stress fractures in runners. Clin Sports Med 31:291–306
100. Borens O, Sen MK, Huang RC, Richmond J, Kloen P, Jupiter JB et al (2006) Anterior tension band plating for anterior tibial stress fractures in high-performance female athletes: a report of 4 cases. J Orthop Trauma 20:425–430
101. Reshef N, Guelich DR (2012) Medial Tibial Stress Syndrome. Clin Sports Med 31:273–290
102. Goh JC, Mech AM, Lee EH, Ang EJ, Bayon P, Pho RW (1992) Biomechanical study on the load-bearing characteristics of the fibula and the effects of fibular resection. Clin Orthop Relat Res:223–228
103. Snyder RA, Koester MC, Dunn WR (2006) Epidemiology of stress fractures. Clin Sports Med 25:37–52. viii
104. Hetsroni I, Mann G (2009) Fibula stress fractures: a treatment review. Oper Tech Sports Med 17:112–114
105. Hoglund LT, Silbernagel KG, Taweel NR (2015) Distal fibular stress fracture in a female recreational runner: a case report with musculoskeletal ultrasound imaging findings. Int J Sports Phys Ther 10:1050–1058
106. DiFiori JP (1999) Stress fracture of the proximal fibula in a young soccer player: a case report and a review of the literature. Med Sci Sports Exerc 31:925–928
107. Crane TP, Spalding T (2009) The management of patella stress fractures and the symptomatic bipartite patella. Oper Tech Sports Med 17:100–105
108. Zaffagnini S, Dejour D, Grassi A, Bonanzinga T, Marcheggiani Muccioli GM, Colle F et al (2013) Patellofemoral anatomy and biomechanics: current concepts. Joints 1:15–20
109. Nelson FR, Brighton CT, Ryaby J, Simon BJ, Nielson JH, Lorich DG et al (2003) Use of physical forces in bone healing. J Am Acad Orthop Surg 11:344–354

110. Wu D, Malda J, Crawford R, Xiao Y (2007) Effects of hyperbaric oxygen on proliferation and differentiation of osteoblasts from human alveolar bone. Connect Tissue Res 48:206–213
111. Bennett MH, Stanford R, Turner R (2005) Hyperbaric oxygen therapy for promoting fracture healing and treating fracture non-union. Cochrane Database Syst Rev:CD004712. https://doi.org/10.1002/14651858.CD004712.pub2
112. Stewart GW, Brunet ME, Manning MR, Davis FA (2005) Treatment of stress fractures in athletes with intravenous pamidronate. Clin J Sport Med 15:92–94
113. Ekenman I (2009) Do not use bisphosphonates without scientific evidence, neither in treatment nor prophylactic, in the treatment of stress fractures. Knee Surg Sports Traumatol Arthrosc 17:433–434
114. Shima Y, Engebretsen L, Iwasa J, Kitaoka K, Tomita K (2009) Use of bisphosphonates for the treatment of stress fractures in athletes. Knee Surg Sports Traumatol Arthrosc 17:542–550
115. Engebretsen L, Steffen K, Alsousou J, Anitua E, Bachl N, Devilee R et al (2010) IOC consensus paper on the use of platelet-rich plasma in sports medicine. Br J Sports Med 44:1072–1081
116. Pereira H, Ripoll L, Oliveira JM, Reis RL, Espregueira-Mendes J, van Dijk C (2016) A Engenharia de tecidos nas lesões do Desporto. In: Pessoa P, Jones H (eds) Traumatologia desportiva. LIDEL, Lisboa, pp 320–335
117. Sanchez M, Anitua E, Cugat R, Azofra J, Guadilla J, Seijas R et al (2009) Nonunions treated with autologous preparation rich in growth factors. J Orthop Trauma 23:52–59
118. Chen D, Zhao M, Mundy GR (2004) Bone morphogenetic proteins. Growth Factors 22:233–241
119. Giannoudis PV, Gudipati S, Harwood P, Kanakaris NK (2015) Long bone non-unions treated with the diamond concept: a case series of 64 patients. Injury 46(Suppl 8):S48–S54
120. Warden SJ, Komatsu DE, Rydberg J, Bond JL, Hassett SM (2009) Recombinant human parathyroid hormone (PTH 1-34) and low-intensity pulsed ultrasound have contrasting additive effects during fracture healing. Bone 44:485–494
121. Barnes GL, Kakar S, Vora S, Morgan EF, Gerstenfeld LC, Einhorn TA (2008) Stimulation of fracture-healing with systemic intermittent parathyroid hormone treatment. J Bone Joint Surg Am 90(Suppl 1):120–127
122. Heckman JD, Ryaby JP, McCabe J, Frey JJ, Kilcoyne RF (1994) Acceleration of tibial fracture-healing by non-invasive, low-intensity pulsed ultrasound. J Bone Joint Surg Am 76:26–34
123. Astur DC, Zanatta F, Arliani GG, Moraes ER, Pochini Ade C, Ejnisman B (2016) Stress fractures: definition, diagnosis and treatment. Rev Bras Ortop 51:3–10
124. Busse JW, Kaur J, Mollon B, Bhandari M, Tornetta P III, Schunemann HJ et al (2009) Low intensity pulsed ultrasonography for fractures: systematic review of randomised controlled trials. BMJ 338:b351
125. Beck BR, Matheson GO, Bergman G, Norling T, Fredericson M, Hoffman AR et al (2008) Do capacitively coupled electric fields accelerate tibial stress fracture healing? A randomized controlled trial. Am J Sports Med 36:545–553
126. Holmes GB Jr (1994) Treatment of delayed unions and nonunions of the proximal fifth metatarsal with pulsed electromagnetic fields. Foot Ankle Int 15:552–556
127. Simonis RB, Parnell EJ, Ray PS, Peacock JL (2003) Electrical treatment of tibial non-union: a prospective, randomised, double-blind trial. Injury 34:357–362
128. Carmont RC, Mei-Dan O, Bennell LK (2009) Stress fracture management: current classification and new healing modalities. Oper Tech Sports Med 17:81–89

Return to Football Following Achilles Tendon Rupture

32

Michael R. Carmont, Jennifer A. Zellers, Maurizio Fanchini, Jon Karlsson, and Karin Grävare Silbernagel

Contents

32.1 Introduction

The incidence of Achilles tendon rupture has been increasing since the 1980s of 18 per 100,000 person years [29]. A much greater appreciation of variations in incidence has occurred with the adoption of nationwide hospital [21, 28, 36] and provider group databases [52, 58, 62] together with the development of Achilles tendon rupture registries [3, 14]. A mean annual increase in rupture rate of 2.4% has been reported [28]. The most recently reported injury rates are of 46 per 100,000 persons in 2013 [53].

The mechanism of injury is typically a rapid eccentric loading of the gastrocnemius-soleus complex. This most commonly occurs during sports activity [24] such as football, particularly 5-a-side and badminton for males and netball for females [8]. Males are more

M.R. Carmont (✉)
Department of Orthopaedic Surgery, Princess Royal Hospital, Shrewsbury & Telford Hospital NHS Trust, Shrewsbury, UK

Department of Neurosciences, Biomedicine and Movement Science, University of Verona, Verona, Italy
e-mail: mcarmont@hotmail.com

J.A. Zellers
The Department of Physiotherapy, University of Delware, Newark, DE, USA

M. Fanchini
Department of Neurosciences, Biomedicine and Movement Science, University of Verona, Verona, Italy

J. Karlsson
The Department of Orthopaedic Surgery, Institute of Clinical Sciences, Sahlgrenska Academy, University of Gothenburg, Gothenburg, Sweden

K.G. Silbernagel
The Department of Physiotherapy, University of Delware, Newark, DE, USA

The Department of Orthopaedic Surgery, Institute of Clinical Sciences, Sahlgrenska Academy, University of Gothenburg, Gothenburg, Sweden

V. Musahl et al. (eds.), *Return to Play in Football*, https://doi.org/10.1007/978-3-662-55713-6_32

frequently affected than females with a ratio of approximately 4–10:1 [8].

32.2 Consequences of Rupture

A rupture of the Achilles tendon has a prolonged recovery and in most studies leaving at least a 10–30% reduction in functional calf strength [42, 43, 54, 63] and endurance [6] despite increased muscle activity [19, 59]. The injury produces long-term limitations [5, 18, 19, 29, 37]—often >10 years—and many (30–40% of patients) fail to return to sports activities at the same level of performance as pre-injury [68].

Fact Box 1
Patients sustaining rupture of the Achilles tendon tend to have 10–30% reduction in functional calf strength.

Large variations exist between individuals, in the performance of specific sports activities, such as those required for return to play (RTP). In a study by Olsson et al. limb symmetry indexes between injured and non-injured sides ranged from 84% to 102% with standard deviations ranging from 15% to 26% during jumping tasks [44]. This variability may be due to several factors—gender, method of management (especially non-operative and operative treatments), plyometric strength deficits, psychological components, and other physical changes indirectly related to injury and recovery course. Patients may be physically able to return to sports activities, but the fear of re-rupture may cause an individual to avoid the sports activity during which the injury occurred.

32.3 Management Options for Achilles Tendon Rupture

The management options for Achilles tendon rupture may be broadly split into non-operative and operative treatments.

Non-operative management now features a temporary or short-term cast followed by functional bracing with early weight-bearing [4, 11] and early functional rehabilitation. For the general population this method produces low re-rupture rates and satisfactory outcomes for activities of daily living [20, 61]. In recent non-operative series RTP percentages have varied with Barfod et al. reporting only 20% of patients RTP to the same level [4], while Ecker et al. reported an 87% return to a recreational level of play [11].

Operative treatment may be divided into percutaneous, minimally invasive, open and augmented repairs. Following repair full weight-bearing as able is encouraged, together with early range of motion training [25, 29, 40, 57].

32.4 Evidence from the Literature

The majority of randomized controlled trials comparing non-operative and operative treatment have shown no significant differences in the primary outcome measure usually the avoidance of re-rupture. The re-rupture rate is approximately 0–3% after surgery and approximately 10–14% after non-operative management. Many studies are adequately powered for current outcome variables (re-rupture), but not for the all the possible confounding factors and as such may not yield accurate information on return to play. In addition many studies include a broad range of patients of different ages, body weights, and physiology that makes them difficult to apply to the competitive sports persons.

The randomized controlled trials do, however, yield the following statistically significant results:

Operative treatment appears to result in superior outcome in calf muscle function, which would be of great importance in athletes such as sprinters [23, 44, 63].

Fact Box 2
Operative treatment appears to result in superior outcome in calf function.

If treatment goes well and without complications, many patients return to their previous level of sports activity [68]. If re-rupture occurs patients rarely return to their previous level of sports activity [40].

Operative repair may be less prone to failure consisting of tendon "non-union" and permanent elongation with interposed scar tissue than non-operative treatment [30, 51].

Patients return to work earlier [12] and have improved early function at 3 months [26] and 6 months after operative treatment.

The literature shows increased re-rupture rate with non-operative treatment compared with operative treatment, but on the other hand, there are fewer overall complications than with surgery. However, if accelerated rehabilitation is used, the risk of re-rupture decreases after non-operative treatment [56].

Minimally invasive and percutaneous surgery improves cosmesis and reduces the risk of wound breakdown and patients have comparable outcome [10, 38, 67] (Fig. 32.1).

The use of a fascial turndown flap to augment repairs compared with a simple end-to-end open repair, neither improves outcome scores nor prevents tendon lengthening and muscle weakness [18, 47].

Another factor of interest is the injurious event. While the majority of Achilles tendon ruptures are sustained during sports or athletic activity, they are not necessarily sustained by patients who would be considered to be athletes. It is common for the patient to be in their mid-forties and have recently returned to sports activity from either a period of work or looking after children during which time the tendon has effectively become de-conditioned.

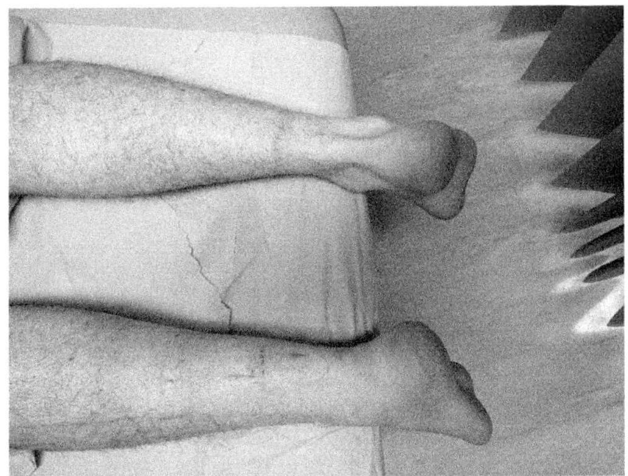

Fig. 32.1 Minimally invasive Achilles repair has good cosmesis, reduced wound breakdown, and comparable outcome to open repair

Given the limited reporting of pre-injury sports participation [68], there are relatively few series of professional and elite athletes who have sustained an Achilles tendon rupture from which it is possible to draw firm conclusions.

32.5 Evidence and Science Specific to Competitive Football and Other Sports

Footballers will have different priorities in terms of treatment compared with the general population. Many patients will accept that an injury such as an Achilles tendon rupture is likely to take the full season to recover and rehabilitate from. Most will wish to avoid the complications, time loss, and reduced functional outcome of re-rupture. Additionally competitive athletes will wish to minimize any functional loss relating to their injury.

Participants in competitive sports activity, such as football, tend to be younger than the typical patient suffering an Achilles rupture and are not usually affected by any medical comorbidity. This means that infection and wound healing problems usually tend not to occur. In terms of factors predicting outcome following treatment, Olsson et al. have determined that a high BMI leads to an increased risk of a poor outcome [46]. This similarly does not apply to most professional sportsmen.

As a result, most players and athletes will choose operative treatment.

How to grade sports activity in cases of Achilles tendon rupture and how do we know that a player has returned to the same level of sports activity?

The ability to return to sport, return to work, and return to sports performance may also be considered to be indicator of a successful outcome. Several scales are commonly used in the literature to compare sports activity.

The Tegner sport and activity scale was devised as a follow-up indicator after knee ligament injuries [60]. The Tegner score has commonly been used in lower limb sports injury surgery and (after 25 years of use) is considered to be an acceptable psychometric parameter of a patient administered score. It also provides an acceptable responsiveness, with an intra-class correlation of 0.8 and minimal detectable change of 1. The Tegner score in its original form has been used for ankle ligament surgery [34], posterior ankle impingement [31], and plantaris [49] injuries. More specifically related to this chapter, the Tegner score has also been used following Achilles tendon injuries [13, 22, 27].

In 2004, Halasi et al. developed a new activity score for the evaluation of ankle instability [17]. This included 53 sports, three working activities, and four general activities inserted into a 0- to 10-point category scoring system. The level of participation is divided into (1) top-level/national team, (2) lower competitive level, and finally (3) recreational level. Halasi's score correlates with the Tegner score ($r = 0.7565$) and is shown to have high reliability. The ankle score differences are spread over a wider range (-1.18 ± 2.12) than the Tegner score differences (-0.68 ± 1.29), and so the new score is considered to have higher sensitivity.

The physical activity score (PAS) has been described by Grimby and Saltin to assess leisure time physical activity and divides the activity into intensity from light, moderate, and hard or very hard exercise [16]. The score has recently been found to have concurrent validity with respect to aerobic capacity and movement analysis. The score also has predictive validity to various risk factors for health conditions.

A simple method of determining whether patients have returned to the same standard of play is to rate their performance on a scale and to compare this rating with that achieved during follow-up.

Another subjective method is to ask patients if they had reached the same level of sports and physical activity or performance as before their injury. Patients can verbally be given the options of not yet, the same, or improved. This terminology was used so that the patient could decide about their own function in respect to their sports. For example, a competitive footballer may return to the same team, play in the same league, and score the same number of goals, but they themselves may feel that they have not yet reached the same level of function.

The suggestion of the answer "not yet" was to encourage patients with strengthening exercises and remind them of the expectation to return to sport.

A systematic review and meta-analysis have been performed to identify return to play (RTP) rates following Achilles tendon rupture and evaluate the measures that are used to determine RTP [68]. A total of 108 studies encompassing 6506 patients were included for review. Eighty-five studies included a measure for determining RTP. The cumulative rate of RTP in all studies was 80% ($CI_{95\%}$: 75–85%). Studies with measures describing determination of RTP reported lower rates compared with those without descriptive methods without metrics described. Eighty percent of patients returned to play following Achilles tendon rupture; however, the return to play rates depend on the determination methods used. To further understand RTP after Achilles tendon rupture, a standardized, reliable, and valid method is required.

Fact Box 3
80% of patients returned to play following Achilles tendon rupture.

A number of authors have published on the outcomes of professional or competitive recreational athletes returning to sport. These are case series rather than randomized controlled trials. Most professional athletes are unlikely to be willing to participate in a randomized controlled trial for risk being randomized to a group with any considered deficiency in outcome.

Similarly Martinelli et al. reported on amateur athletes who undertook regular training sessions for their sport and professional athletes, overall mean age 30.5 years using the TenoLig® device to perform a percutaneous repair [35]. Athletes returned to their pre-injury level of sports at 120–150 days.

On the level of recreational sportsmen, Gigante et al. performed a randomized controlled trial comparing a percutaneous repairs to open repairs performed using an end-to-end Bunnell repair, mean age 41 years ($n = 40$) [15].

Parekh et al. reported a retrospective web-based follow-up of 31 NFL players [48]. Thirty-six percent were unable to return to the same level of play, and of those who were able to return, 50% sustained a 50% drop in performance compared with pre-participation levels.

De Carli et al. reported using Kakiuchi's mini-open technique to repair the Achilles tendons of athletes and found that 76.4% returned to the same sports activity level, but not all returned to their pre-injury level [9].

Maffulli et al. have reported on return to play following Achilles tendon ruptures repaired using a percutaneous technique [32]. In his series of 17 athletes, mean age 34 years (16–41), all were able to weight-bear by the 8th postoperative week, and there was an average RTP of 4.8 ± 0.9 months. Eleven athletes returned without any limitations; however, six either played at a lower level for one season or did not achieve the same level at all. ATRS score at follow-up was 91 ± 11 (79–99) points. Eleven athletes reported swelling around the tendon or ankle at follow-up, and four athletes suffered from calf cramps.

The performance outcomes of NBA players who returned to play were significantly reduced compared with controls following Achilles tendon ruptures in the first ($P = 0.038$) and second seasons ($P = 0.08$) [1]. Eighteen players were followed up; 7 out of 18 never returned to an NBA game; 11 players returned for one season only and 8 for two seasons or more. Notably the injuries were sustained over a 23-year period.

Jallageas et al. performed a 15 months follow-up of 31 athletes, mean age 38 years [23]. Overall, there was a 19% strength deficit; however, those receiving a percutaneous repair returned to play faster (130 days) than those who underwent open surgery. Eighty-one percent of those receiving a percutaneous repair returned to the same level of play, whereas only 73.5% achieved the same level following open repair. The overall return to sport was 153 days (91–246).

Vadala et al. treated 36 professional athletes using a combined percutaneous/mini-open technique; 86% resumed the same level of sports activity within 5 months of repair, another two within 7 months and three within 7–10 months [65].

McCullough et al. reported on a series of NFL players with an average age of 25.6 years [39]. Seventy-eight percent of players returned to NFL competition within an average of 8.9 months. One athlete in this series returned to play in 166 days (5.4 months).

Ververidis et al. also performed a systematic literature review on percutaneous repair in athletes [66]. The most frequent complication was sural nerve injury and the re-rupture rate was low. Ninety-one percent of patients returned to practicing sports, and 78–84% returned to the same or a higher level of sports. From nine studies, the average time to return to sports was 18 weeks.

Byrne et al. reported on a case of an international bobsleigh driver who had a rupture repaired using a minimally invasive technique using locking sutures placed using the PARS device (Arthrex®, Naples, FL) and anchored into the calcaneus using a knotless system [7]. Postoperatively the patient was managed with full weight-bearing, early movement but notably no brace protection. He returned to training at 13 weeks following surgery, won a World Cup silver medal at 18 weeks, and was ultimately 4th at the Winter Olympic Games 2014 at 29 weeks following repair.

32.6 Rehabilitation Following Achilles Tendon Rupture

Rehabilitation following Achilles tendon rupture can be considered in several phases: controlled mobilization, early recovery, late recovery, and return to sport. Despite these distinctions, contributors to return to sport (i.e., strength deficits, psychosocial concerns) should be considered throughout the rehabilitative process [2]. At the later phases of rehabilitation, football-specific guidelines have not been published in the context of Achilles tendon rupture; however, guidelines developed for other orthopedic injuries may be needed to be modified and applied to this population.

32.6.1 Controlled Motion

The controlled mobilization phase begins following injury or surgery. The goal of this phase is to approximate tendon ends and facilitate tendon healing. Of particular concern is the avoidance of tendon elongation. Tendon elongation occurs during the first 8–12 weeks post injury [25, 41] and results in long-term plantar flexor deficits [54] as well as changes in movement biomechanics particularly with running and jumping [64]. Early weight-bearing has been associated with trends toward lower levels of tendon elongation [25, 33]. Early weight-bearing is performed in plantar flexed positions using weight-bearing casts or boots. Later in this phase, the effects of immobilization can be addressed with joint mobilization techniques to the talocrural and subtalar joints, taking care not to put the tendon on stretch. Furthermore, general hypotrophy can be addressed with active range of motion and isometric strengthening avoiding the most extreme dorsiflexion ranges.

32.6.2 Early Recovery

The early recovery stage begins when the patient is able to ambulate in sneakers with a wedge, typically around week 6–8. At this stage, slow, controlled weight-bearing exercises (such as the bilateral heel rise) are initiated to gradually load the tendon. Exercises to address other balance, range of motion, or strength deficits can also be added (Fig. 32.2). The goal of this stage is to walk symmetrically without bracing and perform activities of daily living (stair negotiation, ambulation in community) without compensation [45, 55].

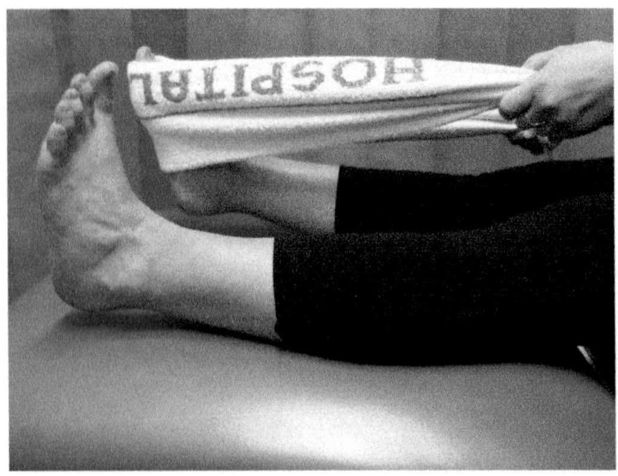

Fig. 32.2 During the early recovery stage, balance, range of motion, and strength deficits can be optimized

32.6.3 Late Recovery

The late recovery stage begins when the patient is able to perform a unilateral heel rise with the goal of gradually progressing strengthening and returning to more dynamic activities, such as running. A running progression can be initiated when the patient is able to complete five unilateral heel rises at 90% of the available height on the ruptured side. If the patient is unable to achieve this milestone by 16 weeks, a running progression can be initiated if the patient is able to raise at least 70% of bodyweight during a unilateral heel rise [55]. Low-speed, low-intensity agility training (i.e., figure-8 jogging, low-speed carioca) can also be initiated during this phase (Fig. 32.3).

The literature comments upon goals to be attained following Achilles tendon rupture. Saxena et al.'s study stated the specific targets to be attained: 5 sets of 25 repetitions. These are introduced over time starting with three sets of ten based upon pain tolerance [50]. The calf circumference, measured 10 cm distal to the inferior pole of the patella, should be comparable to the non-injured limb, and the ankle range of motion should aim to be within 5° of the non-injured side [50]. Return to play was quoted as being between 12 and 26 weeks following Achilles tendon rupture [47].

In Hutchison et al.'s paper on a general population cohort, patients were advised against sports

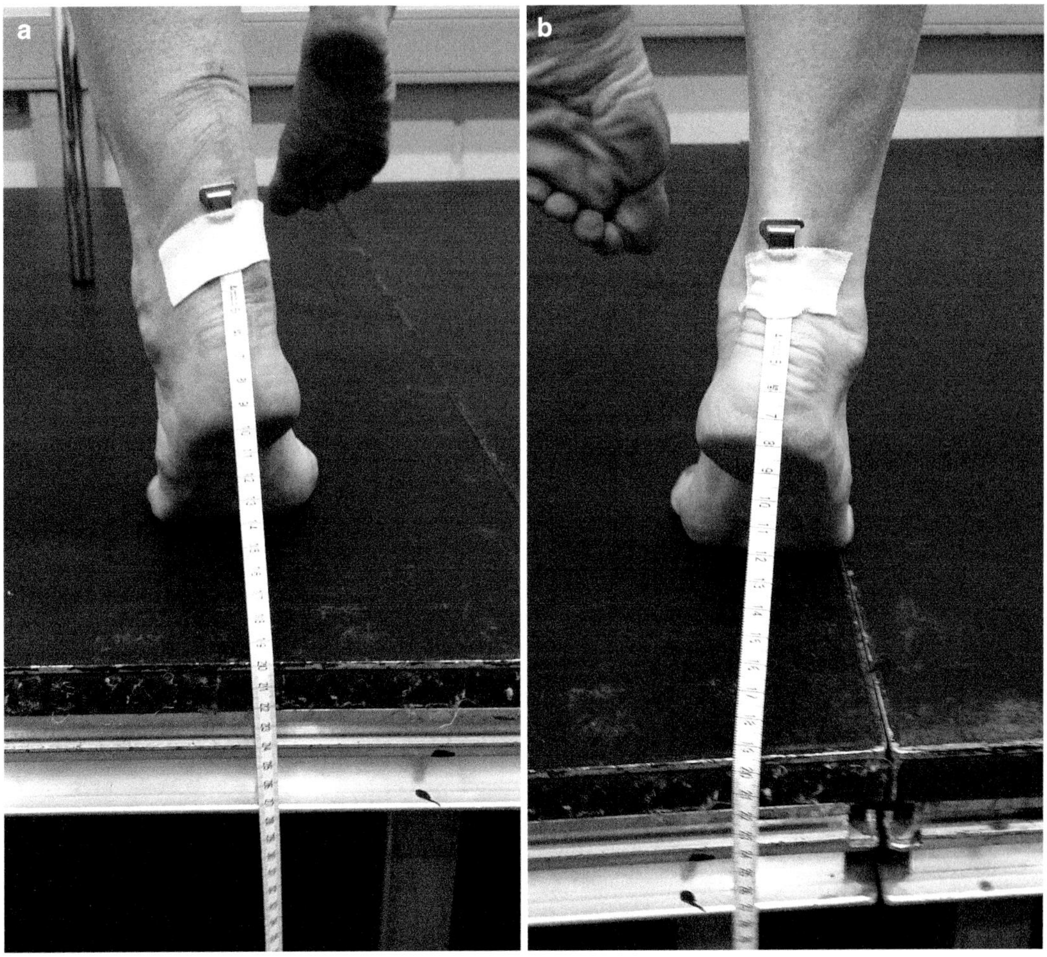

Fig. 32.3 Assessment of single heel rise on the affected side (**a**) can be compared to the non-injured side (**b**)

activity until they could perform a single heel rise, sprint using the toe off phase of gait, perform a horizontal single leg hop 3× for more than 75% of the non-injured leg and lastly perform a vertical hop to >75% of the non-injured side [20].

Goals such as these prepare the player to return to sports activity, training, and ultimately return to team selection. Activity during this program should be organized and prescribed to increase specificity and load in respect to healing of the injury up to competitive matches. During the first weeks of RTP, low and moderate intensity activities with increasing exposure should be pursued. On-field activity may include walking, walking and running alternatively, low agility circuits (as fast feet activities using speed sledge, hurdles, slaloms), and exercises with and without the ball. With time, players should be exposed to high-intensity activities to increase the load on the injured part and to enhance physical performance. Interval training can be used simulating team play. For a load progression through more intense activities, the high-intensity interval method can be used after aerobic interval training. This consists of different running activities performed at high, but not maximal, intensity and short to long sprints (10–30 s) performed at maximal intensity; both spaced out by recovery periods. The high-intensity interval training can be organized as circuits with change of directions and technical exercises to stimulate coordination and agility and to allow the increase of demands on the neuromuscular system and minimize the risk of re-injury. Since high-intensity interval training will produce high neuromuscular stress, its use should be carefully considered especially during early RTP. Nevertheless, before return to team activity (in late RTP), the player should be able to cope with the team's demands, and high-intensity activities provide the metabolic and neuromuscular responses that reproduce soccer-specific demands.

During the return to team phase, the team's session can be considered an additional load for the player. The cognitive (tactical) activity required during a team session places high mental load on the rehabilitating player, and in this manner gradual exposure to team activity is needed. Examples include that during the first week of team training, only low-intensity activity should be allowed (e.g., warm-ups, technical and tactical exercises), whereas in the subsequent week, more intense exercises such as small-sided games are performed on small pitches. In addition, coach encouragement, the presence of goalkeeper, and other influences can change the intensity and should be considered and gradually introduced.

A load monitoring system is costly and is mainly implemented in professional teams; however, alternative strategy can be used in nonprofessional environments. Ratings of perceived exertion (RPE) are less expensive, valid methods to assess training load in soccer. The RPE method is a simple, valid, and cheap method that correlates to heart rate (HR)-based methods in different sports. This is the perceived exercise intensity of the session multiplied by duration. The session-RPE correlates with HR and blood lactate measurement. Indeed, the session-RPE is a global indicator of exercise intensity involving both physiological and psychological factors. For this reason, it may be considered a good integrated marker of internal TL, and it is a method now widespread in professional and amateur level. Even if RPE collection is a simple method, ratings have to be collected confidentially to provide valid and useful ratings.

The implementation of a load monitoring strategy is challenging, and some points should be considered in order to limit the misinterpretation of the outcomes. Different brands and models of GPS tracking systems can provide different reliability so that each player assigned to the same unit is permitted optimal longitudinal assessment (e.g., between days or weeks). Between different metrics, the most frequently used one in football is "the total distance covered." This can be considered both a measure of training volume and a high-intensity running distance.

32.7 When to Return to Competitive Play Following Achilles Tendon Rupture?

The question of when to return to play is frequently considered, even though it is more accurate to consider when to return for training for team selection. Within football most top-level teams will have several players competing for selection for each position, for each game. Given that a player will have a 6 months (or more) lay-off from his/her playing position, it is likely that the replacement player will have become established in that position.

Additionally players will have to have adequate level of psychological recovery to enable play without hesitation.

Psychological aspects are very important during the rehabilitation process and RTP. Information from training load data can be used to provide feedback to the player regarding the ability to cope with on-field specific activities. The sharing of information with athletes can provide consciousness of the ability to RTP and can reduce anxiety and stress and increase their motivation.

32.8 Summary

Achilles tendon ruptures are increasing in number and tend to occur in players at the later stages of their sporting careers. Even when ruptures are "successfully" managed without complication, players will demonstrate objective muscle strength weakness.

In sports, where any loss of muscle strength leads to a considerable disadvantage operative repair, potentially open repair is most probably the management method of choice.

Although return to play at the same level is possible for many recreational athletes, this may be difficult for the professional football player.

Take-Home Message

Operative repair minimizes the strength deficit and optimizes function following an Achilles tendon rupture. Eighty percent of patients returned to play following Achilles tendon rupture. In addition to optimization of calf strength, players will have to have adequate level of proprioceptive calf function as well as psychological recovery to enable RTP without hesitation.

Top Five Evidence Based References

Ardern CL, Glasgow P, Schneiders A, Witvrouw E, Clarsen B, Cools A, Gojanovic B, Griffin S, Khan KM, Moksnes H, Mutch SA, Phillips N, Reurink G, Sadler R, Silbernagel KG, Thorburg K, Wangensteen A, Wilk KE, Bizzini M (2016) 2016 Consensus statement on return to sport from the First World Congress in Physical Therapy, Bern. Br J Sports Med 50(14):853–864

Lantto I, Heikkinen J, Flinkkila T, Ohtonen P, Siira P, Laine V, Leppilahti J (2016) A prospective randomized controlled trial comparing surgical and nonsurgical treatments of acute Achilles tendon ruptures. Am J Sports Med 44(9):2406–2414

Olsson N, Silbernagel KG, Eriksson BI, Sansone M, Brorsson A, Nilsson-Helander K, Karlsson J (2013) Stable surgical repair with accelerated rehabilitation versus non-surgical management for acute Achilles tendon ruptures: a randomized controlled study. Am J Sports Med 41(12):2867–2876

Silbernagel KG, Steele R, Manal K (2012) Deficits in heel rise height and Achilles tendon elongation occur in patients recovering from an Achilles tendon rupture. Am J Sports Med 40(7):1564–1571

Zellers J, Carmont MR, Silbernagel KG (2016) Return to play post Achilles tendon rupture: a systematic review and meta-analysis of rate and measures of return to play. Br J Sports Med 50(21):1325–1332

References

1. Amin NH, Old AB, Tabb LP, Garg R, Toossi N, Cerynik DL (2013) performance outcomes after repair of complete Achilles tendon ruptures in national basketball association players. Am J Sports Med 41(8):1864–1868
2. Ardern CL, Glasgow P, Schneiders A, Witvrouw E, Clarsen B, Cools A, Gojanovic B, Griffin S, Khan KM, Moksnes H, Mutch SA, Phillips N, Reurink G, Sadler R, Silbernagel KG, Thorburg K, Wangensteen A, Wilk KE, Bizzini M (2016) 2016 Consensus statement on return to sport from the First World Congress in Physical Therapy, Bern. Br J Sports Med 50(14):853–864
3. Barfod KW, Nielsen F, Helander KN, Mattila VM, Tingby O, Boesen A, Troelsen A (2013) Treatment of acute Achilles tendon rupture in Scandinavia does not adhere to evidence based guidelines: a cross-sectional questionnaire-based study of 138 departments. J Foot Ankle Surg 52(5):629–633
4. Barfod KW, Bencke J, Lauridsen HB, Ban I, Ebskov L, Troelsen A (2014) Non-operative dynamic treatment of the acute Achilles tendon rupture: the influence of early weight-bearing on clinical outcome: a blinded randomized controlled trial. J Bone Joint Surg Am 96(11):1497–1503
5. Barfod KW, Sveen TM, Ganestam A, Ebskov LB, Troelsen A (2017) Severe functional debilitations after complications associated with acute Achilles tendon ruptures with 9 years of follow up. J Foot Ankle Surg
6. Bostick GP, Jomha NM, Suchak AA, Beaupre LA (2010) Factors associated with calf muscle endurance recovery 1 year after Achilles tendon rupture repair. J Orthop Sports Phys Ther 40(6):345–351
7. Byrne PA, Hopper GP, Wilson WT, Mackay GM (2017) Knotless repair of Achilles tendon rupture in an elite athlete: return to competition in 18 weeks. J Foot Ankle Surg 56(1):121–124
8. Carmont MR, Silbernagel KG, Edge A, Mei-Dan O, Karlsson J, Maffulli N (2013) Functional outcome of percutaneous achilles repair: improvements in achilles tendon total rupture score during the first year. Orthop J Sports Med 1(1):2325967113494584
9. De Carli A, Vadala A, Ciardini R, Iorio R, Feretti A (2009) Spontaneous Achilles tendon ruptures treated with a mini-open technique: clinical and functional evaluation. J Sports Med Phys Fitness 49(3):292–296
10. Del Buono A, Volpin A, Maffulli N (2014) Minimally invasive versus open surgery for acute Achilles tendon rupture: a systematic review. Br Med Bull 109:45–54
11. Ecker TM, Bremer AK, Krause FG, Müller WM (2016) Prospective use of a standardized nonoperative early weight bearing protocol for Achilles tendon rupture: 17 years of experience. Am J Sports Med 44(4):1004–1010
12. Erickson BJ, Masccarenhas R, Saltzman BM, Walton D, Lee S, Cole BJ, Bach BR Jr (2015) Is operative treatment of Achilles tendon ruptures superior to non-operative treatment?: a systematic review of overlapping meta-analyses. Orthop J Sports Med 3(4):2325967115
13. Ferretti A (2014) Functional evaluation of professional athletes treated with mini-open technique for Achilles tendon rupture. Muscles Ligaments Tendons J 4(2):177–181

14. Ganestam A, Kallemose T, Troelsen A, Barfod KW (2016) Increasing incidence of acute Achilles tendon rupture and a noticeable decline in surgical treatment form 1994-2013. A nationwide registry study of 33,160 patients. Knee Surg Sports Traumatol Arthrosc 24(12):370–3737
15. Gigante A, Moschini A, Verdenelli A, Del Torto M, Ulisse S, de Palma L (2008) Open versus percutaneous repair in the treatment of acute Achilles tendon rupture: a randomized prospective study. Knee Surg Sports Traumatol Arthrosc 16(2):204–209
16. Grimby G, Börjesson M, Jonsdottir IH, Schnohr P, Thelle DS, Saltin B (2015) The "Saltin-Grimby Physical Activity Scale" and its application to health research. Scand J Med Sci Sports 25(S4):119–125
17. Halasi T, Kynsburg A, T'allay A, Berkes I (2004) Development of a new activity score for the evaluation of ankle instability. Am J Sports Med 32(4):899–908
18. Heikkinen J, Lantto I, Flinkkilä T, Ohtonen P, Pajala A, Siira P, Leppilahti J (2016) Augmented compared to non-augmented surgical repair after total Achilles rupture: results of a prospective randomized trial with 13 or more years of follow up. J Bone Joint Surg Am 98(2):85–92
19. Horstmann T, Lukas C, Merk J, Brauner T, Mundermann A (2012) Deficits 10 years after Achilles tendon repair. Int J Sports Med 33(6):474–479
20. Hutchison AM, Topliss C, Beard D, Evans RM, Williams P (2015) The treatment of a rupture of the Achilles tendon using a dedicated management programme. Bone Joint J 97-B(4):510–515
21. Huttunen TT, Kannus P, Rolf C, Felländer-Tsai L, Mattila VM (2014) Acute Achilles tendon ruptures: incidence of injury and surgery in Sweden between 2001 and 2012. Am J Sports Med 42(10):2419–2423
22. Ibrahim SA (2009) Surgical treatment of chronic Achilles tendon rupture. J Foot Ankle Surg 48(3):340–346
23. Jallageas R, Bordes J, Daviet JC, Mabit C, Coste C (2013) Evaluation of surgical treatment for ruptured Achilles tendon in 31 athletes. Orthop Traumatol Surg Res 99(5):577–584
24. Józsa L, Kvist M, Bálint BJ, Reffy A, Järvinen M, Lehto M, Barzo M (1989) The role of recreational sport activity in Achilles tendon rupture. A clinical pathoanatomical and sociological study of 292 cases. Am J Sports Med 17(3):338–343
25. Kangas J, Pajala A, Ohtonen P, Leppilahti J (2007) Achilles tendon elongation after rupture repair: a randomized comparison of two post operative regimens. Am J Sports Med 35(1):59–64
26. Keating JF, Will EM (2011) Operative versus non-operative treatment of acute rupture of tendo Achillis: a prospective randomized evaluation of functional outcome. J Bone Joint Surg Br 93(8):1071–1078
27. Kosanovic M, Brilej D (2008) Chronic rupture of Achilles tendon: is the percutaneous technique effective. Arch Orthop Trauma Surg 128(2):211–216
28. Lantto I, Heikkinen J, Flinkkilä T, Ohtonen P, Leppilahti J (2015) Epidemiology of Achilles tendon ruptures: increasing incidence over a 33-year period. Scand J Med Sci Sports 25(1):e133–e138
29. Lantto I, Heikkinen J, Flinkkilä T, Ohtonen P, Kangas J, Siira P, Leppilahti J (2015) Early functional treatment versus cast immobilization in tension after Achilles rupture repair: results of a prospective randomized trial with 10 or more years of follow up. Am J Sports Med 43(9):3020–3029
30. Lantto I, Heikkinen J, Flinkkila T, Ohtonen P, Siira P, Laine V, Leppilahti J (2016) A prospective randomized controlled trial comparing surgical and non-surgical treatments of acute Achilles tendon ruptures. Am J Sports Med 44(9):2406–2414
31. López Valerio V, Sejias R, Alvarez P, Ares O, Steinbacher G, Salient A, Cugat R (2015) Endoscopic repair of posterior ankle impingement syndrome due to os trigonum in soccer players. Foot Ankle Int 36(1):70–74
32. Maffulli N, Longo UG, Maffulli GD, Khanna A, Denaro V (2011) Achilles tendon ruptures in elite athletes. Foot Ankle Int 32(1):9–15
33. Majewski M, Schaeren S, Kohlhaas U, Oschner PE (2008) Postoperative rehabilitation after percutaneous Achilles tendon repair: early functional therapy versus cast immobilization. Disabil Rehabil 30(20-22):1726–1732
34. Matheny LM, Johnson NS, Liechti DJ, Clanton TO (2016) Activity level and function after lateral ankle ligament repair versus reconstruction. Am J Sports Med 44(5):1301–1308
35. Martinelli B (2000) Percutaneous repair of the Achilles tendon in athletes. Bull J Hosp Dis 59(3):149–152
36. Mattila VM, Huttunen TT, Haapasalo H, Sillanpää P, Malmivaara A, Pihlajamäki H (2015) Declining incidence of surgery for Achilles tendon rupture follows publication of major RCTs: evidence influenced change evident using the Finnish registry study. Br J Sports Med 49(16):1084–1086
37. Mavrodontidis A, Lykissas M, Koulouvaris P, Pafilas D, Kontogeorgakos V, Zalavras C (2015) Percutaneous repair of acute Achilles tendon rupture: a functional evaluation study with a minimum 10 year follow up. Acta Orthop Traumatol Turc 49(6):661–667
38. McMahon SE, Smith TO, Hing CB (2011) A meta-analysis of randomized controlled trials comparing conventional to minimally invasive approaches for repair of an Achilles tendon rupture. Foot Ankle Surg 17(4):211–217
39. McCullough KA, Shaw CM, Anderson RB (2014) Min-open repair of Achilles rupture in the National Football League. J Orthop Surg Adv 23(4):179–183
40. Metz R, Verleisdonk EJ, van der Heijden GJ, Clevers GJ, Hammacher ER, Verhofstad MH, van der Werken C (2008) Acute Achilles tendon rupture: minimally invasive surgery versus non-operative treatment with immediate full weight bearing- a randomized controlled trial. Am J Sports Med 36(9):1688–1694
41. Mortensen H, Skov O, Jensen P (1999) Early motion of Achilles after operative treatment of a rupture of the Achilles tendon: a prospective randomized clinical and radiographic study. J Bone Joint Surg Am 81(7):983–990
42. Nilsson-Helander K, Silbernagel KG, Thomeé R, Faxén E, Olsson N, Eriksson BI, Karlsson J (2010)

Acute Achilles Tendon Rupture: a randomized controlled study comparing surgical and non-surgical treatments using validated outcomes measures. Am J Sports Med 38(11):2186–2193
43. Olsson N, Nilsson-Helander K, Karlsson J, Eriksson BI, Thomee R, Faxen E, Silbernagel KG (2011) Major functional deficits persist 2 years after acute Achilles tendon rupture. Knee Surg Sports Traumatol Arthrosc 19:1385–1393
44. Olsson N, Silbernagel KG, Eriksson BI, Sansone M, Brorsson A, Nilsson-Helander K, Karlsson J (2013) Stable surgical repair with accelerated rehabilitation versus non-surgical management for acute Achilles tendon ruptures: a randomized controlled study. Am J Sports Med 41(12):2867–2876
45. Olsson N, Karlsson J, Eriksson BI, Brorsson A, Lundberg M, Silbernagel KG (2014) Ability to perform a single heel rise is significantly related to patient-reported outcome after Achilles tendon rupture. Scand J Med Sci Sports 24(1):152–158
46. Olsson N, Petzold M, Brorsson A, Karlsson J, Eriksson BI, Silbernagel KG (2014) Predictors of clinical outcome after acute Achilles tendon. Am J Sports Med 42(6):1448–1455
47. Pajala A, Kangas J, Siira P, Ohtonen P, Leppilahti J (2009) Augmented compared with non-augmented surgical repair of a fresh total Achilles tendon rupture. A prospective randomized study. J Bone Joint Surg Am 91(5):1092–1100
48. Parekh SG, Wray WH III, Brimmo O, Sennett BJ, Wapner KL (2009) Epidemiology and outcomes of Achilles tendon ruptures in the National Football League. Foot Ankle Spec 2(6):283–286
49. Pollock N, Dijkstra P, Calder J, Chakraverty R (2016) Plantaris injuries in elite UK track and field athletes over a 4 year period: a retrospective cohort study. Knee Surg Sports Traumatol Arthrosc 24(7):2287–2292
50. Saxena A, Ewan B, Maffulli N (2011) Rehabilitation of the operated Achilles tendon: parameters for predicting return to activity. J Foot Ankle Surg 50(1):37–40
51. Schepull T, Kvist J, Aspenberg P (2012) Early E modulus of healing Achilles tendons correlates with late function: similar results with or without surgery. Scand J Med Sci Sports 22(1):18–23
52. Scott A, Grewal N, Guy P (2014) The seasonal variation of Achilles tendon ruptures in Vancouver, Canada: a retrospective study. BMJ 4(2):e004320
53. Sheth U, Wasserstein D, Jenkinson R, Moineddin R, Kreder H, Jaglal SB (2017) The epidemiology and trends in management of acute Achilles tendon ruptures in Ontario, Canada: a population based study of 27607 patients. Bone Joint J 99-B(1):78–86
54. Silbernagel KG, Steele R, Manal K (2012) Deficits in heel rise height and Achilles tendon elongation occur in patients recovering from an Achilles tendon rupture. Am J Sports Med 40(7):1564–1571
55. Silbernagel KG, Brorsson A, Karlsson J (2014) Rehabilitation following Achilles tendon rupture. In: Karlsson J, Calder J, van Dijk CN, Maffulli N, Thermann H (eds) Achilles tendon disorders: a comprehensive overview of diagnosis and treatment. DJO publications, London, pp 151–164
56. Soroceanu A, Sidhwa F, Aarabi S, Kaufman A, Glazebrook M (2012) Surgical versus non-surgical treatment of acute Achilles tendon rupture: a meta-analysis of randomized trials. J Bone Joint Surg Am 94(23):2136–2143
57. Suchak AA, Bostick GP, Beaupré LA, Durand DC, Jomha NM (2008) The influence of early weight bearing compared with non-weight bearing after surgical repair of the Achilles tendon. J Bone Joint Surg Am 90:1876–1883
58. Suchak AA, Bostick G, Reid D, Blitz S, Jomha N (2005) The incidence of Achilles tendon ruptures in Edmonton, Canada. Foot Ankle Int 26(11):932–936
59. Suydam SM, Buchannan TS, Manal K, Silbernagel KG (2015) Compensatory muscle activation caused by tendon lengthening post Achilles tendon rupture. Knee Surg Sports Traumatol Arthrosc 23:868
60. Tegner Y, Lyholm J (1985) Rating systems in the evaluation of knee ligament injuries. Clin Orthop Relat Res 198:43–49
61. Wallace RG, Heyes GJ, Michael AL (2011) The non-operative functional management of patients with a rupture of the tendo Achillis leads to low rates of re-rupture. J Bone Joint Surg 93(11):1362–1366
62. Wang D, Sandlin MI, Cohen JR, Lord EL, Petrigliano FA, SooHoo NF (2015) Operative versus non-operative treatment of acute Achilles tendon rupture: an analysis of 12570 patients in a large healthcare database. Foot Ankle Surg 21(4):250–253
63. Willits K, Amendola A, Bryant D, Mohtadi NG, Giffin JR, Fowler P, Kean CO, Kirkley A (2010) Operative versus non-operative treatment of acute Achilles tendon ruptures: a multicenter randomized trial using accelerated functional rehabilitation. J Bone Joint Surg Am 92:767–775
64. Willy RW, Brorsson A, Powell HC, Wilson JD, Tranberg R, Grävare Silbernagel K (2017) Elevated knee joint kinematics and reduced ankle kinematics are present during jogging and hopping after Achilles tendon ruptures. Am J Sports Med 45:1124
65. Vadalà A, De Carli A, Vulpiani MC, Iorio R, Vetrano SS, Suarez T, Di Salvo F, Ferretti A (2012) Clinical, functional and radiological results of Achilles tenorrhaphy, surgically treated with mini-open technique. J Sports Med Phys Fitness 52(6):616–621
66. Ververidis AN, Kalifis KG, Touzopoulos P, Drosos GI, Tilkeridis KE, Kazakos KI (2015) Percutaneous repair of the Achilles tendon rupture in athletic population. J Orthop 13(1):57–61
67. Yang B, Liu Y, Kan S, Zhang D, Xu H, Liu F, Ning G, Feng S (2017) Outcomes and complications of percutaneous versus open repair of acute Achilles tendon rupture: a meta-analysis. Int J Surg 40:178–186
68. Zellers J, Carmont MR, Grävare-Silbernagel K (2016) Return to play post Achilles tendon rupture: a systematic review and meta-analysis of rate and measures of return to play. Br J Sports Med 50(21):1325–1332

33 Return to Play in Muscle Injuries

Peter Ueblacker
and Hans-Wilhelm Mueller-Wohlfahrt

Contents

33.1 Epidemiology

Muscle injuries constitute more than one-third of all time-loss injuries and cause more than 25% of the total injury absence in high-level European professional football clubs [1, 2]. A football team of 25 players can expect, on average, about 15 muscle injuries over the season; a player sustains 0.6 muscle injuries per season [1].

P. Ueblacker, M.D. (✉)
H.-W. Mueller-Wohlfahrt, M.D.
MW Center of Orthopedics and Sports Medicine, Dienerstrasse 12, 80331 Munich, Germany
e-mail: peter.ueblacker@gmx.net

Ninety-two percent of all *indirect* muscle injuries affect the four major muscle groups of the lower limbs; the hamstring (37%), adductor (23%), quadriceps (19%) and calf (13%) muscles are the most common injury locations [1]. *Direct* muscle injuries involve most likely the intermediate and lateral vastus muscle, the rectus femoris and calf muscles. These five different muscle injury types are among the ten most common injury subtypes in male professional football: hamstring muscle injury, adductor injury, quadriceps muscle injury, calf muscle injury and thigh contusion [3].

Hamstring injury is the most common injury subtype in male professional football, representing 12% of all injuries [2]. The muscle injury rate has remained high and unchanged for more than a decade [4]. Recently, it has been shown that there is even a substantial increase regarding training-related hamstring injury rates since 2001 [2].

Fact Box 1

Epidemiology [1, 5, 6]

- Muscle injuries account for 35% of all injuries in professional football and cause 25% of total absence.
- A male elite football team of 25 players can expect 15 muscle injuries each season.
- On average, every player sustains 0.6 muscle injuries per season.

V. Musahl et al. (eds.), *Return to Play in Football*, https://doi.org/10.1007/978-3-662-55713-6_33

- The muscle injury rate has remained high over the last decade.
- *Indirect* time-loss muscle injuries are much more frequent compared to *direct* injuries.
- Ninety-two percent affect the four muscle groups: hamstring, the quadriceps (mainly rectus femoris), the adductor and the calf muscles.
- The most common single type is hamstring injury (86% of these injuries affect the biceps femoris).
- Hamstring injuries are related to high velocity (sprinting).
- Quadriceps injuries are related to shots at goal.
- The risk of injury is six times higher during matches compared to training.

33.2 Definitions

Following definitions are used in this chapter in accordance with previous publications [2, 7, 8]:

Injury: Injury resulting from playing football and leading to a player being unable to fully participate in future training and match play (time-loss injury).

***Indirect* muscle injury**: A muscle injury caused without the influence of a direct external trauma.

***Non-structural (functional)* injury**: Painful muscle injury without macroscopic evidence of muscle fibre damage (seen in ultrasound/MRI).

***Structural* injury**: Any acute indirect muscle injury with macroscopic evidence of muscle fibre damage ("tear", seen in ultrasound/MRI).

***Direct* muscle injury**: A traumatic muscle injury caused by a direct (blunt or sharp) external trauma.

Return to play (RTP): Refers to the time point after injury when the athlete is fully able to participate in training and available for match selection.

Lay-off/absence: Number of days until the player resumed full team training.

Reinjury/recurrency: Injury of the same type and at the same site as an index injury occurring no more than 2 months after a player's return to full participation from the index injury.

(**Strain**: This term should be avoided since it is a biomechanical term which is not defined and used indiscriminately for anatomically and functionally different muscle injuries.)

33.3 Diagnosis and Classification of Muscle Injuries

Athletic muscle injuries present a heterogeneous group and are difficult to define and categorize. However, an accurate diagnosis is the first step towards a specific treatment and usually allows to predict return to play [8–10]. The risks of misdiagnosis are high; it can affect a player's progress in terms of rehabilitation and return to play and can also be expected to affect recurrence and complication rate for the injury. The diagnosis of acute muscle injuries is normally based on medical history and clinical findings with radiological methods such as MRI or ultrasound being used to provide additional information to confirm the diagnosis [11–14]. Physical examination includes inspection (Fig. 33.1), palpation, functional testing, range of motion of the adjacent joints and stretch testing [10].

Many different classification systems are published in the literature with a high number of proposals in recent years [15–22]. However, some of them are lacking diagnostic accuracy and provide limited prognostic validity.

Due to the variety of classification systems, there is still little consistency within studies and in daily practice. In 2012, a comprehensive expert consensus-based classification was published [16]. This categorization defines and subclassifies most types of athletic muscle injuries. In contrast to other recent classifications, it is based on medical history, examination and imaging—and not solely on imaging. The system differentiates between *indirect* and *direct* muscle injuries which is important because these injury types cause different time of absence [6, 9, 10, 16]. The validity of this so-called *Munich classification system* is

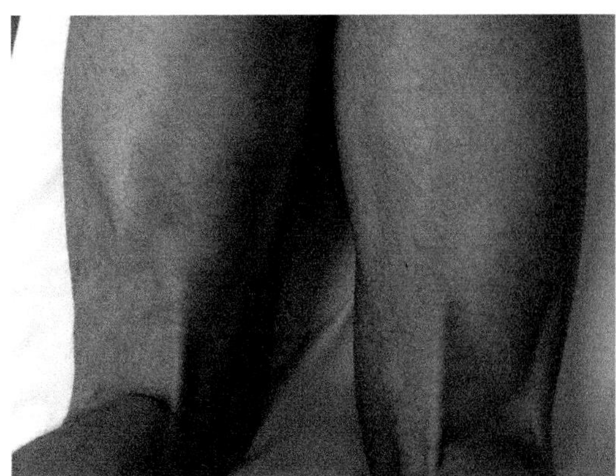

Fig. 33.1 Clinical inspection of an acute *subtotal muscle tear* (distal long head of left biceps femoris) in an elite football player (dynamic inspection—the player contracts the hamstrings against manual resistance). Note the *retracted/proximalized muscle belly* and the *defect zone distally*; the *biceps femoris tendon* is not detectable. Compare the normal *muscle relief* on the right side. The severity of this injury is obvious on inspection and functional testing; however, it was initially underestimated as a *minor partial muscle injury*. The injury was managed conservatively, absence was approximately 5 months, the player returned to preinjury level with unrestricted training and competition, and no reinjury occurred during the following years until today

evaluated for return to play after thigh muscle injury in professional male football players [9]. This is "the first time in over 100 years of muscle injury grading that authors are testing a proposed classification model" [23].

Indirect injuries are differentiated into *functional (non-structural)* and *structural* types. *Functional* injuries/disorders are minor injuries causing swelling, oedema and painful muscle tightness. Players are unable to compete because of *functional* limitations even though muscle fibres are macroscopically intact. *Structural* injuries (tears) are usually induced by eccentric stretching and are caused by a sudden forced lengthening, in excess of the muscle's viscoelastic limits, during a powerful contraction (i.e. an internal force). There are different types and grades of each category [16, 24]. *Structural* injuries, for example, are subclassified according to their size and prognosis into minor and moderate partial and into (sub)total tears.

Direct injuries (i.e. lacerations or contusions) are caused by external forces, e.g. a direct blow from an opponent's knee. Contusion injuries can lead to bleeding, causing pain and a loss of motion, but muscle fibres are usually not torn from longitudinal traction.

The incidence of *indirect* injuries is about eight times higher (1.48/1000 h) compared to *direct* muscle injuries (0.19/1000 h) ($p < 0.01$) [6].

Fact Box 2

Diagnosis and classification [10, 13, 24]

- Diagnosis and classification are based on medical history and clinical examination.
- Imaging (ultrasound and MRI) is indicated in *structural* injuries and provides additional information.
- There are *indirect* ("strains") and *direct* (most of them contusion) injuries.
- *Indirect* injuries are classified into *non-structural* (MRI negative or oedema only) and *structural* (visible tear in MRI) injuries.
- Classification and sub-grouping can have a prognostic validity for RTP.

33.4 Treatment

Current treatment principles have no firm scientific basis; they are practiced largely as empirical medicine due to a lack of prospective randomized studies [24–27].

Immediate treatment. It usually follows the well-known PRICE regimen (protection, rest, ice, compression and elevation), even though there is not a single randomized prospective study to prove its evidence [25, 27]. The aim of the immediate treatment is to minimize bleeding into the injury site. Any larger hematoma is a mechanical barrier for the healing tissue and may lead to scar formation with direct clinical relevance regarding absence. Insufficient acute treatment will not only delay the healing process but also increases the risk of subsequent imaging overestimating the injury owing to the presence of a hematoma or oedema (seen as a bright signal in the MRI). An elastic compression bandage soaked in ice-cold water is a simple and fast immediate treatment for muscle injuries. Even though there is some discussion about cooling and sports injuries [28], its liberal use seems justified even in the presence of uncertainty about the precise diagnosis because of the scarcity of side effects. Early mobilization allows more rapid and intensive capillary ingrowth in the injured area, better regeneration of muscle fibres and a more parallel orientation in the regenerating myofibres and should be aimed in the majority of the cases.

Non-operative treatment versus surgery. As mentioned above, the vast majority of muscle injuries can be resolved with non-operative treatment; only a small number of cases will require surgical intervention [16, 29]. Complete tendinous avulsion/rupture with significant retraction of the muscle (in biomechanical terms, a total tear in the origin or insertion of the muscle) is unlikely to heal spontaneously at the original anatomical localization [30]. Surgical reattachment using suture anchors is usually indicated in these cases, especially on the proximal rectus femoris [30, 31] and the proximal hamstrings [32, 33]. In contrast, complete tendinous avulsions of the proximal adductor longus (an uniarticular muscle) can be managed conservatively with equal results to operative treatment and unrestricted return to play to preinjury level in high-performance athletes [34].

Non-steroidal anti-inflammatory drugs (NSAID). Clinical and basic scientific studies have reported conflicting and even negative effects of NSAIDs on the healing process of muscle injury [35–38]. NSAIDs suppress the perception of pain by inhibiting prostaglandin synthesis, which may create problems, as an accurate and undistorted perception of the state of the injured muscle is of great importance for the player's rapid or progressive rehabilitation [24]. Moreover, NSAIDs can have adverse effects such as fibrosis of the injured muscle [36, 38]. Thus, NSAIDs are not recommended for the treatment of muscle injuries or only for a few days.

Injection therapy. In a number of different variations, it is used frequently, with positive results empirically. Evidence in the form of prospective randomized studies is still needed in order to verify these results and analyse the long-term effects. The aim of injecting therapeutic agents directly into injured muscle tissue is to regulate muscle tone, to create optimum conditions for muscle regeneration and—if there is a hematoma/seroma—to puncture it in the same session. There are several types of medication, such as Actovegin®, a deproteinized hemoderivative (which is not FDA-approved), and autologous serum products (platelet-rich plasma, PRP) that are currently used for injection. Is has been shown that Actovegin® has a positive impact on muscle regeneration after injury, particularly in terms of fibre synthesis, detonization of firm muscle fibres and the shortening of recovery times [39, 40]. New data demonstrate that Actovegin® activates satellite cells and supports the differentiation of myotubes [41]. However, more objective evidence is needed before any definitive conclusions can be drawn.

PRP is increasingly being used in situations that require a rapid RTP, and more and more data are reported on effects on muscle injuries with controversial results [42, 43]. PRP has not yet been systematically studied and questions remain as to when and how PRP should be used in muscle injuries [44]. PRP may contain deleterious cytokines and growth factors, such as TGF-β1, that can cause fibrosis and inhibit optimal muscle healing [45, 46]. Thus, *non-structural* and smaller *structural* muscle injuries should not be treated with PRP in order to avoid scarring.

Stem cell treatment. It has been proposed as another option for the treatment of muscle injuries [47–49]. However, clinical studies are needed before definitive conclusions can be drawn.

Corticosteroids. These should never be used locally or systemically in the treatment of muscle injuries. They can delay healing by suppressing physiological responses to injury, reduce biomechanical strength of injured muscle and increase the risk of a soft tissue infection and/or local soft tissue necrosis [25, 50, 51]. Positive reports in the literature [52] can definitely not be confirmed.

Appropriate physical therapy, rehabilitative exercises and training therapy are essential components of the rehabilitation of an injured muscle.

Table 33.1 Example of a *rehabilitation programme* including a passive, semi-active and active phase with *gradual increasing load*

Week	Principle	ROM	Basic content
1–3	Passive	Hip abduction/adduction limited to 10°–0°–10° No active abduction and stretching until week 7	Gentle lymphatic drainage Passive mobilization of the hip in flexion/extension
4–5	Semi-active	Hip abduction/adduction limited to 20°–0°–20°	Exercises against body weight Cycling and unidirectional aquajogging
6	Active, increasing intensity	Free	Running training unidirectional within aerobic intensity starting with 20 min Training of basic fitness Careful manually guided stretching
7	Active	Free	Careful start with strengthening exercises Activation of adductor longus muscle Coordinative exercises in more complex movement patterns
8–10	Active	Free	Running training with increasing intensity, multidirectional, start of sport-specific training
10+	Active	Free	Sprints and multidirectional running Training with ball, back to team

This particular programme was developed for conservative management after complete proximal adductor longus avulsion (adapted from Ueblacker et al. [34])

Regular follow-up examinations on the current muscle status are crucial to evaluate the progress made in terms of healing and to determine when the injured muscle can be exposed to the next step of load. A precise rehabilitation programme should be developed for each athletic muscle injury, including recommendations for sport-specific training with gradually increasing intensity (Table 33.1). Comprehensive rehabilitation programmes for all specific athletic muscle injuries can be found in [10].

33.5 Return to Play/Absence After Various Types of Muscle Injury

The most important question to physicians and the medical team after an injury is: "when will the player be back safely?"—particularly in elite athletes, where return to play and player availability have significant financial or strategic consequences for the player and the team. For example, the absence of an injured football player can generate costs for the club of 30,000 euro per day (player salary of 5 million euro, transfer amount of 30 million euro and a 5-year contract assumed) [8].

The biology of muscle healing is well described in the current literature [25, 53]. Healing of muscle tears is a gradual process, and time is needed depending on injury type and the size of the tissue defect to restore the function of the muscle to the preinjury level [8, 10, 25, 54]. Muscle tissue can heal *ad integrum* without an obvious remaining scarring/fibrosis depending on the muscle tissue defect and involvement of intramuscular connective tissue, tendons, and fascia. Usually *minor partial muscle tears* heal completely, while *moderate partial tears* or larger injuries result in a defective healing with scarring/fibrosis [53]. Early after injury, the connective tissue scar is the weakest point [25, 55]. At a certain point, depending on the injury size, the maturation of the scar has reached the point at which it no longer is the weakest point of the injured muscle; if loaded to failure, the tissue usually tears within the muscle tissue adjacent to the scar tissue [25]. In more severe injuries, a fibrotic scar can remain, palpable as a rigid mass within the muscle. Fibrosis can impair the function of skeletal muscle; however, many elite athletes play on the highest level with a certain scar tissue in their muscles after more severe muscle injuries. Fibrosis is difficult to quantify [49]; the relationship between fibrosis and increased muscle stiffness remains unclear [56].

Returning to full activity without sufficient healing of the muscle tissue and without a recovery of tensile strength is likely to lead to more severe reinjuries [16, 25]. Thus, an excellent communication between the coaching staff (rehabilitation, fitness and head coach) and the medical team is the essential precondition for a successful RTP after every injury.

Classification and sub-grouping into injury type and dimension of pathology can help to prognosticate RTP after thigh muscle injury in professional male football players [6, 9] (Fig. 33.2). It has been shown that *indirect* muscle injuries cause 19% of total injury-driven absence and *direct* injuries 1%. The mean lay-off time for all *indirect* injuries is 18.5 days what differs significantly from *direct* injuries with 7.0 days ($p < 0.001$) [6].

Muscle contusions. These are usually painful and may cause considerable functional disability in the affected area. However, players with *contusions (direct injuries)* can often continue playing for some time, whereas *indirect structural* injuries most often urge the player to stop at once [24]. It is known that early return to full function and rehabilitative therapy after *direct* injuries can be usually more aggressive to the limit of pain tolerance (Fig. 33.3), which is not the case in *indirect* muscle injuries [6, 57, 58].

Referred pain, spine-related muscle injuries. It is well known that lumbar pathologies such as a disc hernia at the L5/S1 level are very frequent in

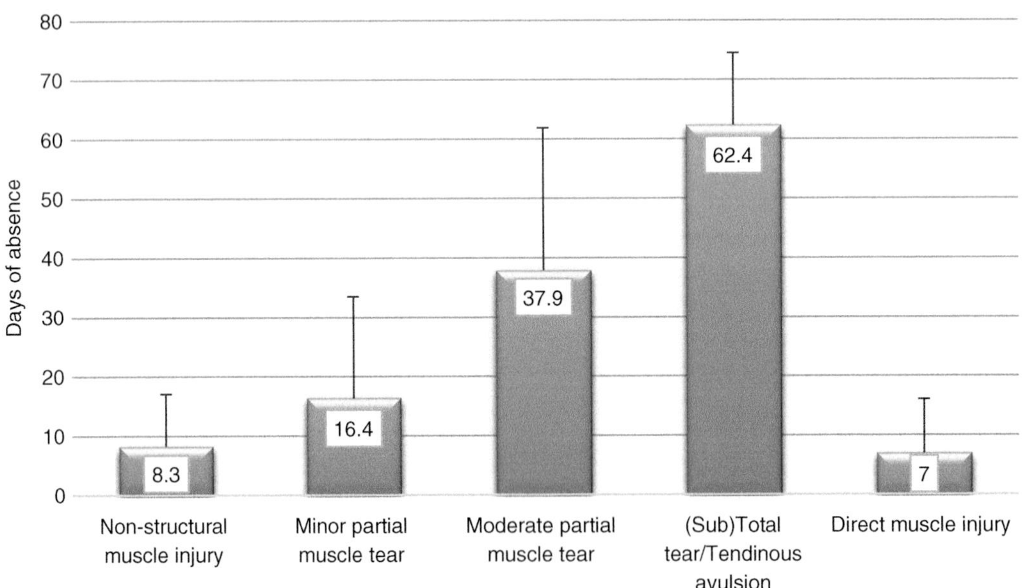

Fig. 33.2 Mean days of *absence* (and standard deviation) after various types and grades of muscle injury (modified from [6, 8, 9]. As the *large standard deviations* show, there is considerable variation in RTP for all muscle injuries; rehabilitation can proceed faster or take longer (e.g. if the central tendon is involved, after previous injury, etc.) depending on the individual case. Note: only a few of *direct* muscle injuries (most of them contusions) cause absence; the vast majority of players with these type of injury can continue to play which is not possible after an *indirect* injury, e.g. partial muscle tear

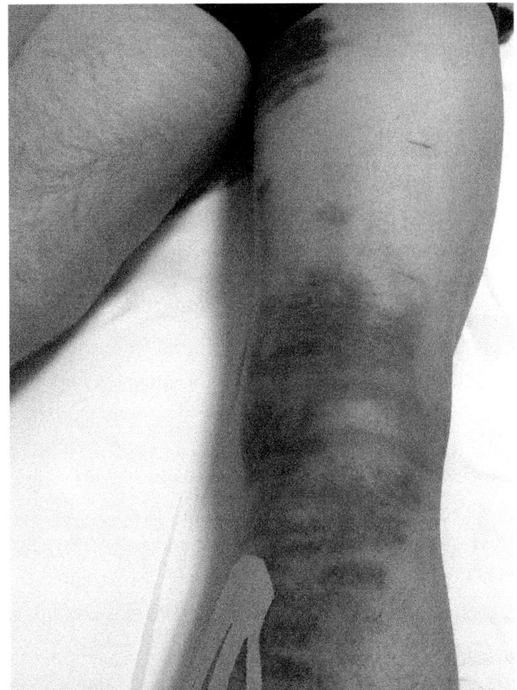

Fig. 33.3 Extensive *muscle contusion* on the dorsal thigh and calf of an elite football player. Clinical examination and imaging demonstrated diffuse hematomas, but no substantial tear; no signs of compartment syndrome. After a *fast 4-day rehabilitation*, the player was asymptomatic and able to fully participate in training. Two days later, he played without complaints in a national league game, no reinjury occurred

elite athletes [59, 60] and may present with hamstring and/or calf pain and limited flexibility. This can result in, or mimic, a muscle injury [61] which can prevent a player from training and competing and will require comprehensive treatment. Differentiation between spine-related injuries and other injuries is important, not only because of the different pathogenesis but also because of the different therapeutic implications [10, 61].

33.6 Risk Factors for Muscle Injury and Preventive Strategies

Previous injury (especially a more severe injury and involvement of the tendon) has been shown to be the highest risk factor for subsequent muscle injury. Other potential risk factors are shown below. The results of recent studies confirm that preventive strategies can reduce the risk of muscle injuries (Table 33.2) [13, 62–67].

Table 33.2 Overview of potential risk factors for muscle injuries and possible preventive strategies

Risk factor	Preventive strategy
Poor strength, hamstring/quadriceps strength ratio imbalance	Balanced muscle strengthening, eccentric muscle exercises (e.g. "Nordic hamstring"), improvement of intermuscular coordination
Limited flexibility	Stretching
Limited ROM of adjacent joints	Joint mobilization
Poor warm up before training/competition	Improvement of warm up methods
Weak core stability	Strengthening of lumbopelvic muscles ("core")
Fatigue	Improvement of basic fitness
Intense training sessions, coaching methods, end of the season	Control of training load, communication between rehabilitation, fitness and head coaches

Exercises to stabilize the lumbopelvic muscles (called also the lumbopelvic-hip complex or "core") have become increasingly popular in recent years for general injury prevention, especially in high-level sports. Deficits in the neuromuscular control of the lumbopelvic region are considered an important predisposing factor for muscle injuries [67]. Many studies confirm that training to improve lumbopelvic stability and strength can influence the function of the lower extremity muscles significantly and that this type of training can also make an important contribution for the prevention of muscle injuries by optimizing the function of the lower extremity muscles [65, 68].

33.7 Return to Play Criteria

It must be emphasized that there are no consensus guidelines or standardized criteria for safe return to sport following muscle injury [8, 10, 66, 69].

The primary aim is a safe RTP with minimal risk of reinjury. But how can this be managed (Table 33.3)?

Table 33.3 An overview of RTP criteria that are discussed in the current literature [8, 13, 66, 70, 71] and their relevance

RTP criteria	Relevance/interpretation
Player is asymptomatic at clinical evaluation	Pain after muscle injury often subsides within a few days. This may tempt the athlete as well as the medical and coaching team to load the injured muscle too early. Absence of pain does not correlate with healing of muscle tissue; pain is not a good indicator during rehabilitation of muscle injuries Muscle tone/tension should be equal to contralateral side; there should be no tenderness on injury site on palpation. However, scar tissue within the muscle can be palpable, especially after more severe muscle injuries
Athletes subjective readiness	Important factor. A recent systematic review demonstrates moderate evidence that visual analogue scale pain at time of injury and predictions for time to RTP by the patient and the clinician are associated with time to RTP [72]
Normalized muscle strength	Controversially discussed, see below
Normal muscle flexibility and ROM of adjacent joints	Easy to determine in clinical examination, important functional factors for RTP and further injury prevention
Normal muscle balance, strong lumbopelvic muscles ("core")	Important functional factors for RTP and further injury prevention but more difficult to determine
Normal basic fitness	Important factor to avoid fatigue (data should be compared with preinjury data)
Ability to complete sport-specific training without pain and symptoms	Important factor, inevitable before team training. Should be performed after progressive rehabilitation programme including running training, sprinting, stop-and-go, etc. and individual non-contact training with the ball
Normalized imaging	Controversially discussed, see below

During rehabilitation, thorough follow-up examinations including palpation, functional testing and imaging (in case of more severe injuries) are crucial to evaluate the progress made in terms of healing and to determine when the injured muscle can be reexposed to the next step of load. If possible, all data should be compared with existing preinjury data (e.g. obtained during preseason testing).

In accordance with others [73], the authors of this chapter recommend a step-by-step algorithm. Progressive exercising of the injured limb in incremental stages not only retrains the muscles in complex movement patterns but also provides valuable feedback for the athletes, the medical and coaching teams. The player is ready to advance to the next stage only when he/she is free of complaints/pain and the tone of the muscle is not elevated. The primary goal is to avoid that players are exposed to high loads too early and thus to avoid reinjury.

Strength testing. The value of strength testing before RTP is still controversially discussed [13, 70, 74, 75]. Less than 10% isokinetic strength deficit was previously described as an acceptable limit. However, a recent study demonstrated that 67% of clinically recovered hamstring injuries showed at least one hamstring isokinetic testing deficit of more than 10% concluding that the normalization of isokinetic strength testing seems not to be a necessary result of the successful completion of a football-specific rehabilitation programme [75]. It remains unknown if an isokinetic strength deficit is associated with an increased risk of reinjury [75]. It has been discussed that muscle function after acute muscle injury is still in question even after an athletes RTP [49]. A study in male semiprofessional football players explored that function improved with time after RTP [49, 76]; injured athletes were slower at sprinting compared to non-injured players at RTP. This study was conducted in semiprofessional players. However, it is debatable whether and how often this occurs on elite level.

It is important to state that no maximal strength tests should be performed before RTP since strength tests represent maximum (and sometimes isolated) load on the injured tissue with a high risk of reinjury.

Imaging. MRI has been the preferred imaging for muscle injuries in recent years [77–80]. Its use in the assessment of muscle injuries is very controversially discussed in the literature [12, 69, 77, 81, 82]. In summary, MRI is partially helpful in grading of injuries, determination of tissue defect size and location of injuries.

During healing and rehabilitation, imaging is especially indicated in the more severe muscle injuries to exclude further retraction of muscle fascicles, to identify hematoma and/or seroma and to assess tissue healing and scarring. However, when imaging is used without concomitant clinical information, it can lead to misinterpretation since there are no specific pathological changes separating *direct* from *indirect* injuries [6, 83]. Moreover, the resolution of the injury as detected by MRI can be delayed compared to functional recovery, in *indirect* injuries [84, 85], as well as in *direct* injuries [57]. Despite markedly abnormal MR images weeks and even months after return to play (i.e. pathological signals resulting from oedema, hematoma, scarring, etc.), athletes can be able to compete at the highest professional level without functional deficit in many cases [57, 82, 84, 85]. Thus, imaging to determine RTP has to be used with caution; its value is very controversially discussed.

33.8 Reinjuries

The recurrence rate in male professional football players amounts to 16% [1]. The greatest risk is during the initial 2 weeks following RTP [54]. Reinjuries are usually more extensive than the initial injury and cause a longer period of absence [1, 5]. Recurrences could be reduced if precise clinical evaluation and diagnosis are performed which are critical for adequate assessment and rehabilitation of a muscle injury. The current discussion about premature RTP after surgery [86] must definitely be expanded to premature RTP after muscle injury.

Fact Box 3

RTP criteria and reinjuries

- Different types and grades of muscle injuries lead to different absence times.
- Biology in terms of tissue healing has to be respected.
- There are no consensus guidelines or standardized criteria.
- The value of strength testing and MR imaging is controversially discussed.
- The highest risk factor for muscle injury is a previous injury (players with a previous hamstring injury have a seven times higher risk for injury); other risk factors are controversially discussed.
- The reinjury rate after muscle injury is 16%.
- Reinjuries cause 30% longer absence.

Take-Home Message

- Muscle injury is the most frequent injury type in professional football.
- RTP/absence following muscle injury depends on the injury type and grade.
- The primary aim is to prevent reinjury.
- A complete risk elimination for recurrence is not possible.
- Diagnosis and classification is based on medical history and clinical examination with additional information gained with imaging.
- *Indirect* injuries ("strains") require a more careful rehabilitation and longer RTP and should be differentiated from *direct* ones ("contusions") with a faster RTP.
- *Non-structural* (MRI negative/MRI oedema only) muscle injuries cause significant shorter absence compared to *structural* muscle injuries (MRI positive, "tears").
- A rehabilitation programme with gradually increasing load should be developed for every individual muscle injury.

- Lumbopelvic muscle ("core") strengthening should be included in daily training before and after RTP to prevent further injuries.
- Running training should be started unidirectionally within aerobic intensity. Muscle fatigue must be strictly avoided.
- Completion of symptom-free individualized sport-specific training including sprinting, shooting, etc. is mandatory before RTP.
- Participation in competition should start with 30–45 min for the first games.
- Regular clinical follow-up examinations are necessary before and after RTP.
- Muscle strength and function may not be 100% at RTP; both usually further improve with time.
- The use of strength tests and imaging as RTP criteria remains questionable.

Top Five Evidence Based References

Bloch W (2013) Muscle healing: physiology and adverse factors. In: Mueller-Wohlfahrt HW, Ueblacker P, Haensel L, Garrett WE (eds) Muscle injuries in sports. Thieme, Stuttgart, NY, pp 105–126

Ekstrand J, Hagglund M, Kristenson K et al (2013) Fewer ligament injuries but no preventive effect on muscle injuries and severe injuries: an 11-year follow-up of the UEFA Champions League injury study. Br J Sports Med 47:732–737

Ekstrand J, Askling C, Magnusson H et al (2013) Return to play after thigh muscle injury in elite football players: implementation and validation of the Munich muscle injury classification. Br J Sports Med 47:769–774

Reurink G, Verhaar JA, Tol JL (2014) More on platelet-rich plasma injections in acute muscle injury. N Engl J Med 371:1264–1265

Tol JL, Hamilton B, Eirale C et al (2014) At return to play following hamstring injury the majority of professional football players have residual isokinetic deficits. Br J Sports Med 48:1364–1369

References

1. Ekstrand J, Hagglund M, Walden M (2011) Epidemiology of muscle injuries in professional football (soccer). Am J Sports Med 39:1226–1232
2. Ekstrand J, Walden M, Hagglund M (2016) Hamstring injuries have increased by 4% annually in men's professional football, since 2001: a 13-year longitudinal analysis of the UEFA Elite Club injury study. Br J Sports Med 50:731–737
3. Ekstrand J (2017) Overview of football injuries. In: Encyclopaedia of football medicine, vol 2. Thieme, Stuttgart, NY, pp 1–13
4. Ekstrand J, Hagglund M, Kristenson K et al (2013) Fewer ligament injuries but no preventive effect on muscle injuries and severe injuries: an 11-year follow-up of the UEFA Champions League injury study. Br J Sports Med 47:732–737
5. Ekstrand J (2013) Epidemiology of muscle injuries in soccer. In: Mueller-Wohlfahrt HW, Ueblacker P, Haensel L, Garrett WE (eds) Muscle injuries in sports. Thieme, Stuttgart, NY, pp 127–134
6. Ueblacker P, Müller-Wohlfahrt HW, Ekstrand J (2015) Epidemiological and clinical outcome comparison of indirect ('strain') versus direct ('contusion') anterior and posterior thigh muscle injuries in male elite football players: UEFA Elite League study of 2287 thigh injuries (2001-2013). Br J Sports Med 49:1461–1465
7. Fuller CW, Ekstrand J, Junge A et al (2006) Consensus statement on injury definitions and data collection procedures in studies of football (soccer) injuries. Clin J Sport Med 16:97–106
8. Ueblacker P, Haensel L, Mueller-Wohlfahrt HW (2016) Treatment of muscle injuries in football. J Sports Sci 34:2329–2337
9. Ekstrand J, Askling C, Magnusson H et al (2013) Return to play after thigh muscle injury in elite football players: implementation and validation of the Munich muscle injury classification. Br J Sports Med 47:769–774
10. Mueller-Wohlfahrt HW, Ueblacker P, Binder A et al (2013) Terminology, classification, patient history, and clinical examination. In: Mueller-Wohlfahrt HW, Ueblacker P, Haensel L, Garrett WE (eds) Muscle injuries in sports. Thieme, Stuttgart, NY, pp 135–167
11. Askling CM, Tengvar M, Saartok T et al (2008) Proximal hamstring strains of stretching type in different sports: injury situations, clinical and magnetic resonance imaging characteristics, and return to sport. Am J Sports Med 36:1799–1804
12. Ekstrand J, Healy JC, Walden M et al (2012) Hamstring muscle injuries in professional football: the correlation of MRI findings with return to play. Br J Sports Med 46:112–117
13. Kerkhoffs GM, Van Es N, Wieldraaijer T et al (2012) Diagnosis and prognosis of acute hamstring injuries in athletes. Knee Surg Sports Traumatol Arthrosc 21:500–509
14. Noonan TJ, Garrett WE Jr (1999) Muscle strain injury: diagnosis and treatment. J Am Acad Orthop Surg 7:262–269
15. Chan O, Del Buono A, Best TM et al (2012) Acute muscle strain injuries: a proposed new classification system. Knee Surg Sports Traumatol Arthrosc 20:2356–2362
16. Mueller-Wohlfahrt HW, Haensel L, Mithoefer K et al (2013) Terminology and classification of muscle injuries in sport: the Munich consensus statement. Br J Sports Med 47:342–350
17. O'Donoghue DO (ed) (1962) Treatment of injuries to athletes. WB Saunders, Philadelphia, PA

18. Pollock N, James SL, Lee JC et al (2014) British athletics muscle injury classification: a new grading system. Br J Sports Med 48:1347–1351
19. Ryan AJ (1969) Quadriceps strain, rupture and charlie horse. Med Sci Sports 1:106–111
20. Stoller DW (ed) (2007) MRI in orthopaedics and sports medicine. Wolters Kluwer/Lippincott, Philadelphia, PA
21. Takebayashi S, Takasawa H, Banzai Y et al (1995) Sonographic findings in muscle strain injury: clinical and MR imaging correlation. J Ultrasound Med 14:899–905
22. Valle X, Alentorn-Geli E, Tol JL et al (2016) Muscle injuries in sports: a new evidence-informed and expert consensus-based classification with clinical application. Sports Med 47:1241. https://doi.org/10.1007/s40279-016-0647-1
23. Hamilton B, Valle X, Rodas G et al (2015) Classification and grading of muscle injuries: a narrative review. Br J Sports Med 49:306
24. Ueblacker P, Hänsel L, Müller-Wohlfahrt H (2017) Muscle injuries - examination and treatment. In: Encyclopaedia of football medicine, vol 2. Thieme, Stuttgart, NY, pp 32–49
25. Jarvinen TA, Jarvinen TL, Kaariainen M et al (2005) Muscle injuries: biology and treatment. Am J Sports Med 33:745–764
26. Orchard JW, Best TM, Mueller-Wohlfahrt HW et al (2008) The early management of muscle strains in the elite athlete: best practice in a world with a limited evidence basis. Br J Sports Med 42:158–159
27. Reurink G, Goudswaard GJ, Tol JL et al (2012) Therapeutic interventions for acute hamstring injuries: a systematic review. Br J Sports Med 46:103–109
28. Bleakley CM, Glasgow P, Webb MJ (2012) Cooling an acute muscle injury: can basic scientific theory translate into the clinical setting? Br J Sports Med 46:296–298
29. Brophy RH, Wright RW, Powell JW et al (2010) Injuries to kickers in American football: the National Football League experience. Am J Sports Med 38:1166–1173
30. Ueblacker P, Müller-Wohlfahrt HW, Hinterwimmer S et al (2015) Suture anchor repair of proximal rectus femoris avulsions in elite football players. Knee Surg Sports Traumatol Arthrosc 23:2590–2594
31. Garcia VV, Duhrkop DC, Seijas R et al (2012) Surgical treatment of proximal ruptures of the rectus femoris in professional soccer players. Arch Orthop Trauma Surg 132:329–333
32. Cohen S, Bradley J (2007) Acute proximal hamstring rupture. J Am Acad Orthop Surg 15:350–355
33. Harris JD, Griesser MJ, Best TM et al (2011) Treatment of proximal hamstring ruptures - a systematic review. Int J Sports Med 32:490–495
34. Ueblacker P, English B, Mueller-Wohlfahrt HW (2016) Nonoperative treatment and return to play after complete proximal adductor avulsion in high-performance athletes. Knee Surg Sports Traumatol Arthrosc 24:3927–3933
35. Obremsky WT, Seaber AV, Ribbeck BM et al (1994) Biomechanical and histologic assessment of a controlled muscle strain injury treated with piroxicam. Am J Sports Med 22:558–561
36. Paoloni JA, Milne C, Orchard J et al (2009) Non-steroidal anti-inflammatory drugs in sports medicine: guidelines for practical but sensible use. Br J Sports Med 43:863–865
37. Shen W, Li Y, Tang Y et al (2005) NS-398, a cyclooxygenase-2-specific inhibitor, delays skeletal muscle healing by decreasing regeneration and promoting fibrosis. Am J Pathol 167:1105–1117
38. Ziltener JL, Leal S, Fournier PE (2010) Non-steroidal anti-inflammatory drugs for athletes: an update. Ann Phys Rehabil Med 53(278-282):282–278
39. Lee P, Rattenberry A, Connelly S et al (2011) Our experience on Actovegin, is it cutting edge? Int J Sports Med 32:237–241
40. Pfister A, Koller W (1990) Treatment of fresh muscle injury. Sportverletz Sportschaden 4:41–44
41. Reichl FX, Holdt LM, Teupser D, Schütze G, Metcalfe AJ, Hickel R, Högg C, Bloch W (2017) Comprehensive analytics of actovegin® and its effect on muscle cells. Int J Sports Med 38(11):809–818. doi:10.1055/s-0043-115738. Epub 2017 Sep 11
42. A Hamid MS, Mohamed Ali MR, Yusof A et al (2014) Platelet-rich plasma injections for the treatment of hamstring injuries: a randomized controlled trial. Am J Sports Med 42:2410–2418
43. Reurink G, Verhaar JA, Tol JL (2014) More on platelet-rich plasma injections in acute muscle injury. N Engl J Med 371:1264–1265
44. Harmon KG (2010) Muscle injuries and PRP: what does the science say? Br J Sports Med 44:616–617
45. Andia I, Abate M (2015) Platelet-rich plasma in the treatment of skeletal muscle injuries. Expert Opin Biol Ther 15:987–999
46. Li H, Hicks JJ, Wang L et al (2016) Customized platelet-rich plasma with transforming growth factor beta1 neutralization antibody to reduce fibrosis in skeletal muscle. Biomaterials 87:147–156
47. Ota S, Uehara K, Nozaki M et al (2011) Intramuscular transplantation of muscle-derived stem cells accelerates skeletal muscle healing after contusion injury via enhancement of angiogenesis. Am J Sports Med 39:1912–1922
48. Quintero AJ, Wright VJ, FH F et al (2009) Stem cells for the treatment of skeletal muscle injury. Clin Sports Med 28:1–11
49. Wong S, Ning A, Lee C et al (2015) Return to sport after muscle injury. Curr Rev Musculoskelet Med 8:168–175
50. Beiner JM, Jokl P, Cholewicki J et al (1999) The effect of anabolic steroids and corticosteroids on healing of muscle contusion injury. Am J Sports Med 27:2–9
51. Kary JM (2010) Diagnosis and management of quadriceps strains and contusions. Curr Rev Musculoskelet Med 3:26–31
52. Levine WN, Bergfeld JA, Tessendorf W et al (2000) Intramuscular corticosteroid injection for hamstring injuries. A 13-year experience in the National Football League. Am J Sports Med 28:297–300

53. Bloch W (2013) Muscle healing: physiology and adverse factors. In: Mueller-Wohlfahrt HW, Ueblacker P, Haensel L, Garrett WE (eds) Muscle Injuries in Sports. Thieme, Stuttgart, NY, pp 105–126
54. Orchard JW, Best TM (2002) The management of muscle strain injuries: an early return versus the risk of recurrence. Clin J Sport Med 12:3–5
55. Hurme T, Kalimo H, Lehto M et al (1991) Healing of skeletal muscle injury: an ultrastructural and immunohistochemical study. Med Sci Sports Exerc 23:801–810
56. Lieber RL, Ward SR (2013) Cellular mechanisms of tissue fibrosis. 4. Structural and functional consequences of skeletal muscle fibrosis. Am J Physiol Cell Physiol 305:C241–C252
57. Diaz JA, Fischer DA, Rettig AC et al (2003) Severe quadriceps muscle contusions in athletes. A report of three cases. Am J Sports Med 31:289–293
58. Trojian TH (2013) Muscle contusion (thigh). Clin Sports Med 32:317–324
59. Ong A, Anderson J, Roche J (2003) A pilot study of the prevalence of lumbar disc degeneration in elite athletes with lower back pain at the Sydney 2000 Olympic Games. Br J Sports Med 37:263–266
60. Ozturk A, Ozkan Y, Ozdemir RM et al (2008) Radiographic changes in the lumbar spine in former professional football players: a comparative and matched controlled study. Eur Spine J 17:136–141
61. Orchard JW, Farhart P, Leopold C (2004) Lumbar spine region pathology and hamstring and calf injuries in athletes: is there a connection? Br J Sports Med 38:502–504. discussion 502-504
62. Arnason A, Andersen TE, Holme I et al (2008) Prevention of hamstring strains in elite soccer: an intervention study. Scand J Med Sci Sports 18:40–48
63. Askling C, Karlsson J, Thorstensson A (2003) Hamstring injury occurrence in elite soccer players after preseason strength training with eccentric overload. Scand J Med Sci Sports 13:244–250
64. Brukner P (2015) Hamstring injuries: prevention and treatment-an update. Br J Sports Med 49: 1241–1244
65. Hrysomallis C (2013) Injury incidence, risk factors and prevention in Australian rules football. Sports Med 43:339–354
66. Orchard J, Best TM, Verrall GM (2005) Return to play following muscle strains. Clin J Sport Med 15:436–441
67. Schlumberger A (2013) Prevention of muscle injuries. In: Mueller-Wohlfahrt HW, Ueblacker P, Haensel L, Garrett WE (eds) Muscle injuries in sports. Thieme, Stuttgart, NY, pp 365–380
68. Sherry MA, Best TM (2004) A comparison of 2 rehabilitation programs in the treatment of acute hamstring strains. J Orthop Sports Phys Ther 34:116–125
69. Reurink G, Brilman EG, De Vos RJ et al (2015) Magnetic resonance imaging in acute hamstring injury: can we provide a return to play prognosis? Sports Med 45:133–146
70. Creighton DW, Shrier I, Shultz R et al (2010) Return-to-play in sport: a decision-based model. Clin J Sport Med 20:379–385
71. Delvaux F, Rochcongar P, Bruyere O et al (2014) Return-to-play criteria after hamstring injury: actual medicine practice in professional soccer teams. J Sports Sci Med 13:721–723
72. Schut L, Wangensteen A, Maaskant J et al (2016) Can clinical evaluation predict return to sport after acute hamstring injuries? A systematic review. Sports Med 47:1123. https://doi.org/10.1007/s40279-016-0639-1
73. Mendiguchia J, Brughelli M (2011) A return-to-sport algorithm for acute hamstring injuries. Phys Ther Sport 12:2–14
74. Croisier JL, Forthomme B, Namurois MH et al (2002) Hamstring muscle strain recurrence and strength performance disorders. Am J Sports Med 30: 199–203
75. Tol JL, Hamilton B, Eirale C et al (2014) At return to play following hamstring injury the majority of professional football players have residual isokinetic deficits. Br J Sports Med 48:1364–1369
76. Mendiguchia J, Samozino P, Martinez-Ruiz E et al (2014) Progression of mechanical properties during on-field sprint running after returning to sports from a hamstring muscle injury in soccer players. Int J Sports Med 35:690–695
77. Hallen A, Ekstrand J (2014) Return to play following muscle injuries in professional footballers. J Sports Sci 32:1229–1236
78. Koulouris G, Connell DA, Brukner P et al (2007) Magnetic resonance imaging parameters for assessing risk of recurrent hamstring injuries in elite athletes. Am J Sports Med 35:1500–1506
79. Schneider-Kolsky ME, Hoving JL, Warren P et al (2006) A comparison between clinical assessment and magnetic resonance imaging of acute hamstring injuries. Am J Sports Med 34:1008–1015
80. Slavotinek JP (2010) Muscle injury: the role of imaging in prognostic assignment and monitoring of muscle repair. Semin Musculoskelet Radiol 14:194–200
81. Moen MH, Reurink G, Weir A et al (2014) Predicting return to play after hamstring injuries. Br J Sports Med 48:1358–1363
82. Reurink G, Whiteley R, Tol JL (2015) Hamstring injuries and predicting return to play: 'bye-bye MRI? Br J Sports Med 49:1162–1163
83. Boeck J, Mundinger P, Luttke G (2013) Magnetic resonance imaging. In: Mueller-Wohlfahrt HW, Ueblacker P, Haensel L, Garrett WE (eds) Muscle injuries in sports. Thieme, Stuttgart, NY, pp 203–225
84. Reurink G, Goudswaard GJ, Tol JL et al (2014) MRI observations at return to play of clinically recovered hamstring injuries. Br J Sports Med 48:1370–1376
85. Sanfilippo JL, Silder A, Sherry MA et al (2013) Hamstring strength and morphology progression after return to sport from injury. Med Sci Sports Exerc 45:448–454
86. Araujo PH, Rabuck SJ, Fu FH (2012) Are we allowing patients to return to participation too soon? Am J Sports Med 40:NP5. author reply NP5-6

34 Return-to-Play After Minor Overuse or Traumatic Injury: 'Stay and Play on Field'

Werner Krutsch, Klaus Eder, and Hauke Mommsen

Contents

W. Krutsch, M.D. (✉)
Department of Trauma Surgery, FIFA Medical Centre of Excellence, University Medical Centre Regensburg, Franz-Josef-Strauss-Allee 11, 93053 Regensburg, Germany
e-mail: werner.krutsch@ukr.de

K. Eder
Eden Reha Rehabilitation Centre, Eden-Reha, Lessingstraße 39, 93093 Donaustauf, Germany
e-mail: klaus.eder@eden-reha.de

H. Mommsen, M.D.
Endo-Reha Zentrum, Holstenstraße 7, 22767 Hamburg, Germany
e-mail: hauke.mommsen@fh-kiel.de

V. Musahl et al. (eds.), *Return to Play in Football*, https://doi.org/10.1007/978-3-662-55713-6_34

34.1 Introduction

Evidence-based data on the return-to-play process after football injuries mostly refer to surgically treated injuries such as anterior cruciate ligaments, ankle injuries, Achilles tendon injuries or severe injuries of the upper extremities [12, 18, 20, 34]. Other well-documented injuries are severe injuries necessitating long absence from football such as groin pain because of osteitis pubis [38]. Injuries associated with short absence from football training and fast recovery are classified as minor injuries [16]. Minor football injuries have a high incidence and lack sufficient evidence-based data with regard to treatment options. The most important reason for the lack of standards for minor overuse and traumatic injuries is the wide variety of conservative treatment options and pain management available. Thus, the success of the healing and return-to-play process after injury depends on the experience of the responsible medical team. The main criteria for a successful return after minor injury are the exclusion of severe injury and symptom-adapted treatment.

Emergency managements use the term 'stay and play', which comprises all steps of medical treatment of the injured body site [39]. In the context of sports traumatology and injuries sustained on a football field, the term 'stay and play' refers to the different steps of treatment provided by the medical staff on field that enable slightly injured players to stay in the match.

34.2 Injury Profiles in Football

Football is a contact sport with frequent rotational movements and abrupt stopping manoeuvres; therefore, football players are susceptible to injuries caused by contact and non-contact mechanisms [16]. A few years ago, partial or indirect contact mechanisms were established as a third possibility [7]. Such injuries are caused by direct contact to anybody site but the injured one immediately before the injury in contrast to injuries caused by direct contact to the injured body site. The mechanisms of non-contact injuries are still being investigated. First results have shown that non-contact injuries do usually not occur because players are inattentive but because of the presence of internal and external risk factors or specific injury situations during a match [1] that challenge the neurocognitive conception of the players.

Typical injury patterns in football have been well described in the literature [2]. In scientific football publications, injuries are divided into time-loss and non-time-loss injuries [16]. This definition is fundamental for epidemiological statistics on football injuries and has often been used successfully in the literature [13, 27, 28]. However, this injury definition may result in the underestimation of non-time-loss injuries that involve a specific trauma or symptom but not time away from official football matches. The frequent failure to include such injuries in scientific injury reports has led to a lack of knowledge about frequency, diagnostics, treatment and return-to-play procedures after non-time-loss injuries.

A further definition by Fuller et al. is the classification of injury severity according to the time away from football [16]. The classification into minor, moderate and severe injuries is well accepted in the literature and represents an important foundation for scientific injury reports in football. Particularly professional football players are under severe pressure to stay on field, to ignore minor injuries and complaints or take painkillers for competition or training [35]. Thus, a detailed classification may be essential to quantify and qualify the minor injuries in detail. Non-time-loss injuries are frequently ignored in scientific publications but represent an important cause of chronic complaints or the development of severe injuries [14, 38]. An injury classification should include all consequences and return-to-play procedures after football injuries, particularly time away from football and other medical consequences (Table 34.1).

Particularly team coaches have to know as early as possible, how long an injured player will

Fact Box 1

- The scientific literature on football medicine and orthopaedics comprises many publications and detailed illustrations about injury patterns in football.
- However, despite the high frequency of minor injuries that only involve short-term absence from football or no absence at all, there is a lack of evidence-based data on treatment outcome and return-to-play procedures.
- New detailed definitions of return-to-play procedures for minor injuries are necessary, in particular in the case of return-to-play within 1 week termed 'stay and play'.

Table 34.1 Injury definition and return-to-play decision

Injury definition	Time away from football	Importance of return-to-play
Non-time-loss injury	Missing no match	Non-time-loss → 'Stay and play' decision
Time-loss injury	Missing at least one match	Relevant loss of athletic skills → 'Return-to-play' decision

Table 34.2 Injury information details to the team coach

Time of information to the coach	Reason for the information to the coach
During the match	→ To substitute the injured player
Until the next match	→ To plan the team configuration for the next match
During the next weeks	→ To plan the change of general tactics in the team
Within the half-season	→ To plan to take on a new player
Within the running season	→ To plan to take on a new player
In general	→ To mentally support the injured player

be away from football and if the player will be able to play again at all (Table 34.2).

34.3 Minor Non-time-loss Injuries in Football

The definition of non-time-loss injuries needs to be clearly established within a team. The term 'non-time-loss' includes minor injuries that do not result in any time away from football so that the players may proceed with their training as planned. The other definition is 'time away from football for at least one training session' but planned participation in the next match. The first situation may only require 'stay and play' steps such as taping the ankle, but the second situation will already require specific medical treatment by the physiotherapist or the medical physician. After successful treatment and participation in the last team training before competition, the return-to-play process of the player needs to be planned. A potential classification for non-time-loss and minor injuries including potential 'stay and play' procedures may look as follows (Table 34.3):

'Stay and play' procedures lack so far sufficient scientific evidence despite the high incidence of non-time-loss injuries in football. For this reason, the above classification is based on the practical expertise of physicians experienced in the treatment of football players. The most important factor for using 'stay and play' proce-

Table 34.3 Stay and play procedure in minor football injuries

1. Minor injury, type I
All minor injuries with immediate return-to-play during the same match (no player substitution)
→ *'Stay and play' procedure I*: first aid on field
2. Minor injury, type II
All minor injuries involving a player's substitution but no further time away from next football training
→ *'Stay and play' procedure II*: first aid on field + clinical diagnosis + symptomatic therapy
3. Minor injury, type III
All minor injuries involving a few days' absence from football training but return-to-play in the next match
→ *'Stay and play' procedure III*: first aid on field + clinical diagnosis + exclusion of more severe injuries (imaging) + conservative treatment + return-to-play test in the last team training

dures I–III is a sufficient clinical diagnosis on the field, the entire range of conservative treatment provided by the medical staff as well as close cooperation of the injured player.

34.3.1 Traumatic Injuries in Football

Traumatic football injuries with low severity and non-time-loss are a frequent occurrence in training and matches [12, 28]. Typical injuries with low severity and generally without any time away from football are [9, 24, 25]:

- Bone contusions
- Skin lacerations
- Joint sprains
- Muscle strains

These types of injury may affect all body sites of the upper and lower extremities, the trunk and the back. Only the head and neck are specific body sites that may require alternative assessment after a low-severity injury. A skin laceration on the head is principally a minor injury but may be associated with a brain injury with neurological symptoms [29].

Frequent minor football-specific injuries requiring 'stay and play' procedures on football field are:

- Ankle sprains
- Thigh muscle strains
- Knee and shank contusion
- Finger sprains
- Head contusion and skin lacerations
- Cervical sprains
- Foot contusion

Sometimes, players who have sustained a severe traumatic injury, for instance, a joint dislocation or fracture, are able to 'stay and play' on the field. One typical example for this situation is a joint dislocation of a finger or a fracture of one of the bones in the hand. Of course, 'stay and play' in such a situation is only possible for field players but not goalkeepers. Field players may wear protective equipment on the injured hand to protect the fracture or joint dislocation from further damage during competition (Fig. 34.1).

34.3.2 Overuse Injuries in Football

Overuse injuries are defined as injuries without any traumatic injury mechanism [16]. These injuries are typically expressed by symptoms such as pain, swelling or restriction of joint movement. Overuse injuries are a frequent occurrence in football because of the specific movements required in this type of sports [12, 26, 34]. In contrast to severe traumatic injuries such as ruptures, fractures or dislocations that are associated with tissue damage, overuse injuries represent chronically developed tissue changes with a variety of symptoms. The main localisations of overuse complaints in football are [14, 38]:

- Lower back
- Sacroiliac joints
- Os pubis
- Patella and proximal ventral tibia
- Achilles tendon
- Sole of the foot

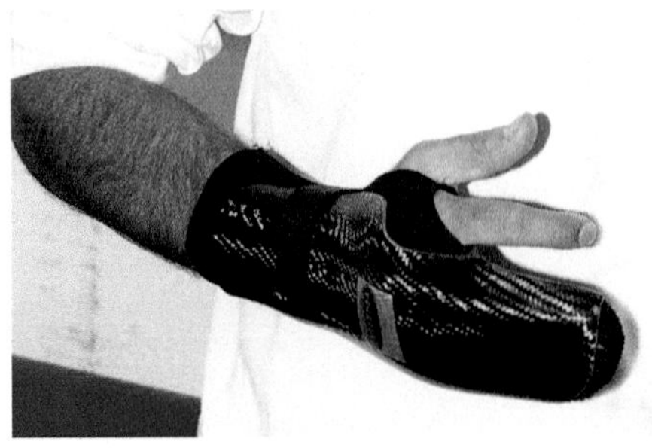

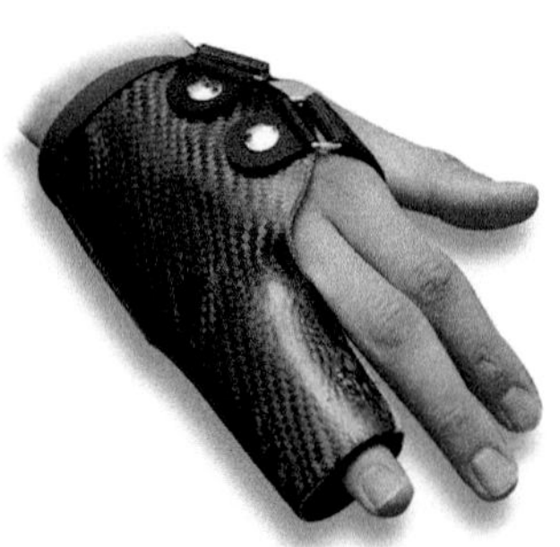

Fig. 34.1 Protection equipment for bone fractures of the hand and fingers to enable 'stay and play' on field (thank you to Hartmut Semsch/Ortema)

The problem with overuse injuries is that the origin of the symptoms is rarely known at the beginning [38]. Similar to traumatic injuries, severe and minor overuse complaints are also classified according to the time away from football [16]. In contrast to traumatic injuries, overuse complaints show the following characteristics:

- Mainly no knowledge of the trigger situation
- Only minor injury at the beginning
- Moderate pain at the beginning
- Only unspecific clinical diagnostics possible in most cases
- Missing consecutive therapy
- Partial disappearance of symptoms by use of painkillers
- Mainly no time away from football after the start of the first symptom
- Players trying to continue playing football by taking painkillers
- Possible chronic aggravation of symptoms by continuation in football activity

A further problem of overuse complaints is moderate pain at the beginning, so that players try to 'stay and play' on field without any medical diagnostics and treatment, particularly in amateur football. Aggravation of symptoms may result in more serious problems, such as muscles ruptures or tissue irritation of another body region. Typical examples are [14, 36]:

1. Rupture of muscle fibres of the thigh after previous muscle strain
2. Osteitis pubis after irritation of the adductor attachment
3. Neurogenic muscle complaints in the thigh after long-term low back pain
4. Jumpers' knee after overstressing the quadriceps muscle

An additional problem of overuse complaints is that continuous pain while playing football may have a negative influence on the neuromotorical adaptation and proprioception of the player. In the case of a previous minor and not fully healed injury of the same body site [18] or another body region [28], such negative influence may result in the occurrence of a severe joint injury of the lower extremities (ankle and knee) after jumping, landing and running movements. Unpublished data obtained from the 'German ACL registry in football' showed minor pre-injury as an influencing factor in one third of ACL injuries of football players. This high percentage indicates that insufficient recovery from minor injuries and persistent pain affect the neuromotorical adaption or trunk muscle strength of football players.

Fact Box 2

- Football is associated with specific minor traumatic and overuse injuries as a result of the sports-specific physical demands on the players in training sessions, the surface of the football pitch, the weather and several other external factors.
- Internal factors such as insufficient regeneration, inadequate preparation or previous and not fully healed injuries influence the incidence of injury.
- The scientific literature comprises many respected publications on the treatment and return-to-play procedures after typical severe football injuries, while non-time-loss injuries are much less documented.
- Standardised procedures for quick return-to-play within 1 week or 'stay and play' on field are essential in football.

34.4 The Healing Process of Different Tissues

Symptom-adapted treatment of overuse and traumatic injuries in football requires detailed knowledge on tissue regeneration and healing potentials. Different body sites have different types of tissue and thus vary in healing and regeneration but also in vulnerability after hits. To understand the healing processes of each body region after injury, the fundamental knowledge about tissue regeneration after injuries is essential for sports physicians to guide the injured player through the rehabilitation process to a fast return-to-play. Physicians have to know that healing process of bone needs immobilisation of the broken body region and a certain axial compression to the fracture. Other tissues like tendons or muscles need also certain immobilisation, but in modern rehabilitation procedures, early functional mobilisation is the main aim of the treatment [8, 12, 13, 18, 20, 34, 36]. Tissue with fast healing potential within few days is cutis and subcutis. In contrast, other tissues like meniscus or articular cartilage have a delayed healing or regeneration potential, and in case of frequent stress on the tissue, meniscus and cartilage may show no regeneration potential after an injury.

The completion of the healing process—which often takes a long time depending on the age of the football player, the gender and other health aspects—is not the most important aim of 'stay and play on field' procedures. The healing process of different tissues also depends on the affected body site and the demands on this particular body region. Immediate- or short-term return-to-play after injuries, which is the main reason for 'stay and play', does not require full tissue regeneration. The 'stay and play' process only includes tissue regeneration in the following types of minor injuries:

- Partial tissue damage (e.g. ligaments and muscles)
- Tissue irritation (e.g. tendons and joint capsules)
- Tissue inflammation (e.g. tendons and bursa)

In the case of complete tissue damage, continuation of sports activity and 'stay and play' depends on the body region. For example, bone fractures or joint ligament injuries of the lower extremities are mainly not compatible with 'stay and play' in football. Injuries that may allow 'stay and play' are fractures and ruptures in the upper extremities, typically fractures of the wrist, hands and fingers of field players or the head after facial fractures. Wearing protective equipment on the face or hands is essential for ensuring 'stay and play' in such cases [29]. The team physician and physical therapist have to understand generally healing process of all tissues to know where the healing process may be expected within few days to allow 'stay and play' by specific treatment steps or to find alternative ways to protect the injured body region in a 'stay and play' decision.

Fact Box 3

- Understanding the different recovery periods and injury types requires knowledge on the healing process of the affected tissue. Complete ruptures of ligaments and tendons or bone fractures are associated with long recovery times and do not allow any 'stay and play' procedures.
- Different body sites are subject to different 'stay and play' procedures.
- The most common minor traumatic and overuse injuries in football are damages at the macroscopic and microscopic level or just irritations of the tissue. The healing process of such damages should be the focus of 'stay and play' procedures in minor injuries.

34.5 'Stay and Play' Procedures After Minor Injuries

After an overuse and traumatic injury, the treatment process starts with adequate first aid on field. In this situation, adherence to the PRICE (protection, rest, ice, compression and elevation) rule by both medical and non-medical staff as well as suitable first aid equipment is essential for the initial treatment of any injury [27], which has to be adapted to the specific type of overuse or traumatic injury. For example, acute traumatic injuries of a joint of the lower extremities or a hit on the back require immediate cooling with ice and further PRICE steps. At the same time, overuse complaints in these body regions, particularly muscular complaints, require heat therapy for tissue relaxation and pain reduction. Choice of the

Table 34.4 Stay and play procedures in football

1. First aid on field [5, 6, 27, 32]
2. Interdisciplinary pain management [35]
3. Various conservative treatment options (medial staff) [31, 32, 36]
4. Rehabilitation strategies (physio) [3, 17]
5. Medical training therapy (athletic coach) [32, 36]

respective treatment option depends on the injury mechanism and the experience of the staff managing first aid. Management of 'stay and play' procedures includes a series of treatments up to the time of return-to-play on field, which includes the complete medical staff and all team coaches (Table 34.4).

Important aspects for a stay and play procedure is the experience in the handling with football players. The body language is in general both for the team coach and the medical staff an important aspect to recognise, how the players feel and if complaints are present. A second aspect with need for experience is the palpation of the players' body. Palpation findings after injuries occur lead the medical staff to the right indication for further diagnostics, further treatment or the decision to proceed football playing. A special aspect after injuries is vegetative escalation of the player, which shows that players do not tolerate pain or the occurred injury. In this situation is a stop in playing football recommendable.

Treatment options for minor injuries and 'stay and play' procedures depend on the extent of medical service available in a football team. In professional football, medical teams include a physician, at least two physiotherapists, an osteopath, a rehabilitation coach and an athletic coach as well as several medical consultants for specific injuries. The 'stay and play' process after minor injuries is mainly managed by the team staff, and medical consultants are only called in for chronic or persistent problems involving a possible time away from football. Interaction among the different members of the medical staff in a professional football team needs to be clearly defined with regard to the workflow after minor injury and the potential start of the 'stay and play' process. The diagnosis needs to be confirmed by the physician in cooperation with the physiotherapist followed by the required treatment depending on the type of injury and the medical setting:

'Stay and play' stage I: If a player sustains a hit, sprain or strain in a match, the medical staff on field have to analyse the body site and severity of the complaint. If movement and function of the affected extremity are normal and if the player is able to carry out a few football-specific movements without restriction, first aid on field may be completed so that the player can continue playing.

'Stay and play' stage II: If a player is limping, shows restricted joint movement or any other signs of injury that necessitates discontinuation in the match, the player has to be substituted and requires a full examination and diagnostics after the match. If pain reduction with or without any relevant therapy is possible after the match, the player has to be evaluated with regard to the possibility of immediate reintegration before the next training. If this short-term return-to-play is possible, different football-specific movements should be attempted on field before the next training.

'Stay and play' stage III: If the medical examination after the match shows that the injured player will be unable to participate in the next training session, detailed diagnostics should take place over the next few days, including imaging diagnostics. If a severe traumatic or overuse injury can be excluded, the injury has no consequences even in the case of highly damaged tissue because symptoms may be expected to abate after a few days. The player should undergo a treatment programme developed by the medical staff with the aim of reintegration into the next match. Parallel to medical treatment, the player should start a step-by-step reintegration to the training process. To achieve the aim of return-to-play until the next official match, reintegration into the last team training before the match is essential to test the skills and readiness of the player for competition.

The last team training should generally represent the situation for the team coach to test their players and evaluate the fitness level of the players. All long-term and short-term injured players should participate in at least in the last team training before competition to show their readiness and to evaluate any other problems. A direct return-to-play to the match without any team training evaluation should be avoided to protect the injured player for unexpected and dangerous situations. Only in professional football may this situation occur, if time pressure and important matches are upcoming, but these situations should represent exceptional cases in a team.

In the case of a clear diagnosis or suspicion of a more severe injury, the player and medical staff have time for diagnostics over the next few days. In general, 'stay and play' procedures on field require medical staff [3, 17, 31], who are knowledgeable and experienced in:

- Individual characteristics of the different players of the team
- Specific requirements of football players
- Individual situation of the injured player within the team
- First aid in sports injuries
- Clinical diagnostics of sports injuries
- Ultrasound diagnostics
- Conservative treatments
- Rehabilitation programmes
- Reintegration training exercises

In modern football, professional teams have the capacity to manage all 'stay and play' procedures, which requires frequent and close communication between the different staff members of the medical team. In junior or amateur football teams, only the team coach and sometimes the physiotherapist are present on the football field. In such situations, many steps of the 'stay and play' process have to be adapted by the physiotherapist or are not practicable at all at these levels of football. The success of each 'stay and play' procedure depends on the skill of the person providing the service. In amateur football, 'stay and play' after minor injuries is frequently not achieved, which results in symptom-adapted time-loss for one training session or match or even longer.

Fact Box 4

- The success of 'stay and play' procedures after non-time-loss injuries requires highly experienced medical staff with a wide knowledge on football, conservative treatment options and pain management.
- In the absence of any evidence-based guideline for first aid on field or other 'stay and play' procedures, football medicine has to rely on the reports of experienced medical staff.
- Based on these reports, further research with a higher evidence level is needed.
- Interaction and close communication among the medical staff is essential for managing small football injuries.

34.6 Symptomatic and Conservative Therapy After Minor Injuries

Conservative therapy consists of many different treatment strategies, which cannot be provided at the highest level by just one physician. To offer professional football players with the highest standard of conservative treatment, the medical staff have to handle basic treatments for a safe and sufficient 'stay and play' process on field that may be summarised in seven main groups of conservative treatment options with a selection of principle conservative treatment strategies.

34.6.1 Clinical Diagnostic and Manual Therapeutic Manoeuvres [11, 14, 31–33, 36, 40]:

- Chiropractic care
- Osteopathy
- Trigger-point therapy

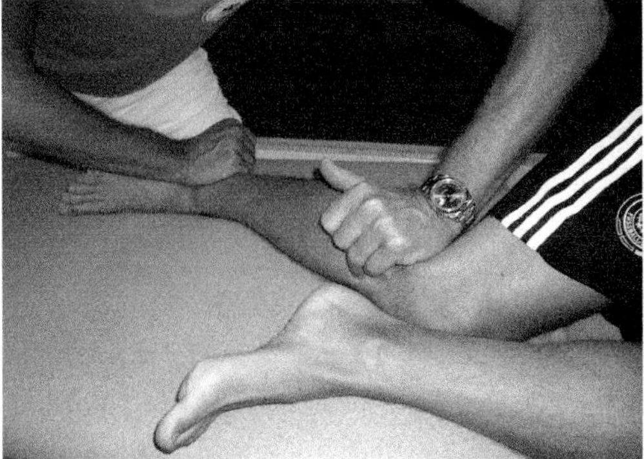
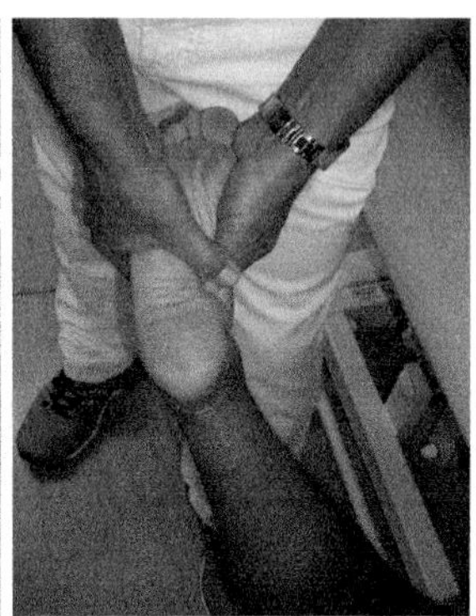

Fig. 34.2 Mobilisation of the fibula and the tarsal (thank you to Klaus Eder/Eden-Reha)

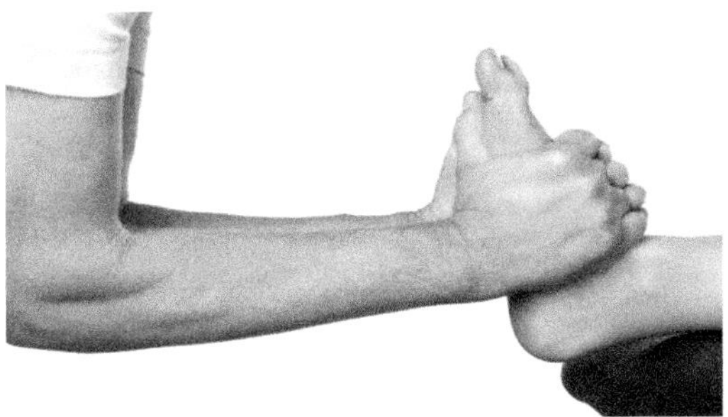

Fig. 34.3 Traction technique on the lower extremity (thank you to Klaus Eder/Eden-Reha)

- Fascial techniques and fascia distorsion model
- Assisted stretching and mobilisation (Fig. 34.2)
- Traction techniques (Fig. 34.3)

34.6.2 Oral Medication [22, 32, 35]:

- Pain management
- Antiphlogistic therapy
- Supplements
- Homeopathy

34.6.3 Invasive Treatment (Needles and Injections) [14, 19, 21, 22, 32]:

- PRP/ACP
- Natural blood products
- Antiphlogistic and biologic substances
- Dry needling
- Analgesic substances
- Acupuncture

34.6.4 Non-invasive Treatment [14, 32, 36, 38, 40]:

- Electrotherapy
- Shock wave therapy
- Ultrasound therapy
- Magnetic therapy
- Cold laser therapy

34.6.5 Unguents and Lotions [6, 32, 36, 42]:

- Thermotherapy
- Cryotherapy
- Antiphlogistics

34.6.6 Tapes and Bandages [4, 11, 30, 32]:

- Elastic tapes (Fig. 34.4)
- Classic tapes (Fig. 34.5
- Elastic bandages
- Medical flossing
- Compression socks

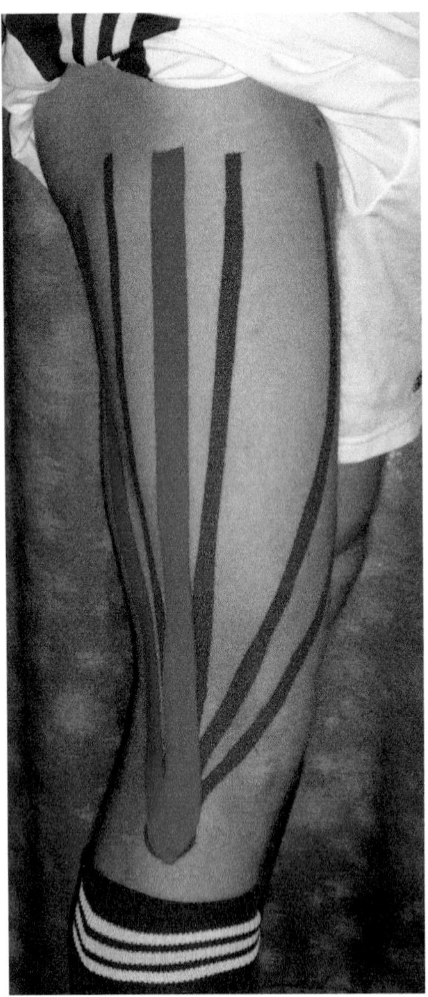

Fig. 34.4 Elastic taping (kinesio taping) to address muscular overuse complaints

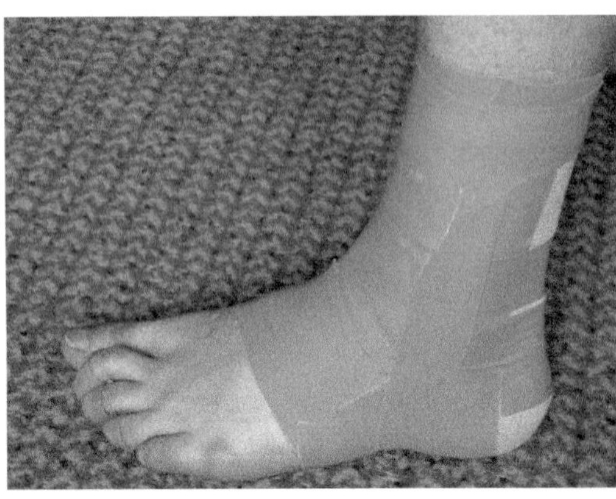

Fig. 34.5 Classic taping for different indications of 'stay and play': secondary prevention after ankle sprain and toe blister

34.6.7 Physical Therapy/Lymphatic Drainage/Physiotherapy [32, 36]

One of the most important steps of conservative treatment strategies is the exclusion of a surgical indication at the beginning of therapy and directly after completion of diagnostics. In today's modern sports therapy, conservative therapy does not represent the first step of a healing attempt that—if not successful—may be rectified by surgical treatment. On the contrary, conservative treatment in modern football medicine is an independent means of treating injuries successfully, particularly in the case of frequent minor injuries. Conservative treatment should start immediately after occurrence of injuries and before establishment of the diagnosis. The different main groups of treatment options may either start in consecutive order or may be combined and started together.

During clinical diagnostics, both the team physician and the physiotherapists should perform manual therapy to remove blockages, reset joints of the spine and the sacroiliac joints and down-regulate hypertension of the muscles. Initial clinical diagnostics and the first manual manoeuvres usually show the type of injury, thus determining the necessary treatment. The physiotherapist and the team physician need to establish a working diagnosis to make sure they talk about the 'same medical condition'. Treatment should start with oral medication followed by further manual techniques and injections or needling, if required. In the intervals between active treatment phases, superficial unguents and tapes may passively support the medical treatment, if indicated also overnight.

Intervals between active treatment phases depend on the specific injury and the expected time of return-to-play. Some treatment options may be repeated daily or sometimes several times per day, for instance, manual manoeuvres or stretching and taping techniques. Other treatment steps such as shock wave therapy or injections require a few days in between.

The scientific literature comprises many details on the indication or use of specific conservative treatment options; however, little information with low evidence is available on the combination of different therapeutic strategies to achieve early return-to-play, as expected in professional football [29]. The medical staff of a football team should consider the combination of all indicated and practicable conservative treatment options. Professional football clubs should ensure that their medical team is put together according to the practical skills and knowledge on football medicine of their individual staff members.

When treating professional athletes, physicians should generally be very careful with regard to any type of treatment including injections and oral medications. Drugs and medications may be in conflict with the anti-doping list of the WADA, and prevention of such conflicts is one of the most important jobs of a team physician [10].

Irrespectively of the elected treatment, a detailed documentation of the complete injury history and the follow-up is essential.

Fact Box 5

- Symptomatic conservative treatment of minor football injuries resulting in 'stay and play on field' is based on the correct clinical diagnosis immediately after injury.
- Correct diagnostics depend on the education of the medical staff and their experience in football medicine.
- Conservative treatment consists of many different options that have to be combined by the medical staff to achieve early return-to-play.
- The formation of a medical team in professional football should be based on their different education and skills, while the scientific evidence is low

34.7 Decisions on 'Stay and Play' Procedures

Minor injuries may result in relevant time away from football but may also be successfully managed by medical staff as an injury without any time-loss. Minor injuries are defined as injuries without any time-loss that result in 'stay and play on field' procedures I, II or III (Chap. III).

34.7.1 Decision-Making on 'Stay and Play'

Both the injured player and the medical staff have to differentiate between and decide on the different 'stay and play' stages. The following principles for the 'stay and play' process are reasonable (Table 34.5).

34.7.2 Time Line of the 'Stay and Play' Process

The 'stay and play' process may be defined by specific time points to provide a guideline for the player, team coach and the medical staff for a better understanding of the principles. The classification of the 'stay and play' process (Table 34.6) and the earliest possible return-to-play time point after injury without any time-loss is based on the classification of injury severity by Fuller et al. [16].

34.7.3 Testing for 'Stay and Play'

The return-to-play process in modern football medicine is based on a sufficient number of tests,

Table 34.5 Decision-making in 'stay and play' on field

'Stay and play' stage I: Player as the main decision-maker to proceed the match
'Stay and play' stage II: Player as the main decision-maker plus agreement by the medical staff
'Stay and play' stage III: Decision of the team coach after one team training test, readiness of the player plus agreement by the medical staff

Table 34.6: Time line in 'stay and play' decision

'Stay and play' stage I: No absence from football (no absence and no substitution in matches)
'Stay and play' stage II: 1–2 days absence from football (absence until next team training)
'Stay and play' stage III: Absence from football of <1 week (until next official match)

Table 34.7 Selection of Return-to-play testings after minor injuries

1. Jumping and landing tests (drop jump and side hop)
2. Balancing tests (balance board)
3. Agility tests (different complex running exercises with side- and backwards runs and rotational movements)

in particular after severe injuries and long time away from sports [7, 17]. Minor injuries associated with only short or no absence from football require adequate medical examinations and tests to evaluate the healing process of the injury. Differences between 'stay and play' tests and return-to-play tests are naturally based on the respective affliction of the player. Typical tests regarding strength, endurance and psychological aspects that are essential after severe injuries such as ACL ruptures [7] are not necessary in 'stay and play' evaluations. Minor injuries rather require evaluation of a pain-free situation and the ability to smoothly perform all football-specific movements on field. The most important step for assessing the readiness of a football player to participate in the next competition is full integration into the last team training before the next match. In addition, players may be tested for specific neuromotorical exercises, especially during the 'stay and play' procedure III (Table 34.7).

The authors of this chapter suggest the use of standardised tests for the 'stay and play' process that imitate typical football movements but also have sufficient comparability to return-to-play tests for severe injuries such as ACL ruptures [7]. 'Stay and play' tests should compare differences between the injured and the healthy leg but—even more importantly in professional football—also consider pre-injury and pre-seasonal data.

Fact Box 6

- The decision on 'stay and play' procedures requires experienced medical staff and adequate tests.
- The decision on possible early return-to-play necessitates close communication and trust between the injured player, the medical staff and the team coach.
- The two pillars of 'stay and play' after minor injuries are coexistence of conservative treatment and reintegration into individual and team training.
- The last step of a short-term return-to-play process is reintegration into team training, at least into the last team training before the next match.

34.8 Influencing Factors on 'Stay and Play' After Minor Injuries

34.8.1 Differences in Age and Skill Level

Minor injuries with the potential of 'stay and play on field' affect football players of all age groups and at all skill levels [26–28]. Medical support in football depends on the appropriate equipment on field and thus on the financial support provided. Beginning with adequate first aid equipment on field [27], all sectors of the 'stay and play on field' process require specific medication and medical devices as well as the knowledge and experience of the medical staff. These skills are more likely to be available in professional football teams than in amateur or junior football teams. There is less pressure to 'stay and play' in junior football because diagnostics and treatment of injured junior players should not be rushed to avoid further or chronic complaints or complications.

34.8.2 Player Susceptibility to Injury and Injury Causation

Both the susceptibility to sustaining a traumatic injury or overuse complaint and pain perception tend to vary widely among football players. Some players may 'stay and play' on field after sustaining a minor injury, while other players with a similar complaint leave the pitch and want a break from football. Team coaches and medical staff have to know and understand the character of their players to be able to support them in different injury situations. The time point of an injury in the football season may also influence return-to-play decisions. Injuries sustained directly before the winter break less frequently involve 'stay and play' or the potential risk of returning to play as quickly as possible. In contrast, minor injuries at the end of the season or before a final cup match are typical situations leading to extended 'stay and play' decisions in several types of injury.

Fact Box 7

- To achieve 'stay and play' after minor injuries depends on various factors.
- The main influencing factors for successful 'stay and play on field' and quick return-to-play after minor injuries are the susceptibility and willingness of the injured player, the decision by the team coach, experienced medical staff and appropriate medical equipment, the time of injury in the football season and financial pressure.

34.9 Specific Steps of the 'Stay and Play' Process After Minor Football Injuries

Apart from the main aim of 'stay and play' after injury, it is also important for players that minor injuries do not result in other problems such as:

→ Becoming chronic complaints

→ Developing into an injury with tissue damage of the same body site

→ Developing into an injury affecting another body region

'Stay and play' after football injuries includes injury-specific aspects, which are unique for each specific injury.

34.9.1 Ankle Sprains

First aid and joint protection until diagnosis; ankle tapes to improve the return-to-play process [4]; understanding of the healing potential of the ligament, no trivialisation; knowing the risk of chronic instability and relevance of preventive neuromotorical exercises.

34.9.2 Muscle Strains and Contusion

Detailed diagnosis of the injury structure or functional disturbance of the muscle [32, 36]; detection of haematoma; first aid and physiotherapy, symptomatic therapy and functional training [3, 42].

34.9.3 Bone Contusion

Immediate clinical exclusion of a fracture; pain management and protection (equipment) against recurrent contusion.

34.9.4 Head Contusion (and Cervical Sprains)

The concussion return-to-play protocol and other protocols for specific head injuries provide guidelines for all types of head injuries; cervical spine protection after head injury and facial masks (Fig. 34.6) [15, 37].

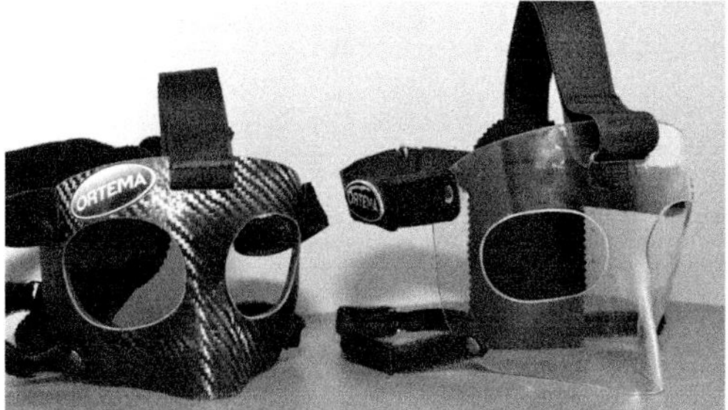

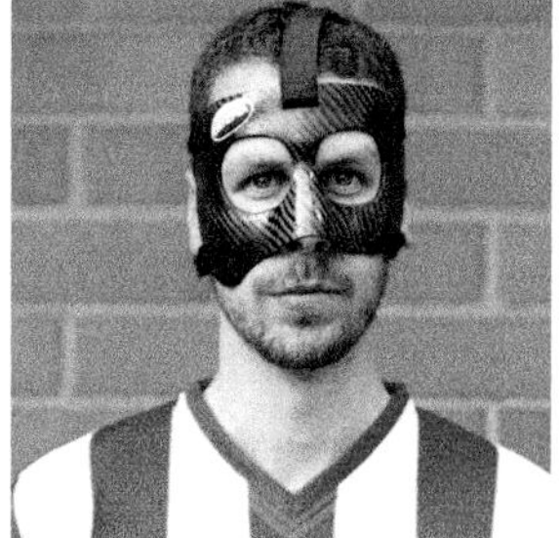

Fig. 34.6 Anatomical facial masks for 'stay and play' on football field and the protection of recurrent facial injuries (thank you to Hartmut Semsch/Ortema)

34.9.5 Skin Lesions and Lacerations

Consideration of affected body site and the healing potential; water permeability of skin and protection plaster.

34.9.6 Low Back Pain

Exclusion of neurological or structural damage by clinical examination; physical therapy and pain management.

34.9.7 Groin Pain

Adjoining symptoms on proximate body sites; exclusion of hernia or urologic problems and adduction test of the hip as recommended return-to-play and 'stay and play' test [23].

34.9.8 Ingrown Toenails

Complete analgesia for the 'stay and play' decision; short-term plan to reduce pain and inflammation; midterm plan to 'stay and play' but planning definite treatment (e.g. surgery) and healing process in the summer or winter break of the season.

34.9.9 Foot Blisters

Early detection of blisters on the foot; sterile puncture to reduce pressure and pain; taping or blister plaster; analgesia for the 'stay and play' decision; prevention of further blisters by wearing adequate shoes and podiatry (Fig. 34.7).

34.9.10 Fractures of the Phalanxes

Immediate splinting and protection in case of a suspected fracture; phalanx fractures of the foot less often result in 'stay and play' because of the pain during running; phalanx fractures of the hand may only negatively affect goalkeepers and after treatment decision (conservative or surgical), wearing of protection equipment to achieve a safe 'stay and play' process. Wearing of appropriate equipment to protect the fracture of the phalanx, but endangering opponent players should be avoided.

Fact Box 8

- Typical football injuries with a high incidence but low evidence of successful treatment and early return-to-play are ankle sprains, muscle strains, bone contusion, head contusion, skin lacerations and pain syndrome of the back and groin. Treatments and early return-to-play after such injuries need to be addressed in more detail in future research.
- Other typical medical problems in football such as ingrown toenails, foot blisters and muscle cramps are frequently trivialised but may be sufficiently managed by the medical staff.

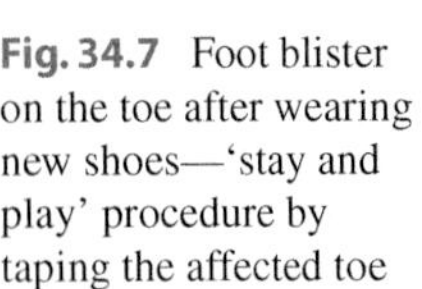
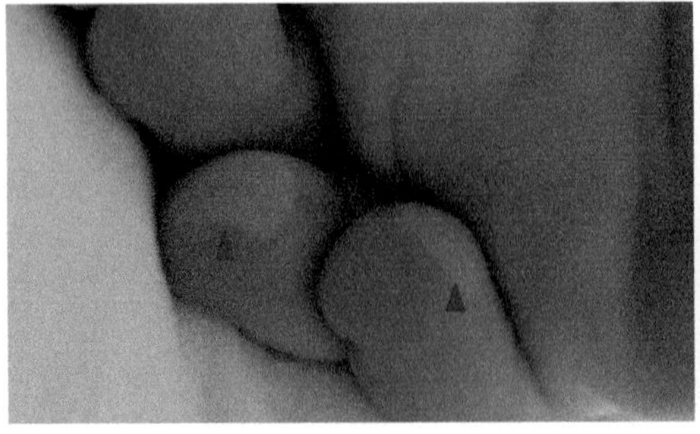
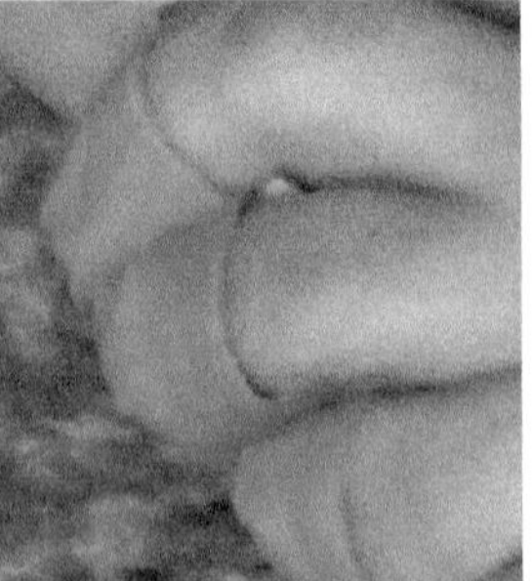

Fig. 34.7 Foot blister on the toe after wearing new shoes—'stay and play' procedure by taping the affected toe

34.10 Exemplary Cases of 'Stay and play' to Achieve a Non-time-loss Injury

This section should illustrate in two common injury types, how conservative treatment strategies are developed in specific steps and with specific staff and equipment, but also how many different approaches are available to treat successfully such sports injuries.

34.10.1 Ankle Sprain

Ankle sprains are a frequent occurrence in football, but adequate 'stay and play' procedures on field are only practicable in professional football. Several steps are essential for achieving an immediate and pain-free situation after an acute injury situation [11]:

1. **First aid on field:**
   - PRICE and pain management
2. **Return-to-structure phase: On field**
   - Body language
   - Recognise the tissue perturbation of the continuum of the injured body region
   - Immediate procedure directly on field conducted by the physiotherapist or physician
   - Correction of trigger bands and continuum disturbance by manual techniques with pressure and traction manipulation
   - Local pain management (lotion or cryotherapy)
3. **Return-to-function phase: Outside the field**
   - Setting of the ankle joint
   - Mobilisation of the proximate joints
   - Elastic taping
   - Checking the arthro-ligamentary function of the muscular synergists and the hyperfunction of the antagonists (reciprocal)
   - Myofascial techniques
   - Immediate break from football in the case of vegetative symptoms
4. **Protection of the structures for the healing process:**
   - Taping and protection equipment
5. **Stay and Play**

Successful 'stay and play' processes require further diagnostics and treatment directly after the match, beginning with first aid on field and PRICE. Quick return-to-play until the next match ('stay and play' III) may necessitate one of the following treatment options within the next few days [11]:

- Osteopathy
- Activation of auto-reparative mechanism by continuous passive motion, biofeedback and isokinetics
- Antagonistic inhibition (reciprocal); PFN and avoidance of overuse of the injured body region
- Return-to-play tests in a rehabilitation setting: Isokinetics and EMG
- Return-to-play decision after functional tests, clinical tests, athletic tests and a last team training before competition
- Besides objective parameters, subjective parameters such as feeling comfortable or analgesia are essential for the decision on 'stay and play' on field

Apart from ankle sprains, muscle strains of the thigh also represent a frequent type of injury associated with an indication for 'stay and play' procedures. Similar to the interdisciplinary and multifaceted approach to treating ankle sprains, muscle strains are also subject to different treatment strategies.

34.10.2 Muscle Injury

Muscular injuries occur frequently in amateur and professional football [26]. Different types of conservative treatment strategies are published in the literature and show the multifaceted approach to these injuries (Table 34.8).

Take-Home Message

'Stay and play on field' procedures after minor injuries are subject to different factors and require highly experienced medical staff. Scientific evidence on this topic has been rather low. The different types of conservative treatment available

Table 34.8 Different therapeutic options for muscle injuries described in the literature

– Stainsby et al. [40]
Cryotherapy + interferential current + cold laser therapy + manual therapy + PNF
– Müller-Wohlfahrt et al. [32]
One option: Puncture + compression bandage + infiltration + medication + supplements
– Valle et al. [42]
PRICE + drugs + biological treatment (PRP) + cooling + therapeutic exercises
– Eder and Hoffmann [11]
First aid + avoid hyperfunction of the antagonists + unguentary bandage + electrotherapy + continuous passive motion for activation + elastic taping

for such injuries should be further investigated in the future. This article illustrates in detail why minor injuries require adequate treatment and safe return-to-play and how these goals may be achieved.

Top Five Evidence Based References

Krutsch V, Gesslein M, Loose O, Weber J, Nerlich M, Gaensslen A, Bonkowsky V, Krutsch W (2017) Injury mechanism of midfacial fractures in football causes in over 40% typical neurological symptoms of minor brain injuries. Knee Surg Sports Traumatol Arthrosc

Krutsch W, Voss A, Gerling S, Grechenig S, Nerlich M, Angele P (2014) First aid on field management in youth football. Arch Orthop Trauma Surg 134(9):1301–1309

Smith RM, Conn AK (2009) Prehospital care - scoop and run or stay and play? Injury 40(Suppl 4):S23–S26

Fuller CW, Ekstrand J, Junge A, Andersen TE, Bahr R, Dvorak J, Hägglund M, McCrory P, Meeuwisse WH (2006) Consensus statement on injury definitions and data collection procedures in studies of football (soccer) injuries. Br J Sports Med 40(3):193–201

Fuller CW, Walker J (2006) Quantifying the functional rehabilitation of injured football players. Br J Sports Med 40(2):151–157

References

1. Alentorn-Geli E, Myer GD, Silvers HJ, Samitier G, Romero D, Lázaro-Haro C, Cugat R (2009) Prevention of non-contact anterior cruciate ligament injuries in soccer players. Part 1: Mechanisms of injury and underlying risk factors. Knee Surg Sports Traumatol Arthrosc 17(7):705–729
2. Angele P, Hoffmann H, Williams A, Jones M, Krutsch W (2016) Specific aspects of football in recreational and competitive sport. In: Mary HO, Zaffagnini S et al (eds) Prevention of injuries and overuse in sports. Directionary for physicians, physiotherapists, sports scientists and coaches. Springer, New York, NY, pp 117–136
3. Askling CM, Tengvar M, Thorstensson A (2013) Acute hamstring injuries in Swedish elite football: a prospective randomised controlled clinical trial comparing two rehabilitation protocols. Br J Sports Med 47(15):953–959
4. Best R, Mauch F, Böhle C, Huth J, Brüggemann P (2014) Residual mechanical effectiveness of external ankle tape before and after competitive professional soccer performance. Clin J Sport Med 24(1):51–57
5. Bleakley CM, Glasgow P, MacAuley DC (2012) PRICE needs updating, should we call the POLICE? Br J Sports Med 46(4):220–221
6. Bleakley CM, O'Connor S, Tully MA, Rocke LG, Macauley DC, McDonough SM (2007) The PRICE study (Protection Rest Ice Compression Elevation): design of a randomised controlled trial comparing standard versus cryokinetic ice applications in the management of acute ankle sprain. BMC Musculoskelet Disord 8:125
7. Bloch H, Klein C, Luig P, Moser N (2015) Return-to-competition. Test-Manual zur Beurteilung der Spielfähigkeit nach Ruptur des vorderen Kreuzbands. VBG, Jedermann-Verlag, Hamburg
8. Deol RS, Roche A, Calder JD (2016) Return to training and playing after acute lisfranc injuries in elite professional soccer and rugby players. Am J Sports Med 44(1):166–170
9. Diaz de leon-Miranda E, Redondo-Aquino G, Bueno-Olmos ME, Arriaga-Paez MA, Rodriguez-Cabrera R, Torres-Gonzalez R (2007) Associated factors to severe sport injuries. Rev Med Inst Mex Seguro Soc 45:47–52
10. Dunn WR, George MS, Churchill L, Spindler KP (2007) Ethics in sports medicine. Am J Sports Med 35(5):840–844
11. Eder K, Hoffmann H (2016) Verletzungen im Fußball. Vermeiden-behandeln-therapieren. Urban & Fischer, München
12. Ekstrand J, Hägglund M, Törnqvist H, Kristenson K, Bengtsson H, Magnusson H, Waldén M (2013) Upper extremity injuries in male elite football players. Knee Surg Sports Traumatol Arthrosc 21(7):1626–1632
13. Ekstrand J, Lee JC, Healy JC (2016) MRI findings and return-to-play in football: a prospective analysis of 255 hamstring injuries in the UEFA Elite Club Injury Study. Br J Sports Med 50(12):738–743

14. Elattar O, Choi HR, Dills VD, Busconi B (2016) Groin Injuries (Athletic Pubalgia) and Return-to-play. Sports Health 8(4):313–323
15. Fowell CJ, Earl P (2013) Return-to-play guidelines following facial fractures. Br J Sports Med 47(10):654–656
16. Fuller CW, Ekstrand J, Junge A, Andersen TE, Bahr R, Dvorak J, Hägglund M, McCrory P, Meeuwisse WH (2006) Consensus statement on injury definitions and data collection procedures in studies of football (soccer) injuries. Br J Sports Med 40(3):193–201
17. Fuller CW, Walker J (2006) Quantifying the functional rehabilitation of injured football players. Br J Sports Med 40(2):151–157
18. Gajhede-Knudsen M, Ekstrand J, Magnusson H, Maffulli N (2013) Recurrence of Achilles tendon injuries in elite male football players is more common after early return-to-play: an 11-year follow-up of the UEFA Champions League injury study. Br J Sports Med 47(12):763–768
19. Garlanger KL, Fredericks WH, Do A, Bauer BA, Laskowski ER (2016) The feasibility and effects of acupuncture in an adolescent nordic ski population. PM R:S1934-1482(16) 31197-2
20. Hart D, Funk L (2015) Serious shoulder injuries in professional soccer: return to participation after surgery. Knee Surg Sports Traumatol Arthrosc 23(7):2123–2129
21. Haser C, Stöggl T, Kriner M, Mikoleit J, Wolfahrt B, Scherr J, Halle M, Pfab F (2017) Effect of dry needling on thigh muscle strength and hip flexion in elite soccer players. Med Sci Sports Exerc 49(2):378–383
22. Horstmann H, Clausen JD, Krettek C, Weber-Spickschen TS (2017) Evidence-based therapy for tendinopathy of the knee joint: which forms of therapy are scientifically proven? Unfallchirurg 120:199
23. Jardí J, Rodas G, Pedret C, Til L, Cusí M, Malliaropoulos N, Del Buono A, Maffulli N (2014) Osteitis pubis: can early return to elite competition be contemplated? Transl Med UniSa 10:52–58
24. Junge A, Langevoort G, Pipe A, Peytavin A, Wong F, Mountjoy M, Beltrami G, Holzgraefe CR, Dvorak J (2006) Injuries in team sport tournaments during the 2004 Olympic games. Am J Sports Med 34:565–576
25. Kerr ZY, Collins CL, Pommering TL, Field S, Comstock RD (2011) Dislocation/separation injuries among US high school athletes in 9 selected sports: 2005-2009. Clin J Sport Med 21:101–108
26. Koch M, Zellner J, Berner A, Grechenig S, Krutsch V, Nerlich M, Angele P, Krutsch W (2016) Influence of preparation and football skill level on injury incidence during an amateur football tournament. Arch Orthop Trauma Surg 136(3):353–360
27. Krutsch W, Voss A, Gerling S, Grechenig S, Nerlich M, Angele P (2014) First aid on field management in youth football. Arch Orthop Trauma Surg 134(9):1301–1309
28. Krutsch W, Zeman F, Zellner J, Pfeifer C, Nerlich M, Angele P (2016) Increase in ACL and PCL injuries after implementation of a new professional football league. Knee Surg Sports Traumatol Arthrosc 24(7):2271–2279
29. Krutsch V, Gesslein M, Loose O, Weber J, Nerlich M, Gaensslen A, Bonkowsky V, Krutsch W (2017) Injury mechanism of midfacial fractures in football causes in over 40% typical neurological symptoms of minor brain injuries. Knee Surg Sports Traumatol Arthrosc
30. Lee SM, Lee JH (2015) Ankle inversion taping using kinesiology tape for treating medial ankle sprain in an amateur soccer player. J Phys Ther Sci 27(7):2407–2408
31. Moen MH, Reurink G, Weir A, Tol JL, Maas M, Goudswaard GJ (2014) Predicting return-to-play after hamstring injuries. Br J Sports Med 48(18):1358–1363
32. Mueller-Wohlfahrt HW, Ueblacker P, Hensel L (2014) Muscle injuries in sports. Thieme Verlag, Stuttgart, NY
33. Nook DD, Nook EC, Nook BC (2016) Utilization of chiropractic care at the world games 2013. J Manipulative Physiol Ther 39(9):693–704
34. Oztekin HH, Boya H, Ozcan O, Zeren B, Pinar P (2009) Foot and ankle injuries and time lost from play in professional soccer players. Foot (Edinb) 19(1):22–28
35. Paoloni JA, Milne C, Orchard J, Hamilton B (2009) Non-steroidal anti-inflammatory drugs in sports medicine: guidelines for practical but sensible use. Br J Sports Med 43(11):863–865
36. Pedret C, Rodas G, Balius R, Capdevila L, Bossy M, Vernooij RW, Alomar X (2015) Return-to-play after soleus muscle injuries. Orthop J Sports Med 3(7):2325967115595802. eCollection 2015
37. Price J, Malliaras P, Hudson Z (2012) Current practices in determining return-to-play following head injury in professional football in the UK. Br J Sports Med 46(14):1000–1003
38. Schöberl M, Prantl L, Loose O, Zellner J, Angele P, Zeman F, Spreitzer M, Nerlich M, Krutsch W (2017) Non-surgical treatment of pubic overload and groin pain in amateur football players: a prospective double-blinded randomised controlled study. Knee Surg Sports Traumatol Arthrosc 25:1958
39. Smith RM, Conn AK (2009) Prehospital care - scoop and run or stay & play? Injury 40(Suppl 4):S23–S26
40. Stainsby BE, Piper SL, Gringmuth R (2012) Management approaches to acute muscular strain and hematoma in National level soccer players: a report of two cases. J Can Chiropr Assoc 56(4):262–268
41. Stanek JM (2016) The effectiveness of compression socks on athletic performance and recovery. J Sport Rehabil 24:1–16
42. Valle X, L Tol J, Hamilton B, Rodas G, Malliaras P, Malliaropoulos N, Rizo V, Moreno M, Jardi J (2015) Hamstring muscle injuries, a rehabilitation protocol purpose. Asian J Sports Med 6(4):e25411

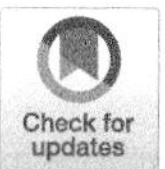

Return to Play with Degenerative Joint Disease

35

Peter Angele, Johannes Zellner, Johannes Weber, and Matthias Koch

Contents

P. Angele (✉)
Department of Trauma Surgery, University Medical Centre Regensburg, Franz-Josef-Strauss-Allee 11, 93053 Regensburg, Germany

Sporthopaedicum Regensburg, Hildegard-von Bingen-Str. 1, 93053 Regensburg, Germany
e-mail: peter.angele@ukr.de

J. Zellner • J. Weber • M. Koch
Department of Trauma Surgery, University Medical Centre Regensburg, Franz-Josef-Strauss-Allee 11, 93053 Regensburg, Germany

35.1 Introduction

Football is one of the most popular sports worldwide [1]. Hundred millions of people play recreational or professional football [1]. It is known that playing football is associated with a high injury risk, and the injury patterns were already analysed in many studies [2–8]. Overall, it was shown that independent of the skill level especially the lower extremities, in particular the knee joint, are affected by injury [3–5, 9]. Own unpublished data concerning the end of career of professional football players of the first and second German football league has shown that around 65% of the football players had to stop playing due to career ending injuries. A further differentiation of these data revealed that around 60% of these players had to retire because of serious knee joint injuries. These career stops were caused by osteoarthritis in almost 70% of the players.

So the early knowledge of osteoarthritis risk factors, as well as the appropriate treatment, guidance and rehabilitation of the football player are crucial for a safe return to sport with no or only minor risk for advanced osteoarthritis in the long term.

35.2 Cartilage Injury

A decisive factor to ensure a suitable treatment of any disease/injury is its clear definition. In terms of cartilage injuries, the chondral or osteochondral

V. Musahl et al. (eds.), *Return to Play in Football*, https://doi.org/10.1007/978-3-662-55713-6_35

defect has to be defined as a focal, non-degenerative, traumatic lesion, as a focal early osteoarthritis defector or as a degenerative lesion at different stages (including diffuse early osteoarthritis and advanced osteoarthritis).

While focal, non-degenerative lesions can successfully be treated by regenerative approaches like microfracturing (MFx), osteochondral autograft transfer (OAT) or autologous chondrocyte implantation (ACI), the treatment of degenerative defects remains challenging [10].

Concerning the surgical management, cartilage repair in focal, traumatic lesions and the return to play following cartilage injuries, the authors refer to Chap. 41 "Return to play following cartilage injuries", Chap. 42 "Surgical management of articular cartilage in football players" and Chap. 43 "Advanced techniques of cartilage repair in football players".

35.3 Osteoarthritis

The status of osteoarthritis is defined by the Osteoarthritis Research Society International (OARSI) as:

> *... a disorder involving movable joints characterized by cell stress and extracellular matrix degradation initiated by micro- and macro-injury that activates maladaptive repair responses including pro-inflammatory pathways of innate immunity. The disease manifests first as a molecular derangement (abnormal joint tissue metabolism) followed by anatomic, and/or physiologic derangements (characterized by cartilage degradation, bone remodeling, osteophyte formation, joint inflammation and loss of normal joint function), that can culminate in illness* [11].

In summary, the development of osteoarthritis is a multistep process. It is initiated by a direct cartilage trauma and/or by recurrent microtrauma based on joint destabilizing injuries. These traumatic insults are accompanied first with a derangement of the micro-environment before a macroscopic progression is replicable. Regarding current treatment options, the extent of the degenerative changes of the articular cartilage remains nowadays the deciding factor. In this context, the status of a focal early osteoarthritis is to differentiate from diffuse early osteoarthritis as well as advanced osteoarthritis, in order to define the period with remaining regenerative potential of the articular cartilage [12].

35.4 Early Osteoarthritis

According to the current literature, the status of early osteoarthritis in comparison to the advanced osteoarthritis is mainly characterized by its partly regenerative qualities.

However, a clear definition of this regenerative status is challenging. While advanced osteoarthritis is easily described by clear signs, i.e. its history, clinical symptoms and the associated radiographic abnormalities, in the early phase of the degenerative process, these characteristics are often limited and sporadically present [12, 13]. The extent of the degenerative process is limited on a tissue-related phenomena leading to a loss of joint homeostasis and consecutively to an established osteoarthritis [13]. Additionally the affected population is different. In contrast to the advanced osteoarthritis, early osteoarthritis is already seen in a high amount of young, sportive people [12, 14], which underlines the urgency to come up with a consensus on definition criteria.

Because of these multiple factors related to early osteoarthritis, isolated clinical and radiographical scores fail to define this period of degeneration. Therefore Luyten et al. described criteria including different diagnostic tools (pain history, standard radiographs, arthroscopy or MRI) that are fulfilled by patients having early osteoarthritis [12, 13].

However, the most informative classification for early osteoarthritis links up with the arthroscopic evaluation due to its direct correlation with the different treatment strategies. Based on the arthroscopical differentiation by Luyten et al. and typical clinical findings, Madry et al. divided the arthroscopic classification for early osteoarthritis in two parts: a peri-lesional centred, focal early osteoarthritis and a diffuse early osteoarthritis [12] (Fig. 35.1).

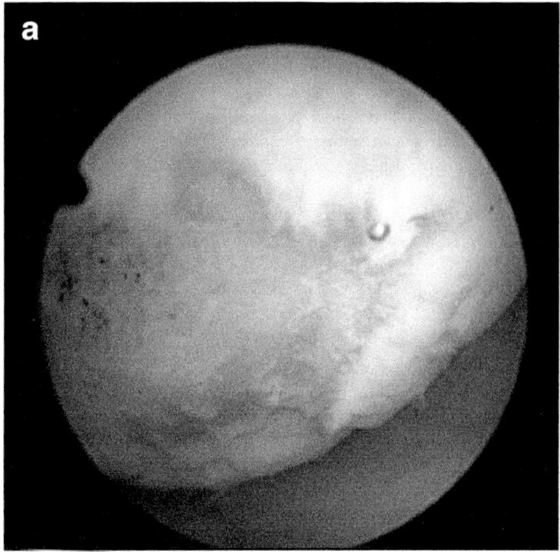
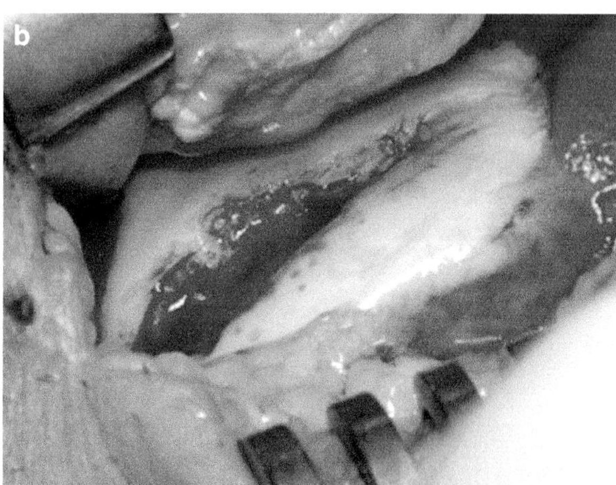

Fig. 35.1 Focal early osteoarthritis defects. (**a**) Arthroscopical view on a femoral condyle with a focal degenerative lesion with rounded edges as well as swelling and fibrillation of the surrounding cartilage; (**b**) direct view on a focal degenerative defect after arthrotomy before matrix-assisted autologous chondrocyte implantation is performed

In case of focal early osteoarthritis, a regenerative potential can be observed. Therefore, the articular surface has to be analysed separately, and any injured area has to be classified according to the ICRS scoring system (grades 1–4) (www.cartilage.org/_files/contentmanagment/ICRS_evaluation.pdf). In contrast to traumatic, focal lesions, the defect edges are mainly rounded. The surrounding peri-lesional degeneration area (characterized by softening, swelling as well as fibrillation of the cartilage surface) has to be staged and graded according to the histomorphometrical OARSI criteria as long as lesions are not deeper than ICRS stage 2. Any further defect (ICRS stage > 2) has to be included into the main defect as long as it touches the defect area. Otherwise, it has to be assessed separately. Knowing the influential effect of additional cartilage lesions, defects on the opposite surface as well as in the other compartments have to be included in the staging analysis (see table "focal early osteoarthritis").

Fact Box 1
Early osteoarthritis has to be differentiated in focal early osteoarthritis and diffuse early osteoarthritis.

In contrast to the peri-lesional centred, focal early osteoarthritis, focal lesions are missing in the diffuse early osteoarthritis, and this degeneration area extends to a minimum of two compartments. According to the QARSI criteria, diffuse cartilage injury needs to be limited to ICRS stage ≤ 2, because progressed degeneration (ICRS stage 3/4) corresponds to advanced osteoarthritis [15] (see table "diffuse early osteoarthritis"). Due to the defect morphology and extension within the joint, regenerative potential in diffuse early osteoarthritis is strongly reduced, so that regenerative treatment approaches are not indicated [16]. The treatment as well as the recommendation to return to sport correspond to the advices of advanced osteoarthritis (Figs. 35.2 and 35.3).

35.4.1 Treatment

In order to find the best treatment option, it is important to know more about etiopathology as well as injury mechanisms. Comorbidities and risk factors have to be requested, too. Dependant on that, surgical and non-surgical options can be applied.

35.4.1.1 Non-operative Treatment

The non-operative treatment strategies include the patient's physical profile as well as functional

Fig. 35.2 Classification of focal early osteoarthritis according to Madry et al. [12]

	focal cartilage defect (ICRS 3/ 4) with perilesional degeneration (ICRS 1/2)
Stage	
0	
1	≤ 25%
2	> 25 % to ≤ 50%
3	> 50 % to ≤ 75%
4	> 75%
Grade	
A	Stages 1-4 with additional cartilage degeneration (ICRS 1/ 2) - **same** compartment - contralateral joint surface
B	Stages 1-4 with additional cartilage degeneration (ICRS 1/ 2) - **other** compartment
C	Stages 1-4 with additional cartilage degeneration (ICRS 3/ 4) - **same** compartment - contralateral joint surface
D	Stages 1-4 with additional cartilage degeneration (ICRS 3/ 4) - **other** compartment

Fig. 35.3 Classification of diffuse early osteoarthritis according to Madry et al. [12]

	Extend of degeneration
Grade	
1	ICRS 1
2	ICRS 2
3	ICRS 3 (probably advanced osteoarthritis)
4	ICRS 4 (probably advanced osteoarthritis)
Stage	
A	- degeneration ≤ **25%** of the main compartment - two joint compartments are involved
B	- degeneration **> 25 % to ≤ 50%**of the main compartment - two joint compartments involved
C	- degeneration **> 50 % to ≤ 75%**of the main compartment - two joint compartments are involved
D	- degeneration **> 75%** of the main compartment - two joint compartments are involved
E	- three joint compartments are involved independent of stage

and pharmacological treatment approaches, such as weight management, physical therapy, NSAID (non-steroidal anti-inflammatory drug) application and injection therapy [17–19].

Weight Management

Obesity is one of the most important and modifiable risk factors for the development of degenerative joint diseases [19]. Adaption of BMI to an adequate level is one of the most important non-surgical treatment options. Reduced body weight leads to reduced joint loads and, therefore, has a crucial influence on the quality of articular cartilage [12, 18, 20].

Physical Therapy

Physical therapy should be individualized after patient assessment [19]. In general, clinical guidelines recommend land- and water-based exercises as well as strength training in order to reduce adhesions, to improve the range of motion (ROM) and to strengthen the joint-encompassing musculature. It is proven that these kinds of passive and active exercises can interject the inflammatory cycle that is associated with the progression of osteoarthritis [18, 19].

Concerning the knee joint, knowing ROM is known as a key factor in muscular weakness and to impact on the joint function. Therefore joint capsule extensibility as well as quadriceps, hamstrings, hip flexor, gastrocnemius and soleus muscle length changes have to be addressed by physical therapy [18, 19].

Furthermore, knee extensors and hip abductors muscles are recommended to be strengthened to reduce pain and improve function in osteoarthritic changed knee joints [18].

Overall, supervised group and supervised individual training is estimated to be superior to independent home exercise [19].

Pharmacological Therapy

The application of painkillers, such as NSAIDs or paracetamol, on an oral or topical way is limited to a symptom-based effect. In contrast to the above-mentioned approaches, any direct influence on the progress of degenerative changes remains unknown [19]. According to the adverse drug reactions of an oral application, topical application has to be taken into account since its therapeutic effect is known to be comparable to the oral application [21]. However, the current literature shows a persisting high abuse of painkillers in football [22, 23]. A dramatic finding in this field is the fact that even in youth football players the use of painkillers is already widespread [24].

Injection Therapy

Although the actual injection therapy seems to have a growing market in the context of osteoarthritis therapy, its use is still limited to a symptom-based effect.

Currently, there are mainly two agents used in clinical practice: corticosteroids and hyaluronic acid. Which substance is injected is based on the present symptoms. Whereas corticosteroids are advocated for the therapy of active synovitis and effusion, hyaluronic acid is considered to be the first-line treatment if effusion is missing and the symptoms persist [18, 21]. Concerning pain relief hyaluronic acid seems to have the potential to provide longer durations of relief [18]. However, the beneficial effect of hyaluronic acid is evaluated to be uncertain according to the OARSI guidelines [25]. Furthermore, frequently repeated injections can result in joint damage as well as increase the risk for infection [19].

In contrast to the established corticosteroids and hyaluronic acid, recently developed blood-derived injectables, such as platelet-rich plasma (PRP), are presumed to act on a bioactive level and to lead to positive effects both at a cartilage level and on the entire joint homeostasis [18]. Nevertheless, there is still no evidence for its superiority in the current literature [18].

35.4.1.2 Operative Treatment

Cartilage Therapy

Cartilage therapy plays a key role in the operative treatment of focal, traumatic lesions as well as focal early osteoarthritis. Initially, regenerative cartilage therapy was limited to traumatic, focal cartilage defects and contraindicated for degenerative defects. However, different studies investigated that up to 60% of the treated lesions were evaluated to already be considered degenerative at the time of therapy [16, 26]. Overall, regenerative cartilage therapy of traumatic focal lesions as well as focal early osteoarthritis defects shows promising results. The failure rate after regenerative therapy with matrix-assisted autologous chondrocyte implantation is described to be 13.9%. In comparison, the failure rate in chondral defects with isolated traumatic origin is 6% [16, 27].

Chondral and osteochondral injuries occur frequently in football players because of primary joint impact and secondary soft tissue injuries resulting in joint instability [18]. Untreated, these defects increase the risk of developing advanced OA compared to the general population [28]. It is well known that these articular cartilage lesions show no spontaneously endogenous healing potential. So, it is crucial to use treatment approaches to effectively and durably restore the joint surface and thus reduce the risk of progression of joint degeneration and enable the athlete to return to sport [18].

Many techniques are already described to enable the athletes to return to high-impact sports. The surgical management of articular cartilage in football players and the strategies to return to play following cartilage injuries are described in detail in Chap. 41 "Return to play following cartilage injuries" and Chap. 42 "Surgical management of articular cartilage in football players".

Microfracture represents the most frequently used treatment approach in clinical practice [16, 18]. This technique enables the athletes to early return to activity. A return rate of 66% at a mean time of 8 months after surgery is reported [29]. Despite short term benefits, this technique fails to provide promising long-lasting results, probably caused by the inferior mechanical properties of the fibrous cartilaginous tissue [16, 18, 30].

Osteochondral transplantation, also known as mosaicplasty, is an alternative treatment approach for small osteochondral lesions [16]. The current literature shows good results with the highest ratio of return to sport with a return rate of 91% within a mean time of 7 months [29]. However, because of donor-site morbidity as well as weak outcomes after the use of more plugs, this technique is critical to discuss for the use in major sized osteochondral defects in active soccer players and thus should just be indicated for small lesions [18, 31].

Autologous chondrocyte implantation as well as matrix-assisted techniques allows the treatment of major sized cartilage defects with good and long-lasting results in athletes [16, 18]. Almost 68% of athletes treated by autologous chondrocyte implantation returned to sport at a mean time of 18 months. However, frequent reverse events were reported [29]. So, the initial limits of the autologous chondrocyte implantation were improved by the matrix-assisted techniques [18]. Also in the group of high-level athletes, a rate of 86% returned to competition within 1 year, and good results are documented over time [18, 30].

However, these results were mainly reported for traumatic lesions in young athletes. Studies focusing on return to sport in early osteoarthritis are still missing. According to the literature there are many factors influencing the ability to return to sport after cartilage therapy: age, longer duration of symptoms and chronic lesions with radiographic signs of degeneration [29]. Since these factors were frequently found in early osteoarthritis patients and weak results are documented in progressed degenerative cases, further studies have to evaluate the outcome of those techniques in early osteoarthritis patients [18, 32].

Treatment approaches specialised for focal early osteoarthritis and respecting the altered joint environment as well as the cartilage and subchondral bone unit are still in a preliminary stage.

Independent of the chosen surgical strategy, an appropriate postoperative rehabilitation programme is a crucial factor for the outcome [18]. It is known to enhance cartilage repair and maturation and additionally improves the functional outcome and also prevents the risk of re-injury [18, 33].

Meniscus Therapy

Meniscal injuries are among the most frequently soft tissue injuries within the knee joint. Loss of meniscal continuity is an essential factor in the development and progression of degenerative changes within the knee joint. Thus, the appropriate therapy is crucial for the athlete's career. The correct choice of treatment options and return to play following meniscal injuries is described in detail in Chap. 40 "Return to play following meniscus injuries".

Regarding the predisposing role of meniscal lesions in the development of early osteoarthritis and its progression towards advanced osteoarthritis, in the treatment of meniscal lesions, there is a consensus to preserve as much meniscal tissue as possible. So, the first line of choice in the treatment of meniscal injuries has shifted from partial meniscectomies to meniscal repair, whenever feasible [34] (Fig. 35.4).

Even if partial meniscectomy means a faster recovery time for the athlete, in case of existing early osteoarthritis a regenerative approach is recommended with respect to the meniscal lesion.

Regenerative approaches are the meniscal suturing and the use of meniscal scaffolds. If there is no indication for meniscal repair, the use of meniscal allograft transplantation in symptomatic patients, who had a previous subtotal/total meniscectomy, remains an alternative reparative strategy [18].

The outcome after meniscal suturing over time shows a success rate above 85% concerning

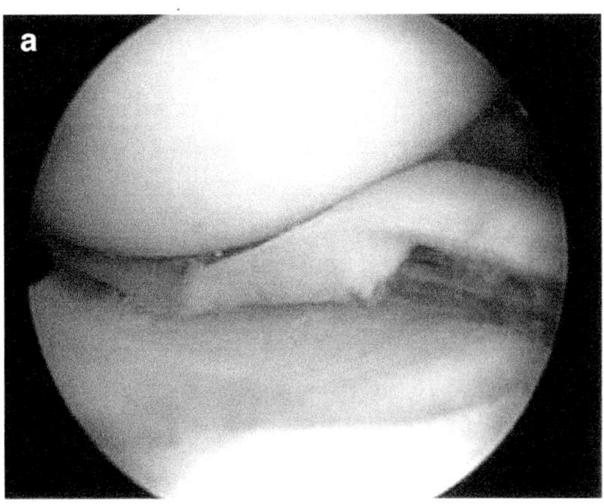

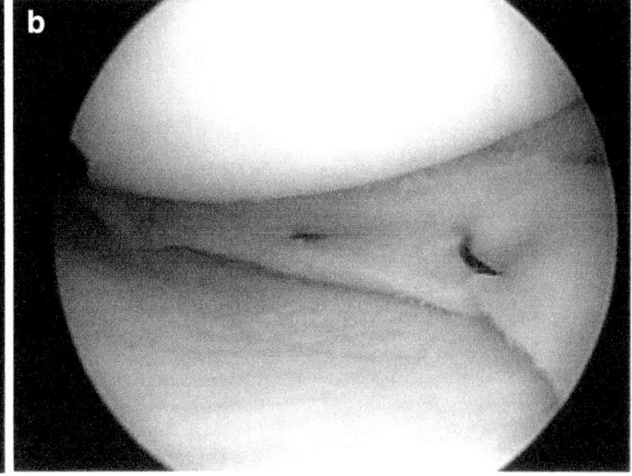

Fig. 35.4 Luxated bucket handle tear and meniscus suture. (**a**) Arthroscopical view on a luxated bucket handle tear; (**b**) refixation of the bucket handle tear by one all-inside suture for the posterior horn and two outside-inside meniscus sutures for the pars intermedia

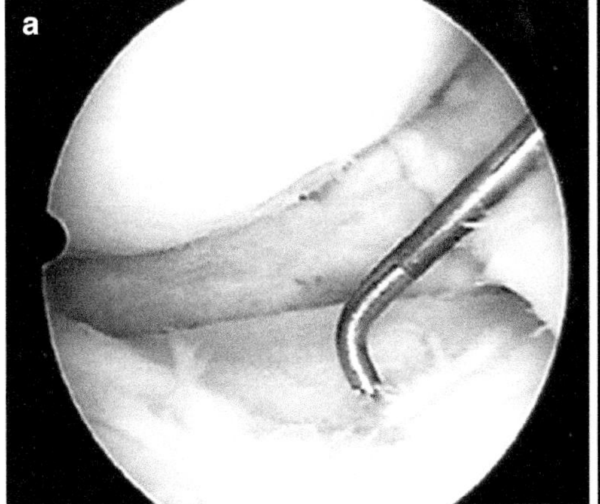

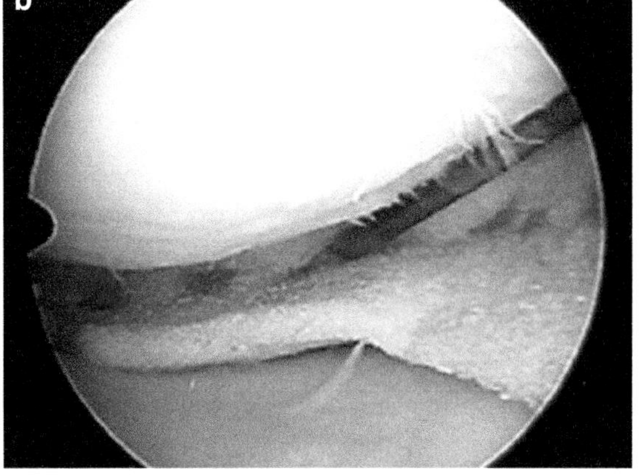

Fig. 35.5 Meniscus defect and defect filling with an artificial meniscus supplement. (**a**) Arthroscopical view on a subtotal meniscus defect with a stable rim and the meniscus basis; (**b**) filling of the meniscus defect with an artificial meniscus supplement and fixation of the meniscal scaffold by suturing (Images taken from [37])

relief of symptoms and function [18, 35]. In the group of competitive football players, a return to play rate of 90% to the pre-injury competition level after recovering from surgery is described [18, 36].

Meniscal scaffolds are an alternative treatment option in patients with a symptomatic partial meniscal lesion in whom meniscal suturing is not indicated [18]. Nowadays, there are two scaffolds available in clinical practice that can be implanted arthroscopically (Fig. 35.5):

- Collagen scaffold (CMI, Collagen Meniscus Implant, CMI-Ivy Sports Medicine GmbH, Germany)
- Polyurethane scaffold (Actifit, Orteq, UK)

Overall, good results with a low cumulative failure rate are reported for both scaffolds [38]. The current literature supports the use of these scaffolds following previous meniscectomy [39]. However, there is no evidence for an implantation in acute meniscal injuries that would especially be relevant to patients with already apparent early osteoarthritis.

Meniscal allografts are indicated for symptomatic patients after total/subtotal meniscectomy [18]. Long-term results show a significant improvement in pain relief and functional outcomes [40]. Furthermore, mid-term results report a 75% return to play rate in professional football players after meniscal allograft implantation when considering the pre-injury level [41]. Although meniscal allografts are associated with a poor outcome in advanced osteoarthritis, positive results at earlier stages of degenerative joint changes as the early osteoarthritis are documented [18].

ACL Therapy

ACL injuries result in an increased anteroposterior translation between the femur and tibia, consecutively causing enhanced shear forces on the articular surface and following predisposing to the development of degenerative changes. The treatment and return to sport after ACL injuries are extensively described in Chap. 37.

If instability impairs the football player, ACL reconstruction is indicated to restore the normal knee joint kinematics. Therefor different grafts (autograft vs. allograft) from different locations (hamstrings, quadriceps tendon, bone patella, tendon bone) are used in clinical practice. All these operative treatment approaches are accompanied with a high rate of return to sports, even to return to competition [18], as long as they are performed before the development of degenerative changes.

However, even with reconstruction of the ACL, an impairment of proprioception and balance due to changed strength and neuromuscular pattern remains, which is accompanied by an increased risk of re-injury [42] and which further influences the progress of degenerative changes.

Alignment Therapy

A deviation of the normal loading axis leads to an increased loading pressure within the particular joint compartment. The shift of the axis according to a valgus or varus deviation defines whether the lateral or medial compartment is affected. Based on an increased loading during sportive activity, the valgus/varus deviation predisposes for the progress of degenerative changes after any previously occurred joint injury. Furthermore, repair strategies after joint injury have to include any axis deviation because of the fact that the increased loading force negatively influences and risks the regenerative approach.

In recent years, osteotomies, such as the proximal tibial or distal femoral osteotomy for the knee joint, developed to a routine strategy to reduce the load of symptomatic degenerative joint compartments. However, for the treatment success an intact contralateral joint compartment is required [18].

Overall, the clinical outcome is good. Most of the affected patients are able to maintain or even improve their sport activities and return to soccer after having realignment procedures [43, 44].

35.4.2 Return to Sport in Early Osteoarthritis: Authors' Recommendation

The early osteoarthritis staging is the key factor in the treatment of osteoarthritis. Based on the preserved regenerative potential according to the injury patterns, different treatment strategies exist. According to the current literature, there are no explicit studies concerning the return to play of football players with early osteoarthritis.

However, regarding the current literature, a high number of regenerative treated cartilage lesions have to be assessed as early osteoarthritic defects [16, 26].So, recommendations concerning return to sport have to be deduced from available data until now.

The crucial questions for the consultation of the athletes are:

- Is any regeneration of the cartilage defect achievable?
- Is any restoration of the causing problem achievable?
- Does the athlete's level justify a return to competitive football even if the causative problem was not solved sufficiently?

In case of a successful cartilage treatment and no further existing concomitant osteoarthritis promoting injuries, like meniscal lesions, joint instability or malalignment, a return to sport and return to competition can be recommended after an appropriate rehabilitation programme. A neuromuscular testing according to Chap. 9 and meeting the validated physiotherapy discharge criteria are recommended before return to high-level sports. However, the athletes have to be informed about the potential re-injury risks and the lack of scientific literature on cartilage repair in early osteoarthritis for elite sports.

If there are concomitant pathologies beside the cartilage defect, it has to be evaluated if a regenerative approach is achievable. If a regenerative treatment strategy (e.g. meniscal suturing or realignment) is successful, a return to sport and return to competition analogous to isolated early osteoarthritis cartilage defects can be recommended.

In cases of an incomplete recovering of the injured joint (e.g. after partial meniscectomy or known increased risk for degenerative changes progression following a procedure as seen after ACL reconstruction), the return to sport depends on the pre-injury level (recreational football player or professional football player). Recreational football players have to be advised against returning to competition and even returning to high joint demanding sports, like for example downhill skiing, tennis, squash or badminton. However, low joint-straining sports, such as cycling, swimming or trekking, have to be recommended.

In contrast, in professional football players, the professional career has to be considered. From a scientific point of view, the current literature lacks data on the return to competition of professional football players having a regenerative therapy of early osteoarthritic cartilage lesions and ACL repair or even partial meniscectomy. From a clinical point of view (adding the risk of osteoarthritis after ACL reconstruction and/or partial meniscectomy together with the longevity of cartilage repair products), a return to competition should not be recommended. If the professional player decides to return to high-level soccer and competition, a realistic overview concerning the risk of advanced osteoarthritis including persistent pain, effusion and functional impairment is recommended. Furthermore, continuous check-ups and an intensive rehabilitation programme for neuromuscular joint stabilization have to be offered.

35.5 Advanced Osteoarthritis

35.5.1 Definition

Within the process of joint degeneration, advanced osteoarthritis as a final status succeeds the status of early osteoarthritis. From a clinical point of view, the advanced osteoarthritis, similar to status of diffuse early osteoarthritis before, is characterized by the loss of regenerative potential as well as a significant progress of symptoms and functional impairments.

Fact Box 2
Advanced osteoarthritis allows no regenerative therapy.

35.5.2 Treatment

35.5.2.1 Conservative Treatment

Conservative treatment options of the advanced osteoarthritis conform to the conservative treatment options of the early osteoarthritis. The main goal is both the relief of symptoms and the functional preservation and improvement during the process of joint degeneration.

35.5.2.2 Operative Treatment

The operative treatment strategies of the advanced osteoarthritis encompass the realignment as well as the unicompartmental and total joint replacement.

Alignment Therapy

Similar to the alignment therapy in early osteoarthritis, the osteotomy in advanced osteoarthritis is performed to unload the medial or lateral compartment in athletes having an unicompartmental osteoarthritis in combination with a valgus or varus axis deviation.

While this therapy option enables regenerative therapy in patients with unicompartmental (osteo-) chondral defects in an early osteoarthritis status, realignment is just a symptomatic therapy in advanced osteoarthritis due to the lost regenerative potential. Its aim is to relief the symptoms, such as pain and functional impairment, and to slow down the progress of degeneration within the affected compartment [45, 46]. So, according to the current literature, the time until a conversion to joint replacement becomes necessary can be prolonged up to an average time of 9.7 years [46].

Therefore, the osteotomy is appropriate especially for younger patients accepting a slight decrease in their physical activity and a longer rehabilitation period in compare to a joint replacing approach [46].

An intact contralateral joint compartment is required as already described for early osteoarthritic defects.

Concerning the postoperative sport activity, the majority of the athletes undergoing osteotomy return to work and sport [43]. Above all, most of the affected patients (78.6%) were able to return to an equal or higher level compared to the level they participated preoperatively, and 54% of the competitive athletes were also able to return to competition [43]. However, the rehabilitation period endured up to 1 year in most patients before they were able to return to work and sport [43] (Fig. 35.6).

Unicompartmental Knee Arthroplasty

An alternative promising option in the treatment of unicompartmental advanced knee osteoarthritis is the implantation of a unicompartmental knee arthroplasty. By this treatment strategy, the affected joint surface is reconstructed by a replacement of the degenerated parts and preservation of the unaffected joint [46]. But, malalignment cannot be addressed according to technical limitations of this treatment approach. Overall, similar to the alignment therapy, just the affected compartment is addressed in terms of pain relief and functional improvement. So, this approach is

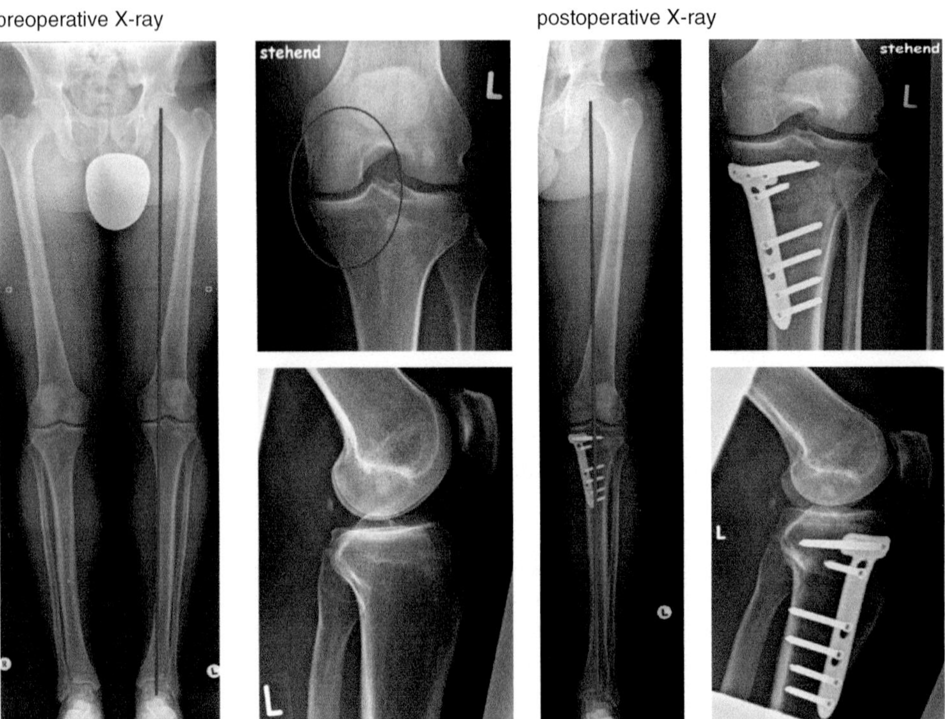

Fig. 35.6 High tibial osteotomy in varus malaligned lower extremity, pre- and postoperative X-ray

limited by the progress of osteoarthritis within the whole joint thus possibly leading to loosening of the prosthesis.

However, introduced in the early 1970s, the technique and durability were improved over the past decades [47]. Nowadays it is characterized by a minimal invasive implantation technique and short postoperative rehabilitation but restricted physical activity afterwards [46]. Anyhow, the postoperative results are good. The average survivorship after 15 years is described with 88.9% for medial and 89.4% for lateral unicompartmental arthroplasties. Regarding medial unicompartmental arthroplasties, additional long-term studies over a period of 25 years showed an average survivorship of 80% [48, 49].

Concerning postoperative physical activity and return to sport, a current review shows excellent rates [50]. The percentage of athletes returning to sport ranged from 75% to more than 100%, meaning that even already retired athletes were able to return to sport after having a unicompartmental arthroplasty. Sport activity was almost regained after a rehabilitation period of around 12 weeks. Some athletes were even able to return to high-impact sports. However, most of the athletes returned to low- and mid-impact sports, like hiking, cycling or swimming [50–52]. Regarding literature, the data do not differ between the medial and lateral site [53] (Fig. 35.7).

Total Joint Replacement

The total knee arthroplasty is the treatment of choice for athletes, in whom osteoarthritic changes include all joint compartments. By the replacement of the whole femoral and tibial parts of the joint, an improved outcome in terms of pain, symptoms, activities of daily living, sport activity and quality of life can be achieved compared with preoperative status [54].

In contrast to the unicompartmental knee arthroplasties, axis deviation as well as instability can be additionally treated by certain implantation techniques and special types of prosthesis in total knee arthroplasty.

Overall, the postoperative clinical outcome shows good to excellent results [55–59]. Especially in young patients (≤55 years) promising results were shown. The activity after total knee arthroplasty, scored by Tegner and Lysholm, was clearly improved postoperative. At least 24% had an activity score of 5 points that means a regular participation in high-demanding sports such as tennis or skiing [57].

Concerning the sport activity of patients having total knee arthroplasty, a high rate of return to sport is documented. However, a shift from high-impact sport to low-impact sport similar to the unicondylar prosthesis is described even if the prosthesis would facilitate higher sports levels [60]. Similar to the unicompartmental arthroplasties, most patients return to sport after a rehabilitation period of 3–6 months [50, 60].

Fact Box 3

Differentiation of low- and high-impact sports according to [60]

Low-impact sport	High-impact sport
Walking	Tennis (single)
Hiking	Squash
Swimming	Soccer
Cycling	Handball
Dancing	Basketball
Golf	Volleyball
Cross-country skiing	Downhill skiing
Tennis (double)	Jogging

35.5.3 Return to Play in Advanced Osteoarthritis: Authors' Recommendation

According to the current literature, there are no studies or recommendations concerning the return to football after having advanced osteoarthritis therapy.

In total three different treatment approaches are used in clinical practice: the conservative therapy, the operative therapy in terms of realignment and the operative therapy in terms of joint replacement.

The non-operative treatment strategy is a symptom-based approach. The aim of this therapy is an appropriate pain relief and functional improvement without directly addressing the cartilage degeneration. The return to sport depends

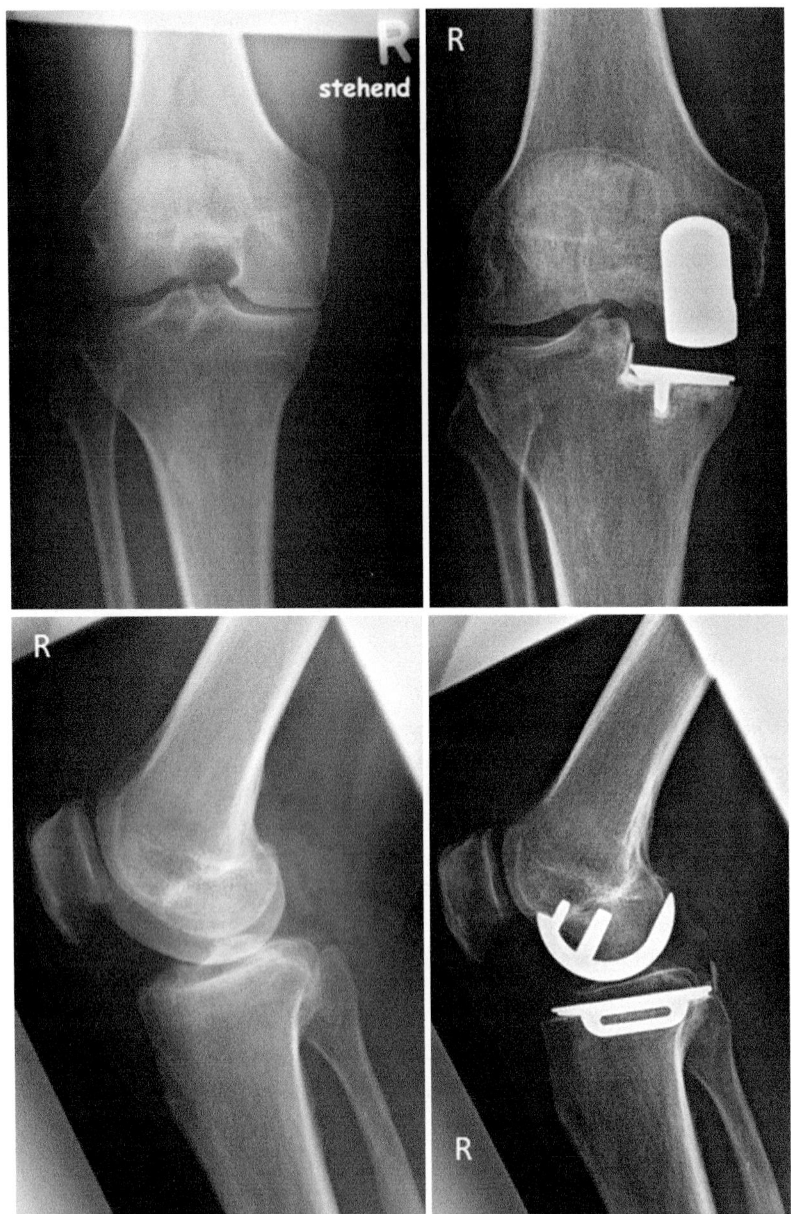

Fig. 35.7 Unicompartmental arthroplasty for medial varus gonarthrosis, pre- and postoperative X-ray

on the remaining symptoms. As long as the athletes feel no impairment, the return to high-impact sport, such as football, is possible. However, to of degeneration and prolong the time to conversion to an operative approach, a downgrading of loading intensity to a recreational basis or a transition to a low-impact sport is recommended.

The operative therapy in terms of a realignment is also a symptom-related strategy. After bony consolidation, a return to play guided by the clinical symptoms is possible. Similar to the non-operative treatment, a reduction of the sports intensity and change to a low-impact sport should be pursued in accordance with the athlete's career.

In contrast to the above-mentioned strategies, arthroplasty is considered as a causally based treatment. By resurfacing the degenerated parts, a relief of symptoms and reconstruction of the joint is obtained. In unicompartmental knee arthroplasties a possible progress of degeneration in the contralateral compartment as well as femoro-patellar compartment has to be taken into account. In contrast, in total knee arthroplasties the whole joints are replaced. Current recommendations concerning a return to sport are mainly based upon experts' opinion and not on evidence-based guidelines [60]. Considering the long-term outcome of arthroplasties, there is a consensus to reduce sportive activity to a low-impact sport after having knee arthroplasty even if the prosthesis would facilitate higher levels of sport [54, 60]. According to two studies, a successful return to high-impact sport (judo, tennis) after total knee arthroplasty is described [60–62]. However, up to now the effects of such activity levels on the long-term outcome are still unknown [60].

In summary, a return to sport should be recommended to every athlete having advanced osteoarthritis, based on the fact that physical activity is recommended in general because of its influence for general health and bone quality [63]. An adaption of intensity and impact has to be realized according to athletes' symptoms as well as skill level and career [60]. Technically demanding sports should not be started after joint replacement because of the increased joint loading and raised risk for injuries during the learning phase for unskilled athletes [63].

Take-Home Message

- A clear differentiation of the stages of osteoarthritis is crucial for an appropriate athletes guidance.
- Treatment of all stages includes both non-operative and operative strategies.
- Focal early osteoarthritis allows a regenerative approach.
- From a clinical point of view, the recommendation to return to pre-injury level should be limited to regenerative approaches in focal early osteoarthritis.
- If no regeneration can be obtained, individualized downgrading of intensity and impact in accordance to the athletes' career has to be recommended.
- After replacement therapy low-impact sport has to be recommended.
- Continuing playing soccer at different levels is possible at all stages of osteoarthritis. However, risking a progress of degeneration with all concomitant symptoms and complications has to be taken into account.

Top Five Evidence Based References

Vannini F, Spalding T, Andriolo L, Berruto M, Denti M, Espregueira-Mendes J et al (2016) Sport and early osteoarthritis: the role of sport in aetiology, progression and treatment of knee osteoarthritis. Knee Surg Sports Traumatol Arthrosc 24:1786–1796

Madry H, Kon E, Condello V, Peretti GM, Steinwachs M, Seil R et al (2016) Early osteoarthritis of the knee. Knee Surg Sports Traumatol Arthrosc 24:1753–1762

Filardo G, Kon E, Longo UG, Madry H, Marchettini P, Marmotti A et al (2016) Non-surgical treatments for the management of early osteoarthritis. Knee Surg Sports Traumatol Arthrosc 24:1775–1785

Angele P, Niemeyer P, Steinwachs M, Filardo G, Gomoll AH, Kon E et al (2016) Chondral and osteochondral operative treatment in early osteoarthritis. Knee Surg Sports Traumatol Arthrosc 24:1743–1752

Papalia R, Del Buono A, Zampogna B, Maffulli N, Denaro V (2012) Sport activity following joint arthroplasty: a systematic review. Br Med Bull 101:81–103

References

1. Koch M, Zellner J, Berner A, Grechenig S, Krutsch V, Nerlich M et al (2015) Influence of preparation and football skill level on injury incidence during an amateur football tournament. Arch Orthop Trauma Surg. https://doi.org/10.1007/s00402-015-2350-3
2. Aus der Funten K, Faude O, Lensch J, Meyer T (2014) Injury characteristics in the German professional male soccer leagues after a shortened winter break. J Athl Train 49:786–793
3. Ekstrand J, Gillquist J (1983) Soccer injuries and their mechanisms: a prospective study. Med Sci Sports Exerc 15:267–270
4. Ekstrand J, Hagglund M, Walden M (2011) Injury incidence and injury patterns in professional football: the UEFA injury study. Br J Sports Med 45:553–558
5. Hagglund M, Walden M, Ekstrand J (2009) Injuries among male and female elite football players. Scand J Med Sci Sports 19:819–827

6. Hagglund M, Walden M, Ekstrand J (2005) Injury incidence and distribution in elite football--a prospective study of the Danish and the Swedish top divisions. Scand J Med Sci Sports 15:21–28
7. Hawkins RD, Fuller CW (1999) A prospective epidemiological study of injuries in four English professional football clubs. Br J Sports Med 33:196–203
8. Junge A, Dvorak J (2004) Soccer injuries: a review on incidence and prevention. Sports Med 34:929–938
9. John R, Dhillon MS, Syam K, Prabhakar S, Behera P, Singh H (2016) Epidemiological profile of sports-related knee injuries in northern India: an observational study at a tertiary care centre. J Clin Orthop Trauma 7:207–211
10. de Girolamo L, Kon E, Filardo G, Marmotti AG, Soler F, Peretti GM et al (2016) Regenerative approaches for the treatment of early OA. Knee Surg Sports Traumatol Arthrosc 24:1826–1835
11. Kraus VB, Blanco FJ, Englund M, Karsdal MA, Lohmander LS (2015) Call for standardized definitions of osteoarthritis and risk stratification for clinical trials and clinical use. Osteoarthritis Cartilage 23:1233–1241
12. Madry H, Kon E, Condello V, Peretti GM, Steinwachs M, Seil R et al (2016) Early osteoarthritis of the knee. Knee Surg Sports Traumatol Arthrosc 24:1753–1762
13. Luyten FP, Denti M, Filardo G, Kon E, Engebretsen L (2012) Definition and classification of early osteoarthritis of the knee. Knee Surg Sports Traumatol Arthrosc 20:401–406
14. Felson DT, Hodgson R (2014) Identifying and treating preclinical and early osteoarthritis. Rheum Dis Clin North Am 40:699–710
15. Madry H, Luyten FP, Facchini A (2012) Biological aspects of early osteoarthritis. Knee Surg Sports Traumatol Arthrosc 20:407–422
16. Angele P, Niemeyer P, Steinwachs M, Filardo G, Gomoll AH, Kon E et al (2016) Chondral and osteochondral operative treatment in early osteoarthritis. Knee Surg Sports Traumatol Arthrosc 24:1743–1752
17. Demange MK, Sisto M, Rodeo S (2014) Future trends for unicompartmental arthritis of the knee: injectables & stem cells. Clin Sports Med 33:161–174
18. Vannini F, Spalding T, Andriolo L, Berruto M, Denti M, Espregueira-Mendes J et al (2016) Sport and early osteoarthritis: the role of sport in aetiology, progression and treatment of knee osteoarthritis. Knee Surg Sports Traumatol Arthrosc 24:1786–1796
19. SP Y, Hunter DJ (2015) Managing osteoarthritis. Aust Prescr 38:115–119
20. Arokoski JP, Jurvelin JS, Vaatainen U, Helminen HJ (2000) Normal and pathological adaptations of articular cartilage to joint loading. Scand J Med Sci Sports 10:186–198
21. Filardo G, Kon E, Longo UG, Madry H, Marchettini P, Marmotti A et al (2016) Non-surgical treatments for the management of early osteoarthritis. Knee Surg Sports Traumatol Arthrosc 24:1775–1785
22. Tscholl PM, Dvorak J (2012) Abuse of medication during international football competition in 2010 - lesson not learned. Br J Sports Med 46:1140–1141
23. Vaso M, Weber A, Tscholl PM, Junge A, Dvorak J (2015) Use and abuse of medication during 2014 FIFA World Cup Brazil: a retrospective survey. BMJ Open 5:e007608
24. Tscholl P, Feddermann N, Junge A, Dvorak J (2009) The use and abuse of painkillers in international soccer: data from 6 FIFA tournaments for female and youth players. Am J Sports Med 37:260–265
25. McAlindon TE, Bannuru RR, Sullivan MC, Arden NK, Berenbaum F, Bierma-Zeinstra SM et al (2014) OARSI guidelines for the non-surgical management of knee osteoarthritis. Osteoarthritis Cartilage 22:363–388
26. Niemeyer P, Feucht MJ, Fritz J, Albrecht D, Spahn G, Angele P (2016) Cartilage repair surgery for full-thickness defects of the knee in Germany: indications and epidemiological data from the German Cartilage Registry (KnorpelRegister DGOU). Arch Orthop Trauma Surg 136:891–897
27. Angele P, Fritz J, Albrecht D, Koh J, Zellner J (2015) Defect type, localization and marker gene expression determines early adverse events of matrix-associated autologous chondrocyte implantation. Injury 46(Suppl 4):S2–S9
28. Flanigan DC, Harris JD, Trinh TQ, Siston RA, Brophy RH (2010) Prevalence of chondral defects in athletes' knees: a systematic review. Med Sci Sports Exerc 42:1795–1801
29. Mithoefer K, Hambly K, Della Villa S, Silvers H, Mandelbaum BR (2009) Return to sports participation after articular cartilage repair in the knee: scientific evidence. Am J Sports Med 37(Suppl 1):167S–176S
30. Kon E, Filardo G, Berruto M, Benazzo F, Zanon G, Della Villa S et al (2011) Articular cartilage treatment in high-level male soccer players: a prospective comparative study of arthroscopic second-generation autologous chondrocyte implantation versus microfracture. Am J Sports Med 39:2549–2557
31. Filardo G, Kon E, Perdisa F, Tetta C, Di Martino A, Marcacci M (2015) Arthroscopic mosaicplasty: long-term outcome and joint degeneration progression. Knee 22:36–40
32. Filardo G, Di Matteo B, Di Martino A, Merli ML, Cenacchi A, Fornasari P et al (2015) Platelet-rich plasma intra-articular knee injections show no superiority versus viscosupplementation: a randomized controlled trial. Am J Sports Med 43:1575–1582
33. Della Villa S, Kon E, Filardo G, Ricci M, Vincentelli F, Delcogliano M et al (2010) Does intensive rehabilitation permit early return to sport without compromising the clinical outcome after arthroscopic autologous chondrocyte implantation in highly competitive athletes? Am J Sports Med 38:68–77
34. Giuliani JR, Burns TC, Svoboda SJ, Cameron KL, Owens BD (2011) Treatment of meniscal injuries in young athletes. J Knee Surg 24:93–100

35. Kotsovolos ES, Hantes ME, Mastrokalos DS, Lorbach O, Paessler HH (2006) Results of all-inside meniscal repair with the FasT-Fix meniscal repair system. Arthroscopy 22:3–9
36. Alvarez-Diaz P, Alentorn-Geli E, Llobet F, Granados N, Steinbacher G, Cugat R (2016) Return to play after all-inside meniscal repair in competitive football players: a minimum 5-year follow-up. Knee Surg Sports Traumatol Arthrosc 24:1997–2001
37. Angele P, Kujat R, Koch M, Zellner J (2014) Role of mesenchymal stem cells in meniscal repair. J Exp Orthopaed 1:12
38. Filardo G, Andriolo L, Kon E, de Caro F, Marcacci M (2015) Meniscal scaffolds: results and indications. A systematic literature review. Int Orthop 39:35–46
39. Rodkey WG, DeHaven KE, Montgomery WH III, Baker CL Jr, Beck CL Jr, Hormel SE et al (2008) Comparison of the collagen meniscus implant with partial meniscectomy. A prospective randomized trial. J Bone Joint Surg Am 90:1413–1426
40. Vundelinckx B, Vanlauwe J, Bellemans J (2014) Long-term subjective, clinical, and radiographic outcome evaluation of meniscal allograft transplantation in the knee. Am J Sports Med 42:1592–1599
41. Marcacci M, Marcheggiani Muccioli GM, Grassi A, Ricci M, Tsapralis K, Nanni G et al (2014) Arthroscopic meniscus allograft transplantation in male professional soccer players: a 36-month follow-up study. Am J Sports Med 42:382–388
42. Dai B, Mao D, Garrett WE, Yu B (2014) Anterior cruciate ligament injuries in soccer: loading mechanisms, risk factors, and prevention programs. J Sport Health Sci 3:299–306
43. Ekhtiari S, Haldane CE, de Sa D, Simunovic N, Musahl V, Ayeni OR (2016) Return to work and sport following high tibial osteotomy: a systematic review. J Bone Joint Surg Am 98:1568–1577
44. Voleti PB, Degen R, Tetreault D, Krych AJ, Williams RJ (2016) Successful return to sport following distal femoral varus osteotomy. Orthop J Sports Med 4:2325967116S00132
45. Brouwer RW, Huizinga MR, Duivenvoorden T, van Raaij TM, Verhagen AP, Bierma-Zeinstra SM et al (2014) Osteotomy for treating knee osteoarthritis. Cochrane Database Syst Rev:Cd004019. https://doi.org/10.1002/14651858.CD004019.pub4
46. Spahn G, Hofmann GO, von Engelhardt LV, Li M, Neubauer H, Klinger HM (2013) The impact of a high tibial valgus osteotomy and unicondylar medial arthroplasty on the treatment for knee osteoarthritis: a meta-analysis. Knee Surg Sports Traumatol Arthrosc 21:96–112
47. Berger RA, Della Valle CJ (2010) Unicompartmental knee arthroplasty: indications, techniques, and results. Instr Course Lect 59:47–56
48. Naouar N, Kaziz H, Mouelhi T, Bouattour K, Mseddi M, Ben Ayeche ML (2016) Evaluation at long term follow up of medial unicompartmental knee arthroplasty in young patients. Tunis Med 94:66–71
49. van der List JP, McDonald LS, Pearle AD (2015) Systematic review of medial versus lateral survivorship in unicompartmental knee arthroplasty. Knee 22:454–460
50. Witjes S, Gouttebarge V, Kuijer PP, van Geenen RC, Poolman RW, Kerkhoffs GM (2016) Return to sports and physical activity after total and unicondylar knee arthroplasty: a systematic review and meta-analysis. Sports Med 46:269–292
51. Naal FD, Fischer M, Preuss A, Goldhahn J, von Knoch F, Preiss S et al (2007) Return to sports and recreational activity after unicompartmental knee arthroplasty. Am J Sports Med 35:1688–1695
52. Waldstein W, Kolbitsch P, Koller U, Boettner F, Windhager R (2016) Sport and physical activity following unicompartmental knee arthroplasty: a systematic review. Knee Surg Sports Traumatol Arthrosc. https://doi.org/10.1007/s00167-016-4167-1
53. Walker T, Gotterbarm T, Bruckner T, Merle C, Streit MR (2015) Return to sports, recreational activity and patient-reported outcomes after lateral unicompartmental knee arthroplasty. Knee Surg Sports Traumatol Arthrosc 23:3281–3287
54. Papalia R, Del Buono A, Zampogna B, Maffulli N, Denaro V (2012) Sport activity following joint arthroplasty: a systematic review. Br Med Bull 101:81–103
55. Bade MJ, Kohrt WM, Stevens-Lapsley JE (2010) Outcomes before and after total knee arthroplasty compared to healthy adults. J Orthop Sports Phys Ther 40:559–567
56. Baldini A, Castellani L, Traverso F, Balatri A, Balato G, Franceschini V (2015) The difficult primary total knee arthroplasty: a review. Bone Joint J 97-b:30–39
57. Diduch DR, Insall JN, Scott WN, Scuderi GR, Font-Rodriguez D (1997) Total knee replacement in young, active patients. Long-term follow-up and functional outcome. J Bone Joint Surg Am 79:575–582
58. Meding JB, Meding LK, Ritter MA, Keating EM (2012) Pain relief and functional improvement remain 20 years after knee arthroplasty. Clin Orthop Relat Res 470:144–149
59. Pavone V, Boettner F, Fickert S, Sculco TP (2001) Total condylar knee arthroplasty: a long-term followup. Clin Orthop Relat Res:18–25
60. Oehler N, Schmidt T, Niemeier A (2016) Total Joint Replacement and Return to Sports. Sportverletz Sportschaden 30:195–203
61. Lefevre N, Rousseau D, Bohu Y, Klouche S, Herman S (2013) Return to judo after joint replacement. Knee Surg Sports Traumatol Arthrosc 21:2889–2894
62. Mont MA, Rajadhyaksha AD, Marxen JL, Silberstein CE, Hungerford DS (2002) Tennis after total knee arthroplasty. Am J Sports Med 30:163–166
63. Kuster MS (2002) Exercise recommendations after total joint replacement: a review of the current literature and proposal of scientifically based guidelines. Sports Med 32:433–445

36 Return to Sports, the Use of Test Batteries

Alli Gokeler, Stefano Zaffagnini, Caroline Mouton, and Romain Seil

Contents

36.1 Introduction

Athletes, in particular young athletes, have high demands in terms of return to sports (RTS) after an ACL reconstruction (ACLR), with 91% of them expecting return to their pre-injury level and doing so without restrictions or symptoms [1].

Walden and colleagues published the results of a 15-year prospective study, examining RTS rates following ACL injury in professional football players [2]. In their study, RTS was defined as the number of days from injury or reconstruction to full training with the team without restrictions (return to training) and to the first match appearance with the first team, reserve team, under-21 team, or a national team (return to match play). A total of 157 ACL injuries in 149 players were recorded during the study period. Although there is an initial high rate of RTS (>90%) at 1 year after ACLR, a pertinent finding from their study was that only 65% of athletes were playing at their highest

A. Gokeler (✉)
University of Groningen, University Medical Center Groningen, Center for Human Movement Sciences, Groningen, The Netherlands
e-mail: a.gokeler@rug.nl

S. Zaffagnini
Rizzoli Orthopaedic Institute, University of Bologna, Bologna, Italy
e-mail: stefano.zaffagnini@unibo.it

C. Mouton • R. Seil
Department of Orthopedic Surgery, Centre Hospitalier de Luxemburg, Luxembourg City, Luxembourg

Sports Medicine Research Laboratory, Department of Population Health, Luxembourg Institute of Health, Luxembourg City, Luxembourg
e-mail: mouton.Caroline@chl.lu; rseil@yahoo.com

V. Musahl et al. (eds.), *Return to Play in Football*, https://doi.org/10.1007/978-3-662-55713-6_36

pre-injury level at 3 years post-ACL rupture. A same trend was found by Zaffagnini et al., and they reported that 95% of professional male football players returned to the same activity level 1 year after ACLR [3]. At follow-up 4 years after ACLR, 15 patients (71%) were still playing competitive football, 13 (62%) at the same pre-injury professional division, and 2 (9%) in a lower division compared to the pre-injury status, due to issues not related to knee performance. Of the six patients that abandoned their football career, the main reason was related not to knee status but to personal issues. In contrast to the findings of Walden et al. [2], the age at final follow-up of retired athletes was significantly higher compared to active players (30.4 years ± 7.2 vs. 25.5 years ± 4.0). Brophy and colleagues contacted football players included in the Multicenter Orthopaedic Outcomes Network (MOON) after ACLR [4]. Initially, 72% of the players RTS at an average of 12.2 months after surgery; however, the standard deviation was 14.3 months indicating the large range in time taken for players to achieve RTS level. A sharp decline was noted at follow-up at 7.2 years, as only 36% were still playing football [4]. Men were more likely (56%) to attribute their ACL injury as the primary reason they were no longer playing football [4].

Patient's general expectations after ACLR are high, with 94% expecting a return to sports (RTS) to the same level as prior to injury [1]. This poses the question as to how clinicians determine when an athlete is ready for RTS in light of associated of risk involved [5]. Clinicians and researchers have become increasingly aware of the high incidence of second ACL injury. Injury rates for a second injury exceed 23% for young highly active RTS athletes [6]. Data from the Swedish ACL Registry revealed that 22% of 15- to 18-year-old female football players reported a revision or contralateral ACLR during a 5-year period [7]. Of note, only those who underwent surgery were accounted for in the registry, indicating that even higher rates of second ACL injury may be possible. Unfortunately, it appears that current ACLR rehabilitation programs are not effective in addressing deficits related to the initial ACL injury and the subsequent surgical intervention [8].

Fact Box
- 62–65% of professional football players are still playing at the pre-injury level 3–4 years after ACLR.
- Second ACL injury exceeds 23% in the first year after RTS.

The reasons for such high reinjury rates warrant further investigation. The relatively high failure rate may be related to closure of developmental physes and lack of compliance to the postoperative rehabilitation [9]. The second injury rate following ACLR is significantly higher in young athletes compared with athletes over the age of 18 years [10].

In addition, deficits in the neuromuscular control of both lower extremities following ACLR have been directly associated with the risk for second ACL injury [11, 12]. These deficits may have been present prior to injury and exacerbated by the surgical procedure. It has been shown that girls throughout the growth spurt display a decrease in knee flexion in combination with an increase in knee abduction moments during a horizontal landing task [13]. In agreement with previous studies summarized in a review, the lack of control of lower limb movements due to rapid growth changes is linked to their increased risk for ACL injuries [14] Therefore, identification and subsequent targeted treatment of aberrant post-ACLR movement patterns are critical not only to maximize functional recovery but also to reduce the risk for a second ACL injury [15]. Another concern is that current RTS test batteries may not be sensitive enough to detect subtle but relevant impairments in physical function, which in turn may affect RTS rates. The decision when an athlete is allowed to RTS is multifactorial, difficult, and challenging [16]. The ability to decide whether an athlete is ready to safely RTS is further compromised by the paucity of prospective studies in the literature validating current RTS criteria [17].

The authors of this chapter propose a comprehensive multifactorial test battery that encompasses factors that are related to enhance performance necessary for an injured football player to integrate into football competition. Moreover the test battery should be sensitive to detect risk factors for a second ACL injury or any other injury. Only factors that are modifiable either though intervention or through healing processes will be discussed.

36.2 Definitions

A recent consensus statement on RTS presented the following operational definitions of the three elements of the RTS continuum (*) [18]:

1. **Return to participation (RTPa)**. The athlete may be participating in rehabilitation, training (modified or unrestricted), or sport but at a level lower than his or her RTS goal. The athlete is physically active but not yet "ready" (medically, physically, and/or psychologically) to RTS. It is possible to train to perform, but this does not automatically mean RTS.
2. **Return to sport (RTS)**. The athlete has returned to his or her defined sport but is not performing at his or her desired performance level. Some athletes may be satisfied with reaching this stage, and this can represent successful RTS for that individual.
3. **Return to performance (RTP)**. This extends the RTS element. The athlete has gradually returned to his or her defined sport and is performing at or above his or her pre-injury level. For some athletes, this stage may be characterized by personal best performance or expected personal growth as it relates to performance.

(*) In this chapter, only the use of test batteries related to RTS and RTP is presented (Fig. 36.1).

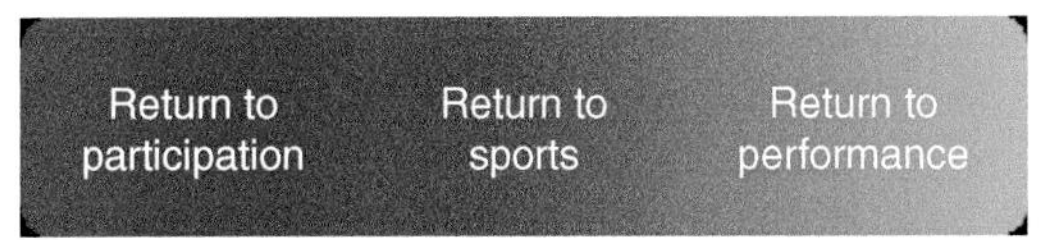

Fig. 36.1 The three elements of return to sports continuum

36.3 Key Items to Aid in Decision-Making Process to Return to Sports

Since the systematic review by Barber-Westin and Noyes in 2011 [17], various prospective studies have been published. Delaying RTS until 9 months after surgery and a more symmetrical quadriceps strength prior to return to level 1 sport were associated with a reduced secondary knee injury risk [19]. Of the 74 patients who returned to level 1 sports, 51 patients did not sustain a second knee injury. Interstingly, those patients had a mean quadriceps limb symmetry index (LSI) of 84.4%, which was below the recommended limb symmetry index (LSI) of >90% [19]. Another recent prospective study of 158 professional male football players who returned to football after ACLR determined risk factors for a second ACL injury [20]. Those players failing to achieve the proposed RTS criteria were four times more likely to sustain a secondary ACL injury compared to those who met all six proposed criteria (LSI > 90% for quadriceps and hamstrings muscle strength tests and three hop tests; *t*-test <11 s and the completion of on-field sport-specific rehabilitation) [20]. However, 12 of the 26 players with a second ACL injury met the RTS criteria, while 28 of the 132 players with no second ACL injury were not discharged by the RTS criteria, leading to a sensitivity of 53% and a specificity of 79%. This raises the question whether the current RTS tests address relevant factors for safe RTS, if cutoff values are appropriate or whether they are sensitive or demanding enough to elucidate clinically relevant differences. Nonetheless, we feel that the work of Kyritsis et al. [20] is important as they included on-field tests that may be more specific compared to standardized test like hop tests as usually performed in a physical therapy clinic. Despite the development of RTS guidelines over recent years, there are still more questions than answers on the most optimal RTS criteria after ACLR. In the following section, we will present a critical appraisal of current RTS criteria after ACLR and present recommendations for future optimizations.

36.3.1 Strength

Although there is a lack of scientific consensus on the criteria to clear an athlete for RTS, achieving appropriate level of strength is often mentioned by clinicians [17].

More stringent recommendations which were categorized based on the type of sports activity have been presented [21]. A combination of strength and hop test assessment was used. For the purpose of this section, a 100% LSI for knee extensor and knee flexor muscle strength was proposed for the pivoting/contact/competitive group [21]. A few major issues arise when using these criteria: (1) only 23% of all patients achieved the abovementioned [21] test battery at 2 years after ACLR, questioning whether this is feasible in daily practice; (2) the LSI is based on the assumption that the uninjured leg can be used as a reference for strength; (3) is it acceptable to have a 10% deficit between limbs? Larsen et al. cautioned that deficits are underestimated when using the uninvolved limb as reference [22]. Their results show that, not only patients after ACLR exhibit side to side deficits, but the uninvolved limb of ACLR is also significantly weaker to a matched limb of a control group. This implies that the uninvolved limb is significantly affected by the ACL injury questioning to use the LSI as a criterion for RTS [22]. A successful outcome for a strength or power test should be a symmetrical level of performance between limbs, which also matches the level of performance within their peer group [23]. A systematic review by Undheim and colleagues revealed that isokinetic knee strength has not been sufficiently validated as a useful criterion measure for RTS [24]. Most studies have exclusively focused on the evaluation of knee muscle strength, but deficits in hip muscle strength have been found after ACLR [25]. Clinicians should pay more attention to the hip muscles as decreased hip external rotator and abductor strength have been associated with increased primary non-contact ACL injury risk [26]. In addition, second ACL injury risk has also been linked to a decreased hip external rotation moment [11].

36.3.2 Hop Tests

Functional performance tests (FPT) are popular due to their ability to quantify knee function. Hop tests are the preferred type of FPT due to utilization of the uninjured limb as a control for between-limb comparisons. Frequently used hop tests are the single hop for distance, triple hop for distance, triple crossover hop, and 6-m timed hop. Researchers have recommended that FPT should also include an endurance hop test like the side hop [21]. LSI criteria >90% are often used as cutoff scores for RTS [21, 27]. As with the LSI for strength, there are some concerns regarding the use of the uninvolved limb as a reference for the involved limb. Even though a more symmetrical hopping performance has been related to returning to pre-injury sport level [28], this symmetry-based approach is debatable and may lead to underestimations of clinical relevant deficits, as bilateral neuromuscular, biomechanical, and functional performance deficits have been demonstrated after unilateral ACLR [29–32].

First, changes in the sensorimotor system need to be considered. It has been shown that an ACL injury causes direct changes in the CNS. Recent studies have shown that altered activity of the motor cortex is present both in ACL-deficient patients as well after ACLR [33–36]. Hence, a bilateral deficit may lead to a falsely high LSI, since LSI is calculated as a ratio between the values of the limbs.

This was confirmed in a recent unpublished work by the authors. When compared to normative data, patients who were tested at 7 months after ACLR had significant and clinically relevant shorter jump distances for the triple leg hop for distance (involved limb males 125.7 cm, females 43.5 cm; uninvolved limb males 104.1 cm, females 30.8 cm). These findings highlight that athletes who have undergone an ACLR demonstrate bilateral deficits on hop tests in comparison to age- and sex-matched data of healthy controls. Using the LSI may underestimate performance deficits and should therefore be used with caution as a criterion for RTS after ACLR. We recommend that football players achieve hop test performance within the SEM of matched uninjured peers. Normative data for collegiate football players have been presented for the single-leg hop (192 cm for males and 149 cm for females), triple leg hop (632 cm males, 470 cm females), and 6-m timed hop (1.74 s males and 2.13 s for females) [37].

Secondly, another disadvantage of the traditional outcomes of hop tests is the strict focus on quantitative outcomes (distance, time, and limb symmetry), while outcomes related to the quality of movement are not captured [38]. Hence, the authors advise to use RTS test that also includes assessment of movement quality. Gokeler and colleagues recently presented a new RTS test battery that included strength tests, hop tests, jump-landing task, and questionnaires [39]. The Landing Error Scoring System (LESS) score was used to determine movement asymmetry during a jump-landing task [40]. Briefly, the subject stands on a 30-cm-high box, jumps forward at a distance half the body height, and jumps for maximal height immediately after landing. The landing is videotaped with two video cameras that have frontal plane and sagittal plane views of the jump landing [40]. Three jumps are performed, and each jump is scored using the LESS score form [40]. A higher LESS score indicates a greater number of landing errors and consequently poorer jump-landing technique. At 6.5 months after ACLR, 30% of patients demonstrated aberrant movement patterns indicated by a LESS > 5 that may predispose them to increased second ACL injury risk [39].

36.3.3 Movement Quality

An increased knee valgus movement, a greater asymmetrical internal knee extensor moment, a decreased contralateral hip external rotation moment during a drop vertical jump and postural stability deficits were associated with increased second ACL injury in athletes who returned to sport after ACLR [11]. These findings are in line with the trend in the current literature to emphasize the importance of movement quality during rehabilitation of ACLR patients [41]. Recently there has been considerable interest in quantification of the pivot-shift test, with the development of methods using, for example, accelerometers, image-based software, tablets, and an iPad application to measure acceleration or tibial translation during the pivot-shift maneuver [42, 43]. Although currently not in use, this technology is very promising to assess movement quality on the field which may enhance validity.

36.3.4 Fatigue

Commonly RTS tests are performed under non-fatigued conditions. This is somewhat in contrast to the clinical situation during rehabilitation. It has been recommended to perform neuromuscular control drills toward the end of a rehabilitation session, after cardiovascular training, to challenge neuromuscular control of the knee joint when the dynamic stabilizers are fatigued [44]. Fatigue has been shown repeatedly to have negative effects on lower extremity biomechanics. A systematic review recently examined the literature pertaining to lower extremity biomechanics and neuromuscular fatigue during single-leg landings [45]. The kinematic data revealed greater knee and hip flexion and increased dorsiflexion post-fatigue. However, as anticipated/practiced, drop landings are performed primarily in the sagittal plane; these specific procedures may not be sufficient to determine movement patterns during athletic competition. When an unanticipated landing was used, the results were drastically different with a significant increase in peak knee valgus angle post-fatigue compared to pre-fatigue. This unanticipated landing would seem to represent the demands of athletic competition more accurately and thus demonstrates an increased risk of injury with neuromuscular fatigue.

A recent systematic review including 4927 patients revealed that a LSI > 90% on standard hop tests (single-leg, crossover, triple, and 6-m timed hop tests) is achieved at 6–9 months postoperatively [46]. Of interest, although the number of studies reporting results of endurance hop tests is limited, the results of the fatigue single-leg hop and side hop in 30 s showed lower LSI values as compared with the standard hop testing regimen [46]. In the context of RTS tests, Augustsson et al. noted that all ACLR patients met the RTS criteria (LSI > 90% single-leg hop test) in a non-fatigued state, while 68% showed an abnormal LSI when fatigued [47]. Similarly, Gokeler et al. determined that 6 months after ACLR, between 78% and 85% of patients passed the LSI > 90% for the single-leg for distance and triple leg hop, but only 50% passed the side hop test [48]. In addition, previous work already indicated the profound effect fatigue has on movement quality in patients after ACLR and uninjured control subjects [48]. The initial median score pre-fatigue for ACLR patients was 6.5 (poor) and 7.0 following fatigue, whereas the uninjured control subjects scored 2.5 (excellent) pre-fatigue and drastically increased to 6.0 (poor) post-fatigue. This shows an obvious decline in movement quality following fatigue, which may place both post-ACLR patients and uninjured controls at risk for injury [48].

Based on the current literature, it seems plausible that testing athletes in a sport-specific fatigued state may enhance the ability to detect clinically relevant deficits after ACLR. Hence, assessment of lower extremity biomechanics in a fatigue state of the player should be an integral part of a RTS test battery.

36.3.5 Patient-Reported Outcome Measures

Patient-reported outcome measures (PROMs) are self-report questionnaires that measure an individual's perception of symptoms, function, activity, and participation [49]. In a survey, specific to ACL injuries, sent to members of international sports medicine associations, including the European Society of Sports Traumatology, Knee Surgery, and Arthroscopy, the American Orthopaedic Society for Sports Medicine, and the American Physical Therapy Association, consensus was reached to use the following PROMs: the KOS-ADLS, Knee Outcome Survey-Sports Activities Scale (KOS-SAS), global rating of perceived function (GRS), Lysholm score, International Knee Documentation Committee (IKDC) Subjective Knee Form, Cincinnati Knee Score, Knee Injury and Osteoarthritis Outcome Score (KOOS), Tegner activity scale, and Marx activity rating scale [49]. The decision to allow RTS after ACLR solely based on PROMs has been questioned [27]. In a prospective cohort study, Logerstedt et al. determined whether IKDC could identify patients who would pass a battery of functional assessment tests after an ACLR [27]. The 15th percentile from the normative data from uninjured individuals was chosen as the cutoff score to ensure that patients who scored below the cutoff were differentiated from those who scored within the normal variance of IKDC scores [50]. They found that patients who scored below the normal values on the IKDC were over four times more likely to fail the RTS tests. Interestingly, for those athletes who scored well on the IKDC, nearly 50% overestimated their recovery as they didn't pass the RTS test battery [27]. In other words, normal IKDC scores do not necessarily mean the patients would pass the RTS tests.

36.3.6 Physiological and Contextual Factors

Traditional rehabilitation after ACLR and subsequent RTS criteria have predominantly focused on the recovery of the physical capacity to cope with the physical demands of a specific sport, maximize performance, and decrease reinjury risk [5]. During recent years, it has become clear that physical recovery alone is not sufficient to ensure successful RTS as many athletes with good physical function do not RTS after ACLR [51]. In a study of female collegiate football players, 85% of the players RTS after ACLR with a median time for clearance for unrestricted game play between 3.9 and 33.2 months [52]. The RTS rate was higher for those in their earlier years of study and for those who had a scholarship (91% RTS rate) [52]. The rate of RTS was not related to surgical factors such as drilling method, graft selection and fixation, or concomitant knee procedures. These findings suggest that personal factors may be stronger indicators of RTS than surgical or physical factors [52].

A recent review on contextual factors affecting RTS after ACLR identified that lower fear of reinjury, greater psychological readiness, and a more positive subjective assessment of knee function favored a return to pre-injury level of sport after ACLR [53]. The ACL-Return to Sport Index (ACL-RSI) has been developed as a condition-specific scale which measures the psychological impact of returning to sport after ACLR [54]. The 12-item scale measures 3 specific psychological constructs—emotions, confidence in performance, and risk appraisal—on a scale of a minimum of 0 to a maximum of 100 [54]. Lentz and co-workers noticed that patients who were unable to return to sports had a mean score of 20 points on the Tampa Scale for Kinesiophobia (TSK-11), while their counterparts who were able to return to sports had a mean score of 15 points [35]. Sonesson et al. found that higher motivation during rehabilitation was associated with returning to pre-injury sport activity [55]. Another study showed that patients who had returned to knee-strenuous sports after ACLR reported higher self-efficacy, evaluated with the Knee Self-efficacy Scale (K-SES), compared with those who had not returned [56, 57].

It is recommended that clinicians screen for contextual factors, particularly psychological factors, early after ACL injury to identify athletes who could be at risk of not returning to the pre-injury level of sport [53]. The Tampa Scale for Kinesiophobia (TSK-11), ACL-RSI, and K-SES have clinical merit to identify athletes at risk. Subsequently, interventions including motivational interviewing, imagery, and goal setting could be added to common rehabilitation regimen to enhance self-efficacy and reduce reinjury anxiety in athletes with sports injury [53].

36.4 On-Field Rehabilitation

The final phases of rehabilitation are performed on the football field. Key factor is to integrate sports-specific elements within the rehabilitation that reflects neuromuscular, physiological, and psychological demands [58].

36.4.1 The Interval Kicking Program

Arundale and co-workers have outlined a detailed interval kicking program [59]. The program consists of 15 steps of which the first 12 steps gradually introduce a player to the loading and impact of kicking. The progression increases kicking distance (using the markings of a soccer field as a guide), volume, and intensity and uses proposed soreness rules, effusion guidelines, and player feedback in order to assist clinicians in determining readiness for advancement through the stages [59]. The authors use the following criteria for football players to enter the program: no pain, full range of motion, no effusion, and thigh strength >LSI 80% (Table 36.1).

36.4.2 On-Field Rehabilitation Program

Della Villa and colleagues referred to this phase as "on-field rehabilitation" (OFR) and [60]. In their hands, OFR is allowed if the patient presents no knee laxity, no giving-way episodes during previous phases, minimal pain (VAS < 3), absence or minimal effusion, complete or nearly complete ROM (full extension, <10° flexion deficit vs. contralateral limb), LSI > 80% isokinetic maximal peak torque for hamstrings and quadriceps and the ability to run on the treadmill at 8 km/h for more than 10 min (Fig. 36.2) [60].

OFR for football players is divided in five phases, and the progression is based on when exercises of each phase were comfortable, well coordinated performed, tolerated well and without adverse effect such as swelling. This allows for a gradual progression of each part and thus ensures correct function and that no adverse knee reaction is noted before moving on to the next level [60]. Rehabilitation programs may fail due to a rapid increase in exercise load. Blanch and Gabbett proposed the inclusion of the acute/chronic workload ratio in the RTS decision-making process

Table 36.1 The interval kicking program

Step 1	Step 2	Step 3
Basic kicking and passing		
• Warm-up dribbling or juggling (5 min) • Two touch passing, 5.5 m (5 min) • Rest (5 min) • Warm-up dribbling or juggling, performing opposite activity from start (5 min) • One touch passing, 5.5 m (5 min)	• Warm-up dribbling or juggling (5 min) • Two touch passing, maximum 16.5 m (5 min) • Rest (5 min) • Warm-up dribbling or juggling, performing opposite activity from start (5 min) • One touch passing, maximum 16.5 m (5 min)	• Warm-up dribbling or juggling (5 min) • Two touch passing, maximum 16.5 m (5 min) • Rest (5–10 min) • Warm-up dribbling or juggling (5 min) • One touch passing, maximum 16.5 m (5 min) • Rest (5–10 min) • Warm-up dribbling or juggling (5 min) • One or two touch passing with a maximum 16.5 m (5 min)
Passing and basic shooting		
Step 4	Step 5	Step 6
• Warm-up dribbling or juggling (5 min) • Two touch passing, maximum 36 m (5 min) • Rest (5 min) • Warm-up dribbling or juggling, performing opposite activity from start (5 min) • One touch passing, maximum 36 m (5 min)	• Warm-up dribbling or juggling (5 min) • Two touch passing, maximum 36 m (5 min) • Rest (5–10 min) • Warm-up dribbling or juggling (5 min) • One touch passing, maximum 36 m (5 min) • Rest (5–10 min) • Warm-up dribbling or juggling (5 min) • One or two touch passing with a maximum 36 m (5 min)	• Warm-up dribbling or juggling (5 min) • One or two touch passing, maximum 36 m (5 min) • Rest (5–10 min) • Warm-up dribbling or juggling, (5 min) • Shooting (10 shots) and chipped/lofted balls, maximum 11 m (2–3 min) • Rest (5–10 min) • Warm-up dribbling or juggling, (5 min) • One or two touch passing, maximum 36 m (5 min)
Advanced shooting		
Step 7	Step 8	Step 9
• Warm-up dribbling or juggling (5 min) • One or two touch passing, maximum 36 m (5 min) • Rest (5–10 min) • Warm-up dribbling or juggling (5 min) • Shooting (10 shots) and chipped/lofted balls, maximum 11 m (2–3 min) • Rest (5–10 min) • Warm-up dribbling or juggling (5 min) • Shooting (10 shots) and chipped/lofted balls, maximum 11 m (2–3 min)	• Warm-up dribbling or juggling (5 min) • One or two touch passing, maximum 36 m (5 min) • Rest (5–10 min) • Warm-up dribbling or juggling (5 min) • Shooting (10 shots) and chipped/lofted balls, maximum 16.5 m (2–3 min) • Rest (5–10 min) • Warm-up dribbling or juggling (5 min) • One or two touch passing with a maximum 36 m (5 min)	• Warm-up dribbling or juggling (5 min) • One or two touch passing, maximum 36 m (5 min) • Rest (5–10 min) • Warm-up dribbling or juggling (5 min) • Shooting (10 shots) and chipped/lofted balls, maximum 16.5 m (2–3 min) • Rest (5–10 min) • Warm-up dribbling or juggling (5 min) • Shooting (10 shots) and chipped/lofted balls, maximum 16.5 m (2–3 min)

Table 36.1 (continued)

Increased intensity and distance		
Step 10[a] • Warm-up dribbling or juggling (5 min) • One or two touch passing, maximum 36 m (5 min) • Rest (5–10 min) • Warm-up dribbling or juggling (5 min) • Shooting (10 shots) and chipped/lofted balls, maximum 36 m (2–3 min) • Rest (5–10 min) • Warm-up dribbling or juggling (5 min) • Shooting (10 shots) and chipped/lofted balls max 16.5 m (2–3 min) *or* one or two touch passing, maximum 36 m (5 min)	Step 11 • Warm-up dribbling or juggling (5 min) • One or two touch passing, maximum 36 m (5 min) • Rest (5–10 min) • Warm-up dribbling or juggling (5 min) • Shooting (10 shots) and chipped/lofted balls, maximum 36 m (2–3 min) • Rest (5–10 min) • Warm-up dribbling or juggling (5 min) • Shooting (10 shots) and chipped/lofted balls, maximum 36 m (2–3 min)	Step 12 • Warm-up dribbling or juggling (5 min) • One or two touch passing, maximum 36 m (5 min) • Rest (5–10 min) • Warm-up dribbling or juggling (5 min) • Lofted driven ball maximum 45 m (25 times) • Rest (5–10 min) • Warm-up dribbling or juggling (5 min) • Shooting (10 shots) and chipped/lofted balls, maximum 36 m (2–3 min) or one or two touch passing, maximum 36 m (5 min)
Initiating return to sport		
Step 13 • At this point goalkeepers should begin their work on punting and drop kicking • Field players may begin to perform >20-min technical portions of practices with their teams as well as shooting and other drills	Step 14[b] • When cleared by medical team, player may begin full practices with their team, initially non-contact and progressing to contact	Step 15[c] • Reintroduce gameplay first through scrimmages in practice and then with gradually increasing periods of game time

The distances listed in each of these steps are maximum distances. Clinicians and players should not spend the entire time passing or shooting at this maximum distance but rather vary the passing/shooting distances throughout the allotted time

Used with permission. Copyright 2015, Int J Sports Phys Ther. 2015 Feb;10(1):114–27. An interval kicking progression for return to soccer following lower extremity injury. Arundale A, Silvers H, Logerstedt D, Rojas J, Snyder-Mackler L

[a]Alternatively, once a player reaches step 10 (if cleared by the medical team), a percentage of time spent in warm-up dribbling/juggling and one or two touch passing drills (maximum 20 min) may be spent working on technical drills with their team, followed by performing the shooting or lofted/driven ball practice defined by the progression (with appropriate rest in between). This alternative should only be used if the medical team is confident that both player and coach are cognizant of all precautions such as only performing small sided technical drills involving passing and dribbling and avoiding player contact

[b]Unlike steps 1–13, steps 14 and 15 require more than 1 day in between. It is at the rehabilitation team's discretion to progress a player through these stages

[c]A gradual increase in game time will allow a player to adjust to the intensity and speed of play while reducing the amount of time they are exposed to the higher-risk game environment

[61]. This ratio describes the relation between the workload of the last week (acute workload) and the rolling average workload of the last 4 weeks (chronic workload). This concept can be applied to a wide range of individually functional relevant training variables representing external workload (e.g., number of jumps or high-speed running covered) or internal workload (e.g., rating of perceived exertion). Rapid spikes in acute/chronic workload ratios during the RTS and RTP process should be avoided. For a clinician, it is therefore important to know the physical demands of football and to gradually expose a player to the football-specific workloads in order to successfully integrate a player back into the game. The workload ratio allows staff involved with RTP to quantify a player's risk for subsequent injury [61]. For example, if a player has a chronic workload of 40% and increases that to 100% within a week, the player has a 28% risk to sustain an injury in the following week [61].

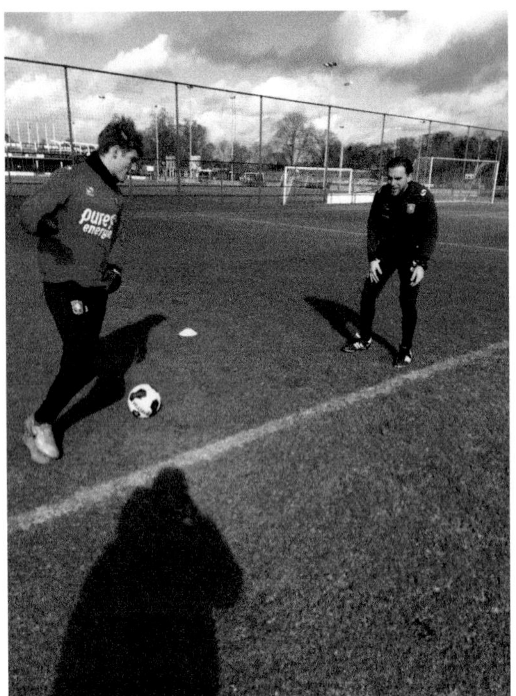

Fig. 36.2 On-field rehabilitation program under supervision of a sports physical therapist assessing movement quality and checks for compensation strategies to unload the injured extremity

In a study of 50 football players, Della Villa and co-workers noted that the OFR program was successfully completed on average at 138 ± 33 (range 74–204) days after ACLR [60]. Professional players followed a daily rehabilitation program, while amateur players did so three times per week [60].

Bizzini et al. proposed a four-phase progression from training to playing matches [58]:

- Return to reduced team training practice (no contact)
- Return to full (normal) team training practice (with contact)
- Return to "friendly" games (initially not over the full duration of a match)
- Return to competitive match (initially not over the full duration of a match)

Following these guidelines, the football player is gradually progressed from individual training to team training [58].

36.4.2.1 Agility Drills

Agility drills serve as an important component in the functional rehabilitation of the lower extremity (hip, knee, and ankle). The drills are designed to replicate the movement demands of the sport and to promote confidence in the returning athlete.

Agility is defined as "a rapid whole body movement with change of direction of speed or direction in response to a stimulus" [62]. According to Young et al., agility consists of two components: (1) change of direction speed and (2) perceptual and decision-making [63]. The latter involves processing of visual information, anticipation, response selection, and motor programming [64]. In football, a change in direction is initiated in response to a stimulus, such as an opponent's actions, and is therefore influenced by perceptual and decision-making skills. Clinicians should therefore be aware that most agility drills are preplanned and therefore only assess a player's ability to change direction (and not respond to a sport-specific stimulus) (Fig. 36.3).

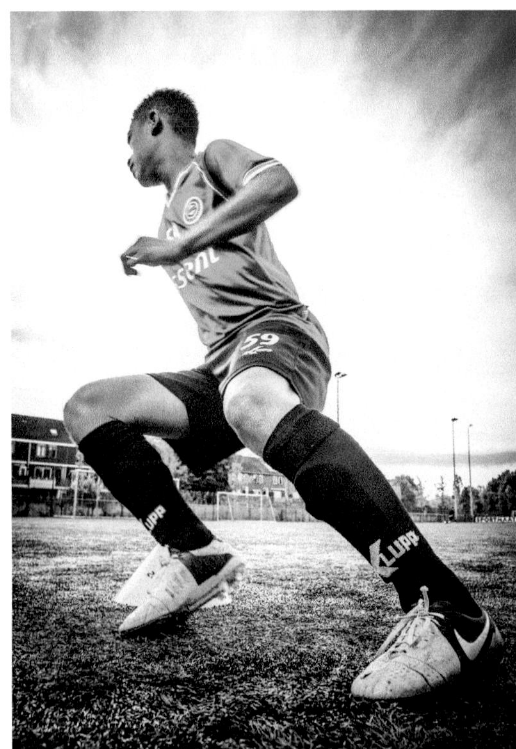

Fig. 36.3 Football player performing the agility T-test

For this reason, the ability to change direction and velocity in a preplanned movement, such as that demonstrated in certain agility tests (e.g., agility T-test), may be better described as change of direction speed and may not replicate on-field situations. Nonetheless, agility tests may provide important information to determine physical readiness regarding the final RTS phases or may be used for RTP enhancement. Agility tests that are frequently used in football are the agility T-test and the Illinois agility test [62]:

- Agility T-test: This assessment requires the player to move in a T-shaped pattern. It requires lateral and front-to-back movements. The clinician gives the signal to "Go" and starts the stopwatch, and the player commences the test. The player runs to and touches the middle cone, side steps 5 m to the left cone and touches it, side steps 10 m to the far cone and touches it, side steps 5 m back to the middle cone and touches it, and then runs 10 m backward to the base of the "T" and touches that cone. The coach stops the stopwatch and records the time when the athlete touches the cone at the base of the "T." The test score is the best time of three trials.
- Illinois agility test: The length of the course is 10 m, and the width (distance between the start and finish points) is 5 m. Four cones are used to mark the start, finish, and two turning points. Another four cones are placed down the center an equal distance apart. Each cone in the center is spaced 3.3 m apart. The player should lie on their front (head to the start line) and hands by their shoulders. On the "Go" command, the stopwatch is started, and the player gets up as quickly as possible and runs around the course in the direction indicated, without knocking the cones over, to the finish line, at which the timing is stopped. The average of three trials is calculated. In the age range of 16–19 years, an excellent score is under 15.2 s for a male and <17 s for a female.

The Illinois agility test has recently been critiqued as it is an asymmetrical test because the numbers of changes of direction performed to the right and to the left are unequal [65]. These authors had football players perform the test in two directions. They found that 52% of the players had a significant better performance—faster time—in the inverted test compared to the standard test [65].

The results of the agility tests after injury should be compared to baseline measures so that progress may be tracked over time.

These are crucial steps in the transition from the usually controlled situations during rehabilitation sessions to team training. During team training, the player has to visually perceive the constantly and quickly changing, unpredictable environment (e.g., movement of another player, opponent, or a ball), quickly process these situational-specific visual-spatial cues within the central nervous system, and develop an appropriate physical response while maintaining dynamic stability of the body. Several studies have shown that experimentally visually cued temporal constraints can affect whole body kinematics and knee loading during athletic activities such as cutting [66, 67]. Therefore, we contend that these four phases as outlined by Bizzini et al. [58] should be successfully completed and are part of the RTS test battery prior to clearance for unrestricted sports activity.

Fact Box

- Prior to entering the RTS phase, the injured football player should progress through a criterion-based rehabilitation program.
- Elements within the rehabilitation should be specific to football that reflects neuromuscular, physiological, and psychological demands.
- There is a lack of a "gold standard" for RTS criteria.

36.5 Time After Anterior Cruciate Ligament Reconstruction

Time after ACLR is the most used criterion to assess RTS readiness with the allowed RTS after 6 months [17]. Grindem et al. recently recommend that RTS should be delayed until 9 months after ACLR [68]. Unfortunately, the risk of sustaining a second ACL injury is still high during the early period after RTS (6–12 months) [20, 68–71].

36.6 Laxity and Biological Assessment of the Graft

Graft maturation is a slow process that is individually different from person to person an can take more than 2 years. It consists of four phases: the initial avascular necrosis, revascularization, cellular proliferation, and finally remodelling [72]. This process could be indirectly monitored through MRI, as it has been proved that poor biomechanical properties and an incomplete graft maturation are related to a hyperintense graft signal on MRI [73]. Weiler et al. demonstrated in an animal model that a significantly elevated graft signal was present between the 6th and 12th weeks, and this condition was correlated to the lowest tensile stress of the graft (estimated around the 7–16% of the initial values) [74]. In clinical practice, graft maturation could be monitored with the Figueroa's score, which accounts for graft signal (hypointensity, isointensity, or hyperintensity) and presence of synovial fluid within tunnel-graft interface [75]. Alternatively, a quantitative measurement with software of graft corrected for background signal (SNQ, signal/noise quotient) could be used. However, the MRI evaluation of graft signal still represents a controversial issue, since Biercevicz et al. [76] reported a correlation between signal intensity and hop test and KOOS score at 3 years and 5 years, respectively, while Li et al. [77] did not find any correlations with IKDC, Lysholm, and Tegner at 3, 6, and 12 months. Therefore, a routinely MRI assessment of graft maturity does not provide solid insights for RTS (Fig. 36.4).

Regarding knee laxity, a successful ACLR is able to restore stability in most of the cases [78]. Static anteroposterior laxity, besides manual tests, could be easily evaluated and quantified with popular instruments such as Rolimeter and KT-1000/2000 arthrometer. Differently, the eval-

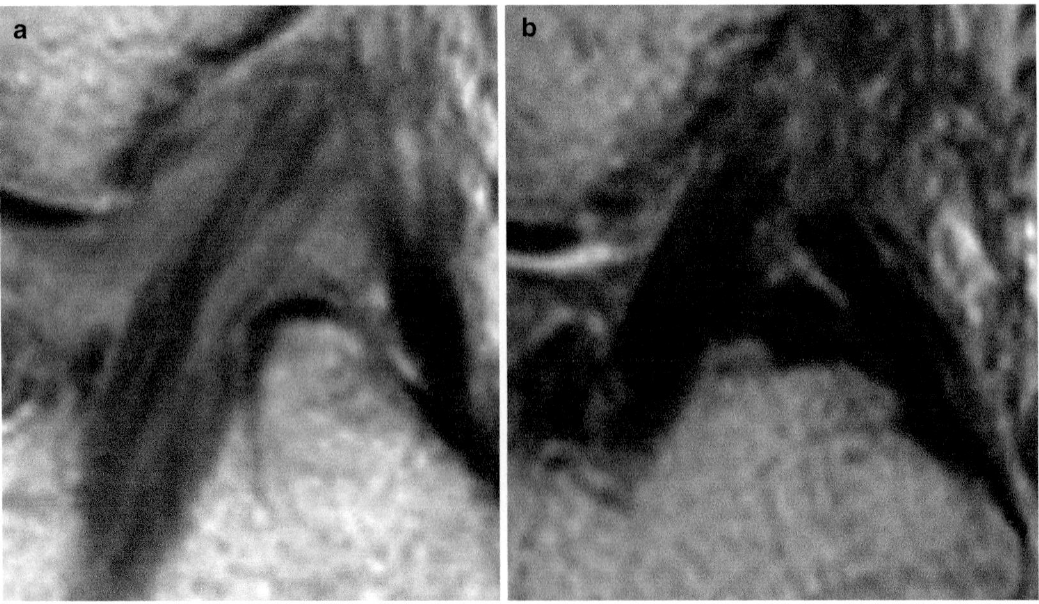

Fig. 36.4 (**a**) ACL graft with high-intensity or (**b**) low-intensity signal

uation of dynamic rotatory laxity—which strongly correlated with instability symptoms—[79] relies on examiner's feeling during the pivot-shift maneuver. Therefore, non-invasive devices for pivot-shift assessment have been developed in the last 10 years [80], in order to both diagnose ACL injury and detect residual rotatory laxity after ACL reconstruction. Zaffagnini et al. [81] proposed a triaxial accelerometer for pivot-shift quantification, which showed a good inter- and intra-rater reliability and correlation with clinical grading. Therefore, such technologies could represent a potential aid in the follow-up evaluation of patients undergoing ACLR and in the RTS decision algorithm, since both anteroposterior and rotatory stability is required to safely RTS.

This issue is relevant since Mouton and colleagues determined that both anterior and rotational knee laxity appears to be greater in the contralateral, non-injured knees of ACL-injured patients than in healthy controls [82], suggesting that increased physiological laxity could be a risk factor for (second) ACL injuries [83]. Increased laxity is associated with more hip adduction and knee valgus during drop landings in females [84]. Baumgart et al. demonstrated that playing football and stretching lead to significant increases in anterior translation which in turn may influence the mechanical properties of the ACL [85]. Summarizing, the recent development of rotational laxity measurement devices has added significant knowledge to the field. The high variability between individuals as well as the ability to identify knees with increased physiological knee laxity may improve screening and prevention programs for athletes [83]. In Table 36.2, the final criteria for RTS are summarized.

Table 36.2 Test battery for return to sport in football

Strength knee	100% limb symmetry index (LSI) on knee extensor and knee flexor strength evaluated with concentric isokinetic dynamometry at 60°/s, 180°/s, and 300°/s
Hop tests	LSI 100% single hop distance, triple hop for distance, triple crossover hop, 6-m timed hop and side (endurance) hop
Movement quality	Landing Error Scoring System LESS < 5, evaluation of multisegmental movement quality during double- and single-leg dynamic activities: individual assessment with advanced clinical reasoning
Patient-reported outcome measures	KOS-ADLS, Knee Outcome Survey-Sports Activities Scale (KOS-SAS), global rating of perceived function (GRS), Lysholm score, International Knee Documentation Committee Subjective Knee Form (IKDC), Cincinnati Knee Score, Knee Injury and Osteoarthritis Outcome Score (KOOS), Tegner activity scale, and Marx activity rating scale
Psychological factors	ACL-Return to Sport Index (ACL-RSI), Tampa Scale for Kinesiophobia (TSK-11), Knee Self-efficacy Scale (K-SES)
Fatigue	Functional tests (like hop tests) should also be tested under football-specific fatigue conditions. In addition movement quality should be assessed
Interval kicking program	Successful completion of all steps without adverse reactions
Agility tests	Player has practiced and displays no hesitation or compensation strategies during agility drills (particularly when decelerating) when performed at 100% effort
On-field rehabilitation	Successful completion of all steps without adverse reactions and feeling of instability
Completed full practice	Assess tolerance of sport-specific training: no pain, swelling, stiffness, giving way
Time after surgery	RTS > 9 months (professional players?)
Laxity and biological assessment graft	No abnormal laxity: KT-1000 arthrometer <3 mm increased anterior laxity compared with the contralateral side, <3 mm Lachman test, grade 0 pivot-shift test. Biological assessment of the graft with MRI

36.7 Return to Performance

Is it a successful outcome after ACLR if a football player has passed the RTS tests and formally discharged from rehabilitation? Can we therefore assume that a player is performing at the pre-injury level? Success means different things to different people and is context-dependent and outcome-dependent [18]. Much of the variability in RTS and RTP rates may be because of a lack of standardization in the definition of "return to sport." The use of the term RTS must be accompanied by a detailed description of the individual characteristics of the athletes being studied (e.g., sex and age); the use of protective equipment (e.g., ankle bracing); the intensity, duration, and frequency of each exposure; the type of activity (e.g., pivoting or non-pivoting, contact or non-contact sports); the level of activity (e.g., elite, competitive, or recreational); the performance level (e.g., match statistics); as well as the timing and duration of sport participation after ACLR.

There is a lack of a comprehensive overview in football that may indicate whether the player has indeed reached pre-injury performance level. Kester et al. identified the impact of ACLR on performance and career length for National Basketball Association (NBA) players [86]. The outcomes included seasons played, games played, games started, minutes per game, points per game, field goals, 3-point shots, rebounds, assists, steals, blocks, turnovers, personal fouls, usage percentage, and player efficiency ratings and were compared with uninjured controls. In their first full season after ACLR, players started in 15.5 fewer games, played in 17.3 fewer games and had combined player efficiency ratings 2.35 points lower when compared to matched controls. Over the length of the careers, players competed in 22.2 fewer games per season.

According to the definition of RTP, this is a continuum from RTS; although the football player may have been discharged from rehabilitation, this does not mean the player is back on pre-injury level. Too often, the end phase of the rehabilitation is not extensive or specific enough, thereby exposing athletes to specific training loads and training characteristics that they cannot handle from a physical, physiologically, neurocognitive as well as psychological perspective. Returning an athlete to participation should be a graduated continuum that progresses from the least demanding to most demanding activities, not a single test or set of tests that releases an athlete to return to participation at one single point in time [44].

Unfortunately, there are no validated sports-specific tests to determine readiness to return to full participation in team practice and competitive matches for football players after ACLR [58]. Data are available for different players' roles (defender, full-back, midfielder, and forward) that, even if cutoff values do not exist, may help in judging the performance and RTP readiness of the player [58].

An analysis of UEFA professional male football players showed a mean time to return to official match of 224 ± 75 days after ACLR [87]. Interestingly this study reported also the "return to train" outcome, which was 201 ± 68 days [87]. Hence, this implies that football players recovering from ACLR who were cleared to training had on average 23 days to progress to match level. Such a short time frame may question whether this is feasible from a medical and/or exercise physiology point of view. The influence of other influencing factors may be at stake here.

Shrier recently proposed the Strategic Assessment of Risk and Risk Tolerance (StARRT) framework for RTS decisions, where factors affecting injury risk are grouped in the assessment of health risk, activity risk, and risk tolerance [88]. The StARRT model is a three-step model that helps estimate the risks of different short-term and long-term outcomes associated with RTS and factors that may affect what should be considered an acceptable risk within a particular context. Step 1 (tissue health) of the StARRT framework synthesizes information relevant to the load (stress) the tissue can absorb before injury. Step 2 (tissue stresses) synthesizes information relevant to the expected cumulative load (stress) on the tissue. Step 3 (risk tolerance modifiers) synthesizes information relevant to the contextual factors that influence the RTS decision-maker's tolerance for risk (Fig. 36.5) [88].

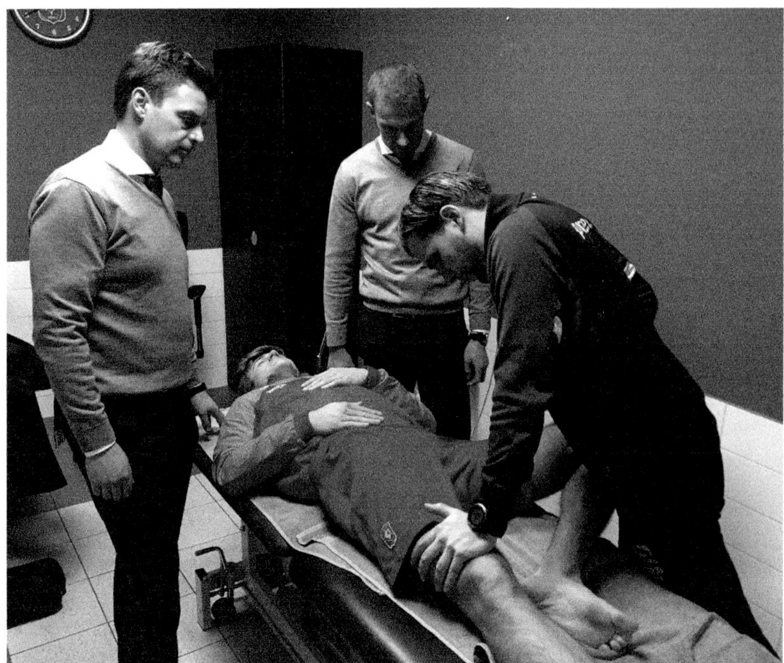

Fig. 36.5 Shared decision process in terms of risk management by orthopedic surgeon, sports medicine physician, and sports physical therapist of an injured professional football player

In medicine there is mainly a focus on the first two steps within this framework (the risk assessment process). However, as the UEFA study indicated, professional football players have a relatively short amount of time to transfer from training to playing the first match [2]. Subsequently, a sudden increase in load may predispose the player to further or recurrent injury.

Take-Home Message

Based on the recent literature, no gold standard exists when evaluating RTS readiness after ACLR. Therefore, the authors propose a multifactorial RTS test battery. A combination of both physical and psychological elements is included in the RTS test battery. The concept presented in this chapter highlights a close cooperation between all members within a multidisciplinary team, facilitating a shared decision-making process.

Acknowledgments The authors would like to thank Dr. Bart Dingenen and PhD cand. Wouter Welling for their scholarly discussions in preparation for this chapter. We would also like to show our gratitude to Dr. Roy Hoogeslag for providing two photographs, sharing his experience in professional football as his comments greatly improved the manuscript.

Top Five Evidence Based References

Ardern CL, Glasgow P, Schneiders A, Witvrouw E, Clarsen B, Cools A, Gojanovic B, Griffin S, Khan KM, Moksnes H, Mutch SA, Phillips N, Reurink G, Sadler R, Gravare Silbernagel K, Thorborg K, Wangensteen A, Wilk KE, Bizzini M (2016) 2016 Consensus statement on return to sport from the First World Congress in Sports Physical Therapy, Bern. Br J Sports Med 50(14):853–864

Dingenen B, Gokeler A (2017) Optimization of the return-to-sport paradigm after anterior cruciate ligament reconstruction: a critical step back to move forward. Sports Med. https://doi.org/10.1007/s40279-017-0674-6

Gokeler A, Benjaminse A, Hewett TE, Paterno MV, Ford KR, Otten E, Myer GD (2013) Feedback techniques to target functional deficits following anterior cruciate ligament reconstruction: implications for motor control and reduction of second injury risk. Sports Med 43(11):1065–1074

Walden M, Hagglund M, Magnusson H, Ekstrand J (2016) ACL injuries in men's professional football: a 15-year prospective study on time trends and return-to-play rates reveals only 65% of players still play at the top level 3 years after ACL rupture. Br J Sports Med 50(12):744–750

Zaffagnini S, Grassi A, Marcheggiani Muccioli GM, Tsapralis K, Ricci M, Bragonzoni L, Della Villa S, Marcacci M (2014) Return to sport after anterior cruciate ligament reconstruction in professional soccer players. Knee 21(3):731–735

References

1. Feucht MJ, Cotic M, Saier T, Minzlaff P, Plath JE, Imhoff AB, Hinterwimmer S (2016) Patient expectations of primary and revision anterior cruciate ligament reconstruction. Knee Surg Sports Traumatol Arthrosc 24(1):201–207
2. Walden M, Hagglund M, Magnusson H, Ekstrand J (2016) ACL injuries in men's professional football: a 15-year prospective study on time trends and return-to-play rates reveals only 65% of players still play at the top level 3 years after ACL rupture. Br J Sports Med 50(12):744–750
3. Zaffagnini S, Grassi A, Marcheggiani Muccioli GM, Tsapralis K, Ricci M, Bragonzoni L, Della Villa S, Marcacci M (2014) Return to sport after anterior cruciate ligament reconstruction in professional soccer players. Knee 21(3):731–735
4. Brophy RH, Schmitz L, Wright RW, Dunn WR, Parker RD, Andrish JT, McCarty EC, Spindler KP (2012) Return to play and future ACL injury risk after ACL reconstruction in soccer athletes from the Multicenter Orthopaedic Outcomes Network (MOON) group. Am J Sports Med 40(11):2517–2522
5. Ardern CL, Bizzini M, Bahr R (2015) It is time for consensus on return to play after injury: five key questions. Br J Sports Med 50(9):506–508
6. Wiggins AJ, Grandhi RK, Schneider DK, Stanfield D, Webster KE, Myer GD (2016) Risk of secondary injury in younger athletes after anterior cruciate ligament reconstruction: a systematic review and meta-analysis. Am J Sports Med 44(7):1861–1876
7. Ahlden M, Samuelsson K, Sernert N, Forssblad M, Karlsson J, Kartus J (2012) The Swedish national anterior cruciate ligament register: a report on baseline variables and outcomes of surgery for almost 18,000 patients. Am J Sports Med 40(10):2230–2235
8. Simoneau GG, Wilk KE (2012) The challenge of return to sports for patients post-ACL reconstruction. J Orthop Sports Phys Ther 42(4):300–301
9. Fabricant PD, Jones KJ, Delos D, Cordasco FA, Marx RG, Pearle AD, Warren RF, Green DW (2013) Reconstruction of the anterior cruciate ligament in the skeletally immature athlete: a review of current concepts: AAOS exhibit selection. J Bone Joint Surg Am 95(5):e28
10. Webster KE, Feller JA (2016) Exploring the high reinjury rate in younger patients undergoing anterior cruciate ligament reconstruction. Am J Sports Med 44(11):2827–2832
11. Paterno MV, Schmitt LC, Ford KR, Rauh MJ, Myer GD, Huang B, Hewett TE (2010) Biomechanical measures during landing and postural stability predict second anterior cruciate ligament injury after anterior cruciate ligament reconstruction and return to sport. Am J Sports Med 38(10):1968–1978
12. Sward P, Kostogiannis I, Roos H (2010) Risk factors for a contralateral anterior cruciate ligament injury. Knee Surg Sports Traumatol Arthrosc 18(3):277–291
13. Wild CY, Munro BJ, Steele JR (2016) How young girls change their landing technique throughout the adolescent growth spurt. Am J Sports Med 44(5):1116–1123
14. Wild CY, Steele JR, Munro BJ (2012) Why do girls sustain more anterior cruciate ligament injuries than boys?: a review of the changes in estrogen and musculoskeletal structure and function during puberty. Sports Med 42(9):733–749
15. Di Stasi S, Myer GD, Hewett TE (2013) Neuromuscular training to target deficits associated with second anterior cruciate ligament injury. J Orthop Sports Phys Ther 43(11):777–792
16. Zaffagnini S, Grassi A, Serra M, Marcacci M (2015) Return to sport after ACL reconstruction: how, when and why? A narrative review of current evidence. Joints 3(1):25–30
17. Barber-Westin SD, Noyes FR (2011) Factors used to determine return to unrestricted sports activities after anterior cruciate ligament reconstruction. Arthroscopy 27(12):1697–1705
18. Ardern CL, Glasgow P, Schneiders A, Witvrouw E, Clarsen B, Cools A, Gojanovic B, Griffin S, Khan KM, Moksnes H, Mutch SA, Phillips N, Reurink G, Sadler R, Gravare Silbernagel K, Thorborg K, Wangensteen A, Wilk KE, Bizzini M (2016) 2016 Consensus statement on return to sport from the First World Congress in Sports Physical Therapy, Bern. Br J Sports Med 50(14):853–864
19. Grindem H, Snyder-Mackler L, Moksnes H, Engebretsen L, Risberg MA (2016) Simple decision rules can reduce reinjury risk by 84% after ACL reconstruction: the Delaware-Oslo ACL cohort study. Br J Sports Med. https://doi.org/10.1136/bjsports-2016-096031
20. Kyritsis P, Bahr R, Landreau P, Miladi R, Witvrouw E (2016) Likelihood of ACL graft rupture: not meeting six clinical discharge criteria before return to sport is associated with a four times greater risk of rupture. Br J Sports Med 50(15):946–951
21. Thomee R, Kaplan Y, Kvist J, Myklebust G, Risberg MA, Theisen D, Tsepis E, Werner S, Wondrasch B, Witvrouw E (2011) Muscle strength and hop performance criteria prior to return to sports after ACL reconstruction. Knee Surg Sports Traumatol Arthrosc 19(11):1798–1805
22. Larsen JB, Farup J, Lind M, Dalgas U (2015) Muscle strength and functional performance is markedly impaired at the recommended time point for sport return after anterior cruciate ligament reconstruction in recreational athletes. Hum Mov Sci 39:73–87
23. Herrington L (2013) Functional outcome from anterior cruciate ligament surgery: a review. OA Orthop 01(2):12
24. Undheim MB, Cosgrave C, King E, Strike S, Marshall B, Falvey E, Franklyn-Miller A (2015) Isokinetic muscle strength and readiness to return to sport following anterior cruciate ligament reconstruction: is there an association? A systematic review and a protocol recommendation. Br J Sports Med 49(20):1305–1310

25. Petersen W, Taheri P, Forkel P, Zantop T (2014) Return to play following ACL reconstruction: a systematic review about strength deficits. Arch Orthop Trauma Surg 134(10):1417–1428
26. Khayambashi K, Ghoddosi N, Straub RK, Powers CM (2016) Hip muscle strength predicts noncontact anterior cruciate ligament injury in male and female athletes: a prospective study. Am J Sports Med 44(2):355–361
27. Logerstedt D, Di Stasi S, Grindem H, Lynch A, Eitzen I, Engebretsen L, Risberg MA, Axe MJ, Snyder-Mackler L (2014) Self-reported knee function can identify athletes who fail return-to-activity criteria up to 1 year after anterior cruciate ligament reconstruction: a Delaware-oslo ACL cohort study. J Orthop Sports Phys Ther 44(12):914–923
28. Ardern CL, Taylor NF, Feller JA, Webster KE (2014) Fifty-five per cent return to competitive sport following anterior cruciate ligament reconstruction surgery: an updated systematic review and meta-analysis including aspects of physical functioning and contextual factors. Br J Sports Med 48(21):1543–1552
29. Clagg S, Paterno MV, Hewett TE, Schmitt LC (2015) Performance on the modified star excursion balance test at the time of return to sport following anterior cruciate ligament reconstruction. J Orthop Sports Phys Ther 45(6):444–452
30. Dingenen B, Janssens L, Claes S, Bellemans J, Staes FF (2015) Postural stability deficits during the transition from double-leg stance to single-leg stance in anterior cruciate ligament reconstructed subjects. Hum Mov Sci 41:46–58
31. Dingenen B, Janssens L, Luyckx T, Claes S, Bellemans J, Staes FF (2015) Lower extremity muscle activation onset times during the transition from double-leg stance to single-leg stance in anterior cruciate ligament injured subjects. Hum Mov Sci 44:234–245
32. Urbach D, Nebelung W, Ropke M, Becker R, Awiszus F (2000) Bilateral dysfunction of the quadriceps muscle after unilateral cruciate ligament rupture with concomitant injury central activation deficit. Unfallchirurg 103(11):949–955
33. Baumeister J, Reinecke K, Schubert M, Weiss M (2011) Altered electrocortical brain activity after ACL reconstruction during force control. J Orthop Res 29(9):1383–1389
34. Baumeister J, Reinecke K, Weiss M (2008) Changed cortical activity after anterior cruciate ligament reconstruction in a joint position paradigm: an EEG study. Scand J Med Sci Sports 18(4):473–484
35. Kapreli E, Athanasopoulos S, Gliatis J, Papathanasiou M, Peeters R, Strimpakos N, Van Hecke P, Gouliamos A, Sunaert S (2009) Anterior cruciate ligament deficiency causes brain plasticity: a functional MRI study. Am J Sports Med 37(12):2419–2426
36. Valeriani M, Restuccia D, Di Lazzaro V, Franceschi F, Fabbriciani C, Tonali P (1999) Clinical and neurophysiological abnormalities before and after reconstruction of the anterior cruciate ligament of the knee. Acta Neurol Scand 99(5):303–307
37. Myers BA, Jenkins WL, Killian C, Rundquist P (2014) Normative data for hop tests in high school and collegiate basketball and soccer players. Int J Sports Phys Ther 9(5):596–603
38. Xergia SA, Pappas E, Georgoulis AD (2015) Association of the single-limb hop test with isokinetic, kinematic, and kinetic asymmetries in patients after anterior cruciate ligament reconstruction. Sports Health 7(3):217–223
39. Gokeler A, Welling W, Zaffagnini S, Seil R, Padua D (2017) Development of a test battery to enhance safe return to sports after anterior cruciate ligament reconstruction. Knee Surg Sports Traumatol Arthrosc 25(1):192–199
40. Padua DA, Marshall SW, Boling MC, Thigpen CA, Garrett WE Jr, Beutler AI (2009) The Landing Error Scoring System (LESS) Is a valid and reliable clinical assessment tool of jump-landing biomechanics: the JUMP-ACL study. Am J Sports Med 37(10):1996–2002
41. Engelen-van Melick N, van Cingel RE, Tijssen MP, Nijhuis-van der Sanden MW (2013) Assessment of functional performance after anterior cruciate ligament reconstruction: a systematic review of measurement procedures. Knee Surg Sports Traumatol Arthrosc 21(4):869–879
42. Hoshino Y, Araujo P, Ahlden M, Samuelsson K, Muller B, Hofbauer M, Wolf MR, Irrgang JJ, FH F, Musahl V (2013) Quantitative evaluation of the pivot shift by image analysis using the iPad. Knee Surg Sports Traumatol Arthrosc 21(4):975–980
43. Zaffagnini S, Lopomo N, Signorelli C, Marcheggiani Muccioli GM, Bonanzinga T, Grassi A, Raggi F, Visani A, Marcacci M (2014) Inertial sensors to quantify the pivot shift test in the treatment of anterior cruciate ligament injury. Joints 2(3):124–129
44. Wilk KE, Arrigo CA (2017) Rehabilitation principles of the anterior cruciate ligament reconstructed knee: twelve steps for successful progression and return to play. Clin Sports Med 36(1):189–232
45. Santamaria LJ, Webster KE (2010) The effect of fatigue on lower-limb biomechanics during single-limb landings: a systematic review. J Orthop Sports Phys Ther 40(8):464–473
46. Abrams GD, Harris JD, Gupta AK, McCormick FM, Bush-Joseph CA, Verma NN, Cole BJ, Bach BR Jr (2014) Functional performance testing after anterior cruciate ligament reconstruction: a systematic review. Orthop J Sports Med 2(1):23
47. Augustsson J, Thomee R, Linden C, Folkesson M, Tranberg R, Karlsson J (2006) Single-leg hop testing following fatiguing exercise: reliability and biomechanical analysis. Scand J Med Sci Sports 16(2):111–120
48. Gokeler A, Eppinga P, Dijkstra PU, Welling W, Padua DA, Otten E, Benjaminse A (2014) Effect of fatigue on landing performance assessed with the landing error scoring system (LESS) in patients after ACL reconstruction. A pilot study. Int J Sports Phys Ther 9(3):302–311

49. Lynch AD, Logerstedt DS, Grindem H, Eitzen I, Hicks GE, Axe MJ, Engebretsen L, Risberg MA, Snyder-Mackler L (2015) Consensus criteria for defining 'successful outcome' after ACL injury and reconstruction: a Delaware-Oslo ACL cohort investigation. Br J Sports Med 49(5):335–342
50. Anderson AF, Irrgang JJ, Kocher MS, Mann BJ, Harrast JJ (2006) The international knee documentation committee subjective knee evaluation form: normative data. Am J Sports Med 34(1):128–135
51. Ardern CL, Webster KE, Taylor NF, Feller JA (2011) Return to sport following anterior cruciate ligament reconstruction surgery: a systematic review and meta-analysis of the state of play. Br J Sports Med 45(7):596–606
52. Howard JS, Lembach ML, Metzler AV, Johnson DL (2016) Rates and determinants of return to play after anterior cruciate ligament reconstruction in national collegiate athletic association Division I soccer athletes: a study of the Southeastern Conference. Am J Sports Med 44(2):433–439
53. Ardern CL (2015) Anterior cruciate ligament reconstruction-not exactly a one-way ticket back to the preinjury level: a review of contextual factors affecting return to sport after surgery. Sports Health 7(3):224–230
54. Webster KE, Feller JA, Lambros C (2008) Development and preliminary validation of a scale to measure the psychological impact of returning to sport following anterior cruciate ligament reconstruction surgery. Phys Ther Sport 9(1):9–15
55. Sonesson S, Kvist J, Ardern C, Osterberg A, Silbernagel KG (2016) Psychological factors are important to return to pre-injury sport activity after anterior cruciate ligament reconstruction: expect and motivate to satisfy. Knee Surg Sports Traumatol Arthrosc. https://doi.org/10.1007/s00167-016-4294-8
56. Hamrin Senorski E, Samuelsson K, Thomee C, Beischer S, Karlsson J, Thomee R (2016) Return to knee-strenuous sport after anterior cruciate ligament reconstruction: a report from a rehabilitation outcome registry of patient characteristics. Knee Surg Sports Traumatol Arthrosc. https://doi.org/10.1007/s00167-016-4280-1
57. Thomee P, Wahrborg P, Borjesson M, Thomee R, Eriksson BI, Karlsson J (2006) A new instrument for measuring self-efficacy in patients with an anterior cruciate ligament injury. Scand J Med Sci Sports 16(3):181–187
58. Bizzini M, Hancock D, Impellizzeri F (2012) Suggestions from the field for return to sports participation following anterior cruciate ligament reconstruction: soccer. J Orthop Sports Phys Ther 42(4):304–312
59. Arundale A, Silvers H, Logerstedt D, Rojas J, Snyder-Mackler L (2015) An interval kicking progression for return to soccer following lower extremity injury. Int J Sports Phys Ther 10(1):114–127
60. Della Villa S, Boldrini L, Ricci M, Danelon F, Snyder-Mackler L, Nanni G, Roi GS (2012) Clinical outcomes and return-to-sports participation of 50 soccer players after anterior cruciate ligament reconstruction through a sport-specific rehabilitation protocol. Sports Health 4(1):17–24
61. Blanch P, Gabbett TJ (2016) Has the athlete trained enough to return to play safely? The acute:chronic workload ratio permits clinicians to quantify a player's risk of subsequent injury. Br J Sports Med 50(8):471–475
62. Sheppard JM, Young WB (2006) Agility literature review: classifications, training and testing. J Sports Sci 24(9):919–932
63. Young WB, James R, Montgomery I (2002) Is muscle power related to running speed with changes of direction? J Sports Med Phys Fitness 42(3):282–288
64. Schmidt RAWC (2005) Motor learning and performance. Human Kinetics, Champaign, IL
65. Rouissi M, Chtara M, Berriri A, Owen A, Chamari K (2016) Asymmetry of the modified Illinois change of direction test impacts young elite soccer players' performance. Asian J Sports Med 7(2):e33598
66. Almonroeder TG, Garcia E, Kurt M (2015) The effects of anticipation on the mechanics of the knee during single-leg cutting tasks: a systematic review. Int J Sports Phys Ther 10(7):918–928
67. Brown SR, Brughelli M, Hume PA (2014) Knee mechanics during planned and unplanned sidestepping: a systematic review and meta-analysis. Sports Med 44(11):1573–1588
68. Grindem H, Snyder-Mackler L, Moksnes H, Engebretsen L, Risberg MA (2016) Simple decision rules can reduce reinjury risk by 84% after ACL reconstruction: the Delaware-Oslo ACL cohort study. Br J Sports Med 50(13):804–808
69. Laboute E, Savalli L, Puig P, Trouve P, Sabot G, Monnier G, Dubroca B (2010) Analysis of return to competition and repeat rupture for 298 anterior cruciate ligament reconstructions with patellar or hamstring tendon autograft in sportspeople. Ann Phys Rehabil Med 53(10):598–614
70. Paterno MV, Rauh MJ, Schmitt LC, Ford KR, Hewett TE (2014) Incidence of second ACL injuries 2 Years after primary ACL reconstruction and return to sport. Am J Sports Med 42(7):1567–1573
71. Schlumberger M, Schuster P, Schulz M, Immendörfer M, Mayer P, Bartholomä J, Richter J (2015) Traumatic graft rupture after primary and revision anterior cruciate ligament reconstruction: retrospective analysis of incidence and risk factors in 2915 cases. Knee Surg Sports Traumatol Arthrosc. https://doi.org/10.1007/s00167-015-3699-0
72. Janssen RP, Scheffler SU (2014) Intra-articular remodelling of hamstring tendon grafts after anterior cruciate ligament reconstruction. Knee Surg Sports Traumatol Arthrosc 22(9):2102–2108
73. Grassi A, Bailey JR, Signorelli C, Carbone G, Tchonang Wakam A, Lucidi GA, Zaffagnini S (2016) Magnetic resonance imaging after anterior cruciate ligament reconstruction: a practical guide. World J Orthop 7(10):638–649
74. Weiler A, Peters G, Maurer J, Unterhauser FN, Sudkamp NP (2001) Biomechanical properties and vascularity of an anterior cruciate ligament graft can be predicted by contrast-enhanced magnetic

resonance imaging. A two-year study in sheep. Am J Sports Med 29(6):751–761
75. Figueroa D, Melean P, Calvo R, Vaisman A, Zilleruelo N, Figueroa F, Villalon I (2010) Magnetic resonance imaging evaluation of the integration and maturation of semitendinosus-gracilis graft in anterior cruciate ligament reconstruction using autologous platelet concentrate. Arthroscopy 26(10):1318–1325
76. Biercevicz AM, Akelman MR, Fadale PD, Hulstyn MJ, Shalvoy RM, Badger GJ, Tung GA, Oksendahl HL, Fleming BC (2015) MRI volume and signal intensity of ACL graft predict clinical, functional, and patient-oriented outcome measures after ACL reconstruction. Am J Sports Med 43(3):693–699
77. Li H, Chen J, Li H, Wu Z, Chen S (2016) MRI-based ACL graft maturity does not predict clinical and functional outcomes during the first year after ACL reconstruction. Knee Surg Sports Traumatol Arthrosc. https://doi.org/10.1007/s00167-016-4252-5
78. Urhausen A, Mouton C, Krecké R, Seil R (2016) Anterior cruciate ligament clinical pathway. Sports Orthop Traumatol 32(2):196–197
79. Lopomo N, Zaffagnini S, Amis AA (2013) Quantifying the pivot shift test: a systematic review. Knee Surg Sports Traumatol Arthrosc 21(4):767–783
80. Grassi A, Lopomo NF, Rao AM, Abuharfiel AN, Zaffagnini S (2016) No proof for the best instrumented device to grade the pivot shift test: a systematic review. J ISAKOS Joint Disord Orthop Sports Med. https://doi.org/10.1136/jisakos-2015-000047
81. Zaffagnini S, Lopomo N, Signorelli C, Marcheggiani Muccioli GM, Bonanzinga T, Grassi A, Visani A, Marcacci M (2013) Innovative technology for knee laxity evaluation: clinical applicability and reliability of inertial sensors for quantitative analysis of the pivot-shift test. Clin Sports Med 32(1):61–70
82. Mouton C, Theisen D, Meyer T, Agostinis H, Nuhrenborger C, Pape D, Seil R (2015) Noninjured knees of patients with noncontact ACL injuries display higher average anterior and internal rotational knee laxity compared with healthy knees of a noninjured population. Am J Sports Med 43(8):1918–1923
83. Mouton C, Theisen D, Seil R (2016) Objective measurements of static anterior and rotational knee laxity. Curr Rev Musculoskelet Med 9(2):139–147
84. Shultz SJ, Schmitz RJ (2009) Effects of transverse and frontal plane knee laxity on hip and knee neuromechanics during drop landings. Am J Sports Med 37(9):1821–1830
85. Baumgart C, Gokeler A, Donath L, Hoppe MW, Freiwald J (2015) Effects of static stretching and playing soccer on knee laxity. Clin J Sport Med 25(6):541–545
86. Kester BS, Behery OA, Minhas SV, Hsu WK (2016) Athletic performance and career longevity following anterior cruciate ligament reconstruction in the National Basketball Association. Knee Surg Sports Traumatol Arthrosc. https://doi.org/10.1007/s00167-016-4060-y
87. Walden M, Hagglund M, Magnusson H, Ekstrand J (2011) Anterior cruciate ligament injury in elite football: a prospective three-cohort study. Knee Surg Sports Traumatol Arthrosc 19(1):11–19
88. Shrier I (2015) Strategic assessment of risk and risk tolerance (StARRT) framework for return-to-play decision-making. Br J Sports Med 49(20):1311–1315

Part V

Return to Play After Complex Knee Injuries

Return to Play After Complex Knee Injuries: Return to Play After Medial Collateral Ligament Injuries

37

Marcin Kowalczuk, Markus Waldén, Martin Hägglund, Ricard Pruna, Conor Murphy, Jonathan Hughes, Volker Musahl, and Matilda Lundblad

Contents

M. Kowalczuk • C. Murphy • J. Hughes
V. Musahl, M.D. (✉)
Department of Orthopaedic Surgery, University of Pittsburgh,
3200 S Water St., Pittsburgh, PA 15203, USA
e-mail: musahlv@upmc.edu

M. Waldén • M. Hägglund
Football Research Group, Department of Medical and Health Sciences, Linköping University, Linköping, Sweden

R. Pruna
FC Barcelona Medical Services, FIFA Medical Centre of Excellence, Barcelona, Spain

M. Lundblad
Football Research Group, Department of Medical and Health Sciences, Linköping University, Linköping, Sweden

Department of Orthopaedics, Sahlgrenska University, Gothenburg, Sweden

37.1 Introduction

Medial collateral ligament (MCL) injuries are a common and debilitating injury in football players. Time lost to injury is significant and contributes to the overall success of the football club [1]. Understanding the anatomy, appropriate clinical

V. Musahl et al. (eds.), *Return to Play in Football*, https://doi.org/10.1007/978-3-662-55713-6_37

examination technique, and accurate imaging workup are paramount to diagnosis and subsequent treatment. Clinical suspicion for concomitant injury to other knee structures must be high. Once the full extent of the injury has been assessed and treatment provided, return to play (RTP) algorithms can be initiated.

37.2 Epidemiology

The MCL is the most commonly injured knee ligament in professional football with an injury rate of approximately 0.33 injuries per 1000 player hours [2, 3]. This correlates to two MCL injuries every season in a 25-player squad. Fifty-seven percent of all football injuries occur during match play and 43% during training, with an overall injury rate seven times greater during match play compared to training [4, 5].

Notably, injuries to the MCL occur at a rate of nine times greater during match play when compared to training, and the median layoff is 16 days until a player is in full training and available for match play [3]. Furthermore, previous injury to the knee is associated with an increased risk of new knee injury and threefold greater risk of identical injury to the same knee [6, 7]. Fortunately, the MCL injury rate has decreased over the last 11 years, while injury rates for muscles, other soft tissues, and overall injuries have remained constant despite increases in total exposure hours due to increased amounts of training relative to match play [3, 4, 8]. This decrease could possibly be explained by improvements in treatment and rehabilitation as well as preventative neuromuscular training methods. Given that MCL injuries are usually the result of a contact mechanism, this decrease may also be in part due to stricter officiating or a shift in football tactics that emphasize a technical as opposed to physical style of play.

37.3 Anatomy

The medial collateral ligament is a static stabilizer to the knee and is the largest structure on its medial aspect (Fig. 37.1). It is composed of two portions, the superficial MCL (sMCL) and deep MCL (dMCL). Medial stability is also conferred by the posterior oblique ligament which is intimately associated with the MCL insertion on the tibia [9].

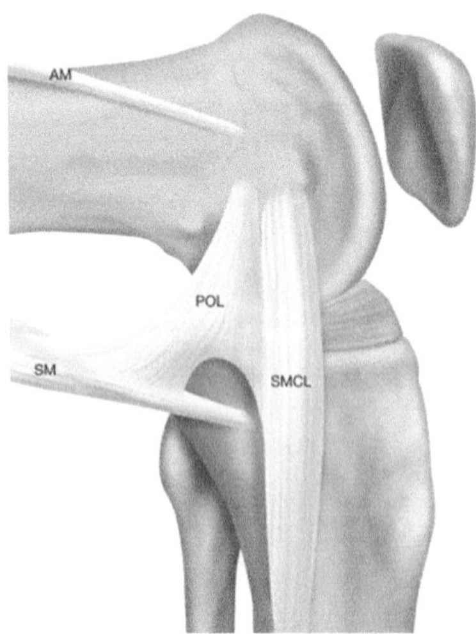

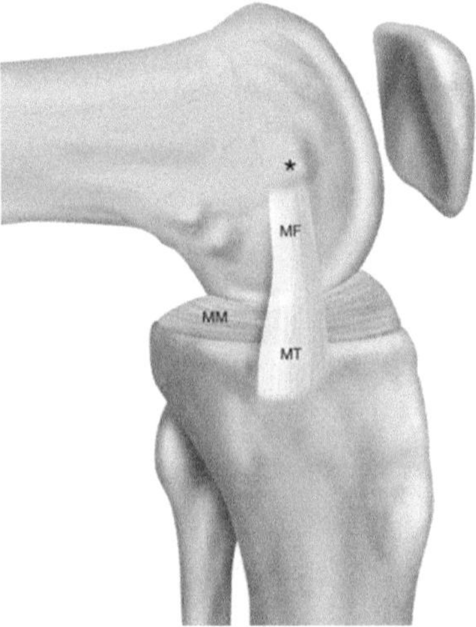

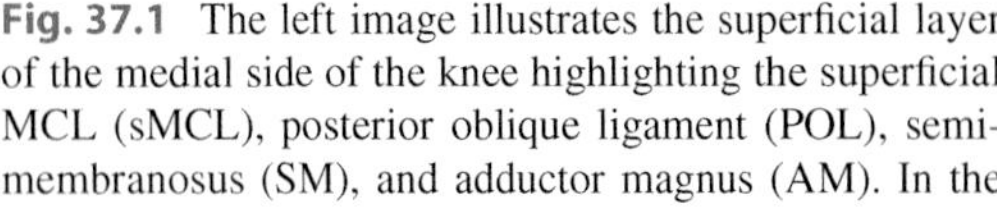

Fig. 37.1 The left image illustrates the superficial layer of the medial side of the knee highlighting the superficial MCL (sMCL), posterior oblique ligament (POL), semimembranosus (SM), and adductor magnus (AM). In the right image, the sMCL has been removed revealing the medial epicondyle (*), medial meniscus (MM), as well as the meniscofemoral (MF) and meniscotibial (MT) portions of the deep MCL

37.3.1 Superficial Medial Collateral Ligament

The sMCL has one femoral attachment and two tibial attachment sites. Recent quantitative anatomic studies have found the femoral origin to be slightly oval in shape and located 3.2 mm proximal and 4.8 mm posterior to the medial epicondyle [9]. The proximal aspect of the tibial insertion site attaches to the anterior aspect of the semimembranosus tendon approximately 12 mm distal to the tibial joint line, while the distal aspect attaches directly to bone approximately 46–60 mm distal to the tibial joint line [9, 10]. The inferior medial geniculate artery and vein course between the proximal and distal attachment sites [9–11].

37.3.2 Deep Medial Collateral Ligament (Mid-third Medial Capsular Ligament)

The deep fibers of the MCL are confluent with the medial joint capsule and medial meniscus and are comprised of two components, the meniscotibial and meniscofemoral ligaments [11].

The meniscofemoral ligament attaches approximately 10–13 mm distal and deep to the sMCL, while the meniscotibial ligament, which is thicker and shorter than the meniscofemoral ligament, attaches 3–4 mm distal to the medial tibial joint line [9, 12].

37.3.3 Posterior Oblique Ligament

There is wide variation in the literature regarding the femoral attachment site of the posterior oblique ligament (POL), ranging from the adductor tubercle to slightly distal to the gastrocnemius tubercle [9, 13, 14]. Distally the POL has three fascial attachments, the central, capsular, and peripheral, which help stabilize the posteromedial aspect of the knee. The central portion attaches to the posterior edge of the tibia and the upper edge of the semimembranosus tendon. The capsular portion blends with the posteromedial capsule and a portion of the oblique popliteal ligament, forming the posteromedial corner. The peripheral portion attaches the semimembranosus sheath and to the tibia distal to the semimembranosus tendon insertion [9, 13, 15, 16].

37.3.4 Healing Potential

The sMCL has an abundant vascular supply, and healing follows the model of hemorrhage, inflammation, repair, and remodeling [17, 18]. Rabbit studies have shown an increase in vascularity 16 weeks after partial transection of the MCL [19, 20]. Additionally, animal models have demonstrated that the MCL healing is location dependent. Midsubstance tears heal quicker than tears near the insertion sites [21]. Immobilization also plays a role in healing potential of the sMCL. Recent animal models have demonstrated increased collagen degradation and reduction of collagen mass after 12 weeks of immobilization [22]. Another study demonstrated that an immobilized MCL failed to increase in mass, and demonstrated declining collagen synthetic rates, as compared to a non-immobilized MCL [23].

37.4 Mechanism of Injury

Injury to the MCL most commonly stems from a valgus moment applied to the lateral knee or a combination of valgus force and external rotation of the tibia [24, 25]. Biomechanical studies confirm that the sMCL experiences the greatest load with valgus and external rotation moments, while internal rotation near full extension results in maximal load of the POL [26]. Approximately 70% of injuries to the MCL during football result from direct contact with another player or object [3]. This is in contrast to anterior cruciate ligament (ACL) injuries where 63% are noncontact in nature [27]. Colliding with an opponent, tackling, and blocking are the most commonly described mechanisms for MCL injury [2, 3].

The rate of MCL injuries increases significantly during the final 15 min of each half during competition suggesting either the additive effects of fatigue render players unable to react to contact with the same quickness or an elevated competition intensity instigates more player contact during the closing minutes [3]. Successful injury prevention through the implementation of neuromuscular training warm-ups and multimodal interventions in youth and female football players implies that there is an internal biomechanical or muscular contribution to injury risk [28–31]. But, these interventions have not been specifically studied with respect to MCL injury, nor have they been studied in the elite football player population. It is possible that movement patterns and neuromuscular conditioning have already been well established in the elite playing population such that these interventions may not be effective [4].

37.5 Clinical Presentation

37.5.1 History

Patients presenting with MCL injury may report feeling a pop and present with localized pain and tenderness along the medial aspect of the knee. Localized swelling and bruising can occur, especially with higher-grade injuries, but normally no early intra-articular effusion is present. Patients will often complain of side-to-side instability, especially during cutting or pivoting exercises.

37.5.2 Physical Examination

Initial management of acute injuries includes a physical examination that should be carried out as soon as possible after the injury occurs. This allows for an accurate examination before any swelling and muscle spasms commence. Any open wounds, erythema, and localized swelling or ecchymosis about the medial aspect of knee should be noted. Palpation may elicit pain about the femoral and tibial attachment sites or along the midsubstance of the ligament. A neurovascular examination is also critical to rule out a complex knee injury or knee dislocation in more severe injuries.

Applying a valgus stress to the knee in maximum extension and 30° of flexion can help classify an MCL injury and possibly concomitant cruciate ligament injuries. There should be no laxity to valgus stress in full extension with an isolated sMCL injury. Valgus stress at 30° of flexion can detect an MCL injury, and has been historically classified as grade I with opening <5 mm, grade II with opening between 5 and 10 mm, and grade III with opening >10 mm [32]. Increased medial joint line opening with valgus stress at 0° and 30° of extension indicates an injury to the MCL and cruciate ligaments [13, 33, 34]. In all footballers with acute knee trauma, the examiner should perform the Lachman, pivot shift, anterior drawer, and posterior drawer tests to further delineate the extent of the injury.

Injury to multiple structures on the medial side of the knee can cause anteromedial rotatory instability, which is defined as anterior translation and external rotation of the tibia with respect to the femur [35]. This rotational instability is magnified as knee flexion increases [36]. However, it is important to note that this external rotational instability is often confused with a posterolateral corner injury, especially with a concomitant ACL injury. Therefore, a detailed physical examination must be performed to ascertain to the source of the injury.

Rotational stability can be assessed with the anteromedial drawer test, also known as the Swain test [37]. The knee is placed into 90° of flexion with an external rotation torque applied to the knee, thus placing the collateral ligaments on stretch. Pain, or increased external rotation as compared to the contralateral knee, is considered a positive test and can indicate an injury to the POL or posteromedial capsule [13].

37.6 Diagnostic Imaging

Imaging in the setting of MCL injury plays a key role not only in determining injury severity but also aids physicians in identifying other concomitant knee injuries. Both of these factors are important in dictating treatment for the injured athlete. Plain radiographs and magnetic resonance imaging (MRI) are the chief imaging modalities used, but computed tomography (CT) and ultrasound (US) are indicated in specific instances.

37.6.1 Radiographs

Evaluation of the injured athlete should always begin with plain radiographs, as they are generally easy to obtain, low cost, and can provide a wealth of information. If tolerated a standard weight-bearing anteroposterior (AP) view, lateral view in 30° of flexion, and Merchant view of the patella are obtained. Plain radiographs in the setting of suspected isolated MCL injury are frequently normal, but subtle findings maybe present which indicate more significant injury.

The clinician should closely scrutinize radiographs for any evidence of bony avulsions, associated tibial plateau or distal femur fractures, a nonconcentric tibiofemoral articulation, and joint space widening medially. At times, a "reverse Segond" fracture may be seen, which is characterized by a small, elliptical fragment of the bone at the proximal medial tibial plateau [38]. This represents an avulsion of the deep capsular component of the MCL and although rare, when seen, injury to the medial meniscus and posterior cruciate ligament (PCL) should be suspected [39, 40]. Furthermore, small avulsion fractures may also occur posteromedially off the tibial plateau and appear as a small bony fragment displaced posterosuperiorly on lateral knee radiographs [41]. This represents avulsion of the semimembranosus tendon, raising suspicion for anteromedial rotatory instability of the knee [39].

In contrast to conventional radiographs, stress radiographs provide additional insight into the severity of injury to the medial structures of the knee. While physical examination allows subjective grading of medial gapping, stress radiographs allow for objective measurements to be taken. Attempts have been made to standardize how stress radiographs are performed, but currently no universal standard has been agreed upon [42–44]. In cadaver studies under clinician-applied valgus stress, in comparison to the contralateral knee, medial joint space widening of >1.7 mm and >3.2 mm at 0° and 20° of flexion is indicative of an isolated complete rupture of the sMCL [45]. Further widening of >6.5 mm and >9.8 mm at 0° and 20° of flexion, respectively, signals complete rupture of the sMCL, dMCL, and POL [45].

Stress radiographs are also useful when assessing the pediatric athlete with suspected medial-sided knee injury. In the setting of open physes, Salter-Harris I or II injuries can be easily misdiagnosed as MCL injury [42]. In addition to subtle physeal widening on conventional radiographs, stress radiographs can be used to discern between these injuries, which differ significantly in terms of treatment and prognosis [46, 47].

37.6.2 Magnetic Resonance Imaging

MRI given its ability to visualize soft tissue structures in great detail, is a valuable tool in evaluating MCL injuries and ruling out other associated injuries such as ACL rupture or tearing of the menisci. The MCL is best evaluated on T2-weighted coronal images such that the entire sMCL can be visualized from its origin near the femoral epicondyle to its attachment approximately 6 cm distal to joint line on the tibia [48]. When evaluating the MCL, it is important to discern the sMCL, the dMCL (with associated meniscotibial and meniscofemoral ligaments), and the interposed bursa [12]. It is also prudent to closely scrutinize the structures of the posteromedial corner, namely, the semimembranosus, POL, and posteromedial capsule [49].

The severity of the injury should be graded, and whether the injury is a tibial or femoral avulsion versus a midsubstance rupture should be noted (Fig. 37.2). It is also critical to remember that MRI is not a substitute for a detailed physical examination, as the correlation between radiographic severity and clinical laxity is inconsistent. Grade I MCL injuries on MRI are characterized by intact fibers with surrounding edema. Progressive injury with partial ligament

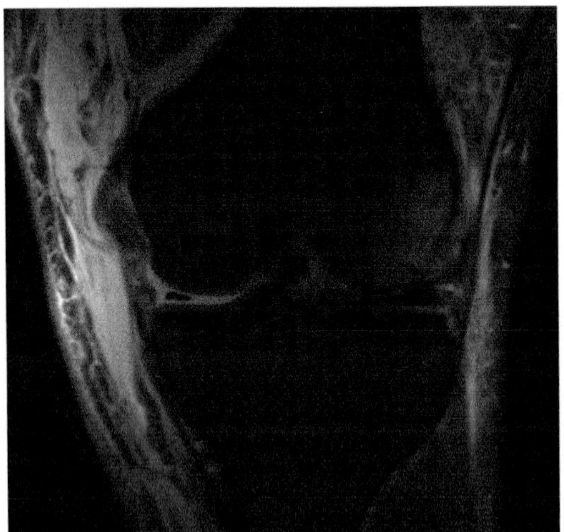

Fig. 37.2 Coronal T2 fat-saturated MRI image of right knee. Grade III midsubstance rupture of the sMCL is noted with overlying soft tissue edema. Grade III injury of the dMCL is also present. Note bony edema of the lateral femoral condyle secondary to concurrent Grade II ACL injury

disruption is consistent with grade II injury, while complete disruption of the ligament is indicative of grade III injury [48].

Several injury patterns on MRI warrant special mention and the clinician should maintain a high index of suspicion as their management differs from that of standard MCL injuries. The first of these are grade III tibial avulsions of both the sMCL and dMCL. These injuries are characterized by disruption of the meniscotibial portion, and non-operative treatment has frequently resulted in poor results [50]. In another subset of tibial-sided sMCL avulsions, if sufficient proximal ligament retraction is present, interposition of the overlying pes anserine tendon may occur. This characteristic injury pattern has been termed the "Stener lesion of the knee" [51]. The final pattern of injury that warrants special attention is isolated grade III disruption of the femoral attachment of the dMCL with an overlying grade I/II femoral-sided sMCL injury. This injury pattern is commonly seen in professional footballers that present with chronic medial-sided knee symptoms after an initial diagnosis of a grade I/II MCL injury [52].

37.6.3 Computerized Tomography and Ultrasound

CT in the setting of MCL injury is rarely utilized. When additional fractures to the tibial plateau or distal femur are suspected, a CT can provide valuable additional information. The use of US to assess in the integrity of the MCL and other ligaments of the knee has noted some recent renewed interest [42, 53]. Given the detail and availability of MRI, coupled with the lack of familiarity many medical practitioners have with US, its use in the setting of MCL injury currently remains limited.

Fact Box 1

Evaluation should always be with standard anteroposterior, 30° lateral flexion, and Merchant patellar knee radiographs.

Stress radiographs are performed at 0° and 20° of flexion. When compared to the contralateral knee medial joint space widening of:

- >1.7 mm and >3.2 mm indicates isolated complete sMCL injury.
- >6.5 mm and >9.8 mm indicates complete injury to the sMCL, dMCL, and POL.

sMCL and dMCL injury location and grade should be evaluated on MRI with increased severity raising the suspicion for concurrent ACL and POL injury.

37.7 Treatment

37.7.1 Grade I and Grade II Injuries

The treatment of MCL injury is often dictated by the clinical severity. Isolated and combined grade I and grade II injuries have historically been treated non-operatively. In contrast to the ACL, the MCL is extra-articular and well vascularized, which is a favorable environment for healing with non-operative treatment [24, 54]. Based on multiple animal studies, the healing of the MCL can be broken down in to four overlapping phases: hemorrhage, inflammation, repair, and remodeling [54–58].

Generally, athletes require a short period of rest followed by a structured and staged rehabilitation program. The use of a hinged brace is not supported by high-quality evidence but may facilitate early motion in the acute post-injury period, especially in grade II injuries [24, 34, 54, 59].

Within the literature, excellent results have been reported consistently with non-operative treatment of isolated grade I and grade II MCL injuries. Kannus, in a retrospective review of 54 partial MCL injuries at 9 years, reported a mean Lysholm score of 94 among patients.[60] In a prospective cohort of 37 patients, Lundberg and Messner reported median Lysholm scores of 96.5 and 100 at 3-month and 4-year follow-up, respectively [61]. At 10-year follow-up, the median Lysholm score was significantly lower at 95, but this is likely clinically insignificant, as patients were still performing at high levels of activity.

Although the vast majority of grade I and grade II MCL injuries respond well to non-operative treatment, a specific subcategory of injuries can at times be recalcitrant to non-operative treatment and cause persistent symptoms. An injury pattern frequently encountered in footballers that requires particular attention presents with pain that is localized just inferior to the femoral epicondyle. Occasionally a palpable thickening of the proximal MCL is also present [52]. Cutting drills, cross-field passing, and any activities where an external rotation type force was applied to the tibia were reported as painful, while straight-line running and simple forceful striking of the ball with the dorsum of the foot was well tolerated. MRI findings in these patients demonstrated grade I or grade II injury to the sMCL but complete rupture of the dMCL from its femoral origin. Although successful treatment of this injury pattern with US-guided cortisone injections has been reported among mainly recreational athletes, results maybe more variable for higher level athletes [62]. In a case series of 15 professional athletes (the majority being professional footballers) that were initially treated with US-guided injection, all had recurrent symptoms at 4 weeks and went on to have surgical treatment [52, 62]. Twelve weeks after operative repair, all patients were asymptomatic and returned to full training. All patients remained asymptomatic at a final mean follow-up of 48 weeks.

37.7.2 Grade III Injury

Treatment of isolated grade III MCL injury should begin with a trial of non-operative treatment [24, 54, 59]. Indelicato was the first to report equivalent patient outcomes with operative repair and non-operative treatment, and since then, multiple authors have reported similar success with non-operative treatment [54, 63–67]. The principals of early weight bearing and range of motion exercises cannot be overemphasized [34]. Athletes should be counseled that although RTP is expected, residual laxity when compared to the contralateral uninjured knee is commonplace. Bracing in the setting of isolated grade III injuries remains controversial, and some authors suggest it may be beneficial in the setting of tibial-sided lesions given their lower propensity to heal [50, 68].

In some instances, operative treatment of isolated grade III MCL injuries is required (Fig. 37.3). The first of these instances is with the aforementioned "Stener lesion of the knee" [51, 68]. Early operative repair is required to remove the interposed tissue before the residual MCL can be reattached to its tibial insertion, usually with a screw and soft tissue washer-type construct. The second case in which surgical treatment is warranted is if chronic pain or instability persists after non-operative treatment [24, 34, 68, 69]. This is more likely to occur in cases of repeat injury or grade III tibial-sided injuries where both the sMCL and dMCL are completely avulsed [50, 69]. In the acute or subacute setting, tissue can be robust enough to allow primary repair, but surgeons should have a low threshold to consider augmentation with allograft or autograft

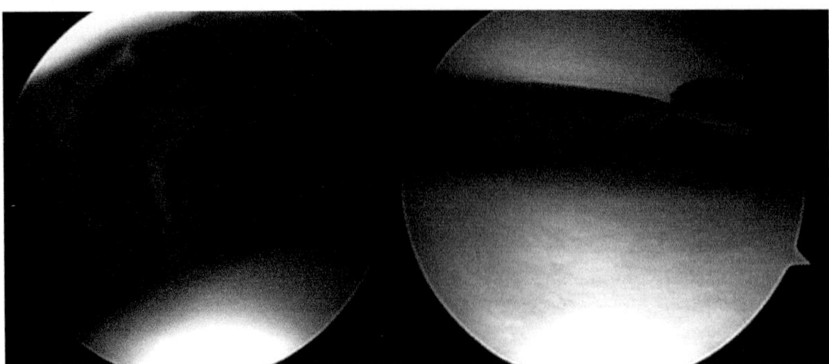

Fig. 37.3 After failure of non-operative management of Grade III tibial-sided MCL avulsion with significant retraction, open repair was performed. Note the arthroscopic "drive-through sign" present in the medial compartment and the sutures placed in remnant MCL tissue. The image on the right was taken after tibial fixation of MCL tissue. The medial compartment has been closed down, and the "drive-through sign" has been eliminated

reconstruction if tissue quality is a concern [68]. It is also important to counsel patients that irrespective of non-operative or operative treatment, residual valgus laxity will always remain after grade III MCL injury [59].

37.7.3 Concurrent ACL Injury

Concurrent ACL ruptures in the setting of MCL injury have generally been treated either with immediate ACL reconstruction coupled with MCL repair/reconstruction or with non-operative treatment of the MCL injury via dedicated rehabilitation protocol and delayed ACL reconstruction [24, 54, 68].

Proponents of immediate surgical treatment cite that the increased valgus laxity present in MCL-deficient patients' places increased forces across the newly reconstructed ACL and therefore may predispose it to failure [54, 70–72]. Residual laxity after ACL reconstruction in patients who did and did not have concurrent MCL injury at the time of surgery has been studied in detail [73]. Despite increased anterior, posterior, and valgus laxity noted in patients with concurrent injury, the clinical significance of these findings remains unclear, as to date increased ACL re-rupture rates in the setting of MCL injury have not been reported.

On the contrary, those favoring ACL reconstruction after healing of the MCL injury fear the higher rates of arthrofibrosis reported with combined ACL/MCL procedures [54, 74]. A recent randomized control trial of operative repair versus non-operative treatment of grade III MCL injury in the setting of ACL reconstruction found that in 47 patients, there was no difference in Lysholm or IKDC functional scores, range of motion, or side-to-side difference of medial joint space gapping on stress radiography [75].

Given the quality of this evidence, many authors now agree that in the setting of grade III ACL/MCL injury, a 6-week trial of non-operative treatment for the MCL is warranted while concurrently undergoing preoperative rehabilitation for eventual ACL reconstruction [24, 49, 54, 68]. At the time of ACL reconstruction, an examination under anesthesia is critical. If the MCL remain incompetent at 30° of flexion with no end point, a concomitant MCL repair or reconstruction is performed. Furthermore, following conservative management of a high-grade MCL injury, the use of hamstring tendon autograft for ACL reconstruction should be approached with caution. Significant scarring can obscure tissue planes rendering dissection of the gracilis and semitendinosus tendons difficult and increasing the risk of graft truncation during harvest.

37.7.4 Anteromedial Rotatory Instability and Multiligamentous Knee Injury

When diagnosing an athlete with a grade III MCL injury, it is important to always consider the presence of anteromedial rotatory instability and multiligamentous knee injury. In the setting of acute anteromedial rotatory instability, early aggressive surgical treatment is recommended by most authors [49, 54, 68]. This can be repaired or reconstructed depending on tissue quality. A detailed discussion of multiligamentous knee injury in football players is beyond the scope of this chapter.

37.7.5 Emerging Treatments

Treatment of ligament and tendon injuries in the field of sports medicine with injection of platelet-rich plasma (PRP) is an emerging treatment. With regard to the MCL, there is currently conflicting animal evidence to suggest efficacy. A histological examination of full-thickness MCL injuries in rabbits treated with a single dose of PRP, found increased blood vessel density at 3 weeks while at 6 weeks collagen alignment was improved when compared to controls [76]. In contrast in a study performed on rats, no difference in histologic or biomechanical properties was noted at 3 weeks between treatment and controls after a single PRP or saline injection in the setting of a full-thickness MCL injury [77].

To date a single case report is published of a 27-year-old professional football player with a grade III femoral-sided MCL injury [78]. Treatment involved a single injection of PRP performed within 48–72 hours of injury without image guidance. Treatment also consisted of a standardized rehabilitation protocol. Training resumed 18 days post-injury, and the patient was able to play in a match at 25 days with no symptoms or functional deficits.

While treatment of MCL injuries with PRP is promising, caution should be exercised. Currently high-level evidence in regards to PRP preparation, injection number, injection timing, and overall efficacy is lacking.

Fact Box 2

Grade I and II as well as isolated grade III MCL injuries generally respond well to non-operative management.

Concurrent ACL/MCL injury should initially be treated with 6 weeks of non-operative treatment after which the integrity of the MCL on examination under anesthesia dictates whether repair or reconstruction of the ligament is warranted.

Anteromedial rotatory instability, grade III tibial-sided avulsions, grade III femoral-sided dMCL with overlying grade I/II sMCL, and "Stener lesions of the knee" require special attention.

37.8 Rehabilitation

37.8.1 Rehabilitation After Non-operative Treatment

Isolated grade I and II MCL injuries can be treated non-operatively, with a concentration on early rehabilitation. Functional bracing of the extremity is utilized as it assists with stability while also allowing full range of motion (ROM) of the knee. Weight bearing is encouraged once pain subsides, with full ROM exercises and progressive strengthening exercises. Optimal loading of injured tissues even in the acute phase is important as it results in improved long-term strength and morphological characteristics of collagenous tissues [79]. Numerous rehabilitation protocols have been described, but they all follow the same general principles: early weight bearing and ROM, followed by progressive strengthening of the quadriceps and hamstrings, and finally RTP [54, 80].

Grade III MCL injuries can also be successfully treated with non-operative management with good long-term results [3]. Historically, treatment consisted of a longer period of immobilization than grade I and II, mostly due to injury of both the superficial and deep portions of the MCL. However, many authors advise against prolonged immobilization due to the detrimental effects on ligament healing [19, 20, 23]. Similar to the treatment of lower-grade injuries, immediate ROM and aggressive early rehabilitation is now advocated [65]. Although timelines are useful to coaches and players as estimates for RTP, it should be emphasized that staged, goal-oriented rehabilitation protocols are recommended and require the injured athlete to meet certain criteria before progressing and ultimately returning to play [81, 82]. A protocol for rehabilitation and RTP after MCL injury adapted from studies by Kim et al. and Logan et al. is depicted in Table 37.1 [82, 83].

37.8.2 Rehabilitation After Operative Treatment

Treatment protocols after MCL surgery varies depending on the severity of the injury and is heavily influenced by concomitant cruciate ligament reconstruction. However, most postoperative programs for surgically treated MCL injuries follow the same general protocol as those treated non-operatively except for several modifications.

37.8.2.1 Phase I Modifications

The knee is placed into a hinged knee brace locked in extension for the first 4–6 weeks with the exception of immediate passive ROM exercises performed with a therapist. Range of motion is generally limited to 0–90° for the first 3 weeks before being progressed to as tolerated [34]. The goal is active ROM from 0° to 120° by 6 weeks.

Table 37.1 Three-phase rehabilitation protocol for medial collateral ligament injuries of the knee

Phase I (acute phase) treatment goal	Intervention
Protect injury and promote healing	Bracing: although evidence is lacking, use of a hinged knee brace with unrestricted ROM can be used to prevent further valgus stress until quadriceps function and gait normalize
	Rest and education: the injured player should be educated on what a valgus knee force is and how it can be avoided during activities of daily living. A common example is dragging the foot of the injured extremity during the initial swing phase of gait
Limit swelling and inflammation	Cryotherapy: (cold whirlpool immersion, intermittent application of ice, application of commercially available joint-specific compression sleeves which cycle cold water)
	Modalities: neuromuscular electrical stimulation, ultrasound
	Elevation, elastic compression wraps
Progression to full weight bearing, regaining ROM, and muscle activation	Progressively wean from all gait aids. Begin with passive ROM progressing to active assisted ROM and finally active ROM. Initiate training on stationary bike as this will also aid in maintaining stamina
Normalizing gait	Gait training which can be initiated in a low resistance aquatic environment
Criteria for progression to phase II: • Minimal effusion • AROM from 0° to 120° • Ability to straight-leg raise without quadriceps lag • Normalized gait	
Phase II (motor control phase) goals	Intervention
Initiate strengthening	Strength training: progress gradually from closed chain to open chain increasing resistance. Exercises should focus on dynamic knee stabilizers especially the quadriceps and hamstring
	Strengthening of additional lower extremity stabilizers such as gluteal musculature, gastrocnemius, and soleus should be initiated

Table 37.1 (continued)

Address causative factors	Full assessment of the athlete should be performed looking for weak hip abductors/external rotators, foot pronation, weak core musculature, or abnormal running mechanics. Review video of the injury identifying means to avoid repeated injury in future
Straight-line jogging	Initiate straight-line jogging first in an aquatic environment or harness supported treadmill. Can progress to normal flat soft surfaces such as a rubberized track, artificial turf, or grass
	Can use alternating jogging, rapid walking to work on cardiorespiratory fitness. Focus also on jogging distance common in football such as 20–30 min at a time
Criteria for progression to phase III: • Comparable strength to unaffected lower extremity on manual muscle tests • No symptoms with straight-line jogging • Potential additional causative factors identified and being actively addressed	
Phase III (return to sport phase)	
Progress from jog to spring	Interval training (sprinting followed by jogging) with focus on sprinting distances common in football such 15–20 m. Gradually increase repetition as speed and if progressing well introduce straight-line ball control/passing and shooting drills
Incorporate football-specific training	Proprioception and plyometric exercises (e.g., single-leg lateral jump) can be initiated with introduction of gentle cutting and change in direction. If progressing well can introduce ball control/passing and shooting drills which involve lateral movement and cutting
Frequent reassessment and careful progression	Ensure to reassess the footballer for symptoms with each step up in activity and intensity Persistent or new symptoms should be carefully evaluated and appropriately treated
Perform performance tests to judge RTP	See Sect. 9 below

ROM range of motion, *RTP* return to play

The patient however is toe-touch weight bearing for the first 6 weeks and is then progressed to weight bearing as tolerated with gradual weaning from gait aids. Patellar mobilization should also begin immediately after surgery to avoid the development of fibrosis in the suprapatellar pouch and to facilitate quadriceps activation [82]. Close attention should also be paid to the surgical wounds ensuring appropriate healing with no signs of infection. Aquatic therapy should not be initiated until all wounds are closed, and clearance is obtained from the treating surgeon. Strengthening in the form of quadriceps sets, straight-leg raises, and ankle pumps should also be initiated within the first week of surgery. Typically the patient can be transitioned from a long postoperative hinged brace to a short functional hinged brace when a straight-leg raise can be performed without quadriceps lag [83]. The use of anti-inflammatory medications postoperatively is controversial and surgeon specific. In order to progress to phase 2 of the rehabilitation protocol, operatively treated patients must meet all the criteria outlined in the phase I nonoperative rehabilitation protocol but also be fully weight bearing without any gait aids [82].

37.8.2.2 Phase II and Phase III Modifications

Both phase II and phase III are expected to be prolonged in the surgically treated patient. This is due to the greater degree of muscle atrophy and proprioceptive dysfunction experienced by these patients [83]. As a result, the benefit of aquatic or harness-based treadmill jogging exercises also increases as it allows for safer correction of asymmetric running [82]. Although evidence is lacking, functional brace use can be discontinued during phase III of the rehabilitation process. Once RTP guidelines are met, there is no evidence that continued bracing prevents future injury in football [54, 82]. Bracing can, however, be indicated during the final sports specific on field rehabilitation stage before full release to RTP.

Fact Box 3

The pillars of non-operative treatment of MCL injuries:

- Early weight bearing
- Aggressive ROM exercises
- Quadriceps and hamstring strengthening

Return to play should be considered when quadriceps and hamstring strength has reached at least 90% of the contralateral side, physical exam demonstrates a stable ligament with a firm end point, and the player has regained physical function and psychological readiness to return.

37.9 Return to Play

Final RTP occurs once patient can practice without pain, quadriceps and hamstring strength has reached that of the contralateral side, and physical examination demonstrates a stable and essentially non-tender ligament with a firm end point [24, 54, 80, 82]. Multiple tests have been proposed to assess muscle strength, proprioception, and neuromuscular control. These include quadriceps index dynamometer testing, the Y-balance test, single-legged hop for distance, and single-legged triple hop for distance [82]. In all instances a value of at least 90% (preferably 100%) compared to the opposite uninjured limb indicates an injured player can RTP. Evidence however is lacking as to which test is best at assessing RTP or predicting reinjury rates [84].

It is important to note that meeting full RTP criteria indicates that a footballer may return to full training including tackling with their respective team. At this point the ultimate decision as to what level a player may return to is at the discretion of the coaching staff. Communication between the medical and coaching staff however is paramount in ensuring safe RTP. At the youth or amateur level, involvement of the coaching staff in simple stepwise protocol where increased stress is placed on the injured knee has been shown to lower reinjury rates [81]. According to the protocol drafted by Hägglund et al., following mild injuries (4–7 day of absence), two full training sessions without subsequent pain or swelling were required before a player was deemed fit for match selection. For moderate (8–28 day absence) and severe (>28 day absence) injuries, three and four such training sessions were required, respectively [81]. Such an algorithm seems therefore reasonable to apply for most coaches acting without any club medical support in the RTP process after grade I and II MCL injuries.

Timelines for RTP are highly variable and dependent on factors such as history of previous injury, injury severity, and presence of other concomitant knee injuries such as ACL rupture or meniscal pathology. A recent study that reported on 346 MCL injuries among 27 professional European football teams over 11 seasons demonstrated that the mean time from injury to RTP was 23 days [3]. Layoff times however were not separated based on injury grade, and therefore the median time of 16 days suggests a preponderance of grade I and uncomplicated grade II injuries in their sample. Another study looking at high school American football players demonstrated that those with grade I MCL injuries returned 10.6 days after injury, while those with grade II MCL injuries returned 19.5 days after injury [85]. In a study of collegiate American football players, a mean RTP time of 10.6 days and 19.5 days was reported for grade I and grade II MCL injuries, respectively [85]. Similar results were found in another prospective cohort of collegiate American football players with grade I or II injuries where a mean RTP time of 21 days was observed [86]. Based on this evidence, we estimate that footballers with grade I MCL injuries that are treated non-operatively can safely RTP after 2–3 weeks, while those with grade II injuries require 3–6 weeks.

The reported timelines for both non-operative and operatively treated grade III injuries are more variable. American football players at the high school level treated non-operatively were reported to RTP at mean time of 34 days [64]. In a cohort of collegiate American football players, full contact play was permitted at a mean of 9.2 weeks [63]. When looking at athletes other than American football players, recovery after non-operative treatment in the order of 8–12 weeks has been reported [65]. RTP in operatively treated patients with either MCL repair or reconstruction is even more variable but is estimated at 6–9 months [68]. Based on the current evidence, football players treated non-operatively with grade III injuries can be expected to RTP at 10–12 weeks. The role of systematic stepwise goal-oriented rehabilitation programs becomes increasingly important with higher-grade injuries. In contrast to those with grade I/II injuries, long-term follow-up has shown that those with grade III injuries irrespective of treatment will have some residual laxity and possibly an increased risk of premature knee osteoarthritis [60, 65].

Take-Home Message An accurate history and physical examination are cornerstones to accurate diagnosis of MCL injuries with radiographic studies used to augment clinical findings.

- Given its extra-articular location, the MCL in the vast majority of cases when injured in isolation or on conjunction with the ACL responds well to non-operative treatment, but with higher-grade MCL injuries, clinicians should remain highly suspicious for multiligamentous knee injury and anteromedial rotatory instability.
- The principles of non-operative treatment include early weight bearing, aggressive range of motion exercises, and progressive strengthening of the quadriceps and hamstrings muscles in the context of a staged goal-oriented rehabilitation protocol.
- Final RTP is recommended once the patient can practice without pain, quadriceps and hamstring strength has reached at least 90% of the contralateral side, physical examination demonstrates a stable ligament with a firm end point, and physical and psychological function is restored.

Top Five Evidence Based References

Lundblad M, Walden M, Magnusson H, Karlsson J, Ekstrand J (2013) The UEFA injury study: 11-year data concerning 346 MCL injuries and time to return to play. Br J Sports Med 47:759–762

Kim C, Chasse PM, Taylor DC (2016) Return to play after medial collateral ligament injury. Clin Sports Med 35:679–696

Wijdicks CA, Griffith CJ, Johansen S, Engebretsen L, LaPrade RF (2010) Injuries to the medial collateral ligament and associated medial structures of the knee. J Bone Joint Surg Am 92:1266–1280

Marchant MH Jr, Tibor LM, Sekiya JK, Hardaker WT Jr, Garrett WE Jr, Taylor DC (2011) Management of medial-sided knee injuries, part 1: medial collateral ligament. Am J Sports Med 39:1102–1113

Halinen J, Lindahl J, Hirvensalo E, Santavirta S (2006) Operative and nonoperative treatments of medial collateral ligament rupture with early anterior cruciate ligament reconstruction: a prospective randomized study. Am J Sports Med 34:1134–1140

References

1. Hagglund M, Walden M, Magnusson H, Kristenson K, Bengtsson H, Ekstrand J (2013) Injuries affect team performance negatively in professional football: an 11-year follow-up of the UEFA Champions League injury study. Br J Sports Med 47:738–742
2. Arnason A, Gudmundsson A, Dahl HA, Johannsson E (1996) Soccer injuries in Iceland. Scand J Med Sci Sports 6:40–45
3. Lundblad M, Walden M, Magnusson H, Karlsson J, Ekstrand J (2013) The UEFA injury study: 11-year data concerning 346 MCL injuries and time to return to play. Br J Sports Med 47:759–762
4. Ekstrand J, Hagglund M, Kristenson K, Magnusson H, Walden M (2013) Fewer ligament injuries but no preventive effect on muscle injuries and severe injuries: an 11-year follow-up of the UEFA Champions League injury study. Br J Sports Med 47:732–737
5. Ekstrand J, Hagglund M, Walden M (2011) Injury incidence and injury patterns in professional football: the UEFA injury study. Br J Sports Med 45:553–558
6. Hagglund M, Walden M, Ekstrand J (2006) Previous injury as a risk factor for injury in elite football: a prospective study over two consecutive seasons. Br J Sports Med 40:767–772

7. Walden M, Hagglund M, Ekstrand J (2006) High risk of new knee injury in elite footballers with previous anterior cruciate ligament injury. Br J Sports Med 40:158–162
8. Hagglund M, Walden M, Ekstrand J (2003) Exposure and injury risk in Swedish elite football: a comparison between seasons 1982 and 2001. Scand J Med Sci Sports 13:364–370
9. LaPrade RF, Engebretsen AH, Ly TV, Johansen S, Wentorf FA, Engebretsen L (2007) The anatomy of the medial part of the knee. J Bone Joint Surg Am 89:2000–2010
10. Warren LF, Marshall JL (1979) The supporting structures and layers on the medial side of the knee: an anatomical analysis. J Bone Joint Surg Am 61:56–62
11. Last R (1948) Some anatomical details of the knee joint. J Bone Joint Surg Br 30:683–688
12. De Maeseneer M, Van Roy F, Lenchik L, Barbaix E, De Ridder F, Osteaux M (2000) Three layers of the medial capsular and supporting structures of the knee: MR imaging-anatomic correlation. Radiographics 20:Spec No:S83-89
13. Hughston JC, Andrews JR, Cross MJ, Moschi A (1976) Classification of knee ligament instabilities. Part I. The medial compartment and cruciate ligaments. J Bone Joint Surg Am 58:159–172
14. Loredo R, Hodler J, Pedowitz R, Yeh LR, Trudell D, Resnick D (1999) Posteromedial corner of the knee: MR imaging with gross anatomic correlation. Skeletal Radiol 28:305–311
15. Hughston JC (1994) The importance of the posterior oblique ligament in repairs of acute tears of the medial ligaments in knees with and without an associated rupture of the anterior cruciate ligament. Results of long-term follow-up. J Bone Joint Surg Am 76:1328–1344
16. Robinson JR, Bull AM, Amis AA (2005) Structural properties of the medial collateral ligament complex of the human knee. J Biomech 38:1067–1074
17. Creighton RA, Spang JT, Dahners LE (2005) Basic science of ligament healing: medial collateral ligament healing with and without treatment. Sports Med Arthrosc 13:145–150
18. Weiss JA, Woo SLY, Ohland KJ, Horibe S, Newton PO (1991) Evaluation of a new injury model to study medial collateral ligament healing: primary repair versus nonoperative treatment. J Orthop Res 9:516–528
19. Bray RC, Leonard CA, Salo PT (2002) Vascular physiology and long-term healing of partial ligament tears. J Orthop Res 20:984–989
20. Frank C, Woo SL, Amiel D, Harwood F, Gomez M, Akeson W (1983) Medial collateral ligament healing. A multidisciplinary assessment in rabbits. Am J Sports Med 11:379–389
21. Frank CB, Loitz BJ, Shrive NG (1995) Injury location affects ligament healing. A morphologic and mechanical study of the healing rabbit medial collateral ligament. Acta Orthop Scand 66:455–462
22. Amiel D, Akeson WH, Harwood FL, Frank CB (1983) Stress deprivation effect on metabolic turnover of the medial collateral ligament collagen. A comparison between nine- and 12-week immobilization. Clin Orthop Relat Res:265–270
23. Walsh S, Frank C, Hart D (1992) Immobilization alters cell metabolism in an immature ligament. Clin Orthop Relat Res:277–288
24. LaPrade RF, Wijdicks CA (2012) The management of injuries to the medial side of the knee. J Orthop Sports Phys Ther 42:221–233
25. Peterson L, Junge A, Chomiak J, Graf-Baumann T, Dvorak J (2000) Incidence of football injuries and complaints in different age groups and skill-level groups. Am J Sports Med 28:S51–S57
26. Griffith CJ, Wijdicks CA, LaPrade RF, Armitage BM, Johansen S, Engebretsen L (2009) Force measurements on the posterior oblique ligament and superficial medial collateral ligament proximal and distal divisions to applied loads. Am J Sports Med 37:140–148
27. Walden M, Hagglund M, Magnusson H, Ekstrand J (2011) Anterior cruciate ligament injury in elite football: a prospective three-cohort study. Knee Surg Sports Traumatol Arthrosc 19:11–19
28. Ekstrand J, Gillquist J, Liljedahl SO (1983) Prevention of soccer injuries. Supervision by doctor and physiotherapist. Am J Sports Med 11:116–120
29. Junge A, Rosch D, Peterson L, Graf-Baumann T, Dvorak J (2002) Prevention of soccer injuries: a prospective intervention study in youth amateur players. Am J Sports Med 30:652–659
30. Soligard T, Myklebust G, Steffen K, Holme I, Silvers H, Bizzini M et al (2008) Comprehensive warm-up programme to prevent injuries in young female footballers: cluster randomised controlled trial. BMJ a2469:337
31. Walden M, Atroshi I, Magnusson H, Wagner P, Hagglund M (2012) Prevention of acute knee injuries in adolescent female football players: cluster randomised controlled trial. BMJ 344:e3042
32. Association AM (1966) Committee on the medical aspects of sports, Subcommittee on classification of sports injuries. Standard nomenclature of athletic injuries. AMA, Chicago, IL, p 126
33. Griffith CJ, LaPrade RF, Johansen S, Armitage B, Wijdicks C, Engebretsen L (2009) Medial knee injury: Part 1, static function of the individual components of the main medial knee structures. Am J Sports Med 37:1762–1770
34. Wijdicks CA, Griffith CJ, Johansen S, Engebretsen L, LaPrade RF (2010) Injuries to the medial collateral ligament and associated medial structures of the knee. J Bone Joint Surg Am 92:1266–1280
35. Norwood LA Jr, Hughston JC (1980) Combined anterolateral-anteromedial rotatory instability of the knee. Clin Orthop Relat Res 147:62–67
36. Robinson JR, Bull AM, Amis AA (2006) The role of the medial collateral ligament and posteromedial capsule in controlling knee laxity. Am J Sports Med 34:1815–1823

37. Lonergan KT, Taylor DC (2002) Medial collateral ligament injuries of the knee: an evolution of surgical reconstruction. Techniques in Knee. Surgery 1:137–145
38. Escobedo EM, Mills WJ, Hunter JC (2002) The "reverse Segond" fracture: association with a tear of the posterior cruciate ligament and medial meniscus. AJR Am J Roentgenol 178:979–983
39. Gottsegen CJ, Eyer BA, White EA, Learch TJ, Forrester D (2008) Avulsion fractures of the knee: imaging findings and clinical significance. Radiographics 28:1755–1770
40. Lee CH, Tan CF, Kim O, Suh KJ, Yao MS, Chan WP et al (2016) Osseous injury associated with ligamentous tear of the knee. Can Assoc Radiol J 67:379–386
41. Chan KK, Resnick D, Goodwin D, Seeger LL (1999) Posteromedial tibial plateau injury including avulsion fracture of the semimembranous tendon insertion site: ancillary sign of anterior cruciate ligament tear at MR imaging. Radiology 211:754–758
42. Craft JA, Kurzweil PR (2015) Physical examination and imaging of medial collateral ligament and posteromedial corner of the knee. Sports Med Arthrosc 23:e1–e6
43. James EW, Williams BT, LaPrade RF (2014) Stress radiography for the diagnosis of knee ligament injuries: a systematic review. Clin Orthop Relat Res 472:2644–2657
44. Sawant M, Narasimha Murty A, Ireland J (2004) Valgus knee injuries: evaluation and documentation using a simple technique of stress radiography. Knee 11:25–28
45. LaPrade RF, Bernhardson AS, Griffith CJ, Macalena JA, Wijdicks CA (2010) Correlation of valgus stress radiographs with medial knee ligament injuries: an in vitro biomechanical study. Am J Sports Med 38:330–338
46. Chen J, Abel MF, Fox MG (2015) Imaging appearance of entrapped periosteum within a distal femoral Salter-Harris II fracture. Skeletal Radiol 44:1547–1551
47. Veenema KR (1999) Valgus knee instability in an adolescent: ligament sprain or physeal fracture? Phys Sportsmed 27:62–75
48. Sanders TG, Miller MD (2005) A systematic approach to magnetic resonance imaging interpretation of sports medicine injuries of the knee. Am J Sports Med 33:131–148
49. Tibor LM, Marchant MH Jr, Taylor DC, Hardaker WT Jr, Garrett WE Jr, Sekiya JK (2011) Management of medial-sided knee injuries, part 2: posteromedial corner. Am J Sports Med 39:1332–1340
50. Wilson TC, Satterfield WH, Johnson DL (2004) Medial collateral ligament "tibial" injuries: indication for acute repair. Orthopedics 27:389–393
51. Corten K, Hoser C, Fink C, Bellemans J (2010) Case reports: a Stener-like lesion of the medial collateral ligament of the knee. Clin Orthop Relat Res 468:289–293
52. Narvani A, Mahmud T, Lavelle J, Williams A (2010) Injury to the proximal deep medial collateral ligament: a problematical subgroup of injuries. J Bone Joint Surg Br 92:949–953
53. De Maeseneer M, Marcelis S, Boulet C, Kichouh M, Shahabpour M, de Mey J et al (2014) Ultrasound of the knee with emphasis on the detailed anatomy of anterior, medial, and lateral structures. Skeletal Radiol 43:1025–1039
54. Marchant MH Jr, Tibor LM, Sekiya JK, Hardaker WT Jr, Garrett WE Jr, Taylor DC (2011) Management of medial-sided knee injuries, part 1: medial collateral ligament. Am J Sports Med 39:1102–1113
55. Hart DP, Dahners LE (1987) Healing of the medial collateral ligament in rats. The effects of repair, motion, and secondary stabilizing ligaments. J Bone Joint Surg Am 69:1194–1199
56. Lechner CT, Dahners LE (1991) Healing of the medial collateral ligament in unstable rat knees. Am J Sports Med 19:508–512
57. Woo SL, Inoue M, McGurk-Burleson E, Gomez MA (1987) Treatment of the medial collateral ligament injury. II: structure and function of canine knees in response to differing treatment regimens. Am J Sports Med 15:22–29
58. Wright RW, Parikh M, Allen T, Brodt MD, Silva MJ, Botney MD (2003) Effect of hemorrhage on medial collateral ligament healing in a mouse model. Am J Sports Med 31:660–666
59. Smyth MP, Koh JL (2015) A review of surgical and nonsurgical outcomes of medial knee injuries. Sports Med Arthrosc 23:e15–e22
60. Kannus P (1988) Long-term results of conservatively treated medial collateral ligament injuries of the knee joint. Clin Orthop Relat Res:103–112
61. Lundberg M, Messner K (1996) Long-term prognosis of isolated partial medial collateral ligament ruptures: a ten-year clinical and radiographic evaluation of a prospectively observed group of patients. Am J Sports Med 24:160–163
62. Jones L, Bismil Q, Alyas F, Connell D, Bell J (2009) Persistent symptoms following non operative management in low grade MCL injury of the knee - the role of the deep MCL. Knee 16:64–68
63. Indelicato PA (1983) Non-operative treatment of complete tears of the medial collateral ligament of the knee. J Bone Joint Surg Am 65:323–329
64. Jones RE, Henley MB, Francis P (1986) Nonoperative management of isolated grade III collateral ligament injury in high school football players. Clin Orthop Relat Res:137–140
65. Reider B, Sathy MR, Talkington J, Blyznak N, Kollias S (1994) Treatment of isolated medial collateral ligament injuries in athletes with early functional rehabilitation: a five-year follow-up study. Am J Sports Med 22:470–477
66. Sandberg R, Balkfors B, Nilsson B, Westlin N (1987) Operative versus non-operative treatment of recent

injuries to the ligaments of the knee. A prospective randomized study. J Bone Joint Surg Am 69:1120–1126
67. Shelbourne KD, Porter DA (1992) Anterior cruciate ligament-medial collateral ligament injury: nonoperative management of medial collateral ligament tears with anterior cruciate ligament reconstruction. A preliminary report. Am J Sports Med 20:283–286
68. Roth J, Taylor DC (2015) Management of acute isolated medial and posteromedial instability of the knee. Sports Med Arthrosc 23:71–76
69. Jiang KN, West RV (2015) Management of chronic combined ACL medial posteromedial instability of the knee. Sports Med Arthrosc 23:85–90
70. Battaglia MJ II, Lenhoff MW, Ehteshami JR, Lyman S, Provencher MT, Wickiewicz TL et al (2009) Medial collateral ligament injuries and subsequent load on the anterior cruciate ligament: a biomechanical evaluation in a cadaveric model. Am J Sports Med 37:305–311
71. Carson EW, Anisko EM, Restrepo C, Panariello RA, O'Brien SJ, Warren RF (2004) Revision anterior cruciate ligament reconstruction: etiology of failures and clinical results. J Knee Surg 17:127–132
72. Ichiba A, Nakajima M, Fujita A, Abe M (2003) The effect of medial collateral ligament insufficiency on the reconstructed anterior cruciate ligament: a study in the rabbit. Acta Orthop Scand 74:196–200
73. Zaffagnini S, Bignozzi S, Martelli S, Lopomo N, Marcacci M (2007) Does ACL reconstruction restore knee stability in combined lesions?: an in vivo study. Clin Orthop Relat Res 454:95–99
74. Robins AJ, Newman AP, Burks RT (1993) Postoperative return of motion in anterior cruciate ligament and medial collateral ligament injuries. The effect of medial collateral ligament rupture location. Am J Sports Med 21:20–25
75. Halinen J, Lindahl J, Hirvensalo E, Santavirta S (2006) Operative and nonoperative treatments of medial collateral ligament rupture with early anterior cruciate ligament reconstruction: a prospective randomized study. Am J Sports Med 34:1134–1140
76. Yoshioka T, Kanamori A, Washio T, Aoto K, Uemura K, Sakane M et al (2013) The effects of plasma rich in growth factors (PRGF-Endoret) on healing of medial collateral ligament of the knee. Knee Surg Sports Traumatol Arthrosc 21:1763–1769
77. Amar E, Snir N, Sher O, Brosh T, Khashan M, Salai M et al (2015) Platelet-rich plasma did not improve early healing of medial collateral ligament in rats. Arch Orthop Trauma Surg 135:1571–1577
78. Eirale C, Mauri E, Hamilton B (2013) Use of platelet rich plasma in an isolated complete medial collateral ligament lesion in a professional football (soccer) player: a case report. Asian J Sports Med 4:158–162
79. Bleakley CM, Glasgow P, MacAuley DC (2012) PRICE needs updating, should we call the POLICE? Br J Sports Med 46:220–221
80. Lundberg M, Messner K (1996) Long-term prognosis of isolated partial medial collateral ligament ruptures. A ten-year clinical and radiographic evaluation of a prospectively observed group of patients. Am J Sports Med 24:160–163
81. Hagglund M, Walden M, Ekstrand J (2007) Lower reinjury rate with a coach-controlled rehabilitation program in amateur male soccer: a randomized controlled trial. Am J Sports Med 35:1433–1442
82. Kim C, Chasse PM, Taylor DC (2016) Return to play after medial collateral ligament injury. Clin Sports Med 35:679–696
83. Logan CA, O'Brien LT, LaPrade RF (2016) Post operative rehabilitation of grade III medial collateral ligament injuries: evidence based rehabilitation and return to play. Int J Sports Phys Ther 11:1177–1190
84. Hegedus EJ, McDonough S, Bleakley C, Cook CE, Baxter GD (2015) Clinician-friendly lower extremity physical performance measures in athletes: a systematic review of measurement properties and correlation with injury, part 1. The tests for knee function including the hop tests. Br J Sports Med 49:642–648
85. Derscheid GL, Garrick JG (1981) Medial collateral ligament injuries in football. Nonoperative management of grade I and grade II sprains. Am J Sports Med 9:365–368
86. Holden DL, Eggert AW, Butler JE (1983) The nonoperative treatment of grade I and II medial collateral ligament injuries to the knee. Am J Sports Med 11:340–344

38 Managing Chronic Medial Collateral Injuries

Peter B. Gifford and Fares S. Haddad

Contents

P.B. Gifford, BSc (PT), MBBS, FRACS (Orth) (✉)
F.S. Haddad, BSc MCh, FRCS, FRCS Dip, Sp Med
University College Hospital, 235 Euston Road, London NW1 2BU, UK
e-mail: pbgifford@email.com

38.1 Introduction

The medial collateral ligament (MCL) is commonly injured in sport, occupying approximately 30% of isolated knee ligament injuries and an additional 13% of combined injuries [1]. Of all knee injuries in soccer, the medial collateral ligament is the most frequently injured structure among all levels of play and all age groups. The blood supply is extensive, dwindling proximal to distal, commonly leading to primary healing and effective resolution of the instability [2]. Chronic symptoms may develop due to laxity and instability, or alternatively the primary symptom may be persistent pain. Persistent pain may develop due to pathological scar, calcification or bursitis. High-grade injuries, especially in setting of combined ligament injury, are more likely to heal with persistent laxity.

38.2 Epidemiology

Knee instability often occurs in multiple planes with rotational and translational instability in addition to valgus instability. Football players are often exposed to MCL injuries due to the nature of the sport. Frequent valgus forces stress the knee during contact made in tackles, especially when the foot is planted, and also landing

V. Musahl et al. (eds.), *Return to Play in Football*, https://doi.org/10.1007/978-3-662-55713-6_38

under pressure from aerials or making rapid changes in direction. Depending on the degree of flexion of the knee, there may be a various component of torsional stress to the valgus force. External rotation of the tibia creates stress in the MCL rather than internal rotation [3]. Chronic medial instability can also result from failed ACL/PCL or combined ligament reconstructions [4].

Injuries to the MCL are common, occupying over 40% of acute knee ligament injuries of the knee [1]. Roach examined data from 17,000 army recruits with MCL injury and noted cadets lost time due to injury, with an average of 23 days, remarkably the same as the results gathered from the UEFA 11-year data review of MCL injuries [5]. The UEFA study also reveals the MCL is the sixth most commonly injury in elite footballers. Injury was nine times more common during match play than practice. At the professional level, a team with a roster of 25 players can expect two MCL injuries per season.

The ligament often heals reliably with non-operative management; however, up to 20% have been speculated to have persistent symptoms [6]. Chronic valgus instability is more likely after severe (grade III) MCL injuries but may develop also in repetative low-grade injuries. Footballers have greater susceptibility to chronic symptoms in lesser grade injuries due to repetitive inside boot kicking and side to side movements.

38.3 Pathoanatomy

Classically the medial side of the knee is divided into three structures. The first layer, of the sartorius and its fascia wrap around the knee. The second layer, or superficial MCL, that starts medial and posterior to the medial epicondyle remains extracapsular and then inserts on soft tissue approximately 4.5 cm below the articular surface of the tibia. The broad insertion site continues distally, approximately 7 cm, eventually blending with the periosteum beneath the pes anserinus (Fig. 38.1). Layer III is the medial joint capsule which thickens to forms the deep MCL. The capsule thickens into a vertically oriented band of short fibres representing the dMCL which forms directly under the parallel fibres of the superficial MCL [7]. The deep structure is a distinct but inseparable layer to the joint capsule. The deep MCL is divided into meniscofemoral and meniscotibial ligaments which insert directly onto the edge of the tibial plateau and medial meniscus. The superficial and deep MCL are separated by a bursa, though not routinely seen on imaging [8] (Fig. 38.2). This is biomechanically important for excursion of the ligaments during flexion and extension. Posteriorly the proximal portion

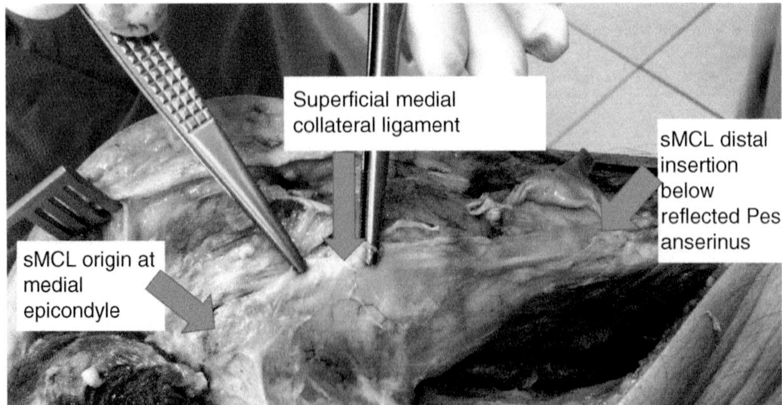

Fig. 38.1 Superficial MCL with origin at the medial epicondyle and long distal insertion below the pes anserinus

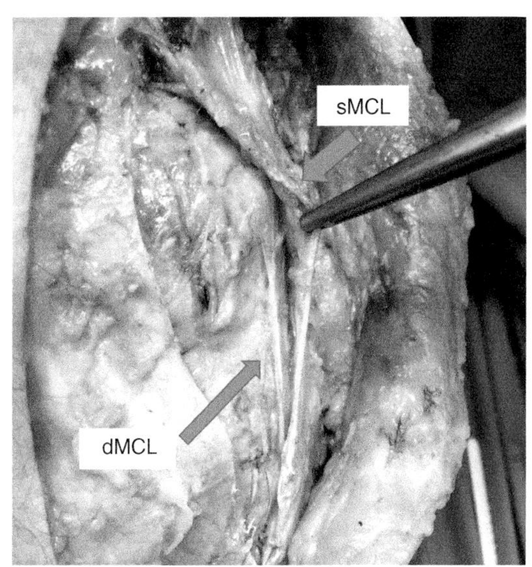

Fig. 38.2 Deep and superficial MCL with bursal space in between. Note also the attachment of the dMCL to the medial meniscus

Fact Box 1
MCL is the most common structure injured in the knee of footballers.

MCL trauma is the second most serious injury to footballers after hamstring trauma.

MCL is weaker than the lateral collateral and cruciate ligaments.

MCL injury occurs in the dominant leg 60% of time.

MCL injuries on average take 23 days for player to RTP.

extends distally, blending with the posteromedial capsule. The medial side of the knee is protected with dynamic stabilisers including the pes anserinus when the knee is in terminal degrees of extension. The MCL is also supported by the vastus medialis with its attachments to the superficial MCL [9].

Persistent pain arising from low-grade injuries has been hypothesised to arise from the deep MCL [10]. The superficial MCL has a well-described progression in healing as an extra-articular ligament. The deep MCL injury may be seen arthroscopically and theoretically may be compromised in healing if synovial fluid interrupts haematoma and progression of maturing collagen [11] (Fig. 38.3). Healing of the MCL following injury is optimal when the torn ends are in contact, but accumulation of large proteoglycans in the healing tissue has been implicated in ongoing inflammation. Pathological scar formation has poorer collagen fibre properties with narrower fibrils, in a thicker healing MCL. This leads to weaker tissue, with up to half the tensile strength of the normal MCL up to 2 years post injury, leaving vulnerability to further injury [4].

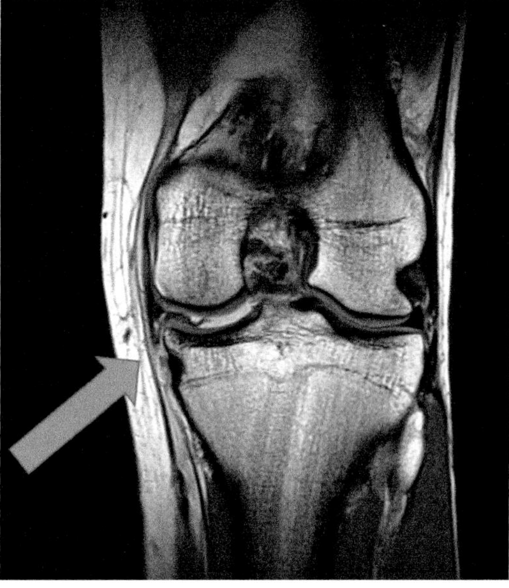

Fig. 38.3 T1-weighted MRI coronal image of high-energy MCL injury with picture demonstrating displacement of sMCL and dMCL into the joint space

38.4 Assessment

The key elements of chronic MCL history include persistent isolated medial knee pain with dynamic activities. There is pain with running, change of direction, pivoting and catching the foot. The most common subjective pain is from the passing action of the football player with short stabbing passes with the knee flexed 15–30° and a sudden external rotation. The player may present after completing the standard bracing and rehabilitation protocol, but attempts to progress dynamic activities reveal disabling pain medially. Diagnosis of a chronic condition can be considered with persistent symptoms after 2 months of conventional treatment [10].

More commonly than pain alone, failure of return to play is due to dynamic instability which may have demonstrable laxity with stress testing. Stability of the medial structures is important for football players to generate power kicking off the inside boot and changing direction with acceleration. The high incidence of MCL injuries in football reflects the uniquely high demand of the ligament complex in this sport.

MCL injuries are traditionally classified according to the criteria of Bergfield [12] with grade I strains consisting of tenderness over the MCL with no instability to valgus stress in full extension or at 25–30° of flexion, grade II consisting of tenderness over the MCL with no instability in extension but greater than 10° in 25–30° flexion with a definite end point and grade III injuries demonstrating laxity in both extension and slight flexion. Any asymmetry should be considered a positive finding. Increase of 3–5 mm compared to the normal side signifies an injury to the superficial MCL. Laxity of 5–7 mm may suggest further injury to the deep MCL, posterior oblique ligament and/or posteromedial corner [13]. More than 7 mm laxity is thought to indicate additional injury to the ACL and up to 20 mm of laxity is seen with bicruciate injury [14].

On examination the player will have isolated pain on palpation of the meniscofemoral component of the deep MCL. The ligament may feel thickened rolling the finger over it. MCL laxity tests may be negative for gapping but provocative of the pain. This may be combined with rapid external rotation of the tibia with the valgus knee stress at 30° of flexion.

The Swain test described by Lonergan and Taylor [15] isolates the MCL and is useful in diagnosing chronic MCL injuries. With the knee flexed to 90°, the tibia is externally rotated. When the knee is externally rotating in flexion, the collateral ligaments are tightened, while the cruciates are relatively lax. Many patients with chronic medial-sided laxity after injury have pain along the medial joint line with this manoeuver. The test is useful to identify the MCL as the source of the persistent medial-sided pain and useful examination to measure response to treatment and determine when the athlete is ready to return to play [9].

Other sources of pain should be considered and excluded, including medial meniscus instability, chondral damage, bone contusion, saphenous nerve entrapment and of course referred pain [16].

Medial collateral ligament bursitis has been described in adults and children as a distended and inflamed bursa between the superficial and deep portions of the MCL. Kerlan and Glousman [17] considered MCL bursitis to be an important cause of chronic medial knee pain, which should be differentiated from other more common medial knee condition. Bursitis may develop secondary to trauma, but also osteophytes, friction, genu valgus knees and planovalgus feet have all been suggested as possible exacerbates. The bursa of the pes anserinus or semimembranosus should also be considered.

38.5 Imaging

Plain radiographs will identify ossification of the proximal superficial MCL known as the Pellegrini-Stieda lesion. This is often an incidental finding, and many believe this is part of an alternate process that does not need surgical intervention [18, 19].

Valgus stress tests radiographs with the knee in 25–30 flexion may be useful to document variation in laxity between the affected side and the normal side.

Ultrasound can identify an inflamed and torn ligament showing thickened and heterogeneous tissue or inflamed bursa. A normal MCL on ultrasound will appear as an elongated band, 1–3 mm thick. The meniscofemoral and meniscotibial structures are hyperechoic, separated by the hypoechoic fat layer.

Magnetic resonance imaging (MRI) is useful to determine extent and location of injury to the MCL. Location of the injury is important for prognosis; femoral avulsions typically healing well, mid-substance injuries may have variable degrees of laxity, and tibial insertional injuries may be complicated by 'Stener'-type lesions, leaving the distal MCL blocked from the tibial periosteum by the pes anserinus. It is crucial in the work up of chronic conditions to exclude other potential confounding sources of pain. Consideration must be given to the medial meniscus, osteo or chondral lesions, a superficial nerve compression or tendinopathy.

Fact Box 2

MRI classification of MCL injury uses the same scale as other ligament injuries.

Grade I injury: High signal is seen superficial to the ligament, which looks normal.
Grade II injury: High signal is seen superficial and within the ligament.
Grade III injury: Complete disruption of the ligament [20].

Schweitzer et al. [20] also accepted there was poor correlation between clinical and radiological classification. They suggested that the key reporting information should be simply 'complete' vs 'incomplete' injury to ligament.

38.6 Treatment

38.6.1 Non-operative

Injection with steroid and local anaesthetic has been shown to be effective for persistent pain in the low-grade MCL tear. Jones [10] described a technique using 2 ml of bupivacaine and 40 mg of Triamcinolone injected with ultrasound guidance deep and superficial to the deep MCL, combined with deep needling of the affected ligament. The players were immediately re-enrolled in active rehabilitation and excluding loss to follow-up, all returned to preinjury level of activity.

Autologous blood and platelet-rich plasma (PRP) have been used to promote healing of tendons and ligaments by the introduction of blood products. These constituents have both anti-inflammatory and pro-inflammatory effects that depend on the degree of platelet activation. Anecdotal evidence for the use of PRP in MCL injuries has been described [21], and there have been mixed results in animal studies [22].

Proliferative injection therapy has also gained popularity in the sports medicine world. This describes the application of an irritant substance, most commonly hyperosmolar dextrose, to stimulate growth factor production and fibroblast proliferation. The theory for its use is that fibroblasts promote extracellular matrix production and healing of disrupted collagen fibres. There is conflicting evidence regarding the efficacy of this technique. It has been described for sprains of the anterior talofibular ligament. A recent animal study has shown the dextrose injection increases the cross-sectional area of the injured MCL but does not improve the mechanical qualities or the laxity of the ligament [23].

38.6.2 Operative

Persistent pain that fails to respond to non-surgical rehabilitation, then also refractory to injections may ultimately require surgery. Surgeon A. Williams describes a series of 17 elite athletes which required surgical intervention at an average of 24 post weeks post injury due to pain after failing functional rehabilitation. Fifteen of the 17 patients in his series did also have an US-guided injection of steroid and local anaesthetic, which failed to cure the persisting symptoms. The authors reported a consistent surgical finding, a failure of healing of a tear of the deep MCL at its femoral origin which could be repaired. Williams describes a layered dissecting and repair of the dMCL and sMCL with 'double-breasting' technique to remove ligament laxity.

Corten [8] describes a technique for players with chronic medial knee pain. The technique involves dissection of the chronic medial inflammatory tissue and then followed by repair. The patient is supine with the affected limb in Fig. 38.4. The approach requires careful exposure of the three layers of the medial knee to identify the pathological tissue and to allow suitable repair. The layers are opened with vertical incisions, and the chronic inflammatory tissue is excised in an ellipse. The remaining tissue is then used to close the interval in layers with absorbable braided sutures.

The players were immobilised in a brace at 30° for 5 weeks with immediate isometric quadriceps and hamstring exercises. Weight-bearing began after 3 weeks to allow PWB to 5 weeks, then FWB. At 12 weeks the players full training activities and allowed to return to play when deemed match fit.

Repair of existing local medial tissue has been shown to be effective in improving medial stability of the knee [24]. Repair of the local tissues alone however may not be adequate to restore stability of the knee [15]. The compromise in structurally sound collagen due to the injury leaves insufficient patent local tissue available for an effective repair at times. Several techniques are described using either local autograft or allograft to reconstruct the medial stabilisers of the knee.

LaPrade and co-authors [7, 14, 25] have extended our knowledge of the posterior oblique ligament (POL) and its anatomy and role in the stability of the knee in extension and rotation. In their technique, allograft is placed in very specific points referencing the adductor tubercle and joint line. Two separate independent grafts are positioned and secured with soft tissue anchors and bioabsorbable screws to reconstruct the POL and sMCL. Their study of 28 patients, with mix of acute and chronic injuries, demonstrated effective elimination of medial opening with stress testing up to 24 months post-operatively [25].

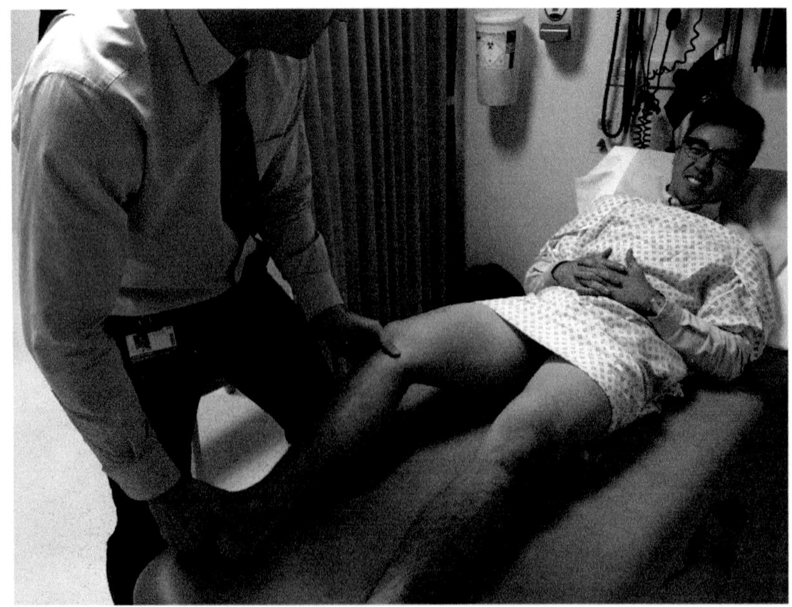

Fig. 38.4 Combined valgus stress test—valgus stress with external rotation of tibia to detect irritability of deep MCL

The semitendinosus tendon is popular as autograft for its location and dimensions. It may be released distally to attempt an entirely anatomical reconstruction or left attached distally to take advantage of its native attachment site. Lind et al. [26] describe their technique of reconstruction of the MCL and posteromedial corner in chronic injury cases. All cases were at least 2 months post injury and had failed non-operative management. The semitendinosus was left attached at the pes anserinus and fixed on the femur at the isometric point and then also to the posteromedial corner of the tibia, deep and posterior to the insertion of the semimembranosus. For isolated MCL reconstruction procedures, a hinged brace was used for 6 weeks. During the first 2 weeks, partial weight-bearing and 0°–90° of motion were allowed. From week 3 to 6, free range of motion and free weight-bearing during standing and walking were permitted. After 6 weeks, free activity was allowed without the brace. Controlled sports activities were allowed after 3 months and contact sports after 6 months. They had follow-up of more than 24 months in 50 patients. In these patients, follow-up demonstrated 10 point improvement in KOOS scores, all but two returned to recreational sport or better [26].

The semitendinosus, as part of the pes anserinus, forms part of the dynamic stabilisation of medial knee, which is lost when used for reconstruction. Augmentation may be achieved with allograft or synthetic graft instead, to protect the native medial structures. The author has demonstrated an effective and safe technique using the 'ligament augmentation and reconstruction system' (LARS®) artificial ligament (Surgical Implants and Devices, Arc-sur-Tille, France) to augment repair. Thirty elite athletes who failed non-operative management with bracing and all but two functional rehabilitation underwent surgical reconstruction and augmentation with synthetic graft. The players were followed up for 1–2 years, and all but two successfully returned to their previous level of sport with an average Tegner score of 9.5.

This chapter has focused on isolated MCL injuries; however chronic instability may be due to combined ligament deficiencies also (Fig. 38.5). When medial collateral injury is combined with anterior cruciate deficiency, significant anterior, valgus and rotatory laxity of the knee occurs [27]. Combined ACL/MCL/PMC injury has an estimated frequency of 6.7% [28]. The anterior cruciate ligament primarily controls anterior translation, but when disrupted, the medial side of the knee contributes significantly. The sMCL contributes at 90° of flexion and the dMCL and POL stabilises in all angles of flexion. The question of whether a low-grade MCL deficiency should be reconstructed in the setting of an acute ACL injury has not been definitively answered [27]. Although biomechanical studies have shown increased stress transferred to ACL grafts when the medial side laxity is not addressed surgically, this has not been shown to have clinical significance in short-term studies [29, 30]. Zhang et al. published their series of 21 patients who underwent ACL-MCL reconstruction for chronic ACL and grade III MCL injuries. At an average of 3.4-year follow-up, the International Knee Documentation Committee was significantly improved from 45 to 87, and 95% patients had normal or near-normal knee ROM. They concluded that combined reconstruction of ACL and all but two MCL can significantly improve stability and clinical outcomes in the short term for chronic combined ACL-MCL injuries.

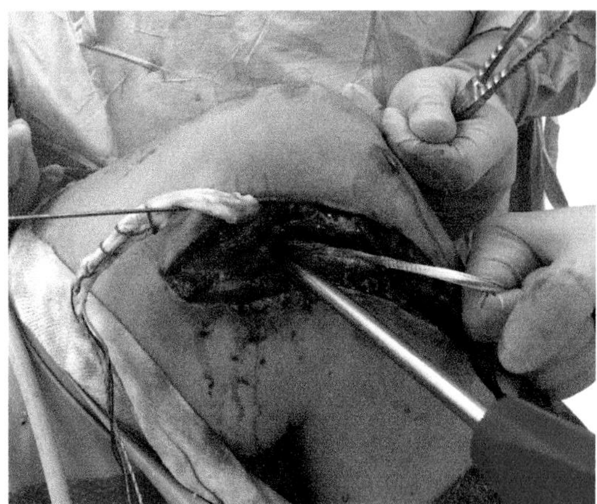

Fig. 38.5 MCL augmentation with LARS® in combined PCL and MCL reconstruction

Jiang and West describe their preference for using a medial closing-wedge distal femoral osteotomy with a blade plate in patients with chronic medial-sided laxity and valgus malalignment. Osteotomies are performed in the setting of chronic medial-sided laxity and valgus malalignment as seen on 3-joint standing x-rays. Excessive valgus malalignment is defined as the weight-bearing line falling lateral to lateral tibial spine into the lateral compartment or >10° of valgus malalignment of the mechanical axis [27].

38.7 Return-to-Play Guidelines

- Full range of motion
- No instability (firm end feel of valgus stress)
- Player confidence
- Muscle strength 85% of the contralateral side
- Proprioception ability is satisfactory
- No tenderness over the medial collateral ligament
- No effusion
- Quadriceps strength; torque/body weight
- Satisfactory in sport specific training and metric assessment of knee function

Take-Home Message

- The medial collateral ligament is the key stabiliser to valgus stress.
- Medial collateral injuries are common and result in missed training and play.
- Incomplete injuries are usually self-limiting but may develop into dynamic instability and chronic medial knee pain.
- In chronic pain, examination is the key element of assessment, supported with imaging.
- Risk of chronic symptoms increases when there is associated injury to cruciates or posterior oblique ligament.
- Mainstay of treatment in chronic pain cases is non-surgical, with novel ultrasound injection therapies. Some refractory cases will respond to surgery.
- Chronic dynamic instability cases recover well after reconstruction with demonstrated return to play.

Top 5 Best Evidence References

Jones L, Bismil Q, Alyas F, Connell D, Bell J (2009) Persistent symptoms following non operative management in low grade MCL injury of the knee – the role of the deep MCL. Knee 16(1):64–68

LaPrade RF, Engebretsen AH, Ly TV, Johansen S, Wentorf FA, Engebretsen L (2007) The anatomy of the medial part of the knee. J Bone Joint Surg Am 89(9):2000–2010

Lind M, Jakobsen BW, Lund B, Hansen MS, Abdallah O, Christiansen SE (2009) Anatomical reconstruction of the medial collateral ligament and posteromedial corner of the knee in patients with chronic medial collateral ligament instability. Am J Sports Med 37(6):1116–1122

Lundblad M, Waldén M, Magnusson H, Karlsson J, Ekstrand J (2013) The UEFA injury study: 11-year data concerning 346 MCL injuries and time to return to play. Br J Sports Med 47(12):759–762

Narvani A, Mahmud T, Lavelle J, Williams A (2010) Injury to the proximal deep medial collateral ligament: a problematical subgroup of injuries. J Bone Joint Surg Br 92(7):949–953

References

1. Bollen S (2000) Epidemiology of knee injuries: diagnosis and triage. Br J Sports Med 34(3):227–228
2. Indelicato PA (1995) Isolated medial collateral ligament injuries in the knee. J Am Acad Orthop Surg 3(1):9–14
3. Griffith CJ, LaPrade RF, Johansen S, Armitage B, Wijdicks C, Engebretsen L (2009) Medial knee injury: part 1, static function of the individual components of the main medial knee structures. Am J Sports Med 37(9):1762–1770
4. Heybeli N, Komur B, Yilmas B, Guler O (2016) Tendons and ligaments. In: Korkusuz F (ed) Musculoskeletal research and basic science. Springer, Cham, pp 465–482
5. Lundblad M, Waldén M, Magnusson H, Karlsson J, Ekstrand J (2013) The UEFA injury study: 11-year data concerning 346 MCL injuries and time to return to play. Br J Sports Med 47(12):759–762
6. Holden DL, Eggert AW, Butler JE (1983) The nonoperative treatment of grade I and II medial collateral ligament injuries to the knee. Am J Sports Med 11(5):340–344
7. LaPrade RF, Engebretsen AH, Ly TV, Johansen S, Wentorf FA, Engebretsen L (2007) The anatomy of the medial part of the knee. J Bone Joint Surg Am 89(9):2000–2010
8. Corten K, Vandenneucker H, Van Lauwe J, Bellemans J (2009) Chronic posttraumatic bursitis of

the medial collateral ligament: surgical treatment in 2 high-level professional athletes. Am J Sports Med 37(3):610–613
9. Marchant MH, Tibor LM, Sekiya JK, Hardaker WT, Garrett WE, Taylor DC (2011) Management of medial-sided knee injuries, part 1: medial collateral ligament. Am J Sports Med 39(5):1102–1113
10. Jones L, Bismil Q, Alyas F, Connell D, Bell J (2009) Persistent symptoms following non operative management in low grade MCL injury of the knee – the role of the deep MCL. Knee 16(1):64–68
11. Bollen S (1999) Sports medicine handbook. Blackwell BMJ Books, London, pp 214–215
12. Bergfeld J (1979) Symposium: functional rehabilitation of isolated medial collateral ligament sprains. First-, second-, and third-degree sprains. Am J Sports Med 7(3):207–209
13. Grood ES, Noyes FR, Butler DL, Suntay WJ (1981) Ligamentous and capsular restraints preventing straight medial and lateral laxity in intact human cadaver knees. J Bone Joint Surg Am 63(8):1257–1269
14. Laprade RF, Bernhardson AS, Griffith CJ, Macalena JA, Wijdicks CA (2010) Correlation of valgus stress radiographs with medial knee ligament injuries: an in vitro biomechanical study. Am J Sports Med 38(2):330–338
15. Lonergan K, Taylor D (2002) Medial collateral ligament injuries of the knee: an evolution of surgical reconstruction. Tech Knee Surg 36(1):137–145
16. Jacobson KE, Chi FS (2006) Evaluation and treatment of medial collateral ligament and medial-sided injuries of the knee. Sports Med Arthrosc 14(2):58–66
17. Kerlan RK, Glousman RE (1988) Tibial collateral ligament bursitis. Am J Sports Med 16(4):344–346
18. Mendes LF, Pretterklieber ML, Cho JH, Garcia GM, Resnick DL, Chung CB (2006) Pellegrini-Stieda disease: a heterogeneous disorder not synonymous with ossification/calcification of the tibial collateral ligament-anatomic and imaging investigation. Skelet Radiol 35(12):916–922
19. Wang JC, Shapiro MS (1995) Pellegrini-Stieda syndrome. Am J Orthop (Belle Mead NJ) 24(6): 493–497
20. Schweitzer ME, Tran D, Deely DM, Hume EL (1995) Medial collateral ligament injuries: evaluation of multiple signs, prevalence and location of associated bone bruises, and assessment with MR imaging. Radiology 194(3):825–829
21. Campbell RS, Dunn AJ (2012) Radiological interventions for soft tissue injuries in sport. Br J Radiol 85(1016):1186–1193
22. Amar E, Snir N, Sher O, Brosh T, Khashan M, Salai M, Dolkart O (2015) Platelet-rich plasma did not improve early healing of medial collateral ligament in rats. Arch Orthop Trauma Surg 135(11):1571–1577
23. Jensen KT, Rabago DP, Best TM, Patterson JJ, Vanderby R (2008) Response of knee ligaments to prolotherapy in a rat injury model. Am J Sports Med 36(7):1347–1357
24. DeLong JM, Waterman BR (2015) Surgical techniques for the reconstruction of medial collateral ligament and posteromedial corner injuries of the knee: a systematic review. Arthroscopy 31(11):2258–2272
25. Laprade RF, Wijdicks CA (2012) Surgical technique: development of an anatomic medial knee reconstruction. Clin Orthop Relat Res 470(3):806–814
26. Lind M, Jakobsen BW, Lund B, Hansen MS, Abdallah O, Christiansen SE (2009) Anatomical reconstruction of the medial collateral ligament and posteromedial corner of the knee in patients with chronic medial collateral ligament instability. Am J Sports Med 37(6):1116–1122
27. Jiang KN, West RV (2015) Management of chronic combined ACL medial posteromedial instability of the knee. Sports Med Arthrosc 23(2):85–90
28. Jari S, Shelbourne KD (2001) Nonoperative or delayed surgical treatment of combined cruciate ligaments and medial side knee injuries. Sports Med Arthrosc Rev 9:185–192
29. Shelbourne KD, Nitz P (1992) Accelerated rehabilitation after anterior cruciate ligament reconstruction. J Orthop Sports Phys Ther 15:256–264
30. Zaffagnini S, Bonanzinga T, Marcheggiani Muccioli GM (2011) Does chronic medial collateral ligament laxity influence the outcome of anterior cruciate ligament reconstruction? A prospective evaluation with a minimum three-year follow-up. J Bone Joint Surg Br 93:1060–1064
31. DeLong JM, Waterman BR (2015) Surgical repair of medial collateral ligament and posteromedial corner injuries of the knee: a systematic review. Arthroscopy 31(11):2249–2255
32. Narvani A, Mahmud T, Lavelle J, Williams A (2010) Injury to the proximal deep medial collateral ligament: a problematical subgroup of injuries. J Bone Joint Surg Br 92(7):949–953

39 Return to Play Following Anterior Cruciate Ligament Injury

Simon Ball, Nathan White, Etienne Cavaignac, Vincent Marot, Jacques Ménétrey, and Andy Williams

Contents

S. Ball (✉) • N. White
Fortius Clinic, 17 Fitzardinge Street, London, W1H 6EQ, UK

Chelsea and Westminster Hospital, London, UK
e-mail: simon.ball@fortiusclinic.com

E. Cavaignac • V. Marot
Département de Chirurgie Orthopédique, CHU Toulouse, Toulouse, France

J. Ménétrey
Department of Surgery, University of Geneva, Geneva, Switzerland

A. Williams
Fortius Clinic, London, UK

39.1 Introduction

Anterior cruciate ligament (ACL) rupture is a devastating injury for the player. However, with advances in technology and improved understanding of the condition over recent decades, most players will make a good recovery and return to play.

In spite of these advances, a review of the literature [1] found that only 65% of athletes returned to their previous level and 55% resumed competition. This highlights the difficulty of defining the term "return to sports" [2]. It seems a priority to define this term accurately, as it can vary from simple return to recreational activity to return to high-level competition [3].

The primary goal when treating any patient with an ACL rupture is to ensure that the patient has a stable knee, which allows them to perform their desired activities safely. For some, this may be achieved without surgery, and patients may choose to modify their activities to avoid surgery. This is certainly an option for the recreational sports person, and it should be noted that non-surgical management has been successful even in the elite athlete [4]. However, it must not be forgotten that ongoing instability and giving way of the knee will lead to secondary meniscal and chondral pathology, with the inevitable onset of early osteoarthritis.

Patient education is an essential part of healthcare, and it is essential to the development of a consensus treatment plan between surgeon and

V. Musahl et al. (eds.), *Return to Play in Football*, https://doi.org/10.1007/978-3-662-55713-6_39

patient. This is particularly true in the management of ACL rupture, where there are multiple described treatment options. Many patients now present having done a literature search and are acutely aware of the risks and benefits of each pathway! Patient expectation has also changed, and very few patients are willing to adjust their activities to accommodate what they consider is a treatable injury. Even relatively sedentary patients may take the view that something has broken and they would like it fixed. In the elite athlete, activity modification is not an option. The goal is not just to return to sport but to return to peak performance.

Once the decision to proceed with surgery has been made, professional athletes want to know when they can anticipate returning to play. This is important from both a team strategy and an individual psychology point of view. The advice to any medical team faced with this question is to present a conservative, reliable time frame to the athlete and coaching staff. Although it may seem desirable to promise a rapid return to play, this may prove unachievable for the athlete in question and must be avoided. However, strategies to optimize management should be emphasized, thus enabling the most efficient return to play.

The process of return to play begins immediately following the injury, and it is essential to "get a good start". There should be an emphasis on swelling management, range of motion, quadriceps activation, patella mobilization and reinstating load if appropriate (dependent on chondral and meniscal damage). Once the swelling is under control and the knee is moving freely, a decision can be made regarding surgery.

As with all surgery, preparation is essential, and it is important that surgeons strive to achieve excellence in the operating theatre by executing a well-thought-out surgical plan in a time-efficient manner. Following surgery there should again be a focus on recovery from the trauma. It is essential early rehabilitation respects the surgery and not too much is done in the first 2 weeks.

During the postoperative period, it is essential for the player and medical team to understand that a biological process is taking place within the knee. While the healing environment can be optimized, the underlying biological process is essential to recovery and requires time. It cannot be beaten and must be respected. Inappropriate rehabilitation can adversely affect this process, which may not only increase the time to return to play but may also have a negative impact on the long-term outcome.

Research on injury prevention has highlighted the consequences of playing sport with neuromuscular deficits [5, 6]. It is recognized that failure to achieve appropriate strength and conditioning during rehabilitation can increase the risk of repeat injury. It is therefore essential that in the middle phase of ACL rehabilitation, players develop a foundation of strength and aerobic fitness, to prepare for the sport-specific return to play program.

Although there are multiple assessment tools to guide decision-making on return to play, the ultimate decision is often made empirically according to the teams between 3 and 12 months [7, 8].

Optimal return to play involves optimization of every aspect of the treatment pathway. In the following chapter, we describe how to get a good start following surgery, the biological process, the importance of strength and conditioning and the program for graduated return to play.

39.2 Getting a Good Start Following Surgery

Among high-level athletes, the main issue now is reducing the period away from competition to a minimum. The progress made in both the surgical technique and rehabilitation has made it possible to reduce the recovery time of more than 1 year in the 1970s to between 4 and 9 months today [9]. It is only with attention to detail at every stage, commencing when return to play seems furthest away and the athlete is at their most dejected, is such a timeline possible.

A good start in the context of ACL reconstruction means building a foundation upon which subsequent phases of rehabilitation will be built and which return to sport ultimately depends. The importance of managing pain and swelling, regaining neuromuscular control and range of movement cannot be overstated. Each of these domains is closely linked, and a deficit in one makes it difficult to achieve the others. As such, an attempt to return to higher levels of activity before these fundamentals have been addressed is generally futile and ultimately counterproductive or even dangerous.

39.2.1 Preoperative Phase

Management of ACL injury begins immediately after the initial trauma. The immediate cessation of physical activity is a prerequisite to any subsequent care. Prompt clinical assessment of the knee is important to identify the ligament injury, before haemarthrosis makes physical examination less reliable. Once the diagnosis has been made, on either clinical or radiological grounds, preoperative rehabilitation should commence. The term "prehab" effectively communicates the goals of this phase to the athlete.

In the days following injury, the patient must be actively encouraged and guided to manage pain, reduce swelling, restore movement and minimize the loss of muscle condition. The goal is to limit the magnitude of the initial inflammatory response and to return the knee to a quiescent state and thus prepare it for surgery. Pain management, cryotherapy, compression and elevation are simple but essential [10].

A program of ongoing supervised physiotherapy attendances has not shown its superiority over a properly followed program of self-rehabilitation [11]. However, it is reasonable that a degree of anxiety will be present after such a significant injury, and education and support should be available.

Risk factors for postoperative difficulty include persistent effusion, which inhibits muscle recruitment, muscle atrophy and loss of joint range [12]. However, there is also evidence that surgery before complete resolution of the initial trauma, and return of function, is not always detrimental [13–15]. Surgery before the knee is entirely quiescent may even be advantageous, by minimizing muscular atrophy. In some instances, it may be reasonable to operate when extension to neutral and flexion beyond 90° is achieved. In selected cases, aspiration of the haemarthrosis may expedite this process. Furthermore, indications for early surgery, such as a locked knee due to a meniscal tear, should be considered.

It is also important to consider the psychological factors involved during recovery from ACL injury. Motivation and determination have been found in several studies as potentially protective factors [16] and clearly have the potential to determine whether a player wishes to return to sport.

39.2.2 Postoperative Phase

In the immediate postoperative period, the objectives are substantially the same as in the preoperative phase. Surgery itself is a form of trauma, and the principles and techniques used after the initial injury remain relevant. Effusion must be managed, optimal joint range must be recovered and good patellar mobility should be achieved by the fourth week. Crutches and knee immobilizers may be used in the first few days for preemptive analgesia before recovery of normal ambulation [17].

It has long been recognized that early mobilization is preferable where possible. In 1990, Shelbourne and Nitz [18] documented their experience that routine restriction of weight bearing and range of movement were both unnecessary and associated with increased risk of arthrofibrosis requiring surgery. They referred to this as accelerated rehabilitation, and their message has become a standard practice.

Immediately after surgery, self-rehabilitation for 20 min, two to three times per day, must be incorporated in order to manage oedema, restore joint range and stimulate muscle fibres in the quadriceps, with supervised physiotherapy from approximately 8 days onwards.

We have found the "prone hang" to be particularly useful in regaining early extension. This consists of the patient, lying prone on a bed with the postoperative limb unsupported below the distal thigh, allowing gravity to assist knee extension [11]. Although passive extension is helpful and "buys time", the key is restoration of active extension with good isometric quadriceps contraction.

Throughout rehabilitation, the contributions to performance of proprioception, core stability, pelvic and gluteal control, as well as whole body strength and fitness should be recognized. This is covered further in Sect. 39.4. Although safety of the recovering knee must take priority, a comprehensive approach to these areas can begin early and will help minimize deconditioning.

39.2.3 Resumption of Training and Beyond

Rehabilitation specifically targeting return to activity should begin around 3 months postoperatively [11]. During this period, a mild intra-articular effusion will not be tolerated in response to resuming exercise. A progressive program of squats, lunges and plyometrics as well as agility drills including shuffling, hops, vertical jumps and running patterns is favoured, culminating in return to sport.

At the present time, no gold standard exists to validate or not the return to competition. Commonly, postoperative time is viewed as the overriding consideration, with an average of 6 months without any consensus [19]. However, this decision should be multifactorial and ideally based primarily on scientific fact. It should take into account not only the time period from surgery but also a range of complex subjective and objective assessments (Limb Symmetry Index, single-leg hop, 6-m timed hop, triple single-leg hop, crossover single-leg hop, and single-leg vertical hop) [19].

The Strategic Assessment of Risk and Risk Tolerance (StARRT) framework is designed to assist in managing the complex information which is involved in return to play [20]. Importantly, this framework recognizes that return to play by necessity involves risk, which may be viewed differently by the multiple stakeholders in the context of professional sport, and thus becomes a source of differing opinion and conflict.

Some authors propose also to assess the possibility of return to competition individually, considering things such as a player's morphology (e.g. genu valgum or relative hamstring weakness), the sport in question and the position played [19].

Rehabilitation following ACL reconstruction is frequently conceptualized as having four phases, culminating in return to play. Progress from resumption of training through return to sport can be described as having four phases also:

Fact Box 1: Progression from individual training through return to play [3]

1. Individual training without interference
2. Team training
3. Participation in a friendly or with a second team
4. Competition

To move from one phase to another, it is necessary to make an objective and subjective assessment, including an assessment of function. However, there are no validated scores specific to a given sport to guide this decision [3].

Simple clinical elements seem important to monitor before progressing: little or no pain, no effusion, symmetrical joint range, limb symmetry, hop testing [21] and the athlete's perceived psychological and physical preparedness [3].

Some authors propose side-to-side comparison of the hamstring/quadriceps ratio as the main criteria for returning to activities, with the postoperative side being >85% of the healthy limb considered acceptable [22].

It is recommended to continue monitoring and follow-up for a deficiency in the lower limb up to 1 year postoperative, even after returning to activities [3].

It would be interesting to continue preventive neuromuscular training for new injuries throughout an athlete's career [3, 23]. KOS-ADLS, KOS-SAS, global rating of perceived function (GRS), Lysholm score, International Knee Documentation Committee 2000 Subjective Knee Form

(IKDC2000), Cincinnati Knee Score, Knee Injury and Osteoarthritis Outcome Score (KOOS), Tegner Activity Scale and Marx Activity Rating Scale are scores frequently found in studies, providing significant assistance in making this decision.

39.3 The Biological Timeline of Reconstruction

The ACL and its reconstruction have been, and continue to be, extensively investigated. Despite this, there is a paucity of high-quality research with regard to the biological process that takes place after reconstruction. This reflects the difficulty in performing such studies, and, as a consequence, the data that is available is from animal studies and human biopsy studies. Information from animal studies is not directly transferrable but is important in aiding the formation of hypotheses and the interpretation of human biopsy studies. Despite being of low-level evidence, it can enable us to challenge previously held hypotheses and assumptions. Due to the limited evidence available, it is also important to use basic orthopaedic principles and logic to guide decision-making.

Graft "healing" can be divided into intra-osseous and intra-articular.

39.3.1 Intra-osseous Healing

Immediately following reconstruction, the graft has been shown to be stronger than the native ACL under load, and hence the fixation points are considered weakest link in the first few weeks. The reconstruction then "heals" to the bone over the course of several weeks. The exact time frame is unknown, but there has been a reported case where the tibial screw fixation was removed at 6 weeks with no subsequent loss of tension of the graft [24].

39.3.2 Intra-articular Healing

This process is often referred to as "ligamentization" of the graft [25] and takes place from the time of graft implantation until quiescence when it is hypothesized that the graft would histologically and biomechanically be more like a native ACL than tendon. It is unlikely that "complete" ligamentization occurs.

The process of ligamentization is a continuum of biological change, and the exact timeline is unknown. For the purposes of return to play and rehabilitation guidelines, it is useful to break down the ligamentization process into phases. Three distinct phases have been described in both the human and animal model as shown.

Fact Box 2: The three phases of the ligamentization process

Early
Remodelling
Maturation

In the animal model, the process of ligamentization has been shown to be more rapid than that in the human. The early phase starts within 2–4 weeks of implantation and is characterized by hypocellularity and central necrosis. This is followed by a period of intense remodelling during which there is hypercellularity, hypervascularity and replacement of the graft with longitudinally orientated collagen. The maturation stage commences at around 12–20 weeks during which the graft slowly becomes similar to that of a native ACL [26–28].

Human biopsy studies demonstrate that the process in humans is much slower. The central necrosis in the early phase has not been demonstrated in human biopsy studies or in non-biopsy studies using human gadolinium-enhanced MRI [29]. The human graft appears to be viable at all stages following implantation. In the early phase, there is synovial healing on the periphery of the graft, while the graft retains a tendon-like structure. In the remodelling phase, there is increased vascularity and cellularity and reorganization of the collagen that appears more regularly orientated and aligned than in the early phase. During the remodelling phase, the cell density and myofibroblast density decreases but never reaches that of a native ACL. Similarly, vascularity increases but never reaches that of a native ACL. There is a well-orientated mature collagen matrix that is similar to, but not the same as, the native ACL.

There is no agreed timeline for the ligamentization process with huge variations for the start and end of each phase. This reflects the very limited data that is available from the studies.

39.3.3 Interaction Between Healing and Rehabilitation Progression

There is no data available with regard to the tensile strength of the reconstruction during each phase of the healing process. It is however important to recognize that there is a biological process that takes place that is dependent on the patients' genetic make-up and the biological environment. This process cannot be speeded up by rehabilitation but can certainly be adversely affected by a program that involves inappropriate exercises.

It is thought that application of a small load to the ACL reconstruction may be important during the remodelling phase and may stimulate the reorientation of collagen fibres and the acquisition of the tensile properties that enable it to function more like a ligament. However, excessive load may lead to graft "stretch" or graft "slippage" in the bone tunnel. This can result in an elongated and nonfunctional but intact ACL reconstruction.

Most rehabilitation protocols will have a timeline that many patients and medical staff will refer to. It must be recognized that this refers to the biological process and is the fastest time frame by which patients can be rehabilitated. It is essential that progression through the program is based on achieving milestones and is not based on the timeline of the protocol. Only a very few elite athletes achieve the appropriate milestones to progress at the fastest rate, and understandably nearly all amateur athletes need longer. For example, return to running is often documented as 3 months. Running is however a series of hops done at high speed with control. In order to do this, patients should be able to single-leg press 1.5 times their body weight (0–60°) and be able to execute a single-leg squat and hop with perfect technique. Many amateur players are unable to achieve this until 6 months post surgery!

In summary, there is very little known about the biological process that takes place in the knee following reconstruction. However, we must recognize that a biological process does take place. Our rehabilitation program must be designed to respect and work with the biological process. This is essential for an optimal return to play and low failure rate.

39.4 The Importance of Strength and Conditioning

Strength and conditioning is a very important part of ACL rehabilitation. It essentially lays the foundations for the athlete to be able to commence a sport-specific program involving more dynamic and complex drills. Strength and conditioning work should commence immediately post injury. In the immediate post-injury phase, the aim should be to aid recovery from injury, prepare the leg for surgery and reduce the deconditioning. During the post-surgery phase, when the knee needs to be rested, players should be encouraged to work on their core stability and upper body strength. While there is an absolute requirement to not jeopardize the healing knee, a role for strength and conditioning can be found throughout all stages of recovery. When optimized, this approach may allow some athletes to return with better strength, core stability and cardiovascular fitness than before injury.

It is immediately clear that this will help minimize deconditioning, fatigue and further injury to the knee. But it could also reduce the risk of remote injury to deconditioned body parts, during what is known to be a vulnerable time. Exceptional neuromuscular control means little if fatigue sets in prematurely, leading to poor technique and the associated risk of injury.

At-risk sports involve bounding, hopping, jumping and landing on one leg. Put simply, players are not kangaroos and they will often be loading and turning off one leg! As the rehabilitation program is designed to return players to these at-risk sports, it is important to isolate each leg when performing strength exercises. It is also essential that "control" is maintained throughout the program. If players are allowed to do exercises where they lack control, they are not only at risk of injury but will put excessive load through the graft. For example, many patients will be encouraged to perform a single-leg squat as part of their rehabilitation program; however, in the early phases of rehabilitation, many patients lack the strength and control to do this properly and therefore drop into a dynamic valgus position.

The role for strength and conditioning may be thought of as relating to the injured limb, to the remainder of the body including the trunk and pelvis, and the cardiovascular system. The overall goal is to enable the player to return to their best in the safest, most time-efficient manner possible. The condition of both the knee and the athlete as a whole must be simultaneously brought to the correct level at the appropriate time to ensure the player is available to play [10].

There is considerable skill involved in appropriately matching strength and conditioning training to the stage of recovery, the sport, and the position played in the team. It is therefore difficult to develop entirely prescriptive guidelines, and literature in this field remains scarce. As with other concepts of progression in ACL rehabilitation, principles of strength and conditioning may be considered in terms of phases [30]. In the absence of compelling evidence, a tailored and collaborative approach is to be encouraged.

It is often in the area of strength and conditioning, and during the later stages of rehabilitation, that an athlete's sense of frustration with time away from sport is encountered. Particularly in the high-level sporting environment, it is important that any enthusiasm for unsafe progression to high-level training be managed with sensitivity and be tempered with discussion of lessons learned from past similar experience. Safe creativity in rehabilitation, and conscious emphasis on what an athlete can do rather than what they cannot, will allow variation in training and a sense of progress towards return. A skilful program should be challenging but also safe and stave off boredom at the same time.

During the strength and conditioning phase of rehabilitation, it is useful to define the strength targets. The aim of rehabilitation is to enable the player to move at speed, jump, land and change direction. In order to achieve this, it is logical to expect players to be able to single-leg press 1.5 times their body weight between 0 and 60° of flexion with perfect technique. Many recreational and amateur sports people will find this difficult to achieve, and this in part reflects their pre-injury conditioning, which is often poor. This target is however achievable, and players should achieve this level of strength before starting running.

In recent years, there has been a lot of work on injury prevention [23]. By identifying and addressing neuromuscular deficits of players, one may reduce the risk of injury. This trend has been shown in the literature. It is also logical, and one may even expect performance levels of athletes to improve as these deficits are addressed.

Within elite sports, there are many examples of the importance of strength and conditioning. One only has to look at gymnasts. They have a finely balanced strength-weight ratio, which enables them to control the skeleton with precision resulting in excellent balance and ability to perform very complex movements. Dedication to conditioning is likely to help the greatest players in the world perform to their abilities and means that in turn they are rarely injured during their careers.

39.5 Graduated Return to Play

39.5.1 Rehabilitation Basics

There are many components that may be part of a rehabilitation program following ACL reconstruction in athletes. However, evidence to support a few with certainty stands out when reviewing the literature. This is summarized below.

Rehabilitation programs must be supervised by a physiotherapist, but continuous monitoring is not necessary. Several physiotherapy sessions seem important enough to assess, train, instruct, and adjust the rehabilitation programs for progress, although the optimal number has not been quantified [11]. Immediate full weight bearing after ACL reconstruction is recommended, as it would seem to decrease the patellofemoral pain and has been shown to be safe [30]. Early mobilization is safe and reduces the risk of late arthrofibrosis [31].

The literature emphasizes the early use of closed chain exercises, by selecting knee joint range movements less than 60° and then open chain exercises with knee angles greater than 40° of flexion for quadriceps strengthening without increasing the pressure on the ACL and without increased stress on the patellofemoral joint. Open chain exercises of 40–90° of flexion, beginning on the sixth postoperative week, seem favourable to increasing quadriceps muscle strength and can be recommended [32].

It has been proven that high-intensity neuromuscular electrical stimulation at 65° of flexion, in addition to volitional exercises, improves the isometric strength of the quadriceps [33].

The results of pool-based rehabilitation programs must be confirmed, but in patients where joint effusion hampers progress, hydrotherapy may be useful [31].

Accelerated rehabilitation (19 weeks instead of 32) seems to be without danger according to a study evaluating anterior-posterior knee laxity, clinical assessment, patient satisfaction, functional performance and cartilage metabolism [34].

39.5.2 Tracking Recovery: Assessment Tools

The date of return to competitive sports, although often recommended between 6 and 9 months postoperative, must be dictated by assessment and not solely as a function of time. Assessments on an athletic level during rehabilitation should be considered as a small step towards the return to sports. The decision to return to sports should be the result of a joined reflection between the various members of a multidisciplinary team, as previously mentioned [35]. To support this decision, the medical team can rely upon several assessment scales [19]:

Fact Box 3: Tracking recovery

Recovery should be monitored through assessment, not solely time.

The decision to return to play should be made as a team.

A range of assessment scales can be used to support this decision.

- *Symptoms, function, activity, participation*:
  - IKDC2000: 18–24 years (>89.7 men, >83.9 women); 25–34 years (>86.2 men, >82.8 women); 35–50 years (>85.1 men, >78.5 women); 51–65 years (>74.7 men, >69.0 women) [36]
  - Tegner Activity Scale: according to the desired level of activity
- *Psychological factors*:
  - ACL-RSI >56 [37]
  - K-SES: men >7.2, women >6.8 [38]
- *Muscular strength* [39]:
  - Competitive pivot-contact sports: LSI (Limb Symmetry Index) = 100% knee extensor and flexor strength, assessed with isokinetic concentric dynamometry at 60°/s, 180°/s, and 300°/s
  - Non-pivot, non-contact, recreational sports: LSI (Limb Symmetry Index) > 90% knee extensor and flexor strength, assessed with isokinetic concentric dynamometry at 60°/s, 180°/s, and 300°/s
  - Hamstring/quadriceps strength ratio > 58% assessed with isokinetic concentric dynamometry at 60°/s [38]

39.5.3 Gradual Return to Sports

A gradual training schedule should be set up to allow for a smooth transition from a clinically controlled environment to a moderately controlled environment and to full athletic activities during rehabilitation [19]. One may be aware that multiple preoperative, operative and postoperative factors can affect the return to sports during rehabilitation.

The return to sports without complete rehabilitation after ACL reconstruction or based on non-specific criteria without gradual reintegration to sports can lead to a lack of confidence in athletes, fear of injury recurrence, and persistence of risk factors that increase the likelihood of a new injury [48]. Furthermore, the return of an athlete with his team must be done according to the following steps [40]:

1. Return to team practice without contact (distinctive jersey)
2. Return to full team practice with contact
3. Return to friendly games/B team (initially not for a full game time)
4. Return to competitive games (initially not for a full game time)

An athlete must successfully pass the functional tests for considering a return to sports; these tests should be well scheduled in time and individualized according to the level of rehabilitation and physical conditioning. It allows for the prevention of a new knee and/or a muscle injury.

To better structure the planning, one can include the acute-chronic workload ratio in the process of returning to sports [41]. This ratio describes the relationship between the workload performed during the previous week (acute workload) and the average workload performed during the past 4 weeks (chronic workload). Sudden peaks in this ratio should be avoided.

39.5.4 Biopsychosocial Factors

39.5.4.1 Alterations of Movements and Risk of Reinjury

When comparing the affected limb to the healthy limb, or injured ACL patients to healthy patients, several authors have identified altered biomechanics in ACL reconstructed patients [42]. These alterations in movement control may persist for up to 2 years postoperatively, even in athletes initially considered suitable to resume sports. Four factors have been identified as being predictive for recurrent injury in postoperative patients [43]. It has also been demonstrated that specific neuromuscular training can improve one or more of these risk factors.

Fact Box 4: Predictive factors for recurrent injury in postoperative patients [43]

1. Increased valgus alignment
2. Asymmetry in internal knee extensor moment on initial contact
3. Monopodal support of postural instability
4. Contralateral hip rotation moment

39.5.4.2 Neurological Effects of the ACL Injury

An ACL injury leads to mechanical instability of the knee, due in part to the alteration of neuromuscular control secondary to signal interruption from damaged mechanoreceptors in the torn ligament. The alteration of the somatosensory message decreases the signals relating to the central nervous system. It results in a reduction of proprioception and an increase in nociceptive activity, provoked by the instability due to the anterior shift of the tibia, that distorts motor control. It is postulated that ACL injury can cause a reorganization of the central nervous system at the sensorimotor cortex level [44]. New studies are required to develop rehabilitation techniques that would alter neuroplasticity and motor control changes in order to improve ACL reconstruction outcomes.

39.5.4.3 Pain

It has been shown that the motor unit activity of the quadriceps was negatively affected not only by the pain but also by the anticipation of pain [45].

39.5.4.4 Fatigue

The ability to maintain a quality of movement throughout all sports activities and to avoid postures at risk of ACL reinjury due to fatigue is a key point of the rehabilitation program. Endurance training to prevent muscle fatigue is paramount in the rehabilitation planning to limit the risk of reinjury in ACL-reconstructed patients. Indeed, it has been reported that fatigue negatively affects postural stability, neuromuscular control, and biomechanics of the lower limb during sporting activities in postoperative ACL patients [46].

39.5.4.5 Psychology

The most common reason cited in case of failure to return to sports is the fear of a new injury. It has been shown that preoperative psychological responses were associated with the probability of returning to pre-injury levels 12 months after ACL reconstruction [37]. This suggests that psychological factors play an important role in the return to sport process. So far, these factors have been largely ignored in the rehabilitation context, and future research is required in this field. Currently, the ACL-Return to Sports after Injury (ACL-RSI) questionnaire can be used, as a survey tool, to determine the psychological state of an athlete and help in the decision-making process of returning to play.

39.5.4.6 Social Pressure

The ever-present socio-economic pressures (i.e. club, coaches, parents, sponsors, etc.) in high-level sports may erroneously lead to a premature return to sports, including at the competitive level [47]. Various stakeholders may need to be reminded that a player represents an asset for the club, sponsors, managers and relatives. In this respect, prioritizing safe recovery over haste will help durability of performance.

The medical team must be aware of this environment and of all these factors when taking care of a player with an ACL injury. To support the RTP decision-making process, each step forwards must be validated by adjusted tests. It should only be possible to move on to the next one if specific tests have been passed with success. Timing, especially extrinsic factors such as competition dates, should not be used as the central variable driving the return to sports.

This review highlights that a successful return to sport is influenced by multiple factors, many of which are not quantifiable. The literature is still sparse in this field, and future research to improve assessment tools will be valuable to guide a safe return to play for our athletes.

Take-Home Messages

- The return to sports must be progressive.
- Capacities must be assessed through appropriate tests.
- The return to sports is influenced by several factors including some nonorganic (psychological/socio-economic).
- Time is not a reliable variable to estimate the return to sports.

Top 5 Evidence Based References

Beynnon B, Uh B, Johnson R (2005) Rehabilitation after anterior cruciate ligament reconstruction: a prospective, randomized, double-blind comparison of programs administered over 2 different time intervals. Am J Sports Med 33(3):347–359

Blanch P, Gabbett T (2016) Has the athlete trained enough to return to play safely? The acute: chronic workload ratio permits clinicians to quantify a player's risk of subsequent injury. Br J Sports Med 50(8):471–475

Hamrin Senorski E, Samuelsson K, Thomee C (2017) Return to knee-strenuous sport after anterior cruciate ligament reconstruction: a report from a rehabilitation outcome registry of patient characteristics. Knee Surg Sports Traumatol Arthrosc 25(5):1364–1374

Hewett T, Di Stasi S, Myer G (2013) Current concepts for injury prevention in athletes after anterior cruciate ligament reconstruction. Am J Sports Med 41(1):216–224

Kyritsis P, Bahr R, Landreau P (2016) Likelihood of ACL graft rupture: not meeting six clinical discharge criteria before return to sport is associated with a four times greater risk of rupture. Br J Sports Med 50(15):946–951

References

1. Ardern C, Taylor N, Feller J (2014) Fifty-five per cent return to competitive sport following anterior cruciate ligament reconstruction surgery: an updated systematic review and meta-analysis including aspects of physical functioning and contextual factors. Br J Sports Med 48(21):1543–1552

2. Warner S, Smith M, Wright R (2011) Sport-specific outcomes after anterior cruciate ligament reconstruction. Arthroscopy 27(8):1129–1134
3. Bizzini M, Silvers H (2014) Return to competitive football after major knee surgery: more questions than answers? J Sports Sci 32(13):1209–1216
4. Weiler R (2016) Unknown unknowns and lessons from non-operative rehabilitation and return to play of a complete anterior cruciate ligament injury in English Premier League football. Br J Sports Med 50(5):261–262
5. Hewett T, Myer G, Ford K (2005) Biomechanical measures of neuromuscular control and valgus loading of the knee predict anterior cruciate ligament injury risk in female athletes a prospective study. Am J Sports Med 33(4):492–501
6. Junge A, Lamprecht M, Stamm H (2010) Countrywide campaign to prevent soccer injuries in Swiss amateur players. Am J Sports Med 39(1):57–63
7. Sterett W, Hutton K, Briggs K (2003) Decreased range of motion following acute versus chronic anterior cruciate ligament reconstruction. Orthopedics 26(2):151–154
8. Shelbourne K, Patel D (1995) Timing of surgery in anterior cruciate ligament-injured knees. Knee Surg Sports Traumatol Arthrosc 3(3):148–156
9. Harner C, Fu F, Irrgang J (2001) Anterior and posterior cruciate ligament reconstruction in the new millennium: a global perspective. Knee Surg Sports Traumatol Arthrosc 9(6):330–336
10. Roi G, Creta D, Nanni G (2005) Return to official Italian First Division soccer games within 90 days after anterior cruciate ligament reconstruction: a case report. J Orthop Sports Phys Ther 35(2):52–61-66
11. Malempati C, Jurjans J, Noehren B (2015) Current rehabilitation concepts for anterior cruciate ligament surgery in athletes. Orthopedics 38(11):689–696
12. De Carlo M, Shelbourne K, Oneacre K (1999) Rehabilitation program for both knees when the contralateral autogenous patellar tendon graft is used for primary anterior cruciate ligament reconstruction: a case study. J Orthop Sports Phys Ther 29(3):144–153–159
13. Graf B, Ott J, Lange R (1994) Risk factors for restricted motion after anterior cruciate reconstruction. Orthopedics 17(10):909–912
14. Howell S, Hull M (1998) Aggressive rehabilitation using hamstring tendons: graft construct, tibial tunnel placement, fixation properties, and clinical outcome. Am J Knee Surg 11(2):120–127
15. Shelbourne K, Gray T (1997) Anterior cruciate ligament reconstruction with autogenous patellar tendon graft followed by accelerated rehabilitation. A two- to nine-year followup. Am J Sports Med 25(6):786–795
16. Paulos L, Wnorowski D, Beck C (1991) Rehabilitation following knee surgery. Recommendations. Sports Med 11(4):257–275
17. Wright R, Haas A, Anderson J (2015) Anterior cruciate ligament reconstruction rehabilitation: MOON guidelines. Sports Health 7(3):239–243
18. Shelbourne K, Nitz P (1990) Accelerated rehabilitation after anterior cruciate ligament reconstruction. Am J Sports Med 18(3):292–299
19. Adams D, Logerstedt D, Hunter-Giordano A (2012) Current concepts for anterior cruciate ligament reconstruction: a criterion-based rehabilitation progression. J Orthop Sports Phys Ther 42(7):601–614
20. Shrier I (2015) Strategic assessment of risk and risk tolerance (StARRT) framework for return-to-play decision-making. Br J Sports Med 49(20):1311–1315
21. Noyes F, Barber S, Mangine R (1991) Abnormal lower limb symmetry determined by function hop tests after anterior cruciate ligament rupture. Am J Sports Med 19(5):513–518
22. Van Grinsven S, Van Cingel R, Holla C (2010) Evidence-based rehabilitation following anterior cruciate ligament reconstruction. Knee Surg Sports Traumatol Arthrosc 18:1128–1144
23. Hewett T, Di Stasi S, Myer G (2013) Current concepts for injury prevention in athletes after anterior cruciate ligament reconstruction. Am J Sports Med 41(1):216–224
24. Logan M, Williams A, Myers P (2003) Is bone tunnel osseointegration in hamstring tendon autograft anterior cruciate ligament reconstruction important? Arthroscopy 19(8):85–87
25. Amiel D, Kleiner J, Roux R (1986) The phenomenon of "ligamentization": anterior cruciate ligament reconstruction with autogenous patellar tendon. J Orthop Res 4(2):162–172
26. Goradia V, Rochat M, Kida M (2000) Natural history of a hamstring tendon autograft used for anterior cruciate ligament reconstruction in a sheep model. Am J Sports Med 28(1):40–46
27. Kondo E, Yasuda K, Katsura T (2012) Biomechanical and histological evaluations of the doubled semitendinosus tendon autograft after anterior cruciate ligament reconstruction in sheep. Am J Sports Med 40(2):315–324
28. Scheffler S, Unterhauser F, Weiler A (2008) Graft remodeling and ligamentization after cruciate ligament reconstruction. Knee Surg Sports Traumatol Arthrosc 16:834–842
29. Howell S, Knox K, Farley T (1995) Revascularization of a human anterior cruciate ligament graft during the first two years of implantation. Am J Sports Med 23(1):42–49
30. Reiman M, Lorenz D (2011) Integration of strength and conditioning principles into a rehabilitation program. Int J Sports Phys Ther 6(3):241–253
31. Wright R, Preston E, Fleming B (2008) A systematic review of anterior cruciate ligament reconstruction rehabilitation: part II: open versus closed kinetic chain exercises, neuromuscular electrical stimulation, accelerated rehabilitation, and miscellaneous topics. J Knee Surg 21(3):225–234
32. Tyler T, McHugh M, Gleim G (1998) The effect of immediate weightbearing after anterior cruciate ligament reconstruction. Clin Orthop Relat Res 357:141–148
33. Snyder-Mackler L, Delitto A, Bailey S (1995) Strength of the quadriceps femoris muscle and functional recovery after reconstruction of the anterior cruciate ligament. A prospective, randomized clinical

trial of electrical stimulation. J Bone Joint Surg Am 77(8):1166–1173
34. Beynnon B, Uh B, Johnson R (2005) Rehabilitation after anterior cruciate ligament reconstruction: a prospective, randomized, double-blind comparison of programs administered over 2 different time intervals. Am J Sports Med 33(3):347–359
35. Ardern C, Bizzini M, Bahr R (2016) It is time for consensus on return to play after injury: five key questions. Br J Sports Med 50(9):506–508
36. Logerstedt D, Di Stasi S, Grindem H (2014) Self-reported knee function can identify athletes who fail return-to-activity criteria up to 1 year after anterior cruciate ligament reconstruction: a Delaware-Oslo ACL cohort study. J Orthop Sports Phys Ther 44(12):914–923
37. Ardern C, Taylor N, Feller J (2013) Psychological responses matter in returning to preinjury level of sport after anterior cruciate ligament reconstruction surgery. Am J Sports Med 41(7):1549–1558
38. Hamrin Senorski E, Samuelsson K, Thomee C (2017) Return to knee-strenuous sport after anterior cruciate ligament reconstruction: a report from a rehabilitation outcome registry of patient characteristics. Knee Surg Sports Traumatol Arthrosc 25(5):1364–1374
39. Thomeé R, Kaplan Y, Kvist J (2011) Muscle strength and hop performance criteria prior to return to sports after ACL reconstruction. Knee Surg Sports Traumatol Arthrosc 19(11):1798–1805
40. Bizzini M, Hancock D, Impellizzeri F (2012) Suggestions from the field for return to sports participation following anterior cruciate ligament reconstruction: soccer. J Orthop Sports Phys Ther 42(4):304–312
41. Blanch P, Gabbett T (2016) Has the athlete trained enough to return to play safely? The acute: chronic workload ratio permits clinicians to quantify a player's risk of subsequent injury. Br J Sports Med 50(8):471–475
42. Bien D, Dubuque T (2015) Considerations for late stage acl rehabilitation and return to sport to limit re-injury risk and maximize athletic performance. Int J Sports Phys Ther 10(2):256–271
43. Paterno M, Schmitt L, Ford K (2010) Biomechanical measures during landing and postural stability predict second anterior cruciate ligament injury after anterior cruciate ligament reconstruction and return to sport. Am J Sports Med 38(10):1968–1978
44. Kapreli E, Athanasopoulos S, Gliatis J (2009) Anterior cruciate ligament deficiency causes brain plasticity: a functional MRI study. Am J Sports Med 37(12):2419–2426
45. Tucker K, Larsson A, Oknelid S (2012) Similar alteration of motor unit recruitment strategies during the anticipation and experience of pain. Pain 153(3):636–643
46. Gokeler A, Eppinga P, Dijkstra PU (2014) Effect of fatigue on landing performance assessed with the landing error scoring system (less) in patients after ACL reconstruction. A pilot study. Int J Sports Phys Ther 9(3):302–311
47. Ekstrand J (2011) A 94% return to elite level football after ACL surgery: a proof of possibilities with optimal caretaking or a sign of knee abuse? Knee Surg Sports Traumatol Arthrosc 19(1):1–2
48. Kyritsis P, Bahr R, Landreau P (2016) Likelihood of ACL graft rupture: not meeting six clinical discharge criteria before return to sport is associated with a four times greater risk of rupture. Br J Sports Med 50(15):946–951

Philosophical and Practical Approach to Dealing with Knee Injuries in Elite Football: Experience Based Rather than Evidence Based

40

Simon Ball, Nathan White, and Andy Williams

Contents

S. Ball • A. Williams (✉)
Fortius Clinic, 17 Fitzardinge Street, London, W1H 6EQ, UK

Chelsea and Westminster Hospital, London, UK

N. White
Fortius Clinic, 17 Fitzardinge Street, London, W1H 6EQ, UK
e-mail: williams@fortiusclinic.com

40.1 Introduction

Whether one likes it or not, sport is important. It is a subject that interests millions across the world, and no sport is more significant than football. It employs thousands of people not including the players themselves. The pursuit of football encourages fitness of the human population, general wellbeing, teamwork, discipline, and for individuals to value their personal health.

Two hundred and sixty-five million people worldwide play football. That equates to 4% of the world's population [1]. It is a multimillion pound entertainment industry. The latest deal for the TV rights for the English Premiership to cover the period of 2016–2019 has seen a 71% increase in the payment made by a TV company compared with that for the period of 2013–2016 [2]. The average wage in the English Premiership for a first team player is £2.3 million a year, which is equivalent to £44,000 a week [3].

The products which the TV companies buy are the matches, of which there are around 60 per season covering all competitions. The pressure to play, win, and reward the TV companies for their investment is ever increasing. In each game, on average, players will run 10 km. It is not surprising that knee injuries are common due to frequent exposure to trauma and attrition overload.

The senior author has been treating professional athletes for nearly 20 years. Currently 60% of all his practice is made up of professional sportsmen and

V. Musahl et al. (eds.), *Return to Play in Football*, https://doi.org/10.1007/978-3-662-55713-6_40

women, and they account for half of the ACL reconstructions he does a year. He currently is involved with the care of 75% of the English Premiership League football teams as well as teams from other levels and different sports. It is a great field of work to be involved in. Athletes test judgement and surgery. Even minor failures can lead to significant interference with athletic performance. It is challenging, but this leads to improvement in the care that can be offered to patients in general.

Whilst this patient group represents a great challenge, the rewards for the treating clinician are worthwhile. Footballers enhance the quality of a surgeon's practice. For example, they allow to study conditions rare in the general population, because they sustain these more frequently. Also, common conditions often pose more of a problem in treatment due to their loading and performance demands. Exposure of the clinician to this benefits the nonsporting population too as well as the athlete. In addition, due to their media exposure, it is relatively easy to follow up patients with coarse outcomes such as graft re-rupture rates and return to play. This can be invaluable in assessing treatments that are frequently undertaken in the normal population. For example, with regard to anterior cruciate ligament reconstruction graft choice, there is considerable controversy, as different grafts seem to work in the general population. In professional football, however, any small issue is exaggerated, and it has become clear to the senior author that patellar tendon grafts have around 50% the re-rupture rate of hamstring grafts (see below), for example.

Fact Box 1

The challenge of dealing with professional footballers' injuries and the pressure to deliver players back from injury quicker and healthier benefit the care of the general population.

Most would agree that evidence-based medicine is generally preferable to experience-based practice. Whilst this seems logical, unfortunately, there are a number of conditions and fields of medicine in which it will never be possible to achieve. The subject matter of this chapter is an example. Whilst we strongly advocate scientific evaluation of conditions and treatment outcomes whenever possible, a lot of elite sports knee practice has to be based on the application of basic scientific knowledge, such as functional anatomy, and past clinician experience. Much in the practice can never be subject to a prospective randomised controlled trial! Many of the conditions treated in this field are occurring in such small numbers that it is impossible to apply rigorous scientific evaluation to them, and in any case, there will never scientific trials of treatment in professional sport. Athletes need to believe that there is only one answer for their problem and they would certainly not wish to be 'randomised' to treatment. In addition, the psychology of treatment of athletes is so powerful that the effect of placebo is enormous. Like it or not, experience-based, rather than evidence-based, practice in treating elite footballers will be a significant part of the whole. The reader needs to take this into account for this chapter. Nevertheless, as experienced-based is often the best one can have, it warrants serious consideration rather than being dismissed.

There is no doubt that professional football players are special, but it should be borne in mind that they are of course human. You cannot therefore speed up nature! Despite what the players, coaching staff and all manners of non-medical 'medical experts' at clubs say, this is a fact. At times even their joints need a rest! This atmosphere poses a considerable challenge.

40.2 Examples of What Has Been Learned from an Experience-Based Perspective

40.2.1 Natural Selection

The average human will put approximately million cycles of movement through their lower limb joints in a year [4]. The number for a professional footballer will be very many times greater than this. Therefore, if they have any 'weakness', it will be demonstrated. Players are thus prone to overuse injuries related to anatomic variations such as malalignment. Furthermore, the forces going through their lower limbs are also much greater than the average population, and any underlying vulnerability to injury due to substandard collagen or joint anatomy is problematic. Put simply, football applies Darwinian pressure so that only the 'fittest will survive'. When a footballer reaches around 20 years of age and they have established themselves, then they have clearly been 'put together properly'. An ACL rupture in a first team player is relatively rare [5].

For the same team, there will be many ACL ruptures each year in the youth players. This is presumably due to lack of neuromuscular control, joint mal-orientation, such as an increased tibial slope laterally, or soft tissue laxity/weakness. In the vast majority of these players, reconstructive surgery is successful and they will return to play. However, despite this, the player under 18 years old at the time of ACL reconstruction will rarely achieve a professional footballing career. In those under 16, it is almost unheard of. The reason for this is interesting. We used to think it was part of the 'natural selection' process or, simply put, that there was something wrong in the players' make-up. Whilst this is true for the reason they ruptured their ACL, once reconstructed it is probably not the reason for failing to progress with a career in football. The problem is almost certainly the fact that these players have effectively missed a year of football, and they can never catch up with their peers. In addition, for an unproven young player, the situation is very different to an established first team player, in whom the club has invested a great deal and will wait. This is not the case for a youngster. This situation underlines the huge pressure on a young professional footballer.

40.3 Examples of What Has Been Learned from an Evidence-Based Perspective

40.3.1 A Common Condition: Meniscal Tears

Early on in our experience of treating professional footballers, it became very clear that a pattern emerged when meniscectomy was undertaken. The footballers having partial lateral meniscectomy regularly had problems with swelling and a slow return to play, unlike those who had a medial meniscus resection. In the longer term, players who had previous lateral meniscal resection would, unlike their medial meniscectomy counterparts, return with repeated problems related to chondral breakdown, and they would frequently require premature retirement for this. As a result of this observation, a formal study was undertaken of 90 professional footballers who had undergone lateral meniscectomy (42 cases) or medial meniscectomy (48 cases). The median time to return to play to the nearest week was longer in the lateral group compared with the medial group (seven versus five $P < 0.001$). At all times after surgery, the cumulative probability of returning to play was nearly six times greater (5.99: 95% confidence interval, 3.34–10.74; $P < 0.001$) after medial meniscectomy. More lateral meniscectomy cases experienced adverse effects related to pain and particularly swelling (69% versus 4% $P < 0.001$). Seven percentage of the lateral meniscectomy cases required a second arthroscopy [6].

Fact Box 2
Loss of lateral meniscus is very problematic in football compared to medial meniscal loss.

It is interesting to note that compared with other running sports such as rugby, lateral meniscectomy seemed to be particularly badly tolerated in football. This is particularly odd when one considers that most professional footballers have varus alignment (that, and pes planus are associated with fast running) when many rugby players are actually in valgus alignment. The answer is not immediately obvious because orthopaedic surgeons tend to think of lower limb alignment not only purely in the coronal plane but also as a static examination on x-ray. Going to a live football match makes it obvious that despite the natural varus stance in full extension, there is an immense amount of time spent with dynamic valgus loading as a player twists and turns. Football is a multidirectional sport, whereas rugby involves much less changing of direction. The concept of dynamic alignment change is one of the important lessons we have learned from dealing with athletes.

Fact Box 3
Treating elite footballers teaches an appreciation of the big difference between static limb alignment, which is assessed clinically and on radiograph, and the variation from this in 'dynamic' alignment that occurs on the pitch during play.

40.3.2 A Common Condition: ACL Ruptures

The first consultation with a player has to be undertaken with great attention to detail. It is essential that the treating doctor realises that the professional footballer is indeed 'special'. It is not the players' fault that they earn a very good living, as well as having the gift to play professional football. In the context of having an injury, they are sad, scared and often suspicious of treatment advice. The clinician must understand this and show empathy, as well as confidence and great attention to detail. The surgeon also has to consider the pressures on the player: they fear losing their place in the team and will have timescales and deadlines to meet such as contract issues and major tournaments.

Even prior to seeing the player, the surgeon concerned should plan ahead. For example, when surgery is needed, as soon as the consultation finishes, the player will want to know when the operation. The surgeon should know their availability.

The timing of ACL reconstruction is important. Frequently, it is safe to undertake surgery within a matter of a few days of injury, but that is not always the case. As already stated, football players are humans and so 'nature rules'. The knee needs to be quiet with little swelling, full active extension, and bending freely to over 90°. The average time to surgery for our professional footballers is around 7–10 days from injury. On occasion, according to the circumstances, it is worth considering sterile aspiration of the joint haemarthrosis to allow prompt restoration of quadriceps activation and full active extension more quickly than waiting for spontaneous resolution of the haemarthrosis.

Individualised graft choice is important and needs to be tailored to the sport concerned. Generally hamstring grafts are our first choice for most people including professional athletes. In professional rugby in the senior author's series, graft re-rupture occurs in 5.6% of cases. In football, the situation is different however. From January 2001 to June 2013, he undertook 212 isolated (no other ligament injury or meniscal pathology) ACL reconstructions in professional footballers. Six of these were excluded (two had patellar tendon allograft—both of which re-ruptured; four patellar tendon grafts were combined with a lateral tenodesis, all of which survived and made a full recovery). At a minimum 2-year follow-up, the rupture rates were compared between four-strand hamstring grafts and middle-third patellar tendon grafts. Obviously with time more re-ruptures will occur, but in professional football, a re-rupture almost exclusively occurs within the first year from surgery. The overall re-rupture rate was 8.6% (7 of 81) for patellar tendon graft and 11% (14 of 125) for quadrupled hamstring grafts. Further analysis was undertaken comparing femoral tunnel position, and the findings were stark. In all cases in the series, the tibial tunnel was drilled to emerge in the centre of the tibial ACL 'footprint'. The femoral tunnel, however, varied from a central 'anatomic' femoral ACL footprint or the anteromedial bundle position within the ACL footprint. The patellar tendon graft re-rupture rate for AM femoral bundle position was 4.5% but more than doubled to 10.2% when placed in the central footprint position on the femur. For hamstring graft, the increasing re-rupture rate was even more dramatic to approximately 2.5 times as much in the central femoral footprint position (17% re-ruptured) compared to 6.9% in the AM bundle position [7]. It is clear that first-choice graft for professional football should be middle-third patellar tendon autograft.

Fact Box 4
Patellar tendon autografts for ACL reconstruction have a much lower re-rupture rate than hamstring autografts.

We are in an era of a return to additional lateral extra-articular tenodeses (LET). Additional LETs have been undertaken in players who are thought to be at a higher than average risk of graft re-rupture, and out of 38 elite athletes, there has so far been only one re-rupture. It is obviously wrong to conclude that the additional procedure is necessary without more rigorous study. Further clinical follow-up is needed to establish true rates of intra-articular ACL graft re-rupture and potential adverse effects such as osteoarthritis. Nevertheless, the laboratory data [8, 9] shows logic for this additional technique. Since there is no evidence base, we add a lateral tenodesis in those who are at particular risk of graft re-rupture such as those with significant malalignment with more than 10° varus or more than 5° valgus alignment, those with marked hyperextension of more than 10°, a history of previous ACL rupture in the contralateral limb or family members with ACL tears, all juvenile cases and in all revision cases. Whilst randomisation would be possible in the general population, it cannot be undertaken in a trial of athletes—they simply will not accept being involved in such studies.

Rehabilitation following ACL reconstruction needs to be taken very seriously in elite footballers. It is important from the start for a surgeon to advise the player that rehabilitation is a long program. Previously there was an attempt to reduce the rehabilitation times to less than 6 months (hence, the term 'aggressive rehabilitation', which we dislike strongly preferring 'intensive rehabilitation')! However, in respect of the re-rupture data above, our view is that this is inappropriate. We prefer a minimum return to play time of 6 months that are more relaxed with slowing down rehabilitation towards 9 months in professional sport. Even longer time frames may be better. The pressure to return early can be immense, but it must be resisted by the surgeon in charge. It is wise to embrace rehabilitation and communicate freely with the therapist involved in it.

40.3.3 An Unusual Condition: 'Non-union' of MCL Tears

Another pattern that emerged early in our experience with professional footballers was that there was a small group of medial collateral ligament injuries which characteristically were minor at presentation (usually only grade 0 or 1) that apparently recovered quickly at first but then developed persisting and disabling pain. The pain is typically felt close to the femoral attachment of the MCL and occurs when a player makes a long crossfield pass or kicks a 'dead ball' such as a free kick when they need to 'bend' the ball in flight. They can kick the ball as hard as they want 'off the laces' such as with shooting or volleying and can perform anything else but nonetheless are disabled from football. Typical examination revealed tenderness at the site of pain, minimal laxity, and pain on rapid external rotation of the knee at 30° flexion. Valgus stress does not particularly cause pain. A consecutive series of 17 of our cases was published [10]. None of these patients had responded to non-surgical treatment, such as ultrasound-targeted injection, and required surgery. The characteristic lesion is found: the superficial MCL is intact at its femoral origin, but the deep MCL is found to have failed to heal at its femoral origin. With surgical repair in all cases, a return to full activity was possible. Since that publication, it has become evident that on occasion there is less commonly a failure of the MCL to heal on the tibial side and that on one occasion, rather than the deep MCL at the femur, it was the posterior oblique ligament attachment to the femur that had not healed which had a very specific presentation—the player could do everything apart from a 'Cruyff turn'. This manoeuvre was first used by the Dutch footballing legend Johan Cruyff who would pull the football back behind the stance leg to change direction of running and 'wrong foot' an opponent. The kicking leg was forced into quick internal rotation to achieve this.

40.4 Treating Footballers Differently

40.4.1 The Service

The service required to treat professional footballers properly reflects the demands and environment of their profession. Clearly, not all doctors would be prepared to offer the level of service required as they feel they could not justify it. A prerequisite for a doctor involved in treating athletes is that they feel that the athletes are indeed special and that they are reconciled to deliver the necessary service. Many knee surgeons seem envious of the work that surgeons such as the senior author undertake with professional footballers' care, but we doubt that few realise the hours involved!

The first requirement is total availability and the discipline to communicate. With advances in information technology, not only are we available on the phone but also with email, and MRI scans can be reviewed remotely via the Internet. Instant response is required, and indeed expected, from the players and club. To achieve this, a surgeon has to have a sympathetic attitude to the requirements of players and therefore an ability to deliver without begrudging it. The willingness to make oneself available and the discipline of making telephone calls and sending text messages and emails are only sustainable if the surgeon has a well-organised and willing office. The office must have the ability to differentiate between patients from the general population that can wait against sometimes less serious professional football cases that require urgent attention. Both the surgeon and office staff need to be able to 'think ahead', so that demands can be answered. This is particularly so for arranging appointments, when often there are never scheduled appointments available to see a busy surgeon! The same applies to surgery dates.

It is pertinent to give an example of 'the service'. By way of illustration, the senior author took a call from an English Premier League team doctor at noon on a Saturday: a young, unestablished player twisted his knee and had locked it in training that morning. The player was admitted to hospital and had an MRI, and an arthroscopic medial meniscectomy was undertaken. The surgeon drove home 5 h after the initial call. To ensure everything occurred smoothly, without any undue stress to the player, in the 5-h period, the senior author made 30 phone calls! These were to organise the admission to hospital and the MRI scan, to brief the staff at the hospital reception not to make the player wait in reception nor to ask for proof of payment (the senior author had to give his own credit card details and guarantee payment!), and to call the club physio and doctor post-MRI and postoperative.

40.4.2 The Consultation

Confidence in the clinician is essential. Just as a player on the pitch assesses the quality of their opponent, they will have a sixth sense for any lack of confidence/competence in the doctor they are seeing. To build confidence, the atmosphere must be unhurried, and the player should be given all the time they require. Consultations of over an hour are required at times. It is essential that the doctor can empathise, and they can only do it if they believe that football is a serious/important business and realise that there are huge pressures on the player. One of the first questions is usually 'when does your contract expire'? An ACL rupture in the last year of a contract is associated with unavoidable increased pressure. Thoroughness is vital. Listen carefully as the player will usually give you the answer just as any patient would. Examination needs to be comprehensive. The whole of the club medical team (doctors, physios, etc.) need to be involved in the decision-making progress too.

Unfortunately, at times the prognosis for a player is poor, and the bad news related to this has to be communicated with sensitivity. It should not be hidden, but the transmission of the information is important. The bad news needs to be stated as soon as possible, but a positive delivery all the same can be helpful; a negative and depressing outlook can be disastrous. The truth needs to be stated from the beginning, but even when faced with an obviously terrible injury, nobody can really be certain that failure is inevitable. If there is a treatment option, it should be undertaken, and it is important that whilst the player knows the severity of the problem, they proceed positively with good psychology. This is obviously a philosophical view, but over the years of experience, we have been endlessly surprised by how awful injuries do not preclude a return to play. When asked the question 'do you know that he is not going to make it'? The answer is no. Therefore, positivity is not necessarily misleading.

40.4.3 The Treatment

It is hugely reassuring to a player to have a clear treatment plan, outlining the steps of surgery and rehabilitation, as well as possible preparation for surgery. Time frames are essential. Most professional footballers, like athletes in general, are very robust and when given a plan will work hard to achieve the goal.

When it comes to surgery, one of the most important guiding principles is for the surgeon to undertake as small an operation as possible to obtain the desired result. It is often better to do less, accepting the risk of potential failure and the need for a second operation, than to undertake excessive surgery. There is always a 'price' for an operation in the way of pain, swelling, muscle loss and the like. The ability for an athlete to 'cope' with unaddressed structural damage can be extraordinary, and the apparent logic of fixing injured structures does not always equate to a good result. We have never met him, but if Usain Bolt were to have bunions (which he may well have), it would be madness to treat them surgically!

To ensure appropriate surgery is undertaken, preoperative planning in great detail is required. Excellence comes from attention to detail after all. There is no excuse to start an operation and 'see how you get on'. It is essential to have good help in the operating theatre with the best staff available. A surgeon has a lot to think about and has concern over, so a good team helps greatly. Whilst it is relatively straightforward to undertake ACL reconstruction without an assistant, it is so much easier to do so with one. With a professional footballer, why add stress? It is usual when operating on professional footballers that a physiotherapist, doctor, or both are present during the surgery. This adds considerable pressure to the surgeon, but the surgeon must accept that this is now the norm, and accepting observers gives a signal of confidence and openness that is positive. The findings at surgery are witnessed by an independent observer who is representing the player, and this helps to dissolve any feelings of mystery or secrecy. In addition, if surprising findings occur, then they can be discussed at the time during surgery. This is also true for the postoperative rehabilitation. The observers learn a lot by being present, and it makes them more understanding of the necessary rehabilitation process.

It is important to maintain control of the situation, and it is wise to use a hospital stay to ensure this. It is a mistake to discharge professional footballers too soon before being certain that complications such as wound bleeding or failure to fully extend the knee have been avoided.

40.4.4 Rehabilitation

It seems to us that it is often the physiotherapists who make the surgeon look good or, on occasion, bad! It is therefore logical to embrace them and communicate with them. One of the disciplines of dealing with professional footballers is the necessity for the surgeon to learn about neuromuscular control, contracture, synovitis, and swelling. An openness to learn from physiotherapists and about rehabilitation is critical. The achievement of a good result for a football player represents a combination of effort from the wider medical team, including the surgeon, but also critically involving the club doctor and physiotherapy team.

The club medical team are often under huge pressure from the coaching staff at a club and value guidance. Initially this surprised us as we felt that they were the experts in rehabilitation. We rapidly realised that they appreciated a logical plan to deliver to the club coaching staff in the surgeon's name as it takes pressure off them. This is an explanation of not only timelines but also the plan for rehabilitation including weight-bearing status, range of motion allowed, requirement for bracing or not, mobilisation of soft tissue, strengthening, restoration of balance and control, and timing to return of activities.

One of the most important lessons learned is that the surgeon needs to use time appropriately. It is of course a duty to get the player back as soon as it is safe to play again, but frequently at the start of treatment, stating an unpalatably long recovery is important. An inexperienced surgeon will often yield to pressure to offer unrealistically short timelines to return to play. Breaking the bad news early is important. For chondral surgery in particular, we have increased our return to play times over the years so that a microfracture for a tibiofemoral lesion is usually 6–9 months compared to up to 12 months for a patellar lesion.

40.4.5 Nonoperative Treatment

Quite correctly, the vast majority of new consultations do not result in surgery. They are vital to give confidence and certainty that surgery is not required at that time. Of course a warning that if things do not progress as required, surgery may be necessary later is important. Nonetheless, most consultations will result in a nonoperative management plan. This is usually straightforward for an injury such as a medial collateral ligament tear but can be extremely problematic for the treatment of synovitis and swelling when a period of rest/overload is needed but hard to quantify. Part of the surgeon's duty over the years is to educate not only those involved with the care of players, but the players themselves, that swelling is not something that should be tolerated within a knee. An accumulation of fluid inhibits neuromuscular control, and the fluid contains chemicals that soften the articular surface which can then break down with persistent loading. We would say that the biggest problem in dealing with professional footballers is indeed the control of swelling. This often occurs in the postoperative period due to excessively fast and heavy loading in rehabilitation or in players who have chronic joint surface damage who then break down with training loads or injury. It is likely that there is a genetic predisposition to swelling. Those athletes who lack the 'swelling gene' will be expected to make a prompt and safe recovery. The 'swellers' need much longer for their knee to settle and the articular surface to recover before they can play safely. Unfortunately, those involved in the treatment of football players have seen cases where new and significant chondral damage has occurred due to failure to respect swelling, and this is, of course, permanent.

Most orthopaedic surgeons understand the link between mechanical overload, and the occurrence and progression of chondral lesions, which may be exacerbated by malalignment or loss of congruity of a joint following ligament injury. Fewer appreciate the role of humeral elements. For example, in a knee with an ACL rupture, bone bruising in the lateral compartment reflects the area of subluxation that caused the ligament rupture. Yet, if a player persistently loads through swelling in the postoperative period, then a lesion of the trochlear groove will frequently occur. This area of the joint was completely uninjured at the time of the ACL rupture, but due to the loading through swelling, which softens the articular cartilage, it has broken down. This is related to the humeral environment of a swollen joint [11]. With the result of basic science research already mentioned, in time chondro-protectant drugs may allow a more rapid and safe rehabilitation of the injured knee. This time has not yet come, and therefore, the key principle is to appreciate that swelling in a knee is not normal and should be resolved before a return to play. The lesson should have been learnt from the 1970s when intra-articular steroid injections were frequently undertaken, allowing the player to overload an already compromised joint surface, thus accelerating chondral damage and progression to osteoarthritis.

In practice, the control of swelling is usually non-surgical and involves rest, gentle strengthening, cautious use of anti-inflammatory drugs, and intra-articular drainage and injection. It is safe to inject viscosupplement and platelet-rich growth factors/PRP, but the injection of intra-articular steroid has to be extremely carefully considered. It should be viewed as a late option and only be used when the player has agreed to have a prolonged period of weeks off playing after the injection.

40.5 Football Medicine: The Madness

40.5.1 Journalists and the Media in General

Many of the players treated have a big media profile, and their injury will generate a lot of newsprint. The best policy is to never discuss a specific case, or in fact cases in general, with journalists. It is incredibly tempting for a young surgeon, particularly if they are excited to be involved in professional football injury work, to 'try to be helpful' or even self-promoting. To do so compromises the special relationship with the player and can rarely be justified. The confidentiality of the player should be paramount. Things will be said and facts learnt must remain confidential.

40.5.2 Agents

Generally speaking, football agents have earned a bad reputation. Their profile within our work has increased over time. Not all of this is bad. Having been established in treating footballer's knee injuries for nearly 20 years, the senior author has got to know many of the agents who look after his patients. As a result, there is an element of trust, and the working relationship becomes easier. Agents can of course make life difficult, particularly when they wish to interfere with pre-signing medicals for clubs or criticise treatment. They can be difficult when a player's recovery is not going well, and they take the player to another surgeon for a second opinion. It is not only undermining but very stressful. There are, however, agents who generally care about a player, particularly when the player is young, and this is often overlooked by the media and the public too.

40.5.3 Other Doctors

When treating professional footballers, a surgeon will frequently see a player who has previously had treatment with another clinician. In the pressured atmosphere of the consultation, it is very easy to make comments about the previous treatment, and a surgeon should be extremely careful in doing so. What seems to be clear at that moment may not be as the surgeon thinks. Even minor disparaging remarks can be misconstrued by the player and cause tremendous anxiety and stress to the first clinician and even lead to legal action.

Another aspect is that some doctors are envious of a clinician's practice and make unjustified but nonetheless unpleasant comments. The senior author has learnt over the years that there is a lot of jealousy and the best way to deal with it is to ignore it and be above criticism by ensuring that his personal behaviour and practice are of the highest standard; one can do no more than this.

40.5.4 Medicolegal

The potential for lawsuits is increasing, partly due to the attitude of patients and the potential for large financial gains. A surgeon treating professional footballers can be sued by the player, the agent, the sponsor, and the club. The stakes are therefore high.

In a well-documented case in which the senior author was an expert witness, the damages claimed meant that despite the fact that the footballer was awarded much less than he had requested, the two major medical indemnity companies in the UK stopped insuring doctors for dealing with professional sportsmen. In this case, a mid-20s midfielder had an isolated grade II PCL rupture that should have, of course, been treated non-surgically. However, he had an arthroscopy followed a week or 2 later by a PCL reconstruction using allograft. Surgery was performed in such a bad manner that the tibial tunnel appeared to be in the position of an ACL tunnel, and, unfortunately more severe, the femoral tunnel exploded the medial femoral condyle causing an intra-articular fracture. The player subsequently had an osteotomy and recovered well enough to become a football coach but disappointingly lost his footballing career. Despite being a player in an English Championship League team (i.e. the second tier) and being relatively unknown, his claim was for £8.5 million. At that time, the maximum cover from the insurance companies to doctors was £10 million.

With a potential of four lawsuits from various parties affected, clearly, insurance cover was inadequate for any clinician treating professional athletes. As a result of this case, a new insurance scheme has been developed which is more helpful to surgeons involved in treating professional athletes, but unfortunately the cover is still only a maximum of £20 million. Whilst experienced surgeons dealing with large numbers of athletes are at high risk because of the volume of surgery undertaken, those surgeons who infrequently treat athletes are at high risk due to their inexperience with the demands that have to be met. The classic scenario is the tibial fracture in professional footballers. This usually gets treated, like any other patient, via the emergency department, and the on-call surgeon undertakes the surgery. In my experience from dealing with the aftermath of such cases, the complication rates are extremely high. It often relates to simple problems such as prominence of metal work, which requires further intervention. Attention to detail is required to a much greater extent in professional footballers than usual. Unfortunately, this is not always appreciated by those unused to dealing regularly with professional footballers. Thinking ahead and planning customised surgery are keys when dealing with athletes.

40.5.5 Advice on Survival

Necessarily, dealing with elite footballers is a stressful, time-consuming, and energy-sapping activity. To be able to sustain it in the longer term, it is important for the surgeon to have a robust psychology and coping strategies. The level of service required will affect not only the surgeon but also his or her family life. Phone calls at night and over weekends are the norm as well as over the holiday periods.

Of course what we have to say is relevant to us and may or may not be relevant to other people, but here are some thoughts that may be helpful. Firstly, realise that it was your choice to be involved in this work and nobody else's. You could say no, but if you do not, then you must accept the situation. Be aware of the fact that it is a privilege to deal with such a special group of people and that there has to be a personal cost for this. In our experience, an appreciation of being lucky enough to undertake this line of work forces a feeling of positivity about the opportunity and ability to cope with the downsides.

Secondly, surround yourself with a team who look after you. This includes your family; it is fortunate to have a tolerant and understanding spouse! The office must be tuned to provide the highest level of service for football. The secretaries must have a 'sixth sense' to give the 'right answer' to a football team representative, even without referring to the surgeon. Clinical colleagues need to understand what is needed. It is your background team who support you.

Thirdly, you must love sport. If you do not, then you will never understand why the pressures are applied to you to see patients who have seemingly minor problems that appear to be exaggerated compared to normal patients. You should realise that for these patients, these minor problems are actually serious issues. If you do not have a love for sport, you will not find it easy to find the empathy required to treat footballers properly and with the respect they deserve.

Fourthly, you have to realise that even when you do your best, seemingly achieve good results, and give excellent advice, due to the nature of the environment in which the players live, your sensible judgement will be questioned without justification! You must develop a tolerance of players being moved to other specialists, even without you being informed. There is no loyalty in football, and this extends to the medical staff too. People are certainly not always nice. When you realise these facts, it is much less stressful to accept such disappointments.

Fifthly, do not forget that this is fascinating and exciting work and a very good discipline for excellence. It will help you treat your nonsporting patients in a better way. There are also privileged occasions when you can enjoy the success of a player or team. It is important that you enjoy these times, as it energises you for the future, but only in a discrete and private manner. It must not be converted to a public display of self-congratulation or arrogance. You must not forget that in this business, you are only as good as your last case, and failure is not tolerated well.

Sixthly, and finally, you usually have one chance to get the situation right in terms of the quality of consultation with the player, the decision-making process, advice given, or, of course, surgery. Attention to detail with a high level of discipline is required to 'get it right the first time'. As well as medical skills, this includes the highest levels of discipline, self-control, and personal behaviour. Some would describe this as 'soft touch'. Being attuned to behave in an appropriate way is invaluable as it will encourage trust and faith from the player and the club concerned.

Take-Home Message
Whilst treating professional footballers is a challenge and, at times, very stressful, it should not be forgotten that it is also hugely helpful in improving a surgeon's ability to treat the normal population as well as being a privilege. Football has genuinely driven improvements in care for all people.

Top 5 Evidence Based References

Ekstrand J, Bengtsson H, Hallen A et al (2016) .UEFA elite club injury study 2015/2016 season report http://www.uefa.org/MultimediaFiles/Download/uefaorg/Medical/02/40/27/65/2402765_DOWNLOAD.pdf. Accessed 16 Mar 2017

Nawabi D, Crow S, Hamid I et al (2014) Return to play after lateral meniscectomy compared with medial meniscectomy in elite professional soccer players. Am J Sports Med 42:2193–2198

Narvani A, Mahmud T, Lavelle J et al (2010) Injury to proximal deep medial collateral ligament – problematical subgroup of injuries. Bone Joint J 92(7):949–953

Watt F, Paterson E, Freidin A et al (2016) Acute molecular changes in synovial fluid following human knee injury: association with early clinical outcomes. Arthr Rheumatol 68(9):2129–2140

Smigielski U, Zdanowicz M, Drwięga M et al (2016) The anatomy of the anterior cruciate ligament and its relevance to the technique of ACL reconstruction. Bone Joint J 98:1020–1026

References

1. Ekstrand J, Bengtsson H, Hallen A et al (2016) .UEFA elite club injury study 2015/2016 season report http://www.uefa.org/MultimediaFiles/Download/uefaorg/Medical/02/40/27/65/2402765_DOWNLOAD.pdf. Accessed 16 Mar 2017
2. Nawabi D, Crow S, Hamid I et al (2014) Return to play after lateral meniscectomy compared with medial meniscectomy in elite professional soccer players. Am J Sports Med 42:2193–2198
3. Narvani A, Mahmud T, Lavelle J et al (2010) Injury to proximal deep medial collateral ligament – problematical subgroup of injuries. Bone Joint J 92(7):949–953
4. Watt F, Paterson E, Freidin A et al (2016) Acute molecular changes in synovial fluid following human knee injury: association with early clinical outcomes. Arthritis Rheumatol 68(9):2129–2140
5. Smigielski U, Zdanowicz M, Drwięga M et al (2016) The anatomy of the anterior cruciate ligament and its relevance to the technique of ACL reconstruction. Bone Joint J 98:1020–1026
6. FIFA (2006) FIFA big count .2006. http://www.fifa.com/mm/document/fifafacts/bcoffsurv/bigcount.statspackage_7024.pdf. Accessed 16 Mar 2017
7. BBC News (2015) Premier league in record £5.14bn TV rights deal. http://www.bbc.com/news/business-31379128. Accessed 16 Mar 2017
8. Bernstein J (2015) Wayne Rooney will earn around £73million on his current Manchester United deal while five Manchester City players are among the 10 best paid in the Premier League. http://www.dailymail.co.uk/sport/football/article-3227651. Accessed 16 Mar 2017
9. Silva M, Shepherd E, Jackson W et al (2002) Average patient walking activity approaches 2 million cycles per year. J Arthroplast 17(6):693–697
10. Kittl C, Halewood C, Stephen J et al (2015) Length change patterns in the lateral extra-articular structures of the knee and related reconstructions. Am J Sports Med 43(2):354–362
11. Kittl C, El-Daou H, Athwal K et al (2015) The role of the anterolateral structures and the ACL in controlling laxity of the intact and ACL deficient knee. Am J Sports Med 44(2):345–354

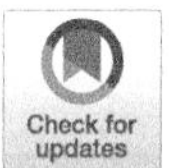

On Field Testing After Anterior Cruciate Ligament Reconstruction

41

Pelin Pişirici, Atakan Çağlayan, Mustafa Karahan, and Michael Hantes

Contents

P. Pişirici
Private Pendik Regional Hospital, Istanbul, Turkey

A. Çağlayan
Sports Sciences, School of Sports Sciences, Duzce University, Duzce, Turkey

M. Karahan, M.D. (✉)
Department of Orthopedic Surgery, Acibadem University, Istanbul, Turkey
e-mail: drmustafakarahan@gmail.com

M. Hantes
Department of Orthopedic Surgery, University of Thessalia, Larissa, Greece

41.1 Introduction

41.1.1 Football and ACL Injuries

Despite the fact that football is played in wide field, most of the action takes place in limited spaces with a high level of combat, physical activities, and technical skills [1]. Aerobic and anaerobic capacity, muscular strength, power, endurance, flexibility, balance, proprioception, speed, agility, and functional movements are the targeted means [2]. Failure to address the requirements of the game may result in an anterior cruciate ligament (ACL) injury.

41.1.2 Treatment of ACL Injuries

It is estimated that 125,000–200,000 anterior cruciate ligament reconstructions (ACLR) are thought to be performed per year in the United States [3]. There are various methods to perform ACLR, and the aim is to stabilize the knee and allow the athlete to return to football at the highest performance [4, 5].

41.1.3 Rehabilitation After ACL Reconstruction

Despite the improved surgical techniques and rehabilitation protocols, approximately two-thirds of

V. Musahl et al. (eds.), *Return to Play in Football*, https://doi.org/10.1007/978-3-662-55713-6_41

the surgically operated athletes are observed not to be able to return to the condition of their pre-injury sports level even after a year [3]. Rerupture rates for the operated knee in athletes who return to their previous sports and competitive level are 3–19%, and rupture for the contralateral side is 9–24% [6].

The rehabilitation program should be well organized and systematic in order to safely guide the athlete back to previous level. The phases are usually acute, subacute, functional, and return to sport. The transition timings should be based on certain criteria (joint range of motion, strength, gaining function); assignments should be intensive but not aggressive and, rather than completing the time given, changing as long as the improvements are done [7, 8]. By the end of the program, the athlete should have regained normal range of motion, muscle strength, balance, and proprioception which is followed by return to sports programs. In the "return to sports" phase, the aim is to prepare the athlete against competitive activities by teaching special movement patterns under a controlled condition [9].

41.1.4 Return to Sport Programs

Before starting the program, the athletes should fulfill the minimum criteria:

- Subjective knee examination of the patient must be at least 70 according to the International Knee Documentation Committee.
- No postsurgical history of giving away or negative pivot shift.
- A minimum baseline strength knee extension peak torque/body mass of at least 40% (male) and 30% (female) at 180°/s [10].

The key for a successful program is one-on-one approach allowing to set the program intensity and content. Compatible movement is another important factor between surgeon, athlete, sports physiotherapist, and athletic trainer.

41.2 Determinative Tests of Return to Sport

41.2.1 Isokinetic Tests

Isokinetic dynamometer tests are often used to assess maximal power production in injured [11] or uninjured legs after surgery. Isokinetic testing is reported to be safe in terms of graft rupture even at 6 months postoperatively [12]. The importance of isokinetic tests for safe return of sports is known, but the correlation between these tests and functional strength tests is questioned [13, 14].

41.2.2 Subjective Assessment Tests

IKDC 2000 is a reliable and valid tool for measuring knee symptoms, function, and sport involvement of patients following knee injury. IKDC is often used to determine the knee function of patients after ACL surgery. It is used to identify knee deficits and physical performance after ACL surgery and to determine successful knee function and to increase knee function with proper rehabilitation use [6, 15, 16].

41.2.3 Functional Performance Tests (FPT)

Functional tests should measure the performance level. Measurements should include both extremities so that operative leg performance can be proportional. This proportion is called the extremity limb symmetry index (LSI). A test battery for a football player who has suffered an ACL injury should include leap, agility, and endurance. Physical resources, such as strength and power, as well as properties such as acceleration, sprinting, jumping, and durability are the determinants for performance in terms of ensuring continuity of these properties [17].

41.2.3.1 Use of Functional Tests in Football

The choice of appropriate FPT requires careful assessment of safety, interest, specificity, and practicality [18]. An aggressive FPT may be performed on injured knees, usually after 12–16 weeks of soft tissue repair [19].

41.2.3.2 Application of Functional Test

Tests should be planned, so those requiring explosive power should be done on the first day, followed by more strenuous aerobic conditions [18, 20]. A standard warming protocol should be applied to athletes before performing functional tests. The purpose of warming is to increase heart rate, blood flow, body temperature, and respiration [21]. Static or dynamic stretches are recommended prior to maximal effort tests to reduce the risk of injury and to prevent muscle stiffness after activity. Experiments should be performed to avoid risky outcomes in functional tests [22, 23]. Performing the tests in a hierarchical order is important to avoid injuries that may occur during testing as depicted in Table 41.1.

41.2.3.3 Frequently Used Functional Performance Tests

Endurance Tests

Yo-Yo Test

In a number of field tests which have been designed for use in soccer for the assessment of aerobic fitness, the Yo-Yo tests have become popular in recent years. Yo-Yo tests have been designed for use in soccer for the assessment of aerobic fitness. There are two versions of the Yo-Yo intermittent test. The Yo-Yo intermittent endurance (YYIE) test allows a recovery period of 5 s, while the Yo-Yo intermittent recovery (YYIR) test allows 10 s. Two levels of each test have been developed, one for young people, amateur athlete elite, or habitually active people (L1) and an advanced one for elite athletes who have progressed through all the level 1 stages (L2) [24].

In the Yo-Yo intermittent recovery test (Fig. 41.1), participants make 2 × 20 m shuttle runs at increasing speeds that are made backward and forward between the start, turn, and finish lines. Each shuttle run has an active recovery period of 10 s, within 5 m of the participants' walking or jogging. The running speed at the test is determined by the automatically controlled warning chimes. The funnel is used to determine

Table 41.1 Commonly used functional performance tests and the components addressed

	Endurance	Agility	Strength	Coordination	Stability
Yo-Yo test	✓				
The shuttle run test		✓			
Modified agility *T* test		✓			
Single-leg hop test			✓		
Single-leg cross hop test		✓		✓	
Square hop test	✓				
Single-legged vertical jump test		✓	✓		
The box landing					
Five-jump test	✓	✓	✓		
Single-leg 6 m timed hop test		✓	✓		
Single-legged squat test		✓	✓	✓	✓

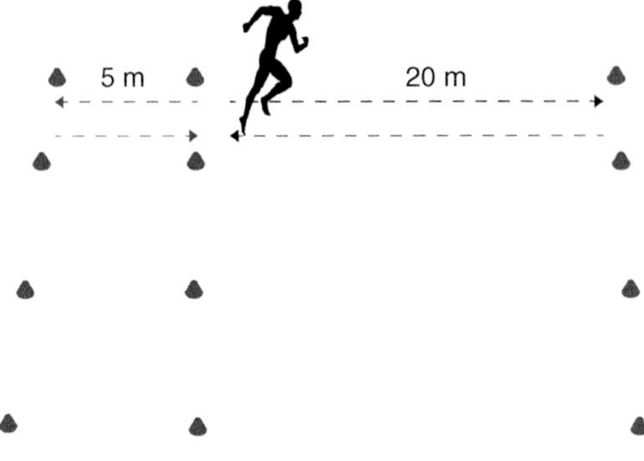

Fig. 41.1 Yo-Yo test

running strips 2 m wide and 20 m long. Each strip has another funnel located 5 m behind the starting line, and this area shows the recovery zone. The test is terminated when the athlete runs out of power or fails to reach the finish line twice, and the total distance run in the test (including the endless last shuttle run) is calculated as the test result [25].

> **Fact Box 1**
> - Testing should be done subsequently.
> - The tests should be planned as tests consisting of explosive power of the first day and then the tests consisting of more tiring aerobic sprints on the other day subsequently.

Agility Tests

Modified Agility *T* Test

Agility *T* test was modified to show lower extremity side-to-side differences in cutting and running maneuvers. This modification, included four 90° directional switches isolated in a single direction throughout the test. The aim is to reach at least 90% symmetry between the two extremities. For the modified *T* test (Fig. 41.2), the starting foot is left to the player. The participant is first directed by the test manager in the direction of shuffling motion throughout the course and not running on the lateral movement parts of the test and not taking cross steps. When they feel that rest is sufficient (about 2 min), the test is applied in the other direction. The test is performed twice for each direction. The best time for each direction is recorded [26, 27].

The Shuttle Run Test

Shuttle run test (Fig. 41.3) measures speed and agility of the athlete while changing direction [28]. This test requires the athlete to run as much as she/he can and turn to the other side on the operated leg at the end of the designated area. Reliability and validity of shuttle run test are acknowledged in the literature [29].

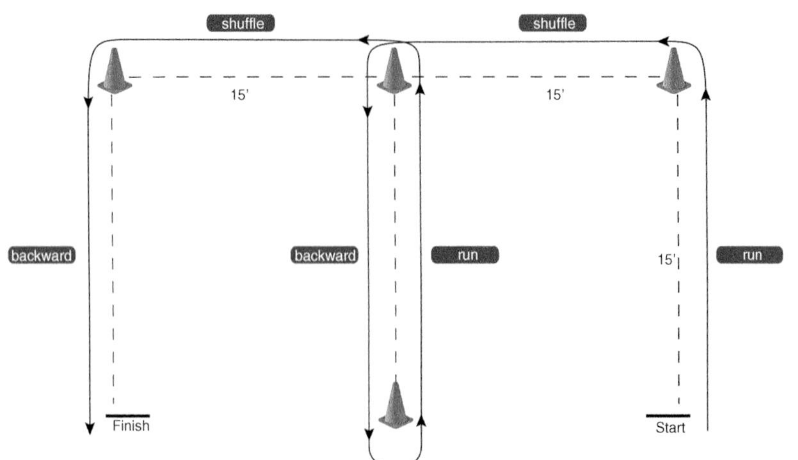

Fig. 41.2 Modified *T* test

Strength Tests

Fact Box 2
In single hop tests, a difference in limb performance greater than 5% is classified as abnormal and may indicate an increased risk for giving away of knee during sport activation.

Single-Leg Hop Test

In single-leg jump test (Fig. 41.4), the athlete stands on her/his single leg, jumps as much as possible, and falls onto the same leg keeping balance for at least 2 s. Total distance is measured as the interval between the starting point and rear heel of the leg on the floor. Each foot is tested twice, the tests are averaged, and this average is used for calculating in accordance with extremity symmetry index [1, 30, 31].

Fig. 41.3 Shuttle run test

Single-Leg Triple Hop Test

In triple jump test (Fig. 41.4), the patient stands on her/his single leg and performs three jumps as much as possible successively. The patient should fall onto the same leg and keep her/his balance for at least 2 s after falling down. Waiting for more than 1s between second and third jumps and loss of balance invalidate the test [32]. Total distance is measured starting from the starting point, and it is measured up to the contact point of heel to the ground after third jump is completed [33]. Each extremity is tested between one and three tries; its average is taken and evaluated according to extremity symmetry index [26, 30].

Single-Leg Cross Hop Test

In single-leg cross jump test (Fig. 41.4), a band with 15 cm width and 6 m length is placed on the center of the ground. The athlete should jump forward on the same leg successively by crossing the band three times. The athlete should keep her/his

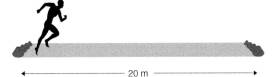

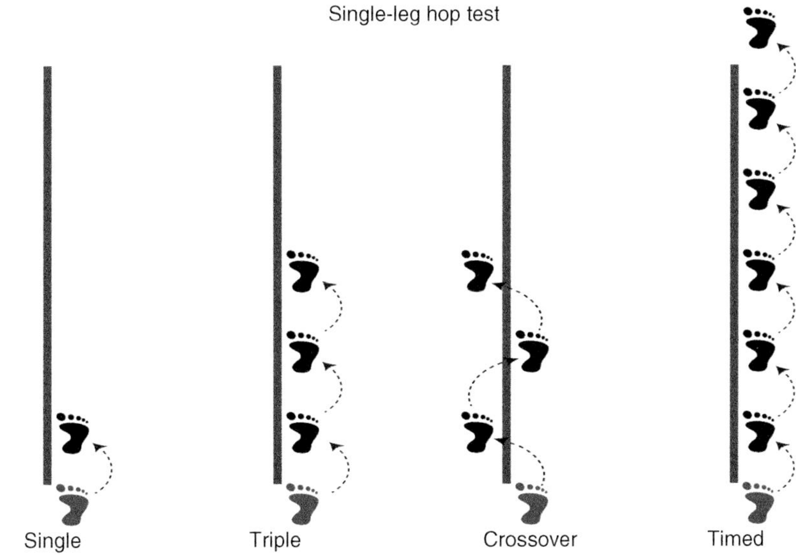

Fig. 41.4 Single-leg hop tests

balance for 2 s during the test and after the last hop. The total distance is calculated and each extremity is tested twice. Their averages are taken, and it is calculated according to LSI (limb symmetry index) [30].

Single-Leg 6 m Timed Hop Test

The 6 m hop test (Fig. 41.4) requires the patient to jump 6 m as fast as possible on single leg. Time is calculated with chronometer. Two measurements are taken for each extremity. Their averages are taken and calculated according to LSI [30].

Single-Legged Vertical Jump Test

Single-legged vertical jump test (Fig. 41.5) can be performed with computer systems or simply by signing the wall with a piece of chalk. At the beginning, patient extends the arm to the point where he/she can extend maximal. Then patient stands on single leg and performs maximal vertical jump and required to land on the same leg. Then, the point where she/he touches is determined again, and the distance between this point and the point determined beforehand is recorded [20]. Patient is asked to try the test three times; the best score is recorded.

Vertical Jump Test Followed by Double Jump

Vertical jump test followed by double jump requires hands are at the back and on the affected leg with 30 cm height. A band 45 cm ahead of the box is placed in a way that will sign the starting point. The athlete jumps without crossing the starting point or contacting the line in a way that she/he will fall onto single leg and instantly performs maximal jumps twice on the same leg. The distance is measured from the starting position till the heel line of the patient's tested leg [34].

Square Hop Test

In square hop test, it should be stood outside of a square area placed on the ground with band in the form of 40 × 40 on the leg to be tested and hands should be backward. And, a 10 cm framework is signed around the square test area. The patients are asked to jump clockwise inward and outward of the square for 30 s for the right leg. If more than 25% of the tests includes fault, another 30 s testing is carried out after resting period of 3 min. On the other hand, a counterclockwise testing is performed for the left leg [34].

Five-Jump Test

Five-jump test requires five jumps performed successively. The athlete jumps forward with her/his single leg from the starting position. After four jumps in which right and left feet change alternatively, the individual should finish the last jump with the starting foot [35].

Stabilization Tests

Single-Legged Squat Test

Patients stand on a box with a height of 20 cm and make squat five times on single leg in a way

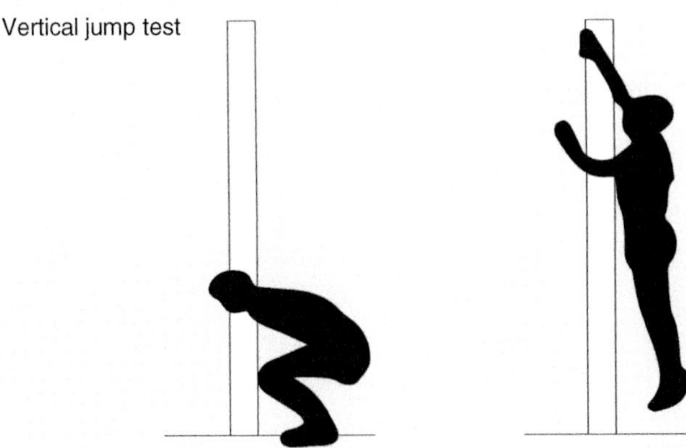

Fig. 41.5 Vertical jump test

that their arms will be cross on the chest and in a slow and controlled way (2 s per squat). The test is evaluated as "good," "sufficient," or "weak." For a test to be acceptable, the patient should make the movement properly, squat should be at least 60°, the patient should be able to keep her/his balance, body movement (lateral deviation, rotation, lateral flexion, forward flexion) and hip movement (lateral displacement, lateral deviation, rotation or tilt) should not be at all, and hip adduction and internal rotation should not be observed at all. Furthermore, it should not be valgus on the knee, and center of the knee should stay over the center of the foot [36].

41.3 Discussion

Functional performance and field tests are crucial for the physiotherapists and athletic trainers to rehabilitate the athlete to her/his previous performance level after ACLR.

The fact that laboratory tests take more time and cost than in field tests and also logistic requirements for taking team to laboratory are important factors in determining the availability and effectiveness of laboratory tests, which are often more reliable and valid, leads to the design of credibility field tests [24]. Although field tests are influenced by environmental factors such as the ground and air conditions, field tests are preferred because of their sport specificity, less time, and equipment requirements [37].

While the athlete continues to be rehabilitated on the field, we are not sure that the tests we run have a combination of different dynamics. The dynamics are meaningful when they come together, because you cannot expect agility when there is lack of strength and you cannot expect full coordination when there is lack of stabilization. For this reason, it is necessary to deal with the athlete in many ways. That is, we should use the most reliable tests in series instead of using field tests separately. Although each test contains several dynamics within itself, it is emphasized that the combined use of the tests gives more sufficient and reliable results.

When evaluating the results between uninjured and injured leg reference is taken as injured side being 90% of the uninjured side. If the uninjured leg performance should be accepted as normal, we need to know its performance before it got injured. So we can say that preseason screening may be essential for future improvement of return to sports.

The relationship among functional testing, clinical evaluation, and subjective evaluation is found to be inadequate, perhaps because each method evaluates the patient in one healing period, and therefore different aspects are missing. It is also stated that the test communities increase the sensitivity [38]. Reliability and repeatability were found to be sufficient in independent tests which are used for testing the reliability of test combinations [39].

In addition to assessing the return of the injured player to the sport, field tests also allow the recovered player to be observed during certain periods of the season and to make program changes if necessary. Field test programs that can be repeated within a day, without interrupting the routine training program, which can be repeated at intervals determined for recovered players during the season, can be planned for athletic specificity [40].

The order of construction of the tests should be based on agility, power and strength, sprints, local muscular endurance, anaerobic capacity, and lastly the order of aerobic capacity testing according to the National Strength and Conditioning Association (NSCA) test sequence, taking into account rest stops and fatigue levels [41].

Considering this ranking, the program that we will play on the recovered player will be completed with a sufficient warm-up phase, and then the agility tests will be completed with the tests such as pro agility test, modified *T* test, and Illinois test with/without ball. In the future, hop and vertical jump tests are used in healthy athletes to determine muscular strength, neuromuscular coordination, and stabilization of the lower extremity joints and to determine abnormal limb symmetry and weakness. Anaerobic evaluation is done by repeated sprint tests (RST). Finally, the

Yo-Yo intermittent test completes the aerobic test [16, 19, 37, 42].

Take-Home Message

- Failure to address the requirements of the game may result in an ACL rerupture.
- By the end of the rehabilitation program, the athlete should have regained normal range of motion, muscle strength, balance, and proprioception which is followed by return to sports programs.
- The key for a successful program is one-on-one approach allowing to set the program intensity and content. Compatible movement is another important factor between surgeon, athlete, sports physiotherapist, and athletic trainer.
- Each test should be applied with utmost attention, and results should be interpreted judiciously.
- Although each test contains unique measurements, it should be kept in mind that the combined use of the tests gives more sufficient and reliable results.
- It should not be forgotten that field tests do not evaluate isolated quadriceps strength.
- The most frequently preferred test combination contains four different hop tests.

Top 5 Evidence Based References

Ardern CL, Taylor NF, Feller JA et al (2014) Fifty-five percent return to competitive sport following anterior cruciate ligament reconstruction surgery: an updated systemic review and meta-analysis including aspects of physical functioning and contextual factors. Br J Sports Med 48:1543–1552

Bizzini M, Hancock D, Impellizzeri F (2012) Suggestions from the field for return to sports participation following anterior cruciate ligament reconstruction: soccer. J Orthop Sports Phys Ther 42(4):304–312

Myer GD, Paterno MV, Ford KR et al (2006) Rehabilitation after anterior cruciate ligament reconstruction: criteria-based progression through the return-to-sport phase. J Orthop Sports Phys Ther 36(6):385–402

Barber-Westin SD, Noyes FR (2011) Factors used to determine return to unrestricted sports activities after anterior cruciate ligament reconstruction. Arthroscopy 27(12):1697–1705

Williams D, Heidloff D, Haglage E et al (2015) Anterior cruciate ligament functional sports assessment. Oper Tech Sports Med 24:59–64

References

1. Hoff J, Helgerud J (2004) Endurance and strength training for soccer players: physiological considerations. Sports Med 34(3):165–180
2. Orishimo KF, Kremenic IJ, Mullaney MJ et al (2010) Adaptations in single-leg hop biomechanics following anterior cruciate ligament reconstruction. Knee Surg Sports Traumatol Arthrosc 18(11):1587–1593
3. Ardern CL, Taylor NF, Feller JA et al (2014) Fifty-five percent return to competitive sport following anterior cruciate ligament reconstruction surgery: an updated systemic review and meta-analysis including aspects of physical functioning and contextual factors. Br J Sports Med 48:1543–1552
4. Myer GD, Schmitt LC, Brent JL et al (2011) Utilization of modified NFL combine testing to identify functional deficits in athletes following ACL reconstruction. J Orthop Sport Phys Ther 41(6):377–387
5. Sendelides T, Kouidi E, Metaxas T et al (2003) Cardiorespiratory adaptations in soccer players. Hung Rev Sports Med 44:141–151
6. Mehran N, Williams PN, Keller RA et al (2016) Athletic performance at the national basketball association combine after anterior cruciate ligament reconstruction. Orthop J Sports Med 4(5):2325967116648083. https://doi.org/10.1177/2325967116648083
7. Bizzini M, Hancock D, Impellizzeri F (2012) Suggestions from the field for return to sports participation following anterior cruciate ligament reconstruction: soccer. J Orthop Sports Phys Ther 42(4):304–312
8. Fitzgerald GK, Lephart SM, Hwang JH et al (2001) Hop tests as predictors of dynamic knee stability. J Orthop Sports Phys Ther 31(10):588–597
9. Souissi S, Wong DP, Dellal A et al (2011) Improving functional performance and muscle power 4-to-6 months after anterior cruciate ligament reconstruction. J Sports Sci Med 10:655–664
10. Myer GD, Paterno MV, Ford KR et al (2006) Rehabilitation after anterior cruciate ligament reconstruction: criteria-based progression through the return-to-sport phase. J Orthop Sports Phys Ther 36(6):385–402
11. Barber SD, Noyes FR, Mangine RE et al (1990) Quantitative assessment of functional limitations in normal and anterior cruciate ligament-deficient knees. Clin Orthop Relat Res 255:204–214
12. Hoff J, Wisløff U, Engen LC, Kemi OJ, Helgerud J (2002) Specific aerobic endurance training. Br J Sports Med 36(3):218–221
13. Davies GJ, Zilmer DA (2000) Functional progression of a patient through a rehabilitation program. Orthop Phys Ther Clin N Am 9:103–118
14. Smaros G (1980) Energy usage during a football match. In: Vecciet L (ed) Proceedings of the 1st international congress on sports medicine applied to football. D. Guanello, Rome, pp 795–801
15. Kollock R, Lunen BLV, Ringleb SI et al (2015) Measures of functional performance and their asso-

ciation with hip and thigh strength. J Athl Train 50(1):14–22
16. Mirkov D, Nedeljkovic A, Kukolj M et al (2008) Evaluation of the reliability of soccer-specific field tests. J Strength Cond Res 22(4):1046–1050
17. Hamilton RT, Shultz SJ, Schmitz RJ (2008) Triple hop distance as a valid predictor of lower limb symmetry and power. J Athl Train 43(2):144–151
18. Nakayama Y, Shirai Y, Narita T et al (2000) Knee functions and a return to sports activity in competitive athletes following anterior cruciate ligament reconstruction. J Nippon Med Sch 67(3):172–176
19. Castagna C, Impellizzeri FM, Belardinelli R et al (2006) Cardiorespiratory responses to Yo-yo intermittent endurance test in nonelite youth soccer players. J Strength Cond Res 20:326–330
20. Lephart SM, Kocher MS, Harner CD et al (1993) Quadriceps strength and functional capacity after anterior cruciate ligament reconstruction: patellar tendon autograft versus allograft. Am J Sports Med 21:738–743
21. Paterno MV, Schmitt LC, Ford KR et al (2010) Biomechanical measures during landing and postural stability predict second anterior cruciate ligament injury after anterior cruciate ligament reconstruction and return to sport. Am J Sports Med 38(10):1968–1978
22. Gokeler A, Welling W, Zaffagnini S et al (2017) Development of a test battery to enhance safe return to sports after anterior cruciate ligament reconstruction. Knee Surg Sports Traumatol Arthrosc 25:192–199
23. Reiman MP, Manske RC (2009) Functional testing in human performance. Human Kinetics, Champaign, IL
24. Thacker SB, Gilchrist J, Stroup DF et al (2004) The impact of stretching on sports injury risk: a systematic review of the literature. Med Sci Sports Exerc 36(3):371–378
25. Manske R, Reiman M (2013) Functional performance testing for power and return to sports. Sports Health 5(3):244–250
26. Hall MP, Paik RS, Ware AJ et al (2015) Neuromuscular evaluation with single leg-leg squat test at 6 months after anterior cruciate ligament reconstruction. Orthop J Sports Med 3(3):2325967115575900. https://doi.org/10.1177/2325967115575900
27. Metaxas TI, Koutlianos NA, Kouıdi EJ et al (2005) Comparative study of field and laboratory tests for the evaluation of aerobic capacity in soccer players. J Strength Cond Res 19(1):79–84
28. Logerstedt D, Grindem H, Lynch A et al (2012) Single-legged hop tests as predictors of self-reported knee function after anterior cruciate ligament reconstruction: the Delaware-Oslo ACL cohort study. Am J Sports Med 40(10):2348–2356
29. Keays SL, Bullock-Saxton J, Keays AC (2000) Strength and function before and after anterior cruciate ligament reconstruction. Clin Orthop Relat Res 373:174–183
30. Brotzman SB, Wilk KE (2007) Handbook of orthopaedic rehabilitation. Elsevier, Atlanta, GA
31. Gustavsson A, Neeter C, Thomeé P et al (2006) A test battery for evaluating hop performance in patients with an ACL injury and patients who have undergone ACL reconstruction. Knee Surg Sports Traumatol Arthrosc 14:778–788
32. Sporıs G, Jukıc I, Milanovıc L et al (2010) Reliability and factorial validity of agility tests for soccer players. J Strength Cond Res 24(3):679–686
33. Bolgla LA, Keskula DR (1997) Reliability of lower extremity functional performance tests. J Orthop Sports Phys Ther 26(3):138–142
34. Gremion G (2005) Is stretching for sports performance still useful? A review of the literature. Rev Med Swiss 1(28):1830–1834
35. Ostenberg A, Roos E, Ekdahl C et al (1998) Isokinetic knee extensor strength and functional performance in healthy female soccer players. Scand J Med Sci Sports 8(5 Pt 1):257–264
36. Crossley KM, Zhang WJ, Schache AG et al (2011) Performance on the single-leg squat task indicates hip abductor muscle function. Am J Sports Med 39(4):866–873
37. Walker S, Turner A (2009) A one-day field test battery for the assessment of aerobic capacity, anaerobic capacity, speed, and agility of soccer players. Strength Cond J 31(6):52–60
38. Jamshidi AA, Olyaei GR, Heydarian K, Talebiana S (2005) Isokinetic and functional parameters in patients following reconstruction of the anterior cruciate ligament. Isokinet Exerc Sci 13(4):267–272
39. Harman E (2008) Principles of test selection and administration. In: Baechle TR, Earle RW (eds) Essentials of strength training and conditioning. Human Kinetics, Champaign, IL, pp 237–247
40. Barber-Westin SD, Noyes FR (2011) Factors used to determine return to unrestricted sports activities after anterior cruciate ligament reconstruction. Arthroscopy 27(12):1697–1705
41. Wilk KE, Macrina LC, Cain EL et al (2012) Recent advances in the rehabilitation of anterior cruciate ligament injuries. J Orthop Sports Phys Ther 42(3):153–171
42. Williams D, Heidloff D, Haglage E et al (2015) Anterior cruciate ligament functional sports assessment. Oper Tech Sports Med 24:59–64

Return to Play After Posterolateral Corner Injuries

42

Pablo E. Gelber, Magnus Forssblad, and Dani Romero-Rodríguez

Contents

P.E. Gelber, M.D., Ph.D. (✉)
Orthopaedic Surgery, Hospital de la Santa Creu i Sant Pau, ICATME-Hospital Universitari Dexeus, ReSport Clinic, Universitat Autònoma de Barcelona, Barcelona, Spain
e-mail: pablogelber@gmail.com

M. Forssblad, M.D., Ph.D.
Karolinska Institutet, Karolinska University Hospital, Stockholm, Sweden
e-mail: magnus@forssblad.se

D. Romero-Rodríguez
EUSES (University School of Health and Sport, University of Girona), Barcelona, Spain

42.1 Introduction

Injuries to the posterolateral corner (PLC) of the knee are infrequently seen but can lead to chronic disability due to persistent instability and articular cartilage degeneration if not appropriately treated [1]. Successful treatment of these lesions requires a detailed understanding of the anatomical complexity and biomechanics of the region. Injuries are graded according to the structural involvement and the resulting patterns of instability. Although some mild PLC injuries can be treated nonoperatively, most require surgery [2]. Reconstruction techniques vary widely depending on the severity of the injury and personal preferences and differ in their ability to recreate the biomechanics of the region. Approaches to reconstruction range from open surgery to minimally and arthroscopically assisted techniques. Depending on each specific case, therefore, postoperative rehabilitation protocols and return to play vary greatly. This chapter gives an overview of current scientific evidence and recommendations to successfully approach return to play after PLC injuries of the knee.

The PLC of the knee consists of multiple anatomic structures that are responsible for the posterolateral stabilization. While many components of the posterolateral corner have been identified [2–5], three main structures provide most of the functional mechanics of the region, particularly from a surgical reconstruction perspective: the

V. Musahl et al. (eds.), *Return to Play in Football*, https://doi.org/10.1007/978-3-662-55713-6_42

fibular collateral ligament (FCL), the popliteus tendon (PLT), and the popliteofibular ligament (PFL). These elements prevent varus angulation, posterior tibial shift, and excessive external rotation of the knee [6].

Several series have reported outcomes following PLC reconstructions, but data on long-term results of PLC reconstructions are limited. Prospective randomized studies are lacking, and the few studies published to date are case-control cohort studies or case series. Notwithstanding, the results in most short-term studies and the few long-term studies available are positive [7–10]. It is difficult to effectively compare clinical outcomes; however, because the rates of associated injuries are high, acute and chronic cases are mixed, and treatment outcome measurements are inconsistent. Furthermore, research regarding return to play in football and other similarly demanding sports after PLC injuries is limited. Few series, for example, have reported Tegner scores or the KOOS subscale function in sport, and detailed and individual information is lacking.

42.2 Grading and Classification of PLC Injuries

It is necessary to differentiate mild from moderate/severe PLC injuries. Although scientific evidence is lacking, it is logical that expectations differ regarding return to play in football. First, it is mandatory to rule out associated injuries, specifically those involving the cruciate ligaments. The second crucial step to treat these injuries properly is to grade the severity and then tailor the reconstruction to the grade.

Fact Box 1

There are two critical issues to determine when facing PLC injuries:

- Are the injuries isolated or are concomitant cruciate ligament injuries present?
- What is the degree of PLC injury?

Table 42.1 Fanelli classification of PLC injuries

Fanelli A	Fanelli B	Fanelli C
Increased external rotation	Increased external rotation and mild varus instability	Significant rotational and varus instability
Isolated injury to PFL	Injury to PFL and partial FCL	Complete injury to PFL, FCL, and cruciate ligaments

For a grading system to be considered optimal in PLC injuries, it must include assessment of both varus and rotational stabilities. The grading system described by Fanelli and Larsen [11] fulfills this requisite. It classifies PLC injuries as types A, B, and C (Table 42.1).

42.2.1 FCL Injuries

Fibular collateral ligament (FCL) injuries are not common among footballers. In a study published by Majewski et al. [12], it was found that it only occurred in 1.1% of 17,397 sport injuries. The activities leading to most injuries were soccer (35%) and skiing (26%). Fibular collateral ligament injuries were more associated with tennis and gymnastics rather than with football. In the Swedish ACL registry during the period 2005–2015, there were 226 FCL operated on with other concomitant procedures, while only one FCL was reconstructed as an isolated surgical technique.

LCL injuries can be divided in minimal (grade 1), partial (grade 2), and complete tears (grade 3). The clinical evaluation is based on varus stress tests where 0–5 mm represents a minimal tear, 5–10 mm a partial tear, and >10 mm probably a total tear. Final diagnosis can be done with both plain radiographs (with varus stress) and MRI.

For minimal and partial tears, we recommend nonoperative treatment such as physiotherapy with different modalities. The recovery time is probably the same as a MCL injury with return-to-sport within 4–6–10 weeks depending on the degree of injury.

On the other hand, a grade 3 tear is almost always in combination with cruciate ligament tears. Thus, it is mandatory to rule out other injuries when a total FCL tear is diagnosed.

When facing a grade 3 FCL injury, surgical treatment is recommended [13]. In case of an avulsion fracture from the fibular head, fixation with bone sutures, bone anchor, or a less recommended screw is usually enough. However, intrasubstance tears require reconstruction in most cases. The author's preference is the use of an Achilles tendon allograft with the bone plug fixed in the fibular side with an interference screw. It is also advisable to perform the fibular tunnel under fluoroscopic control. There is a natural tendency to perform this tunnel excessively superficial, which could lead to lateral cortex breakage.

42.2.2 Isolated PLC Injuries

Isolated PLC injuries make up less than 2% of all acute knee ligament injuries [14]. Following the Fanelli classification described above [11], grade C is automatically excluded from this scenario.

Conservative treatment for isolated PLC injuries is reported to achieve successful outcomes only in cases of the not-so-common grade A lesions after 4 weeks of cast immobilization in knee extension or after early mobilization. Although Kannus [15] also reported acceptable functional results after nonoperative treatment for grade B injuries, persistent instability was observed, making this option suitable only in low-demand patients. In football players, therefore, only rare, isolated injuries of the popliteofibular ligament might undergo conservative treatment.

In a series of 27 patients with isolated PLC injuries that were treated surgically, Jakobsen et al. [14] noted that the injury was due to a sports accident in 53% of cases. They noted that half of these patients were able to return to high-level sport, but they also observed that the KOOS subscale for sport/recreation was one of the most affected items. Although it was not specified, the surgical technique performed and the fact that both the popliteus complex and FCL were torn preoperatively suggest that all the cases had at least a moderate PLC injury.

42.2.2.1 Postoperative Rehabilitation

The recommended treatment after surgery is stabilization of the knee in an unlocked hinged knee brace, allowing a passive range of motion from 0° to 90° for 2–4 weeks. For the first 4–6 weeks, protected weight-bearing of the limb is also recommended to minimize stress on the graft. A normal gait pattern is usually achieved 8 weeks after surgery, and the brace can then be discontinued. A progressive rehabilitation program with emphasis on regaining full motion of the knee includes quadriceps-strengthening and progressive resistance exercises. Strength is regained by the use of close kinetic chain exercises as well as open kinetic chain knee extension exercises from 0° to 60°. Balance and proprioceptive activities are initiated once the patient is fully weight-bearing in order to regain neuromuscular control of the knee. As strength improves, reaching up to 70% of that of the non-injured knee, sport-specific drills may be started and gradually progressed. In cases of isolated PLC injuries, full activities and return to sport may begin 4–6 months after surgery [16].

42.2.3 PLC Injuries Associated with Cruciate Ligament Injuries

Magnetic resonance has shown that 16% of all knee ligament injuries involve the PLC [17]. Most PLC injuries occur concomitantly with cruciate ligaments tears and especially posterior cruciate ligament (PCL) (from 43 to 80%) tears [18].

As expected, the rehabilitation protocol and the functional outcome will be influenced by these concomitant injuries.

42.2.3.1 Fanelli Grade A

When facing reconstruction of the ACL concomitantly with reconstruction of the popliteofibular ligament, a return to play football at the pre-injury level can be reliably expected. Postoperatively, some surgeons advocate protection of the PFL reconstruction by means of a locked hinged knee brace for 1 month and protected weight-bearing for the first 10–12 weeks [19]. However, this conservative rehabilitation protocol is not based on any scientific evidence, and a more aggressive rehabilitation protocol can be safely followed. It is the author's opinion that postoperative care can follow the rehabilitation protocol of an isolated anterior cruciate ligament (ACL) reconstruction, particularly if the PFL was reconstructed using mini-open or arthroscopically assisted technique [8, 20]. In any case, sporting activities are not recommended for the first 6–10 months after surgery.

Successful return to play in football is less likely, however, if the posterior cruciate ligament is reconstructed concomitantly with a PFL. This situation, however, is rare. Surgical treatment of such injuries can provide sufficient function for standard daily activities but not for sports activities [10]. Again, neither functional nor sport-related outcomes have been reported in athletes in these specific injuries.

42.2.3.2 Fanelli Grade B

These injuries are far more commonly diagnosed. A level III case-control study compared isolated transtibial ACL reconstructions versus ACL and PLC reconstruction with a nonanatomic biceps tendon split [7]. The authors of the study observed worse results in the ACL and PLC reconstruction group regarding KOOS Sport subscale at 1 and 2 years, but patients with combined injuries had much lower mean preoperative scores. Conversely, KOOS Sport subscale showed a tendency to be comparable in both groups at the 5-year follow-up assessment. This infers that although a much longer recovery might be expected due to greater morbidity and a lower preoperative score, functional improvements can still be expected even 2 years after surgery.

A recent systematic review reported the outcomes of surgical treatment for acute PLC injuries [21]. The authors included 8 studies with a total of 134 patients, most of whom had an evidence level 4. They reported that reconstruction of the PLC was clearly superior to isolated repair of the PLC. Unfortunately, the activity level was rarely included in these studies. Two of included studies reported grossly that the postoperative Tegner score was between 3 and 7. They did not specify the pre-injury level of each individual or provide any data regarding return to play scales. Another recent review concluded that most of the available literature consists of low level 4 case series combining different mechanisms of injury and different patterns of multiligamentous injury into single cohorts [8]. Although none of these series focused on return to play, the few studies that reported on activity and sport scores suggest that a return to high-level sport is rarely possible.

42.2.3.3 Fanelli Grade C

These injuries are more properly considered knee dislocations, and they are far more severe than a simple PLC injuries entity. They are frequently a consequence of car accidents or high-energy trauma rather than sport accidents. Although they are further detailed in another chapter, return to play football after this devastating knee injury is seldom achieved. Overall functional results are highly dependent on the results of central pivot reconstruction [22], which rarely allows a successful return to pivoting sports.

In the last 10 years, the authors have treated nine football players with PLC injuries. None of these has been an isolated PLC injury. In two patients, a Fanelli grade C with both cruciate ligaments concomitantly injured led to the end of their careers. Although both cruciates and a Laprade technique in the PLC were performed in both players, they could not even get close to their pre-injury activity level. The remaining seven patients had a Fanelli grade A or B concomitantly with an ACL tear. While the ACLs were reconstructed either with patellar or quadriceps tendons autografts, the PLC corner were reconstructed with a mini-open technique to address the PFL or the PFL and the FCL injuries [23]. In all these cases, the patients were able to resume their sport activity after 8–10 months. All but one of these seven patients could restore exactly the same pre-injury level of activity.

42.2.4 Recommended Postoperative Rehabilitation

When concomitant reconstruction of the ACL is required, postoperative rehabilitation must consider preventing anterior tibial translation, especially in open kinetic actions where coactivation is more difficult to achieve. Similarly, when facing associated PCL reconstruction, posterior tibial forces must be specifically restricted. In both cases and specifically during the first 12–16 weeks, the rehabilitation protocol should be addressed to protect the reconstructed cruciate ligament.

PLC prevents both varus and external rotation of the tibia. Rehabilitation must therefore consider protecting these movements when programming exercise in order to progress in basic and specific sport skills.

The rehabilitation program can be divided in two main periods:

42.2.4.1 0–12 Weeks

In the first 4 months, rehabilitation should follow the parameters determined by the concomitant ACL/PCL/ACL + PCL reconstruction. It should only add a hinged knee brace used 24/7 to prevent excessive tibial rotation and varus forces, without any restriction in the ROM. However, some surgeons advocate maintaining the knee in full extension for the first 4 weeks. Restricted weight-bearing of 5–10 kg is recommended for the first 4–8 weeks, depending on the strength of the reconstruction. During this period, intensive physical therapy treatment is carried out with periods of restricted mobility varying according to concomitant injuries. Therapy should focus on improving ROM, muscle activation, strength, and balance, not on specific football skills.

42.2.4.2 After 12 Weeks

At this point, the player is usually allowed to start greater weight-bearing activities (between 12 and 16 weeks). After 16 weeks, therapy to address recovery of basic skills is initiated.

The rehabilitation program should follow three steps:

- Basic motor skills
- Football-specific skills
- Consideration of neuromuscular and biomechanical key points when designing and performing a task

This return to play methodology progresses from basic to specific sport skills [24, 25].

Figure 42.1 shows the progression of basic skills from linear running action to complex actions of turning while pivoting on the operated knee (when a considerable knee varus moment is elicited) and changing direction with impulsion of the injured knee (when high external rotation is involved). Both tasks severely stress the knee and are carried out with the foot on the ground. This represents a closed kinetic action, with multiple combinations of rotational moments.

This Fig. 42.1 shows exercises performed with inertial and elastic resistances. Inertial training creates high resistances, and it has provided notable improvements in strength and power both in healthy [3, 26, 27] and injured sport players [28, 29]. It also allows several high demanding strength and balance tasks. On the other hand, elastic resistance work emphasizes more functional tasks, improving action speed and coordination.

Figure 42.2 shows the progression of both inertial and elastic exercises. Football-specific skills are now included, starting with ball control moves and progressing to dribbling moves while under attack. Perceptive and cognitive processes should also be included in order to reach maximum performance before return to play. After all the phases described are successfully performed, the footballer is allowed to train with the team on the field, gradually decreasing the limitations.

A footballer's gradual and safe return to play is achieved at approximately 8 to 12 months postoperatively. However, a return to previous sporting level in these complex injuries is to some degree unpredictable and depends considerably on the degree of PLC injury and the associated lesions. In the most severe cases, when three or four of the major ligaments of the knee require surgery, return to play to the pre-injury level is highly unlikely.

BASIC SKILLS			
SKILL	**Neuromuscular-biomechanical key points**	**Low demanding exercise**	**High demanding exercise**
Running forward and backward	- First impact action - Light anterior translation of the tibia - Moderate stress on frontal and transversal planes of the knee - Greater activation of hamstring muscles and external rotators of the knee (running backward)	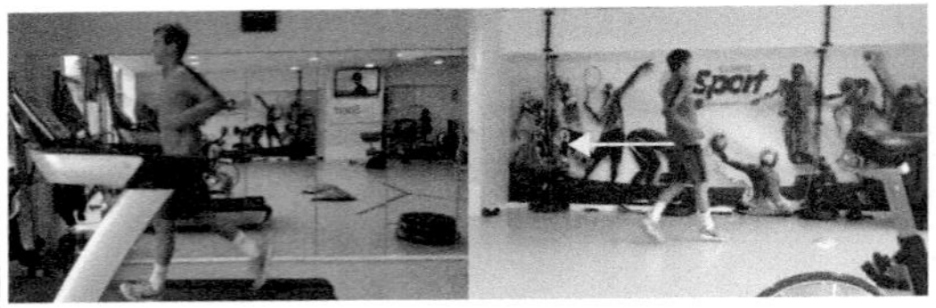	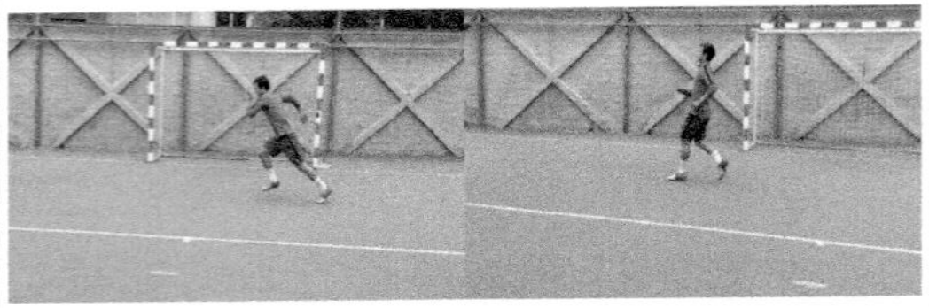
Forward acceleration	- Explosive quadriceps action - Moderate stress on frontal and transversal planes of the knee - Great quadriceps-hamstring coactivation - Implication of core stability in the breaking action - Speed work	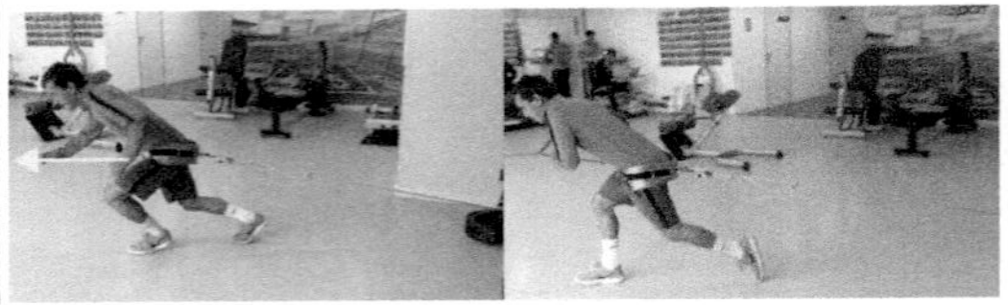	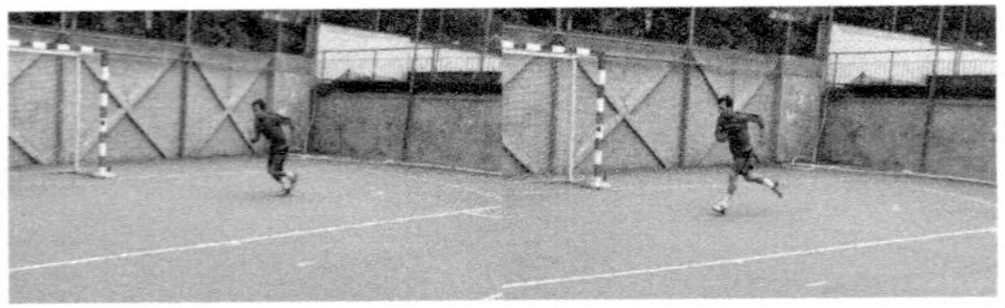
Breaking action	- Great eccentric quadriceps action - Big amount of anterior shear forces of the tibia - Greater Q-H coactivation - Higher stress on the hamstring muscles (also at the postero-lateral corner) - Higher stress and functionality when breaking after sprinting	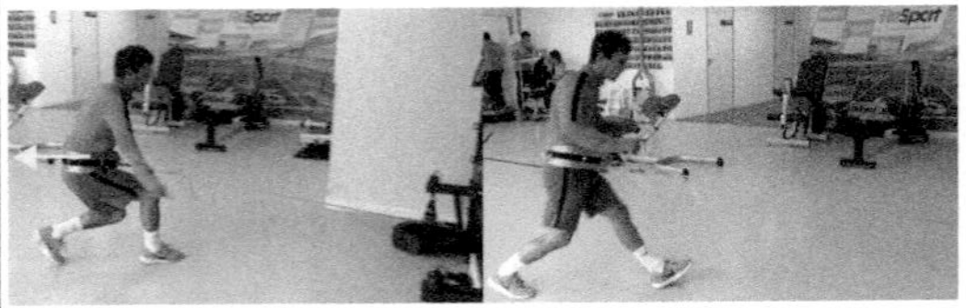	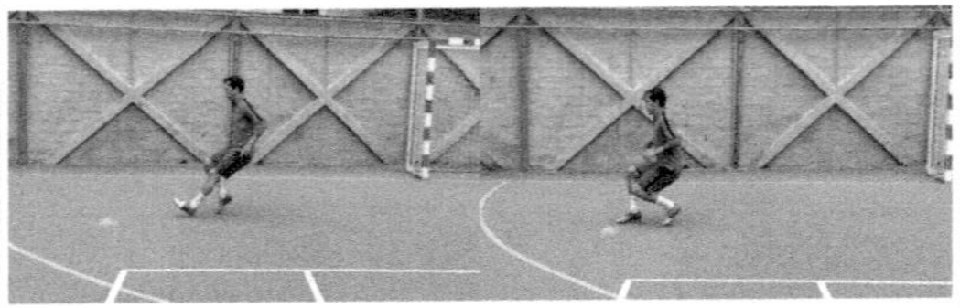
Jumping vertical direction (from leg press exercise to vertical jump)	- Increase of quadriceps strength - Need of reciprocal inhibition to jump (vertical axe) - Increase of explosive quadriceps activation in vertical direction - Need of Q-H coactivation when landing - Explosive extension torque in the knee	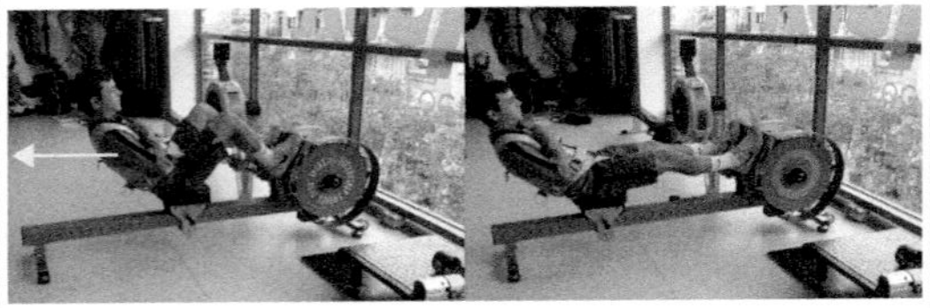	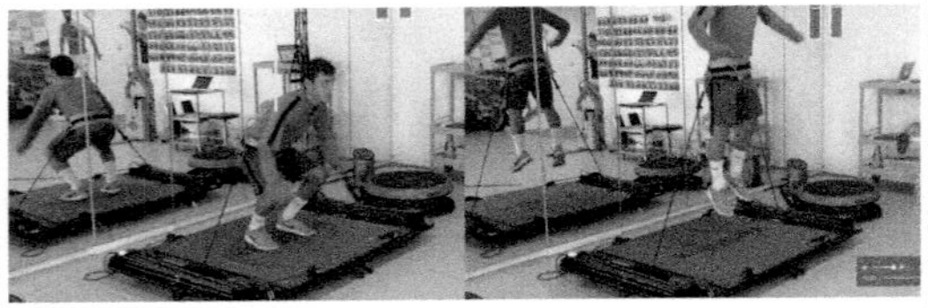

Jumping lateral direction (from lateral lunge to lateral jump)	- Great tension in the frontal plane: high demanding stabilization by the lateral complex of the knee - High Q-H coactivation in both actions - Initial knee varus action in the jumping leg (greater need of balance) - Forced varus-valgus when landing	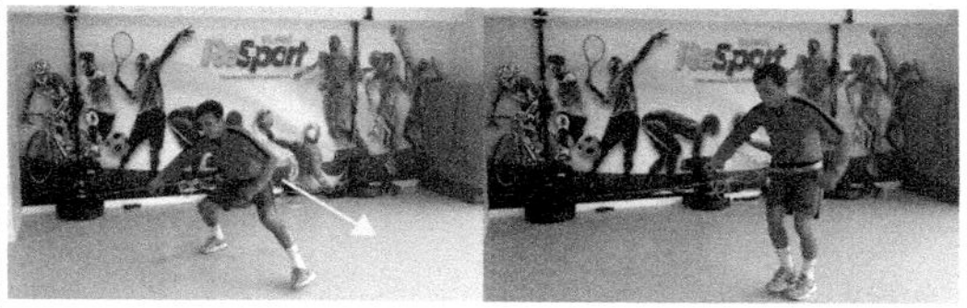	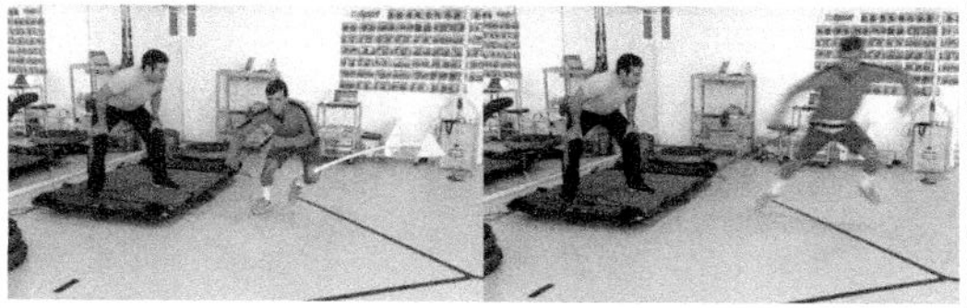
Jumping forward direction (working on the landing)	- Increase of anterior shear forces when landing - Increase of Q-H coactivation to stabilize the sagittal plane - Controlled initial work of rotational moments depending of the foot landing position - Need of reciprocal inhibition to jump (sagittal plane)	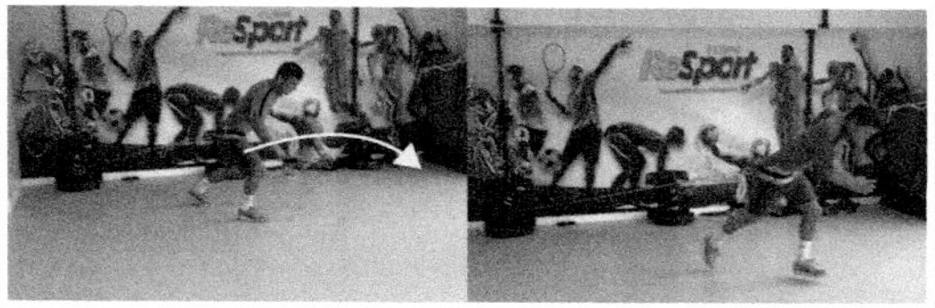	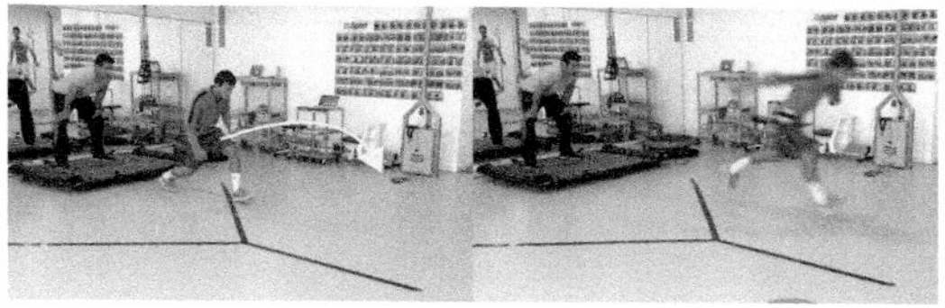
Change of direction pivoting on the non-injured side (right side). The injured side is provoking impulsion (rigt side).	- High demanding coactivation Q-H adding a rotational moment - Stabilization with the tibia usually in external rotation - High demanding control of varus-valgus (frontal plane) - Explosive action of the quadriceps - Introduction of perturbation in basic skills	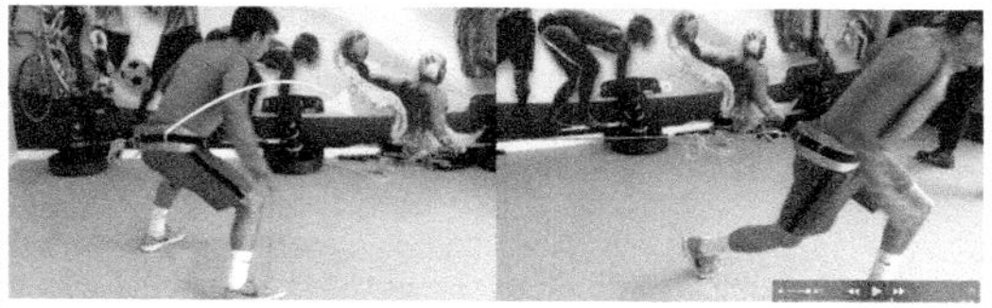	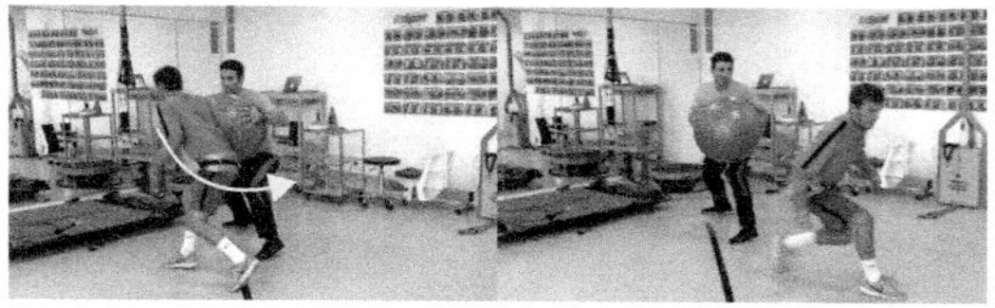
Change of direction pivoting on the injured side (left side). The pivoting action is done by the injured side.	- Light stabilization role - Great rotational ROM of the knee - Greatexternal rotation of the tibia (impulse moment) - Important joint stress (depending of the position of this pivoting leg) - Explosive action of the quadriceps - Introduction of perturbation in basic skills	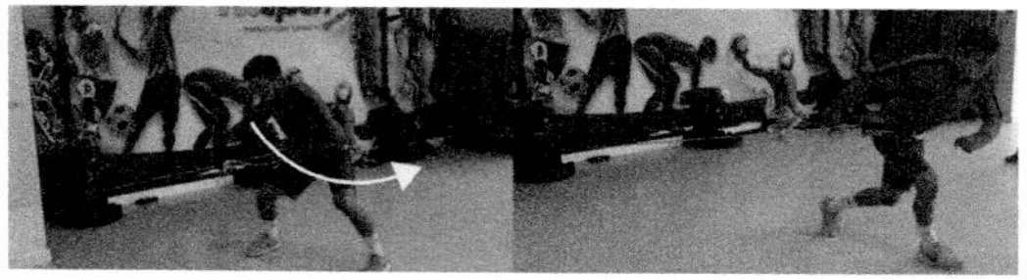	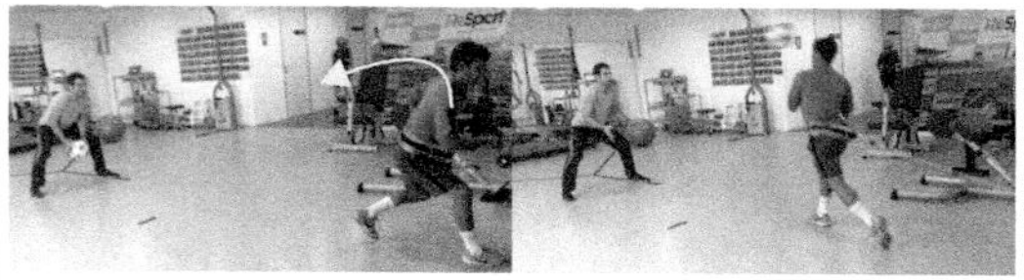

Fig. 42.1 Exercises performed with inertial and elastic resistances have both a central role in the rehabilitation

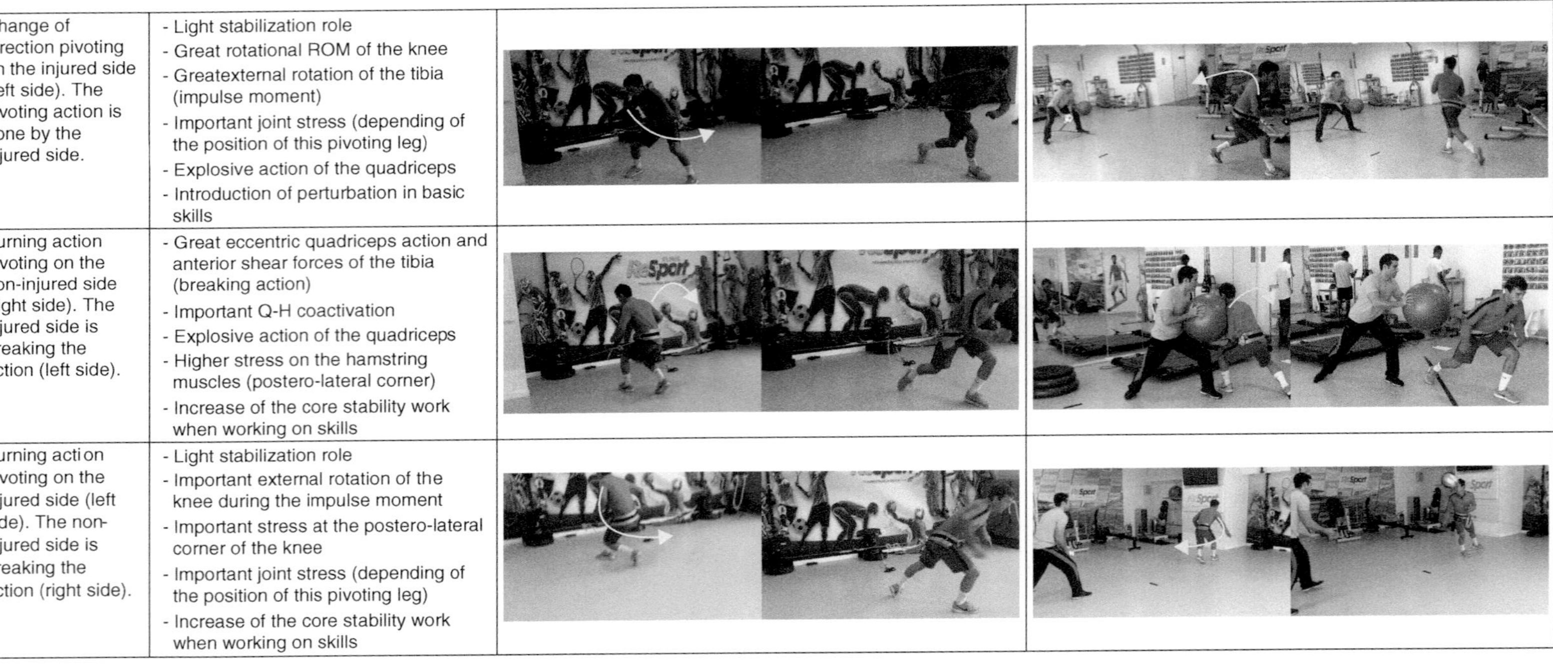

Change of direction pivoting on the injured side (left side). The pivoting action is done by the injured side.	- Light stabilization role - Great rotational ROM of the knee - Greatexternal rotation of the tibia (impulse moment) - Important joint stress (depending of the position of this pivoting leg) - Explosive action of the quadriceps - Introduction of perturbation in basic skills		
Turning action pivoting on the non-injured side (right side). The injured side is breaking the action (left side).	- Great eccentric quadriceps action and anterior shear forces of the tibia (breaking action) - Important Q-H coactivation - Explosive action of the quadriceps - Higher stress on the hamstring muscles (postero-lateral corner) - Increase of the core stability work when working on skills		
Turning action pivoting on the injured side (left side). The non-injured side is breaking the action (right side).	- Light stabilization role - Important external rotation of the knee during the impulse moment - Important stress at the postero-lateral corner of the knee - Important joint stress (depending of the position of this pivoting leg) - Increase of the core stability work when working on skills		

Fig. 42.1 (continued)

FOOTBALL SPECIFIC SKILLS		
SKILL	Neuromuscular-biomechanical key points	
Ball control actions	- When receiving in a frontal position (A), knee is suffering mild stress - Increase of the stress when the injured leg (left side) is working as the supporting leg (CKC) (B) - Mild-moderate varus and external rotation (B and C when landing) - Mild stress when the injured leg is controlling the ball	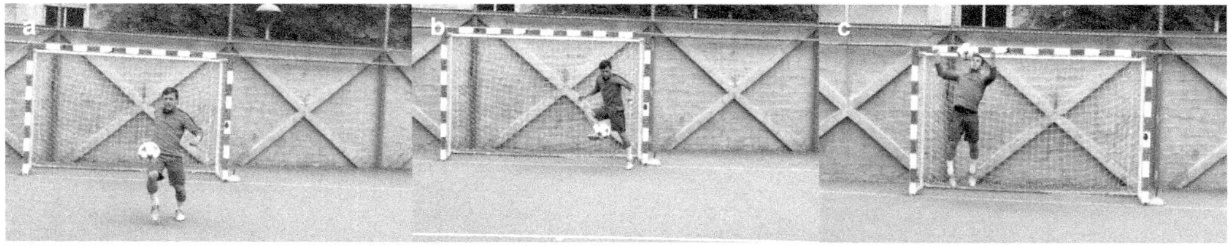 a b c
Passing the ball	- Injured leg (A) is the supporting leg: moderate stress by knee rotation (CKC) - Injured leg (B) passing the ball: more external rotation in OKC - More general stress in CKC - Progression of passing the ball by increasing the distance (C,) and accuracy (more coactivation)	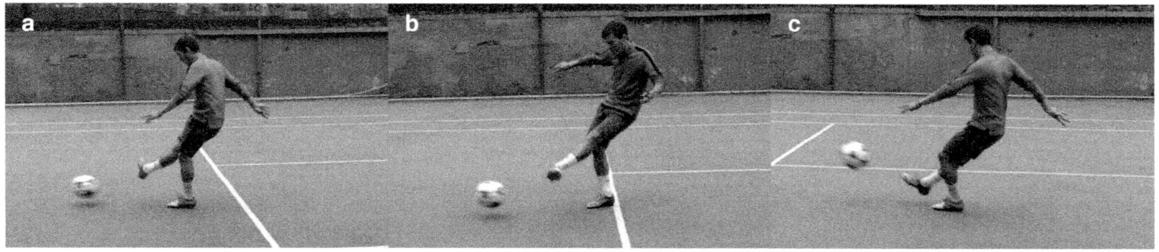 a b c
Dribbling without opponent (running with the ball)	- Progression with speed (B) and different directions of the action(C) - Dribbling: first action to increase the activity of mild changes of direction, creating circuits to develop it - Mild change of direction provokes an increase varus-valgus and rotations of the knee(C)	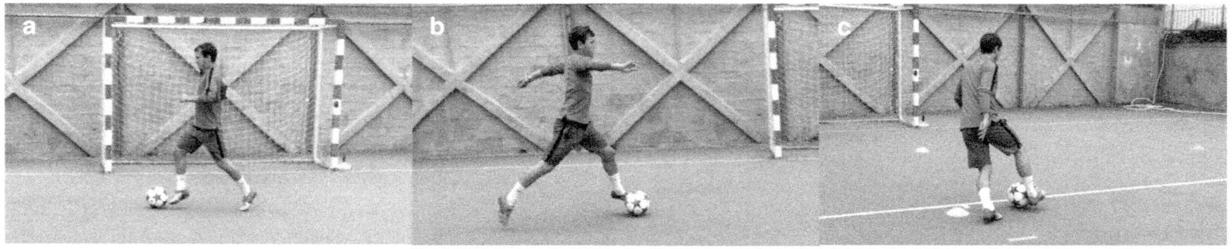 a b c
Heading (jumping action is associated)	- Increase of explosive action to the knee - Vertical jump (A and B): moderate stress in rotation when landing - Jumping in a forward displacement(C): increase of rotational and varus-valgus moment in the knee when landing; increase of anterior shear forces of the tibia	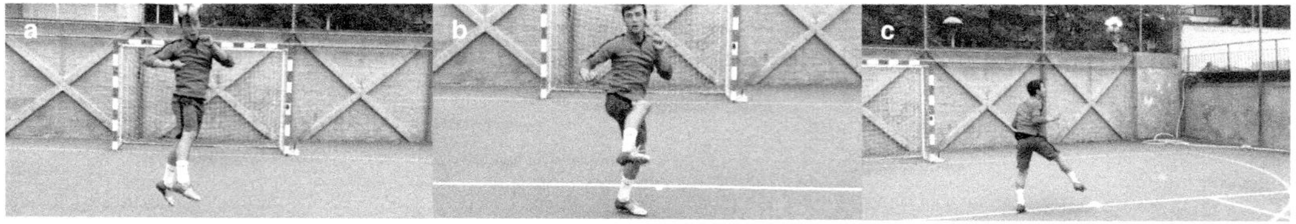 a b c

Fig. 42.2 Progression of both inertial and elastic exercises. Football specific skills are now included

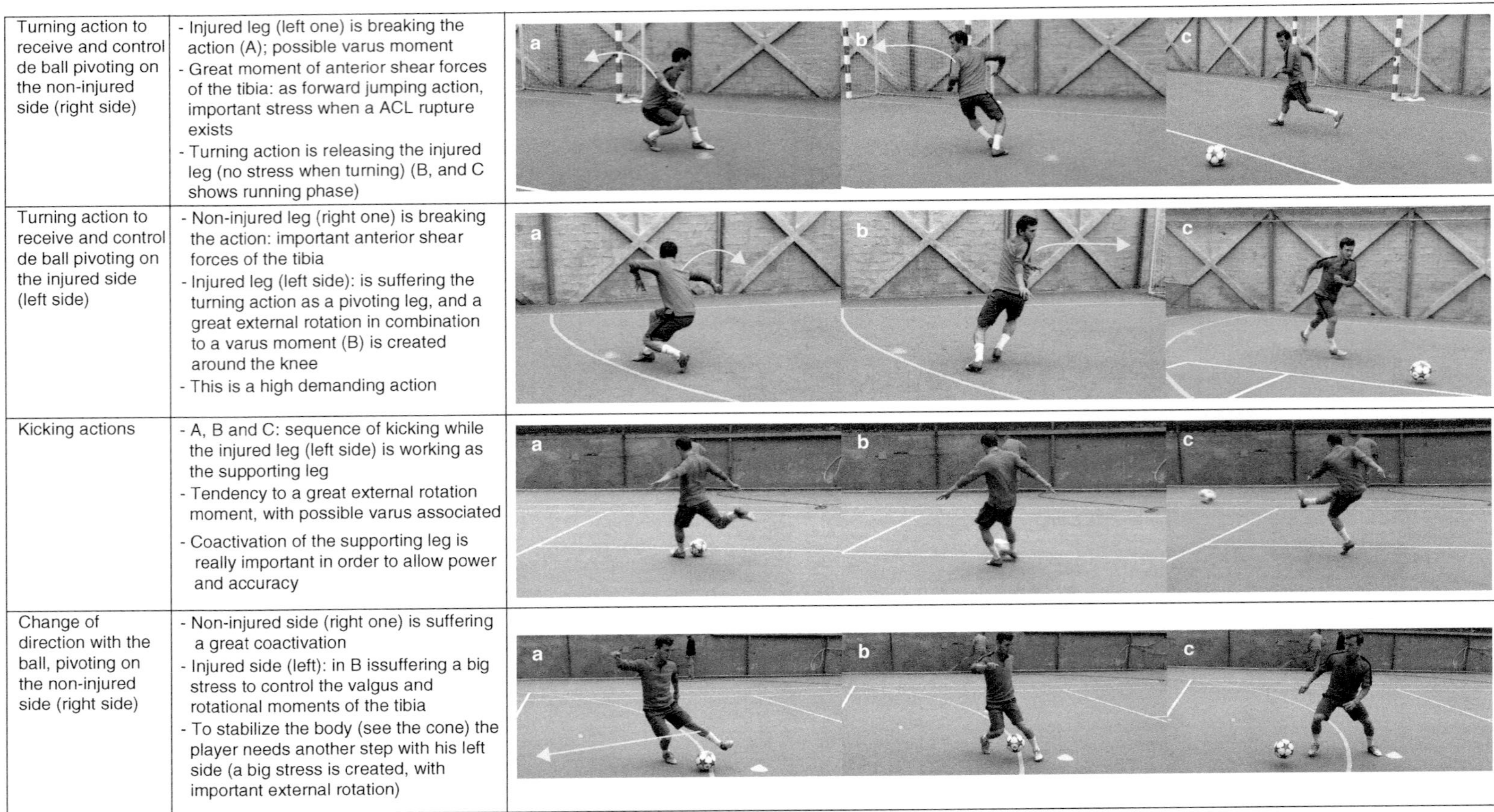

Turning action to receive and control de ball pivoting on the non-injured side (right side)	- Injured leg (left one) is breaking the action (A); possible varus moment - Great moment of anterior shear forces of the tibia: as forward jumping action, important stress when a ACL rupture exists - Turning action is releasing the injured leg (no stress when turning) (B, and C shows running phase)	a b c
Turning action to receive and control de ball pivoting on the injured side (left side)	- Non-injured leg (right one) is breaking the action: important anterior shear forces of the tibia - Injured leg (left side): is suffering the turning action as a pivoting leg, and a great external rotation in combination to a varus moment (B) is created around the knee - This is a high demanding action	a b c
Kicking actions	- A, B and C: sequence of kicking while the injured leg (left side) is working as the supporting leg - Tendency to a great external rotation moment, with possible varus associated - Coactivation of the supporting leg is really important in order to allow power and accuracy	a b c
Change of direction with the ball, pivoting on the non-injured side (right side)	- Non-injured side (right one) is suffering a great coactivation - Injured side (left): in B issuffering a big stress to control the valgus and rotational moments of the tibia - To stabilize the body (see the cone) the player needs another step with his left side (a big stress is created, with important external rotation)	a b c

Change of direction with the ball, pivoting on the injured side (left side)	- Injured side (left) is suffering a great coactivation action to keep balance and giving the right direction to the body - The injured side is suffering a great rotational moment in the knee (A) - The injured side is also suffering great tension from pivoting to impulsion action (C)	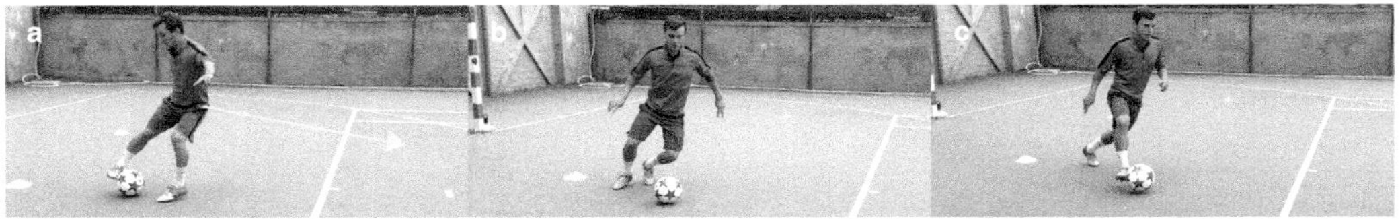 a b c
Dribbling with a close opponent (free actions with continuous perturbations)	- 1x1: previous task to the team work - Multiple combinations of rotational and varus-valgus loads in the knee - Figure A and B shows the injured side (left) working to stabilize the body and protect the ball - The player incorporates to the task perturbations and perceptual and decision-making contentas well	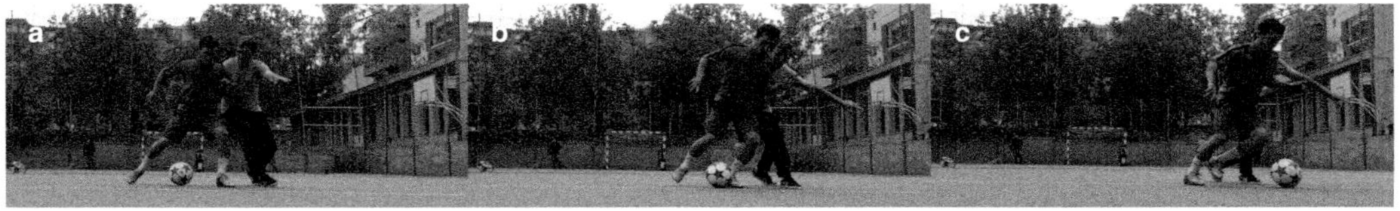 a b c

Fig. 42.2 (continued)

Fact Box 2

- Restoring the previous football level in these complex injuries largely depends on the degree of PLC injury and associated lesions.
- In the most severe cases, return to play at the same pre-injury level is highly unlikely.

Take-Home Message

- FCL and PLC injuries are not very common in football players.
- Most posterolateral corner injuries occur concomitantly with cruciate ligament tears.
- Although no evidence is available in the literature regarding return to play in football players after posterolateral corner injuries, surgical reconstructions of mild injuries should allow a successful restoration to the pre-injury sport level.
- Return to play after treatment of moderate to severe PLC injuries, however, is more unlikely.

Top Five Evidence-Based References

Cartwright-Terry M, Yates J, Tan CK, Pengas IP, Banks JV, McNicholas MJ (2014) Medium-term (5-Year) comparison of the functional outcomes of combined anterior cruciate ligament and posterolateral corner reconstruction compared with isolated anterior cruciate ligament reconstruction. Arthroscopy 30(7):811–817

Spitzer E, Doyle JB, Marx RG (2015) Outcomes for surgical treatment of posterolateral instability of the knee. J Knee Surg 28(6):471–474

Moulton SG, Geeslin AG, LaPrade RF (2015) A Systematic review of the outcomes of posterolateral corner knee injuries, part 1: surgical treatment of acute injuries. Am J Sport Med 44(5):1616–1623

Wajsfisz A, Christel P, Djian P (2010) Does combined posterior cruciate ligament and posterolateral corner reconstruction for chronic posterior and posterolateral instability restore normal knee function? Orthop Traumatol Surg Res 96(4):394–399

Saenz I, Pelfort X, LaPrade RF, Fritsch BA, Gelber PE, Karl-Heinz F (2016) Posterolateral corner reconstruction: approach to treatment including mini-open and arthroscopic techniques. In: Becker R, Kerkhoffs G, Gelber PE, Denti M, Seil R (eds) ESSKA ICL book. Springer, London

References

1. Cooper JM, McAndrews PT, LaPrade RF (2006) Posterolateral corner injuries of the knee: anatomy, diagnosis, and treatment. Sports Med Arthrosc 14(4):213–220
2. Davies H, Unwin A, Aichroth P (2004) The posterolateral corner of the knee. Anatomy, biomechanics and management of injuries. Injury 35(1):68–75
3. de Hoyo M, Pozzo M, Sañudo B, Carrasco L, Gonzalo-Skok O, Domínguez-Cobo S, Morán-Camacho E (2015) Effects of a 10-week in-season eccentric-overload training program on muscle-injury prevention and performance in junior elite soccer players. Int J Sports Physiol Perform 10(1):46–52
4. LaPrade RF, Morgan PM, Wentorf FA, Johansen S, Engebretsen L (2007) The anatomy of the posterior aspect of the knee. An anatomic study. J Bone Joint Surg Am 89(4):758–764
5. Raheem O, Philpott J, Ryan W, O'Brien M (2007) Anatomical variations in the anatomy of the posterolateral corner of the knee. Knee Surg Sports Traumatol Arthrosc 15(7):895–900
6. Veltri DM, Warren RF (1995) Posterolateral instability of the knee. Instr Course Lect 44:441–453
7. Cartwright-Terry M, Yates J, Tan CK, Pengas IP, Banks JV, McNicholas MJ (2014) Medium-term (5-Year) comparison of the functional outcomes of combined anterior cruciate ligament and posterolateral corner reconstruction compared with isolated anterior cruciate ligament reconstruction. Arthroscopy 30(7):811–817
8. Spitzer E, Doyle JB, Marx RG (2015) Outcomes for surgical treatment of posterolateral instability of the knee. J Knee Surg 28(6):471–474
9. Strobel MJ, Schulz MS, Petersen WJ, Eichhorn J (2006) Combined anterior cruciate ligament, posterior cruciate ligament, and posterolateral corner reconstruction with autogenous hamstring grafts in chronic instabilities. Arthroscopy 22(2):182–192
10. Yung Y, Jung H, Kim S, Park S, Song K, Lee Y, Lee S (2008) Posterolateral corner reconstruction for posterolateral rotatory instability combined with posterior cruciate ligament injuries: comparison between fibular tunnel and tibial tunnel techniques. Knee Surg Sports Traumatol Arthrosc 16(3):239–248
11. Fanelli GC, Larson RV (2002) Practical management of posterolateral instability of the knee. Arthroscopy 18(2 Suppl 1):1–8

12. Majewski M, Susanne H, Klaus S (2006) Epidemiology of athletic knee injuries: a 10-year study. Knee 13(3):184–188
13. Krukhaug Y, Molster A, Rodt A, Strand T (1998) Lateral ligament injuries of the knee. Knee Surg Sports Traumatol Arthrosc 6(1):21–25
14. Jakobsen BW, Lund B, Christiansen SE, Lind MC (2010) Anatomic reconstruction of the posterolateral corner of the knee: a case series with isolated reconstructions in 27 patients. Arthroscopy 26(7):918–925
15. Kannus P (1989) Nonoperative treatment of grade II and III sprains of the lateral ligament compartment of the knee. Am J Sports Med 17(1):83–88
16. Irrgang JJ, Fitzgerald GK (2000) Rehabilitation of the multiple-ligament-injured knee. Clin Sports Med 19:545–571
17. LaPrade RF, Wentorf FA, Fritts H, Gundry C, Hightower CD (2007) A prospective magnetic resonance imaging study of the incidence of posterolateral and multiple ligament injuries in acute knee injuries presenting with a hemarthrosis. Arthroscopy 23(12):1341–1347
18. Covey DC (2001) Injuries of the posterolateral corner of the knee. J Bone Joint Surg Am 83-A(1):106–118
19. Zhang H, Feng H, Hong L, Wang XS, Zhang J (2009) Popliteofibular ligament reconstruction for posterolateral external rotation instability of the knee. Knee Surg Sports Traumatol Arthrosc 17(9):1070–1077
20. Frosch KH, Akoto R, Heitmann M, Enderle E, Giannakos A, Preiss A (2015) Arthroscopic reconstruction of the popliteus complex: accuracy and reproducibility of a new surgical technique. Knee Surg Sports Traumatol Arthrosc 23(10):3114–3120
21. Moulton SG, Geeslin AG, LaPrade RF (2015) A Systematic review of the outcomes of posterolateral corner knee injuries, Part 1: Surgical treatment of acute injuries. Am J Sport Med 44(5):1616–1623
22. Wajsfisz A, Christel P, Djian P (2010) Does combined posterior cruciate ligament and posterolateral corner reconstruction for chronic posterior and posterolateral instability restore normal knee function? Orthop Traumatol Surg Res 96(4):394–399
23. Saenz I, Pelfort X, LaPrade RF, Fritsch BA, Gelber PE, Karl-Heinz F (2016) Posterolateral corner reconstruction: approach to treatment including mini-open and arthroscopic techniques. In: Becker R, Kerkhoffs G, Gelber PE, Denti M, Seil R (eds) ESSKA ICL book. Springer, London
24. Fort-Vanmeerhaeghe A, Romero-Rodríguez D, Lloyd RS, Jusher A, Myer GD (2016) Integrative neuromuscular training in youth athletes. Part II: strategies to prevent injuries and improve performance. Strength Cond J 38(4):9–27
25. Fort-Vanmeerhaeghe A, Romero-Rodriguez D, Montalvo A, Kiefer AW, Lloyd RS, Myer GD (2016) Integrative neuromuscular training and injury prevention in youth athletes. Part I: identifying risk factors. Strength Cond J 38(3):36–48
26. Gonzalo-Skok O, Tous-Fajardo J, Valero-Campo C, Berzosa C, Bataller AV, Arjol-Serrano JL, Moras G, Mendez-Villanueva A (2016) Eccentric overload training in team-sports functional performance: constant bilateral vertical vs. variable unilateral multidirectional movements. Int J Sports Physiol Perform 14:1–23
27. Tous-Fajardo J, Gonzalo-Skok O, Arjol-Serrano JL, Tesch P (2016) Enhancing change-of-direction speed in soccer players by functional inertial eccentric overload and vibration training. Int J Sports Physiol Perform 11(1):66–73
28. Gual G, Fort-Vanmeerhaeghe A, Romero-Rodríguez D, Tesch PA (2016) Effects of in-season inertial resistance training with eccentric overload in a sports population at risk for patellar tendinopathy. J Strength Cond Res 30(7):1834–1842
29. Romero-Rodriguez D, Gual G, Tesch PA (2011) Efficacy of an inertial resistance training paradigm in the treatment of patellar tendinopathy in athletes: a case-series study. Phys Ther Sport 12(1):43–48

Return to Play Following Meniscal Injuries

43

Cécile Batailler, Elvire Servien, Robert Magnussen, Sébastien Lustig, and Philippe Neyret

Contents

C. Batailler, M.D. (✉) • E. Servien
S. Lustig • P. Neyret
Orthopedic Surgery, Centre Albert Trillat – Croix-Rousse Hospital, 103 Grande rue de la Croix Rousse, 69004 Lyon, France
e-mail: cecile.batailler@chu-lyon.fr

R. Magnussen
Department of Orthopaedics, OSU Sports Medicine, The Ohio State University, Columbus, OH, USA

43.1 Introduction

Soccer involves frequent pivoting and cutting. It is a frequent cause of anterior cruciate ligament (ACL) and meniscal injuries. Studies have shown that 24–40% of soccer knee injuries are ligamentous and 21–31% involve the menisci [1–5]. Chomiak et al. found that the meniscal tears represented 8% of all injuries sustained over a season in professional soccer [1]. Up to 75% of ACL injuries of soccer players are associated with a meniscal tear [6].

The menisci play an essential role in knee function, including shock absorption, load bearing, knee stability, as well as lubrication and nutrition of articular cartilage. The presence of an unstable meniscal tear can be disabling and painful for the patient, with a risk that the tear progresses. However, removal of portions of the meniscus significantly alters the load-bearing and shock-absorbing capabilities of the knee. Management of meniscal tears thus involves a delicate balance, particularly in athletes.

In particular, professional players have different expectations compared to recreational players and the general population. A fast return to pre-injury level of play level is the main concern of players and teams. The goal of a fast recovery is not always associated with the best long-term outcomes. The treatment of each meniscal tear must be individualized

V. Musahl et al. (eds.), *Return to Play in Football*, https://doi.org/10.1007/978-3-662-55713-6_43

based on the pattern of the tear, the presence of associated injuries, the age and goals of the patient, and the level of competition. The surgeon must then have a lengthy discussion with the athlete about the implications of the various treatment options before surgery. In this chapter, we will discuss the potential surgical treatments of meniscal injuries in the football players and their consequences for return to play.

43.2 Meniscal Repair

43.2.1 Indications

Meniscal repair has two potential advantages compared to partial meniscectomy: prevent the occurrence of osteoarthritis and increase the stability of the knee. The surgeon must consider the characteristics of the tear (size, tear pattern, acuity, location) and more general factors (age, activity level, stability of the knee, alignment). The theoretical indications in soccer players remain the same as for other patients, and meniscal repairs should generally be performed for tears with a high healing potential. Repairs with a low chance of success must be avoided to decrease the risk of reoperation and prolonged recovery.

43.2.1.1 Stable or Stabilized Knee

Meniscal repair in athletes should be considered only in the stable knee. In athletes, isolated meniscal repair in an ACL-deficient knee has a high failure risk. No study, to our knowledge, specifically reports outcomes of meniscal repair in an unstable knee in athletes. However, several studies have reported poor results that precluded sport participation in young patients who underwent meniscal repair in ACL-deficient knees [7, 8]. In contrast, meniscal repair in conjunction with ACL reconstruction has good to excellent clinical results in more than 80% of patient in the short term, with a satisfactory return to play [9, 10]. The knee must thus be either stable or stabilized to consider a meniscal repair [7, 11–13].

43.2.1.2 Medial Versus Lateral Meniscus

Lateral meniscal repair has generally had better clinical outcomes and knee function than medial meniscal repair. The healing rate is also higher for the lateral meniscus, with a lower rate of secondary meniscectomy [10].

43.2.1.3 Tear Type

The ideal tear for meniscal repair is an unstable, longitudinal tear in the peripheral region of the meniscus (Fig. 43.1). If the meniscal tissue quality allows, meniscal repair is recommended to stabilize the unstable tear [14]. Longitudinal tears of more than 10 mm in length are easy to reduce and are well suited for the placement of vertical mattress sutures. Radial tears that extend to the periphery disrupt the meniscus' ability to contain hoop stresses and are biomechanically similar to a complete meniscectomy. Although technically difficult to reduce and repair, we believe the surgeon should attempt to repair these lesions in some cases, even in soccer players [15, 16]. If large radial tears are treated with meniscectomy or neglect, weight bearing will result in extrusion of the meniscus and result in markedly altered contact stresses and probable early osteoarthritis [17]. Complex meniscal tears, defined as a tear in two or more planes, are generally characterized as not repairable. They are treated with partial meniscectomy, because the failure risk is too high.

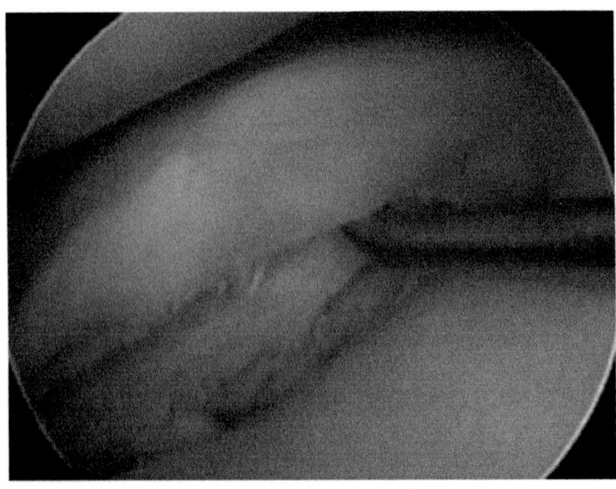

Fig. 43.1 A pattern of meniscal tear favorable for a meniscal repair: unstable, vertical longitudinal tear in the peripheral region of the medial meniscus

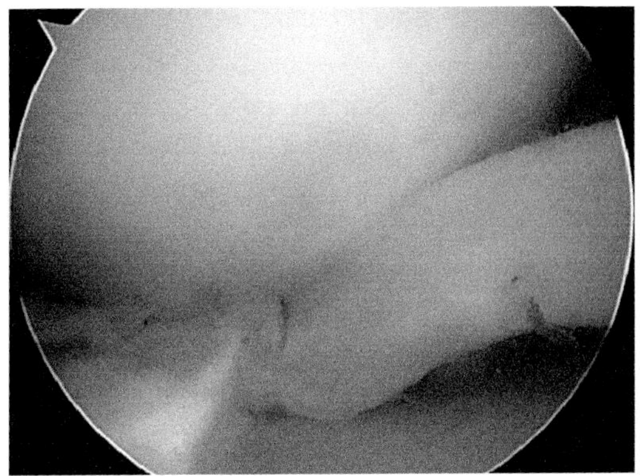

Fig. 43.2 A displaced bucket-handle tear of the medial meniscus of a right knee

Bucket-handle tears are large unstable longitudinal tears (Fig. 43.2) and are commonly seen in ACL-deficient knees. Meniscectomy for these lesions involves removing a large amount of meniscal tissue and should be avoided, except in the presence of meniscal degenerative changes. Shelbourne and Carr treated 155 medial bucket-handle tears at the time of ACL reconstruction, with either repair or partial meniscectomy according to tissue quality. Using these criteria, only 9% of meniscal repairs failed [18]. For bucket-handle tears, if the meniscus does not show degenerative changes, meniscal repair should be attempted.

The acuity of the meniscal tear may have a role in predicting healing. Most authors have shown that acute tears (<12 weeks) have a better prognosis [19, 20].

43.2.1.4 Location of the Meniscal Tear

Location of the tear is another critical factor. Only the peripheral 10–25% of the meniscus is vascularized in adults [21]. Therefore meniscal tears in the peripheral (red-red) zone have the best potential for healing. Several clinical studies have demonstrated good long-term survivorship of meniscal repair in red-white zone and even in white-white zone of meniscus [18, 22]. However for professional players, the meniscal suture must be limited to peripheral (red-red) zone to decrease the failure risk. In very young players, one can consider discussing a meniscal repair in more central regions of the meniscus with the understanding that the risk of failure and secondary meniscectomy is increased with such repairs.

In the professional football player, the therapeutic choice can be difficult if the player needs very early to return to play and doesn't accept a meniscal repair. These difficult situations must be discussed at length with the player and his coach, according to the player's age and the period in football season. We will perform then a partial meniscectomy with expanded indications to favor the rapidity to return to play, in particular for a player at the end of his career. Nevertheless if the tear is large, in peripheral zone, and should require a large meniscectomy, we warn the player and his team that a meniscal repair must be and will be performed, particularly for a young player. A large meniscectomy would induce an early osteoarthritis but also a shorter soccer career.

43.2.2 Rehabilitation and Return to Sport

Significant variability exists in rehabilitation protocols after meniscal repair according to surgeon discretion. Nevertheless the rehabilitation principles are the same.

The rehabilitation time is long after a meniscal repair, even without surgical complications or repair failure. Early weight bearing is often allowed for most repairs, but squatting is prohibited in many cases due to increased stress on the repaired posterior horn of the meniscus. Some surgeons recommend partial weight bearing for 4 weeks [9]. Low-impact exercises can be performed early but running is not allowed for the first 3 months. Once the athlete is running well, agility drills can begin followed by sport-specific skills. Return to sports is generally permitted in the absence of knee inflammation or effusion, lack of pain, and restoration of complete knee range of motion (0–135°) and adequate muscle strength [23, 24]. Usually the return to high-level football competition can take 6–8 months. Repair of tears that involve disruption of circumferential meniscal fibers (radial tears and root avulsions) requires protected weight bearing for 6 weeks to avoid hoop stresses and generally leads to slower return to sport than more traditional repair indication of longitudinal tears.

43.2.3 Complications and Surgical Revisions

The reoperation rate following meniscal repair is higher than that reported following partial meniscectomy (20.7 versus 3.9%) [25]. In a 2003 symposium at the French Arthroscopic Society, 25% of patients who underwent meniscal repair were reported to require subsequent partial meniscectomy. Repairs of the medial meniscus were more prone to failure and many occurred in the first 2 years after the repair [10]. The risk of reoperation after medial meniscal repair has been reported as more than twice as high as that for the lateral meniscus [10, 26]. In athletes, studies have reported reoperation risk due to pain between 21% and 29% after meniscal repair [23, 24, 26] and a subsequent meniscectomy risk between 7.6% and 24% [23, 24, 26–29]. The risk of meniscal repair failure remains high and thus problematic for soccer players who require a fast recovery without recurrence [30].

43.2.4 Outcomes

Alvarez-Diaz et al. [9] studied outcomes of 29 soccer players who underwent meniscal repair with or without ACL reconstruction at a mean follow-up of 6 years. There were no significant differences in outcomes based on the presence of an associated ACL reconstruction. Two patients (6.7%) required secondary meniscectomy, delaying return to sport. Twenty-six patients (89.6%) returned to the same level of competition after recovering from the surgery. Return to sports in the short term in competitive soccer players after meniscal repair is generally between 80% and 90% across studies [9, 26, 31].

At long-term follow-up, meniscal repair has been associated with better clinical results and less radiologic evidence of degeneration than partial meniscectomy [25, 32, 33]. In the study of Alvarez-Diaz et al., 13 patients (45%) were still playing football at any level and eight (28%) of them were still competing at their pre-injury level 6 years postoperative [9]. Stein et al. [33] reported on 81 medial menisci (42 meniscal repairs and 39 partial meniscectomies) at a follow-up of 8.8 years. They noted progression osteoarthritis in only 19% of patients in the repair group but 60% of patients in the partial meniscectomy group. They described that 96% of patients in the repair group reached the pre-injury activity level, in contrast to only 50% in the partial meniscectomy group.

Fact Box

Despite the delayed recovery time and the risk of reoperation, meniscal repair should be the primary method of treatment of repairable meniscal tears and in young athletes in order to maximize clinical results and minimize osteoarthritis in the long term.

43.3 Partial Meniscectomy

Partial meniscectomy is a fast and easy procedure (Fig. 43.3) that is frequently used to treat irreparable and degenerative menisci. Failure risk and reoperation rates following partial meniscectomy are low in the short term. The procedure allows fast recovery, with minimal limitations during rehabilitation. Nevertheless, several factors must be considered before performing a partial meniscectomy in a young athlete.

43.3.1 Indications

43.3.1.1 Medial or Lateral Meniscus

Excision of significant portions of the lateral meniscus typically results in poorer outcomes than excisions on the medial side and often results in a longer time to return to play [34, 35]. Chatain et al. found that athletes had a lower chance of returning to the same sports level after partial lateral meniscectomy than after partial medial meniscectomy [36].

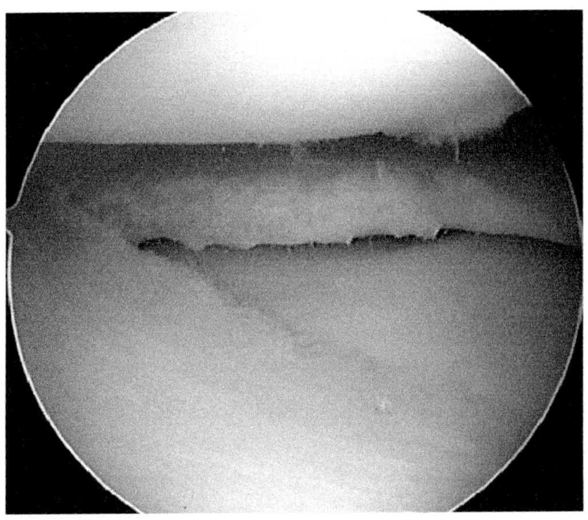

Fig. 43.3 Partial meniscectomy performed for a medial meniscal tear in the white-white region of a stable knee

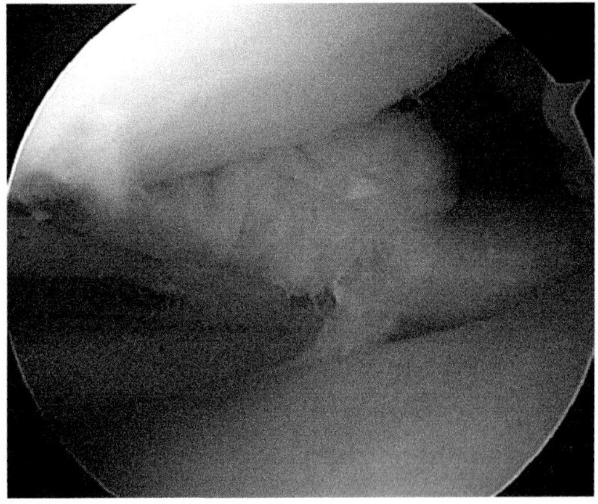

Fig. 43.4 A complex tear of the medial meniscus with a high risk of failure of meniscal repair

43.3.1.2 Stable or Stabilized Knee

In athletes, partial meniscectomy in an ACL-deficient knee is associated with a rapid decrease in function (frequently leading to discontinuation of high-level sport participation) and a high risk of osteoarthritis development and progression [37, 38]. In athletes, the knee must be stable or stabilized in the setting of meniscal loss in order to decrease these risks.

43.3.1.3 Type of Meniscal Tear

Currently, the primary indication for partial meniscectomy is a meniscal tear for which other treatment options (benign neglect or meniscal repair) have failed or have a low chance of success [14], in particular when the healing potential is low. Tears that meet these criteria are the tears in the white-white region of the meniscus (rim width greater than 8 mm), degenerative meniscal tears, complex tear patterns (Fig. 43.4), some radial tears, and chronic displaced tears with deformation.

43.3.2 Rehabilitation and Return to Sport

Following partial meniscectomy, patients can be mobilized within the limits of pain rapidly after the surgery. They may return to low-impact exercises within few days and can advance their activities as pain and effusion permit. Most athletes are able to return to full competition between 4 and 6 weeks following surgery with no or minimal symptoms. Lateral meniscectomy tends to be associated with a delayed return to competition compared to medial meniscectomy, particularly in cases of a large resection [34].

43.3.3 Complications and Surgical Revisions

Two potentially related yet independent complications can occur after partial meniscectomy: rapid chondrolysis in the short term and the development of osteoarthritis in the long term. Rapid chondrolysis in the lateral compartment has been described in professional players after a partial lateral meniscectomy [39–41]. The diagnosis is suspected following the development of persistent effusions, limited range of motion, and localized pain and tenderness at the lateral joint line within 3 months following partial lateral meniscectomy. A flexed knee radiograph (schuss view) can show a decrease in the lateral joint space. This complication remains rare in spite of the relatively large number of partial lateral meniscectomies performed in soccer players (22 cases reported in 16 professional athletes in the literature). It is mainly found in professional athletes and could be related to the rapid increase in load on the articular cartilage with a quick return to high-intensity training. After the diagnosis, conservative treatment is initiated to include 4 weeks of non-weight bearing, an intra-articular corticosteroid injection, and a low-impact isokinetic rehabilitation program. If the symptoms continue to progress despite these treatments, some authors have recommended an arthroscopic lavage [41]. Mariani et al. hypothesized that partial lateral meniscectomy may have a role in exacerbating subtle rotatory instability that combined with high stress of sports activity can dramatically increase the susceptibility of joint to chondrolysis. Open surgery correcting the insufficiency of posterolateral corner has been found to be effective in improving knee function and reducing patients' symptoms at a short-term follow-up [40].

After partial meniscectomy, the reported reoperation rate is variable but generally quite low. Nawabi et al. [34] reported 7% risk of repeat arthroscopy after lateral meniscectomy at a median of 10 weeks but no reoperation after medial meniscectomy in 90 soccer players.

43.3.4 Outcomes

The prognosis of an isolated partial meniscectomy is good in the short term, with a fast recovery without specific rehabilitation, but do vary by location. Partial lateral meniscectomies have longer recovery periods and poorer difficult outcomes than partial medial meniscectomies. Servien et al. [35] found that after a lateral meniscectomy, 6 months are necessary to return to preoperative activity level. In a series of 104 lateral meniscal lesions treated with partial meniscectomy, only 30% were able to resume light physical activity on the IKDC scale at 1 month. In another study of 90 soccer players [34], 69% of players who underwent partial lateral meniscectomy had adverse events during the early recovery phase (persistent effusions, lateral joint line pain) compared to 8% of players who underwent medial meniscectomy. Nawabi et al. [34] found the median time to return to play after a partial lateral meniscectomy to be longer than after a partial medial meniscectomy (7 versus 5 weeks) in a series of 42 partial lateral meniscectomies and 48 partial medial meniscectomies. They noted the cumulative probability of returning to play was six times greater for players with a partial medial versus partial lateral meniscectomy. Aune et al. reported that non-speed position players were four times more likely to return to play than those in speed positions after lateral meniscectomy [42].

In the long term, the risk of osteoarthritis after partial meniscectomy is higher than the following repair. Removal of 50% of the meniscus has been demonstrated to double contact pressures on the articular cartilage [43]. These alterations in loading patterns may predispose to early osteoarthritis [6, 44–48]. Neyret et al. [6] described the outcomes of 72 soccer players among 167 patients who underwent partial meniscectomy, including 42 with and 30 without ACL deficiency at a mean follow-up of 26 years. The functional level 5 years after meniscectomy was excellent for 92% in the ACL-intact group and 51% of patients in the ACL-deficient group. At the last follow-up, these numbers were 68% in the ACL-intact groups and 31% in the ACL-deficient group. Five years postoperatively, 31% of patients with ACL deficiency gave up sports altogether, compared to only 5% of patients with an intact ACL. The incidence of osteoarthritis for patients with ACL deficiency was about 65% at 27 years, and 86% 30 years after meniscectomy, compared to 34% and 50% for patients with an intact ACL. Other authors have described similar results [47, 49]. Clearly, meniscectomy has negative effects on the knee joint in the long term that are magnified in athletes—particularly in the setting of ACL deficiency [50].

Fact Box
Partial meniscectomy is a fast and easy procedure, allowing an early return to sport without symptoms in many cases. Outcomes are more variable following partial lateral meniscectomy, with early functional decline possible. There is a relatively high risk of symptomatic osteoarthritis at long-term follow-up, particularly in the setting of an ACL-deficient knee.

43.4 Benign Neglect

Some meniscal tears can spontaneously heal [48]. The meniscal tears with the greatest potential for healing with nonoperative treatment are short (<1 cm), longitudinal, stable, asymptomatic, and in the lateral meniscus. These indications must be respected to avoid progression of the meniscal tear. In professional soccer players, the risk of tear progression is high. These injuries can become symptomatic and could eventually require a partial meniscectomy. This option is thus rarely used in high-level athletes, due to the risk of failure and reoperation. To our knowledge, there are no recommendations available for return to sport after meniscal tears left in situ. Usually, rehabilitation proceeds in a similar fashion as to a meniscal repair. Full weight bearing is allowed immediately, and low-impact exercises are performed early. Squatting and running are prohibited during the first 3 months. Return to sports is adapted to symptoms, and the return to the competition is often possible at 6 months.

43.5 Meniscal Replacement

Meniscal allograft transplantation or synthetic meniscal scaffolds can be surgically implanted into a meniscus-deficient knee and can be a viable solution to relieve pains and improve function. Its indication is mainly for a symptomatic knee after total or subtotal meniscectomy.

Few studies report the results of this technique in high-demand populations and only at midterm. Marcacci et al. [51] described the outcomes of 12 professional soccer players treated with meniscal allograft transplantation. At 12-month follow-up, all scores improved significantly from baseline, and 67% of the patients returned to playing soccer at the same activity level as before injury. At 36-month follow-up, 75% of the patients played as professionals and 17% as semiprofessionals. The mean duration of rehabilitation was 7 months, and the mean time to return to official competition was 10 months, without difference between lateral or medial meniscus. Other studies found similar results in competitive soccer players [52] and other active populations [53].

The rehabilitation protocol is usually organized as follows after meniscal transplant [54–56]:

- During the two first weeks, no weight bearing and immobilization.
- Between 2 and 6 weeks, toe-touch weight bearing, restriction of range of motion (0–90° for 4 weeks and then free range of motion), isometric exercises, and closed-chain strengthening.
- At 6 weeks postoperatively, full weight bearing and full flexion.
- At 3 months, sport-specific exercises can start and, at 4 months, return to noncontact activities. Before 6 months, running is not advised.
- After 8–9 months, return to soccer.

These operations are considered "salvage" procedures and still have a 10–29% failure risk [57–60].

43.6 Rehabilitation and Return to Sport

43.6.1 Rehabilitation

The postoperative physical therapy program has several goals: (1) minimize the postoperative effusion, (2) achieve full range of motion, (3) prevent muscular atrophy, (4) normalize gait, (5) maintain proprioception, and (6) maintain cardiovascular fitness.

The early phase range of motion that is allowed depends on the treatment rendered (repair versus partial meniscectomy). Quadriceps and hamstring exercises help maintain muscle strength and protect the knee joint. During rehabilitation and return to play, if the athlete complains of swelling or pain recurrence, the rehabilitation must be slowed or backed off until the symptoms have resolved.

There is no evidence-based research surrounding return-to-play criteria following meniscal injury and treatment. We recommend criteria for return to sport to include a painless knee, full range of motion, no effusion, and restoration of strength and sport-specific function as well as confidence in the knee sufficient to play effectively.

Fact Box

Positive prognostic factors of successful return to competition in soccer players after meniscal injuries are (1) short duration of symptoms (<3 months prior to surgery), (2) tears in the vascular area, (3) medial meniscal injury, (4) no degenerative articular damage, and (5) a stable knee (no associated ACL tear).

43.6.2 Prevention

Given the traumatic nature of meniscal tears in many athletes, complete prevention of these injuries is impossible. However, one of the major risks factors for sustaining a meniscal tear is having an ACL-deficient knee. Stabilizing these knees by an ACL reconstruction will decrease the risk of further meniscal injuries—particularly medially. Neuromuscular deficits may also contribute to meniscal injuries. The FIFA 11+ program was originally designed to decrease the risk of ACL injuries in football players. This program may also reduce the risk of meniscal tears. Medical personnel should encourage this program for athletes at all levels.

Some players can develop degenerative tears of the medial meniscus by an overstressing of the medial compartment of the knee with a varus alignment or due to frequent movements with the ball between the legs, typical for football players. An open-wedge high tibial osteotomy can be discussed on a varus knee with medial meniscal tears, to avoid the stage of degenerative meniscus.

Take-Home Message

- The choice of meniscal tear management must be tailored to the tear type and to the individual athlete's situation.
- Preserving as much of the meniscus as possible is crucial, especially in young patient.
- The rehabilitation time is long after a meniscal repair, with a return to sport typically between 4 and 6 months following surgery. Repair is also associated with increased risk of tear recurrence and a reoperation. However, the meniscal repair may facilitate preservation of high-level sport participation in the long term as well as reduce osteoarthritis risk.
- Partial meniscectomy allows an early return to high-level sport (between 4 and 6 weeks). Nevertheless some complications can occur, particularly with partial lateral partial meniscectomy. Long-term clinical outcomes are less satisfying than those following repair.
- The surgeon must have a lengthy discussion with the athlete about the implications of the various treatment options before surgery and come to an informed decision regarding how to proceed.

Top 5 Evidence-Based References

Neyret P, Donell ST, Dejour H (1993) Results of partial meniscectomy related to the state of the anterior cruciate ligament. Review at 20 to 35 years. J Bone Joint Surg Br 75(1):36–40

Nawabi DH, Cro S, Hamid IP, Williams A (2014) Return to play after lateral meniscectomy compared with medial meniscectomy in elite professional soccer players. Am J Sports Med 42(9):2193–2198

Alvarez-Diaz P, Alentorn-Geli E, Llobet F, Granados N, Steinbacher G, Cugat R (2016) Return to play after all-inside meniscal repair in competitive football players: a minimum 5-year follow-up. Knee Surg Sports Traumatol Arthrosc 24(6):1997–2001

Sonnery-Cottet B, Archbold P, Thaunat M, Carnesecchi O, Tostes M, Chambat P (2014) Rapid chondrolysis of the knee after partial lateral meniscectomy in professional athletes. Knee 21(2):504–508

Marcacci M, Marcheggiani Muccioli GM, Grassi A, Ricci M, Tsapralis K, Nanni G, Bonanzinga T, Zaffagnini S (2014) Arthroscopic meniscus allograft transplantation in male professional soccer players: a 36-month follow-up study. Am J Sports Med 42(2):382–388

References

1. Chomiak J, Junge A, Peterson L, Dvorak J (2000) Severe injuries in football players. Influencing factors. Am J Sports Med 28(5 Suppl):S58–S68
2. Kujala UM, Kaprio J, Sarna S (1994) Osteoarthritis of weight bearing joints of lower limbs in former elite male athletes. BMJ 308(6923):231–234

3. Nielsen AB, Yde J (1989) Epidemiology and traumatology of injuries in soccer. Am J Sports Med 17(6):803–807
4. Sandelin J, Santavirta S, Kiviluoto O (1985) Acute soccer injuries in Finland in 1980. Br J Sports Med 19(1):30–33
5. Turner AP, Barlow JH, Heathcote-Elliott C (2000) Long term health impact of playing professional football in the United Kingdom. Br J Sports Med 34(5):332–336
6. Neyret P, Donell ST, Dejour H (1993) Results of partial meniscectomy related to the state of the anterior cruciate ligament. Review at 20 to 35 years. J Bone Joint Surg Br 75(1):36–40
7. Koukoulias N, Papastergiou S, Kazakos K, Poulios G, Parisis K (2007) Mid-term clinical results of medial meniscus repair with the meniscus arrow in the unstable knee. Knee Surg Sports Traumatol Arthrosc 15(2):138–143
8. Steenbrugge F, Van Nieuwenhuyse W, Verdonk R, Verstraete K (2005) Arthroscopic meniscus repair in the ACL-deficient knee. Int Orthop 29(2): 109–112
9. Alvarez-Diaz P, Alentorn-Geli E, Llobet F, Granados N, Steinbacher G, Cugat R (2016) Return to play after all-inside meniscal repair in competitive football players: a minimum 5-year follow-up. Knee Surg Sports Traumatol Arthrosc 24(6):1997–2001
10. Beaufils P, Cassard X (2007) Meniscal repair—SFA 2003. Rev Chir Orthop Reparatrice Appar Mot 93(8 Suppl):5S12–5S13
11. Dejour H, Walch G, Deschamps G, Chambat P (1987) Arthrosis of the knee in chronic anterior laxity. Rev Chir Orthop Reparatrice Appar Mot 73(3):157–170
12. Hanks GA, Gause TM, Handal JA, Kalenak A (1990) Meniscus repair in the anterior cruciate deficient knee. Am J Sports Med 18(6):606–611. discussion 603–12
13. Steenbrugge F, Verdonk R, Verstraete K (2002) Long-term assessment of arthroscopic meniscus repair: a 13-year follow-up study. Knee 9(3):181–187
14. Beaufils P, Hulet C, Dhenain M, Nizard R, Nourissat G, Pujol N (2009) Clinical practice guidelines for the management of meniscal lesions and isolated lesions of the anterior cruciate ligament of the knee in adults. Orthop Traumatol Surg Res 95(6):437–442
15. Noyes FR, Barber-Westin SD (2000) Arthroscopic repair of meniscus tears extending into the avascular zone with or without anterior cruciate ligament reconstruction in patients 40 years of age and older. Arthroscopy 16(8):822–829
16. Yoo JC, Ahn JH, Lee SH, Lee SH, Kim JH (2007) Suturing complete radial tears of the lateral meniscus. Arthroscopy 23(11):e1241–e1247
17. Starke C, Kopf S, Petersen W, Becker R (2009) Meniscal repair. Arthroscopy 25(9):1033–1044
18. Shelbourne KD, Carr DR (2003) Meniscal repair compared with meniscectomy for bucket-handle medial meniscal tears in anterior cruciate ligament-reconstructed knees. Am J Sports Med 31(5):718–723
19. DeHaven KE, Lohrer WA, Lovelock JE (1995) Long-term results of open meniscal repair. Am J Sports Med 23(5):524–530
20. Eggli S, Wegmuller H, Kosina J, Huckell C, Jakob RP (1995) Long-term results of arthroscopic meniscal repair. An analysis of isolated tears. Am J Sports Med 23(6):715–720
21. Arnoczky SP, Warren RF (1982) Microvasculature of the human meniscus. Am J Sports Med 10(2):90–95
22. Melton JT, Murray JR, Karim A, Pandit H, Wandless F, Thomas NP (2011) Meniscal repair in anterior cruciate ligament reconstruction: a long-term outcome study. Knee Surg Sports Traumatol Arthrosc 19(10):1729–1734
23. Barber FA, Schroeder FA, Oro FB, Beavis RC (2008) FasT-Fix meniscal repair: mid-term results. Arthroscopy 24(12):1342–1348
24. Haas AL, Schepsis AA, Hornstein J, Edgar CM (2005) Meniscal repair using the FasT-Fix all-inside meniscal repair device. Arthroscopy 21(2):167–175
25. Paxton ES, Stock MV, Brophy RH (2011) Meniscal repair versus partial meniscectomy: a systematic review comparing reoperation rates and clinical outcomes. Arthroscopy 27(9):1275–1288
26. Logan M, Watts M, Owen J, Myers P (2009) Meniscal repair in the elite athlete: results of 45 repairs with a minimum 5-year follow-up. Am J Sports Med 37(6):1131–1134
27. Kalliakmanis A, Zourntos S, Bousgas D, Nikolaou P (2008) Comparison of arthroscopic meniscal repair results using 3 different meniscal repair devices in anterior cruciate ligament reconstruction patients. Arthroscopy 24(7):810–816
28. Kotsovolos ES, Hantes ME, Mastrokalos DS, Lorbach O, Paessler HH (2006) Results of all-inside meniscal repair with the FasT-Fix meniscal repair system. Arthroscopy 22(1):3–9
29. Krych AJ, McIntosh AL, Voll AE, Stuart MJ, Dahm DL (2008) Arthroscopic repair of isolated meniscal tears in patients 18 years and younger. Am J Sports Med 36(7):1283–1289
30. Nepple JJ, Dunn WR, Wright RW (2012) Meniscal repair outcomes at greater than five years: a systematic literature review and meta-analysis. J Bone Joint Surg Am 94(24):2222–2227
31. Tucciarone A, Godente L, Fabbrini R, Garro L, Salate Santone F, Chillemi C (2012) Meniscal tear repaired with Fast-Fix sutures: clinical results in stable versus ACL-deficient knees. Arch Orthop Trauma Surg 132(3):349–356
32. Shelbourne KD, Dersam MD (2004) Comparison of partial meniscectomy versus meniscus repair for bucket-handle lateral meniscus tears in anterior cruciate ligament reconstructed knees. Arthroscopy 20(6):581–585
33. Stein T, Mehling AP, Welsch F, von Eisenhart-Rothe R, Jager A (2010) Long-term outcome after arthroscopic meniscal repair versus arthroscopic partial meniscectomy for traumatic meniscal tears. Am J Sports Med 38(8):1542–1548

34. Nawabi DH, Cro S, Hamid IP, Williams A (2014) Return to play after lateral meniscectomy compared with medial meniscectomy in elite professional soccer players. Am J Sports Med 42(9):2193–2198
35. Servien E, Acquitter Y, Hulet C, Seil R, French Arthroscopy S (2009) Lateral meniscus lesions on stable knee: a prospective multicenter study. Orthop Traumatol Surg Res 95(8 Suppl 1):S60–S64
36. Chatain F, Adeleine P, Chambat P, Neyret P, Societe Francaise dA (2003) A comparative study of medial versus lateral arthroscopic partial meniscectomy on stable knees: 10-year minimum follow-up. Arthroscopy 19(8):842–849
37. Brophy RH, Gill CS, Lyman S, Barnes RP, Rodeo SA, Warren RF (2009) Effect of anterior cruciate ligament reconstruction and meniscectomy on length of career in National Football League athletes: a case control study. Am J Sports Med 37(11):2102–2107
38. Neyret P, Walch G, Dejour H (1988) Intramural internal meniscectomy using the Trillat technic. Long-term results of 258 operations. Rev Chir Orthop Reparatrice Appar Mot 74(7):637–646
39. Ishida K, Kuroda R, Sakai H, Doita M, Kurosaka M, Yoshiya S (2006) Rapid chondrolysis after arthroscopic partial lateral meniscectomy in athletes: a case report. Knee Surg Sports Traumatol Arthrosc 14(12):1266–1269
40. Mariani PP, Garofalo R, Margheritini F (2008) Chondrolysis after partial lateral meniscectomy in athletes. Knee Surg Sports Traumatol Arthrosc 16(6):574–580
41. Sonnery-Cottet B, Archbold P, Thaunat M, Carnesecchi O, Tostes M, Chambat P (2014) Rapid chondrolysis of the knee after partial lateral meniscectomy in professional athletes. Knee 21(2):504–508
42. Aune KT, Andrews JR, Dugas JR, Cain EL Jr (2014) Return to play after partial lateral meniscectomy in national football league athletes. Am J Sports Med 42(8):1865–1872
43. Pena E, Calvo B, Martinez MA, Doblare M (2006) A three-dimensional finite element analysis of the combined behavior of ligaments and menisci in the healthy human knee joint. J Biomech 39(9):1686–1701
44. Aglietti P, Zaccherotti G, De Biase P, Taddei I (1994) A comparison between medial meniscus repair, partial meniscectomy, and normal meniscus in anterior cruciate ligament reconstructed knees. Clin Orthop Relat Res 307:165–173
45. Ait Si Selmi T, Fithian D, Neyret P (2006) The evolution of osteoarthritis in 103 patients with ACL reconstruction at 17 years follow-up. Knee 13(5):353–358
46. Bolano LE, Grana WA (1993) Isolated arthroscopic partial meniscectomy. Functional radiographic evaluation at five years. Am J Sports Med 21(3):432–437
47. Hazel WA Jr, Rand JA, Morrey BF (1993) Results of meniscectomy in the knee with anterior cruciate ligament deficiency. Clin Orthop Relat Res (292):232–238
48. Lynch MA, Henning CE, Glick KR Jr (1983) Knee joint surface changes. Long-term follow-up meniscus tear treatment in stable anterior cruciate ligament reconstructions. Clin Orthop Relat Res (172):148–153
49. Aglietti P, Buzzi R, Bassi PB (1988) Arthroscopic partial meniscectomy in the anterior cruciate deficient knee. Am J Sports Med 16(6):597–602
50. Roos H, Lindberg H, Gardsell P, Lohmander LS, Wingstrand H (1994) The prevalence of gonarthrosis and its relation to meniscectomy in former soccer players. Am J Sports Med 22(2):219–222
51. Marcacci M, Marcheggiani Muccioli GM, Grassi A, Ricci M, Tsapralis K, Nanni G et al (2014) Arthroscopic meniscus allograft transplantation in male professional soccer players: a 36-month follow-up study. Am J Sports Med 42(2):382–388
52. Alentorn-Geli E, Vazquez RS, Diaz PA, Cusco X, Cugat R (2010) Arthroscopic meniscal transplants in soccer players: outcomes at 2- to 5-year follow-up. Clin J Sport Med 20(5):340–343
53. Zaffagnini S, Grassi A, Marcheggiani Muccioli GM, Benzi A, Roberti di Sarsina T, Signorelli C et al (2016) Is sport activity possible after arthroscopic meniscal allograft transplantation? Midterm results in active patients. Am J Sports Med 44(3):625–632
54. Getgood A, LaPrade RF, Verdonk P, Gersoff W, Cole B, Spalding T et al (2016) International meniscus reconstruction experts forum (IMREF) 2015 consensus statement on the practice of meniscal allograft transplantation. Am J Sports Med pii:0363546516660064
55. Lee SR, Kim JG, Nam SW (2012) The tips and pitfalls of meniscus allograft transplantation. Knee Surg Relat Res 24(3):137–145
56. Rodeo SA (2001) Meniscal allografts—where do we stand? Am J Sports Med 29(2):246–261
57. Elattar M, Dhollander A, Verdonk R, Almqvist KF, Verdonk P (2011) Twenty-six years of meniscal allograft transplantation: is it still experimental? A meta-analysis of 44 trials. Knee Surg Sports Traumatol Arthrosc 19(2):147–157
58. Rosso F, Bisicchia S, Bonasia DE, Amendola A (2015) Meniscal allograft transplantation: a systematic review. Am J Sports Med 43(4):998–1007
59. Samitier G, Alentorn-Geli E, Taylor DC, Rill B, Lock T, Moutzouros V et al (2015) Meniscal allograft transplantation. Part 2: systematic review of transplant timing, outcomes, return to competition, associated procedures, and prevention of osteoarthritis. Knee Surg Sports Traumatol Arthrosc 23(1):323–333
60. Smith NA, MacKay N, Costa M, Spalding T (2015) Meniscal allograft transplantation in a symptomatic meniscal deficient knee: a systematic review. Knee Surg Sports Traumatol Arthrosc 23(1):270–279

Return to Play Following Cartilage Injuries

44

Renato Andrade, Rogério Pereira, Ricardo Bastos, Hélder Pereira, J. Miguel Oliveira, Rui L. Reis, and João Espregueira-Mendes

Contents

44.1 Introduction

Football (soccer) is the most played sport worldwide, practiced by more than 300 million people [1]. It is a high-impact contact sport, and with the increasing competitive level, it often results in sports-related damage of the knee structures, including articular cartilage injuries [2–4]. These articular cartilage injuries can also be caused by forceful and repetitive mechanical stresses on the

R. Andrade
Clínica do Dragão, Espregueira-Mendes Sports Centre – FIFA Medical Centre of Excellence, Porto, Portugal

Dom Henrique Research Centre, Porto, Portugal

Faculty of Sports, University of Porto, Porto, Portugal

R. Pereira
Clínica do Dragão, Espregueira-Mendes Sports Centre – FIFA Medical Centre of Excellence, Porto, Portugal

Dom Henrique Research Centre, Porto, Portugal

Faculty of Sports, University of Porto, Porto, Portugal

Faculty of Health Science, University Fernando Pessoa, Porto, Portugal

R. Bastos
Clínica do Dragão, Espregueira-Mendes Sports Centre – FIFA Medical Centre of Excellence, Porto, Portugal

Dom Henrique Research Centre, Porto, Portugal

Universidade Federal Fluminense, Nirteói, Rio de Janeiro, Brazil

H. Pereira
Dom Henrique Research Centre, Porto, Portugal

3B's Research Group – Biomaterials, Biodegradables and Biomimetics, University of Minho, Headquarters of the European Institute of Excellence on Tissue Engineering and Regenerative Medicine, AvePark, Parque de Ciência e Tecnologia, Zona Industrial da Gandra, 4805-017 Barco, Guimarães, Portugal

V. Musahl et al. (eds.), *Return to Play in Football*, https://doi.org/10.1007/978-3-662-55713-6_44

knee joint during the football practice [5–8]. When the cartilage damage reaches the subchondral bone, it often results in knee complaints [9], including pain, swelling, catching, and locking [3, 10, 11]. Nonetheless, articular cartilage injuries may be present in asymptomatic athletes which, if not treated properly, may lead to an early onset of knee osteoarthritis [12–14]. Moreover, it may lead to activity-related symptoms and lifestyle modifications and, eventually, the football player may never recover his previous level of performance which can result into an early career ending [15–17].

ICVS/3B's – PT Government Associate Laboratory, Braga/Guimarães, Portugal

Ripoll y De Prado Sports Clinic – FIFA Medical Centre of Excellence, Murcia-Madrid, Spain

Orthopedic Department Centro Hospitalar Póvoa de Varzim, Vila do Conde, Portugal

J. Miguel Oliveira
3B's Research Group – Biomaterials, Biodegradables and Biomimetics, University of Minho, Headquarters of the European Institute of Excellence on Tissue Engineering and Regenerative Medicine, AvePark, Parque de Ciência e Tecnologia, Zona Industrial da Gandra, 4805-017 Barco, Guimarães, Portugal

ICVS/3B's – PT Government Associate Laboratory, Braga/Guimarães, Portugal

Ripoll y De Prado Sports Clinic – FIFA Medical Centre of Excellence, Murcia-Madrid, Spain

R.L. Reis
3B's Research Group – Biomaterials, Biodegradables and Biomimetics, University of Minho, Headquarters of the European Institute of Excellence on Tissue Engineering and Regenerative Medicine, AvePark, Parque de Ciência e Tecnologia, Zona Industrial da Gandra, 4805-017 Barco, Guimarães, Portugal

ICVS/3B's – PT Government Associate Laboratory, Braga/Guimarães, Portugal

J. Espregueira-Mendes (✉)
Clínica do Dragão, Espregueira-Mendes Sports Centre – FIFA Medical Centre of Excellence, Porto, Portugal

Dom Henrique Research Centre, Porto, Portugal

3B's Research Group – Biomaterials, Biodegradables and Biomimetics, University of Minho, Headquarters of the European Institute of Excellence on Tissue Engineering and Regenerative Medicine, AvePark, Parque de Ciência e Tecnologia, Zona Industrial da Gandra, 4805-017 Barco, Guimarães, Portugal

ICVS/3B's – PT Government Associate Laboratory, Braga/Guimarães, Portugal

Department of Orthopaedic, Minho University, Braga, Portugal
e-mail: espregueira@dhresearchcentre.com

Football involves high financial impact and heavy social media coverage, comprising high pressure from the football club stakeholders, resulting in an increased onus of the healthcare professionals that are involved in the player's recovery. Thus, it is crucial to perform the injury clinical reasoning with great scrutiny, taking into account important factors including age, level of completion, timing within the season, and career status [2].

Intact knee articular cartilage has optimal load-bearing features which constantly adjust to the imposed loading stresses [18]. However, high-impact loads may overcome the articular cartilage capabilities and, consequently, decrease the cartilage proteoglycan levels and increase degradative enzyme levels, which eventually may result in chondrocyte apoptosis [19, 20]. This process will result in loss of articular cartilage volume and stiffness, higher contact pressures and, ultimately, in the development of cartilage defects [18]. Moreover, due to its isolation from vessels and nerve supply, the articular cartilage shows limited capacity to potentially heal [17, 21–23]. Hence, the functional long-term restoration of the articular surface is still a tough challenge within the orthopedic community.

44.1.1 Epidemiology

Prevalence of articular cartilage injuries in athletic populations has been reported to be higher than that found in the general population [2, 3, 24, 25]. Flanigan et al. [3] systematized the occurrence of articular cartilage injuries in a cohort of 931 athletes (989 knees), involving 732 men and 199 women, with a mean age of 33 years old. Overall, 40% were professional athletes, but none comprised football players. The sample comprised a total of 883 full-thickness chondral defects from 355 athletes (with 335 of them with more than one chondral defect), representing an overall prevalence of 0.89 articular cartilage lesions per each knee assessed. The articular cartilage injuries were distributed by the femoral condyles (35%), the patellofemoral joint (37%), and the tibial plateaus (25%). From the total cohort of athletes, 132 (14%) were asymptomatic with a calculated pooled prevalence of knee full-thickness chondral defects of 59% (ranging from 18% up to 63%).

Concerning specifically football, a systematic review [2] reported 217 articular cartilage injuries in a total cohort of 183 football players (158 male and 25 female), with a mean age of 26 years old. Eighty-two percent of the players played professional football. The overall prevalence was 1.19 articular cartilage lesions per each knee assessed. Opposing to the overall athletic population reported above, the football players had the majority of the chondral lesions at the femoral condyles (medial femoral condyle, 51%; and lateral femoral condyle, 27%), followed by patellofemoral joint (18%) and the tibial plateaus (4%). The defect size varied across the included cohort (from 0.6 up to 7.0 cm^2). A smaller defect size (<2.0 cm^2) has shown to provide higher rate of return to high-impact competition [26, 27].

The UEFA Elite Club Injury Study reports the exposure and incidence of injuries in 29 elite European football clubs [28]. In the football season of 2015/2016, the clubs reported on average 20 training sessions and 5.4 matches per each month. When considering the type of injury, it was reported a total of 43 cartilage/meniscus injuries, accounting for 3.7% of all injuries. These injuries, beyond the layoff time from training and match competition, may lead to a high injury burden which influences negatively the team's performance [29]. Moreover, Drawer and Fuller [30] reported that 32% of retired English professional football players had osteoarthrosis diagnosis when they retired.

44.1.2 Treatment

The treatment of articular cartilage injuries is complex and multifactorial [31]. In an athletic population, the treatment goal is to provide the player a long-standing cartilage restoration which can bear the high-impact mechanical stresses that are often imposed to the player's knee joint [2]. This may be accomplished by providing to the damaged defect hyaline-like cartilage or fibrocartilage, with full integration into the adjacent cartilage and underlying bone. Hence, it is possible to reestablish the physiological properties of all the osteochondral unit and obtain a normal knee function [6, 32]. In this sense, chondrofacilitation (facilitate intrinsic repair of damaged articular cartilage) and chondrorestoration (prevent loss of existing cartilage) and resurfacing (chondral surface replacement) techniques have been developed [33].

Nonoperative treatment of knee articular cartilage lesions in football players may only be considered when there is a small and superficial focal lesion in early stages (Outerbridge levels I and II). Football players that present with high-grade articular cartilage injuries (Outerbridge levels III and IV) and need to proceed playing throughout the rest of the season can also be managed through symptomatic nonoperative treatment. However, success is less likely and operative interventions may be required. Nonoperative options include chondroprotective pharmacotherapy (glucosamines, chondroitin, diacerein, hyaluronic acid, platelet-rich plasma, and gene therapy), nonsteroidal anti-inflammatory medication and tramadol, physiotherapy, and hydrotherapy [16, 34, 35]. The nutritional supplements and viscosupplementation can be a valuable clinical recommendation when envisioning managing the symptoms and ultimately can help prevent further damage of the cartilage [35, 36]. Nevertheless, there is still a lack of evidence for these therapies in focal articular cartilage lesions of the professional football player. Intra-articular injection therapy (hyaluronic acid and platelet-rich plasma) for knee articular cartilage lesions in professional athletes still requires more research as only preliminary results have been reported [37]. A recent study has also investigated the effect of both intra-articular injection therapies in end career professional football players, reporting significant clinical improvement for both therapies [38].

Nowadays, several surgical techniques are available to approach articular cartilage injuries in the football player. The most commonly used surgical techniques for the treatment of these lesions include microfracture, mosaicplasty or osteochondral autograft transplantation (OAT), autologous chondrocyte implantation (ACI), and matrix-induced autologous chondrocyte implantation (MACI) [2, 23, 39, 40]. More recently, new biological cartilage repair techniques have emerged as potential solutions to restore the articular cartilage defects. Nevertheless, clinical outcomes in football players are not available yet. Some of these emerging techniques include autologous matrix-induced chondrogenesis (AMIC™ Geistlich Pharma AG) [41, 42], concentrated bone marrow aspirate and mesenchymal stem cell-induced chondrogenesis (MCIC™) [43–45], autologous collagen-induced chondrogenesis (ACIC™) [46, 47], minced cartilage repair (DeNovo NT, ISTO Technologies, St. Louis, MO, United States; and CAIS, DePuy/Mitek, Raynham, MA, United States) [48–50], osteochondral biomimetic scaffolds (*MaioRegen*®, Fin-Ceramica Faenza S.p.A., Faenza, Italy) [51–54], and implantable liquid scaffolds (BTS-CarGel®, Smith & Nephew, Andover, MA, United States) [55–58].

Timing of the surgery is important once athletes which performed the surgery within 1 year from the injury are three- to fivefold more likely to return to sports [27, 59–61]. Additionally, performing the surgery as soon as possible will decrease the risk of further cartilage injury and development of knee osteoarthritis [4, 8, 17, 61–64].

The microfracture technique is frequently used as first-line treatment and involves the micro-perforation of the subchondral bone (after the defect is properly debrided) aiming to release mesenchymal stem cells, forming a stable clot which fills the chondral defect [65–67]. Good short-term outcomes have been reported with this technique [68, 69], however, with deterioration of the clinical outcomes at long term, requiring in some cases further surgery [70, 71]. The final tissue obtained is fibrocartilage—and not hyaline cartilage (as the native tissue)—which yields mechanical properties that are not prepared to handle the long-term loading demands due to its softness and decreased capability to withstand the joint shear stress [72–74]. In this sense, enhanced microfracture techniques have been developed with good reported short-term outcomes [73, 75, 76].

The OAT technique is used to transfer autologous hyaline articular cartilage to the defect, providing a stable size-matched osteochondral autograft. For small defects, the single plug transfer may be used to fill the defect. However, for larger defects, the mosaicplasty is the most adequate technique as it transfers multiple cylinders (osteochondral plugs) to the defect [65, 66]. Nevertheless, the restricted graft availability and donor site-related morbidity are concerns to be taken into account [77]. To mitigate these disadvantages, the upper tibiofemoral joint has been proposed as a potential donor site, which provides the possibility to transfer up to 5 cm^2 of osteochondral graft, without additional iatrogenic complications [78]. Transplantation of osteochondral allograft is a viable option to manage larger osteochondral injuries, including those that involve an entire compartment [65, 66, 79].

The ACI approach is a two-stage procedure which involves implanting autologous chondrocyte cells to the articular cartilage defect aiming to regenerate hyaline-like cartilage [65, 66, 80, 81]. Nevertheless, a hyaline-like cartilage is not consistently achieved in all patients, as some patients still develop fibrocartilage [82, 83]. This procedure has the advantages of providing longevity of the healed cartilage tissue and good long-term clinical and functional outcomes [61, 84]. In turn, the MACI technique is an attractive alternative which involves culturing the chondrocytes cells into a biodegradable scaffold which is after implanted into the defect [65, 66]. The MACI sandwich technique involves the implantation of a two-membrane custom-made (bottom membrane facing up and top membrane facing down) with the advantage of reducing the operation time and exposure, while avoiding periosteal harvesting [85]. The reported short- to midterm outcomes show promising results of this technique in articular cartilage injuries of the knee joint [86–88].

Evidence-based treatment of articular cartilage injuries is mainly based on the defect's size and involvement of the entire osteochondral unit

[89]. In this sense, several clinical treatment algorithms have been developed [23, 33, 89–93]. However, when dealing with high-level athletes, important factors such as timing within the season and player's career status must be taken into account and discussed with the patient. Hence, Beckers et al. [39] proposed a clinical treatment algorithm for articular cartilage injuries, adapted professional football players (Fig. 44.1).

44.1.2.1 Treatment of Associated Lesions

Articular cartilage injuries of the knee are often associated to other knee injuries including ligament deficiency, meniscus damage, and lower limb malalignments. These associated lesions must be treated concomitantly [5, 16, 90, 95–100] as it has been reported to improve the overall cartilage repair and avoids the need for further surgical interventions without negatively influencing the return to sports [8, 61, 64, 101].

Knee articular cartilage associated injuries are frequently seen in athletes. In this sense, Flanigan et al. [3] identified a total of 850 concomitant injuries in 931 athletes (883 defects) including meniscal tears ($n = 441$), anterior cruciate ligament ruptures ($n = 282$), and medial or lateral collateral ligament tears ($n = 127$). In addition, Andrade et al. [2] reported 101 concomitant knee surgeries in 168 football players with articular cartilage injuries of the knee. Most common procedures comprised anterior cruciate ligament reconstruction ($n = 54$), meniscectomy ($n = 19$) and meniscal repair ($n = 4$), high tibial osteotomy ($n = 9$), and tibial tubercle osteotomy ($n = 5$).

44.1.3 *Post*operative Rehabilitation and Return to Play Criteria

The postoperative rehabilitation is of upmost importance to return the player as fast and as safe as possible to sports competition within the preinjury level and prevent reinjury and long-term sequelae [31, 39]. In this sense, the rehabilitation focuses in providing the mechanical environment to promote the adaptation and remodeling of the repair tissue [18]. The rehabilitation progression should respect the biology related to the repair technique, characteristics of the defect, symptomatology, and level of competition. Thus, the rehabilitation should be a step-wise and individualized program according to the repair technique, according to the athlete's specific demands, following criteria-based progression through the different phases (Fig. 44.2). Additionally, the rehabilitation process is also important for the athletes to acquire self-confidence and sport-specific self-efficacy, which will play a crucial role in the return to competition within the preinjury level [18].

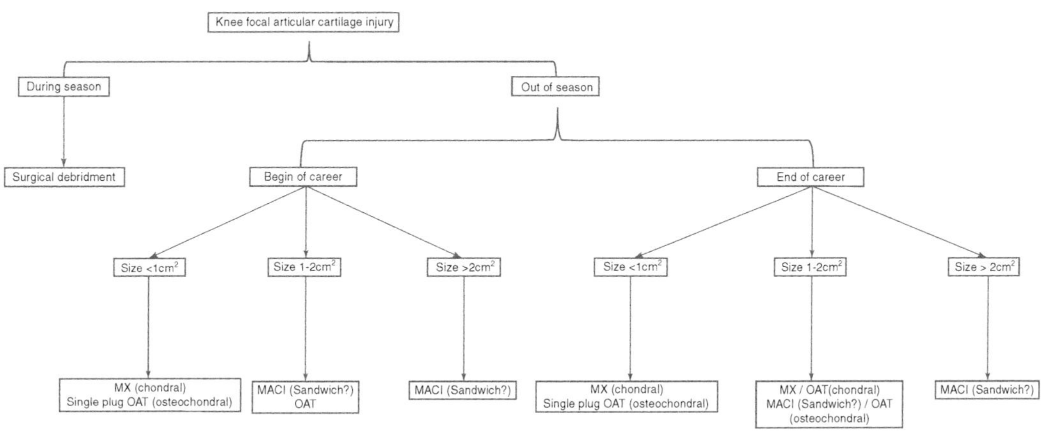

Fig. 44.1 Clinical treatment algorithm for articular cartilage injuries of professional football players, adapted from Beckers et al. [94]

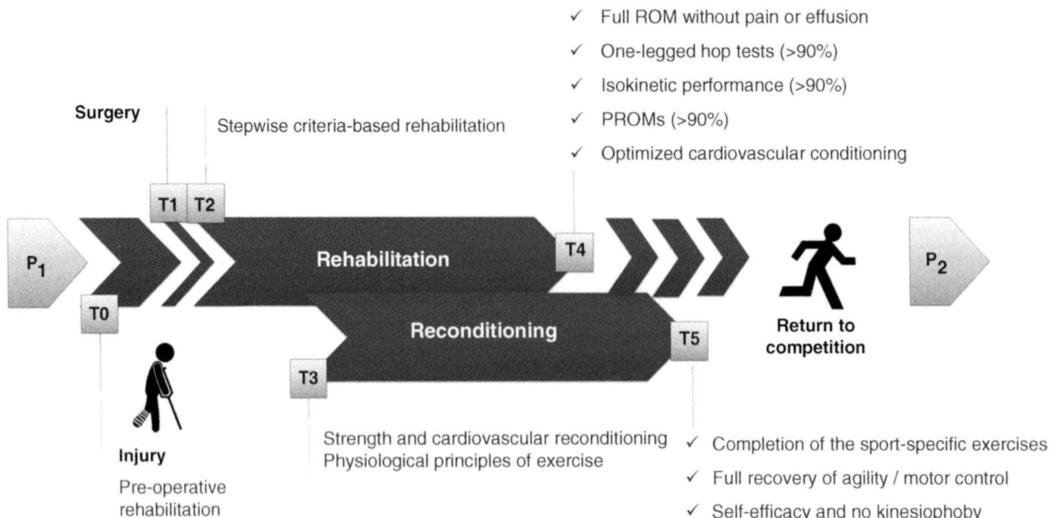

Fig. 44.2 Progressive stepwise criteria-based diagram, from injury to return to play (*P_1* primary prevention, *T0* injury occurrence, *T1* articular cartilage repair/restoration, *T2* beginning of postoperative rehabilitation, *T3* beginning of physical reconditioning, *T4* criteria to return to training, *T5* criteria to return to competition, P_2 secondary prevention)

When concomitant surgical procedures were performed (such as meniscal repair or anterior cruciate ligament reconstruction), special attention should be taken, and a slower rehabilitation progression may be required [102, 103]. Moreover, the location of the defect may influence the rehabilitation program since trochlear defects may require adjustments [104].

The rehabilitation process of knee articular cartilage repair of the athlete is based on three criteria-based progressive biologic-rehabilitation phases (Table 44.1). It is essential for the physiotherapist to monitor the athlete symptomatology (pain and swelling) during the rehabilitation once it may be indicative of overload of the healing cartilage tissue [18].

Table 44.1 Biologic and rehabilitation phases after articular cartilage repair/restoration

	Biologic phase	Rehabilitation phase
Phase 1	Graft integration and stimulation (proliferation)	Joint protection and activation
Phase 2	Extracellular matrix production and cartilage organization (transition)	Progressive loading and functional joint restoration
Phase 3	Repair cartilage maturation and adaptation (remodeling and maturation)	Activity restoration

In phase 1 (graft stimulation and integration at the defect) allows the athlete to adapt to the postoperative effects, while protecting the repair tissue [31]. In this sense, the envisioned goals are the progressive reestablishment of range of movement and weight bearing and address muscle impairment and neuromuscular control while controlling knee pain and swelling [18, 104–109]. Within this phase, the procedures may differ between reparative (ACI/MACI/microfracture) and restorative (OAT/mosaicplasty) techniques [18, 31]. In the reparative approach, the physiotherapist must be aware to avoid the mechanical overload of the repaired tissue which may hamper the tissue integration into the defect bed and surrounding noninjured articular cartilage tissue [110, 111]. Accelerated weight-bearing rehabilitation protocols have been proposed, with full weight-bearing at 6–8 weeks [112, 113]. However, caution should be taken concerning the graft protection in the early initial phase once it is vulnerable [106]. Further high-quality research is needed to evaluate the benefits of accelerated weight-bearing rehabilitation after microfracture surgery [114]. During the restorative approach in the first phase, bone-to-bone healing is expected, and thus, there is less limitation in the weight-bearing progression [18]. Within this line, correct management of rehabilitation loads is crucial because too much load may be detrimental as it may lead to reduction of chondrocyte metabolic rate, but if the correct load stimulation is provided, it will favor the new cartilage formation and nutrition and, at the same time, bone-to-bone healing [115–118]. Performing rehabilitation in the swimming pool in early stages (from the second week) allows to take advantage of the therapeutic effect provided by physics of aquatic environment (e.g., temperature, hydrostatic pressure, fluctuation) creating low-impact conditions, allowing partial weight-bearing and management of the axial load, enabling to perform sport-specific movement patterns safely without compromising the repair tissue. It is possible to gradually progress the compressive knee loading by means of taking the advantage of the features of the antigravity treadmill (from 20% up to 80% of body weight reduction), providing the most suitable mechanical stimulus for safe tissue repair enhancement (Fig. 44.3). In order to progress into the second phase, the athlete must achieve full passive knee range of motion, present minimal pain and effusion, and regain muscle activation and normal gait [18, 105].

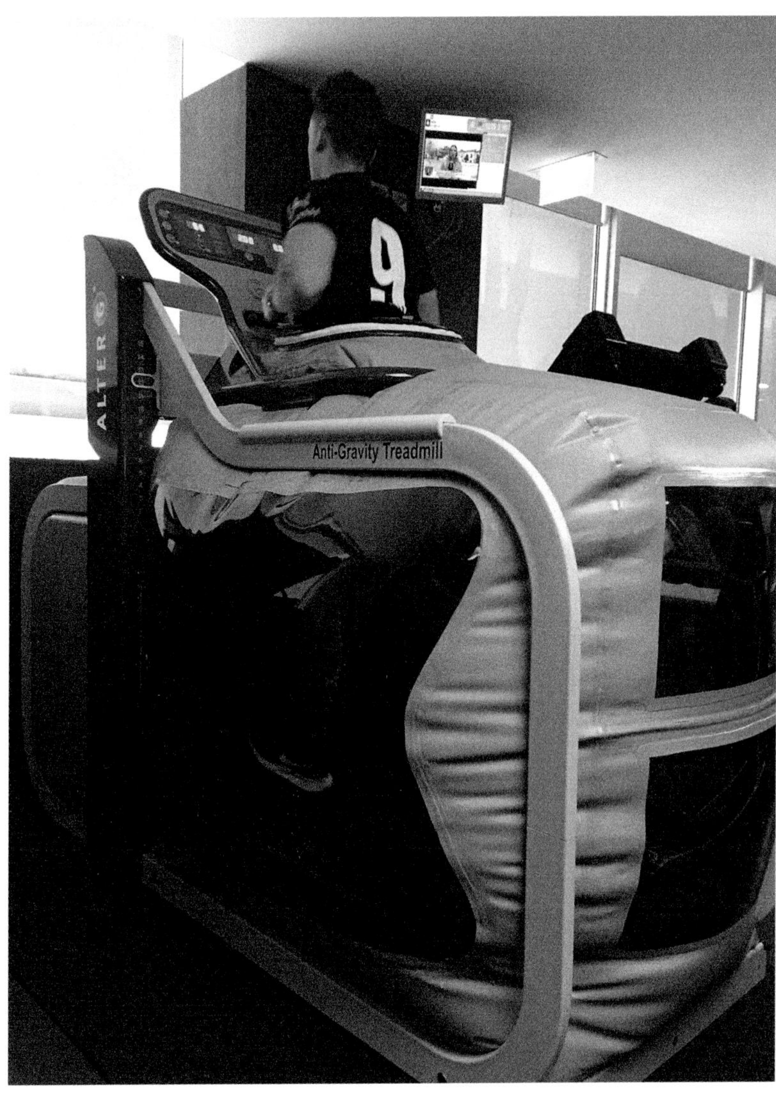

Fig. 44.3 Football player running at the antigravity treadmill (Alter-G®)

In phase 2 (extracellular matrix production and cartilage organization), the main rehabilitation goal is to manage joint load and neuromuscular control in order to provide the athlete a pain-free normal running, without effusion or locking, and reestablishment of sport-specific movement patterns [18, 105]. Hence, the athlete performs progressive controlled mechanical stresses (compressive and shear stress) to the joint in order to stimulate the cellular metabolism of the repair joint [18, 119]. Progression to the subsequent phase is allowed when the athlete is able to run at 8 km/h for more than 15 minutes (without pain or joint effusion), one-legged hop tests and isokinetic performance with side-to-side difference below 20%, and patient-reported outcomes measures with the limb asymmetry index greater than 90% [18, 105]. Moreover, if possible, the athlete should perform a cartilage-sensitive magnetic resonance imaging exam to evaluate the integrity of the repaired tissue (Fig. 44.4) [18].

The phase 3 (repaired cartilage maturation and adaptation) comprises the on-field rehabilitation which is of paramount importance before the player return to competition. In this phase, the main goal is to restore any physical and psychological impairment related to muscle power and coordination, neuromuscular control, speed and endurance performance, metabolic capacity, self-efficacy, and sport-specific movement patterns, aiming to reestablish the preinjury level of sports performance, with minimal risk of reinjury [18, 120]. The joint stress demands (without overloading) are gradually increased, progressing to high-speed pivoting and cutting activities, plyometrics, acceleration and deceleration drills, and sport-specific skills replicating the complex interactions of sports [18, 94, 120]. In addition, training in sand may be more

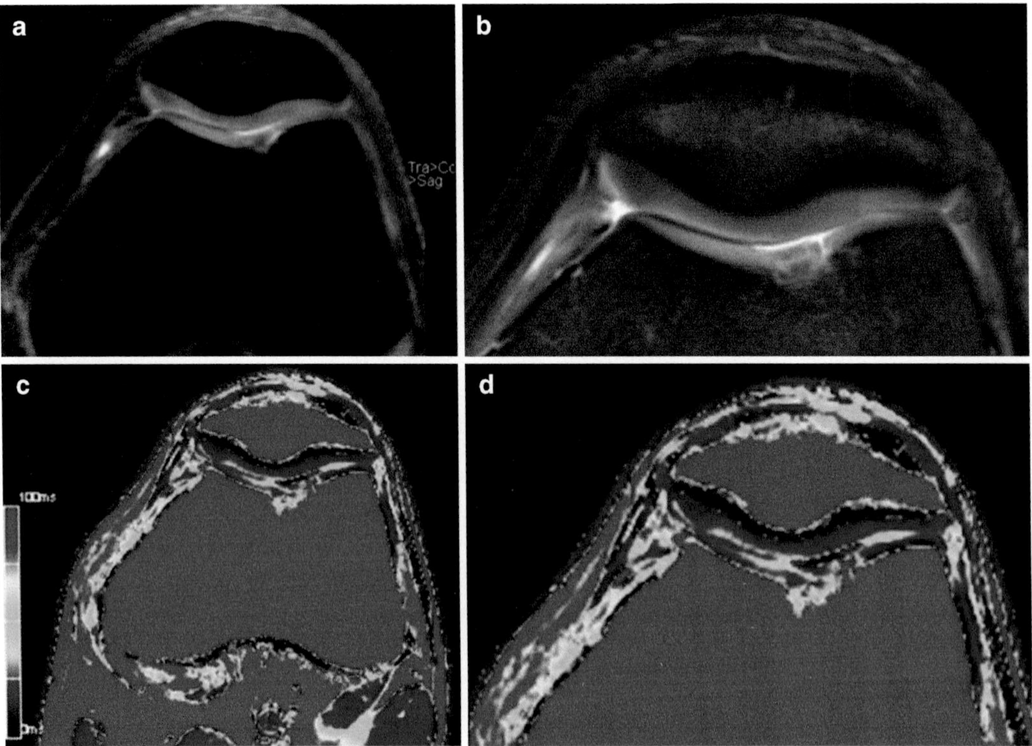

Fig. 44.4 MRI scanning of a football player knee 2 months after microfracture procedure. (**a**) Double-echo steady-state MRI sequence showing appearance of fibrocartilage following the microfracture procedure; (**b**) fast spin-echo diffusion-prepared fat saturation MRI sequence showing increased signal revealing discontinuity on the fibrocartilage of the repaired tissue; (**c**) T2 mapping MRI sequence confirming the fibrocartilage discontinuity; (**d**) closeup T2 mapping image

physically demanding (i.e., greater energy expenditure and metabolic power) being associated with greater deceleration values and smaller joint compressive stress [121–126]. Moreover, the use of novel global positioning systems (GPS) may be employed to enable further individualization of training load monitoring and optimal periodization and, ultimately, develop rehabilitation and return-to-running protocols specific to the player position, optimizing a safe return to play decision making [127–131]. Monitoring the training loads through the acute-chronic workload ratio (acute, current week; chronic, preceding four training weeks) for optimal loading may be a useful tool to plan and manage the load progression in this last phase before the return to competition [132].

Fact Box 1

- Antigravity treadmill provides an early and safe mechanical stimulus to the joint.
- Sand training (later phases) provides a more physically demanding training without compromising the graft biological healing.
- GPS allows the individualization of the training load monitoring and optimal training periodization.

Return to play at preinjury level as fast as possible represents the most important outcome for the injured football player [12]. Nevertheless, returning to high-impact activities (such as football) is often delayed to decrease the risk of overloading and consequently damage the repaired tissue [31, 133, 134]. Moreover, when the ACI or MACI technique was employed, further caution regarding the graft maturation should be taken [135]. Hence, the criteria to allow the player to return to unrestricted training is the following: completion of the sport-specific exercises and one-on-one opposed practice of sport-specific skills, without pain or joint effusion; one-legged hop tests (Fig. 44.5) and isokinetic performance with side-to-side difference below 10%; patient-reported outcome measures greater than 90%; and no kinesiophobia or fear of reinjury (Tampa Scale of Kinesiophobia) [18, 105].

Fact Box 2

Allowance for unrestricted training and competition should follow specific evidence-based criteria:

- Completion of the sport-specific exercises and one-on-one opposed practice of sport-specific skills
- Without pain or joint effusion at rest or during the exercises
- One-legged hop tests with side-to-side difference below 10%
- Isokinetic performance with side-to-side difference below 10%
- Patient-reported outcome measures greater than 90%
- No kinesiophobia or fear of reinjury

The best strategy for secondary prevention to avoid further cartilage damage may be to maintain the knee as stable as possible and correct any lower limb malalignments. Nonetheless, secondary prevention exercise-based programs should be employed as soon as the player returns to training and throughout his career to avoid further knee damage (ligaments, meniscus, or cartilage defects) and the development/progression of knee osteoarthritis.

44.2 Outcome Scores and Return to Play Considerations

The accurate identification, extent, location and classification of an articular cartilage injury is of upmost importance to correctly address the defect. In this sense, the International Cartilage Repair Society (ICRS) cartilage injury evaluation package is the most commonly classification system used to characterize macroscopically the articular cartilage defect [137]. Regarding the outcome scores, there is substantial variability in outcome reporting after knee articular cartilage

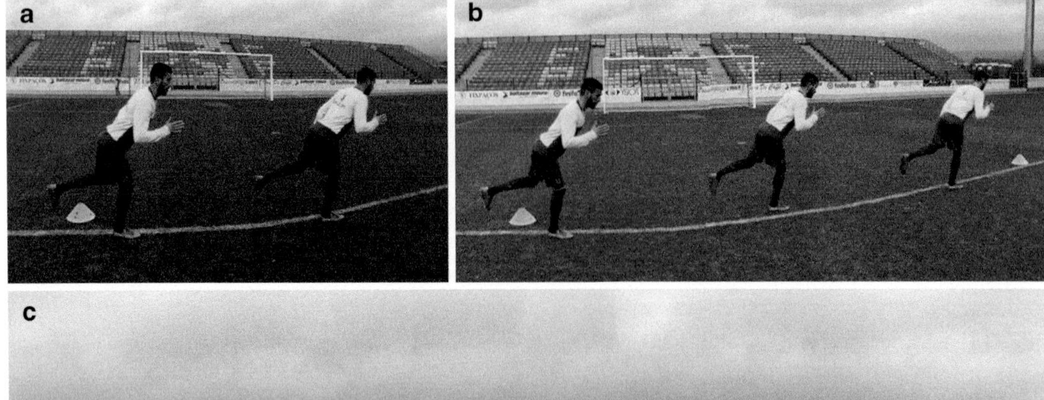

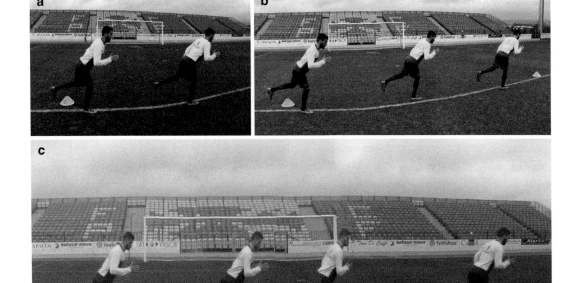

Fig. 44.5 Performance of one-leg hop tests to assess the limb symmetry index: (**a**) single hop for distance; (**b**) cross-over hop for distance; (**c**) triple hop for distance and 6-meter timed hop test [136]

Table 44.2 Suggested disease- and joint-specific, activity-related, associated quality of life and psychological outcome scores for athletes following articular cartilage surgery [18, 66, 139–145]

Common outcome scores for athletes following articular cartilage surgery			
Joint-specific	Activity-related	Quality of life	Psychological
KOOS	Tegner	SF-12/SF-36	Tampa scale
IKDC	Marx	EQ-5D	Knee Self-Efficacy Scale
Lysholm			Injury-Psychological Readiness to Return to Sport Scale

KOSS Knee Injury and Osteoarthritis Outcome Score, *IKDC* International Knee Documentation Committee, *SF-12* short-form 12 items, *SF-36* short-form 36 items, *EQ-5D* EuroQoL-5 dimensions

surgery [138]. Nevertheless, there are some disease- and joint-specific, activity-related, associated quality of life and psychological evaluation outcome scores that may be suggested to be used in athletes following articular cartilage injuries (Table 44.2) [18, 66, 139–145].

Return to sports should be a shared decision between all the involved sports medicine professionals and the stakeholders directly involved (coach, club directors, and the player itself), with well-defined roles in the return to play process [146–149]. Moreover, the combination of high-quality research evidence, clinical expertise, intensive rehabilitation, and player motivation are the keystones to the optimal return to competition [150–153]. In addition, several return to play decision-making models have been proposed to assist the sports medicine professionals to make a safe decision, including the Strategic Assessment of Risk and Risk Tolerance (StARRT) [154] and the biopsychosocial model [155–157].

Table 44.3 Return to sports (%) and (months) following articular cartilage surgery for football players and general athletic population, based on results of systematic reviews

	Football			Athletic population		
	OAT	MF	ACI	OAT	MF	ACI
Rate	87%	88%	85%	89–93%	58–75%	67–84%
Time to RTP	4.5 mo.	8 mo.	13.1 mo.	5.2–7.1 mo.	8–9.1 mo.	11.8–18 mo.

MF microfracture; *mo.* months, *RTP* return to play

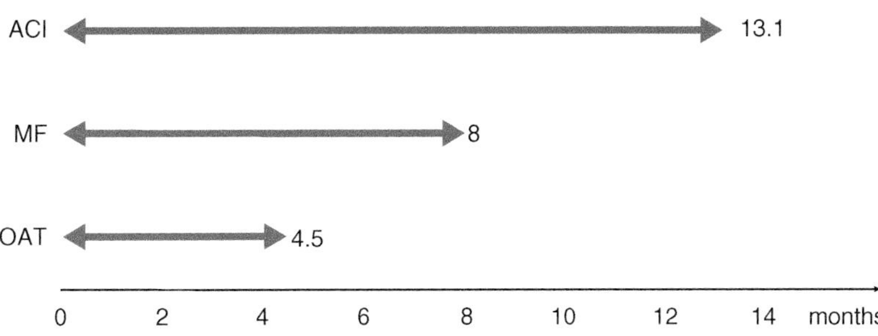

Fig. 44.6 Reported mean return to play in football players following articular cartilage surgery according technique

Regarding articular cartilage lesions of the knee, the scientific literature reports good return to play rates following OAT/mosaicplasty, microfracture, and ACI surgical techniques in athletic populations [8, 158, 159]. When focusing football players [2], the return to play rate seems to be higher, taking less time to return to play (Table 44.3). For football players, the results were pooled for each technique and presented according to the weighted mean [2]. Note that the return to play rate for ACI procedure was recalculated from the original study to exclude the recreational football players, which would lower return to play rate otherwise [60]. For the general athletic population, it is presented the range of means reported within the systematic reviews [8, 158, 159]. In the case of football players, the OAT procedure provides a faster return to competition (4.5 months), followed by microfracture (8 months) and ACI (13.1 months) (Fig. 44.6) [77]. Still, when considering amateur football players, the return to play rate may be under the expected (only 16% returned to football) [60]. This may be explained by the fact that recreational football players aim for pain relief and recover the joint functionality while safeguarding the possibility of some sports participation, without the need for returning to high-level sports activity. In contrast, professional football players require a fast return to competition, preferably at the preinjury sports activity level. In addition, professional players may have access to higher-quality rehabilitation clinical facilities and more experienced sports medicine professionals, providing the ideal opportunity to apply a more aggressive rehabilitation aiming a faster return to play. Nevertheless, it must be highlighted that these players also require good quality chondral repair to avoid compromising the player's long-term functionality and quality of life [39].

The microfracture procedure is the most commonly treatment employed in professional football players with the belief that it provides a safe option that will result in a faster return to competition. Nevertheless, this common assumption is not accurate as it often takes longer rehabilitation and may be longer than OAT procedures (Table 44.3). Moreover, microfracture seems to have higher clinical deterioration overtime and, subsequently, lower clinical durability compared to OAT and ACI procedures [40, 160].

In-season and early career injuries often require prompt clinical decisions, once the player needs to return to competition as soon as possible and still play the rest of the season. Thus, time into the season and career status play a crucial role in the decision of the surgical technique. In this sense, it may be opted for microfracture or OAT procedure or even a simple surgical debridement if the injury is small (<2 cm^2). Nevertheless, the ACI/MACI technique should be considered as first-line option as it provides a more durable cartilage repair, especially in early career football players. In case of in-season players, the orthopedic surgeon may opt by debriding the cartilage defect to provide symptomology relief and collect a cartilage biopsy concomitantly to perform an ACI in the off-season period. Similarly, if the football player is reaching his career ending, the microfracture/OAT may provide a fast pain relief to play the rest of his career and perform an ACI/MACI procedure once the player retires [39].

The size of the lesion plays an important role as greater articular cartilage defects (>2 cm^2) would benefit from ACI/MACI surgical procedures (Fig. 44.1) once it provides higher clinical and functional outcomes [160].

Fact Box 3

- Surgical technique decision may vary depending on player's age, defect size, levels of competition, career status, and time into the season.
- OAT/mosaicplasty and microfracture allow a faster return to sports; however, they have lower durability.
- ACI/MACI has a delayed return to sports, but provides a durable and higher-quality repaired tissue.
- Large articular cartilage defects (>2cm^2) benefit the most from ACI/MACI procedures.

Take-Home Message

The ultimate goal for the football player is to return to play at the preinjury sports activity level as fast as possible. Nevertheless, the sports medicine professional must always ensure a safe return to play—primum non nocere.

The clinical decision making regarding the surgical technique and rehabilitation procedure must be customized according to the defect and the football player's individual characteristics (age, defect size, levels of competition, career status, and time into the season).

The OAT/mosaicplasty and microfracture surgical techniques provide a faster return to competition than ACI/MACI procedures, however, that display a less durable and lower-quality repaired tissue.

Top 5 Evidence-Based References

Andrade R, Vasta S, Papalia R, Pereira H, Oliveira JM, Reis RL et al (2016) Prevalence of articular cartilage lesions and surgical clinical outcomes in football (soccer) players' knees: a systematic review. Arthroscopy 32:1466–1477

Bekkers J, de Windt TS, Brittberg M, Saris D (2012) Cartilage repair in football (soccer) athletes what evidence leads to which treatment? A critical review of the literature. Cartilage 3:43S–49S

Hambly K, Silvers HJ, Steinwachs M (2012) Rehabilitation after articular cartilage repair of the knee in the football (soccer) player. Cartilage 3:50S–56S

Mithoefer K, Della Villa S (2012) Return to sports after articular cartilage repair in the football (soccer) player. Cartilage 3:57S–62S

Reinold MM, Wilk KE, Macrina LC, Dugas JR, Cain EL (2006) Current concepts in the rehabilitation following articular cartilage repair procedures in the knee. J Orthop Sports Phys Ther 36:774–794

References

1. Mithoefer K, Peterson L, Saris D, Mandelbaum B, Dvorák J (2012) Special issue on articular cartilage injury in the football (soccer) player. Cartilage 3:4S–5S
2. Andrade R, Vasta S, Papalia R, Pereira H, Oliveira JM, Reis RL et al (2016) Prevalence of articular cartilage lesions and surgical clinical outcomes in football (soccer) players' knees: a systematic review. Arthroscopy 32:1466–1477
3. Flanigan DC, Harris JD, Trinh TQ, Siston RA, Brophy RH (2010) Prevalence of chondral defects in athletes' knees: a systematic review. Med Sci Sports Exerc 42:1795–1801
4. Mithoefer K, Steadman RJ (2012) Microfracture in football (soccer) players a case series of professional athletes and systematic review. Cartilage 3:18S–24S

5. Gomoll A, Filardo G, De Girolamo L, Esprequeira-Mendes J, Marcacci M, Rodkey W et al (2012) Surgical treatment for early osteoarthritis. Part I: cartilage repair procedures. Knee Surg Sports Traumatol Arthrosc 20:450–466
6. Krych AJ, Robertson CM, Williams RJ (2012) Return to athletic activity after osteochondral allograft transplantation in the knee. Am J Sports Med 40:1053–1059
7. Mithoefer K, Della Villa S (2012) Return to sports after articular cartilage repair in the football (soccer) player. Cartilage 3:57S–62S
8. Mithoefer K, Hambly K, Della Villa S, Silvers H, Mandelbaum BR (2009) Return to sports participation after articular cartilage repair in the knee scientific evidence. Am J Sports Med 37:167S–176S
9. Dvorak J, Peterson L, Junge A, Chomiak J, Graf-Baumann T (2000) Incidence of football injuries and complaints in different age groups and skill-level groups. Am J Sports Med 28:51–57
10. Messner K, Maletius W (1996) The long-term prognosis for severe damage to weight-bearing cartilage in the knee: a 14-year clinical and radiographic follow-up in 28 young athletes. Acta Orthop 67:165–168
11. Piasecki DP, Spindler KP, Warren TA, Andrish JT, Parker RD (2003) Intraarticular injuries associated with anterior cruciate ligament tear: findings at ligament reconstruction in high school and recreational athletes. An analysis of sex-based differences. Am J Sports Med 31:601–605
12. Arendt E, Dick R (1995) Knee injury patterns among men and women in collegiate basketball and soccer NCAA data and review of literature. Am J Sports Med 23:694–701
13. Heijink A, Gomoll AH, Madry H, Drobnič M, Filardo G, Espregueira-Mendes J et al (2012) Biomechanical considerations in the pathogenesis of osteoarthritis of the knee. Knee Surg Sports Traumatol Arthrosc 20:423–435
14. Vannini F, Spalding T, Andriolo L, Berruto M, Denti M, Espregueira-Mendes J et al (2016) Sport and early osteoarthritis: the role of sport in aetiology, progression and treatment of knee osteoarthritis. Knee Surg Sports Traumatol Arthrosc 24:1786–1796
15. Engström B, Forssblad M, Johansson C, Tornkvist H (1990) Does a major knee injury definitely sideline an elite soccer player? Am J Sports Med 18:101–105
16. Pánics G, Hangody LR, Baló E, Vásárhelyi G, Gál T, Hangody L (2012) Osteochondral autograft and mosaicplasty in the football (soccer) athlete. Cartilage 3:25S–30S
17. Steinwachs M, Engebretsen L, Brophy R (2012) Scientific evidence base for cartilage injury and repair in the athlete. Cartilage 3:11S–17S
18. Mithoefer K, Hambly K, Logerstedt D, Ricci M, Silvers H, Villa SD (2012) Current concepts for rehabilitation and return to sport after knee articular cartilage repair in the athlete. J Orthop Sports Phys Ther 42:254–273
19. Kiviranta I, Tammi M, Jurvelin J, Arokoski J, Säuäumäunen A-M, Helminen HJ (1992) Articular cartilage thickness and glycosaminoglycan distribution in the canine knee joint after strenuous running exercise. Clin Orthop Relat Res 283:302–308
20. Stefan Lohmander L, Roos H, Dahlberg L, Hoerrner LA, Lark MW (1994) Temporal patterns of stromelysin-1, tissue inhibitor, and proteoglycan fragments in human knee joint fluid after injury to the cruciate ligament or meniscus. J Orthop Res 12:21–28
21. Buckwalter JA (1998) Articular cartilage: injuries and potential for healing. J Orthop Sports Phys Ther 28:192–202
22. Gomoll AH, Minas T (2014) The quality of healing: articular cartilage. Wound Repair Regen 22:30–38
23. McAdams TR, Mithoefer K, Scopp JM, Mandelbaum BR (2010) Articular cartilage injury in athletes. Cartilage 1:165–179
24. Årøen A, Løken S, Heir S, Alvik E, Ekeland A, Granlund OG et al (2004) Articular cartilage lesions in 993 consecutive knee arthroscopies. Am J Sports Med 32:211–215
25. Curl WW, Krome J, Gordon ES, Rushing J, Smith BP, Poehling GG (1997) Cartilage injuries: a review of 31,516 knee arthroscopies. Arthroscopy 13: 456–460
26. Marcacci M, Kon E, Zaffagnini S, Iacono F, Neri MP, Vascellari A et al (2005) Multiple osteochondral arthroscopic grafting (mosaicplasty) for cartilage defects of the knee: prospective study results at 2-year follow-up. Arthroscopy 21:462–470
27. Mithoefer K, Williams RJ, Warren RF, Wickiewicz TL, Marx RG (2006) High-impact athletics after knee articular cartilage repair a prospective evaluation of the microfracture technique. Am J Sports Med 34:1413–1418
28. Ekstrand J. (2016) UEFA elite club injury study report 2015/16.. http://www.uefa.org/MultimediaFiles/Download/uefaorg/Medical/02/40/27/65/2402765_DOWNLOAD.pdf
29. Hägglund M, Waldén M, Magnusson H, Kristenson K, Bengtsson H, Ekstrand J (2013) Injuries affect team performance negatively in professional football: an 11-year follow-up of the UEFA Champions League injury study. Br J Sports Med 47:738–742
30. Drawer S, Fuller C (2001) Propensity for osteoarthritis and lower limb joint pain in retired professional soccer players. Br J Sports Med 35: 402–408
31. Hambly K, Silvers HJ, Steinwachs M (2012) Rehabilitation after articular cartilage repair of the knee in the football (soccer) player. Cartilage 3:50S–56S
32. Verdonk P, Dhollander A, Almqvist K, Verdonk R, Victor J (2015) Treatment of osteochondral lesions in the knee using a cell-free scaffold. Bone Joint J 97:318–323
33. Murray IR, Benke MT, Mandelbaum BR (2016) Management of knee articular cartilage injuries in athletes: chondroprotection, chondrofacilitation, and

resurfacing. Knee Surg Sports Traumatol Arthrosc 24:1617–1626
34. Erggelet C, Mandelbaum BR (2008) Principles of cartilage repair. Springer, New York, NY
35. Gorsline RT, Kaeding CC (2005) The use of NSAIDs and nutritional supplements in athletes with osteoarthritis: prevalence, benefits, and consequences. Clin Sports Med 24:71–82
36. Clark KL (2007) Nutritional considerations in joint health. Clin Sports Med 26:101–118
37. Tamburrino P, Castellacci E (2016) Intra-articular injections of HYADD4-G in male professional soccer players with traumatic or degenerative knee chondropathy. A pilot, prospective study. J Sports Med Phys Fitness 56:1534
38. Papalia R, Zampogna B, Russo F, Vasta S, Tirindelli M, Nobile C et al (2016) Comparing hybrid hyaluronic acid with PRP in end career athletes with degenerative cartilage lesions of the knee. J Biol Regul Homeost Agents 30:17
39. Bekkers J, de Windt TS, Brittberg M, Saris D (2012) Cartilage repair in football (soccer) athletes what evidence leads to which treatment? A critical review of the literature. Cartilage 3:43S–49S
40. Harris JD, Brophy RH, Siston RA, Flanigan DC (2010) Treatment of chondral defects in the athlete's knee. Arthroscopy 26:841–852
41. Gille J, Schuseil E, Wimmer J, Gellissen J, Schulz A, Behrens P (2010) Mid-term results of autologous matrix-induced chondrogenesis for treatment of focal cartilage defects in the knee. Knee Surg Sports Traumatol Arthrosc 18:1456–1464
42. Lee YHD, Suzer F, Thermann H (2014) Autologous matrix-induced chondrogenesis in the knee. A review. Cartilage 5:145–153
43. Gobbi A, Karnatzikos G, Sankineani SR (2014) One-step surgery with multipotent stem cells for the treatment of large full-thickness chondral defects of the knee. Am J Sports Med 42:648–657
44. Gobbi A, Karnatzikos G, Scotti C, Mahajan V, Mazzucco L, Grigolo B (2011) One-step cartilage repair with bone marrow aspirate concentrated cells and collagen matrix in full-thickness knee cartilage lesions results at 2-year follow-up. Cartilage 2:286–299
45. Huh SW, Shetty AA, Ahmed S, Lee DH, Kim SJ (2016) Autologous bone-marrow mesenchymal cell induced chondrogenesis (MCIC). J Clin Orthop Trauma 7:153–156
46. Shetty AA, Kim SJ, Shetty V, Jang JD, Huh SW, Lee DH (2016) Autologous collagen induced chondrogenesis (ACIC: Shetty–Kim technique)—a matrix based acellular single stage arthroscopic cartilage repair technique. J Clin Orthop Trauma 7:164–169
47. Stelzeneder D, Shetty AA, Kim S-J, Trattnig S, Domayer SE, Shetty V et al (2013) Repair tissue quality after arthroscopic autologous collagen-induced chondrogenesis (ACIC) assessed via T2* mapping. Skelet Radiol 42:1657–1664
48. Farr J, Cole BJ, Sherman S, Karas V (2012) Particulated articular cartilage: CAIS and DeNovo NT. J Knee Surg 25:023–030
49. Farr J, Tabet SK, Margerrison E, Cole BJ (2014) Clinical, radiographic, and histological outcomes after cartilage repair with particulated juvenile articular cartilage. A 2-year prospective study. Am J Sports Med 42:1417–1425
50. Harris JD, Frank RM, McCormick FM, Cole BJ (2014) Minced cartilage techniques. Oper Tech Orthop 24:27–34
51. Brix M, Kaipel M, Kellner R, Schreiner M, Apprich S, Boszotta H et al (2016) Successful osteoconduction but limited cartilage tissue quality following osteochondral repair by a cell-free multilayered nano-composite scaffold at the knee. Int Orthop 40:625–632
52. Delcogliano M, de Caro F, Scaravella E, Ziveri G, De Biase CF, Marotta D et al (2014) Use of innovative biomimetic scaffold in the treatment for large osteochondral lesions of the knee. Knee Surg Sports Traumatol Arthrosc 22:1260–1269
53. Kon E, Delcogliano M, Filardo G, Busacca M, Di Martino A, Marcacci M (2011) Novel nanocomposite multilayered biomaterial for osteochondral regeneration a pilot clinical trial. Am J Sports Med 39:1180–1190
54. Kon E, Delcogliano M, Filardo G, Pressato D, Busacca M, Grigolo B et al (2010) A novel nanocomposite multi-layered biomaterial for treatment of osteochondral lesions: technique note and an early stability pilot clinical trial. Injury 41:693–701
55. Hoemann CD, Tran-Khanh N, Chevrier A, Chen G, Lascau-Coman V, Mathieu C et al (2015) Chondroinduction Is the main cartilage repair response to microfracture and microfracture with BST-CarGel results as shown by ICRS-II histological scoring and a novel zonal collagen type scoring method of human clinical biopsy specimens. Am J Sports Med 43:2469–2480
56. Méthot S, Changoor A, Tran-Khanh N, Hoemann CD, Stanish WD, Restrepo A et al (2015) Osteochondral biopsy analysis demonstrates that BST-CarGel treatment improves structural and cellular characteristics of cartilage repair tissue compared with microfracture. Cartilage 7:16–28
57. Shive MS, Stanish WD, McCormack R, Forriol F, Mohtadi N, Pelet S et al (2015) BST-CarGel® treatment maintains cartilage repair superiority over microfracture at 5 years in a multicenter randomized controlled trial. Cartilage 6:62–72
58. Stanish WD, McCormack R, Forriol F, Mohtadi N, Pelet S, Desnoyers J et al (2013) Novel scaffold-based BST-CarGel treatment results in superior cartilage repair compared with microfracture in a randomized controlled trial. J Bone Joint Surg Am 95:1640–1650
59. Mithöfer K, Minas T, Peterson L, Yeon H, Micheli LJ (2005) Functional outcome of knee articular cartilage repair in adolescent athletes. Am J Sports Med 33:1147–1153
60. Mithöfer K, Peterson L, Mandelbaum BR, Minas T (2005) Articular cartilage repair in soccer players with autologous chondrocyte transplantation

functional outcome and return to competition. Am J Sports Med 33:1639–1646
61. Peterson L, Vasiliadis HS, Brittberg M, Lindahl A (2010) Autologous chondrocyte implantation a long-term follow-up. Am J Sports Med 38:1117–1124
62. Blevins FT, Rodrigo JJ, Silliman J (1998) Treatment of articular cartilage defects in athletes: an analysis of functional outcome and lesion appearance. Orthopedics 21:761
63. Mithoefer K, Minas T, Peterson L, Yeon H, Micheli LJ (2005) Functional outcome of knee articular cartilage repair in adolescent athletes. Am J Sports Med 33:1147–1153
64. Mithoefer K, Peterson L, Mandelbaum BR, Minas T (2005) Articular cartilage repair in soccer players with autologous chondrocyte transplantation functional outcome and return to competition. Am J Sports Med 33:1639–1646
65. Bedi A, Feeley BT, Williams RJ (2010) Management of articular cartilage defects of the knee. J Bone Joint Surg Am 92:994–1009
66. Krych AJ, Gobbi A, Lattermann C, Nakamura N (2016) Articular cartilage solutions for the knee: present challenges and future direction. J ISAKOS 1:93–104
67. Mithoefer K, Williams RJ, Warren RF, Potter HG, Spock CR, Jones EC et al (2005) The microfracture technique for the treatment of articular cartilage lesions in the knee. J Bone Joint Surg Am 87:1911–1920
68. Gobbi A, Nunag P, Malinowski K (2005) Treatment of full thickness chondral lesions of the knee with microfracture in a group of athletes. Knee Surg Sports Traumatol Arthrosc 13:213–221
69. Mithoefer K, McAdams T, Williams RJ, Kreuz PC, Mandelbaum BR (2009) Clinical efficacy of the microfracture technique for articular cartilage repair in the knee an evidence-based systematic analysis. Am J Sports Med 37:2053–2063
70. Bae DK, Song SJ, Yoon KH, Heo DB, Kim TJ (2013) Survival analysis of microfracture in the osteoarthritic knee—minimum 10-year follow-up. Arthroscopy 29:244–250
71. Solheim E, Hegna J, Inderhaug E, Øyen J, Harlem T, Strand T (2016) Results at 10–14 years after microfracture treatment of articular cartilage defects in the knee. Knee Surg Sports Traumatol Arthrosc 24:1587–1593
72. Carey JL (2012) Fibrocartilage following microfracture is not as robust as native articular cartilage: commentary on an article by Aaron J Krych, MD, et al: activity levels are higher after osteochondral autograft transfer mosaicplasty than after microfracture for articular cartilage defects of the knee. A retrospective comparative study. J Bone Joint Surg Am 94:e80
73. Case JM, Scopp JM (2016) Treatment of articular cartilage defects of the knee with microfracture and enhanced microfracture techniques. Sports Med Arthrosc 24:63–68
74. Krych AJ, Harnly HW, Rodeo SA, Williams RJ (2012) Activity levels are higher after osteochondral autograft transfer mosaicplasty than after microfracture for articular cartilage defects of the knee. J Bone Joint Surg Am 94:971–978
75. Koh Y-G, Kwon O-R, Kim Y-S, Choi Y-J, Tak D-H (2016) Adipose-derived mesenchymal stem cells with microfracture versus microfracture alone: 2-year follow-up of a prospective randomized trial. Arthroscopy 32:97–109
76. Sofu H, Kockara N, Oner A, Camurcu Y, Issın A, Sahin V (2016) Results of hyaluronic acid-based cell-free scaffold application in combination with microfracture for the treatment of osteochondral lesions of the knee: 2-year comparative study. Arthroscopy 33:209–216
77. Andrade R, Vasta S, Pereira R, Pereira H, Papalia R, Karahan M et al (2016) Knee donor-site morbidity after mosaicplasty – a systematic review. J Exp Orthop 3:31
78. Espregueira-Mendes J, Pereira H, Sevivas N, Varanda P, Da Silva MV, Monteiro A et al (2012) Osteochondral transplantation using autografts from the upper tibio-fibular joint for the treatment of knee cartilage lesions. Knee Surg Sports Traumatol Arthrosc 20:1136–1142
79. De Caro F, Bisicchia S, Amendola A, Ding L (2015) Large fresh osteochondral allografts of the knee: a systematic clinical and basic science review of the literature. Arthroscopy 31:757–765
80. Brittberg M, Lindahl A, Nilsson A, Ohlsson C, Isaksson O, Peterson L (1994) Treatment of deep cartilage defects in the knee with autologous chondrocyte transplantation. N Engl J Med 331:889–895
81. Roberts S, McCall IW, Darby AJ, Menage J, Evans H, Harrison PE et al (2002) Autologous chondrocyte implantation for cartilage repair: monitoring its success by magnetic resonance imaging and histology. Arthritis Res Ther 5:1
82. Henderson I, Lavigne P, Valenzuela H, Oakes B (2007) Autologous chondrocyte implantation: superior biologic properties of hyaline cartilage repairs. Clin Orthop Relat Res 455:253–261
83. Horas U, Pelinkovic D, Herr G, Aigner T, Schnettler R (2003) Autologous chondrocyte implantation and osteochondral cylinder transplantation in cartilage repair of the knee joint. J Bone Joint Surg Am 85:185–192
84. Tom Minas M, Arvind VKM, Bryant T, Gomoll AH (2014) The John Insall Award: a minimum 10-year outcome study of autologous chondrocyte implantation. Clin Orthop Relat Res 472:41
85. Bartlett W, Gooding C, Carrington R, Skinner J, Briggs T, Bentley G (2005) Autologous chondrocyte implantation at the knee using a bilayer collagen membrane with bone graft. Bone Joint J 87:330–332
86. Basad E, Wissing FR, Fehrenbach P, Rickert M, Steinmeyer J, Ishaque B (2015) Matrix-induced autologous chondrocyte implantation (MACI) in the knee: clinical outcomes and challenges. Knee Surg Sports Traumatol Arthrosc 23:3729–3735

87. Ebert JR, Fallon M, Wood DJ, Janes GC (2017) A prospective clinical and radiological evaluation at 5 years after arthroscopic matrix-induced autologous chondrocyte implantation. Am J Sports Med 45:59
88. Meyerkort D, Ebert JR, Ackland TR, Robertson WB, Fallon M, Zheng M et al (2014) Matrix-induced autologous chondrocyte implantation (MACI) for chondral defects in the patellofemoral joint. Knee Surg Sports Traumatol Arthrosc 22:2522–2530
89. Bekkers JE, Inklaar M, Saris DB (2009) Treatment selection in articular cartilage lesions of the knee. A systematic review. Am J Sports Med 37:148S–155S
90. Cole BJ, Pascual-Garrido C, Grumet RC (2009) Surgical management of articular cartilage defects in the knee. J Bone Joint Surg Am 91:1778–1790
91. de Windt TS, Saris DB (2014) Treatment algorithm for articular cartilage repair of the knee: towards patient profiling using evidence-based tools. In: Shetty A, Kim SJ, Nakamura N, Brittberg M (eds) Techniques in cartilage repair surgery. Springer, New York, NY, pp 23–31
92. Gomoll AH, Farr J, Gillogly SD, Kercher J, Minas T (2010) Surgical management of articular cartilage defects of the knee. J Bone Joint Surg Am 92:2470–2490
93. Tetteh ES, Bajaj S, Ghodadra NS, Cole BJ (2012) The basic science and surgical treatment options for articular cartilage injuries of the knee. J Orthop Sports Phys Ther 42:243–253
94. Della Villa S, Boldrini L, Ricci M, Danelon F, Snyder-Mackler L, Nanni G et al (2012) Clinical outcomes and return-to-sports participation of 50 soccer players after anterior cruciate ligament reconstruction through a sport-specific rehabilitation protocol. Sports Health 4:17–24
95. Brophy RH, Zeltser D, Wright RW, Flanigan D (2010) Anterior cruciate ligament reconstruction and concomitant articular cartilage injury: incidence and treatment. Arthroscopy 26:112–120
96. Indelicato P, Bittar E (1985) A perspective of lesions associated with ACL insufficiency of the knee. A review of 100 cases. Clin Orthop Relat Res 198:77–80
97. Mandelbaum BR, Browne JE, Fu F, Micheli L, Mosely JB, Erggelet C et al (1998) Articular cartilage lesions of the knee. Am J Sports Med 26:853–861
98. Noyes FR, Bassett R, Grood E, Butler D (1980) Arthroscopy in acute traumatic hemarthrosis of the knee. Incidence of anterior cruciate tears and other injuries. J Bone Joint Surg Am 62:687–695
99. Shelbourne KD, Jari S, Gray T (2003) Outcome of untreated traumatic articular cartilage defects of the knee. J Bone Joint Surg Am 85:8–16
100. Widuchowski W, Widuchowski J, Koczy B, Szyluk K (2009) Untreated asymptomatic deep cartilage lesions associated with anterior cruciate ligament injury results at 10-and 15-year follow-up. Am J Sports Med 37:688–692
101. Mithoefer K, Peterson L, Saris DB, Mandelbaum BR (2012) Evolution and current role of autologous chondrocyte implantation for treatment of articular cartilage defects in the football (soccer) player. Cartilage 3:31S–36S
102. Alford JW, Lewis P, Kang RW, Cole BJ (2005) Rapid progression of chondral disease in the lateral compartment of the knee following meniscectomy. Arthroscopy 21:1505–1509
103. Mariani PP, Garofalo R, Margheritini F (2008) Chondrolysis after partial lateral meniscectomy in athletes. Knee Surg Sports Traumatol Arthrosc 16:574–580
104. Stone JY, Schaal R (2012) Postoperative management of patients with articular cartilage repair. J Knee Surg 25:207–212
105. Della Villa S, Kon E, Filardo G, Ricci M, Vincentelli F, Delcogliano M et al (2010) Does intensive rehabilitation permit early return to sport without compromising the clinical outcome after arthroscopic autologous chondrocyte implantation in highly competitive athletes? Am J Sports Med 38:68–77
106. Hambly K, Bobic V, Wondrasch B, Van Assche D, Marlovits S (2006) Autologous chondrocyte implantation postoperative care and rehabilitation science and practice. Am J Sports Med 34:1020–1038
107. Howard JS, Mattacola CG, Romine SE, Lattermann C (2010) Continuous passive motion, early weight bearing, and active motion following knee articular cartilage repair evidence for clinical practice. Cartilage 1:276–286
108. Jakobsen RB, Engebretsen L, Slauterbeck JR (2005) An analysis of the quality of cartilage repair studies. J Bone Joint Surg Am 87:2232–2239
109. Reinold MM, Wilk KE, Macrina LC, Dugas JR, Cain EL (2006) Current concepts in the rehabilitation following articular cartilage repair procedures in the knee. J Orthop Sports Phys Ther 36:774–794
110. Shapiro F, Koide S, Glimcher M (1993) Cell origin and differentiation in the repair of full-thickness defects of articular cartilage. J Bone Joint Surg Am 75:532–553
111. Shortkroff S, Barone L, Hsu H-P, Wrenn C, Gagne T, Chi T et al (1996) Healing of chondral and osteochondral defects in a canine model: the role of cultured chondrocytes in regeneration of articular cartilage. Biomaterials 17:147–154
112. Ebert J, Robertson W, Lloyd DG, Zheng M, Wood D, Ackland T (2008) Traditional vs accelerated approaches to post-operative rehabilitation following matrix-induced autologous chondrocyte implantation (MACI): comparison of clinical, biomechanical and radiographic outcomes. Osteoarthr Cartil 16:1131–1140
113. Wondrasch B, Risberg M-A, Zak L, Marlovits S, Aldrian S (2015) Effect of accelerated weightbearing after matrix-associated autologous chondrocyte implantation on the femoral condyle a prospective, randomized controlled study presenting MRI-based and clinical outcomes after 5 years. Am J Sports Med 43:146–153
114. Thornley P, Niroopan G, Khan M, McCarthy C, Simunovic N, Adamich J et al (2016) No difference

in outcome between early versus delayed weight-bearing following microfracture surgery of the hip, knee or ankle: a systematic review of outcomes and complications. J ISAKOS 1:2–9

115. Arokoski J, Jurvelin J, Väätäinen U, Helminen H (2000) Normal and pathological adaptations of articular cartilage to joint loading. Scand J Med Sci Sports 10:186–198
116. Hinterwimmer S, Krammer M, Krötz M, Glaser C, Baumgart R, Reiser M et al (2004) Cartilage atrophy in the knees of patients after seven weeks of partial load bearing. Arthritis Rheum 50:2516–2520
117. Lane Smith R, Trindade M, Ikenoue T, Mohtai M, Das P, Carter D et al (2000) Effects of shear stress on articular chondrocyte metabolism. Biorheology 37:95–107
118. Mouritzen U, Christgau S, Lehmann H, Tanko L, Christiansen C (2003) Cartilage turnover assessed with a newly developed assay measuring collagen type II degradation products: influence of age, sex, menopause, hormone replacement therapy, and body mass index. Ann Rheum Dis 62:332–336
119. Stoddart MJ, Ettinger L, Häuselmann HJ (2006) Enhanced matrix synthesis in de novo, scaffold free cartilage-like tissue subjected to compression and shear. Biotechnol Bioeng 95:1043–1051
120. Lorenz DS, Reiman MP (2011) Performance enhancement in the terminal phases of rehabilitation. Sports Health 3:470–480
121. Binnie MJ, Dawson B, Arnot MA, Pinnington H, Landers G, Peeling P (2014) Effect of sand versus grass training surfaces during an 8-week pre-season conditioning programme in team sport athletes. J Sports Sci 32:1001–1012
122. Binnie MJ, Dawson B, Pinnington H, Landers G, Peeling P (2013) Part 2: effect of training surface on acute physiological responses after sport-specific training. J Strength Cond Res 27:1057–1066
123. Binnie MJ, Dawson B, Pinnington H, Landers G, Peeling P (2014) Sand training: a review of current research and practical applications. J Sports Sci 32:8–15
124. Binnie MJ, Peeling P, Pinnington H, Landers G, Dawson B (2013) Effect of surface-specific training on 20-m sprint performance on sand and grass surfaces. J Strength Cond Res 27:3515–3520
125. Gaudino P, Gaudino C, Alberti G, Minetti AE (2013) Biomechanics and predicted energetics of sprinting on sand: hints for soccer training. J Sci Med Sport 16:271–275
126. Rago V, Rebelo A, Pizzuto F, Barreira D (2016) Small-sided football games on sand are more physical-demanding but less technical-specific compared to artificial turf. J Sports Med Phys Fitness PMID:27627990
127. Bartlett J, O'Connor F, Pitchford N, Torres-Ronda L, Robertson S (2016) Relationships between internal and external training load in team sport athletes: evidence for an individualised approach. Int J Sports Physiol Perform. https://doi.org/10.1123/ijspp.2016-0300
128. Mara JK, Thompson KG, Pumpa KL, Ball NB (2015) Periodization and physical performance in elite female soccer players. Int J Sports Physiol Perform 10:664–669
129. Reid LC, Cowman JR, Green BS, Coughlan GF (2013) Return to play in elite rugby union: application of global positioning system technology in return-to-running programs. J Sport Rehabil 22:122–129
130. Ritchie D, Hopkins WG, Buchheit M, Cordy J, Bartlett JD (2016) Quantification of training load during return to play following upper and lower body injury in Australian rules football. Int J Sports Physiol Perform. https://doi.org/10.1123/ijspp.2016-0300
131. Shrier I, Clarsen B, Verhagen E, Gordon K, Mellette J (2017) Improving the accuracy of sports medicine surveillance: when is a subsequent event a new injury? Br J Sports Med 51:26–28
132. Blanch P, Gabbett TJ (2016) Has the athlete trained enough to return to play safely? The acute: chronic workload ratio permits clinicians to quantify a player's risk of subsequent injury. Br J Sports Med 50:471–475
133. Grindem H, Snyder-Mackler L, Moksnes H, Engebretsen L, Risberg MA (2016) Simple decision rules can reduce reinjury risk by 84% after ACL reconstruction: the Delaware-Oslo ACL cohort study. Br J Sports Med 50:804–808
134. Nagelli CV, Hewett TE (2017) Should return to sport be delayed until 2 years after anterior cruciate ligament reconstruction? Biological and functional considerations. Sports Med 47(2):221–232
135. Edwards PK, Ackland T, Ebert JR (2014) Clinical rehabilitation guidelines for matrix-induced autologous chondrocyte implantation on the tibiofemoral joint. J Orthop Sports Phys Ther 44:102–119
136. Kyritsis P, Bahr R, Landreau P, Miladi R, Witvrouw E (2016) Likelihood of ACL graft rupture: not meeting six clinical discharge criteria before return to sport is associated with a four times greater risk of rupture. Br J Sports Med 50:946–951
137. Brittberg M, Aglietti P, Gambardella R, Hangody L, Hauselmann H, Jakob R, et al. (2000) ICRS cartilage injury evaluation package. Paper presented at proceedings of 3rd ICRS meeting, Göteborg, Sweden
138. Makhni EC, Meyer MA, Saltzman BM, Cole BJ (2016) Comprehensiveness of outcome reporting in studies of articular cartilage defects of the knee. Arthroscopy 32:2133–2139
139. George SZ, Lentz TA, Zeppieri G Jr, Lee D, Chmielewski TL (2012) Analysis of shortened versions of the Tampa Scale for Kinesiophobia and Pain Catastrophizing Scale for patients following anterior cruciate ligament reconstruction. Clin J Pain 28:73
140. Glazer DD (2009) Development and preliminary validation of the Injury-Psychological Readiness to Return to Sport (I-PRRS) Scale. J Athl Train 44:185–189

141. Hambly K, Griva K (2008) IKDC or KOOS? Which measures symptoms and disabilities most important to postoperative articular cartilage repair patients? Am J Sports Med 36:1695–1704
142. Kanakamedala AC, Anderson AF, Irrgang JJ (2016) IKDC Subjective Knee Form and Marx Activity Rating Scale are suitable to evaluate all orthopaedic sports medicine knee conditions: a systematic review. J ISAKOS 1:25–31
143. Mithoefer K, Acuna M (2013) Clinical outcomes assessment for articular cartilage restoration. J Knee Surg 26:31–40
144. Thomeé P, Währborg P, Börjesson M, Thomeé R, Eriksson BI, Karlsson J (2006) A new instrument for measuring self-efficacy in patients with an anterior cruciate ligament injury. Scand J Med Sci Sports 16:181–187
145. Thomeé P, Währborg P, Börjesson M, Thomeé R, Eriksson BI, Karlsson J (2010) A randomized, controlled study of a rehabilitation model to improve knee-function self-efficacy with ACL injury. J Sport Rehabil 19:200
146. Ardern CL, Bizzini M, Bahr R (2016) It is time for consensus on return to play after injury: five key questions. Br J Sports Med 50:506–508
147. Bizzini M, Silvers HJ (2014) Return to competitive football after major knee surgery: more questions than answers? J Sports Sci 32:1209–1216
148. Elwyn G, Frosch D, Thomson R, Joseph-Williams N, Lloyd A, Kinnersley P et al (2012) Shared decision making: a model for clinical practice. J Gen Intern Med 27:1361–1367
149. Shrier I, Safai P, Charland L (2013) Return to play following injury: whose decision should it be? Br J Sports Med 48:394–401
150. Ardern CL, Glasgow P, Schneiders A, Witvrouw E, Clarsen B, Cools A et al (2016) 2016 Consensus statement on return to sport from the first world congress in sports physical therapy, Bern. Br J Sports Med 50:853–864
151. Ardern CL, Khan KM (2015) The old knee in the young athlete: knowns and unknowns in the return-to-play conversation. Br J Sports Med 50:505–506
152. Grindem H, Risberg M, Eitzen I (2015) Two factors that may underpin outstanding outcomes after ACL rehabilitation. Br J Sports Med 49:1425–1425
153. McCall A, Lewin C, O'driscoll G, Witvrouw E, Ardern C (2016) Return to play: the challenge of balancing research and practice. Br J Sports Med. https://doi.org/10.1136/bjsports-2016-096752
154. Shrier I (2015) Strategic assessment of risk and risk tolerance (StARRT) framework for return-to-play decision-making. Br J Sports Med 49:1311–1315
155. Ardern CL, Kvist J, Webster KE (2016) Psychological aspects of anterior cruciate ligament injuries. Oper Tech Sports Med 24:77–83
156. Ayers DC, Franklin PD, Ring DC (2013) The role of emotional health in functional outcomes after orthopaedic surgery: extending the biopsychosocial model to orthopaedics. J Bone Joint Surg Am 95:e165
157. Wiese-Bjornstal DM, Smith AM, Shaffer SM, Morrey MA (1998) An integrated model of response to sport injury: Psychological and sociological dynamics. J Appl Sport Psychol 10:46–69
158. Campbell AB, Pineda M, Harris JD, Flanigan DC (2016) Return to sport after articular cartilage repair in athletes' knees: a systematic review. Arthroscopy 32:651–668
159. Krych AJ, Pareek A, King AH, Johnson NR, Stuart MJ, Williams RJ (2016) Return to sport after the surgical management of articular cartilage lesions in the knee: a meta-analysis. Knee Surg Sports Traumatol Arthrosc. https://doi.org/10.1007/s00167-016-4262-3
160. Kon E, Filardo G, Berruto M, Benazzo F, Zanon G, Della Villa S et al (2011) Articular cartilage treatment in high-level male soccer players a prospective comparative study of arthroscopic second-generation autologous chondrocyte implantation versus microfracture. Am J Sports Med 39:2549–2557

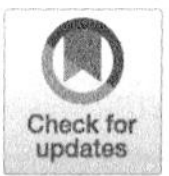

45 Surgical Management of Articular Cartilage in Football Players

Jarret Woodmass, Michael Stuart, and Aaron Krych

Contents

45.1 Introduction

Injury to the articular cartilage in athletes is not uncommon with over one third of patients demonstrating full-thickness defects at the time of diagnostic arthroscopy [1]. Furthermore, articular cartilage lesions have been identified in approximately half of young athletes undergoing primary anterior cruciate ligament (ACL) reconstruction [2]. Not all full-thickness lesions are symptomatic; therefore, an individualized approach to each athlete needs to be considered.

Multiple non-operative techniques can be employed for a symptomatic lesion, including physiotherapy, analgesics, bracing, and injections. However, there is low potential for intrinsic healing, and these cartilage injuries can progress to larger lesions and eventual degenerative joint disease [3]. The main surgical treatment options currently used in the United States include arthroscopic lavage with debridement, microfracture (MF), osteochondral autograft transfer (OAT), osteochondral allograft (OCA) transplantation, and autologous chondrocyte implantation (ACI). Many authors have published outcomes using these techniques, but there is significant heterogeneity in study design, patient demographics, lesion size, and location [4–8]. This heterogeneity in study design makes data interpretation and surgical decision-making difficult. This is complicated further in football players where additional factors including the stage of a player in their career, upcoming events, recovery time, and longevity with high-impact activity must also be considered.

This chapter will review the surgical options, assess their advantages and disadvantages (Table 45.1), and provide an evidence-based algorithm to help guide the treatment of

J. Woodmass, M.D., F.R.C.S.C (✉)
M. Stuart, M.D. • A. Krych, M.D.
Department of Orthopedic Surgery and the Sports Medicine Center, Mayo Clinic and Mayo Foundation, Rochester, MN, USA
e-mail: Woodmass.Jarret@mayo.edu; Krych.Aaron@mayo.edu

V. Musahl et al. (eds.), *Return to Play in Football*, https://doi.org/10.1007/978-3-662-55713-6_45

Table 45.1 Advantages and disadvantages of the surgical procedures currently utilized for treating full-thickness cartilage lesions in football players

	Debridement / chondroplasty	Microfracture	Osteochondral autograft transfer	Osteochondral allograft	Autologous chondrocyte implantation
Advantages	Alleviates mechanical symptoms	Single stage	Normal host cartilage	Can treat large lesions	Can treat large lesions
	Fastest return to sport	Technically reproducible	Relatively fast return to sport	No donor site morbidity	Hyaline-like cartilage
	Inexpensive	Inexpensive	Bone and cartilage transfer	Bone and cartilage transfer	Longevity
Disadvantages		Unable to restore bone stock	Donor site morbidity	Possible disease transmission	Delayed return to sport
	No regenerative potential	Limited to small, contained lesions	Technically challenging	Limited allograft availability	Unable to restore bone stock
		Can compromise future cartilage procedures	Small lesions	Expensive	Expensive

full-thickness articular cartilage lesions in football players. There are ultimately three goals of surgical intervention: (1) enable the player to return to a highly competitive level of activity, (2) provide the player timely return to sport, and (3) deliver longevity for an athlete's career.

45.2 Surgical Interventions

45.2.1 Arthroscopic Debridement and Chondroplasty

Fact Box 1

Chondroplasty provides short-term pain relief and rapid return to activity without disrupting the subchondral bone.

Background: Arthroscopic debridement and chondroplasty allow for removal of loose bodies and unstable cartilage fragments that may be contributing to synovial inflammation and mechanical irritation [4]. Debridement can be performed either by mechanical means with a shaver or using radiofrequency ablation [4]. Chondroplasty has the distinct advantage over other cartilage interventions in that it allows for rapid return to activity and does not disrupt the subchondral bone, potentially altering the outcomes of future cartilage restoration techniques [9].

Surgical technique: Care is taken to debride the damaged cartilage back to a stable peripheral rim. This can be done mechanically (open or arthroscopic) with a shaver and curettes or by radiofrequency ablation. Manual curettage is the preferred debridement technique as the shaver alone can result in crater-like defects while bipolar undermines the cartilage wall [10].

Outcomes: Short-term benefits in both pain relief and symptom improvement have been documented following chondroplasty [11]. However, chondroplasty has never been shown to alter the natural history of arthritis progression [12]. A recent randomized control trial compared no cartilage intervention, chondroplasty, and MF in patients with full-thickness cartilage lesions [13]. They demonstrated no difference in Knee Injury and Osteoarthritis Outcome Scores (KOOS) at 2-year follow-up. This is reassuring to both patients and surgeons as it demonstrates that the potential short-term benefit of removing loose cartilage flaps has no negative effect on intermediate-term outcomes. Conversely, patients who underwent MF showed deteriorating outcomes at 2 years.

Scillia et al. [14] performed arthroscopic debridement and chondroplasty in 52 players in the National Football League. They reported that over two thirds of players were able to return to play at an average of 8.2 months postoperatively. This was in comparison to players who underwent MF who were more than four times less likely to return to sport than those who had debridement alone.

45.2.2 Microfracture (MF)

Background: Pridie et al. first described subchondral drilling for osteoarthritis in 1957 [15]. This was later modified by Steadman et al. [16] in 1997 to reflect the modern MF with marrow stimulation. MF has become the most commonly used restorative technique for treating cartilage lesions [17]. MF is a relatively inexpensive, single-stage procedure that is technically less challenging than more advanced restorative techniques [18]. However, histologic studies have demonstrated that the defect fills contain less durable fibrocartilage [19]. Scaffold augmentation has been used in recent years in an attempt to improve defect fill and induce hyaline-like cartilage rather than fibrocartilage [20, 21].

Surgical technique: The technique for MF has been described in detail [16]. The cartilage lesion is assessed and debrided back to a stable border circumferentially (Fig. 45.1a, b). The calcified cartilage is then carefully removed from between the

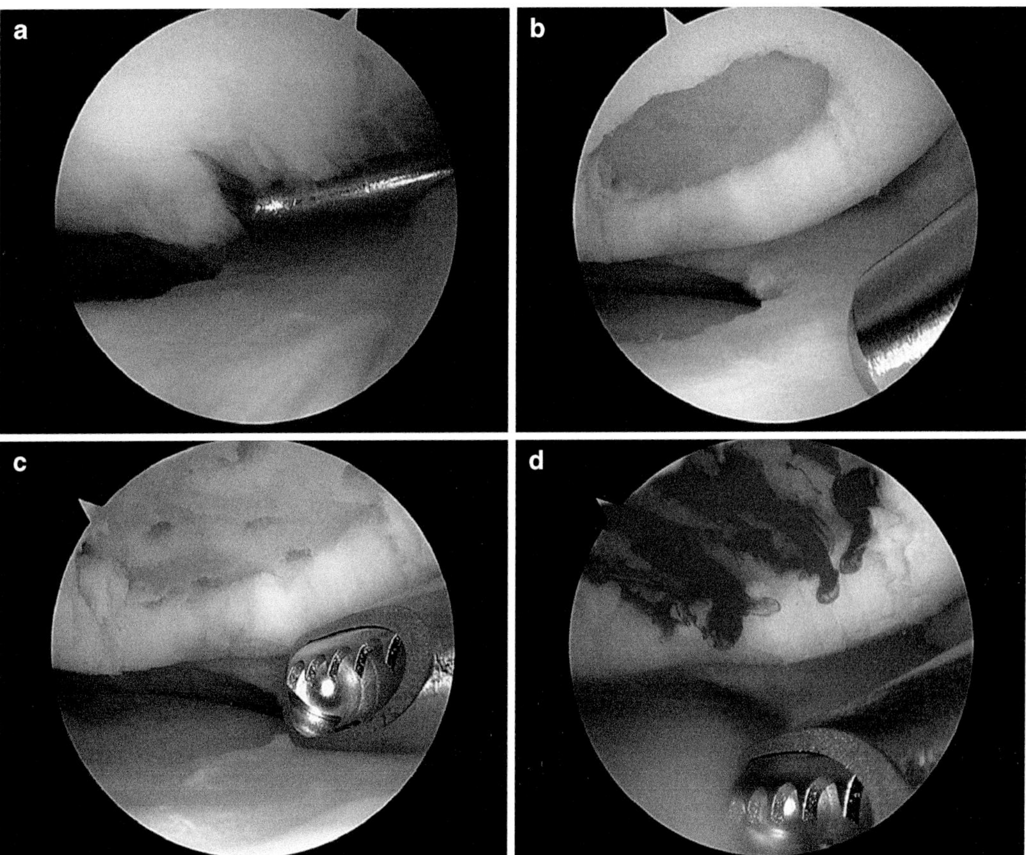

Fig. 45.1 Microfracture. (**a**) Arthroscopic view of a right medial femoral condyle with a 10 × 15 mm full-thickness cartilage lesion. (**b**) Full-thickness cartilage defect after debridement of the calcified cartilage layer with stable vertical borders. (**c**) Microperforations throughout cartilage defect with 3–4 mm of space between each perforation. (**d**) Release of marrow elements following microfracture

deep cartilage and the subchondral bone. Microperforation is then performed using a pick instrument. The perforations begin peripherally and move centrally leaving 3–4 mm bone bridges (Fig. 45.1c). After completion of homogeneous microperforation, the inflow is stopped, and influx of blood and marrow products is confirmed (Fig. 45.1d). If allograft extracellular matrix augmentation is performed, the flow remains off while the particles are applied to the base of the defect.

Outcomes: MF provides the best outcome when performed on small (<2–3 cm^2), full-thickness cartilage lesions. Increased age (over 35–45 years), BMI (>25–30 kg/m^2), and duration of symptoms (>12 months) all lead to worse outcomes [22]. Eighty percent of patients have reported improvement from preoperative pain and function at an average of 11.3 years [23]. MF is also one of few techniques that have been directly studied in football players. Twenty of 21 patients (95%) returned to professional football the following season and continued to play for an average of 5 years (1–13 years) [17]. While these case series have demonstrated promising results, the outcomes of MF in young athletes have been less optimistic in prospective comparative studies [6, 7] with outcomes that deteriorate over time [24]. Long-term outcomes following MF were reported on 63 athletes. While only 14% demonstrated pain and effusions with strenuous activity at 2 years, this increased to over half of patients at final follow-up (average 15 years). In addition, radiographic progression of osteoarthritis had occurred in 40% of knees [25].

Recently, scaffold augmentation of MF has been introduced into clinical practice. A randomized trial compared MF with BST-CarGel scaffold to MF alone [21]. Radiographs at 12 months demonstrated significantly better lesion filling and hyaline-like cartilage signals. However, there was no difference in clinical outcomes as measured by Short Form-36 (SF-36) and the Western Ontario and McMaster Universities Osteoarthritis Index (WOMAC). Animal studies have recently demonstrated increased fill with bone marrow aspirate augmentation [26]. An alternative method for MF augmentation is platelet-rich plasma (PRP) gel [27].

45.2.3 Osteochondral Autograft Transfer (OAT)

Fact Box 2
OAT is best performed for lesions 1–4 cm^2 to reduce the risk of donor site morbidity.

Background: OAT provides immediate restoration of cartilage defects with normal hyaline articular cartilage. The donor tissue is obtained from the healthy host's ipsilateral or contralateral knee in a minimal weight-bearing zone. A single plug can be harvested for a smaller lesion; however, multiple smaller plugs are often required to fill a defect. This process was pioneered by Hangody et al. [28] in the 1990s and is commonly termed mosaicplasty. OAT has the distinct advantage of transferring the bone with each cartilage plug. This allows small defects resulting from an osteochondritis dissecans to be filled during transfer [29]. The main limitation of OAT is defect size. Larger defects make it more difficult to restore the articular surface geometry and also increase donor site morbidity [30]. This technique is best suited for lesions 1–4 cm^2 in size [29].

Surgical technique: The surgical technique for osteochondral autograft transfer has been described [30]. First, the defect size is determined (Fig. 45.2a). The recipient site is then debrided of all non-healthy tissue using a combination of curettes, reamers, and a knife blade down to a healthy subchondral bone. Recipient plugs are obtained from the minimal weight-bearing periphery of the femoral condyles at the level of the patellofemoral joint. The plugs are inserted in succession into the osteochondral defect. A combination of different graft sizes should be used to obtain 90–100% defect fill (Fig. 45.2b). Fibrocartilage is expected to fill any remaining defects and the interstices between the plugs.

Outcomes: The results following OAT are good/excellent in 92% for the femoral condyles, 87% for the tibial plateau, and 74% for the patella and trochlea [29]. Good/excellent results were reported for International Cartilage Repair

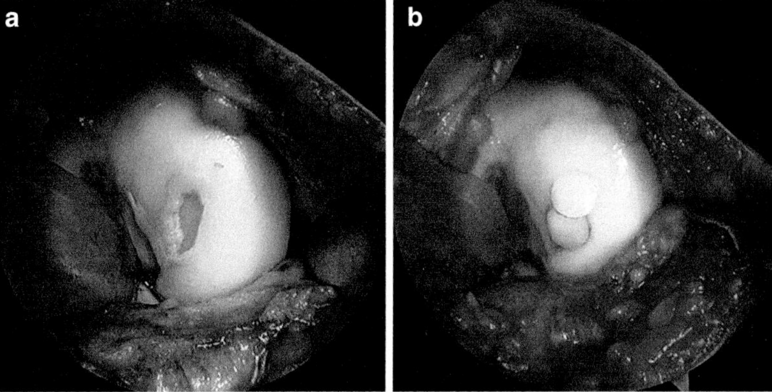

Fig. 45.2 Osteochondral autograft transfer. (**a**) Medial femoral condyle of a right knee with a 5 × 12 mm full-thickness chondral defect observed through a medial parapatellar arthrotomy. (**b**) Right medial femoral condyle with two 7 mm osteochondral autograft plugs after mosaicplasty

Society (ICRS) outcomes (77%) and significant International Knee Documentation Committee (IKDC) subjective scores at 7 years' post-op (71.8) when compared to preoperative scores (34.8) [31]. In a retrospective comparative study, it was shown that patients who underwent OAT had similar SF-36, International Knee Documentation Committee (IKDC), and Knee Outcome Survey activities of daily living scores but significantly higher Marx Activity Rating Scale scores at 2, 3, and 5 years when compared to MF [32]. They attributed these findings to patients modifying their activity levels to one that provides satisfactory knee function and comfort. It was shown that OAT is superior to MF in young active athletes at 3 years' follow-up [33]. A case series of 61 football players was followed for an average of 9.6 years. The International Cartilage Repair Society (ICRS) score was 89% good or excellent with an overall 67% rate of return to the same level of sport. A significantly greater rate of return was observed among elite players (89%) compared to competitive players (62%) [34].

45.2.4 Osteochondral Allograft (OCA) Transplantation

Background: OCA involves transplanting cadaveric tissue to fill cartilage defects. This technique allows for immediate structural restoration of the articular surface and has demonstrated consistent clinical results [35]. OCA has the distinct advantage of filling large bone and cartilage defects with no donor site morbidity. However, to ensure that the articular surface is congruent, donor specimens must be geometrically matched to their recipient. After a match has been identified, the donor tissue undergoes bio-microbial testing for approximately 2 weeks. Ideally, transplantation occurs prior to 28 days to optimize chondrocyte survival [36]. The greatest challenges in OCA cases often relate to timing and logistics for both the surgeon and the patient given the short window of opportunity for transplantation.

Surgical technique: OCA is performed in a similar manner to OAT as discussed above. First the size of the defect is assessed (Fig. 45.3a, b). Commercially available instrumentation is used to remove the damaged cartilage and subchondral bone from the recipient site (Fig. 45.3c). The defect circumference and depth are measured. A donor osteochondral plug is harvested perpendicular to the cartilage surface from the same geographic zone and contoured to the appropriate thickness (Fig. 45.3d). The donor plug is marginally larger in circumference to allow for a compression fit (Fig. 45.3e, f) [37]. Compression screws can be added for additional fixation if there is concern regarding the fragment stability.

Outcomes: Osteochondral allograft transplantation for cartilage and bone defects has shown good long-term survival with 85% survival of femoral grafts and 80% survival for tibial plateau

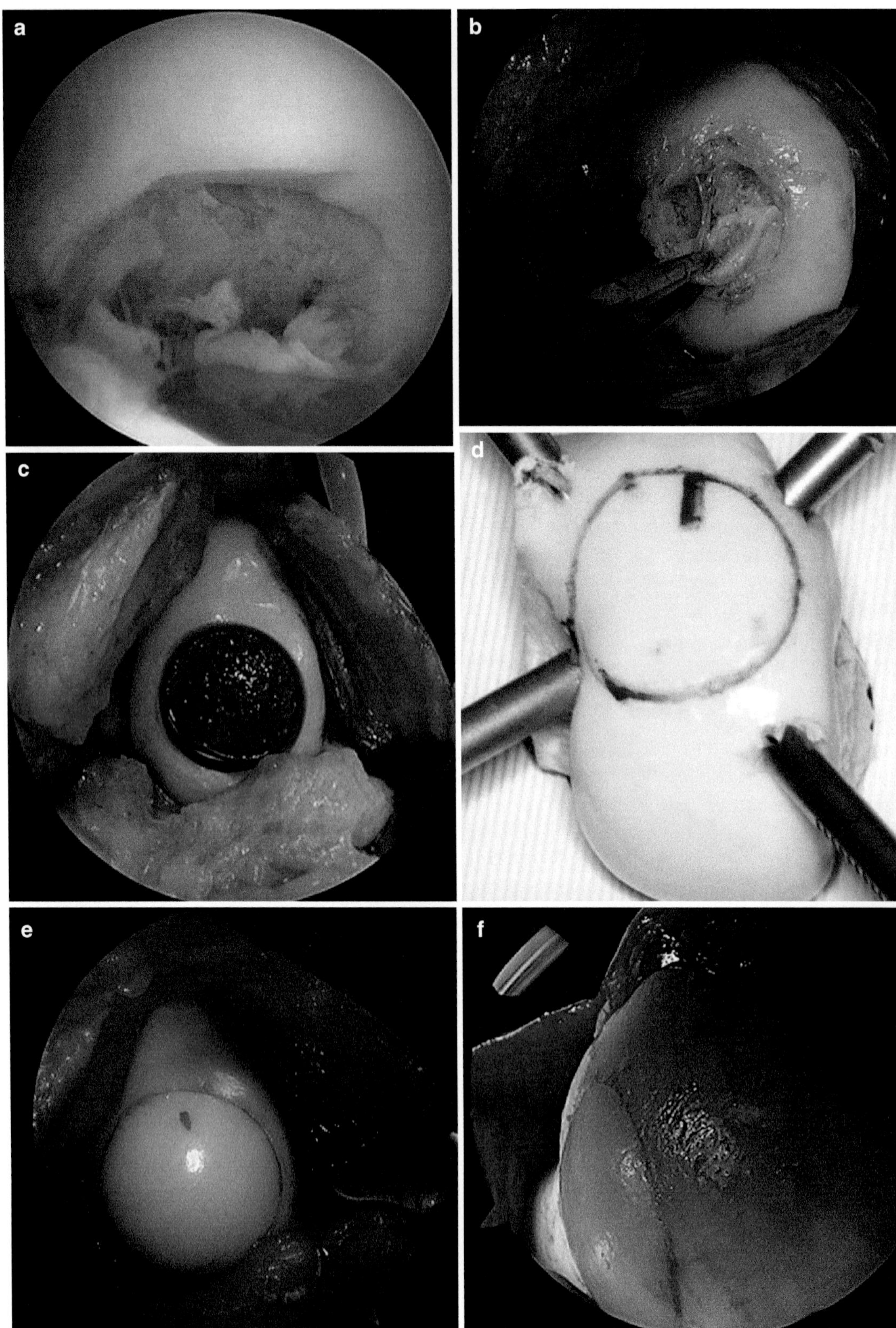
a
b
c
d
e
f

grafts at 10 years' follow-up [38]. OCA provides good to excellent clinical outcomes in 72% of patients [39]. The rate of return to sport following OCA was assessed [7]. Forty-three patients with a mean defect size greater than 7 cm^2 were followed for over 2 years. They demonstrated that 79% of patients were able to return to their preinjury level of activity. No direct comparisons exist for OAT versus OCA in competitive athletes. This is likely because OAT is the preferred procedure for smaller lesions while OCA is performed for larger lesions with concern for donor site morbidity.

45.2.5 Autologous Chondrocyte Implantation (ACI)

Background: In 1994, Peterson and colleagues described autogenous chondrocyte implantation (ACI) as the first cell-based therapy for cartilage restoration [40]. The original two-stage technique implanted cultured autologous chondrocytes under a periosteal sleeve that was sewn over the cartilage defect. The most common complication following this procedure was graft hypertrophy in as many as 36% of patients [41]. Second- and third-generation techniques have since been developed including collagen-covered ACI (C-ACI) and matrix-induced ACI (M-ACI). C-ACI utilizes a collagen membrane instead of a periosteal flap which significantly reduces graft hypertrophy and reoperation [42]. M-ACI utilizes tissue engineering to provide a scaffold for even cell distribution within the graft. In this technique, the chondrocytes are implanted into the collagen membrane matrix in the laboratory and later positioned into the cartilage defect [5]. Histologic analysis at 2 years following ACI has demonstrated 80% hyaline-like cartilage [43]. This is a distinct advantage over MF which produces fibrocartilage [19].

Surgical technique: The surgical technique for ACI has been described in detail [40]. ACI is a two-stage procedure. The first stage allows for a diagnostic arthroscopy to carefully assess the size and depth of the cartilage defect and determine if ACI is indicated (Fig. 45.4a, b). Normal cartilage is then harvested from a minor load-bearing zone such as the upper medial or lateral femoral condyle or the margins of the intercondylar notch. The cartilage (and associated chondrocytes) is then placed in a storage medium and sent to a specialized laboratory for culture proliferation. The patient is scheduled for the second stage in 6–12 weeks after the biopsy. The cartilage defect is identified and debrided back to normal borders. A membrane is sewn to the normal edges around the cartilage defect to provide containment of the chondrocytes which are injected underneath (Fig. 45.4c). The synthetic membrane has decreased hypertrophy rates substantially without compromising fill or integration [42].

Outcomes: The outcomes following ACI have been promising with survivorship of 71% at 10 years and improved function in 75% of patients [44]. Multiple trials have compared ACI to MF demonstrating similar short-term results followed by significantly better functional scores at 2–5 years' follow-up after ACI [45, 46]. Return to sport was reported in a prospective, nonrandomized comparative study of second-generation ACI and MF in patients with grade III/IV cartilage lesions [46]. Both groups had improved IKDC scores when compared to baseline, but the patients who underwent ACI had significantly greater clinical improvement. In addition, patients treated with ACI maintained their 2-year rate of return to sport when assessed again at 5 years' follow-up. This was in contrast to those who underwent MF who demonstrated a decline in sports participation over time. This suggests that intermediate-term clinical improvements

Fig. 45.3 Right medial femoral condyle osteochondral allograft. (**a**) Arthroscopic image of a full-thickness cartilage defect. (**b**) Cartilage defect measuring 20 × 20 mm. (**c**) Recipient site after reamed preparation with 22.5 mm reamer with a stable peripheral rim. (**d**) Size-matched donor graft marked for harvest. (**e**) Post compression fit placement of 22.5 mm allograft plug. (**f**) Lateral view post allograft plug

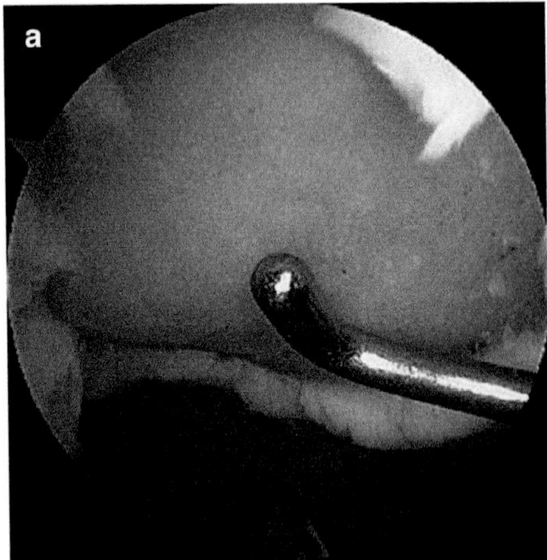

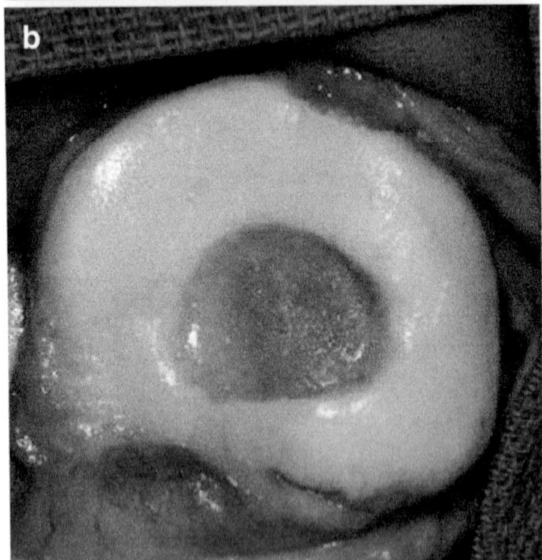

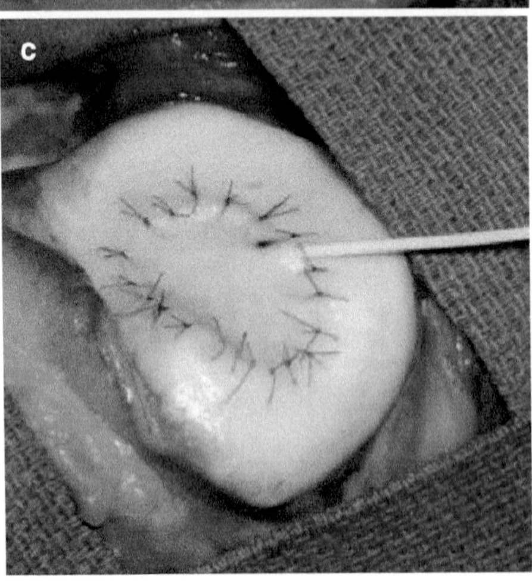

Fig. 45.4 Autologous chondrocyte implantation. (**a**) Arthroscopic view of a patella demonstrating a 20 × 16 mm full-thickness cartilage lesion. (**b**) Cartilage defect after debridement to stable borders. (**c**) Injection of autologous condrocytes under a synthetic membrane flap sewn to the peripheral edge of the cartilage defect

achieved following ACI can be expected to persist through long-term follow-up. These results are supported by Peterson et al. [47] who showed that 50 of 51 patients who had a good to excellent outcome at 2 years had similar outcomes at 5–11 years' follow-up. Return to soccer after ACI in 45 players with full-thickness cartilage lesions showed while only 33% of all players returned, 83% of competitive players return in comparison to only 16% of recreational players. Of those players who returned to soccer, 80% returned at the same skill level and maintained their ability to compete at an average of 52 ± 8 months [48]. They concluded that ACI is successful in highly competitive soccer players with a high rate of return to soccer and durability after return. ACI has also shown improved clinical outcomes when compared to MF in multiple randomized trials.

45.3 Return to Sport Comparison of All Techniques

Fact Box 3

Seventy-six percent of athletes will return to previous level of activity.

OATS = 93%
OCA = 88%
ACI = 82%
MF = 58%

A systematic review for return to sport following cartilage restoration techniques showed an overall return to sport of 73% in 1363 patients [49]. The highest rate of return (91%) and shortest time (7 ± 2 months) to return occurred in patients who underwent OAT. Patients who underwent ACI demonstrated the highest rate (96%) of continued sports participation at 7 years; however, these patients required the longest time to return to sport at an average of 18 ± 4 months. Factors affecting a patient's ability to return to sport included age, duration of preoperative symptoms, level of play, lesion size, and tissue morphology. Since 2009, multiple high-quality studies have been published assessing return to sport. An updated meta-analysis supports the results described above [50]. Forty-four studies met the inclusion criteria with 2549 patients (1756 male, 793 female). The overall rate of return to sport was 76%. The highest rate of return occurred in 93% of patients following OAT, followed by 82% after ACI, and 58% after MF. The fastest time to return to sport was 5.2 ± 1.8 months for OAT, followed by 9.1 ± 2.2 months for MF, 9.6 ± 3.0 months for OCA, and 11.8 ± 3.8 months for ACI ($p < 0.001$). Due to study heterogeneity, a meta-regression was performed to assess factors including patient age, lesion size, and preoperative Tegner scores, none of which were shown to affect the rate of return to sport. This meta-analysis concluded that OAT provided the greatest rate of return to sport and fastest recovery for the treatment of full-thickness cartilage defects in the knee.

45.4 Author's Evidence-Based Approach

The decision-making process for high-demand athletes with full-thickness cartilage defects is complex (Fig. 45.5). Multiple factors should be considered including symptom severity, patient age, career stage, and upcoming competition. In select circumstances where mechanical symptoms are present or expedited return to play is a priority, palliative arthroscopic debridement and chondroplasty can be considered. It is important that the athlete fully understands that chondro-

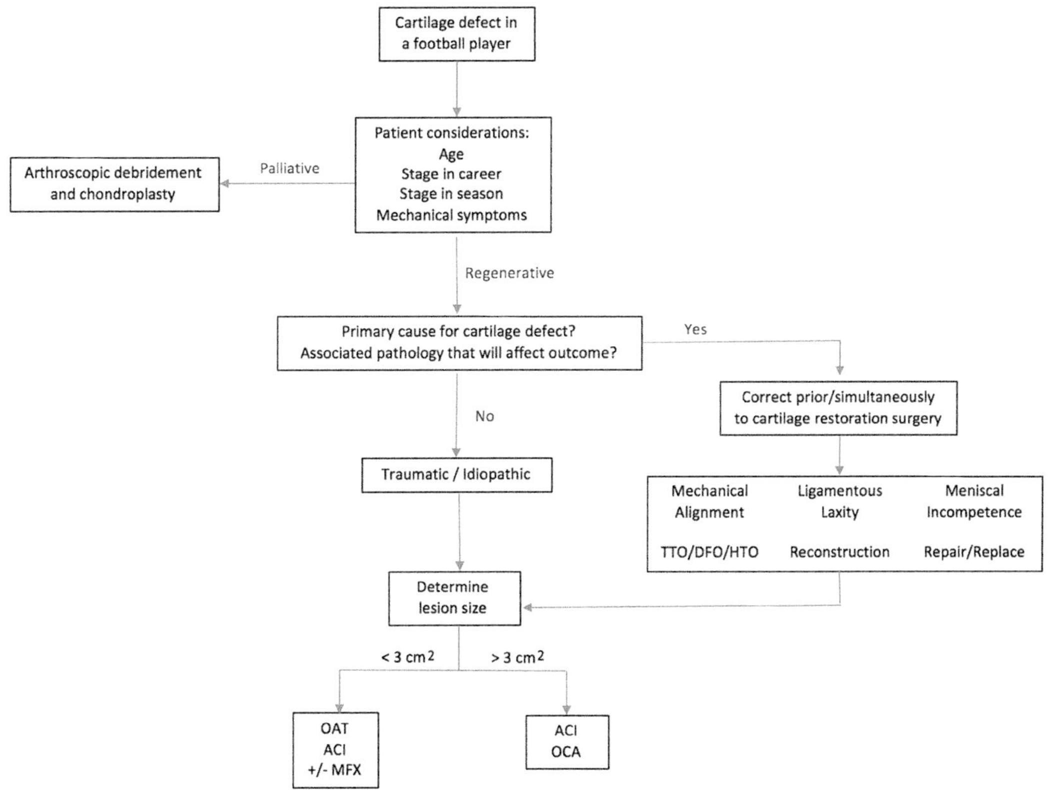

Fig. 45.5 Author's preferred treatment algorithm for symptomatic full-thickness cartilage lesions in the competitive athlete (*TTO* tibial tubercle osteotomy, *DFO* distal femoral osteotomy, *HTO* high tibial osteotomy, *OAT* osteochondral autograft transplantation, *ACI* autologous chondrocyte implantation, *MF* microfracture)

plasty will not provide long-term symptom relief and may place them at risk for further chondral damage before restorative or regenerative options are sought.

Fact Box 4

Always identify and correct the cause for cartilage damage and all concomitant pathology.

If the decision is made to proceed with restorative techniques, the cause for the cartilage lesion and all concomitant pathology should be sought and corrected simultaneously with any cartilage intervention. If the mechanical axis passes through the affected compartment, an osteotomy should be performed to off-load the joint where possible. As a general rule, overcorrection should not be performed in an athlete; therefore, the mechanical axis cutoff is 5 degrees. Ligament deficiencies are corrected with reconstruction, and meniscal pathology is addressed with partial resection, repair, or transplantation.

The size of the cartilage lesion is measured on MRI. Our preferred method of cartilage restoration in high-demand athletes for an isolated lesion measuring less than 3 cm^2 is OAT. Osteochondral autograft provides a durable reconstruction with a demonstrated high rate of return to the same level of sport participation with the shortest recovery time. ACI can be considered for lesions less than 3 cm^2; however, the delayed time to return to sport often excludes this option based on patient preference. MF is no longer performed routinely in young high-demand athletes due to its deteriorating outcomes over time and potential detrimental effect on future regenerative procedures.

If the lesion measures greater than 3 cm^2, the morbidity associated with OAT is considered high. ACI and OCA become the preferred interventions for large chondral defects at our institution with good success. If the lesion involves the patellofemoral joint, ACI is favored. If the subchondral bone is deficient, OCA is favored. Patient preference is also taken into consideration. OCA can provide an expedited return to sport, but allograft availability, patient acceptance of cadaveric tissue, and graft longevity must also be considered. If a patient chooses ACI, we currently practice a second-generation technique using a synthetic membrane in place of a periosteal sleeve. The timeline for return to sport after ACI remains controversial. We restrict competitive sport participation until a minimum of 12 months following the second-stage ACI and OCA.

Take-Home Message

- Each patient must be treated on an individual basis to align their expectations with the potential advantages and disadvantages of the surgical option available.
- Debridement and chondroplasty provide short-term pain relief and rapid return to sport.
- OAT offers the fastest recovery and highest rate of return to sport rate in cartilage restoration surgery (ideal for lesions less than 3 cm^2).
- Larger lesions are amenable to ACI with good outcomes in football players.
- New cell-based and scaffold techniques offer a promising future in cartilage restoration: however, these techniques have not yet been validated in high-demand football players.

Top 5 Evidence-Based References

Steadman JR, Miller BS, Karas SG, Schlegel TF, Briggs KK, Hawkins RJ (2003) The microfracture technique in the treatment of full-thickness chondral lesions of the knee in National Football League players. J Knee Surg 16(2):83–86

Panics G, Hangody LR, Balo E, Vasarhelyi G, Gal T, Hangody L (2012) Osteochondral autograft and mosaicplasty in the football (soccer) athlete. Cartilage 3(1 Suppl):25S–30S

Kon E, Filardo G, Berruto M, Benazzo F, Zanon G, Della Villa S, Marcacci M (2011) Articular cartilage treatment in high-level male soccer players: a prospective comparative study of arthroscopic second-generation autologous chondrocyte implantation versus microfracture. Am J Sports Med 39(12):2549–2557

Mithoefer K, Hambly K, Della Villa S, Silvers H, Mandelbaum BR (2009) Return to sports participation after articular cartilage repair in the knee: scientific evidence. Am J Sports Med 37(1 Suppl):167S–176S

Görtz S, Williams RJ III, Gersoff WK, Bugbee WD (2012) Osteochondral and meniscal allograft transplantation in the football (soccer) player. Cartilage 3(1 Suppl):37S–42S

References

1. Flanigan DC, Harris JD, Trinh TQ, Siston RA, Brophy RH (2010) Prevalence of chondral defects in athletes' knees: a systematic review. Med Sci Sports Exerc 42:1795–1801. https://doi.org/10.1249/MSS.0b013e3181d9eea0
2. Spindler KP, Schils JP, Bergfeld JA, Andrish JT, Weiker GG, Anderson TE, Piraino DW, Richmond BJ, Medendorp SV (1993) Prospective study of osseous, articular, and meniscal lesions in recent anterior cruciate ligament tears by magnetic resonance imaging and arthroscopy. Am J Sports Med 21:551–557
3. Maletius W, Messner K (1996) The effect of partial meniscectomy on the long-term prognosis of knees with localized, severe chondral damage. A twelve- to fifteen-year follow-up. Am J Sports Med 24:258–262
4. Barber FA, Iwasko NG (2006) Treatment of grade III femoral chondral lesions: mechanical chondroplasty versus monopolar radiofrequency probe. Arthroscopy 22:1312–1317. https://doi.org/10.1016/j.arthro.2006.06.008
5. Dewan AK, Gibson MA, Elisseeff JH, Trice ME (2014) Evolution of autologous chondrocyte repair and comparison to other cartilage repair techniques. Biomed Res Int 2014:–272481. https://doi.org/10.1155/2014/272481
6. Gudas R, Gudaite A, Mickevicius T, Masiulis N, Simonaityte R, Cekanauskas E, Skurvydas A (2013) Comparison of osteochondral autologous transplantation, microfracture, or debridement techniques in articular cartilage lesions associated with anterior cruciate ligament injury: a prospective study with a 3-year follow-up. Arthroscopy 29:89–97. https://doi.org/10.1016/j.arthro.2012.06.009
7. Krych AJ, Robertson CM, Williams RJ III, Cartilage Study Group (2012) Return to athletic activity after osteochondral allograft transplantation in the knee. Am J Sports Med 40:1053–1059. https://doi.org/10.1177/0363546511435780
8. Steadman JR, Miller BS, Karas SG, Schlegel TF, Briggs KK, Hawkins RJ (2003) The microfracture technique in the treatment of full-thickness chondral lesions of the knee in National Football League players. J Knee Surg 16:83–86
9. Lee YH, Suzer F, Thermann H (2014) Autologous matrix-induced chondrogenesis in the knee: a review. Cartilage 5:145–153. https://doi.org/10.1177/1947603514529445
10. Drobnic M, Radosavljevic D, Cor A, Brittberg M, Strazar K (2010) Debridement of cartilage lesions before autologous chondrocyte implantation by open or transarthroscopic techniques: a comparative study using post-mortem materials. J Bone Joint Surg Br 92:602–608. https://doi.org/10.1302/0301-620X.92B3.22558
11. Hubbard MJ (1996) Articular debridement versus washout for degeneration of the medial femoral condyle. A five-year study. J Bone Joint Surg Br 78:217–219
12. Grieshober JA, Stanton M, Gambardella R (2016) Debridement of articular cartilage: the natural course. Sports Med Arthrosc 24:56–62. https://doi.org/10.1097/JSA.0000000000000108
13. Rotterud JH, Sivertsen EA, Forssblad M, Engebretsen L, Aroen A (2016) Effect on patient-reported outcomes of debridement or microfracture of concomitant full-thickness cartilage lesions in anterior cruciate ligament-reconstructed knees: a nationwide cohort study from Norway and Sweden of 357 patients with 2-year follow-up. Am J Sports Med 44:337–344. https://doi.org/10.1177/0363546515617468
14. Scillia AJ, Aune KT, Andrachuk JS, Cain EL, Dugas JR, Fleisig GS, Andrews JR (2015) Return to play after chondroplasty of the knee in National Football League athletes. Am J Sports Med 43:663–668. https://doi.org/10.1177/0363546514562752
15. Pridie KH (1959) A method of resurfacing osteoarthritic knee joints. J Bone Joint Surg Br 41B:618–623
16. Steadman JR, Rodkey WG, Briggs KK, Rodrigo JJ (1999) The microfracture technic in the management of complete cartilage defects in the knee joint. Orthopade 28:26–32
17. Mithoefer K, Steadman RJ (2012) Microfracture in football (soccer) players: a case series of professional athletes and systematic review. Cartilage 3:18S–24S. https://doi.org/10.1177/1947603511418960
18. Miller DJ, Smith MV, Matava MJ, Wright RW, Brophy RH (2015) Microfracture and osteochondral autograft transplantation are cost-effective treatments for articular cartilage lesions of the distal femur. Am J Sports Med 43:2175–2181. https://doi.org/10.1177/0363546515591261
19. Nehrer S, Spector M, Minas T (1999) Histologic analysis of tissue after failed cartilage repair procedures. Clin Orthop Relat Res 365:149–162
20. Siclari A, Mascaro G, Gentili C, Kaps C, Cancedda R, Boux E (2014) Cartilage repair in the knee with subchondral drilling augmented with a platelet-rich plasma-immersed polymer-based implant. Knee Surg Sports Traumatol Arthrosc 22:1225–1234. https://doi.org/10.1007/s00167-013-2484-1
21. Stanish WD, McCormack R, Forriol F, Mohtadi N, Pelet S, Desnoyers J, Restrepo A, Shive MS (2013) Novel scaffold-based BST-CarGel treatment results in superior cartilage repair compared with microfracture in a randomized controlled trial. J Bone Joint Surg Am 95:1640–1650. https://doi.org/10.2106/JBJS.L.01345
22. Camp CL, Stuart MJ, Krych AJ (2014) Current concepts of articular cartilage restoration techniques in the knee. Sports Health 6:265–273. https://doi.org/10.1177/1941738113508917

23. Steadman JR, Briggs KK, Rodrigo JJ, Kocher MS, Gill TJ, Rodkey WG (2003) Outcomes of microfracture for traumatic chondral defects of the knee: average 11-year follow-up. Arthroscopy 19:477–484. https://doi.org/10.1053/jars.2003.50112
24. Gudas R, Simonaityte R, Cekanauskas E, Tamosiunas R (2009) A prospective, randomized clinical study of osteochondral autologous transplantation versus microfracture for the treatment of osteochondritis dissecans in the knee joint in children. J Pediatr Orthop 29:741–748. https://doi.org/10.1097/BPO.0b013e3181b8f6c7
25. Gobbi A, Karnatzikos G, Kumar A (2014) Long-term results after microfracture treatment for full-thickness knee chondral lesions in athletes. Knee Surg Sports Traumatol Arthrosc 22:1986–1996. https://doi.org/10.1007/s00167-013-2676-8
26. Fortier LA, Potter HG, Rickey EJ, Schnabel LV, Foo LF, Chong LR, Stokol T, Cheetham J, Nixon AJ (2010) Concentrated bone marrow aspirate improves full-thickness cartilage repair compared with microfracture in the equine model. J Bone Joint Surg Am 92:1927–1937. https://doi.org/10.2106/JBJS.I.01284
27. Milano G, Sanna Passino E, Deriu L, Careddu G, Manunta L, Manunta A, Saccomanno MF, Fabbriciani C (2010) The effect of platelet rich plasma combined with microfractures on the treatment of chondral defects: an experimental study in a sheep model. Osteoarthr Cartil 18:971–980. https://doi.org/10.1016/j.joca.2010.03.013
28. Hangody L, Kish G, Karpati Z, Szerb I, Udvarhelyi I (1997) Arthroscopic autogenous osteochondral mosaicplasty for the treatment of femoral condylar articular defects. A preliminary report. Knee Surg Sports Traumatol Arthrosc 5:262–267. https://doi.org/10.1007/s001670050061
29. Hangody L, Vasarhelyi G, Hangody LR, Sukosd Z, Tibay G, Bartha L, Bodo G (2008) Autologous osteochondral grafting—technique and long-term results. Injury 39(Suppl 1):S32–S39. https://doi.org/10.1016/j.injury.2008.01.041
30. Hangody L, Fules P (2003) Autologous osteochondral mosaicplasty for the treatment of full-thickness defects of weight-bearing joints: ten years of experimental and clinical experience. J Bone Joint Surg Am 85-A(Suppl 2):25–32
31. Marcacci M, Kon E, Delcogliano M, Filardo G, Busacca M, Zaffagnini S (2007) Arthroscopic autologous osteochondral grafting for cartilage defects of the knee: prospective study results at a minimum 7-year follow-up. Am J Sports Med 35:2014–2021. https://doi.org/10.1177/0363546507305455
32. Krych AJ, Harnly HW, Rodeo SA, Williams RJ III (2012) Activity levels are higher after osteochondral autograft transfer mosaicplasty than after microfracture for articular cartilage defects of the knee: a retrospective comparative study. J Bone Joint Surg Am 94:971–978. https://doi.org/10.2106/JBJS.K.00815
33. Gudas R, Kalesinskas RJ, Kimtys V, Stankevicius E, Toliusis V, Bernotavicius G, Smailys A (2005) A prospective randomized clinical study of mosaic osteochondral autologous transplantation versus microfracture for the treatment of osteochondral defects in the knee joint in young athletes. Arthroscopy 21:1066–1075. https://doi.org/10.1016/j.arthro.2005.06.018
34. Panics G, Hangody LR, Balo E, Vasarhelyi G, Gal T, Hangody L (2012) Osteochondral autograft and mosaicplasty in the football (soccer) athlete. Cartilage 3:25S–30S. https://doi.org/10.1177/1947603511408286
35. Meyers MH, Akeson W, Convery FR (1989) Resurfacing of the knee with fresh osteochondral allograft. J Bone Joint Surg Am 71:704–713
36. LaPrade RF, Botker J, Herzog M, Agel J (2009) Refrigerated osteoarticular allografts to treat articular cartilage defects of the femoral condyles. A prospective outcomes study. J Bone Joint Surg Am 91:805–811. https://doi.org/10.2106/JBJS.H.00703
37. Hohmann E, Tetsworth K (2016) Large osteochondral lesions of the femoral condyles: treatment with fresh frozen and irradiated allograft using the mega OATS technique. Knee 23:436–441. https://doi.org/10.1016/j.knee.2016.01.020
38. Gross AE, Shasha N, Aubin P (2005) Long-term followup of the use of fresh osteochondral allografts for posttraumatic knee defects. Clin Orthop Relat Res 435:79–87
39. Emmerson BC, Gortz S, Jamali AA, Chung C, Amiel D, Bugbee WD (2007) Fresh osteochondral allografting in the treatment of osteochondritis dissecans of the femoral condyle. Am J Sports Med 35:907–914. https://doi.org/10.1177/0363546507299932
40. Brittberg M, Lindahl A, Nilsson A, Ohlsson C, Isaksson O, Peterson L (1994) Treatment of deep cartilage defects in the knee with autologous chondrocyte transplantation. N Engl J Med 331:889–895. https://doi.org/10.1056/NEJM199410063311401
41. Niemeyer P, Pestka JM, Kreuz PC, Erggelet C, Schmal H, Suedkamp NP, Steinwachs M (2008) Characteristic complications after autologous chondrocyte implantation for cartilage defects of the knee joint. Am J Sports Med 36:2091–2099. https://doi.org/10.1177/0363546508322131
42. Gomoll AH, Probst C, Farr J, Cole BJ, Minas T (2009) Use of a type I/III bilayer collagen membrane decreases reoperation rates for symptomatic hypertrophy after autologous chondrocyte implantation. Am J Sports Med 37(Suppl 1):20S–23S. https://doi.org/10.1177/0363546509348477
43. Peterson L, Minas T, Brittberg M, Nilsson A, Sjogren-Jansson E, Lindahl A (2000) Two- to 9-year outcome after autologous chondrocyte transplantation of the knee. Clin Orthop Relat Res 374:212–234
44. Minas T, Von Keudell A, Bryant T, Gomoll AH (2014) The John Insall Award: a minimum 10-year outcome study of autologous chondrocyte implantation. Clin Orthop Relat Res 472:41–51. https://doi.org/10.1007/s11999-013-3146-9
45. Basad E, Ishaque B, Bachmann G, Sturz H, Steinmeyer J (2010) Matrix-induced autologous

chondrocyte implantation versus microfracture in the treatment of cartilage defects of the knee: a 2-year randomised study. Knee Surg Sports Traumatol Arthrosc 18:519–527. https://doi.org/10.1007/s00167-009-1028-1

46. Kon E, Gobbi A, Filardo G, Delcogliano M, Zaffagnini S, Marcacci M (2009) Arthroscopic second-generation autologous chondrocyte implantation compared with microfracture for chondral lesions of the knee: prospective nonrandomized study at 5 years. Am J Sports Med 37:33–41. https://doi.org/10.1177/0363546508323256
47. Peterson L, Brittberg M, Kiviranta I, Akerlund EL, Lindahl A (2002) Autologous chondrocyte transplantation. Biomechanics and long-term durability. Am J Sports Med 30:2–12
48. Mithofer K, Peterson L, Mandelbaum BR, Minas T (2005) Articular cartilage repair in soccer players with autologous chondrocyte transplantation: functional outcome and return to competition. Am J Sports Med 33:1639–1646. https://doi.org/10.1177/0363546505275647
49. Mithoefer K, Hambly K, Della Villa S, Silvers H, Mandelbaum BR (2009) Return to sports participation after articular cartilage repair in the knee: scientific evidence. Am J Sports Med 37(Suppl 1):167S–176S. https://doi.org/10.1177/0363546509351650
50. Krych AJ, Pareek A, King AH, Johnson NR, Stuart MJ, Williams RJ III (2016) Return to sport after the surgical management of articular cartilage lesions in the knee: a meta-analysis. Knee Surg Sports Traumatol Arthrosc. https://doi.org/10.1007/s00167-016-4262-3

46 Advanced Techniques of Cartilage Repair in Football Players

Andrea Sessa, Francesco Perdisa, Giuseppe Filardo, and Elizaveta Kon

Contents

A. Sessa (✉) • F. Perdisa • G. Filardo
I Clinic – Nano-Biotechnology Lab,
Rizzoli Orthopedic Institute,
Via di Barbiano n. 1/10, 40136 Bologna, Italy
e-mail: a.sessa86@gmail.com

E. Kon
Department of Biomedical Sciences – Humanitas Clinical and Research Center, Knee Joint Reconstruction Center - 3rd Orthopaedic Division, Humanitas Clinical Institute, Humanitas University, 20089 Rozzano, Milan, Italy

46.1 Introduction

Among all sports disciplines, soccer is the most popular worldwide, with more than 300 million players overall, 200,000 of them being professional/elite athletes [1–3]. As it is a high-speed contact activity, with marked intensity of joint impact and torsional loading [4], soccer is estimated to be responsible for the majority of athletic injuries in Europe [5]. Most soccer injuries occur in the lower extremities (52–95%) and most frequently at knee (16–46%) and ankle (17–40%) joints [6–10]. This forceful and repetitive mechanical stress is also associated with a growing incidence of articular cartilage damage of the knee [11–14].

Traumatic or microtraumatic injury of the articular cartilage and the underlying subchondral bone are frequent conditions in athletes, as reported by a systematic review of the literature performed by Flanigan et al. [11]. They estimated the presence of asymptomatic cartilaginous defects in over 50% of athletes, with a 36% prevalence of full-thickness injuries. These kinds of defect often result in debilitating symptoms, and, since articular cartilage lacks spontaneous self-repair capacity [15–17], if untreated, they can lead to joint degeneration, with an increased risk of developing osteoarthritis (OA) in the long term compared with the

V. Musahl et al. (eds.), *Return to Play in Football*, https://doi.org/10.1007/978-3-662-55713-6_46

general population [11, 18]. Indeed, OA has been reported as the major chronic pathology suffered by professional soccer players [19], eventually leading to an early career ending and to the problem of young patients with old joints [17, 20–22].

All these reasons make it mandatory to address defects of the articular surface in order to restore the correct knee function and allow an early and durable return to sport activity. Young patients with "recent injuries" are factors positively correlated with the clinical outcome of cartilage lesions. Unfortunately, cartilage defects often present a gradual and degenerative onset, so that physicians and surgeons face degenerative lesions secondary to overuse or to progressive injuries. Nonetheless, the high motivation and compliance of this kind of patients may still lead to satisfactory clinical results with the help of recent techniques developed to restore an optimal articular surface (Table 46.1).

The aim of this chapter is to resume the evidence regarding the most advanced treatments for cartilage injuries in high-level athletes, with a specific focus on contact sports such as soccer.

Table 46.1 Factors most commonly associated with better outcomes and with recovery time and level of sport activity after cartilage treatment

Factors	Best outcomes
Age	<25 years
Symptoms duration	<12 months
Sport level	Competitive athletes
Associated procedures	Not influential
Surgical technique	Mini-invasive technique
Rehabilitation	"Step-based" rather than "time-based" rehabilitation protocol

46.2 Principles of Treatment of Cartilage Lesions in Athletes

The treatment of articular cartilage lesions is mainly based on the size of the chondral lesion and any possible bone involvement [23]. Generally, the management of these defects in athletes is complex and multifactorial [24] involving a conservative approach and, once failed, surgical treatments and rehabilitation programs. Briefly, nonsurgical treatments include chondroprotective pharmacotherapy, nonsteroidal anti-inflammatory medication, physiotherapy, and hydrotherapy, which are especially suitable for early stages [22]. However, these are symptomatic and nondisease-modifying approaches, which offer mainly a temporary benefit.

The surgical indication involves a symptomatic full-thickness cartilage defect, with or without involvement of subchondral bone (ICRS grades III–IV), refractory to conservative treatments [23]. Treatment options range from reparative techniques, such as microfractures and drilling; to reconstructive ones, including mosaicplasty, osteochondral autograft transplantation (OAT), and fresh allograft transplantation; and to the more recent regenerative techniques, like autologous chondrocyte implantation (ACI) and/or matrix-induced autologous chondrocyte transplantation (MACT). Finally, one-step techniques like cell-free scaffolds exploiting the self-regenerative potential of damaged tissues have recently been proposed. However, although the literature reports good or excellent results for most athletes with satisfactory rate of return to sports [13, 14, 24–26], no consensus on the best technique has been reached so far, with each procedure carrying its own indications and limitations (Table 46.2).

Table 46.2 Main surgical indications and characteristics of the most studied surgical techniques in athletes

	Microfractures	Mosaicplasty	Allografts	ACI/MACT
Size	<2 cm^2		>2 cm^2	
Depth	Chondral	Osteochondral	Osteochondral	Chondral
Time to return to sport	9 months	7 months	10 months	16 months
Return to sport	75%	89%	88%	84–86%[a]
Return to the same sport level	69%	70%	79%	71–75%[a]

[a]Range of different ACI techniques

46.3 Reparative and Reconstructive Techniques

Microfractures take advantage of the creation of small channels through subchondral bone, allowing progenitor cells and growth factors to migrate from bone marrow into the previously prepared chondral lesion to form a clot, which then differentiate into fibrocartilaginous tissue [27]. It is a relatively cheap mini-invasive technique that can be performed arthroscopically, which allows a relatively short rehabilitation time and early return to sport. For this reason, microfractures are widely used in the common clinical practice as first-line treatment for cartilage injuries in athletic patients [28], and overall, they remain the most widely used surgical approach to treat cartilage lesions [29]. A significant improvement from the preoperative level to early follow-up has been documented, with comparable clinical outcomes between competitive and recreational athletes [30]. However, Gobbi et al. [31] showed that good early clinical results gradually deteriorated at long-term follow-up in a group of 61 athletes evaluated for an average of 15.1 years.

Among reconstructive techniques, mosaicplasty is the most widely investigated. It involves the transplantation of autologous osteochondral cylinders harvested from a nonbearing area of the same knee and press-fit implants into the defect area [32]. Good clinical results have been reported to be stable up to long-term follow-up. Moreover, the rationale of transferring healthy hyaline cartilage directly into the defect, taking advantage of more rapid bone to bone healing in the deeper part of the graft, makes it suitable for an early return to sport [33–36]. Hangody, the main developer of this procedure [22], evaluated the clinical outcomes in 61 elite football players at 2–17 years of follow-up and found 89% good and excellent results. Sixty-seven percent of all players returned to the same level of sport: this ratio was higher in elite players (89%) rather than competitive ones (62%). Moreover, an early return to competition was reported, after a mean of 4.5 months from surgery. This, together with experiences from other authors [37–39], confirmed mosaicplasty to be a suitable option for the treatment of articular cartilage defects in a high-demanding population. On the other hand, a certain degree of morbidity in the donor site remains inevitable, and this issue strongly limits the indication of this technique for the treatment of defects not exceeding 2–3 cm^2, as emphasized by long-term studies [37, 38].

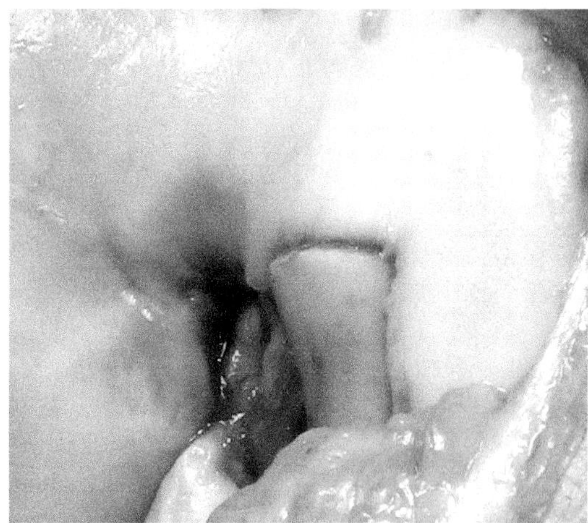

Fig. 46.1 Implantation of osteochondral allograft

A different reconstructive option sharing some characteristic with mosaicplasty involves the use of osteochondral allografts (Fig. 46.1), which on the other hand allow to overcome the limitation of donor site morbidity for the treatment of large lesions. Among different storage conditions, the use of fresh graft is recommended in order to better preserve chondrocyte viability [40]. This procedure can be performed by freehand techniques or using dedicated instruments for the press-fit transfer of appropriately sized osteochondral cylinders [41]. The outcome of this procedure has been investigated also among athletes. Krych et al. [42] observed positive findings in 43 athletes treated with fresh-stored osteochondral allograft transplantation at 2.5-year of follow-up: 79% recovered to unrestricted activity at the same level as before symptoms onset, with a mean time to return to sport of 9.6 ± 3.0 months. Risk factors for not returning to sport included age ≥25 years and preoperative duration of symptoms ≥12 months, which are rather common in soccer players presenting chondral problems. Therefore, together with other evidences showing less satisfactory results [43, 44], these findings highlight some limitations for the treatment of an athletic population and support the need for other techniques able to restore the articular surface.

46.4 Regenerative Techniques

The abovementioned limitations of the "traditional" procedures have powered, in the past two decades, the research on "regenerative" techniques, aiming at improving tissue quality, and offer optimal outcomes with more stable to long-term results [45].

46.4.1 Autologous Chondrocyte Implantation (ACI)

ACI procedure involves the injection of a cell suspension of chondrocytes, previously harvested from the same knee and culture-expanded, under a periosteal flap taken from the ipsilateral tibia and sutured to cover the defect [46]. This technique was introduced over two decades ago and produced positive results in isolated lesions of the femoral condyles, even in case of large size defects, becoming one of the most documented regenerative techniques for the surgical treatment of articular cartilage defects [46]. Recent literature showed stable and satisfactory results in long-term follow-up [47, 48]. Concerning the results obtained for the treatment of athletes, Mithoefer et al. [49] evaluated at 41 months of follow-up 45 young (26 years mean age) soccer players treated with ACI. Besides an overall 72% of good or optimal results, return to soccer was achieved in only 33% of cases, at a mean of 18 months postsurgery. However, high-level players had both higher rate of return (83%) and shorter recovery time (14 months). Conversely, only 16% of amateur athletes returned to practice sports. These findings highlight the importance of pre-injury level of activity, which is a key prognostic factor probably due to both preconditioning and personal motivation. Mithoefer et al. [50] later performed a study on 20 teenager athletes at 47-month follow-up, showing a return to sport rate of 96%, with 60% to a level equal or even higher than before the onset of symptoms. The outcomes were positively correlated with shorter duration (<12 months) of preoperative symptoms and absence of previous surgical treatments. Finally, the intense participation in sporting activities was related to better outcomes, as it was also reported by other authors. Kreuz et al. evaluated 118 athletes based on their level of sport activity and found that those who had higher activity were more likely to be back to their pre-injury level after ACI surgery [51]. The importance of activity level was confirmed also by Van Assche et al. [52], who compared the results obtained in 33 patients treated with ACI, versus 34 treated with microfractures at 24 months of follow-up. They did not find any significant intergroup difference, but they observed better results in patients more compliant to the rehabilitation protocol and in those with higher level of physical activity. These promising yet not optimal results, obtained using ACI, highlight how important it is to identify the ideal patient who can obtain the best benefit using this regenerative procedure. In fact, satisfactory results were observed in young and more active patients, all factor that should be considered when choosing the indication for treatment. However, despite the good results obtained by ACI technique in active patients, this surgical approach remains linked to relatively high complication and reoperation rates, mainly due to hypertrophy of the periosteal graft and the need for arthrotomy [48]. This, together with the progresses obtained in bioengineering, has led to the development of new regenerative procedures.

46.4.2 Second-Generation Autologous Chondrocyte Implantation

These procedures were introduced in 1998, as an evolution of the ACI procedure that was improved using bioengineered matrixes as a scaffold to support the growth of chondrocytes previously expanded in culture (matrix-assisted chondrocyte

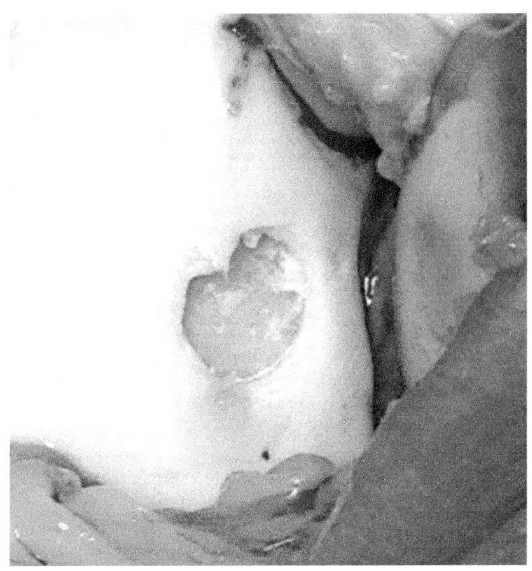

Fig. 46.2 View of the osteochondral lesion before the treatment

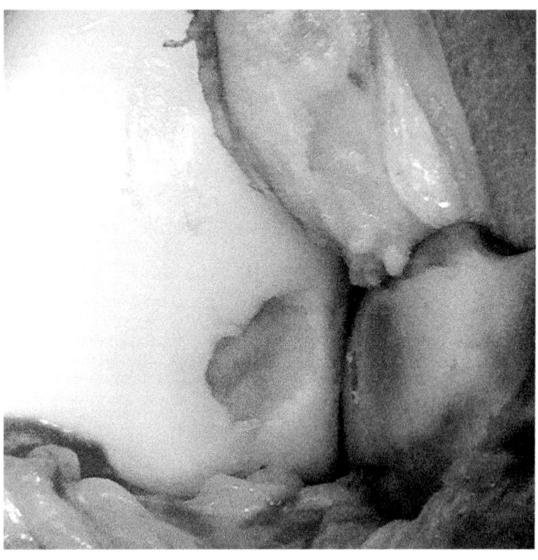

Fig. 46.3 Osteochondral lesion after hyalograft C implantation

transplantation, MACT) [53]. Different biomaterials have been used, but collagen type I/III or hyaluronic acid matrixes were most commonly reported in the clinical setting [45]. The easy handling of bioengineered materials compared to liquid cultures has reduced the procedure invasiveness, and some of these implants can be performed by arthroscopy [54].

Fact Box 1

The use of bioengineered biomaterials seeded with cultured chondrocytes produced excellent and long-lasting clinical results, probably thanks to the hyaline-like characteristics of the regenerated tissue. Unfortunately, the use of cell-based techniques is plagued by issues in terms of costs and the need for two surgical interventions related to procedures of ex vivo processing.

Literature findings showed excellent outcomes for MACT techniques, proven to be durable at to long-term evaluations. Various applications have been investigated, from patellofemoral injuries to degenerative or cartilage defects in arthritic knees [55, 56], and some studies looked specifically at their use in a sport-active population. Filardo et al. [57] evaluated 62 patients at a mean follow-up of 84 months after implantation of hyaluronic acid-based MACT (Hyalograft C®, Fidia, Padova, Italy) for lesions located at the femoral condyles (Figs. 46.2 and 46.3). The significant clinical improvement was stable over time, and better results were obtained in young male patients. A significant positive correlation was also found with the level of physical activity before the accident. Subsequently, Kon et al. published a study on 41 professional or semiprofessional football players evaluated at a mean follow-up of 7.5 years, where results obtained using MACT were compared to those obtained with microfractures (21 and 20 patients, respectively) [58]. Both groups significantly improved and no difference was observed at 24 months of follow-up. However, at the final evaluation microfractures showed a significant deterioration of the results, compared to the stable outcomes of the MACT group. While 80% of patients in the microfractures group returned to their prior activity level at a mean of 8 months after surgery, 86% of those treated with MACT resumed sport activity at a mean of 12.5 months. Thus, this study confirms that microfractures allow a faster but less durable recovery, while MACT requires more time for patient to return to previous activities, but, at the same time, it provides better quality tissue and longer-lasting results. Finally, Pestka et al. [59] recently performed a retrospective study on the return to sport after MACT. Among 130 patients evaluated, 73.1% was able to resume sports activities, independently from lesion site and size. However, duration and frequency of the activity significantly decreased compared to pre-injury: in detail, intense high-impact sports were mostly abandoned in favor of less durable and intense ones, and only 40% of the patients managed to maintain the previous level of activity.

Among the wide literature available on MACT, specific studies are available focusing on the effects of postoperative rehabilitation variables. Ebert et al. tested an accelerated rehabilitation protocol, demonstrating the ability to speed up the recovery of normal walking, in association with a reduction in pain and complications compared to standard rehabilitation protocols [60]. Della Villa et al. also applied an intensive rehabilitation after MACT on 31 athletes, optimizing the results without compromising the integrity of the graft but, at the same time, decreasing complications and leading to a more rapid and efficient recovery, both compared to a control study group and to literature findings: 81% of the patients was back to the previous sports activity within 12 months [61].

The use of bioengineered biomaterials with chondrocytes has shown to ensure excellent long-lasting clinical results, probably thanks to the hyaline-like characteristics of the regenerated tissue [14]. Unfortunately, the use of cell-based techniques is plagued by issues in terms of costs and need for two surgical interventions related to procedures of ex vivo processing [45]; thus, researchers have focused their efforts on the development of alternative solutions, in order to overcome practical, economic, and legislative problems related to cell manipulation.

46.4.3 Acellular Scaffolds

Some biomaterials have shown the ability to promote tissue regeneration by stimulating the self-regenerative potential of the tissue itself. These scaffolds can be used as a "one-step" procedure, since they do not need any supplementation with cells, containing costs and problems due to cell manipulation and double surgical procedure. Several scaffolds were tested at preclinical level, but the use in the clinical practice has been reported for only a few of these [45].

Fact Box 2
The use of cell-free osteochondral scaffold is emerging as possible treatment options. Results are still not definitive, but promising outcomes have been shown in active and young patients, suggesting that this technique may represent an alternative treatment of carefully selected cases in high-demanding population with limited surgical options. Time to return to sport remains a concern.

The AMIC (Autologous Matrix-Induced Chondrogenesis) technique applies a type I/III collagen-based scaffold for the treatment of chondral and osteochondral lesions in young patients, with promising results at short- to medium-term follow-up [62, 63]. Unfortunately, there is still lack of evidence regarding the outcomes offered for the treatment of this kind of lesions in athletic patients. The latest evolution of this surgical approach provides the association with platelet-rich plasma or concentrated autologous bone marrow to increase its regenerative potential, but the results are still preliminary and in neither case there is any evidence on outcomes in the sport population [63].

Among cell-free chondral scaffolds, the growing awareness on the role of subchondral bone in the pathogenesis of joint degenerative processes has led to the development of biphasic constructs, designed to reproduce the different biological and functional characteristics of bone and cartilage tissues. In particular, this strategy plays an important role in the treatment of large lesions [64]. MaioRegen™ (Fin-Ceramica, Faenza, Italy) is a nanostructured scaffold composed of three layers with different percentages of type I

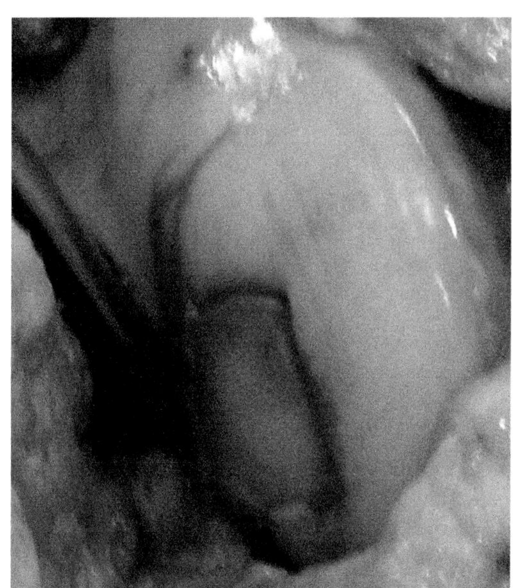

Fig. 46.4 Implant of a cell-free osteochondral scaffold

collagen and hydroxyapatite (Fig. 46.4). After promising preliminary results, positive results have been confirmed on 27 patients up to mid-term follow-up [65], with a satisfactory recovery of their activity level, even if this remained significantly lower than the level before the injury. The clinical efficacy of this approach has also been confirmed in different groups of patients, mostly active, afflicted by complex and/or large-sized lesions [66]. Even if controversial issues have been raised regarding the quality of the regenerated tissue [67], the procedure has been widely used. Besides isolated case reports on active patients, who experienced significant improvement of the clinical scores at short-term follow-ups [68, 69], no literature is available about the rate or the level of return to sports. However, the best overall results were observed in active and young patients [65], suggesting that this technique could represent a viable option for the treatment of selected cases in athletes patients.

Two other bilayer devices documented in clinical literature are TruFit® (Smith & Nephew, Andover, MA), a bilayer scaffold made of a porous polymer PLGA-Ca-sulfate [44, 45], and Agili-C (CartiHeal 2009 Ltd., Israel), made of aragonite in crystalline form with hyaluronic acid on the top layer. Whereas the first device produced mainly unsatisfactory results and it is no longer available, only a case report has been published so far on the second one, reporting on a 37-year-old patient who returned to sports activity within the 24 months of follow-up [64].

Finally, mesenchymal stem cells are gaining increasing attention for the treatment of cartilage lesions, but also in this case, results are still preliminary. Fu et al. reported optimal results at 7.5 years in a lateral trochlea lesion treated with patellar realignment, plus periosteum-covered PBSCs implantation in a kick boxer [70]. While promising results are suggested for cell-free scaffold or for approaches taking advantage of the regenerative potential of concentrated mesenchymal stem cells, more data are needed to prove their outcomes, in particular their ability to restore an optimal articular surface able to allow high-level athletes to return to sport.

Conclusion

High-level athletes are at high risk of knee injuries, ranging from meniscal and ligament tears to damage of the articular surface. An effective surgical treatment should be aimed not only at repairing the defect but also at restoring the correct biomechanics of the knee, by addressing all related comorbidities, including instabilities and meniscal lesions.

Various techniques proposed over the years for the treatment of articular cartilage lesions have shown the ability to successfully return injured athletes back to sports activity, provided that surgery is followed by an early and intensive rehabilitation protocol, tailored on both patient and lesion characteristics. In addition, the appropriate technique must be carefully considered, since demands and timing for rehabilitation can vary accordingly. The indication for surgical treatment of cartilage defects in athletes requires a careful consideration of all these factors.

Regenerative options claim for longer durability of the outcomes over time, but usually require longer time before complete recovery due to the tissue maturation time. Conversely, traditional techniques allow earlier recovery of the activity, but present less predictable outcomes. Thus, the indication should always be carefully evaluated and discussed with the patients, in order to fit their expectations and career perspectives. Finally, since literature shows only limited superiority of few techniques among others, the background and experience of the surgeon with the different procedures still remain central in the decision-making process.

Take-Home Message

The treatment of articular cartilage lesions is mainly based on the size of the chondral lesion defect and on the possible involvement of the subchondral bone. Generally, the management of these defects in athletic patients is complex and multifactorial, ranging from conservative approach to surgical treatments and rehabilitation programs.

An effective surgical treatment should be aimed not only at repairing the defect but also at restoring the correct biomechanics of the knee, by addressing all related comorbidities, including alignment, instabilities, and meniscal lesions.

Traditional techniques, such as microfractures, allow an earlier recovery of the activity, but present less predictable long-term outcomes, while regenerative options claim for longer durability of the results over time, but usually require longer time before complete recovery due to the longer tissue maturation process.

Regardless of the selected surgical approach, an early and intensive rehabilitation program, tailored both on the patient and lesions characteristics, according to the technique performed, is key to reach the best outcomes.

Top 5 Evidence Based References

Della Villa S, Kon E, Filardo G, Ricci M, Vincentelli F, Delcogliano M, Marcacci M (2010) Does intensive rehabilitation permit early return to sport without compromising the clinical outcome after arthroscopic autologous chondrocyte implantation in highly competitive athletes? Am J Sports Med 38(1):68–77

Kon E, Filardo G, Berruto M, Benazzo F, Zanon G, Della Villa S, Marcacci M (2011) Articular cartilage treatment in high-level male soccer players: a prospective comparative study of arthroscopic second-generation autologous chondrocyte implantation versus microfracture. Am J Sports Med 39(12):2549–2557

Mithöfer K, Peterson L, Mandelbaum BR, Minas T (2005) Articular cartilage repair in soccer players with autologous chondrocyte transplantation: functional outcome and return to competition. Am J Sports Med 33(11):1639–1646

Mundi R, Bedi A, Chow L, Crouch S, Simunovic N, SibilskyEnselman E, Ayeni OR (2016) Cartilage restoration of the knee: a systematic review and meta-analysis of level 1 studies. Am J Sports Med 44(7):1888–1895

Steinwachs MR, Engebretsen L, Brophy RH (2012) Scientific evidence base for cartilage injury and repair in the athlete. Cartilage 3(1 Suppl):11S–17S

References

1. Engström B, Johansson C, Törnkvist H (1991) Soccer injuries among elite female players. Am J Sports Med 19(4):372–375
2. Junge A, Dvorak J (2004) Soccer injuries: a review on incidence and prevention. Sports Med 34(13):929–938
3. Mithoefer K, Peterson L, Saris D, Mandelbaum B, Dvorák J (2012) Special issue on articular cartilage injury in the football (soccer) player. Cartilage 3(1 Suppl):4S–5S
4. Neyret P, Donell ST, DeJour D, DeJour H (1993) Partial meniscectomy and anterior cruciate ligament rupture in soccer players. A study with a minimum 20-year followup. Am J Sports Med 21(3):455–460
5. Nielsen AB, Yde J (1989) Epidemiology and traumatology of injuries in soccer. Am J Sports Med 17(6):803–807
6. Giza E, Mithöfer K, Farrell L, Zarins B, Gill T (2005) Injuries in women's professional soccer. Br J Sports Med 39(4):212–216. discussion 212–6
7. Maehlum S, Daljord OA (1984) Football injuries in Oslo: a one-year study. Br J Sports Med 18(3):186–190
8. Morgan BE, Oberlander MA (2001) An examination of injuries in major league soccer. The inaugural season. Am J Sports Med 29(4):426–430
9. Poulsen TD, Freund KG, Madsen F, Sandvej K (1991) Injuries in high-skilled and low-skilled soccer: a prospective study. Br J Sports Med 25(3):151–153
10. Roaas A, Nilsson S (1979) Major injuries in Norwegian football. Br J Sports Med 13(1):3–5
11. Flanigan DC, Harris JD, Trinh TQ, Siston RA, Brophy RH (2010) Prevalence of chondral defects in athletes' knees: a systematic review. Med Sci Sports Exerc 42(10):1795–1801
12. Honnas CM, Liskey CC, Meagher DM, Brown D, Luck EE (1990) Malignant melanoma in the foot of a horse. J Am Vet Med Assoc 197(6):756–758
13. Mithoefer K, Steadman RJ (2012) Microfracture in football (soccer) players: a case series of professional athletes and systematic review. Cartilage 3(1Suppl):18S–24S

14. Mithoefer K, Hambly K, Della Villa S, Silvers H, Mandelbaum BR (2009) Return to sports participation after articular cartilage repair in the knee: scientific evidence. Am J Sports Med 37(Suppl 1):167S–176S
15. Buckwalter JA (1998) Articular cartilage: injuries and potential for healing. J Orthop Sports Phys Ther 28(4):192–202
16. McAdams TR, Mithoefer K, Scopp JM, Mandelbaum BR (2010) Articular cartilage injury in athletes. Cartilage 1(3):165–179
17. Steinwachs MR, Engebretsen L, Brophy RH (2012) Scientific evidence base for cartilage injury and repair in the athlete. Cartilage 3(1 Suppl):11S–17S
18. Kujala UM, Kettunen J, Paananen H, Aalto T, Battié MC, Impivaara O, Videman T, Sarna S (1995) Knee osteoarthritis in former runners, soccer players, weight lifters, and shooters. Arthritis Rheum 38(4):539–546
19. Roos H (1998) Are there long-term sequelae from soccer? Clin Sports Med 17(4):819–831. viii
20. Drawer S, Fuller CW (2001) Propensity for osteoarthritis and lower limb joint pain in retired professional soccer players. Br J Sports Med 35(6):402–408
21. Engström B, Forssblad M, Johansson C, Törnkvist H (1990) Does a major knee injury definitely sideline an elite soccer player? Am J Sports Med 18(1):101–105
22. Pánics G, Hangody LR, Baló E, Vásárhelyi G, Gál T, Hangody L (2012) Osteochondral autograft and mosaicplasty in the football (soccer) athlete. Cartilage 3(1 Suppl):25S–30S
23. Bekkers JE, Inklaar M, Saris DB (2009) Treatment selection in articular cartilage lesions of the knee: a systematic review. Am J Sports Med 37(Suppl 1):148S–155S
24. Hambly K, Silvers HJ, Steinwachs M (2012) Rehabilitation after articular cartilage repair of the knee in the football (soccer) player. Cartilage 3(1 Suppl):50S–56S
25. Harris JD, Brophy RH, Siston RA, Flanigan DC (2010) Treatment of chondral defects in the athlete's knee. Arthroscopy 26(6):841–852
26. Mithoefer K, Della Villa S (2012) Return to sports after articular cartilage repair in the football (soccer) player. Cartilage 3(1 Suppl):57S–62S
27. Steadman JR, Rodkey WG, Rodrigo JJ (2001) Microfracture: surgical technique and rehabilitation to treat chondral defects. Clin Orthop Relat Res 391(Suppl):S362–S369
28. Mithoefer K, Williams RJ III, Warren RF, Potter HG, Spock CR, Jones EC, Wickiewicz TL, Marx RG (2005) The microfracture technique for the treatment of articular cartilage lesions in the knee. A prospective cohort study. J Bone Joint Surg Am 87(9):1911–1920
29. Brophy RH, Rodeo SA, Barnes RP, Powell JW, Warren RF (2009) Knee articular cartilage injuries in the National Football League: epidemiology and treatment approach by team physicians. J Knee Surg 22(4):331–338
30. Blevins FT, Steadman JR, Rodrigo JJ, Silliman J (1998) Treatment of articular cartilage defects in athletes: an analysis of functional outcome and lesion appearance. Orthopedics 21(7):761–767. discussion 767–8
31. Gobbi A, Karnatzikos G, Kumar A (2014) Long-term results after microfracture treatment for full-thickness knee chondral lesions in athletes. Knee Surg Sports Traumatol Arthrosc 22(9):1986–1996
32. Marcacci M, Kon E, Zaffagnini S, Iacono F, Neri MP, Vascellari A, Visani A, Russo A (2005) Multiple osteochondral arthroscopic grafting (mosaicplasty) for cartilage defects of the knee: prospective study results at 2-year follow-up. Arthroscopy 21(4):462–470
33. Bartha L, Vajda A, Duska Z, Rahmeh H, Hangody L (2006) Autologous osteochondral mosaicplasty grafting. J Orthop Sports Phys Ther 36(10):739–750
34. Bedi A, Feeley BT, Williams RJ III (2010) Management of articular cartilage defects of the knee. J Bone Joint Surg Am 92(4):994–1009
35. Moran CJ, Pascual-Garrido C, Chubinskaya S, Potter HG, Warren RF, Cole BJ, Rodeo SA (2014) Restoration of articular cartilage. J Bone Joint Surg Am 96(4):336–344
36. Mundi R, Bedi A, Chow L, Crouch S, Simunovic N, SibilskyEnselman E, Ayeni OR (2016) Cartilage restoration of the knee: a systematic review and meta-analysis of level 1 studies. Am J Sports Med 44(7):1888–1895
37. Filardo G, Kon E, Perdisa F, Tetta C, Di Martino A, Marcacci M (2015) Arthroscopic mosaicplasty: long-term outcome and joint degeneration progression. Knee 22(1):36–40
38. Gudas R, Gudaite A, Pocius A, Gudiene A, Cekanauskas E, Monastyreckiene E, Basevicius A (2012) Ten-year follow-up of a prospective, randomized clinical study of mosaic osteochondral autologous transplantation versus microfracture for the treatment of osteochondral defects in the knee joint of athletes. Am J Sports Med 40(11):2499–2508
39. Hangody L, Dobos J, Baló E, Pánics G, Hangody LR, Berkes I (2010) Clinical experiences with autologous osteochondral mosaicplasty in an athletic population: a 17-year prospective multicenter study. Am J Sports Med 38(6):1125–1133
40. Cook JL, Stannard JP, Stoker AM, Bozynski CC, Kuroki K, Cook CR, Pfeiffer FM (2016) Importance of donor chondrocyte viability for osteochondral allografts. Am J Sports Med 44(5):1260–1268
41. De Caro F, Bisicchia S, Amendola A, Ding L (2015) Large fresh osteochondral allografts of the knee: a systematic clinical and basic science review of the literature. Arthroscopy 31(4):757–765
42. Krych AJ, Robertson CM, Williams RJ III (2012) Cartilage Study Group. Return to athletic activity after osteochondral allograft transplantation in the knee. Am J Sports Med 40(5):1053–1059
43. Gracitelli GC, Meric G, Pulido PA, McCauley JC, Bugbee WD (2015) Osteochondral allograft transplantation for knee lesions after failure of cartilage repair surgery. Cartilage 6(2):98–105
44. Shaha JS, Cook JB, Rowles DJ, Bottoni CR, Shaha SH, Tokish JM (2013) Return to an athletic lifestyle

after osteochondral allograft transplantation of the knee. Am J Sports Med 41(9):2083–2089
45. Kon E, Filardo G, Di Martino A, Marcacci M (2012) ACI and MACI. J Knee Surg 25(1):17–22
46. Brittberg M, Lindahl A, Nilsson A, Ohlsson C, Isaksson O, Peterson L (1994) Treatment of deep cartilage defects in the knee with autologous chondrocyte transplantation. N Engl J Med 331(14):889–895
47. Filardo G, Kon E, Andriolo L, Di Matteo B, Balboni F, Marcacci M (2014) Clinical profiling in cartilage regeneration: prognostic factors for midterm results of matrix-assisted autologous chondrocyte transplantation. Am J Sports Med 42(4):898–905
48. Niemeyer P, Porichis S, Steinwachs M, Erggelet C, Kreuz PC, Schmal H, Uhl M, Ghanem N, Südkamp NP, Salzmann G (2014) Long-term outcomes after first-generation autologous chondrocyte implantation for cartilage defects of the knee. Am J Sports Med 42(1):150–157
49. Mithöfer K, Peterson L, Mandelbaum BR, Minas T (2005) Articular cartilage repair in soccer players with autologous chondrocyte transplantation: functional outcome and return to competition. Am J Sports Med 33(11):1639–1646
50. Mithöfer K, Minas T, Peterson L, Yeon H, Micheli LJ (2005) Functional outcome of knee articular cartilage repair in adolescent athletes. Am J Sports Med 33(8):1147–1153
51. Kreuz PC, Steinwachs M, Erggelet C, Lahm A, Krause S, Ossendorf C, Meier D, Ghanem N, Uhl M (2007) Importance of sports in cartilage regeneration after autologous chondrocyte implantation: a prospective study with a 3-year follow-up. Am J Sports Med 35(8):1261–1268
52. Lawrie GM, Pacifico A, Kaushik R, Nahas C, Earle N (1991) Factors predictive of results of direct ablative operations for drug-refractory ventricular tachycardia. Analysis of 80 patients. J Thorac Cardiovasc Surg 101(1):44–55
53. Krych AJ, Harnly HW, Rodeo SA, Williams RJ III (2012) Activity levels are higher after osteochondral autograft transfer mosaicplasty than after microfracture for articular cartilage defects of the knee: a retrospective comparative study. J Bone Joint Surg Am 94(11):971–978
54. Marcacci M, Filardo G, Kon E (2013) Treatment of cartilage lesions: what works and why? Injury 44(Suppl 1):S11–S15
55. Filardo G, Vannini F, Marcacci M, Andriolo L, Ferruzzi A, Giannini S, Kon E (2013) Matrix-assisted autologous chondrocyte transplantation for cartilage regeneration in osteoarthritic knees: results and failures at midterm follow-up. Am J Sports Med 41(1):95–100
56. Filardo G, Kon E, Di Martino A, Patella S, Altadonna G, Balboni F, Bragonzoni L, Visani A, Marcacci M (2012) Second-generation arthroscopic autologous chondrocyte implantation for the treatment of degenerative cartilage lesions. Knee Surg Sports Traumatol Arthrosc 20(9):1704–1713
57. Filardo G, Kon E, Di Martino A, Iacono F, Marcacci M (2011) Arthroscopic second-generation autologous chondrocyte implantation: a prospective 7-year follow-up study. Am J Sports Med 39(10):2153–2160
58. Kon E, Filardo G, Berruto M, Benazzo F, Zanon G, Della Villa S, Marcacci M (2011) Articular cartilage treatment in high-level male soccer players: a prospective comparative study of arthroscopic second-generation autologous chondrocyte implantation versus microfracture. Am J Sports Med 39(12):2549–2557
59. Pestka JM, Feucht MJ, Porichis S, Bode G, Südkamp NP, Niemeyer P (2016) Return to sports activity and work after autologous chondrocyte implantation of the knee: which factors influence outcomes? Am J Sports Med 44(2):370–377
60. Ebert JR, Robertson WB, Lloyd DG, Zheng MH, Wood DJ, Ackland T (2008) Traditional vs accelerated approaches to post-operative rehabilitation following matrix-induced autologous chondrocyte implantation (MACI): comparison of clinical, biomechanical and radiographic outcomes. Osteoarthr Cartil 16(10):1131–1140
61. Della Villa S, Kon E, Filardo G, Ricci M, Vincentelli F, Delcogliano M, Marcacci M (2010) Does intensive rehabilitation permit early return to sport without compromising the clinical outcome after arthroscopic autologous chondrocyte implantation in highly competitive athletes? Am J Sports Med 38(1):68–77
62. Gille J, Schuseil E, Wimmer J, Gellissen J, Schulz AP, Behrens P (2010) Mid-term results of autologous matrix-induced chondrogenesis for treatment of focal cartilage defects in the knee. Knee Surg Sports Traumatol Arthrosc 18(11):1456–1464
63. Lee YH, Suzer F, Thermann H (2014) Autologous matrix-induced chondrogenesis in the knee: a review. Cartilage 5(3):145–153
64. Kon E, Filardo G, Perdisa F, Venieri G, Marcacci M (2014) Clinical results of multilayered biomaterials for osteochondral regeneration. J Exp Orthop 1(1):10
65. Kon E, Filardo G, Di Martino A, Busacca M, Moio A, Perdisa F, Marcacci M (2014) Clinical results and MRI evolution of a nano-composite multilayered biomaterial for osteochondral regeneration at 5 years. Am J Sports Med 42(1):158–165
66. Berruto M, Delcogliano M, de Caro F, Carimati G, Uboldi F, Ferrua P, Ziveri G, De Biase CF (2014) Treatment of large knee osteochondral lesions with a biomimetic scaffold: results of a multicenter study of 49 patients at 2-year follow-up. Am J Sports Med 42(7):1607–1617
67. Christensen BB, Foldager CB, Jensen J, Jensen NC, Lind M (2016) Poor osteochondral repair by a biomimetic collagen scaffold: 1- to 3-year clinical and radiological follow-up. Knee Surg Sports Traumatol Arthrosc 24(7):2380–2387

68. Kon E, Delcogliano M, Filardo G, Altadonna G, Marcacci M (2009) Novel nano-composite multi-layered biomaterial for the treatment of multifocal degenerative cartilage lesions. Knee Surg Sports Traumatol Arthrosc 17(11):1312–1315
69. Perdisa F, Filardo G, Di Matteo B, Di Martino A, Marcacci M (2014) Biological knee reconstruction: a case report of an Olympic athlete. Eur Rev Med Pharmacol Sci 18(1 Suppl):76–80
70. Fu WL, Ao YF, Ke XY, Zheng ZZ, Gong X, Jiang D, Yu JK (2014) Repair of large full-thickness cartilage defect by activating endogenous peripheral blood stem cells and autologous periosteum flap transplantation combined with patellofemoral realignment. Knee 21(2):609–612

Return to Play After Multiple Knee Ligament Injuries

47

Jorge Chahla, Luke O'Brien, Jonathan A. Godin, and Robert F. LaPrade

Contents

47.1 Introduction

Multiple ligament knee injuries constitute a complex and challenging entity for the orthopedic surgeon not only because of the reconstruction procedure itself but also because of the rehabilitation program after the index procedure. Recovery after a multiligament knee reconstruction surgery typically requires 9–12 months of rehabilitation prior to returning to full activities. This time frame allows for knee homeostasis recovery and ligamentization of the grafts in order to prevent graft failures. Furthermore, a thorough rehabilitation protocol helps allay fatigue and endurance issues that can cause reinjury to the operative knee or the contralateral side.

A well-guided rehabilitation protocol after a multiligament knee reconstruction should focus on a staged intervention with goals for each stage: range of motion recovery and graft protection, muscular endurance, muscular strength, muscular power, and return to play. Full range of motion is especially vital to long-term outcomes, and patients should aim to obtain 0–90° of knee flexion within the first 2 weeks after surgery. The purpose of this chapter is to give a thorough overview of key concepts of rehabilitation after a multiligament knee reconstruction.

47.2 Acute Postoperative Management

Rehabilitation following a multiligament knee reconstruction is a key element of the process of returning a patient to their previous sport activity level. The rehabilitation program should be emphasized in providing a mechanical environment for the local adaptation and remodeling of the graft tissues that will enable the patient to

J. Chahla, M.D., Ph.D. • J.A. Godin, M.D., M.B.A.
R.F. LaPrade, M.D., Ph.D. (✉)
Steadman Philippon Research Institute—The Steadman Clinic, Vail, CO, USA
e-mail: drlaprade@sprivail.org

L. O'Brien, P.T., M.Phty. (Sports), S.C.S.
Howard Head Sports Medicine, Vail, CO, USA

V. Musahl et al. (eds.), *Return to Play in Football*, https://doi.org/10.1007/978-3-662-55713-6_47

safely return to optimal levels of function. The acute management will vary in form and length depending on the associated lesions, soft tissue damage, and general status and demographics of the patient (such as BMI, age, etc.). Thus, every rehabilitation program should be individualized [1]. A structured physical therapy protocol is fundamental to obtaining and maintaining a satisfactory result. Initial management should focus on supportive measures such as pain control, inflammation/effusion control (cryotherapy, elevation, and compression), range of motion reestablishment, patellar mobilization, restoring appropriate muscle firing patterns, and progressive gait training. Soft tissue healing involves a predictable series of phases (inflammation, proliferative and remodeling phases) that should be addressed at a proper time to promote physiologic healing responses, minimize negative changes, and facilitate the proliferation and alignment of collagen fibers [1]. The inflammatory phase occurs from 0 to 3 days, and the primary aim is to decrease inflammation and manage pain. Successively, the repair/proliferation phase takes place between 2 days and 3 weeks. In this phase, collagen stretching (that naturally tends to contract) should be the focus. Finally, in the remodeling/maturation phase (between 3 weeks and 12 months), the emphasis should be placed on more aggressive mobilization [2].

Pharmacological pain management and alternative therapies such as cryotherapy or electromyography (EMG) biofeedback can act as coadjuvants to achieve early neuromuscular control postoperatively. Spencer et al. [3] reported that as little as 20–30 mL of effusion can retard the contraction of the vastus medialis oblique muscle. Residual stiffness is the most common complication after a multiligament knee reconstruction [4], and, therefore, one of the primary goals of rehabilitation is restoration of full range of motion while protecting the grafts [5]. An early start to quadriceps exercises in the postoperative period has been reported to improve early ROM development [6]. Prompt ROM restoration will result in more effective patient participation in subsequent rehabilitation phases [7]. Obtaining extension must take precedence during the initial phases of rehabilitation, and progressive flexion should be achieved with a minimum of 90° of flexion goal at 2 weeks.

Patellar mobilization should be a primary initial focus of the rehabilitation, as hypomobility of the proximal pole of the patella can interfere with the extensor mechanism leading to loss of range of motion and a quadriceps lag [1]. Conversely, flexion can be affected by a diminished patellar inferior glide. The force utilized to produce patellar gliding should be concordant with the degree of inflammation present. Overly

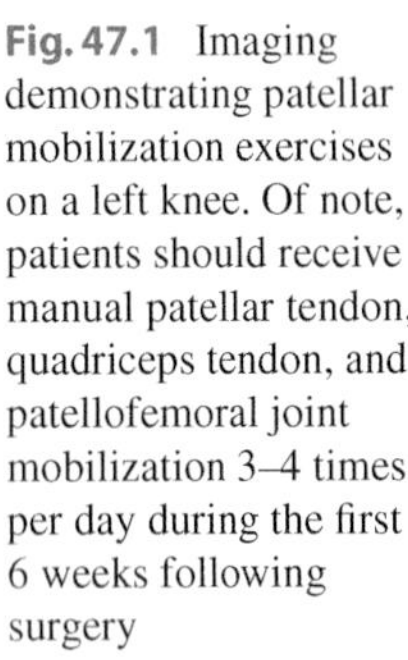

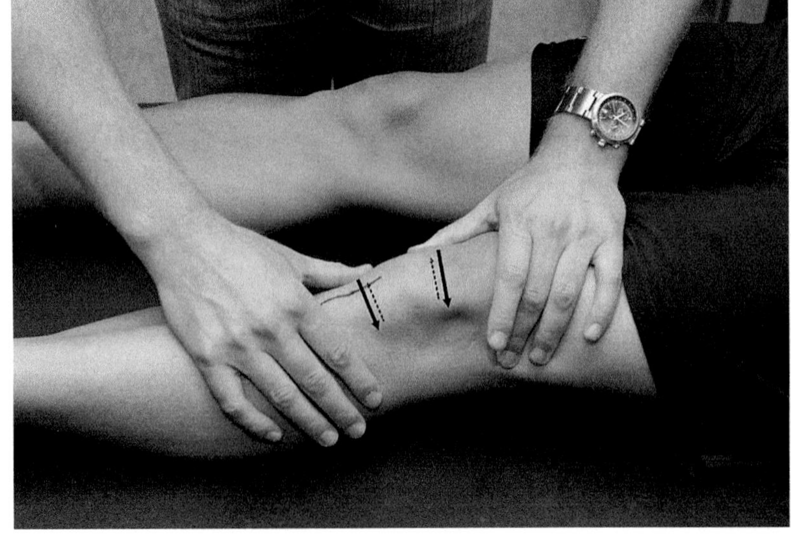

Fig. 47.1 Imaging demonstrating patellar mobilization exercises on a left knee. Of note, patients should receive manual patellar tendon, quadriceps tendon, and patellofemoral joint mobilization 3–4 times per day during the first 6 weeks following surgery

Table 47.1 Early postoperative restrictions, brace utilization, and weight-bearing status

Restrictions	Time frames
Range of motion	0–90 × 2 weeks then FROM
Brace	Immobilizer × 6 weeks PCL Jack brace × 6 months (if PCL is involved)
Weight bearing	NWB × 6 weeks

FROM full range of motion, *PCL* posterior cruciate ligament, *NWB* non-weight bearing

aggressive patellar mobilization in the acute postoperative period could exacerbate pain and swelling, which can contribute to loss of motion (Fig. 47.1).

Fact Box Initial management

- Pain control
- Cryotherapy
- Elevation
- Compression
- Range of motion reestablishment
- Patellar mobilization
- Appropriate muscle firing patterns
- Progressive gait training

With regard to weight bearing, to date there is no randomized clinical trial assessing the effectiveness of early weight bearing after a multiligament knee reconstruction, and therefore protected weight bearing is carried out for the first 6 weeks after which partial weight bearing is allowed (Table 47.1).

47.3 Periodization

Periodization is the division of a training or rehabilitation program into smaller phases (periods) as a means of creating more manageable segments. The scientific foundation of periodization was first described by Hans Selye, who described the body's general adaptation syndrome (GAS) and its three stages [8]. The first stage is the alarm reaction, in which the body responds to the disruption to homeostasis [9]. The second stage is resistance, during which the stress is relatively mild and advantageous [9]. The final stage is exhaustion, during which the stress is chronic and the body cannot adjust [9]. The goal of effective training is to promote increased physiological capacities such as muscular energy stores, strength, and endurance. When applying these principles to athletic training, the goal is to alternate the athlete between stages I and II within the GAS. Stage III is to be avoided, because the athlete's performance will likely regress, and he or she will be more susceptible to injury. It was within this context that periodization emerged as sport scientists and coaches aimed to divide the training plan into smaller, distinct phases [10]. Translating periodization from training to rehabilitation, physical therapists can utilize the same concepts to expedite a patient's return to sport after multiligament knee reconstruction with therapeutic doses of stress reapplied to tissues following surgery in order to take the tissues first to the alarm stage of the GAS, with the goals of progressing the damaged tissue to the stage of resistance while simultaneously avoiding the stage of exhaustion [10]. In sum, periodization manages and optimizes overload.

Several studies have noted the benefit of periodization in the rehabilitation of sport injuries because some form of periodization is needed for maximal strength gains [11]. In addition, periodization may be beneficial by adding variation to workouts, thereby avoiding boredom or training plateaus [12–14]. Periodization can be accomplished by manipulating resistance, repetitions, sets, exercise order, number of exercises, rest periods, type of contractions, and training frequency. There are two primary models for periodization—the classic or linear model and the nonlinear model. The linear model, developed by Leo Matveyev [15] and endorsed by Bompa [16], is based on changing exercise volume and load across several predictable mesocycles (3–4-month periods). Nonlinear periodization (NLP), described by Poliquin [17], employs more frequent volume and load alterations to frequently change stimuli and to allow the neuromuscular system more frequent periods of recovery. In addition, reverse linear periodization

(RLP) modified volume and load in reverse order: increasing volume and decreasing load [18].

Comparisons between linear and nonlinear periodization models are quite limited. Prestes et al. compared linear periodization (LP) and RLP and found that LP presented more positive effects on body composition and maximal strength [19]. On the other hand, Baker et al. compared the effectiveness of three periodization models (non-periodized control, LP, NLP) on maximal strength and vertical jump in 22 athletes performing a 12-week strengthening program and found similar results across the three groups [20]. Rhea et al. compared LP, RLP, and NLP with equated volume and intensity for muscular endurance [18]. All three models increased local muscular endurance, and the RLP group demonstrated greater endurance improvements than did the LP and NLP groups [18]. In the setting of rehabilitation, Wong et al. compared a non-periodized and a periodized program for patellar stabilization [21]. The periodization group displayed greater vastus medialis oblique size, passive patellar stability, and knee extension force [21].

Applying these principles to a postoperative multiligament knee reconstruction rehabilitation program, muscular endurance (Table 47.2), strength (Table 47.3), and power (Table 47.4) phases can be developed based on the patient's return-to-play timelines. In LP, the length of each phase depends on the time frame of the rehabilitation program but should be no shorter than 6 weeks. With ROM restored, the treatment emphasis at week 8 shifts to the development of a muscular endurance base. A transition in training emphasis to the development of muscular strength can be made at week 15 before muscular power is developed at week 21. Three to four sessions a week are appropriate while still providing adequate recovery between sessions [22]. In summary, the concept of periodization in strength training has shown promise in healthy trained and untrained athletes, but there is a paucity of data in periodization use in the rehabilitation setting.

Table 47.2 Muscular endurance sample program

Exercise	Sets + repetitions	Rest (s)
Single-leg press	3 × 15	45
Static lunge hold with medicine ball press	3 × 60s	45
Squat progression (regular squat, squat into calf raise, squat into weight shift) (Fig. 47.2)	3 × 30 (10 each)	45
Single-leg dead lift (Fig. 47.3)	3 × 15	45
Tuck squat	3 × 60s	45

Table 47.3 Muscular strength sample program

Exercise	Sets + reps	Rest (s)
Single-leg press	3 × 12	90
Single-leg squat	3 × max	90
Single-leg dead lift with kettle bell	3 × 12	90
Reverse lunge with dumbbells	3 × 12	90
Tuck squat with sport cord resistance	3 × max	90

Table 47.4 Muscular power sample program

Exercise	Sets + reps	Rest (s)
Single-leg press	3 × 8	180
High-box step-up into hip drive (Fig. 47.4)	3 × 8	180
Double-leg high-box jump up	3 × 8	180
Olympic bar dead lift	3 × 8	180
Split jumps	3 × 8	180

Fact Box Periodization phases

1. Muscular endurance
2. Muscular strength
3. Muscular power

47.4 Load Monitoring

In the last 15 years, the practice of sport science has exploded among professional and collegiate sport teams. The knowledge provided from this field has allowed coaches and medical staffs to gain valuable insight and quantifiable and actionable data on athletes' training and game loads, as well as their ability to recover from those applied loads. Although the rehabilitation of athletes following injury almost always

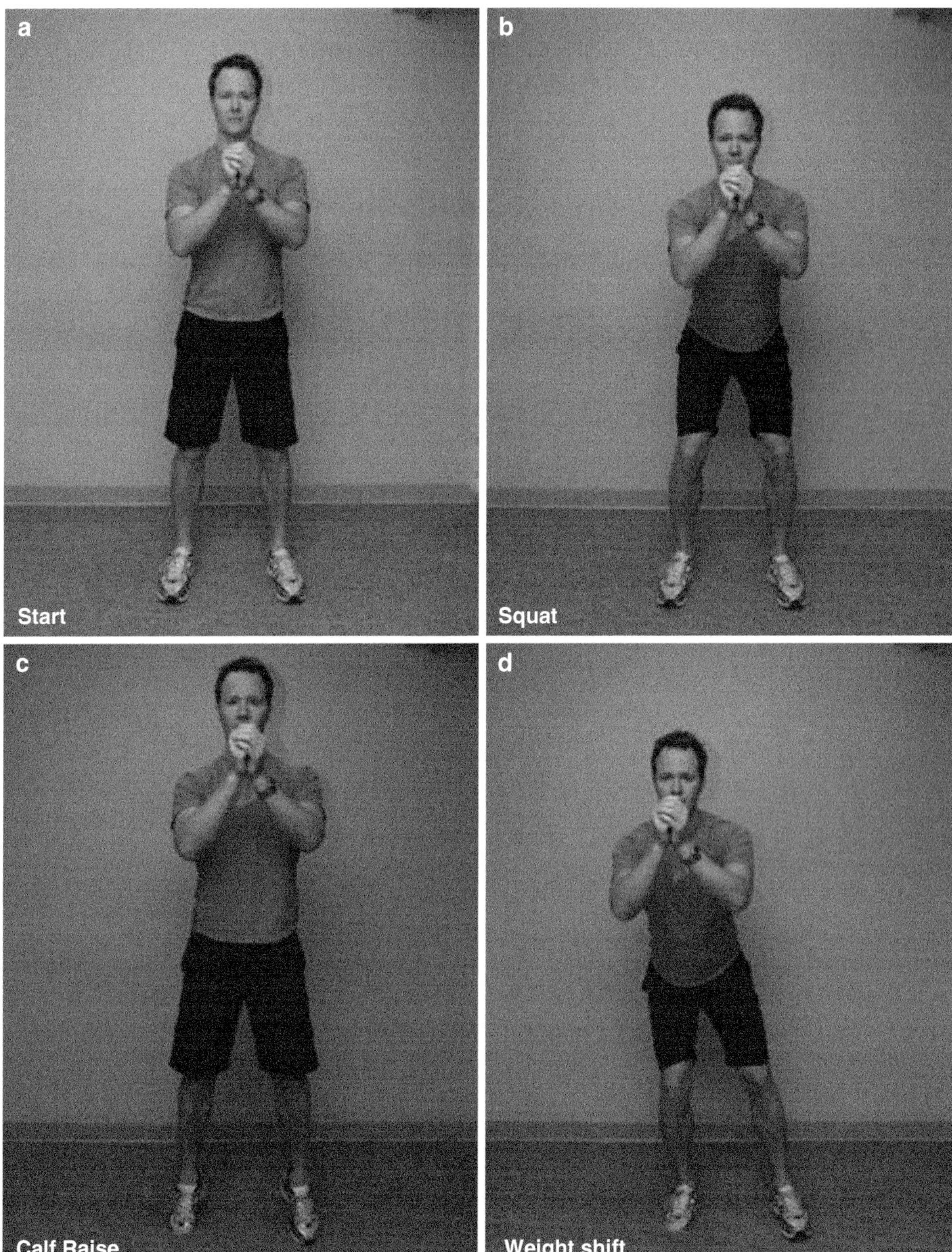

Fig. 47.2 Squat progression sequence demonstrating (**a**) a regular squat starting point, (**b**) a regular squat end point, (**c**) a squat into calf raise, and (**d**) a squat into weight shift

involves components of strength and conditioning in conjunction with various running programs, rehabilitation professionals have been slower to capture and utilize this data.

There exists a large and growing evidence base supporting the role of load monitoring in the prevention of injury. In their paper describing the attempts to reduce tibial stress fracture incidence

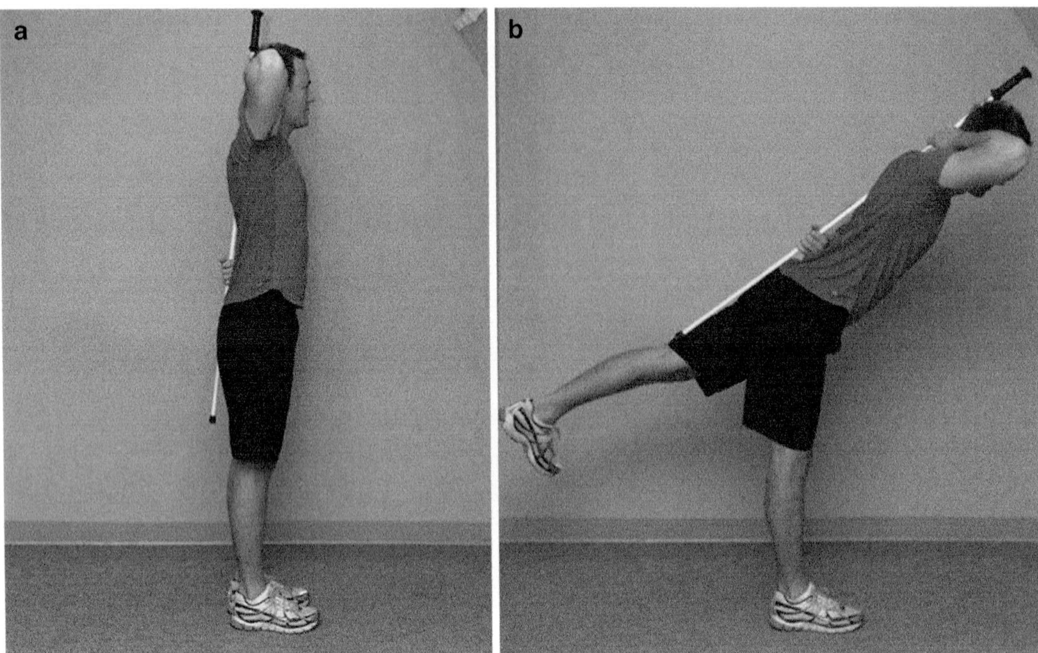

Fig. 47.3 Image showing the (**a**) starting and (**b**) finishing position of a single-leg dead lift

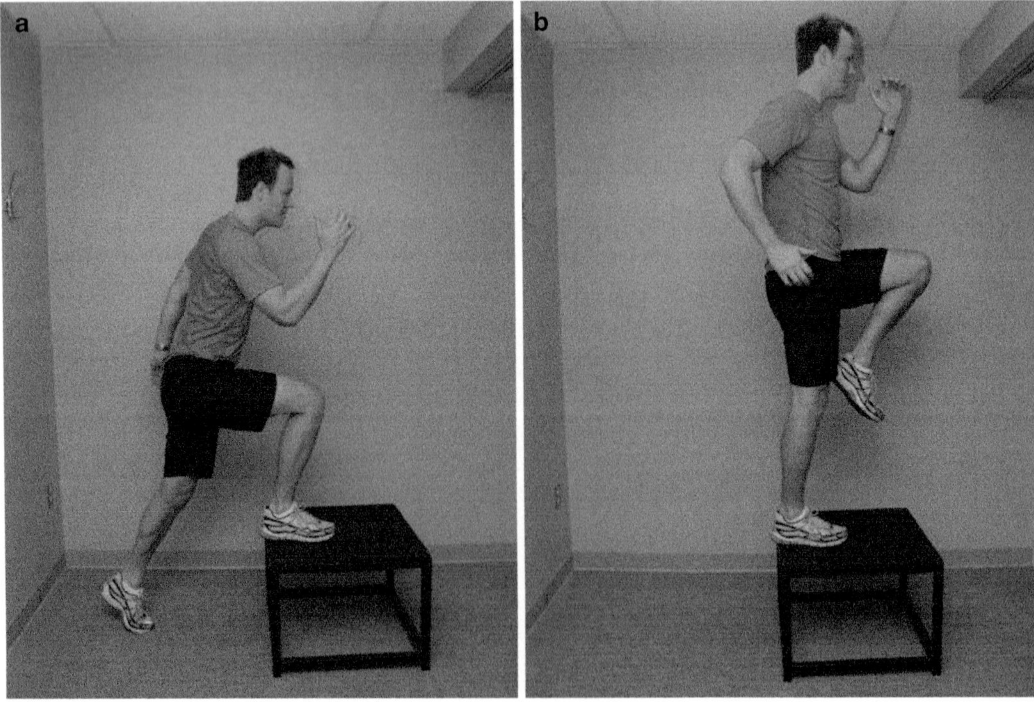

Fig. 47.4 Picture demonstrating the (**a**) starting and (**b**) finishing position of a high-box step-up into hip drive

in new military recruits, Finestone and Milgrom [23] were one of the first to link large increases in training volume combined with limited recovery with increased injury rates. Gabbet et al. [24] have expanded this work and demonstrated that preseason training volume can be used to predict soft tissue injury rates in rugby league players.

This evidence base provides sound rationale for rehabilitation professionals to explore ways to monitor training volume of athletes under their care during the strength and conditioning and return to running phases of rehabilitation.

47.5 How to Measure Training Load

The duration and intensity of training are the primary determinants of training load. Training load can be further divided into "internal" and "external" workloads. Internal workload refers to the athlete's perception of effort (e.g., rate of perceived exertion (RPE) or heart rate), whereas external workload references the quantity of work done by the athlete (distance run by a runner, number of pitches delivered in baseball, etc.). While there are a number of means to measure both internal and external workload, the most common is the product of RPE on a 10-point scale and training session duration [25].

RPE × Training session duration in minutes = Training load unit (TLU).

In isolation, a TLU has little value. However, it can be used to calculate an "acute/chronic workload" ratio, where acute workload is the average daily workload of the last 7-day period compared to the chronic average daily workload over the last 28-day period.

Acute (TLU average last 7 days) : Chronic (TLU average last 28 days).

Murray et al. [26] were able to demonstrate that sharp increases in acute workload increased the risk of injury in both the week the workload was performed and the subsequent week. Hulin et al. [27] demonstrated similar results in cricket players. Hulin et al. [28] concluded that acute workload spikes, acute/chronic workload ratios >1.5, placed rugby players at an increased injury risk.

While there is no current evidence to support acute/chronic workloads in the rehabilitation environment, it does not seem inappropriate to generalize these results to an injured athlete population. It is common practice for patients that have been non-weight bearing for a period of time to be prescribed a graduated walking progression. The evidence surrounding workload ratios would indicate that current best clinical practice would be to begin to quantify the volume and intensity (TLU) of exercise prescription in the later phases of recovery. Once baseline TLUs are captured and acute/chronic workloads are calculated for strength and conditioning sessions and/or running sessions, appropriate steps can be made to plan for exercise progression to meet the volume and intensity demands required to return to training and ultimately play without unnecessarily spiking the athlete's acute workload. Doing so will reduce the chance of injury and allow for more accurate return-to-play prognosis.

47.6 Testing for Return to Play

Given the numerous variables that can interact and play a role in the decision to allow a patient to return to sport, the rehabilitation process and eventual return to sport should be progressive and tailored to the individual patient. A systematic review of 264 studies by Barber-Westin and Noyes reported that the return-to-play decision was based on subjective nonspecific criteria such as "regained full functional stability," "normal knee function on clinical examination," "satisfactory stability," or "nearly full ROM and muscle strength" [29]. Regarding objective criteria, time from surgery, muscle strength, ROM, and effusion were most frequently used [29]. Here, we describe an objective score (the Vail Sport Test) to help guide the decision of return-to-play timing. In addition, patients should demonstrate nearly normal reported outcome scores (SANE/IKDC <5% difference from contralateral side).

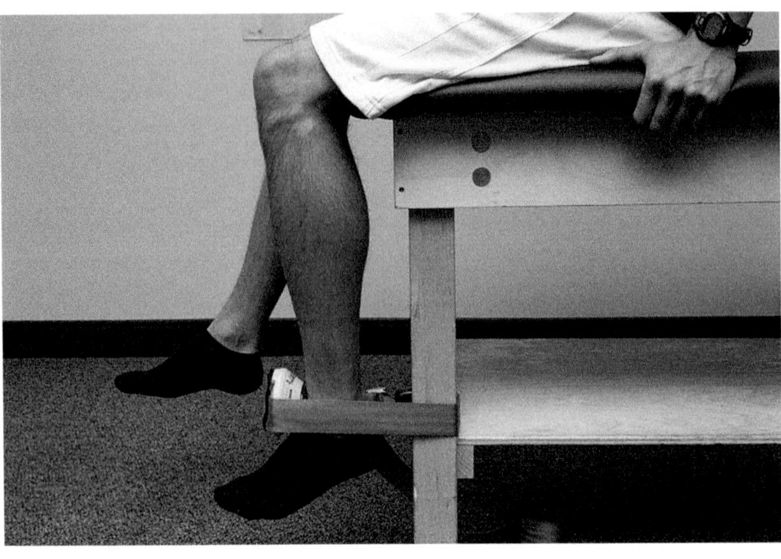

Fig. 47.5 Image showing a dynamometer being applied to a left leg to assess the quad index. Of note, this should be compared to the opposite leg

Table 47.5 Progression criteria for protection/ROM phase

Goals/criteria to progress: protection/ROM phase	Stipulations
Active terminal knee extension >=0	Should be equal to unaffected side
Active knee flexion within 10^0 of opposite side	
Gait without assistive device × 20 min	
Swelling within 1 cm of opposite knee	Measured at joint line

ROM range of motion

Table 47.6 Progression criteria for muscular endurance phase

Goals/criteria to advance: muscular endurance phase	Stipulations
Full active ROM	Equal to nonoperative limb—maintain
10 rep leg press	Weight = 2.5 × body weight
Single-leg squat from 10 in. for 15 reps	Avoidance of excessive trunk lean and knee/hip valgus
Anterior reach within 8 cm	Compared to opposite leg
Quad index >80%	Dynamometer compared to opposite leg
DorsaVi—pass single-leg squat	Valgus $<5^0$

ROM range of motion, *DorsaVi* motion analysis sensors

The development of muscle strength, power, and endurance can be quantified by single hop, box drop, quad index (Fig. 47.5), and RM testing, and these should meet the aforementioned cutoff criteria.

The decision to allow a patient to return to sport following reconstructive knee surgery is challenging for surgeons, physical trainers, athletic trainers, and all other members of an athletes' treatment team. Using the above objective criteria to aid in quantifying and measuring a patient's performance can help determine the readiness of an individual patient with regard to return to sport. Goals/criteria to progress to the protection/ROM phase, muscular endurance phase, muscular strength phase, and muscular power phase are detailed in Tables 47.5, 47.6, 47.7, and 47.8, respectively.

The minimum requirements for postoperative bracing are that patients wear either a dynamic PCL brace (Ossur PCL Rebound brace) (if the PCL was reconstructed) or a hinged ACL brace (Ossur CTi) if the PCL was not reconstructed through the first competitive season for activities. In addition, for revision MLI cases, the use of an ACL-type brace would be recommended indefinitely for sporting activities to protect their collateral reconstruction grafts.

47.7 Running and Speed Agility Program

The construction of a running and speed agility program is highly athlete- and sport-dependent. The position and sport-specific demands of the recovering athlete should be considered when constructing the program to ensure that the volume and intensity of running that the athlete is subjected to once they return to training and game play is matched to the training sessions at the end of the rehabilitation period.

As a general rule, running volume is progressed before intensity. While there are many possible means of constructing such a program, one possible approach include a walk/run program over 3–6 weeks, depending upon the total volume required, with weekly progression of the walk/run ratio (see Table 47.9).

With a running progression completed, the conditioning emphasis shifts to addressing intensity. While there are a multitude of potential drills available to develop speed and agility, the prescription of these drills should first address single-plane agility with a progression to multiplane agility (see Tables 47.10 and 47.11).

Table 47.7 Progression criteria for muscular strength phase

Goals/criteria to advance: muscular strength phase	Stipulations
10 rep leg press	Weight = 2.8 × body weight
Anterior reach within 4 cm	Compared to opposite leg
Quad girth within 1 cm	Compared to opposite leg
Quad index with 90%	Dynamometer compared to opposite
Hamstring/quad ratio >60%	Dynamometer compared to opposite leg
DorsaVi—box drop	Valgus <5^0
Vail Sport Test	Passing score > 46/54

DorsaVi motion analysis sensors
There are a total of four components of the test that include a single-leg squat for 3 min, lateral bounding for 90 s, and forward/backward jogging for 2 min each. After each component, the patient is given 2.5 min to rest prior to proceeding to the next task. The patient is graded based upon the ability to demonstrate strength and muscular endurance and absorb and produce force all while maintaining appropriate movement quality at the trunk and lower extremity. The potential scores for the individual components are as follows: the single-leg squat and the lateral bounding both have a maximum award of 15 points, and the forward and backward jogging have a maximum award of 12 points each for a total composite score of 54 points.

Table 47.8 Progression criteria for muscular power phase

Goals/criteria to advance: muscular power phase	Stipulations
T-Test for agility	Within 90% of time for unaffected side
10 rep leg press	Weight = 3.1 × body weight
Single-leg hop for distance (Fig. 47.6)	Distance within 90% of unaffected side
Single-leg vertical jump with DorsaVi	Flight time within 90% of unaffected side

T test This *test* requires the athlete to touch a series of cones set out in "T" shape, while *DorsaVi* is the motion analysis sensors

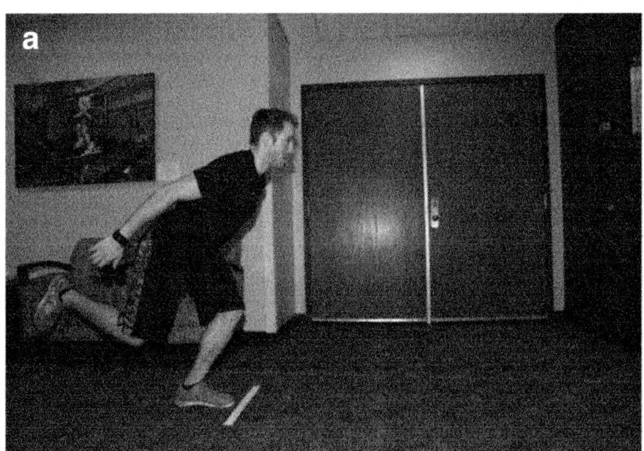

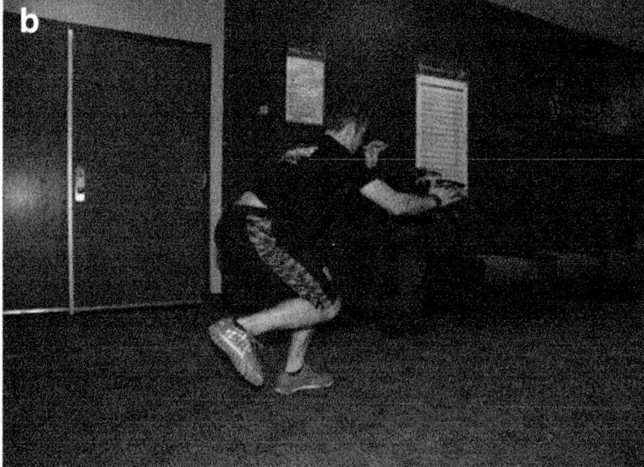

Fig. 47.6 Picture demonstrating the (**a**) starting and (**b**) finishing position of a single-leg hop

Table 47.9 Running progression

	Walk (min)	Run (min)
Week 1	4	1
Week 2	3	2
Week 3	2	3
Week 4	1	4
Week 5	–	20
Week 6		25

Table 47.10 Single-plane speed and agility sample

Week 1	Reps
Weave run	×3
Zigzag shuffle	×3
Dip and touch	×3
Circle around	×3

Table 47.11 Multiplane speed and agility sample

Week 2	Reps
Jump over and sprint	×3
Front/back shuffle	×3
Sprint-shuffle shuttle	×3

Take-Home Message

- Multiligament knee injury prognosis has dramatically improved in recent years due to a better understanding of the pathology and advancements in surgical techniques and instruments.
- Postoperative rehabilitation is of outmost importance to achieve a satisfactory outcome following multiligament knee reconstruction.
- Stepwise rehabilitation phases (periodization) should be followed, including phases focusing on graft protection and regaining of motion, muscular endurance, muscular strength, and muscular power.
- Once a muscular strength foundation with good dynamic neuromuscular control has been established, patients can progress to their functional sport-specific exercises.
- It is important to define phase-specific goals and criteria for progression to the subsequent phase because a staged approach has demonstrated improved outcomes when compared to a single test at the end of the rehabilitation program.
- Using the objective criteria outlined in this chapter can aid providers in assessing a patient's readiness to return to sport following multiligament knee reconstruction.

Top Five Evidence Based References

Medvecky MJ, Zazulak BT, Hewett TE (2007) A multidisciplinary approach to the evaluation, reconstruction and rehabilitation of the multi-ligament injured athlete. Sports Med 37:169–187

Shaw T, Williams MT, Chipchase LS (2005) Do early quadriceps exercises affect the outcome of ACL reconstruction? A randomised controlled trial. Aust J Physiother 51:9–17

Lorenz DS, Reiman MP, Walker JC (2010) Periodization: current review and suggested implementation for athletic rehabilitation. Sports Health 2:509–518

Drew MK, Finch CF (2016) The relationship between training load and injury, illness and soreness: a systematic and literature review. Sports Med 46:861–883

Barber-Westin SD, Noyes FR (2011) Factors used to determine return to unrestricted sports activities after anterior cruciate ligament reconstruction. Arthroscopy 27:1697–1705

References

1. Romeyn RL, Jennings J, Davies GJ (2008) Surgical treatment and rehabilitation of combined complex ligament injuries. N Am J Sports Phys Ther 3:212–225
2. Medvecky MJ, Zazulak BT, Hewett TE (2007) A multidisciplinary approach to the evaluation, reconstruction and rehabilitation of the multi-ligament injured athlete. Sports Med 37:169–187
3. Spencer JD, Hayes KC, Alexander IJ (1984) Knee joint effusion and quadriceps reflex inhibition in man. Arch Phys Med Rehabil 65:171–177
4. Sisto DJ, Warren RF (1985) Complete knee dislocation. A follow-up study of operative treatment. Clin Orthop Relat Res 198:94–101
5. Lachman JR, Rehman S, Pipitone PS (2015) Traumatic knee dislocations: evaluation, management, and surgical treatment. Orthop Clin North Am 46:479–493
6. Shaw T, Williams MT, Chipchase LS (2005) Do early quadriceps exercises affect the outcome of ACL reconstruction? A randomised controlled trial. Aust J Physiother 51:9–17
7. Saka T (2014) Principles of postoperative anterior cruciate ligament rehabilitation. World J Orthop 5:450–459
8. Selye H (1956) The stress of life. McGraw-Hill, New York, NY

9. Selye H (1951) The general-adaptation-syndrome. Annu Rev Med 2:327–342
10. Hoover DL, VanWye WR, Judge LW (2016) Periodization and physical therapy: bridging the gap between training and rehabilitation. Phys Ther Sport 18:1–20
11. Wilk KE, Arrigo C (1993) Current concepts in the rehabilitation of the athletic shoulder. J Orthop Sports Phys Ther 18:365–378
12. Buford TW, Rossi SJ, Smith DB, Warren AJ (2007) A comparison of periodization models during nine weeks with equated volume and intensity for strength. J Strength Cond Res 21:1245–1250
13. Fleck S (1999) Periodized strength training: a critical review. J Strength Cond Res 13:82–89
14. Kraemer WJ, Ratamess NA (2004) Fundamentals of resistance training: progression and exercise prescription. Med Sci Sports Exerc 36:674–688
15. Matveyev L (1982) Fundamentals of sports training. Victor Kamkin, Rockville, MD
16. Bompa TO, Jones D (1983) Theory and methodology of training: the key to athletic performance. Kendall/Hunt Publishing Company, Dubuque, IA
17. Poliquin C (1988) FOOTBALL: five steps to increasing the effectiveness of your strength training program. Strength Cond J 10:34–39
18. Rhea MR, Phillips WT, Burkett LN et al (2003) A comparison of linear and daily undulating periodized programs with equated volume and intensity for local muscular endurance. J Strength Cond Res 17:82–87
19. Prestes J, De Lima C, Frollini AB, Donatto FF, Conte M (2009) Comparison of linear and reverse linear periodization effects on maximal strength and body composition. J Strength Cond Res 23:266–274
20. Baker D, Wilson G, Carlyon R (1994) Periodization: the effect on strength of manipulating volume and intensity. J Strength Cond Res 8:235–242
21. Wong YM, Chan ST, Tang KW, Ng GY (2009) Two modes of weight training programs and patellar stabilization. J Athl Train 44:264–271
22. Lorenz DS, Reiman MP, Walker JC (2010) Periodization: current review and suggested implementation for athletic rehabilitation. Sports Health 2:509–518
23. Finestone A, Milgrom C (2008) How stress fracture incidence was lowered in the Israeli army: a 25-yr struggle. Med Sci Sports Exerc 40:S623–S629
24. Gabbett TJ (2010) The development and application of an injury prediction model for noncontact, soft-tissue injuries in elite collision sport athletes. J Strength Cond Res 24:2593–2603
25. Drew MK, Finch CF (2016) The relationship between training load and injury, illness and soreness: a systematic and literature review. Sports Med 46:861–883
26. Murray NB, Gabbett TJ, Townshend AD, Hulin BT, McLellan CP (2017) Individual and combined effects of acute and chronic running loads on injury risk in elite Australian footballers. Scand J Med Sci Sports 27(9):990–998
27. Hulin BT, Gabbett TJ, Blanch P, Chapman P, Bailey D, Orchard JW (2014) Spikes in acute workload are associated with increased injury risk in elite cricket fast bowlers. Br J Sports Med 48:708–712
28. Hulin BT, Gabbett TJ, Lawson DW, Caputi P, Sampson JA (2016) The acute:chronic workload ratio predicts injury: high chronic workload may decrease injury risk in elite rugby league players. Br J Sports Med 50:231–236
29. Barber-Westin SD, Noyes FR (2011) Factors used to determine return to unrestricted sports activities after anterior cruciate ligament reconstruction. Arthroscopy 27:1697–1705

Return to Soccer Following Acute Patellar Dislocation

48

Robert A. Magnussen, Laura C. Schmitt, and Elizabeth A. Arendt

Contents

R.A. Magnussen, M.D., M.P.H.
Department of Orthopaedics, Ohio State University, Columbus, OH, USA

L.C. Schmitt, P.T., Ph.D.
Division of Physical Therapy, School of Health and Rehabilitation Sciences, Ohio State University, Columbus, OH, USA

E.A. Arendt, M.D. (✉)
Department of Orthopaedic Surgery, University of Minnesota, 2450 Riverside Avenue South, Suite R200, Minneapolis, MN 55454, USA
e-mail: arend001@umn.edu

48.1 Introduction

First-time patellar dislocations are frequent in young, athletic patients, representing the second most common cause of traumatic hemarthrosis of the knee after injuries to the anterior cruciate ligament in all age groups [1] and the most common cause of hemarthrosis in the pediatric population [2, 3]. This injury frequently occurs during rotational sporting activities, with the knee in a position near terminal extension with axial load and valgus stress [4, 5]. Cutting and pivoting sports such as soccer place athletes (particularly females) at high risk for this injury. An analysis of high school epidemiology injury data in 2015 demonstrated the incidence of patellar instability injuries to be 1.22 per 100,000 athletic exposures in males and 2.92 per 100,000 athletic exposures in females [6]. The rate of injuries for females in games (5.80 per 100,000 exposures) placed soccer as the second highest risk sport (behind gymnastics) for patellar instability among females [6].

First-time patellar dislocations have historically been treated nonoperatively, although the risk of recurrent dislocation has been reported to be between 13% and 70% [7]. In addition to recurrent instability risk, the literature also demonstrates a high prevalence of persistent symptoms that limit activity participation and harm quality of life [8]. These findings have led some authors to recommend surgical treatment for first-time patellar instability; however, the question of

V. Musahl et al. (eds.), *Return to Play in Football*, https://doi.org/10.1007/978-3-662-55713-6_48

operative versus nonoperative acute management of first-time patellar dislocations remains controversial [5, 9]. While some studies have evaluated risk factors for recurrent instability [10–12], additional high-level studies are necessary to accurately identify patients who may specifically benefit from early surgery following first-time dislocation events. Nonoperative management remains the standard of care for first-time patellar dislocations at most medical centers. Patients who suffer recurrent instability, those with significant intra-articular cartilage damage or large loose bodies, and other select patients may be treated with patellar stabilization procedures of varying types depending on injury, anatomy, and patient-specific factors. Rehabilitation guidelines and return to activity considerations following surgical procedures are beyond the scope of this work.

Fact Box 1 Key risk factors for recurrent lateral patellar dislocations

- Skeletal immaturity at the time of the first-time dislocation
- Atraumatic first-time dislocation
- Family history of recurrent instability
- Ligamentous laxity
- Patella alta (Fig. 48.1)
- Trochlear dysplasia (Fig. 48.2)

The goals of this chapter are to review published nonoperative treatment regimens for patellar instability and discuss published guidelines and evidence-based rationale for return to soccer following first-time patellar dislocation.

48.2 Mechanisms of Injury

Patellofemoral joint stability is maintained by static and active restraints and by healthy lower extremity biomechanics during dynamic activity [13–19]. The patella is most vulnerable to translational forces during weight bearing in the first 20–30 degrees of knee flexion [13, 14, 20]. Lateral patellar dislocation injuries result from either direct contact with the medial aspect of the knee or through indirect, noncontact mechanisms often related to biomechanical and/or anatomic factors that result in patellar lateralization with respect to the trochlear groove [4]. The bony wall of the trochlear groove is the ultimate stabilizer of the patella guarding against translational forces. Therefore anatomic factors that reduce the bony constraint between the patella and the trochlear groove, such as trochlear and/or patellar dysplasia (more shallow groove) or patella alta (late entry into the groove), increase risk of patellar dislocations [10, 21–24]. During dynamic activity, injuries

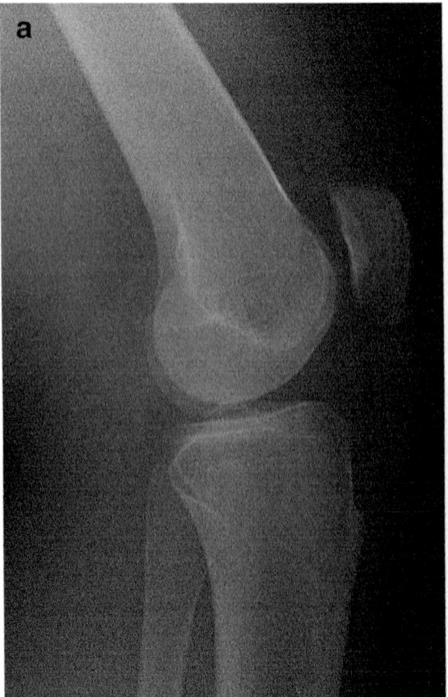

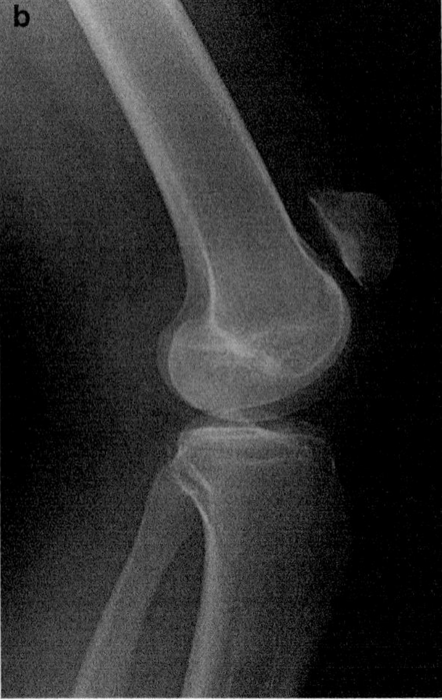

Fig. 48.1 Lateral plain radiographs of a patient with normal patellar height (**a**) and a patient with patella alta (**b**)

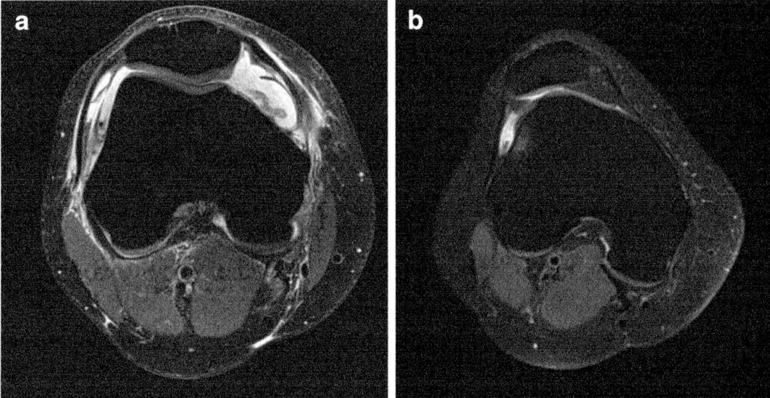

Fig. 48.2 Axial T2 MRI slice of a patient with a normal trochlea (**a**) and a patient with trochlear dysplasia (**b**)

are thought to occur due to abnormal biomechanical forces placed on medial patella restraints, which often occur during cutting and pivoting activities, such as soccer. This at-risk position places high strain on medial restraints of the patella and occurs when the foot is planted on the ground, with the knee in 20–30° of flexion and in a dynamic valgus position, which results, in part, from simultaneous femoral internal and tibial external rotation often observed during cut and pivot maneuvers [25–29]. Injury occurs within this mechanism in over 90% of the cases [30]. Factors associated with altered knee loading and increase risk of patellar instability include proximal (altered trunk, pelvis, hip kinematics, and muscle activation/strength deficits) and distal (excessive subtalar joint pronation) factors. It is thought that these factors should be considered in rehabilitation following first-time dislocation to reduce risk of subsequent dislocations.

48.3 Biology of Healing

Recent years have seen increased scrutiny and improved understanding of the medial soft tissue restraints to lateral patellar dislocation, specifically the medial patellofemoral ligament (MPFL) [31, 32]. The MPFL extends from a point on the femur between the adductor tubercle and the medial epicondyle to the proximal two-thirds of the medial border of the patella and distal quadriceps tendon [33]. The MPFL provides 50–60% of the resisting force to lateral patellar dislocation—particularly with the knee near extension [32, 34]. During the first 20–30° of knee flexion, the MPFL is a primary restraint against patella lateralization and helps guide the patella into the trochlear groove [13, 14, 20, 23, 35]. The MPFL is ruptured in 94–100% of cases of acute patellar dislocation [36].

There is a lack of research into healing of the MPFL following first-time patellar dislocation. It remains unclear whether truly anatomical, functional healing of the MPFL ever occurs in the majority of cases; however, it is prudent for rehabilitation programs to respect the time required to heal medial structures to the extent that they can heal. No studies specific to the cellular and molecular basis of MPFL healing have been performed; however, given the extra-articular nature of the ligament, insight into its healing can likely be gleaned from review of the large body of work evaluating healing of the medial collateral ligament (MCL).

Animal models evaluating MCL injury have found that the ligament undergoes distinct phases during healing: hemorrhage, inflammation, repair (matrix and cellular proliferation), and remodeling and maturation [37, 38]. During the remodeling phase, the ligaments gradually return to a near-normal state, but some differences persist including decreased strength and viscoelasticity [37]. Variables that impact healing appear to be the size of ligamentous disruption, location of injury, and relative motion [37, 39, 40]. In order to apply data from MCL healing to the MPFL, one must consider the impact of lesion location and early immobilization which can influence healing and subsequent outcome following MPFL injury.

Studies of acute MPFL injury often classify tear locations as femoral origin, mid-substance, patellar insertion, or diffuse injuries. Sillanpaa and Maenpaa [41] identified injury location of the MPFL as femoral in 34% of cases, patellar in 54% of cases, and mid-substance in 12% of cases. In a pediatric population, a patella-based injury isolated or as a part of a multifocal injury was present on MRI in 95% of first-time patellar dislocations aged <15 years [35]. In a separate study, Sillanpaa et al. [42] found that avulsion from the femoral origin was associated with increased risk of recurrent instability.

Historically, immobilization was believed to be necessary to protect ligaments from stress while healing [43, 44]; however, more recent basic science work has cast doubt on the utility of immobilization in promoting healing. Immobilization results in less organized collagen, decreased biomechanical ligament strength, and worse knee biomechanics [38]. Improved understanding of the consequences of immobilization has driven contemporary rehabilitation protocols to encourage immediate range-of-motion exercises and early weight bearing as pain and effusion allow [45]. Although definitive data are lacking regarding the influence of bracing on risk of recurrent instability, many clinicians utilize a lateral buttress brace in the early post-injury period to ease patient apprehension and re-dislocation risk. The impact of early bracing on MPFL healing is unknown.

48.4 Nonsurgical Management of Acute Patellar Dislocation

Although nonoperative management is the most common treatment for first-time patellar dislocation, very little data exist to define an optimal rehabilitation protocol. Most published rehabilitation protocols do share aims, but methods for their achievement vary greatly. Many protocols begin with the goals of minimizing effusion, limiting pain, and restoring range of motion. The ultimate goals are to minimize recurrence and restore function, but the literature does not clearly demonstrate the best method to accomplish these goals. There are relatively few studies that compare type or duration of immobilization, investigate the impact of bracing, or compare specific rehabilitation protocols. In addition, literature of current nonoperative outcomes should include detail of known risk factors [21, 46], in particular appropriate imaging risk factors for proper patient stratification. This is necessary to create meaningful clinical algorithms.

48.4.1 Immobilization

Variability exists among studies regarding the technique and duration of initial immobilization. The immobilization period has been reported to range from 0 to 6 weeks and has included splinting, bracing, and cylinder casting among other techniques. Most of the literature suggests that immobilization time does not influence recurrence risk. Cofield and Bryan reported on 48 acute patellar dislocations with a minimum of 5-year follow-up and found no identifiable difference between those not immobilized and those immobilized up to 6 weeks [47]. Similarly, Larsen and Lauridsen treated 79 acute patellar dislocations with either elastic bandage or plaster cast and noted clinical outcome and recurrent dislocation were similar in both groups [48]. A more recent trial randomized 18 patients with first-time dislocation to taping vs. casting for 6 weeks followed by intense rehabilitation in both groups and found greater activity level as judged by Lysholm score in the taped group 5 years after index injury but no re-dislocations [49].

In regard to the degree of knee motion allowed in the early post-injury phase, one must consider the goal of immobilization. If the goal of immobilization is to help the MPFL heal in its most favorable (shortened) length, then it would logically follow that full extension be avoided. The MPFL is in its most lengthened position when the knee is fully extended with the quadriceps muscle activated, as this is when the patella is in its most cephalad position. Knee flexion resists the quadriceps' cephalad pull on the patella and helps to stabilize the patella within the bony restraint of the trochlear groove, giving the soft tissue a less stressful healing environment.

48.4.2 Rehabilitation Considerations and Functional Progression

48.4.2.1 Overall Considerations

An individualized plan of care that considers the individual's unique characteristics, such as anatomic alignment, skeletal age, injury history, and severity of impairments, within the context of their injury will optimize outcomes. Beyond physical characteristics, consideration of psychosocial attributes, such as motivation/self-efficacy, fear avoidance, or kinesiophobia, in the rehabilitation plan of care will foster a comprehensive approach and maximize outcomes. Specific interventions and the pace of progression will be guided by the severity of impairments and functional limitations, as well as by the patient's goals. For athletes returning to soccer in season, communication with other healthcare providers, as well as coaching staff members, will ensure collaboration with the plan of care.

The overall goals of rehabilitation are to protect injured tissues and promote healing, maximize function and return to sport, minimize risk of recurrence, and preserve long-term joint integrity [50]. It should be noted that re-dislocation or recurrent instability can persist in up to 50% of individuals following the primary injury event, particularly in young individuals. Surgical decisions following recurrent lateral dislocations are beyond the scope of this review. However, a recent Cochrane review [7] comparing surgical to non-operative intervention for patellar dislocations concludes, "There is insufficient high quality evidence to confirm any significant difference in outcome between surgical or non-surgical initial management of people following ***primary patellar dislocation***, and none examining this comparison in people with ***recurrent patellar dislocation***. Adequately powered randomized, multi-centre controlled trials, conducted and reported to contemporary standards are recommended."

A comprehensive plan of care that considers time-based and criterion-based functional progression as well as addresses impairments that contributed to the initial injury event will foster successful physical therapy management for both the first-time and recurrent patellar dislocation patient. This approach will ensure adequate tissue healing and promote accommodation by the injured tissues to the forces and loads associated with soccer-specific activities [50]. The plan of care will be guided by a comprehensive history and clinical examination to appropriately gauge severity of impairments and functional limitations.

Following an acute patellar dislocation, several hallmark impairments are observed that should be considered throughout the rehabilitation plan of care. Initially, the dramatic hemarthrosis creates a significant shutdown of the quadriceps femoris (QF) muscles. The QF muscles are a prime mover and dynamic stabilizer of the tibiofemoral and patellofemoral joints. With weakness, dysfunction, and inhibition of the QF muscles, it is logical that the knee is more vulnerable to recurrent injury; therefore, re-training of QF activation and strength should be employed early in the plan of care and throughout the rehabilitation program. In addition to volitional exercise, consideration of neuromuscular electrical stimulation to facilitate QF activation and strength particularly during the early phases of rehabilitation has been shown successful in other similar patient populations [51–53].

Another point of concern following lateral patellar dislocation, particularly in instances of noncontact injury, is faulty kinematics or altered joint biomechanics that contribute to increased lateral patellar translation. As discussed above, altered lower extremity kinematics that result in a dynamic valgus position put increased strain on medial knee joint structures. Addressing these altered kinematic patterns and the contributing factors (such as poor gluteal activation or strength and poor positional control of the femur) during weight-bearing tasks should be addressed early and throughout the plan of care to reduce risk of recurring lateral subluxation.

48.4.2.2 Considerations for the Acute Phase

During the acute phase of rehabilitation, protecting the injured tissues is a primary goal. A knee immobilizer may be given as an ambulatory aide for convenience, rather than for evidence-based reasoning. In order to allow for active knee motion and protect the knee, most often crutches are utilized after an acute PF dislocation with a large effusion until a reasonable gait pattern is achieved. A lateral patellar buttress utilizing a knee sleeve or taping is also common.

Resolution of impairments associated with the injury, such as pain, effusion, and decreased joint range of motion, is a goal of the phase in preparation toward more functional activities. There should be an emphasis on the restoration of QF muscle activation and strength through volitional exercise as well as neuromuscular electrical stimulation, if appropriate. Rehabilitation interventions that promote appropriate movement patterns, joint loading, and lower extremity neuromuscular control should be initiated during this phase. Beyond the restoration of the local impairments directly associated with the injury, other deficiencies should be considered and begin to be addressed, such as gluteal weakness and poor activation, poor core strength, hamstring tightness, or limited ankle dorsiflexion, to name a few [54, 55]. By the end of the initial phase, it is expected that the patient will have met the following criteria: minimal pain, minimal effusion and no reactive effusion, normalized knee range of motion, volitional QF control to perform a straight leg raise with no lag, demonstrate symmetrical weight bearing during double limb stance, and normal walking mechanics without an assistive device, if appropriate [50].

48.4.2.3 Considerations for the Intermediate Phase

The intermediate phase of rehabilitation focuses on strengthening and neuromuscular development. Interventions during this phase should progress lower extremity and core muscle strength, activation, and endurance through open/closed-chain progressive resistive exercise and functional strengthening. Interventions should promote appropriate knee joint loading strategies by progressing neuromuscular control activities that facilitate appropriate and uncompensated movement patterns and lower extremity mechanics. By the end of the intermediate phase, it is expected that patient will have met the following criteria: QF strength >80% of the uninvolved side, good core and lower extremity muscle strength (at least a 4/5 by manual muscle testing), and demonstrate functional movement with appropriate mechanics and joint loading strategies [50].

48.4.2.4 Considerations for the Advanced Phase

The advanced phase of rehabilitation will focus on functional progression toward return to soccer and restore the ability of the patient to return to pre-injury playing levels. Activities in this phase continue to focus on appropriate joint loading and lower extremity neuromuscular control through progressive core and lower extremity functional strengthening as well as initiation and progression of jogging/running and plyometric activities. Specific attention must be paid to not only the movement patterns and postures demonstrated with specific therapy exercises and activities but also the patterns of muscular activation used to achieve the task. This is critical, as dysfunctional gluteal muscle activation and/or recruitment is common in patients with patellofemoral pain [56, 57] and is likely in this patient population, although this has not been studied. Therapeutic activities should include double- and single-leg activities, single- and multiple-plane activities, as well as soccer- and position-specific activities.

The decision to reintegrate into soccer activities and return to play is collaborative with other members of the healthcare team and is based on objective criteria. Considerations should include impairment-level deficits, such as pain, effusion, range of motion, strength (Fig. 48.3), quality of movement assessment (Fig. 48.4), performance-based measures of function, and patient-reported measures of function (assessing knee-related function and psychosocial readiness) (Table 48.1). It is recommended that patients achieve the specific objective criteria outlined in Fact Box 2 for return to play decision-making. A progressive reintegration into sport participation should be considered to minimize risk of subsequent injury and continue to maximize the athlete's knee-related confidence. Initial return to play involves participation in noncontact drills and conditioning activities, progressing toward participation in contact drills and practice, and

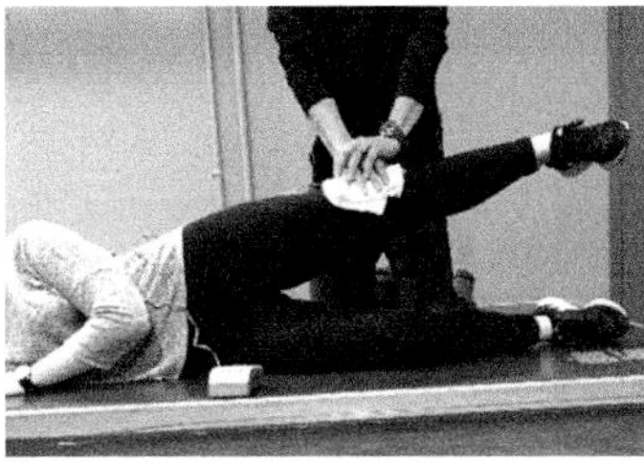
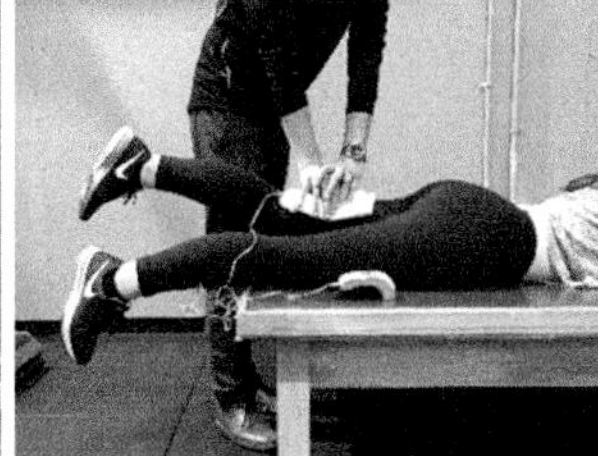
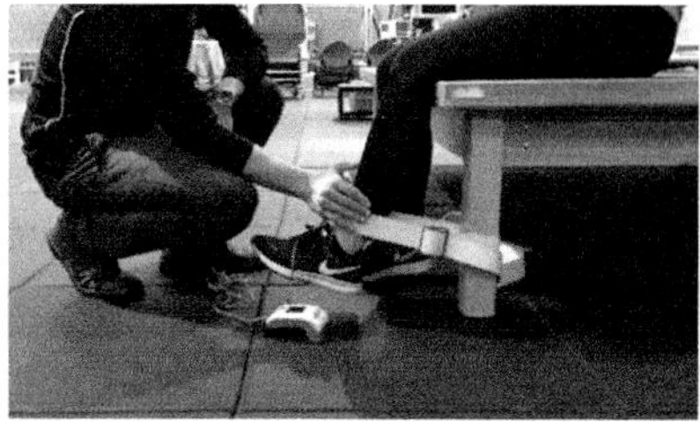

Fig. 48.3 Handheld dynamometry measures for hip abductors (*left*), hip extensors (*center*), and knee extensors (*right*)

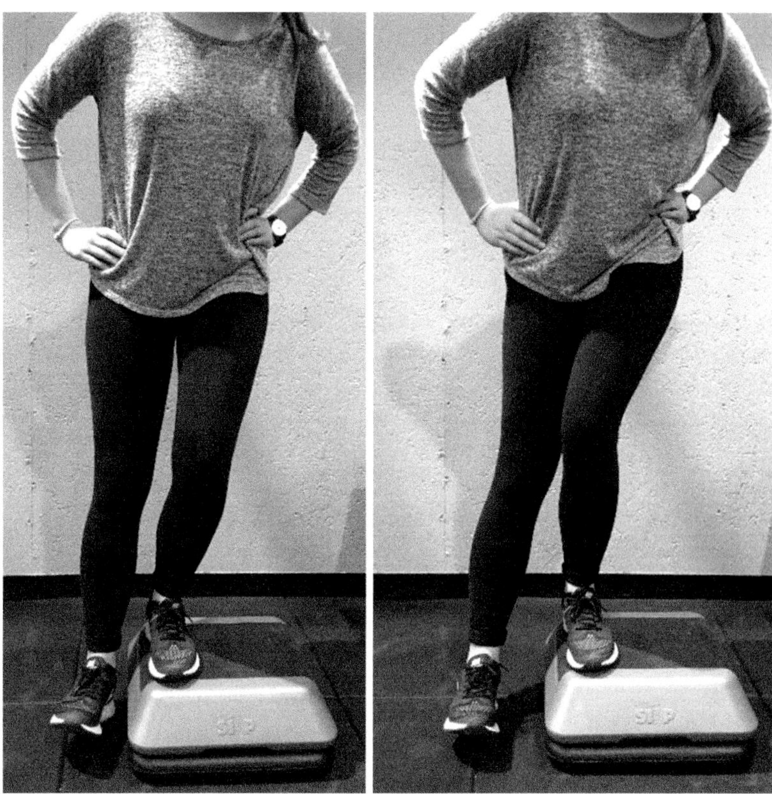

Fig. 48.4 Lateral step-down test [58]. *Left*: Performance demonstrates increased trunk movement, pelvis out of plane, and valgus knee position indicating poor quality of movement. *Right*: Performance demonstrates appropriate arm, trunk, pelvis, knee movement patterns, and steady unilateral stance for good quality of movement

finally progression to scrimmage and competitive game play [59]. Through each transition, modifications to the time of participation and the effort/demand of participation (i.e., 50% effort or speed progressing to full effort/speed) are considered for successful transition to unrestricted sport participation [59].

48.4.2.5 Additional Considerations

Additional treatment considerations are listed in Table 48.2. The challenge and complexity of therapy tasks should be elevated as the patient demonstrates appropriate mastery of foundational components. Core, hip, and quadriceps strength and endurance exercises should be introduced early and are the base upon which other activities build. Low-impact cardiovascular conditioning may be initiated once a baseline of adequate strength and neuromuscular control with closed kinetic chain activities is demonstrated. Regaining muscular strength, building muscular endurance, and restoring appropriate joint loading strategies and good quality of movement are a focus throughout rehabilitation. Continued pain and/or effusion will dictate activity progressions and may warrant referral to referring physician.

Table 48.1 Evaluation components for return-to-sport consideration [59]

Component	Measure
Pain	NPRS
Effusion	Girth Modified stroke test [60]
Range of motion	Goniometry
Strength/endurance	Dynamometer assessment (hip and thigh [61]) (Fig. 48.3)1-repetition maximum test [61] (hip and thigh) Functional endurance tests (core)
Quality of movement	Step-down test [58] (Fig. 48.4) Single-leg squat test (Fig. 48.5)
Performance-based function	Dynamic balance tests (e.g., Y Balance Test [62, 63]) Single-leg hop tests Soccer- and position-specific activities/drills
Reported-based function	Knee-specific instrument (e.g., IKDC Subjective Form, KOOS) Psychosocial readiness instrument

NPRS Numeric Pain Rating Scale, *IKDC* International Knee Documentation Committee, *KOOS* Knee Injury and Osteoarthritis Outcome Score

Fact Box 2 Considerations for return to sport decision-making after lateral patella dislocation

ISAKOS guidelines [64]:

- No complaints of pain or knee instability.
- Full range of motion/no new effusion.
- Test for core strength and endurance.
- Test for dynamic balance activities (e.g., Y Balance Test).
- LSI >85% on single-leg hop tests (+) pivoting/jumping sports.
- Adequate performance in physical therapy with sport-specific drills (simulate the intensity and body movement patterns of the athlete's given sport/activity).
- Athlete demonstrates psychological readiness.

Additional considerations [59]:

- QF strength that is 90% of the uninvolved (LSI ≥90%).
- Hip and other relevant lower extremity muscle strength that is 85–90% of the uninvolved (LSI = 85–90%).
- Demonstrate appropriate joint loading strategies and good quality of movement during neuromuscular control activities and sport-specific activities.
- Score of 85–90 on knee-related patient-reported outcome measure (e.g., IKDC Subjective Form or KOOS).

Abbreviations: LSI, limb symmetry index; QF, quadriceps femoris muscles; IKDC, International Knee Documentation Committee; KOOS, Knee injury and Osteoarthritis Outcome Score

Table 48.2 Additional rehabilitation considerations

Component
Patellar stability maintained – Taping, bracing
Adequate early isolated quadriceps muscle activation – No pattern of hamstring/quadriceps co-contraction
Progression of QF strength with objective assessment throughout plan of care (see Table 48.1)
Restoration of normal gait pattern and speed (attention to sagittal plane knee control with loading response, frontal plane hip control)
Progression of gluteal muscle strength/activation – Repetitions to failure with leg lifting activities – Dynamometry
Core stability progressions
Postural limb stability/proprioceptive control
Demonstration of appropriate joint loading and good quality of movement (Table 48.1, Figs. 48.4 and 48.5) – Focus on eccentric sagittal and frontal plane control of trunk, hips, and knee – Appropriate technique with soccer- and position-specific activities
Increasing exercise intensity (per control and symptoms) – Increased external load (strength, power) – Increased speed of movement (agility, power) – Increased duration/repetitions (endurance) – Increased task complexity and directional challenge (coordination)
Soccer- and position-specific training

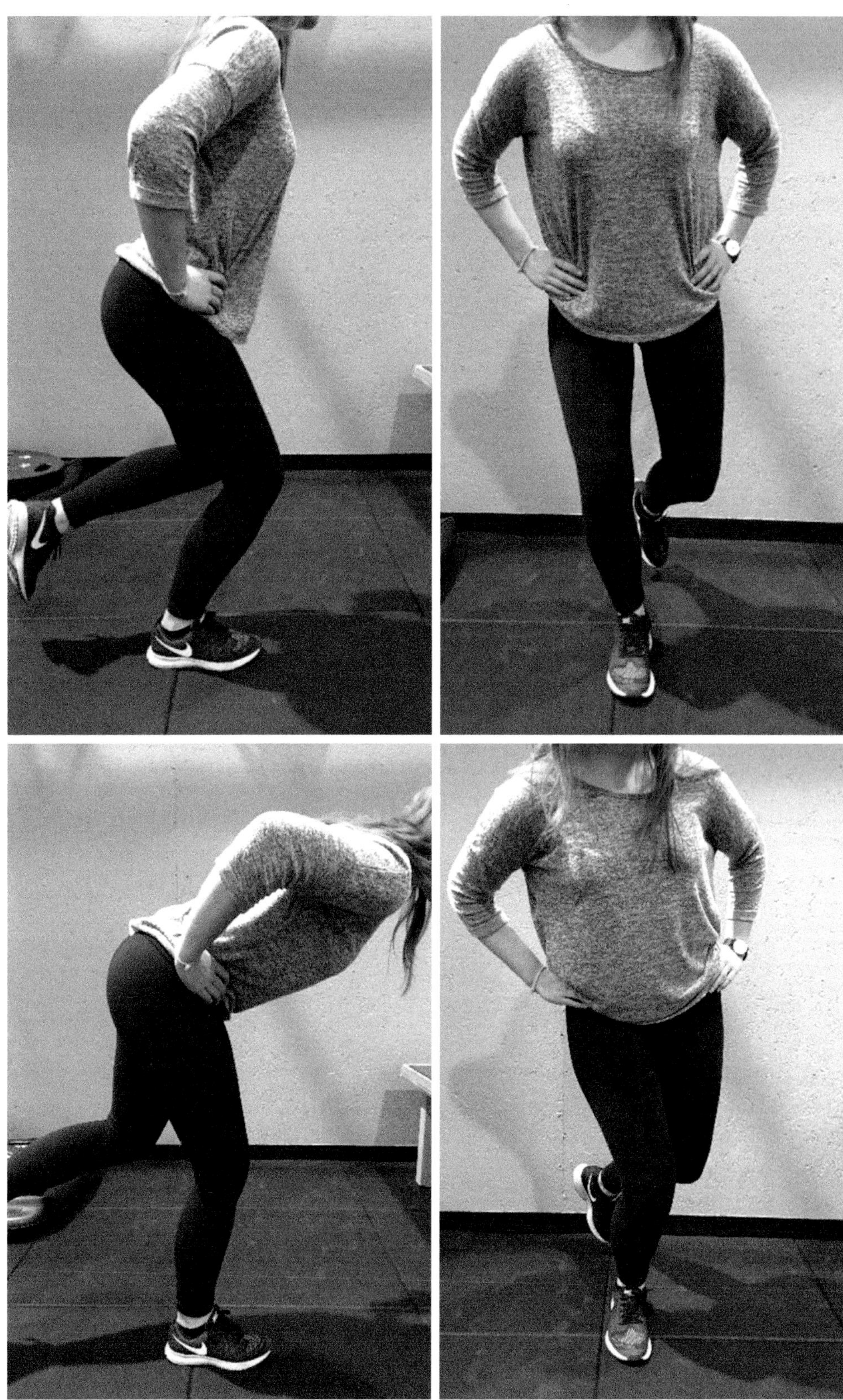

Fig. 48.5 Performance of single-leg squat test with appropriate mechanics (*top*) and with poor mechanics (*bottom*). Note decreased knee excursion and increased trunk excursion (*bottom left*) and increased trunk motion and knee valgus motion (*bottom right*)

Take-Home Message
Nonoperative management remains that standard of care for first-time patellar dislocations at most centers. Specific treatment protocols continue to be highly individualized and vary based on patient factors as well as surgeon and therapist preferences. A comprehensive plan of care, which considers time-based and criterion-based functional progression as well as addresses impairments that contributed to the initial injury event, will foster successful physical therapy management. It is not clear whether there is any benefit from joint immobilization or restriction of joint motion.

Top Five Evidence Based References

Askenberger M, Janarv P-M, Finnbogason T, Arendt EA (2017) Morphology and anatomic patellar instability risk factors in first-time traumatic lateral patellar dislocations. Am J Sports Med 45(1):50–58

Jaquith BP, Parikh SN (2015) Predictors of recurrent patellar instability in children and adolescents after first-time dislocation . J Pediatr Orthop [E-pub ahead of print 21 Oct 2015]

Magnussen RA, Duffee AR, Kalu D, Flanigan DC (2015) Does early operative treatment improve outcomes of primary patellar dislocation? A systematic review. Curr Orthop Pract 26(3):281–286

Monson J, Arendt EA (2012) Rehabilitative protocols for select patellofemoral procedures and nonoperative management schemes. Sports Med Arthrosc 20(3):136–144

ISAKOS Orthopaedic Sports Medicine Committee, Almquist F, Arendt EA, Coolican M, Doral N, Ernlund L (2012) Guidelines for the evaluation, management and safe return to sport after lateral patellar dislocation or surgical stabilization in the athletic population. Paper presented at the ISAKOS return to play consensus meeting. ISAKOS, London

References

1. DeHaven KE (1980) Diagnosis of acute knee injuries with hemarthrosis. Am J Sports Med 8(1):9–14
2. Askenberger M, Ekstrom W, Finnbogason T, Janarv P-M (2014) Occult intra-articular knee injuries in children with hemarthrosis. Am J Sports Med 42(7):1600–1606
3. Nietosvaara Y, Aalto K, Kallio PE (1994) Acute patellar dislocation in children: Incidence and associated osteochondral fractures. J Pediatr Orthop 14(4):513–515
4. Fithian DC, Paxton EW, Stone ML, Silva P, Davis DK, Elias DA, White LM (2004) Epidemiology and natural history of acute patellar dislocation. Am J Sports Med 32(5):1114–1121
5. Smith TO, Song F, Donell ST, Hing CB (2011) Operative versus non-operative management of patellar dislocation. A meta-analysis. Knee Surg Sports Traumatol Arthrosc 19(6):988–998
6. Mitchell J, Magnussen RA, Collins CL, Currie DW, Best TM, Comstock RD, Flanigan DC (2015) Epidemiology of patellofemoral instability injuries among high school athletes in the United States. Am J Sports Med 43(7):1676–1682
7. Hing CB, Smith TO, Donell S, Song F (2011) Surgical versus non-surgical interventions for treating patellar dislocation. Cochrane Database Syst Rev 11:CD008106
8. Magnussen RA, Verlage M, Stock E, Zurek L, Flanigan DC, Tompkins M, Agel J, Arendt EA (2015) Primary patellar dislocations without surgical stabilization or recurrence: How well are these patients really doing? Knee Surg Sports Traumatol Arthrosc. https://doi.org/10.1007/s00167-015-3716-3:1-5
9. Magnussen RA, Duffee AR, Kalu D, Flanigan DC (2015) Does early operative treatment improve outcomes of primary patellar dislocation? A systematic review. Curr Orthop Pract 26(3):281–286
10. Balcarek P, Oberthur S, Hopfensitz S, Frosch S, Walde TA, Wachowski MM, Schuttrumpf JP, Sturmer KM (2014) Which patellae are likely to redislocate? Knee Surg Sports Traumatol Arthrosc 22(10):2308–2314
11. Jaquith BP, Parikh SN (2015) Predictors of recurrent patellar instability in children and adolescents after first-time dislocation. J Pediatr Orthop [E-pub ahead of print 21 Oct 2015] doi:https://doi.org/10.1097/BPO.0000000000000674
12. Lewallen LW, McIntosh AL, Dahm DL (2013) Predictors of recurrent instability after acute patellofemoral dislocation in pediatric and adolescent patients. Am J Sports Med 41(3):575–581
13. Amis AA, Firer P, Mountney J, Senavongse W, Thomas NP (2003) Anatomy and biomechanics of the medial patellofemoral ligament. Knee 10(3):215–220
14. Amis AA, Senavongse W, Bull AMJ (2006) Patellofemoral kinematics during knee flexion-extension: an in vitro study. J Orthop Res 24(12):2201–2211
15. Balcarek P, Jung K, Frosch K-H, Sturmer KM (2011) Value of the tibial tuberosity-trochlear groove distance in patellar instability in the young athlete. Am J Sports Med 39(8):1756–1761
16. Powers CM (2010) The influence of abnormal hip mechanics on knee injury: a biomechanical perspective. J Orthop Sports Phys Ther 40(2):42–51
17. Powers CM, Ward SR, Fredericson M, Guillet M, Shellock FG (2003) Patellofemoral kinematics during weight-bearing and non-weight-bearing knee extension in persons with lateral subluxation of the patella: a preliminary study. J Orthop Sports Phys Ther 33(11):677–685

18. Senavongse W, Amis AA (2005) The effects of articular, retinacular, or muscular deficiencies on patellofemoral joint stability: a biomechanical study in vitro. J Bone Joint Surg Br 87(4):577–582
19. Souza RB, Draper CE, Fredericson M, Powers CM (2010) Femur rotation and patellofemoral joint kinematics: a weight-bearing magnetic resonance imaging analysis. J Orthop Sports Phys Ther 40(5):277–285
20. Philippot R, Boyer B, Testa R, Farizon F, Moyen B (2012) Study of patellar kinematics after reconstruction of the medial patellofemoral ligament. Clin Biomech (Bristol, Avon) 27(1):22–26
21. Askenberger M, Janarv P-M, Finnbogason T, Arendt EA (2017) Morphology and anatomic patellar instability risk factors in first-time traumatic lateral patellar dislocations. Am J Sports Med 45(1):50–58
22. Dejour H, Walch G, Nove-Josserand L, Guier C (1994) Factors of patellar instability: an anatomic radiographic study. Knee Surg Sports Traumatol Arthrosc 2(1):19–26
23. Tompkins MA, Rohr SR, Agel J, Arendt EA (2017) Anatomic patellar instability risk factors in primary lateral patellar dislocations do not predict injury patterns – an MRI based study . Knee Surg Sports Traumatol Arthrosc [E-pub ahead of print 2 Mar 2017] doi:https://doi.org/10.1007/s00167-017-4464-3:1-8
24. Ward SR, Terk MR, Powers CM (2007) Patella alta: association with patellofemoral alignment and changes in contact area during weight-bearing. J Bone Joint Surg Am 89(8):1749–1755
25. Atkin DM, Fithian DC, Marangi KS, Stone ML, Dobson BE, Mendelsohn C (2000) Characteristics of patients with primary acute lateral patellar dislocation and their recovery within the first 6 months of injury. Am J Sports Med 28(4):472–479
26. Fulkerson J (1996) Biomechanics of the patellofemoral joint. In: Cooke DB (ed) Disorders of the patellofemoral joint, 3rd edn. Williams & Wilkins, Baltimore, MD, pp 23–38
27. Hinton RY, Sharma KM (2003) Acute and recurrent patellar instability in the young athlete. Orthop Clin North Am 34(3):385–396
28. Myer GD, Ford KR, Di Stasi SL, Foss KDB, Micheli LJ, Hewett TE (2015) High knee abduction moments are common risk factors for patellofemoral pain (PFP) and anterior cruciate ligament (ACL) injury in girls: is PFP itself a predictor for subsequent ACL injury? Br J Sports Med 49(2):118–122
29. Visuri T, Maenpaa H (2002) Patellar dislocation in army conscripts. Mil Med 167(7):537–540
30. Sillanpaa P, Mattila VM, Iivonen T, Visuri T, Pihlajamaki H (2008) Incidence and risk factors of acute traumatic primary patellar dislocation. Med Sci Sports Exerc 40(4):606–611
31. Conlan T, Garth WP Jr, Lemons JE (1993) Evaluation of the medial soft-tissue restraints of the extensor mechanism of the knee. J Bone Joint Surg Am 75(5):682–693
32. Desio SM, Burks RT, Bachus KN (1998) Soft tissue restraints to lateral patellar translation in the human knee. Am J Sports Med 26(1):59–65
33. Placella G, Tei M, Sebastiani E, Speziali A, Antinolfi P, Delcogliano M, Georgoulis A, Cerulli G (2015) Anatomy of the medial patello-femoral ligament: a systematic review of the last 20 years literature. Musculoskelet Surg 99(2):93–103
34. Hautamaa PV, Fithian DC, Kaufman KR, Daniel DM, Pohlmeyer AM (1998) Medial soft tissue restraints in lateral patellar instability and repair. Clin Orthop Relat Res 349(349):174–182
35. Askenberger M, Arendt EA, Ekstrom W, Voss U, Finnbogason T, Janarv P-M (2016) Medial patellofemoral ligament injuries in children with first-time lateral patellar dislocations: a magnetic resonance imaging and arthroscopic study. Am J Sports Med 44(1):152–158
36. Kang HJ, Wang F, Chen BC, Zhang YZ, Ma L (2013) Non-surgical treatment for acute patellar dislocation with special emphasis on the MPFL injury patterns. Knee Surg Sports Traumatol Arthrosc 21(2):325–331
37. Frank CB, Loitz BJ, Shrive NG (1995) Injury location affects ligament healing. A morphologic and mechanical study of the healing rabbit medial collateral ligament. Acta Orthop Scand 66(5):455–462
38. Woo SL, Vogrin TM, Abramowitch SD (2000) Healing and repair of ligament injuries in the knee. J Am Acad Orthop Surg 8(6):364–372
39. Loitz-Ramage BJ, Frank CB, Shrive NG (1997) Injury size affects long-term strength of the rabbit medial collateral ligament. Clin Orthop Relat Res 337:272–280
40. Nakamura N, Horibe S, Toritsuka Y, Mitsuoka T, Yoshikawa H, Shino K (2003) Acute grade III medial collateral ligament injury of the knee associated with anterior cruciate ligament tear. The usefulness of magnetic resonance imaging in determining a treatment regimen. Am J Sports Med 31(2):261–267
41. Sillanpaa PJ, Maenpaa HM (2012) First-time patellar dislocation: surgery or conservative treatment? Sports Med Arthrosc 20(3):128–135
42. Sillanpaa PJ, Mattila VM, Maenpaa H, Kiuru M, Visuri T, Pihlajamaki H (2009) Treatment with and without initial stabilizing surgery for primary traumatic patellar dislocation. A prospective randomized study. J Bone Joint Surg Am 91(2):263–273
43. Fetto JF, Marshall JL (1978) Medial collateral ligament injuries of the knee: a rationale for treatment. Clin Orthop Relat Res 132:206–218
44. Indelicato PA (1983) Non-operative treatment of complete tears of the medial collateral ligament of the knee. J Bone Joint Surg Am 65(3):323–329
45. Reider B, Sathy MR, Talkington J, Blyznak N, Kollias S (1994) Treatment of isolated medial collateral ligament injuries in athletes with early functional rehabilitation. A five-year follow-up study. Am J Sports Med 22(4):470–477

46. Arendt EA, England K, Agel J, Tompkins MA (2016) An analysis of knee anatomic imaging factors associated with primary lateral patellar dislocations. Knee Surg Sports Traumatol Arthrosc [Epub ahead of print 04 May 2016] doi:https://doi.org/10.1007/s00167-016-4117-y:1-9
47. Cofield RH, Bryan RS (1977) Acute dislocation of the patella: results of conservative treatment. J Trauma 17(7):526–531
48. Larsen E, Lauridsen F (1982) Conservative treatment of patellar dislocations. Influence of evident factors on the tendency to redislocation and the therapeutic result. Clin Orthop Relat Res 171:131–136
49. Rood A, Boons H, Ploegmakers J, van der Stappen W, Koeter S (2012) Tape versus cast for non-operative treatment of primary patellar dislocation: a randomized controlled trial. Arch Orthop Trauma Surg 132(8):1199–1203
50. National Guideline Clearinghouse (2014) Evidence-based care guideline for conservative management of lateral patellar dislocations and instability in children and young adults aged 8–25 years. In: National Guideline Clearinghouse (NGC) [web site]. Agency for Healthcare Research and Quality (AHRQ), Rockville MD, pp 1–30
51. Fitzgerald GK, Piva SR, Irrgang JJ (2003) A modified neuromuscular electrical stimulation protocol for quadriceps strength training following anterior cruciate ligament reconstruction. J Orthop Sports Phys Ther 33(9):492–501
52. Snyder-Mackler L, Delitto A, Bailey SL, Stralka SW (1995) Strength of the quadriceps femoris muscle and functional recovery after reconstruction of the anterior cruciate ligament. A prospective, randomized clinical trial of electrical stimulation. J Bone Joint Surg Am 77(8):1166–1173
53. Snyder-Mackler L, Delitto A, Stralka SW, Bailey SL (1994) Use of electrical stimulation to enhance recovery of quadriceps femoris muscle force production in patients following anterior cruciate ligament reconstruction. Phys Ther 74(10):901–907
54. McConnell J (2007) Rehabilitation and nonoperative treatment of patellar instability. Sports Med Arthrosc 15(2):95–104
55. Monson J, Arendt EA (2012) Rehabilitative protocols for select patellofemoral procedures and nonoperative management schemes. Sports Med Arthrosc 20(3):136–144
56. Brindle TJ, Mattacola C, McCrory J (2003) Electromyographic changes in the gluteus medius during stair ascent and descent in subjects with anterior knee pain. Knee Surg Sports Traumatol Arthrosc 11(4):244–251
57. Cowan SM, Crossley KM, Bennell KL (2009) Altered hip and trunk muscle function in individuals with patellofemoral pain. Br J Sports Med 43(8):584–588
58. Piva SR, Fitzgerald K, Irrgang JJ, Jones S, Hando BR, Browder DA, Childs JD (2006) Reliability of measures of impairments associated with patellofemoral pain syndrome. BMC Musculoskelet Disord 7:33
59. Schmitt L, Byrnes R, Cherny C, Filipa A, Harrison A, Paterno M, Smith T, Cincinnati Children's Hospital Medical Center (2010) Evidence-based clinical care guideline for return to activity after lower extremity injury. Guideline 38:1–13. http://almacen-gpc.dynalias.org/publico/Lower%20extremity%20injury.%20cchmc%202010.pdf
60. Sturgill LP, Snyder-Mackler L, Manal TJ, Axe MJ (2009) Interrater reliability of a clinical scale to assess knee joint effusion. J Orthop Sports Phys Ther 39(12):845–849
61. Sinacore JA, Evans AM, Lynch BN, Joreitz RE, Irrgang JJ, Lynch AD (2017) Diagnostic accuracy of handheld dynamometry and 1-repetition-maximum tests for identifying meaningful quadriceps strength asymmetries. J Orthop Sports Phys Ther 47(2):97–107
62. Hertel J (2008) Sensorimotor deficits with ankle sprains and chronic ankle instability. Clin Sports Med 27(3):353–370. vii
63. Plisky PJ, Rauh MJ, Kaminski TW, Underwood FB (2006) Star Excursion Balance Test as a predictor of lower extremity injury in high school basketball players. J Orthop Sports Phys Ther 36(12):911–919
64. ISAKOS Orthopaedic Sports Medicine Committee, Almquist F, Arendt EA, Coolican M, Doral N, Ernlund L (2012) Guidelines for the evaluation, management and safe return to sport after lateral patellar dislocation or surgical stabilization in the athletic population. Paper presented at the ISAKOS return to play consensus meeting. ISAKOS, London

49 Return to Play Following Tendon Injuries

Mirco Herbort, Christoph Kittl, and Hermann Mayr

Contents

M. Herbort (✉) • C. Kittl
Clinic for Trauma-, Hand- and Reconstructive Surgery, University Clinic Muenster, Muenster, Germany
e-mail: mirco.herbort@gmail.com

H. Mayr
Schoen Clinic Munich-Harlaching, Munich, Germany

49.1 Introduction

Distal quadriceps tendon rupture and patellar tendon rupture are relatively rare injuries most often reported in middle-aged or older persons [1].

A degenerative weakness of the tendon has been postulated as precondition for quadriceps or patellar tendon rupture [2].

Kannus and Józsa showed degenerative changes in 865 of 891 (97%) spontaneous tendon ruptures, while degenerative changes were seen in only 149 of 445 patients in a control group (34%) [2].

Predisposing factors for quadriceps tendon ruptures are different medications like anabolic steroids, statins, and corticosteroids locally injected and for systemic use [3]. Systemic diseases can also predispose to quadriceps or patellar tendon rupture like renal disease, hyperparathyroidism, diabetes mellitus, rheumatoid arthritis, systemic lupus erythematosus, gout, obesity, and various infections [4, 5].

Kuechle et al. reported on six patellar tendon ruptures in five active athletes which were treated during a 10-year period [6]. These ruptures occurred during sporting activity and without any previous signs of degenerative or other concomitant diseases. During the same period, 135 patellar tendon ruptures all caused by non-sport injuries were treated.

Four of the five patients played basketball and one softball when the rupture happened. Three athletes had signs of proximal patellar tendon

V. Musahl et al. (eds.), *Return to Play in Football*, https://doi.org/10.1007/978-3-662-55713-6_49

tendinopathy, and one had received three corticosteroids injections to the proximal patellar tendon.

There are no scientific information regarding incidence of quadriceps or patellar tendon ruptures in football. Boublik et al. analyzed 24 patellar tendon ruptures in 22 NFL players and 14 quadriceps tendon ruptures in 14 NFL players from 1994 to 2004 [7]. The most often encountered injury mechanism of quadriceps or patellar tendon rupture was eccentric overload on a flexed knee [7]. The following injury patterns were also observed in their study: 9/22 patellar tendon ruptures occurred after deceleration while running or jumping, 7/22 during an unspecified overload event, 4/22 while blocking another player, 1/22 player was tackled, and 3/22 sustained a direct blow to the knee [7].

Although quadriceps tendon rupture is a rare injury in football, chronic tendinopathies of the patellar tendon or less frequently of quadriceps tendon are common injuries in football players.

Acute quadriceps or patellar tendon ruptures are rare injuries in young athletes following degenerative changes in.

Hagglund et al. performed a longitudinal study, where they followed 51 European elite soccer clubs (2229 players) between 2001 and 2009 for incidence of patellar tendinopathy [8]. During the study period, 137 patella tendinopathies were reported, accounting for 1.5% of total injuries with an incidence of 0.12 injuries/1000 h. Each season, 2.4% of all players were affected.

Although patellar tendinopathy is frequently mentioned as potential reason for patellar tendon rupture, only two acute-onset partial ruptures and no complete rupture were identified during the whole study period [8]. The authors concluded that these injuries are rare in elite football players. One reason for these injuries being rare could be adequate treatment of early symptoms of patellar tendinopathy [8].

Although more than half of complete ruptures occur without any prior warning signals, in nearly all patients, degenerative tendon changes are found [2].

Histological studies have shown degeneration (mucoid, hyaline) fibrinoid necrosis or pseudocyst change [9, 10].

Currently there is no evidence for acute inflammation [9].

49.2 Tendon Healing

Information about tendon healing is mainly from animal studies. There is, however, limited information about tendon healing processes in degenerative tendons.

The healing process occurs in typical three phases:

49.2.1 Inflammatory Phase

Rupture of the tendon induces a hematoma which activates several chemotactic factors and proinflammatory molecules. Erythrocytes, platelets, neutrophils, monocytes, and macrophages migrate to the ruptured area, and fibroblasts start the synthesis of various components of the extracellular matrix. Chemotactic and vasoactive factors are released following increased vascular permeability activating angiogenesis and tenocytes proliferation. Tenocytes migrate then to the rupture, and type III collagen synthesis is initiated. This phase lasts for up to 5 days [11, 12].

49.2.2 Regenerative Phase

After approximately 5 days, the regenerative phase starts. During this period, type III collagen synthesis is continued. Glycosaminoglycan concentration and water content remain high. This phase lasts up to 6 weeks.

49.2.3 Remodeling Phase

The remodeling phase starts after approximately 6 weeks with decreased cellularity, collagen, and glycosaminoglycan synthesis. The remodeling phase can be divided in two parts: consolidation and maturation phases.

The consolidation stage takes place between 6th and 10th week. During this period, the repair tissue transforms from cellular to fibrous, and

Table 49.1 The three phases of tendon healing

1.	(1–4 days)	Inflammatory phase	Erythrocytes Inflammatory cells (neutrophils)	Vasoactive chemotactic factors are released/ angiogenesis + stimulation of tenocytes
2.	(5 days to 6 weeks)	Regenerative phase	Type III collagen synthesis	High water content and glycosaminoglycan concentration
3.	(6 weeks to 1 year)	Remodeling phase (a) Consolidation phase (6–10 weeks) (b) Maturation phase (10 weeks to 1 year)	Decreased cellularity, collagen, and glycosaminoglycan synthesis	Converting type III collagen into type I collagen

tenocyte metabolism remains high. Tenocytes and collagen fibers follow the direction of stress and become aligned [13].

During this period, the type I collagen synthesis is induced and type III collagen is converted to type I collagen.

After 10 weeks, the maturation phase begins transforming fibrous tissue to scar-like tendon tissue [12]. This process takes up to 1 year. During the second part of this period, both tenocyte metabolism and tendon vascularity decline [14]. Proliferation and migration of tenoblasts initiate the repair process (Table 49.1).

49.3 Limitations of Healing

In animal studies, the healed tendons do not match the structural properties of intact tendons. For example, the spontaneously healed transected sheep Achilles tendons showed tensile strength of 56.7% of intact tendons 1 year after rupture [15] (Fig. 49.1).

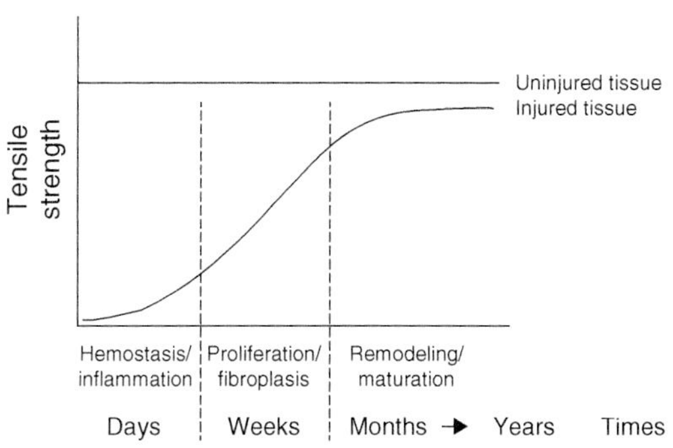

Fig. 49.1 Stress-strain diagram demonstrating the structural properties of a tendon [16]

This could be related to postoperative immobilization and emphasizes the need for early mobilization and adapted strain during rehabilitation phase (Fig. 49.2).

Palmes et al. investigated the effect of immobilization of tendon healing in an animal model. These authors showed that postoperative mobilization resulted in a more rapid restoration of load to failure in comparison with an immobilization group [18].

After 35 days, the mobilized tendons showed equal load to failure compared with the intact tendons.

The immobilized tendon group did not reach a normal load to failure, even after 16 weeks.

After 16 weeks, the mobilized tendon group even regained their original stiffness, whereas the immobilized tendons reached half the amount of stiffness in the same periods of time [18].

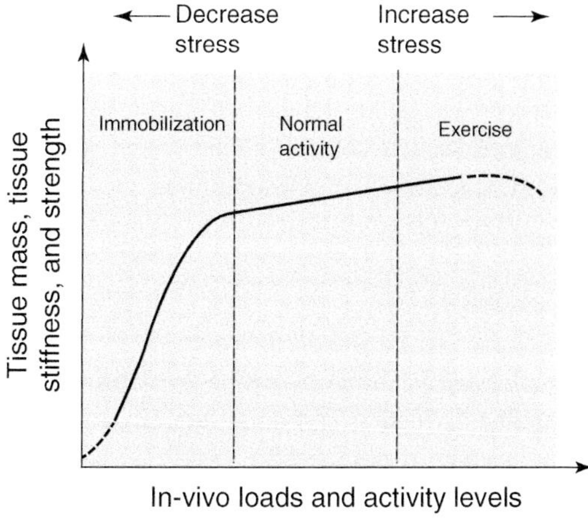

Fig. 49.2 A schematic describing the influence of activity level on the structural properties of tendons and ligaments [17]

Other animal studies have confirmed these results and showed 80–90% restoration of load to failure in ruptured tendons after 12 weeks.

These results from studies in animal models can be transferred into clinical practice for a stage-adapted rehabilitation protocol.

49.4 Rehabilitation Protocol

The goal of an optimized rehabilitation is an individualized compromise between protection of the acutely repaired tendon and prevention of side effects following immobilization, weight-bearing restriction, and general inactivity.

The repaired quadriceps or patellar tendons need protection in the early healing period.

Therefore, the rehabilitation protocol can be divided in two parts:

1. *Early rehabilitation phase*: The primary goal of early rehabilitation is protection of the repair, taking into consideration the primary stability of the fixation before tendon healing. This rehabilitation phase is during the inflammatory and regenerative phases of tendon healing (1 day to 6 weeks, postoperatively).
2. The *late rehabilitation phase* starts approximately 6 weeks after repair during the remodeling phase. During this period, the tendon heals by scar tissue, and the produced collagen fibers must get loaded to induce the remodeling to strong tendon fibers [18, 19]. The second goal of the late rehabilitation phase is to address side effects like muscle hypotrophy and deficits in proprioception, neuromuscular control, balance, and psychological factors like kinesophobia.

Fact Box 1

Rehabilitation should be adapted to the biological healing process of the tendon. It can be divided in early and late rehabilitation phase.

The primary stability of quadriceps or patellar tendon repairs at time zero has been analyzed in biomechanical cadaver studies. A maximum load of approximately 300–800 N depending on the repair technique and rupture configuration was measured [20, 21].

A typical rehabilitation protocol of quadriceps or patellar tendon repair consists of an immobilization in straight-leg brace for 2 weeks followed by a restricted active flexion using a movable brace 2 weeks 0°–0°–30°, 2 weeks 0°–0°–60°, and 2 weeks 0°–0°–90°. The patients partially weight-bear during at least 6 weeks. After 6 weeks, weight-bearing is slowly increased to full weight-bearing after 8–10 weeks.

Other researchers in previous studies recommend a decelerated rehabilitation protocol and immobilize the knee for 4–6 weeks in extension followed by slow increase of range of motion [6, 22, 23].

Marder and Timmerman reported favorable results after accelerated rehabilitation protocol [24]. The patients were allowed to do active flexion to 45° and passive extension to 0° within 1–2 days of surgery.

In conclusion, the rehabilitation includes restriction of weight-bearing, active extension, ROM, and general activity for at least several weeks.

The rehabilitation program should start with isometric muscle exercises and should progress to eccentric training with increasing resistance and weights.

Besides strength rehabilitation, proprioception and neuromuscular training is important.

49.5 Return-to-Sport Criteria (Fig. 49.3)

The risk factors after quadriceps or patellar tendon rupture are twofold.

On the one hand is the compromised tissue strength of the tendon after repair and remodeling with higher risk of rerupture and on the other hand the deficits in muscle strength, proprioception, and neuromuscular control after activity restriction during rehabilitation.

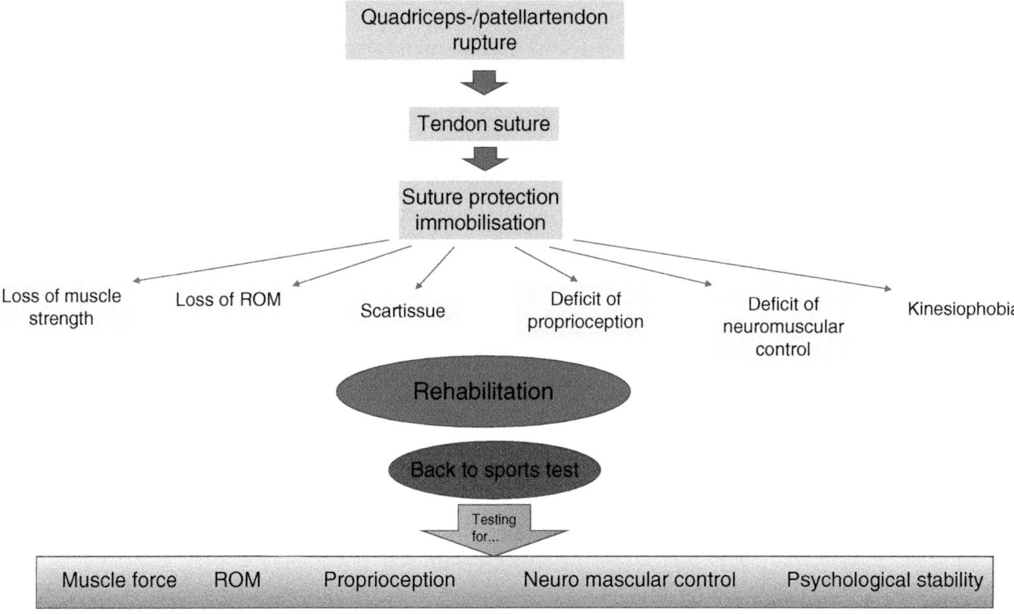

Fig. 49.3 Flowchart showing deficits after tendon rupture and repair and goals of rehabilitation protocols

The time period of healing and remodeling is not yet sufficiently analyzed, but there is some evidence in animal studies that after 12 weeks a stable scar for advanced loading of the tendon has developed [18, 19].

After 6 weeks, slow increase to full weight-bearing is recommended and full weight-bearing after 8 weeks.

Although there is no knowledge about the remodeling time in human tendons, a nearly full loading capacity of the repaired tendon after 4 to 6 months is realistic [18, 19].

Postulating a regular tendon healing, a full loading in sport activity of the tendon after 6–8 months appears to be possible although a remodeling process up to 1 year after rupture can be expected.

Fact Box 2

After regular healing process, return to play after 6–8 months appears to be possible, but a RTP test is highly recommended.

The second important criteria for a safe back-to-sport decision are the general deficits in terms of muscle strength and proprioception of the lower limbs resulting from injury.

The deficits are the same as seen after knee ligament injury and ligament reconstruction (ACL, PCL, etc.):

- Muscle strength
- Proprioception
- Neuromuscular control
- Core stability

49.6 Return-to-Sport Test

Synonymous to other injuries of the lower extremity like ACL rupture, time-related criteria for RTP are not recommended.

The healing process of the ruptured tendon is time depended. Therefor increasing weight-bearing after 6 weeks following regular tendon healing process is supposed to be save. During the next 6 weeks, an increasing loading of the tendon can be done.

The tendon healing process should be monitored by routine clinical investigations.

Muscle strength analysis is an important part of functional evaluation and is important for the decision-making process for RTP.

Muscle strength analysis using an isokinetic measurement is desirable. A test battery like the one presented by Herbst and Hildebrandt et al. can be used to measure muscle deficits [25, 26] (see Chap. 8).

Besides deficits in muscles and strength and neuromuscular control, proprioceptive deficits generally follow after quadriceps or patellar tendon rupture.

The importance of these deficits for RTP decision-making is comparable with ACL ruptures. Moreover, there is a logical connection to the risk for reinjuries after ACL rupture and rehabilitation.

Therefore, a testing battery with analysis of neuromuscular and proprioceptive function is recommended before the patients' return to high-level sport activities like cutting maneuvers and pivoting sports. Testing batteries developed and validated for ACL rupture can be used [25, 26] (see Chap. 8).

49.7 Return to Play and Clinical Results After Patellar Tendon Rupture

Boublik et al. analyzed 24 patellar tendon ruptures in NFL players and reported that one player returned to play after partial patellar tendon rupture missing 12 weeks and another player with a complete tear returned to play after 28 weeks. All other players missed the upcoming or current season [7].

However, in this study, almost 80% of players returned to their previous level of activity.

More than 50% of the players did not show any patellar tendon symptoms upon return to play and no signs of previous tendinopathy either [7].

Kuechle et al. report in collective study of six patellar tendon ruptures in athletes, who were operated on an average of 2.5 days after the injury, good results.

At final follow-up, no patient suffered any knee-related complaints, and all return to previous level of sport activity at an average of 18 months [6].

There were no differences in terms of range of motion or muscular strength compared with the uninjured side.

The rehabilitation protocol included a 6-week plaster cast immobilization and partial weight-bearing. During this period, the patients were allowed to perform isometric quadriceps muscle strengthening. After 6 weeks, they started progressive resistance quadriceps muscle strengthening.

The patients were allowed to perform cutting and pivoting sports at 6 months after surgery.

Fact Box 3
Quadriceps tendon and patellar tendon ruptures in athletes show in literature a high rate of RTP with 80%.

49.8 Return to Play and Clinical Results After Quadriceps Tendon Rupture

Boublik et al. in a case study on NFL (National Football League) players between 1994 and 2004 found 14 quadriceps tendon ruptures in this group [27]. Eleven players suffered total quadriceps tendon rupture while three players suffered from a partial tendon rupture. All patients got surgical treatment with tendon suture. Fifty percent of the players returned to play in regular season NFL games.

De Baere et al. present a study with a mean follow-up of 75 months after quadriceps rupture and repair. The collective of non-sportive patients with a mean age of 58 years presented consistently a quadriceps muscle atrophy. Twelve of 24 patients had normal knee mobility. Three had a flexion deformity of 10°, and two showed a flexion deficit less than 120° [28]. The active knee extension did not show any deficit. Three patients reported about instability of their knee joint. But all patients were subjectively satisfied with the operative result after 75 months. Some patients have been tested with Cybex tests for isokinetic forces and showed approximately a concentric force deficit of 30% for quadriceps muscle and for flexor muscles. The detected deficit of eccentric force was approximately 13% for extensor muscles and 7% for flexor muscles [28].

Take-Home Message

Tendon healing after quadriceps or patellar tendon rupture takes place in three phases: inflammation, proliferation, and remodeling.

The rehabilitation protocol should be adapted to these phases concerning tendon loading, weight-bearing, and patients' mobilization.

There is low evidence about RTP after quadriceps or patellar tendon rupture, but single studies show a high RTP rate of 80% after 6 months.

Performing of a RTP test is highly recommended to analyze functional deficits during rehabilitation process.

Top Five Evidence Based References

Boublik M, Schlegel T, Koonce R, Genuario J, Lind C, Hamming D (2011) Patellar tendon ruptures in national football league players. Am J Sports Med 39:2436–2440

Boublik M, Schlegel TF, Koonce RC, Genuario JW, Kinkartz JD (2013) Quadriceps tendon injuries in national football league players. Am J Sports Med 41:1841–1846

De Baere T, Geulette B, Manche E, Barras L (2002) Functional results after surgical repair of quadriceps tendon rupture. Acta Orthop Belg 68:146–149

Hagglund M, Zwerver J, Ekstrand J (2011) Epidemiology of patellar tendinopathy in elite male soccer players. Am J Sports Med 39:1906–1911

Palmes D, Spiegel HU, Schneider TA, Langer M (2002) Achilles tendon healing: long-term biomechanical effects of postoperative mobilization and immobilization in a new mouse model. J Orthopaed. https://doi.org/10.1016/S0736-0266(02)00032-3

References

1. Rasul T, Fischer DA (1993) Primary repair of quadriceps tendon ruptures: results of treatment, vol 289. Clin Orthop Relat Res, pp 205–207
2. Kannus P, Józsa L (1991) Histopathological changes preceding spontaneous rupture of a tendon – a controlled-study of 891 patients. J Bone Joint Surg Am 73A:1507–1525
3. David HG, Green JT, Grant AJ, Wilson CA (1995) Simultaneous bilateral quadriceps rupture: a complication of anabolic steroid abuse. J Bone Joint Surg Br 77:159–160
4. Konrath GA, Chen D, Lock T, Goitz HT, Watson JT, Moed BR, D'Ambrosio G (1998) Outcomes following repair of quadriceps tendon ruptures. J Orthop Trauma 12:273–279
5. Lee D, Stinner D, Mir H (2013) Quadriceps and patellar tendon ruptures. J Knee Surg Thiem Med Publ 26:301–308
6. Kuechle DK, Stuart MJ (1994) Isolated rupture of the patellar tendon in athletes. Am J Sports Med 22(5):692–695
7. Boublik M, Schlegel T, Koonce R, Genuario J, Lind C, Hamming D (2011) Patellar tendon ruptures in national football league players. Am J Sports Med 39:2436–2440
8. Hagglund M, Zwerver J, Ekstrand J (2011) Epidemiology of patellar tendinopathy in elite male soccer players. Am J Sports Med 39:1906–1911
9. Fredberg U, Bolvig L (2002) Significance of ultrasonographically detected asymptomatic tendinosis in the patellar and achilles tendons of elite soccer players: a longitudinal study. Am J Sports Med 30:488–491
10. Khan KM, Bonar F, Desmond PM, Cook JL, Young DA, Visentini PJ, Fehrmann MW, Kiss ZS, OBrien PA, Harcourt PR, Dowling RJ, OSullivan RM, Crichton KJ, Tress BM, Wark JD (1996) Patellar tendinosis (jumper's knee): findings at histopathologic examination, US, and MR imaging. Radiology 200:821–827
11. James R, Kesturu G, Balian G, Chhabra AB (2008) Tendon: biology, biomechanics, repair, growth factors, and evolving treatment options. J Hand Surg 33:102–112
12. Sharma P, Maffulli N (2005) Basic biology of tendon injury and healing. Surgeon 3:309–316
13. Hooley CJ, Cohen RE (1979) A model for the creep behaviour of tendon. Int J Biol Macromol 1(3):123–132
14. Amiel D, Akeson WH, Harwood FL, Frank CB (1983) Stress deprivation effect on metabolic turnover of the medial collateral ligament collagen. A comparison between nine- and 12-week immobilization. Clin Orthop Relat Res 172:265–270
15. Bruns J, Kampen J, Kahrs J, Plitz W (2000) Achilles tendon rupture: experimental results on spontaneous repair in a sheep-model. Knee Surg Sports Traumatol Arthrosc 8:364–369
16. Gomez M (1995) The physiology and biochemistry of soft tissue healing. In: Griffin L (ed) Rehabilitation of the injured knee, 2nd edn. Mosby Company, St. Louis, MO, pp 34–44
17. Woo S, Gomez MA, Sites TJ, Newton PO, Orlando CA, Akeson WH (1987) The biomechanical and morphological-changes in the medial collateral ligament of the rabbit after immobilization and remobilization. J Bone Joint Surg Am 69A:1200–1211
18. Palmes D, Spiegel HU, Schneider TA, Langer M (2002) Achilles tendon healing: long-term biomechanical effects of postoperative mobilization and

immobilization in a new mouse model. J Orthopaed. https://doi.org/10.1016/S0736-0266(02)00032-3
19. Mass DP, Tuel RJ, Labarbera M, Greenwald DP (1993) Effects of constant mechanical tension on the healing of rabbit flexor tendons. Clin Orthop Relat Res 296:301–306
20. Bushnell BD, Byram IR, Weinhold PS, Creighton RA (2006) The use of suture anchors in repair of the ruptured patellar tendon: a biomechanical study. Am J Sports Med Am Orthopaed Soc Sports Med 34:1492–1499
21. Ettinger M, Dratzidis A, Hurschler C, Brand S, Calliess T, Krettek C, Jagodzinski M, Petri M (2013) Biomechanical properties of suture anchor repair compared with transosseous sutures in patellar tendon ruptures: a cadaveric study. Am J Sports Med Am Orthopaed Soc Sports Med 41:2540–2544
22. Larsen E, Lund PM (1986) Ruptures of the extensor mechanism of the knee-joint – clinical-results and patellofemoral articulation. Clin Orthop Relat Res 213:150–153
23. Siwek CW, Rao JP (1981) Ruptures of the extensor mechanism of the knee joint. J Bone Joint Surg Am 63(6):932–937
24. Marder RA, Timmerman LA (1999) Primary repair of patellar tendon rupture without augmentation. Am J Sports Med 27:304–307
25. Herbst E, Hoser C, Hildebrandt C, Raschner C, Hepperger C, Pointner H, Fink C (2015) Functional assessments for decision-making regarding return to sports following ACL reconstruction. Part II: clinical application of a new test bat. Knee Surg Sports Traumatol Arthrosc 23:1–9
26. Hildebrandt C, Müller L, Zisch B, Huber R, Fink C, Raschner C (2015) Functional assessments for decision-making regarding return to sports following ACL reconstruction. Part I: development of a new test battery. Knee Surg Sports Traumatol Arthrosc 23:1273–1281
27. Boublik M, Schlegel TF, Koonce RC, Genuario JW, Kinkartz JD (2013) Quadriceps tendon injuries in national football league players. Am J Sports Med 41:1841–1846
28. De Baere T, Geulette B, Manche E, Barras L (2002) Functional results after surgical repair of quadriceps tendon rupture. Acta Orthop Belg 68:146–149

Part VI

Concussion

50 Role of Baseline Testing

Philip Schatz

Contents

50.1 Evolution of Baseline Testing

Baseline neurocognitive testing was implemented by Barth and colleagues in the late 1980s [1], in what has been called the landmark "Virginia football study." This was the first multisite study in which college athletes were tested prior to the athletic season, and serially following a concussion, while matched with a non-concussed athlete from the same cohort. Baseline and post-concussion tests were administered using pencil-and-paper (PnP) measures, requiring significant time and resources in the form of trained personnel. This model, or the "Sports as a Laboratory Assessment Model" (or SLAM) [2], was soon adopted by colleges [3, 4] and professional sports leagues [5, 6] (Fig. 50.1).

Along with the increased focus on player safety and use of neuropsychological test measures to supplement clinical evaluation of players with suspected concussions, there was similar growth in the use of personal computers in the 1980s and 1990s. The percentage of US households with a computer rose dramatically across this time period, from only 8.2% in 1984 to 42% in 1998, to 52% in 2000 [7], and finally to 84% in 2013 [8]. As computing devices became more popular, so did the focus on using these devices in clinical assessments, especially since limitations of PnP testing were being recognized. One limitation recognized early in the implementation of "traditional, paper-based" test measures was the inherent practice effects observed when healthy, non-concussed controls completed the measures over several administrations. In fact, researchers documented significant practice effects across only two serial administrations of measures of intelligence in college students [9]. Measurement of reaction time was restricted to the use of stopwatches and, thus, long since recognized as being limited by the subjective response time of the test administrator [10]. This decreases the accuracy of tests which measure timing, as compared to use of electronic timing devices [11]. Computer-based versions of paper-based measures were introduced, with evidence

P. Schatz, Ph.D.
Saint Joseph's University, Philadelphia, PA, USA
e-mail: schatzsju@gmail.com

V. Musahl et al. (eds.), *Return to Play in Football*, https://doi.org/10.1007/978-3-662-55713-6_50

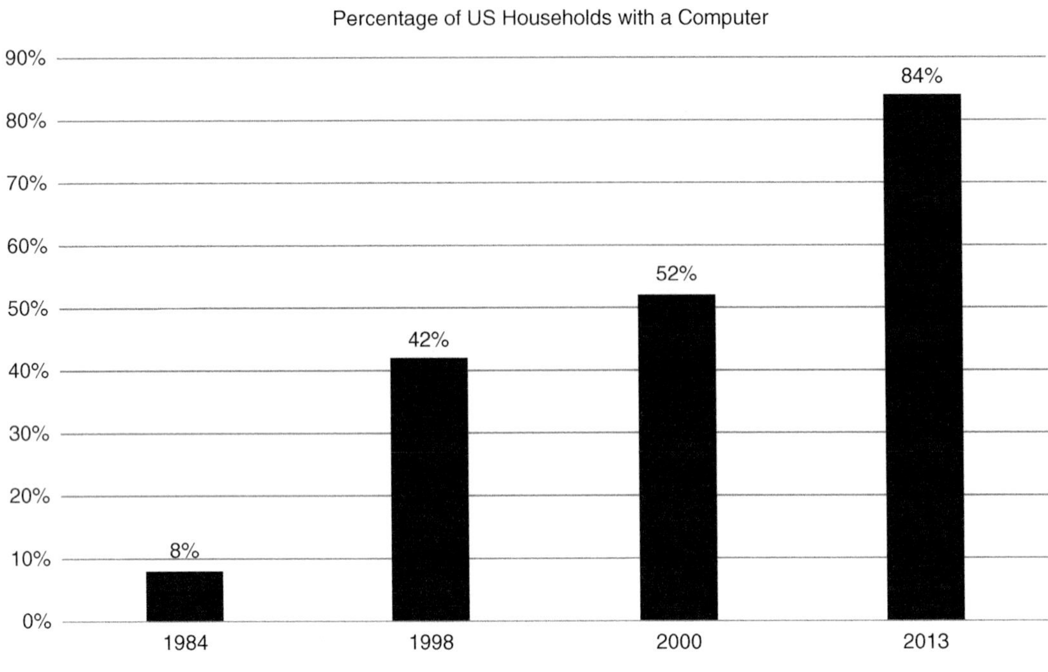

Fig. 50.1 Percentage of US households with a computer, from 1984 to 2013 (Adapted from Newburger [7] and Fine and Ryan [8])

that the computer versions were psychometrically equivalent [12], followed by novel tests developed specifically for computer-based administration. Benefits of computer-based assessment included (1) the freedom to increasingly focus on treatment or qualitative assessment gained by the automation of data collection, (2) more precise measurement of multiple domains of performance (response latency or response time in milliseconds), and more efficient randomization of trials or rapid modification of stimuli [13]. Financially, computer-based assessments were thought to provide cost-benefit gains over traditional administration procedures [14], as well as increased security of test data and patient records through computerized storage [15]. In addition, the time and staffing requirements needed to administer and analyze a battery of PnP measures to a team, school, or league of athletes can be significant, and computer-based measures allow for group administration and automatic scoring. Sports leagues, such as the NFL [16] and NHL [17], included computer-based test measures in their baseline and post-concussion test batteries, and use of computer-based measures has become widespread in high schools and colleges across the United States [18, 19].

50.2 Consensus Expert Views on Baseline Testing

Over the past two decades, there has been increased focus on sports-related concussion, as well as issues regarding the assessment, management, and return to play. In this context, the first of several "Concussion in Sports Group" (CISG) meetings were convened, with a "range of experts" participating in the discussion and drafting of a consensus statement. While the focus of these meetings was broader than the topic of baseline neurocognitive testing, there were discussion and inclusion of recommendations regarding its use. At the first meeting in Vienna in 2001, one of the "overriding principles" recognized as "common to all neuropsychological test batteries" was the "need for and benefit of baseline preinjury testing and serial follow-up" [20]. At that time, neuropsychological assessment was considered to be "one of the cornerstones of concussion evaluation" contributing "significantly" to management of the concussed individual, and baseline testing was "recommended" in order to "maximize the clinical utility" of the neuropsychological assessment.

Fact Box 1

CISG meeting—Vienna, 2001:

- The "need for and benefit of baseline preinjury testing and serial follow-up" is one of the recognized overriding principles common to all neuropsychological test batteries [20].
- Neuropsychological assessment was considered to be "one of the cornerstones of concussion evaluation."
- Neuropsychological assessment contributing "significantly" to management of the concussed individual.
- Baseline testing was "recommended" in order to "maximize the clinical utility" of the neuropsychological assessment.

The CISG convened again in Prague in 2004 and recommended "both a baseline cognitive assessment (such as the Sport Concussion Assessment Tool (SCAT) in the absence of computerized neuropsychological testing) and symptom score" as part of baseline, pre-participation evaluation, especially for participants engaged in "high-risk" sports [21]. In addition, while not specifically related to the "use" of baseline testing, it was noted that severity of concussion could only be determined retrospectively, after symptoms had abated, neurological examination was normal, and "cognitive function has returned to baseline" [22]. The committee acknowledged that athletes may return to baseline on neurocognitive testing while they were still symptomatic but recognized the "need for and benefit of" baseline testing before injury and serial follow-up [21].

Fact Box 2

CISG meeting—Prague, 2004:

- Recommended a baseline cognitive assessment (such as the SCAT) in the absence of computerized neuropsychological testing and also symptom scores as part of baseline, pre-participation evaluation.
  - Especially for participants engaged in "high-risk" sports [23]
- Noted that severity of concussion could only be determined retrospectively, after symptoms had abated, neurological examination was normal, and "cognitive function has returned to baseline" [21].
- Noted that while athletes may return to baseline on neurocognitive testing while they were still symptomatic, there is a "need for and benefit of" baseline testing before injury, and serial follow-up [23] was recognized.

The third CISG meeting took place in Zurich in 2008, and while the focus was not solely on computer-based measures and it was recognized that formal baseline NP screening may be "beyond the resources of many sports or individuals," the CISG again recommended that consideration be given for all participants in high-risk sports to obtain preseason baseline cognitive evaluations [24]. The committee recognized the ongoing cognitive maturity and need for "developmental sensitivity" in assessment measures through the early teen years, limiting the utility of comparing a young athlete's post-concussion data to either normative data or to their own baseline.

Fact Box 3

CISG meeting—Zurich, 2008:

- Formal baseline NP screening may be beyond the resources of many sports leagues or individuals.
- Consideration should be given for all participants in high-risk sports to obtain preseason baseline cognitive evaluations [22].
- Due to ongoing cognitive maturity, there is a need for assessment measures sensitive to development through the early teen years.

At the fourth CISG meeting in Zurich in 2012, baseline neuropsychological testing was considered as "not felt to be required as a mandatory aspect" of every assessment, but it was thought to "be helpful to add useful information to the overall interpretation" of the tests. While baseline testing was thought to provide an "additional educative opportunity for the physician to discuss the significance of this injury with the athlete," the CISG felt there was "insufficient evidence" at the time to recommend the "widespread routine use of baseline neuropsychological testing" [25]. A revision of the SCAT was introduced (the SCAT2), and it was agreed that while "a variety of measures should be employed" as part of a concussion assessment, "important clinical information can be ascertained" through the use of a streamlined multimodal instrument such as the SCAT2, and a "baseline assessment is advised wherever possible."

Fact Box 4

CISG meeting—Zurich, 2012:

- Baseline neuropsychological testing was not considered as mandatory, but it was thought to add useful information to the interpretation of the tests.
- Insufficient evidence at the time to recommend the "widespread routine use of baseline neuropsychological testing" [24].
- SCAT2 introduced a baseline assessment which was advised "wherever possible."

At the fifth CiSG meeting in Berlin in 2016 [26], baseline testing was deemed "useful", but "not necessary for interpreting post-injury scores". The importance of controlling the testing environment was noted, and it was suggested that clinicians "strive to replicate baseline testing conditions" when using baseline test data as a comparator. Given the diversity in availability of economic resources across the globe, baseline or pre-season neuropsychological testing was not felt to be required as a "mandatory aspect of every assessment", but was thought to be "helpful or add useful information" to the interpretation of post-concussion test scores.

Fact Box 5

CISG meeting—Berlin, 2016:

- Baseline testing was deemed "useful", but "not necessary" for interpreting post-injury scores.
- It was recommended that clinicians using baseline test data should "strive to replicate baseline testing conditions".
- Baseline/pre-season testing was not felt to be "required as a mandatory aspect" of every assessment, but "may be helpful or add useful information".

50.3 Reliability Versus Stability of Baseline Testing

Neuropsychological tests have been used as baseline measures of neurocognitive functioning, due to their sensitivity to deficits in attention and concentration, working memory, information processing speed, and reaction time [27–29]. The widely used Immediate Post-concussion Assessment and Cognitive Testing (ImPACT) test battery was developed for the assessment of sports-related concussion in high school, collegiate, and professional athletes [30]. ImPACT is a computer-based program administered via the Internet, which assessed neurocognitive function and concussion symptoms. It consists of a concussion symptom scale, as well as six tests that evaluate attention, working memory, and processing speed. These, in turn, yield composite scores on the areas of verbal memory, visual memory, processing speed, reaction time, and impulse control.

The introduction of baseline and post-injury serial testing of concussed athletes raised immediate questions regarding the temporal stability or test-retest reliability of neuropsychological measures. There has been significant debate regarding the psychometric properties [31, 32], clinical utility [33–35], and ability of baseline testing to reduce risks associated with premature return to play [36]. At the time of Barth et al.'s [1] study, perhaps the greatest concern was that of practice effects, given that "deficits" on post-concussion assessment were identified in concussed athletes in the context of "failure to benefit from repeated administrations," as compared to non-concussed controls [37]. More specifically, non-concussed "matched" controls showed significant improvement on serial assessments, from baseline, whereas concussed athletes showed improvement from baseline but not to the same degree as controls. Among the initial advantages of computer-based neuropsychological assessment was the ability to randomize test stimuli, using multiple test versions, in order to minimize practice effects [30]. It is important to note that while many paper-based measures utilized in early concussion research employed multiple versions, such as the Hopkins Verbal Learning Test (HVLT) and the Brief Visual Motor Test-Revised (BVMT-R), practice effects were still noted using these measures when assessing concussed professional football players [5, 6].

Overt measurement of practice effects involves repeated measures comparison of improvement from baseline (often referred to as Time 1) to post-injury (or Time 2) using a paired sample *t*-test. Test-retest (or practice) effects have been documented in the published literature across intervals as short as 7 days and as long as 2 years (see Table 50.1). Initial evaluation of practice effects with 7 days between assessments, using the ImPACT battery, showed evidence of improvement on the visual motor speed composite score, but not verbal or visual memory or reaction time [38]. Improved performance on visual motor speed has been replicated across intervals of 30 days [39] and 1 year [40], but not 90 days [41] or 2 years [42], suggesting that while athletes may show some improvement in procedural memory or their ability to interact with a computer-based test, there is no commensurate improvement in memory or reaction time performance over time. A lack of evidence of practice effects may be interpreted, as evidence of stability and, thus, reliability.

Traditionally, the reliability of a test measure (specifically temporal stability or test-retest reliability) is often measured using Pearson's product-moment correlation coefficient. Pearson's product-moment correlations are generally thought of as a measure of the strength and direc-

Table 50.1 Comparison of test-retest data from published studies

		Interval between assessments				
Variable		7 days[a]	30 days[b]	90 days[c]	1 year[d]	2 years[e]
Verbal	Time 1	88.7 (9.5)	89.5 (8.8)	89.9 (8.4)	85.6 (9.1)	87.6 (8.3)
Memory	Time 2	88.8 (8.1)	92.5 (7.6)	92.5 (7.6)	86.4 (9.1)	87.8 (9.5)
Visual	Time 1	78.7 (13.4)	69.6 (11.2)	78.8 (13.2)	72.0 (12.7)	75.6 (12.1)
Memory	Time 2	77.5 (12.7)	71.4 (9.8)	82.8 (12.1)	75.5 (14.0)*	78.1 (11.4)
Visual	Time 1	40.5 (7.6)	39.0 (5.8)	40.5 (7.5)	37.5 (6.7)	41.2 (5.9)
Motor speed	Time 2	42.2 (7.1)*	41.8 (6.0)*	41.1 (8.8)	39.8 (6.8)*	42.0 (6.9)
Reaction	Time 1	0.54 (0.09)	0.61 (0.08)	0.55 (07)	0.59 (0.08)	0.54 (0.06)
Time	Time 2	0.54 (0.06)	0.59 (0.06)	0.53 (0.07)	0.57 (0.07)*	0.53 (0.07)

[a]Iverson et al. [38]; $N = 30$; middle school, high school, university
[b]Schatz and Ferris [39]; $N = 25$; university
[c]Miller et al. [41]; $N = 58$; university
[d]Elbin et al. [40]; $N = 369$; high school
[e]Schatz [42]; $N = 95$; university

tion of the relationship or associations between two interval/ratio variables. It is important to note that Pearson's r is considered to be a weak measure of test-retest reliability in situations where (1) coefficients are high and (2) group means are similar, but (3) there is considerable variation in individual scores from Time 1 to Time 2 [43]. For example, research investigating test-retest reliability of immediate repetition of the ImPACT battery [44] revealed that while means from the serial assessments were essentially equivalent (94.5 versus 92.7) with similarly low standard deviations (4.8 versus 5.6), Pearson's correlation coefficient was $r = 0.01$. In this context, given the lack of practice effect but presence of variation within trials, the utility of a correlation coefficient is quite low.

Alternatively, Intraclass Correlation Coefficients (ICCs) have been used as a measure of test-retest reliability. The ICC is considered, by many, as a better measure of association than Pearson's *r*. The ICC was originally developed as a measure of the degree of association of an independent set of raters, for the measurement of inter-rater reliability [45]. In this context, two or more raters are observing the same event, and the ICC measures the agreement of the ratings or observations. Applying ICCs to test-retest reliability treats each assessment and an independent rating of the same event, even though data across assessments may not be identical. However, ICCs are thought to distinguish those sets of scores that are merely ranked in the same order from Time 1 to Time 2 from those that are not only ranked in the same order but are in low, moderate, or complete agreement [46]. Both Pearson's *r* and ICCs have been used as a measure of the reliability of baseline neurocognitive assessments, across intervals ranging from 7 days to 2 years (Table 50.2). A widely accepted classification system for interpreting obtained reliability coefficients identifies a coefficient ≥0.90 as "very high," 0.80–0.89 as "high," 0.70–0.79 as "adequate," 0.60–0.69 as "marginal," and <0.60 as "low," [47], with a 0.70 cutoff often used to denote adequate reliability [48]. As one might expect, coefficients decrease as the time interval increases, and nearly all the time (reaction time and visual motor speed), indices fall above the cutoff of 0.70 within a 1-year range.

Table 50.2 Comparison of Pearson's and intraclass correlation coefficients from published studies

		Interval between assessments				
Variable		7 days[a]	30 days[b]	45 days[c]	1 year[d]	2 years[e]
Verbal memory (ICC)	–	0.79	0.76	0.62	0.46	
	(*r*)	0.70	0.66	–	0.45	0.30
Visual memory	–	0.60	0.72	0.70	0.65	
	(*r*)	0.67	0.43	–	0.55	0.49
Visual motor speed	–	0.88	0.87	0.82	0.74	
	(*r*)	0.86	0.78	–	0.74	0.60
Reaction time	–	0.77	0.67	0.71	0.68	
	(r)	0.79	0.63	–	0.62	0.52

[a]Iverson et al. [38]; $N = 30$
[b]Schatz and Ferris [39]; $N = 25$
[c]Nakayama et al. [49]; $N = 96$
[d]Elbin et al. [40]; $N = 369$
[e]Schatz [42]; $N = 95$

Within the context of serial assessment of an athlete recovering from sport-related concussion, improvement due to practice effects or serial exposure to the test instrument needs to be parsed out, so that the clinician can determine how much improvement has taken place since the time of injury. The psychotherapy literature provided reliable change indices (RCIs), which characterize how much improvement is necessary to establish improvement "beyond chance" [50]. Recognizing that test measures do not have a test-retest reliability of +1.0, the RCU incorporates the test-retest coefficient in the denominator of the ratio between the observed change (numerator) and standard error (denominator), with specific formulas developed to account for practice effects [51]. The RCI places the magnitude of change from Time 1 to Time 2 on a standardized *Z*-score, allowing for identification of cases that fall outside a pre-specified confidence interval (CI), such as 1.28 for an 80% CI, 1.68 for a 90% CI, and 1.96 for a 95% CI. Basic measurement theory tells us that 80% of cases (in a

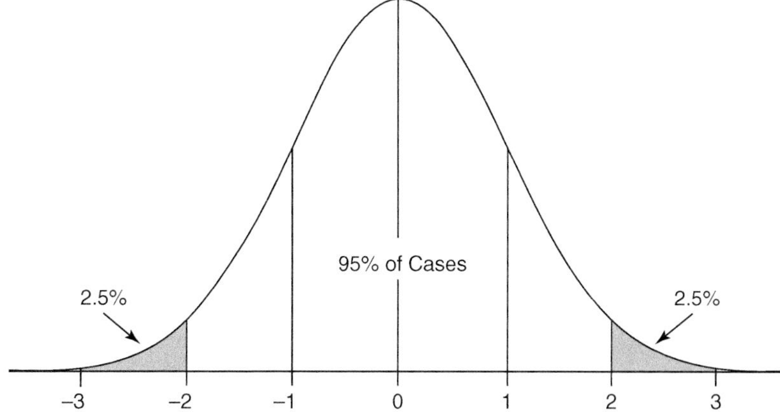

Fig. 50.2 95% confidence interval

Table 50.3 Comparison of rates of decline using reliable change intervals at the 80% CI from published studies

	Interval between assessments			
Variable	7 days[a]	30 days[b]	45 days[c]	1 year[d]
Verbal memory	Δ9/11%	Δ9/0%	Δ12/1%	Δ16/4%
Visual memory	Δ14/11%	Δ14/4%	Δ15/2%	Δ17/3%
Visual motor speed	Δ7/7%	Δ5/4%	Δ7/2%	Δ6/2%
Reaction time	Δ0.06/9%	Δ0.08/4%	Δ0.07/8%	Δ0.09/8%

[a]Iverson et al. [38]; $N = 30$; middle school, high school, university
[b]Schatz and Ferris [39]; $N = 25$; university
[c]Nakayama et al. [49]; $N = 96$; university
[d]Elbin et al. [40]; $N = 369$; high school

normal distribution) should fall within an 80% CI, whereas 20% of cases are expected to fall outside this CI. Using the same logic, 95% of cases should fall within a 95% CI, whereas 5% of cases are expected to fall outside this CI (Fig. 50.2). RCIs also allow for the documentation of the percentage of cases that fall outside the CI as well as the delta or change required to fall outside this interval. Table 50.3 compares four published studies documenting RCI intervals using an 80% CI, across an interval of 7 days to 1 year. There is considerable stability in the delta required for "clinical" change, with some increases noted as the time interval increases. Similarly, Table 50.3 documents the percentage of cases that showed "reliable declines" across the time interval from each study, using an 80% CI. Since these scores can be two-tailed, or bidirectional, one might expect 20% of scores to fall outside an 80% CI, with 10% showing increases (i.e., to the right of the curve) and 10% showing decreases (i.e., to the left of the curve). Rates of "reliable decline" all fall below 10%, except for two scores from the 7-day interval study, demonstrating considerable stability in test scores across "clinically relevant" intervals (i.e., 1 month, 45 days) to longer intervals related to annual baseline assessments.

50.4 Evidence for Baseline Testing Contributing to Return-to-Play Decisions

Traditionally, interpretation of post-injury data, using neuropsychological test batteries, typically involves comparison to normative data. In cases where baseline test data are not available for post-injury comparison, clinicians (e.g., physicians, neuropsychologists, and other sports medicine professionals) would compare a concussed athlete's performance to normative reference values. Early investigations comparing the utility of post-concussion data to baseline data revealed 19%

improved diagnostic accuracy when using neuropsychological test data (83% sensitivity) over subjective symptom reporting (64% sensitivity; see Fig. 50.3) [52]. It is well documented that over 50% of football players participating at the high school [23] and professional levels [53] do not report concussions or concussion-related symptoms. In this regard, in a sample of athletes who were observed to sustain a sport-related concussion, yet denied any post-concussion symptoms, but were suspected of invalid response patterns, neurocognitive testing was shown to have a diagnostic accuracy of 95% [54]. However, these investigations did not systematically evaluate the utility of baseline versus normative comparisons.

Researchers have evaluated the utility of comparing post-concussion neuropsychological data to normative data (i.e., in the absence of baseline data) versus comparing post-concussion data to baseline data. One study comparing post-concussion data to normative cutoffs, versus change from baseline using RCI, concluded that the majority of college athletes who experience clinically meaningful post-concussion cognitive decline can be identified *without* baseline data [55]. Other researchers found mixed results that baseline comparisons identified 2.6× more impaired athletes on simple reaction time performance, whereas normative comparisons identified 7.6× more impaired athletes on mathematical processing [56]. Factors such as history of attention deficit hyperactivity disorder [55] and low or high intellectual capacity [57] have been identified as factors which may moderate post-injury performance. As such, decision-making criteria based on normative comparisons would likely *overlook* a significant change (e.g., from baseline) in high-functioning individuals while overclassifying lower-functioning individuals [58]. Accounting for baseline level of performance by classifying athletes as "above average," "average," or "below average" resulted in significantly fewer "above average" symptomatic concussed athletes being classified as concussed when using

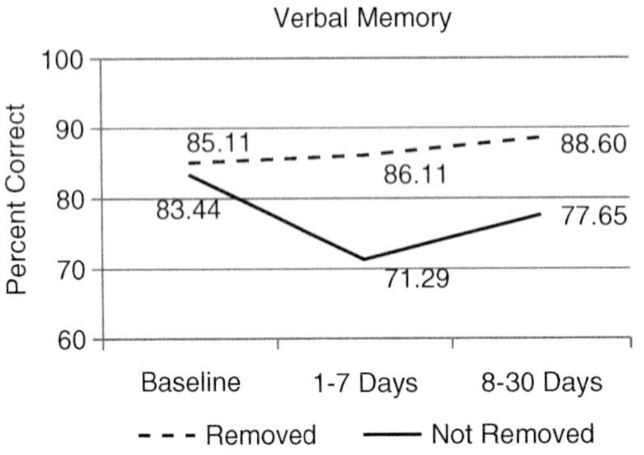

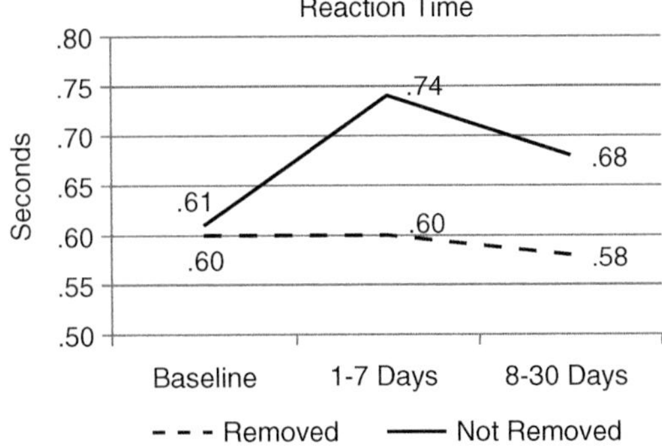

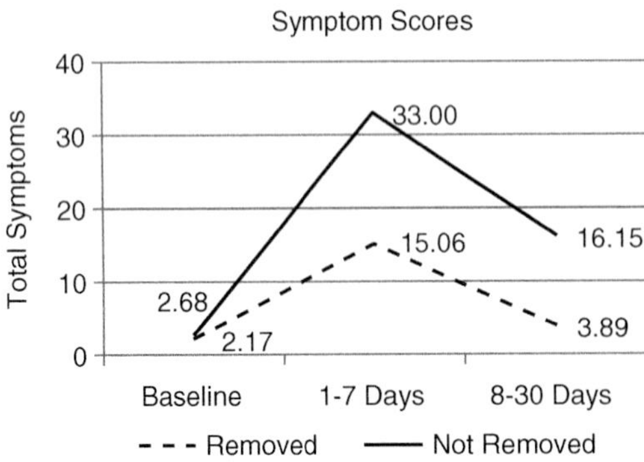

Fig. 50.3 The "value added" of neuropsychological test data over symptom reporting (Adapted from Van Kampen et al. [52])

normative references but significantly more "below average" symptomatic concussed athletes being classified as concussed [59]. However, when using baseline references, these same symptomatic concussed athletes were classified at a similar rate, regardless of whether they were "below average" or "above average."

Fact Box 6

Removal from play:

- Immediate removal for a player with a diagnosed concussion, with no return to play that day [25].
- Delayed removal following suspected sport-related concussion was associated with 14× greater risk of protracted recovery greater than 21 days [60].
- Delayed removal following suspected sport-related concussion was associated with significantly worse neurocognitive performance as compared to their own preinjury baseline [60].

Consensus experts have recommended immediate removal for a player with a diagnosed concussion, with no return to play that day [25]. Delayed removal versus immediate removal from play following suspected sport-related concussion was associated with 14x greater risk of protracted recovery greater than 21 days, as well as significantly worse neurocognitive performance as compared to their own preinjury baseline [60] (see Fig. 50.4). An epidemiological study documenting 1 year of high school concussions revealed that (1) approximately 25% of high school athletes completed preseason, baseline computerized testing and (2) those who completed baseline testing and were then retested after suspected concussion were significantly *less likely* to return to play on the same day or within a week of their injury, as compared to the 75% of concussed athletes who did not complete baseline testing [61]. Computer-based neurocognitive testing is widely used, with 95% of athletic trainers reporting implementation of baseline testing of athletes at high schools and universities in the United States [18] and 96% of those same train-

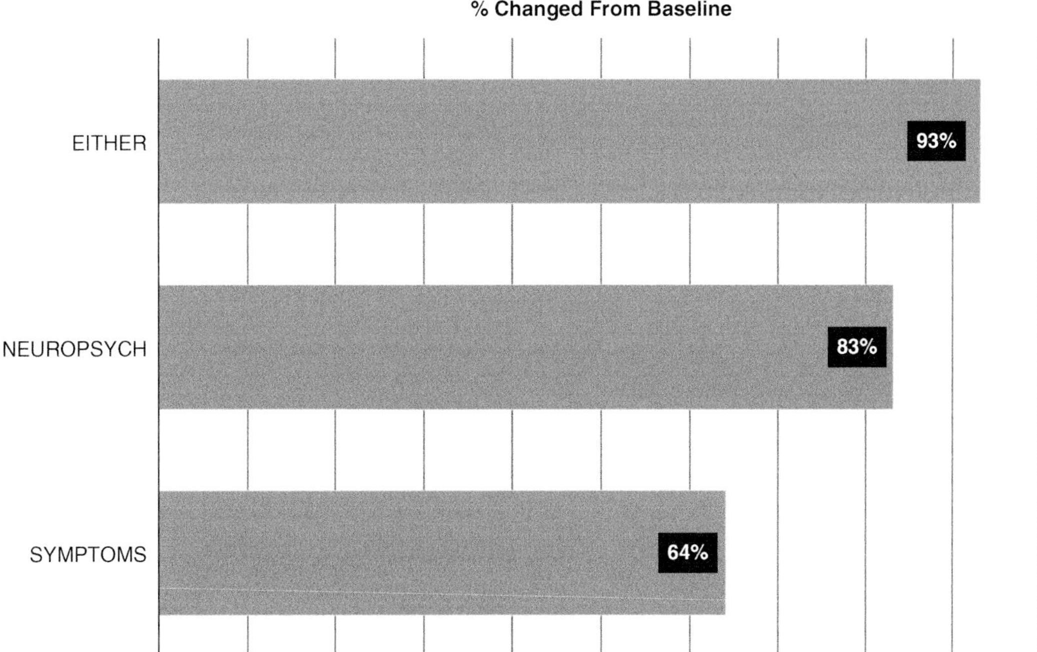

Fig. 50.4 Prolonged symptoms and neurocognitive effects for athletes continuing to play with concussion symptoms (Adapted from Elbin et al. [60])

ers reporting "return to baseline" as a requirement for return to play following a concussion. In fact, nearly 87% reported that they would not return an asymptomatic player back to play if that player had not yet returned to baseline levels of neurocognitive functioning [18].

Take-Home Message

- Baseline neurocognitive testing has been recognized by consensus experts as adding useful information to the overall interpretation of post-concussion test data.
- The reliability of baseline testing has been debated in the literature, but use of reliable change methodologies has demonstrated the stability of baseline testing across intervals of 1 month to 1 year.
- Comparing post-concussion test data to baseline neurocognitive testing has been shown to increase diagnostic accuracy, as opposed to comparing post-concussion test data to normative data, especially for athletes who are above or below average.

Top Five Evidence Based References

Elbin RJ, Schatz P, Covassin T (2011) One-year test-retest reliability of the online version of ImPACT in high school athletes. Am J Sports Med 39(11):2319–2324

Macciocchi SN (1990) 'Practice makes perfect': retest effects in college athletes. J Clin Psychol 46(5):628–631

Miller JR, Adamson GJ, Pink MM, Sweet JC (2007) Comparison of preseason, midseason, and postseason neurocognitive scores in uninjured collegiate football players. Am J Sports Med 35(8):1284–1288

Schatz P, Robertshaw S (2014) Comparing post-concussive neurocognitive test data to normative data presents risks for under-classifying "above average" athletes. Arch Clin Neuropsychol 29(7):625–632

Van Kampen DA, Lovell MR, Pardini JE, Collins MW, Fu FH (2006) The "value added" of neurocognitive testing after sports-related concussion. Am J Sports Med 34(10):1630–1635

References

1. Barth JT, Alves W, Ryan T, Macciocchi SN, Rimel RW, Nelson WE (1989) Mild head injury in sports: neuropsychological sequelae and recovery of function. In: Levin HS, Eisenberg HM, Benton AL (eds) Mild head injury. Oxford University Press, New York, NY, pp 257–275
2. Kelly JC, Amerson EH, Barth JT (2012) Mild traumatic brain injury: lessons learned from clinical, sports, and combat concussions. Rehabil Res Pract 2012:371970
3. Echemendia RJ, Julian LJ (2001) Mild traumatic brain injury in sports: neuropsychology's contribution to a developing field. Neuropsy Rev 11(2):69–88
4. Lovell MR, Collins MW (1998) Neuropsychological assessment of the college football player. J Head Trauma Rehabil 13(2):9–26
5. Lovell MR, Burke CJ (2002) The NHL concussion program. In: Cantu RC (ed) Neurologic athletic head and spine injury. WB Saunders, Philadelphia, pp 32–45
6. Pellman EJ, Lovell MR, Viano DC, Casson IR, Tucker AM (2004) Concussion in professional football: neuropsychological testing—part 6. Neurosurgery 55(6):1290–1303. discussion 1303–1295
7. Newburger EC (2001) Current population reports: home computers and Internet use in the United States, August 2000. U.S. Department of Commerce, US Census Bureau, Washington, DC
8. Fine T, Ryan C (2014) Computer and Internet use in the United States: 2013. American community survey reports, vol ACS-28. U.S. Census Bureau, Washington, DC
9. Macciocchi SN (1990) 'Practice makes perfect': retest effects in college athletes. J Clin Psychol 46(5):628–631
10. Rumberger EK (1927) The accuracy of timing with the stop watch. J Exp Psychol 10(1):60–61
11. Hetzler RK, Stickley CD, Lundquist KM, Kimura IF (2008) Reliability and accuracy of handheld stopwatches compared with electronic timing in measuring sprint performance. J Strength Cond Res 22(6):1969–1976
12. Campbell KA, Rohlman DS, Storzbach D, Binder LM, Anger WK, Kovera CA, Davis K, Grossmann S (1999) Test-retest reliability of psychological and neurobehavioral tests self-administered by computer. Assessment 6:21–32
13. APA (1986) Guidelines for computer-based tests and interpretations. American Psychological Association, Washington, DC
14. French CC, Beaumont JG (1987) The reaction of psychiatric patients to computerized assessment. Br J Clin Psychol 26(4):267–277
15. Barak A (1999) Psychological applications on the Internet: a discipline on the threshold of a new millennium. Appl Prevent Psychol 8(4):231–245
16. Pellman EJ, Lovell MR, Viano DC, Casson IR (2006) Concussion in professional football: recovery of NFL and high school athletes assessed by computerized neuropsychological testing—part 12. Neurosurgery 58(2):263–274. discussion 263–274
17. Echemendia RJ, Bruce JM, Meeuwisse W, Comper P, Aubry M, Hutchison M (2016) Long-term reliability of ImPACT in professional ice hockey. Clin Neuropsychol 30(2):328–337
18. Covassin T, Elbin RJ III, Stiller-Ostrowski JL, Kontos AP (2009) Immediate post-concussion assessment and cognitive testing (ImPACT) practices of sports

medicine professionals. J Athl Train 44(6):639–644
19. Kerr ZY, Snook EM, Lynall RC, Dompier TP, Sales L, Parsons JT, Hainline B (2015) Concussion-related protocols and preparticipation assessments used for incoming student-athletes in national collegiate athletic association member institutions. J Athl Train 50(11):1174–1181
20. Aubry M, Cantu R, Dvorak J, Graf-Baumann T, Johnson K, Kelly J, Lovell M, McCrory P, Meeuwisse W, Schamasch P (2002) Summary and agreement statement of the first international conference on concussion in sport, Vienna 2001. Sports Med Alert 8(3):17–19
21. McCrory P, Johnston K, Meeuwisse W, Aubry M, Cantu R, Dvorak J et al (2004) Summary and agreement statement of the 2nd international conference on concussion in sport, Prague. Br J Sports Med 29:196–204
22. McCrory P, Matser E, Cantu R, Ferrigno M (2004) Sports neurology. Lancet Neurol 3(7):435–440
23. McCrea M, Hammeke T, Olsen G, Leo P, Guskiewicz K (2004) Unreported concussion in high school football players: implications for prevention. Clin J Sport Med 14(1):13–17
24. McCrory P, Meeuwisse W, Johnston K, Dvorak J, Aubry M, Molloy M, Cantu R (2009) Consensus statement on concussion in sport – the 3rd international conference on concussion in sport, held in Zurich, November 2008. J Clin Neurosci 16(6):755–763
25. McCrory P, Meeuwisse WH, Aubry M, Cantu B, Dvorak J, Echemendia RJ, Engebretsen L, Johnston K, Kutcher JS, Raftery M, Sills A, Benson BW, Davis GA, Ellenbogen RG, Guskiewicz K, Herring SA, Iverson GL, Jordan BD, Kissick J, McCrea M, McIntosh AS, Maddocks D, Makdissi M, Purcell L, Putukian M, Schneider K, Tator CH, Turner M (2013) Consensus statement on concussion in sport: the 4th international conference on concussion in sport held in Zurich, November 2012. Br J Sports Med 47(5):250–258
26. McCrory P, Meeuwisse W, Dvořák J et al (2017) Consensus statement on concussion in sport – the 5th international conference on concussion in sport held in Berlin, October 2016. Br J Sports Med 51:838–847
27. Schatz P, Zillmer EA (2003) Computer-based assessment of sports-related concussion. Appl Neuropsy 10(1):42–47
28. Rimel RW, Giordani B, Barth JT, Boll TJ, Jane JA (1981) Disability caused by minor head injury. Neurosurgery 9(3):221–228
29. Collins MW, Grindel SH, Lovell MR, Dede DE, Moser DJ, Phalin BR, Nogle S, Wasik M, Cordry D, Daugherty KM, Sears SF, Nicolette G, Indelicato P, McKeag DB (1999) Relationship between concussion and neuropsychological performance in college football players. JAMA 282(10):964–970
30. Maroon JC, Lovell MR, Norwig J, Podell K, Powell JW, Hartl R (2000) Cerebral concussion in athletes: evaluation and neuropsychological testing. Neurosurgery 47(3):659–669. discussion 669–672
31. Mayers LB, Redick TS (2012) Clinical utility of ImPACT assessment for postconcussion return-to-play counseling: psychometric issues. J Clin Exp Neuropsychol 34(3):235–242
32. Schatz P, Kontos A, Elbin R (2012) Response to Mayers and Redick: "clinical utility of ImPACT assessment for postconcussion return-to-play counseling: psychometric issues". J Clin Exp Neuropsychol 34(4):428–434. discussion 435–442
33. Lovell MR (2006) Letters to the editor. J Athl Train 41(2):137–140
34. Randolph C (2006) Letters to the editor. J Athl Train 41(2):138–140
35. Randolph C, McCrea M, Barr WB (2005) Is neuropsychological testing useful in the management of sport-related concussion? J Athl Train 40(3):139–152
36. Randolph C (2011) Baseline neuropsychological testing in managing sport-related concussion: does it modify risk? Curr Sports Med Rep 10(1):21–26
37. Macciocchi SN, Barth JT, Alves W, Rimel RW, Jane JA (1996) Neuropsychological functioning and recovery after mild head injury in collegiate athletes. Neurosurgery 39(3):510–514
38. Iverson GL, Lovell MR, Collins MW (2003) Interpreting change on ImPACT following sport concussion. Clin Neuropsychol 17(4):460–467. https://doi.org/10.1076/clin.17.4.460.27934
39. Schatz P, Ferris CS (2013) One-month test-retest reliability of the ImPACT test battery. Arch Clin Neuropsychol 28(5):499–504
40. Elbin RJ, Schatz P, Covassin T (2011) One-year test-retest reliability of the online version of ImPACT in high school athletes. Am J Sports Med 39(11):2319–2324
41. Miller JR, Adamson GJ, Pink MM, Sweet JC (2007) Comparison of preseason, midseason, and postseason neurocognitive scores in uninjured collegiate football players. Am J Sports Med 35(8):1284–1288
42. Schatz P (2010) Long-term test-retest reliability of baseline cognitive assessments using ImPACT. Am J Sports Med 38(1):47–53
43. Rodgers JL, Nicewander WA (1998) Thirteen ways to look at the correlation coefficient. Am Stat 42:59–66
44. Schatz P, Cameron N (2011) The effects of technology-related and software-related factors on neurocognitive baseline test performance using ImPACT. Arch Clin Neuropsychol 26:521
45. Bartko JJ (1966) The intraclass correlation coefficient as a measure of reliability. Psychol Rep 19(1):3–11
46. Chicchetti DV (1994) Guidelines, criteria, and rules of thumb for evaluating normed and standardized assessment instruments in psychology. Psychol Assess 6(4):294–290
47. Slick DJ (2006) Psychometrics in neuropsychological assessment. In: Strauss E, Sherman E, Spreen O (eds) A compendium of neuropsychological tests. Oxford University Press, New York, NY
48. Baumgartner TA, Chung H (2001) Confidence limits for intraclass reliability coefficients. Meas Phys Educ Exerc Sci 5:179–188
49. Nakayama N, Covassin T, Schatz P, Nogle S, Kovan J (2014) Examination of test-retest reliability of a com-

puterized neurocognitive test battery. Am J Sports Med 6(42):2000–2005
50. Jacobson NS, Truax P (1991) Clinical significance: a statistical approach to defining meaningful change in psychotherapy research. J Consul Clin Psych 59(1):12–19
51. Chelune GJ, Naugle RI, Lüders H, Sedlak J, Awad IA (1993) Individual change after epilepsy surgery: practice effects and base-rate information. Neuropsychology 7:41–52
52. Van Kampen DA, Lovell MR, Pardini JE, Collins MW, Fu FH (2006) The "value added" of neurocognitive testing after sports-related concussion. Am J Sports Med 34(10):1630–1635
53. SportingNews (2012) NFL concussion poll: 56 percent of players would hide symptoms to stay on field. http://aol.sportingnews.com/nfl/story/2012-11-11/nfl-concussions-hide-symptoms-sporting-news-midseason-players-poll. Accessed 4 Dec 2012
54. Schatz P, Sandel N (2013) Sensitivity and specificity of the online version of ImPACT in high school and collegiate athletes. Am J Sports Med 41(2):321–326
55. Echemendia RJ, Bruce JM, Bailey CM, Sanders JF, Arnett P, Vargas G (2012) The utility of post-concussion neuropsychological data in identifying cognitive change following sports-related MTBI in the absence of baseline data. Clin Neuropsychol 26(7):1077–1091
56. Schmidt JD, Register-Mihalik JK, Mihalik JP, Kerr ZY, Guskiewicz KM (2012) Identifying Impairments after concussion: normative data versus individualized baselines. Med Sci Sport Exer 44(9):1621–1628
57. Rabinowitz AR, Arnett PA (2012) Reading based IQ estimates and actual premorbid cognitive performance: discrepancies in a college athlete sample. J Int Neuropsy Soc 18(1):139–143
58. Lezak MD (2004) Neuropsychological assessment. Oxford University Press, New York, NY
59. Schatz P, Robertshaw S (2014) Comparing post-concussive neurocognitive test data to normative data presents risks for under-classifying "above average" athletes. Arch Clin Neuropsychol 29(7):625–632
60. Elbin RJ, Sufrinko A, Schatz P, French J, Henry L, Burkhart S, Collins MW, Kontos AP (2016) Removal from play after concussion and recovery time. Pediatrics 138(3). https://doi.org/10.1542/peds.2016-0910
61. Meehan WP III, d'Hemecourt P, Comstock RD (2010) High school concussions in the 2008–2009 academic year: mechanism, symptoms, and management. Am J Sports Med 38(12):2405–2409

51 Multimodal Concussion Assessment

Alicia Sufrinko, Daniel Charek, and Brandon Gillie

Contents

A. Sufrinko (✉) • D. Charek • B. Gillie
Sports Concussion Program, Department of Orthopedic Surgery, University of Pittsburgh Medical Center, 3200 S. Water St., Pittsburgh, PA 15203, USA
e-mail: sufrinkoam@upmc.edu

51.1 Introduction

The rate of football-related concussions treated in emergency departments has increased significantly across the past 20 years [1]. Concussion risk is particularly high in female football players [2], especially compared to concussion rates in other female sports [3, 4]. Concussion was defined as a "complex pathophysiological process affecting the brain, induced by biomechanical forces" in the most recent consensus statement on concussion in sports [5]. Concussion is a heterogenous injury that results in a myriad of physical, cognitive, and emotional symptoms and diverse functional impairments (e.g., cognitive, balance, vestibular-ocular) that often manifest in clinical profiles or subtypes that dictate treatment and return to play recommendations [6]. As such, it is important that concussion assessment involves a comprehensive, multimodal battery assessing domains of functioning, including neurocognitive, vestibular, postural stability, oculomotor, and physical exertion tolerance [7]. Many studies have demonstrated that a multimodal or multifaceted test battery is more sensitive than any stand-alone measures in identifying concussion [8–10] and diverse deficits resolve at differing time intervals [11]. Further, a multimodal assessment battery has demonstrated good utility in predicting recovery duration [12]. Certain impairments can evolve or worsen in the days following injury [13], further highlighting the importance of serial or repeat assessment prior to return to play (RTP).

V. Musahl et al. (eds.), *Return to Play in Football*, https://doi.org/10.1007/978-3-662-55713-6_51

51.2 Concussion Diagnosis and Sideline Assessment

Initially, the primary goal of concussion assessment is to identify and accurately diagnose the head injury. Expert consensus for best practice is unanimous in stating all athletes should be removed from play immediately following concussion [5]. Concussions should be diagnosed as soon as possible, to remove the player from the game immediately to prevent further injury and facilitate faster recovery [14]. In some situations, minimal standardized sideline testing is required to diagnose concussion, as overt signs of injury are present, including loss of consciousness, staggering gait, and clear confusion or disorientation. However, a majority of the time, the signs and symptoms of injury are more ambiguous, and brief standardized sideline assessment tools may be used to further clarify diagnosis. The most commonly used sideline tool is the SCAT3, which can be used in athletes 13 years and older and available for public use. Recent review [15] and clinically relevant metrics of the measure [16], including details on sensitivity and normative data in healthy controls, are available elsewhere [15, 16]. This tool includes evaluation of symptoms, cognitive screening, balance examination, neck examination, and coordination examination.

51.3 The Multimodal Battery Administered by a Multidisciplinary Assessment Team

Although sideline assessments can be useful in injury diagnosis, evidence suggests that such assessments are insensitive to identifying deficits in balance beyond 3–5 days and mental status beyond 48 h and should not be relied on for RTP decisions [17, 18]. Once a concussion is diagnosed, it is vital to implement follow-up management to reduce premature RTP, as repeat injury without adequate recovery time is thought to contribute to poor outcomes [19]. Comprehensive evaluation (see Fig. 51.5) through concussion-specialty clinics is becoming more widely appreciated, particularly as clinicians have begun to better understand the diverse nature of concussion symptoms and the possibility of distinct treatment pathways [7, 20]. Ideally, concussion assessment should be implemented in the context of a multidisciplinary team, with team/sports medicine physicians, neuropsychologists, certified athletic trainers, and physical therapists all playing a potential role in the RTP decision for a concussed athlete. For example, neuropsychologists specialize in interpreting cognitive testing post injury, an important assessment component of post-concussion testing. However, many patients will benefit from working with a skilled vestibular therapist or require medication management with a headache specialist. Because it is not always feasible to have a multidisciplinary team evaluate a patient at initial point of contact due to resources (e.g., specialist availability, healthcare costs), many providers rely on using screening tests to determine when referral to other providers is warranted.

Fact Box 1

Research studies suggest that multimodal test batteries have shown high sensitivity (77–100%) in identifying concussion compared to stand-alone measures (<50% sensitivity) due to the heterogenous nature of the injury.

Fact Box 2

Multimodal assessment batteries can predict recovery duration and identify which treatment modalities may be most beneficial for the athlete.

51.4 Components of a Multimodal Concussion Assessment Battery

51.4.1 Symptom Reporting

51.4.1.1 Standardized Symptom Scales

An individual's subjective report of concussion symptoms is the foundation of concussion diagnosis and evaluation. As assessment procedures have evolved, standardized measures of concussion symptoms that demonstrate sound psychometric properties and clinical prognostic utility have emerged and supplemented detailed clinical interviews. There are several different scales that have empirical support for use in children ages 5–19, some of which include parent/teacher report. The content of these instruments often reflects the diverse nature of concussion symptoms, though all self-report scales contain items that assess physical and cognitive symptoms. A recent factor analysis of the Post-Concussion Symptom Scale, one of the most widely used self-report symptom assessment tools, revealed symptom reports for a group of recently concussed athletes that were comprised of a 4-factor solution that included cognitive-fatigue-migraine, affective, somatic, and sleep symptoms [21]. Of note these results also found that throughout the first week of injury, a global cognitive-fatigue-migraine presentation is predominant, with fatigue, cognitive, migraine-related and vestibular-based symptoms occurring in combination [21]. These results, coupled with emerging research suggesting that concussion may exhibit clinical profiles and recovery trajectories [7], highlight the need for clinicians to regularly utilize symptom scales to assess changes in symptom presentation that may occur as injuries transition from acute to subacute to potentially chronic phases.

From a clinical perspective, symptom reports are also useful as prognostic indicators of recovery and as instruments that can help inform the need for targeted and focused treatment plans. For example, evidence suggests that football players who experienced dizziness on the field at the time of injury on average took 21 days longer to recover than those players who did not [22]. Similarly, the presence of other specific symptoms, including post-traumatic migraine [23], has also been associated with delayed recovery. However, it is also worth noting that initial symptom burden plays an important role, as several studies have linked greater initial symptom scores with longer duration of symptoms (>28 days), even after accounting for other confounds such as age, sex, history of previous concussion/migraine, neurocognitive test performance, amnesia, and loss of consciousness at the time of injury [24, 25].

51.4.1.2 Aerobic/Exertion Tolerance and Symptom Provocation

During concussion recovery, many athletes become asymptomatic when resting or lowly exertive but experience provocation of symptoms with physical activity. As such, being "asymptomatic" with physical activity is necessary to be considered "recovered" and consequently a component of international RTP criteria [5]. However, it can be argued that exertion testing does not need to be reserved only for a measure of recovery provided by the growing support for physical activity as a treatment modality following concussion [26]. Authors have suggested that serial assessment of exertion tolerance and symptom provocation with physical activity can be helpful in both determining recovery status [27] and also identifying patients who would benefit from treatment, such as exertion therapy [7]. At present, the field is lacking validated, comprehensive assessments to evaluate exertional tolerance. Graded aerobic treadmill testing has preliminary support [28], although this test only evaluates aerobic exercise tolerance rather than dynamic movement or sport-specific exertional demands [7]. Our group has developed a structured exertion evaluation that includes aerobic testing, dynamic exercises (e.g., push-ups, extended twist and pull) (Fig. 51.1), as well as noncontact sport-specific

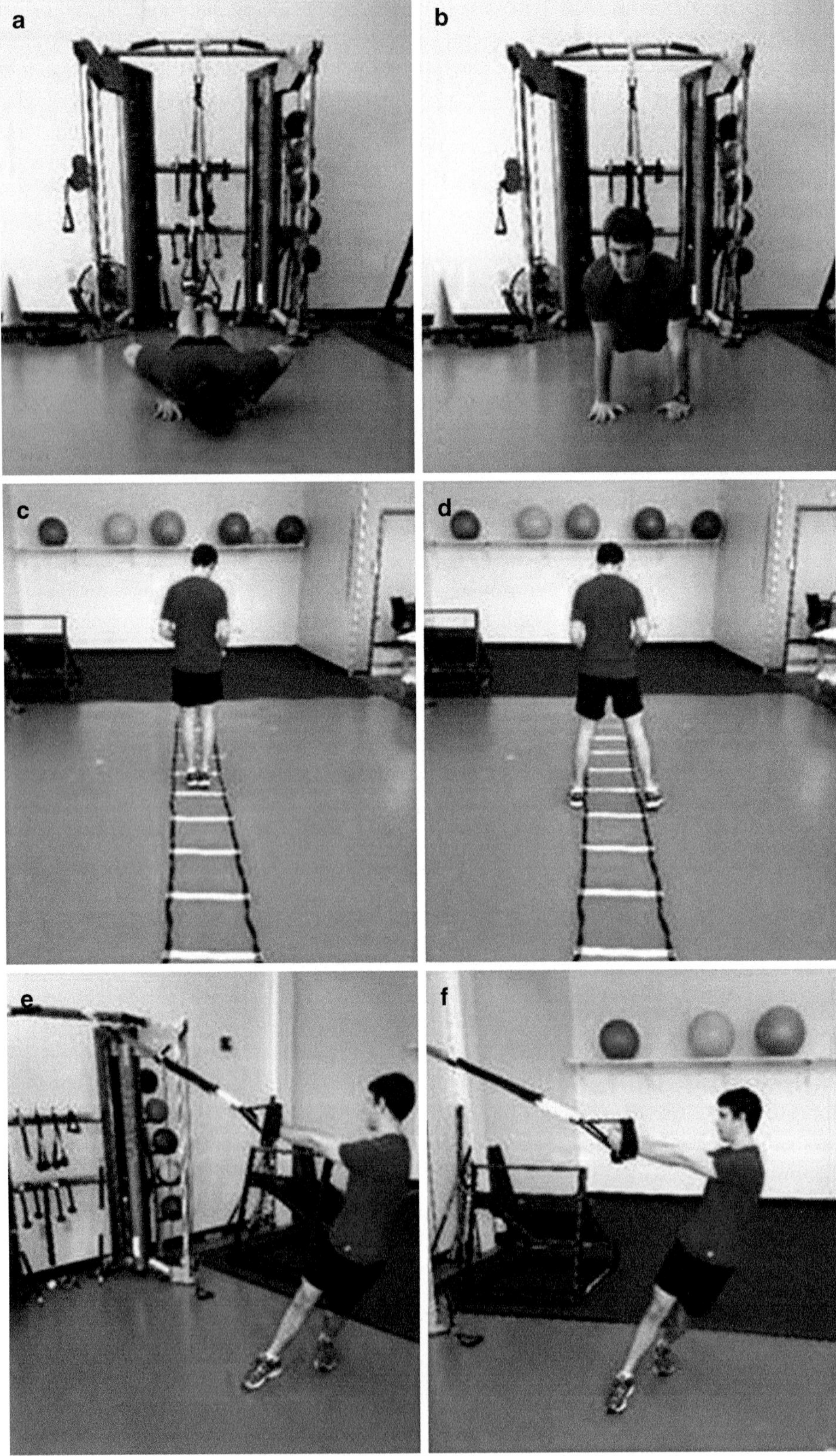

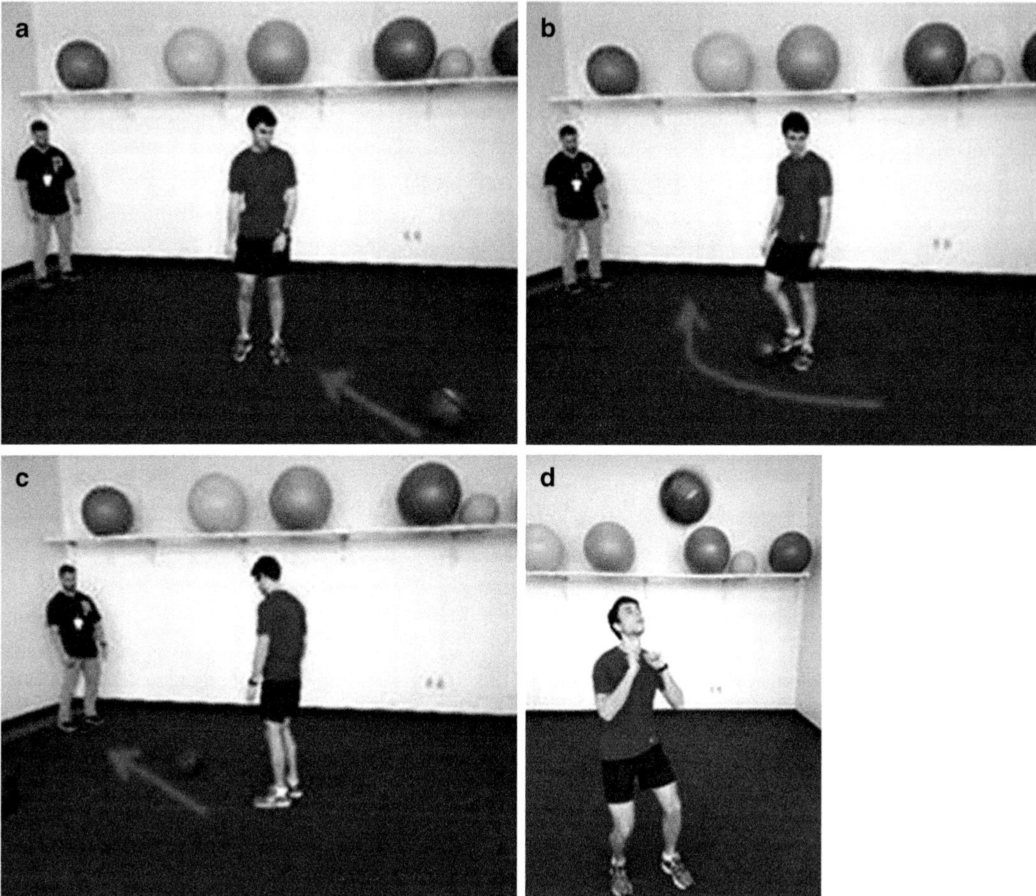

Fig. 51.2 Exit clearance test for concussion—football-specific exercises. (**a**) Receive pass, (**b**) trap ball and turn, (**c**) pass ball, (**d**) heading the ball. Note: steps A–C are repeated several times in a quick, fluid motion

drills (e.g., passing, headers) (Fig. 51.2), although further research is necessary prior to routine use. At this point, experienced athletic trainers, and sometimes physical therapists, often rely on progressive or stepwise return to play protocols [29] that assess symptom provocation but may also be therapeutic to recovery. These protocols lack empirical support despite widespread use.

51.4.2 Neurocognitive Testing

Neurocognitive testing has long played an important role in concussion management, starting with the use of traditional paper and pencil neuropsychological test batteries (i.e., P&P) to more recently developed computerized neurocognitive testing (i.e., CNT). Typically, neurocognitive testing is completed in an office setting and has

Fig. 51.1 Exit clearance test for concussion—non-sport-specific exercises. (**a**, **b**) Push-up with elevated feet, (**c**, **d**) floor ladder agility drill, (**e**, **f**) extended twist and pull. Note: Cardiovascular exercises including treadmill workout not pictured

been shown to be sensitive to deficits acutely (e.g., <24 h following injury) and may detect deficits after an athlete is symptom-free [30–32]. A recent meta-analysis of computerized neurocognitive testing found that concussion had a low to moderate effect on neurocognitive functioning, with variability in effect size attributed to the complex and individualized nature of concussion [33]. CNTs developed for concussion are considered screening tests and can be used by a variety of healthcare professionals with appropriate test-specific training. However, administering and interpreting P&P testing require the expertise of a clinical neuropsychologist. It is important to recognize that extraneous factors such as motivation, effort, sleep, pain, and anxiety can influence neurocognitive test performance [34]. With this in mind, neuropsychologists should play a role in concussion management whenever possible, and it is essential that clinicians maintain up-to-date knowledge regarding neurocognitive assessment, including the strengths and limitations of different testing modalities (i.e., P&P vs. CNT) and specific instruments.

The two modalities of neurocognitive testing have different strengths and weaknesses (see Table 51.1). For example, the use of P&P testing allows for a more flexible, task-specific approach and permits assessment of auditory-based (i.e., nonvisual) tasks as well as observations of test-taking behavior and overall functioning. However, P&P testing tends to be more time intensive, subject to administration/scoring errors, and less sensitive to acute neurocognitive changes in comparison with CNT [8]. On the other hand, CNT tends to be brief, practical, and easily repeatable while also offering standardized administration/scoring. Additionally, CNT has the added benefit of being able to more precisely detect and measure reaction time and processing speed performance [35]. However, given that CNT is more easily administered, it is possible that they exhibit a greater potential for misuse and misinterpretation by underqualified individuals. Both modalities may face a similar challenge in demonstrating adequate test-retest reliability, a fundamental property of neuropsychological tests, with some evidence suggesting that the two approaches have

Table 51.1 Comparison of paper and pencil and computerized neurocognitive testing

	Paper and pencil neurocognitive testing	Computerized neurocognitive testing
Advantages	• Larger normative databases • Test selection flexibility • Can assess neurocognitive functioning in multiple modalities (e.g., auditory and visual)	• Relatively brief • Precise assessment of subtle differences on speeded measures (e.g., reaction time) • Can be administered by a variety of providers, rather than strictly neuropsychologists • Baseline data can be efficiently obtained • Alternate forms reduce practice effects • Rapid computerized scoring • Centralized data repositories are easily accessible
Disadvantages	• Time intensive • Labor intensive • Greater inter-examiner administration and scoring variability • Certain relevant domains not easily assessed (e.g., reaction time) • Shorter time range for sensitivity	• Concerns regarding psychometric properties • Greater potential for misuse (e.g., interpretation by underqualified individuals) • Less direct observation/supervision of examinees performance
Battery/test examples	• NHL Paper and Pencil Battery – Hopkins Verbal Learning Test (HVLT) – Brief Visuospatial Memory Test-Revised (BVMT-R) – Controlled Oral Word Association Test (COWAT) – Color Trail Making Test – PSU Symbol Cancellation Task – Symbol Digit Modalities Test (SDMT)	• Immediate Post-Concussion Assessment and Cognitive Testing (ImPACT) • Automated Neurocognitive Assessment Metrics (ANAM) • Axon Sports Computerized Cognitive Assessment Tool • Concussion Vital Signs (CVS) • HeadMinder CRI

similar test-retest reliability when considering cognitive domain being tested [36], whereas others have expressed concerns about the reliability of CNT, in particular [37, 38]. Although CNT is becoming more utilized than P&P testing, authors of recent review articles have speculated that a hybrid approach that combines both modalities, such as the one currently employed by the National Hockey League, may maximize the strengths and minimize the weaknesses of both approaches [34]. While non-neuropsychologists, such as physicians and certified athletic trainers, can be trained to use cognitive screening tests (e.g., CNT), a neuropsychologist will always need to be consulted in cases wherein more extensive neuropsychological testing is warranted [39].

51.4.2.1 Computerized Neurocognitive Testing (CNT)

Among the many CNTs available, the Immediate Post-Concussion Assessment and Cognitive Testing Test Battery (ImPACT) is the most widely used and researched. ImPACT is a computerized neurocognitive assessment tool that requires approximately 20–25 min to complete and is suitable for ages 10–59. The test battery consists of six individual test modules that measure aspects of cognitive functioning including attention, memory, reaction time, and processing speed. Each test module contributes to one or more composite scores (i.e., verbal memory, visual memory, visual motor speed, and reaction time) that are used to summarize an individual's overall performance. In addition, ImPACT contains an embedded Post-Concussion Symptom Scale [40], a 22-item measure of common concussive symptoms (e.g., headache, dizziness, nausea, etc.), which individuals complete prior to and following completion of neurocognitive testing. The ImPACT test battery has been shown to have good psychometric properties, with several studies demonstrating its concurrent validity, test-retest reliability, and diagnostic sensitivity and specificity [41]. Also of importance is that ImPACT appears to have significant clinical utility. For example, an individual's pattern of performance acutely can predict length of recovery [42].

A number of other used CNTs include Concussion Vital Signs (CNS Vital Signs, LLC, 2012) and the Concussion Resolution Index (CRI), also known as HeadMinder [43]. The CRI is a Web-based computerized neuropsychological assessment battery comprised of subtests that assess memory, reaction time, speed of decision making, and speed of information processing. Similarly, CNS Vital Signs is a computerized neurocognitive test battery that consists of well-known neuropsychological tests including verbal and visual memory, finger tapping, symbol digit coding, the Stroop test, a test of shifting attention, and the continuous performance test. Both CNTs have evidenced adequate levels of reliability, validity, and sensitivity in terms of identifying sports-related concussion (see Table 51.1) [8, 44, 45].

51.4.3 Neuromotor Functioning

51.4.3.1 Vestibular/Balance

The vestibular system is a complex sensorimotor system linking inner ear sensory organs with central nervous system processing areas. Input from the vestibular system is utilized in coordinating gaze, stabilizing eye movements (vestibulo-ocular reflex), and regulating muscular responsivity in order to maintain balance (vestibulospinal reflex). Vestibular dysfunction secondary to concussion is common, with 43% of athletes reporting balance disruption and 50% reporting dizziness during the acute stages of injury [46]. Specific vestibular-associated symptoms following concussion may include dizziness, disrupted balance, motion sensitivity, vertigo, unstable vision, and difficulty in stimulating/busy environments [47, 48].

Recognizing the role of vestibular dysfunction following concussion, balance testing has traditionally been utilized as a proxy for the assessment of post-concussion vestibular deficits. The Balance Error Scoring System (BESS) provides a noninstrumented and efficient protocol for the assessment of balance and is among the more commonly utilized measures, with 16% of certified athletic trainers in the USA reporting regular use of the BESS in concussion evaluations [49]. The BESS involves three stances, a double-leg

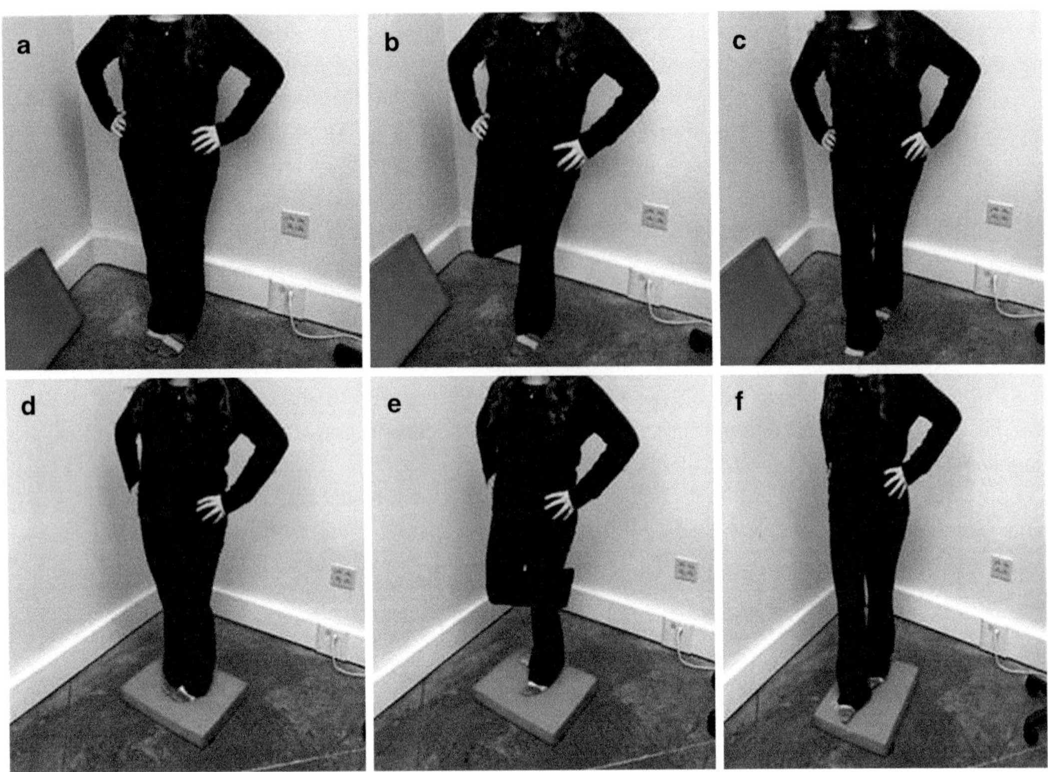

Fig. 51.3 Balance Error Scoring System (BESS) on firm- and medium-density foam surface. (**a**) Double-leg stance (firm surface), (**b**) single-leg stance (firm surface), (**c**) tandem stance (firm surface), (**d**) double-leg stance (foam surface), (**e**) single-leg stance (foam surface), and (**f**) tandem stance (foam surface)

stance with feet placed together, a single-leg stance on the nondominant leg, and a tandem stance with the nondominant foot aligned directly behind the dominant foot (Fig. 51.3). Examinees' hands are positioned on their hips with eyes closed for the duration of each 20-s trial, and the three stances are performed on a firm surface and a medium-density foam surface [50]. Total errors are counted for each trial. An error occurs when the examinee removes their hands from their hips, takes a step, falls from the test position, lifts a foot, abducts greater than 30° at the hips, fails to return to a stance within 5 s, or opens their eyes. The BESS is specific and sensitive for identifying concussed athletes in the acute stages of injury but has limited discriminant utility at longer post-injury durations [17, 51]. More sophisticated methods of balance assessment exist, such as the sensory organization test which utilizes force plates to measure postural sway while systematically disrupting visual and somatosensory information [52]. Such assessments require specialized equipment and are most sensitive in identifying impairments in the very acute stages of injury [52, 53].

While measures of balance offer downstream information regarding vestibular functioning, the vestibular/ocular motor screening assessment (VOMS) was developed to more directly assess vestibular, as well as oculomotor, sequelae of concussion (Fig. 51.4). The VOMS consists of brief screening across five domains, including smooth pursuits, horizontal and vertical saccadic eye movements, near point of convergence, horizontal and vertical vestibulo-ocular reflex (VOR), and visual motion sensitivity (VMS, Fig. 51.4). Prior to assessing these domains, patients subjectively rate the severity of baseline headache, dizziness, nausea, and mental fogginess, utilizing a 0 (none) to 10 (severe) scale. Patients re-rate symptoms after

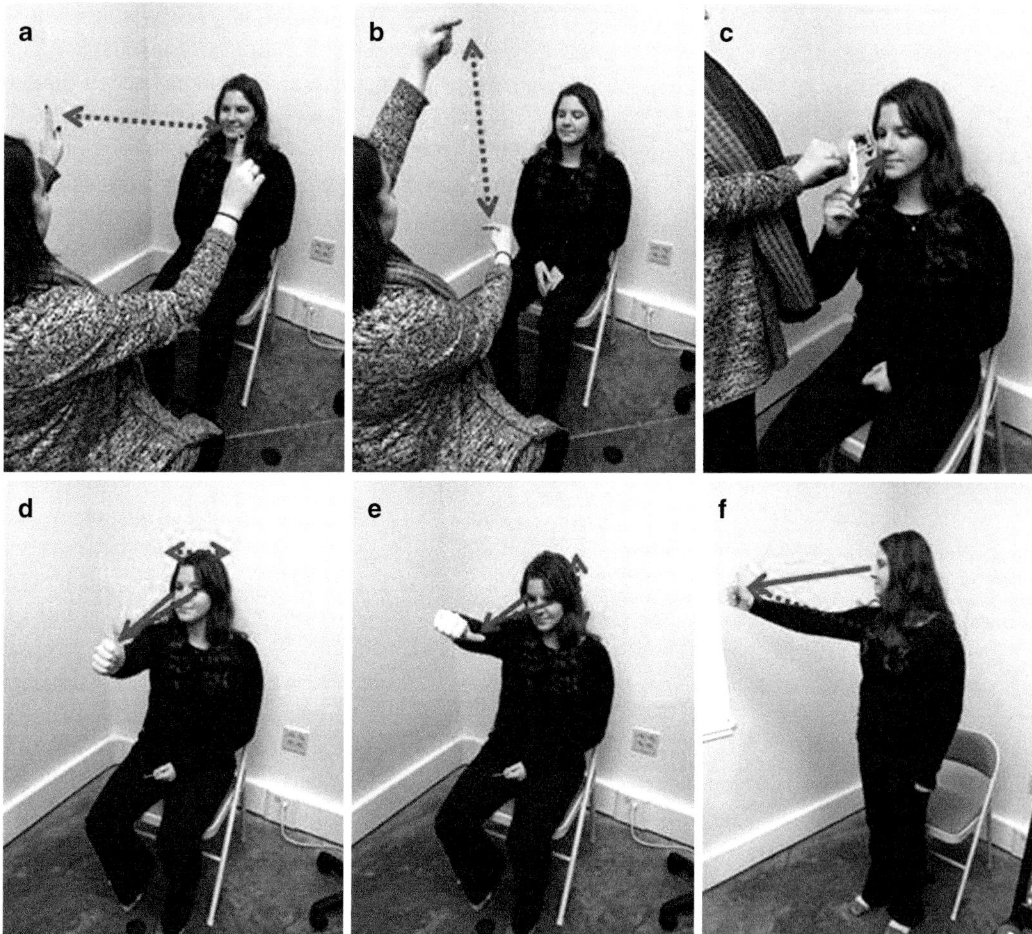

Fig. 51.4 Administration of vestibular/ocular motor screening assessment (VOMS). Smooth pursuits, (**a**) horizontal saccades, (**b**) vertical saccades, (**c**) near point convergence, (**d**) horizontal VOR, (**e**) vertical VOR, (**f**) visual motion sensitivity (note: smooth pursuits not pictured)

assessment of each domain, and clinicians consider areas of symptom exacerbation, average near point of convergence across three trials (normative cutoff is ≤5 cm), and clinically relevant behavioral observations (e.g., hypometric saccades, ocular exodeviation, behavioral avoidance/hesitancy) in drawing clinical inferences. The VOMS is an internally consistent measure with empirically demonstrated utility in differentiating healthy and injured athletes [54, 55].

In cases of concussion with suspected vestibular involvement and positive findings on screening measures such as the VOMS and BESS, consultation with vestibular therapists offering comprehensive assessment of vestibular functioning may be indicated. A comprehensive vestibular evaluation may include examination of oculomotor function, static positioning, postural balance, dynamic movement, peripheral vestibular organ response, gait, and subjective symptoms, with specific batteries constructed on the basis of individual patient presentation [48, 56]. In particular, two objective measures of vestibular functioning are frequently utilized with concussion patients and may be useful in informing return to play decisions, the Gaze Stability Test (GST) and Dynamic Visual Acuity Test (DVAT) [57, 58]. Both tests assess vestibulo-ocular reflex functioning by measuring visual acuity with head movements. The DVAT measures visual acuity with yaw (horizontal plane) and pitch (vertical plane) head movements at a fixed velocity, with the size of visual targets progressively decreasing. The GST assesses the maximum velocity at which an examinee can accurately identify a visual target while performing yaw and pitch head motion. Both measures are sensitive to changes in vestibulo-ocular reflex functioning post concussion [57, 58] and demonstrate adequate test-retest reliability in the empirical literature [59, 60].

> **Fact Box 3**
>
> Abnormal vestibular functioning has been reported in up to 60–80% of patients, while 40–69% of patients have at least one oculomotor abnormality at varying time intervals following sport-related concussion.

51.4.3.2 Oculomotor Assessment

Oculomotor dysfunction, or difficulty with coordinated eye movements, represents another common sequela of concussion, with estimates that 33–65% of patients experience such difficulties post injury [21, 61]. Specific oculomotor deficits may include problems with vergence, accommodation, version, visual alignment, visual pursuit, and saccadic eye movements, of which convergence insufficiency and accommodative insufficiency are most commonly seen in patients with concussion [61–63]. Until recently, the role of oculomotor dysfunction in concussion was not fully appreciated, and as a result, few practical assessment methods exist [7, 55, 64]. The King-Devick test is designed to detect impaired saccadic eye movements thought to reflect suboptimal neurological functioning, and empirical evidence suggests potential utility as an acute screening measure of oculomotor functioning when used in conjunction with other assessment methods [65–67]. The VOMS (previously described in the Vestibular/Balance section) assesses symptom provocation with smooth pursuits, saccadic eye movements, and near point of convergence and has been adapted to include accommodation as well [68]. This offers a more complete screening of oculomotor functioning while also targeting relevant vestibular functions (Table 51.2).

51.4.4 Emotional Functioning

It is common for individuals to experience increased emotional difficulties, such as anxiety and depression, shortly after experiencing a concussion [69]. Additionally, several studies have found that a history of mental health treatment and/or diagnosed mental health condition predicts delayed overall recovery from concussion [70–73]. While symptom checklist measures of concussion commonly include at least a brief assessment of affective symptoms, these tend to be only one or two items that likely fail to capture the full complexity and intensity of the emotional sequelae that may develop following SRC. Accordingly, consensus statements on SRC have called for more research exploring the assessment of affective symptoms that may accompany SRC, as well as how this information may be used to guide management and treatment decisions [5]. As there are countless standardized, self-report clinical measures that assess affective symptoms, it is helpful to distinguish between those that measure state or acute emotional functioning from those that measure more trait-like qualities. Both kinds of measures serve different purposes and provide different types of clinical information. For instance, acute measures of emotional functioning, such as the Beck Depression Inventory-II and the Beck Anxiety Inventory, are best suited to detecting more recent changes in affective symptoms, such as those that are likely to occur more immediately post injury. These measures have the additional advantage of being brief and easily administered by different types of providers (e.g., psychologist, physician), with appropriate training. However, overlap in

Table 51.2 Description of vestibular and oculomotor assessment measures used in the assessment of sports-related concussion

Measure	Vestibular/oculomotor functions assessed	Brief description of measure
Balance Error Scoring System (BESS)	Postural stability/balance	Three stances are performed on a firm- and a medium-density foam surface with hands on hips and eyes closed. Stances are held 20 s and total errors are recorded
Sensory organization test	Postural stability/balance	Subjects stand on dual-force plates in a 3-sided surround. Degree of anterior-posterior sway is recorded. Six conditions are administered with sensory conditions systematically varied. Each condition is comprised of three trials lasting 20 s
Gaze stability test (GST)	Vestibulo-ocular reflex	Patient rotates head in vertical and horizontal plane at progressively increasing velocity, measuring the most rapid velocity at which the patient is able to identify the orientation of a visual target
Dynamic visual acuity test (DVST)	Vestibulo-ocular reflex	Patient's head is rotated in the vertical and horizontal plane at a fixed velocity, with visual acuity for progressively smaller visual target compared to static head movement conditions
Vestibular/ocular motor screening (VOMS)	Smooth pursuits, saccadic eye movements, near point of convergence, vestibulo-ocular reflex, vestibulo-ocular cancellation	Brief screening measure designed to assess vestibular and oculomotor functioning. Patient subjectively rates pre-screening symptoms, and clinician notes neurobehavioral abnormalities during screening while patient subjectively identifies symptom exacerbation
King-Devick test	Saccadic eye movements	A series of numbers are read from left to right, with stimuli becoming progressively more visually challenging to read fluidly. Errors and completion time are recorded

symptom etiology can complicate interpretation of these measures. For example, dizziness and light-headedness are both symptoms of vestibular dysfunction and anxiety. Such issues highlight both the importance of multimodal assessment and the advantage of a psychologist on a multidisciplinary team, who can help to distinguish whether the origin of a symptom is more physiological or psychological.

Besides assessment instruments that assess more acute emotional functioning, there are comprehensive measures that provide an assessment of various psychological concepts that are thought to be long-standing (i.e., personality). Some individuals experience quite prominent post-concussion affective symptoms that may prolong their overall recovery and return to play. In these cases, it may be recommended that individuals seek additional evaluation and possible treatment with a mental health specialist, such as a psychiatrist or clinical psychologist. One way to determine whether such services are needed, as well as the severity of more long-standing affective symptoms, is to utilize more in-depth assessment instruments. Two such measures that provide a more in-depth assessment of emotional functioning are the Minnesota Multiphasic Personality Inventory-II Revised Factor and the Personality Assessment Inventory. These measures are commonly administered and interpreted by a clinical psychologist and are frequently used to support the diagnosis of a mental health condition and/or the need for mental health treatment. Although such measures will not be commonly utilized by most practitioners who

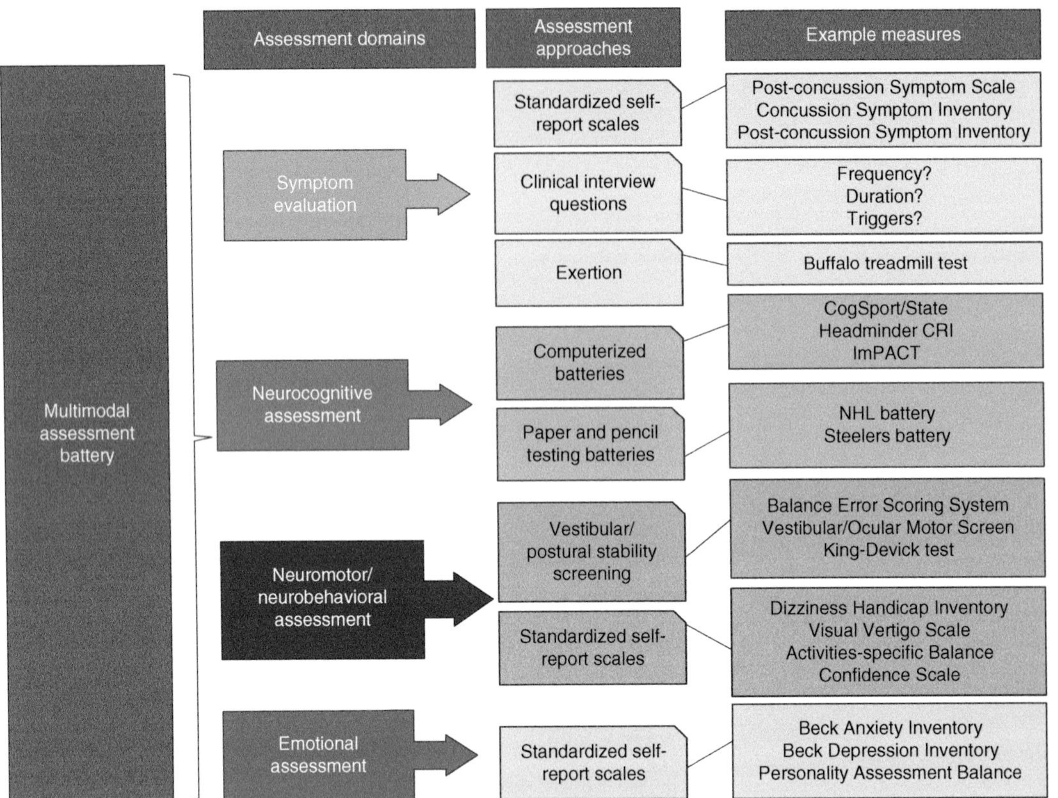

Fig. 51.5 Summary of multimodal assessment and examples of measures

evaluate and manage concussion, it behooves clinicians to closely monitor an individual's emotional functioning throughout the course of concussion management and address more severe emotional difficulties as they present (Table 51.3).

> **Fact Box 4**
> It is estimated that 12–44% of individuals experience some degree of depression or anxiety within the first 3 months following concussion.

51.5 Return to Play Following Concussion

International criteria to return to play following concussion state that an athlete is required to be asymptomatic at rest and with physical activity before return to play consideration [5]. This practice stimulated the development of progressive, staged exertional protocols for athletes to complete as a means to reach a symptom-free status with physical activity. However, international criteria are viewed as the minimal requirements or standard of care, and many experts agree that cognitive performance should be deemed consistent with preinjury expectations, either compared to an individual baseline or normative data. Further, it is important to determine that all deficits that were initially evaluated post injury fully resolved, including any vestibular and oculomotor impairments.

Take-Home Message
Concussion is a complex and heterogenous injury common in football players. Assessment of injury may start with basic diagnostic or sidelines tools, although the gold standard of concussion management requires a comprehensive, multimodal

Table 51.3 Description of emotional/affective measures

Questionnaire	Time frame of assessment	Number of questions	Symptoms assessed
Beck Depression Inventory-II [74]	Acute: past 2 weeks	21	Depression: sadness, anhedonia, fatigue, sleep dysregulation, cognitive difficulties, suicidality, pessimism, changes in appetite, worthlessness
Beck Anxiety Inventory [75]	Acute: past week	21	Anxiety: fearful thoughts, nervousness, and physiological hyperarousal
Personality Assessment Inventory [76]	Trait	344	Somatic concerns, depression, anxiety, mania, paranoia, schizophrenia, borderline features, antisocial features, and alcohol and drug problems (clinical scales)
Profile of Mood States 2nd Edition [77]	Acute and trait	65	Anger-hostility, confusion-bewilderment, depression-dejection, fatigue, friendliness, tension-anxiety, and vigor-activity
Minnesota Multiphasic Personality Inventory-II Restructured Form [78]	Trait	338	Demoralization, somatic complaints, low positive emotions, cynicism, antisocial behavior, ideas of persecution, negative emotions, aberrant experiences, hypomania (restructured clinical scales)
State-Trait Anxiety Inventory [79]	Acute and trait	40	Fear, nervousness, discomfort, physiological hyperarousal; disposition to experience psychological stress and worry

battery that is repeatable to measure progress and guide treatment recommendations and safe return to play.

Top Five Evidence Based References

Elbin R, Sufrinko A, Schatz P, French J, Henry L, Burkhart S, Collins MW, Kontos AP (2016) Removal from play after concussion and recovery time. Pediatr 138(3):e20160910

Henry LC, Elbin R, Collins MW, Marchetti G, Kontos AP (2016) Examining recovery trajectories after sport-related concussion with a multimodal clinical assessment approach. Neurosurgery 78:232–241

Broglio SP, Macciocchi SN, Ferrara MS (2007) Sensitivity of the concussion assessment battery. Neurosurgery 60:1050–1058

Resch JE, Brown CN, Schmidt J, Macciocchi SN, Blueitt D, Cullum CM et al (2016) The sensitivity and specificity of clinical measures of sport concussion: three tests are better than one. BMJ Open Sport Exerc Med 2:e000012

Sufrinko AM, Marchetti GF, Cohen PE, Elbin RJ, Re V, Kontos AP (2017) Using acute performance on a comprehensive neurocognitive, vestibular, and ocular motor assessment battery to predict recovery duration following sport-related concussion (SRC). Am J Sports Med 45(5):1187–1194

References

1. Smith NA, Chounthirath T, Xiang H (2016) Soccer-related injuries treated in emergency departments: 1990–2014. Pediatrics 138(4):e20160346
2. O'Kane JW, Spieker A, Levy MR, Neradilek M, Polissar NL, Schiff MA (2014) Concussion among female middle-school soccer players. JAMA Pediatr 168(3):258–264
3. Marshall SW, Guskiewicz KM, Shankar V, McCrea M, Cantu RC (2015) Epidemiology of sports-related concussion in seven US high school and collegiate sports. Injury Epidemiol 2(1):1
4. Pfister T, Pfister K, Hagel B, Ghali WA, Ronksley PE (2016) The incidence of concussion in youth sports: a systematic review and meta-analysis. Br J Sports Med 50(5):292–297
5. McCrory P, Meeuwisse WH, Aubry M, Cantu B, Dvořák J, Echemendia RJ, Engebretsen L, Johnston K, Kutcher JS, Raftery M (2013) Consensus statement on concussion in sport: the 4th international conference on concussion in sport held in Zurich, November 2012. Br J Sports Med 47(5):250–258
6. Collins MW, Kontos AP, Okonkwo DO, Almquist J, Bailes J, Barisa M, Bazarian J, Bloom OJ, Brody DL, Cantu R (2016) Statements of agreement from the targeted evaluation and active management (TEAM) approaches to treating concussion meeting held in Pittsburgh, October 15–16, 2015. Neurosurgery 79(6):912–929

7. Collins M, Kontos A, Reynolds E, Murawski C, Fu F (2014) A comprehensive, targeted approach to the clinical care of athletes following sport-related concussion. Knee Surg Sports Traumatol Arthrosc 22(2):235–246
8. Broglio SP, Macciocchi SN, Ferrara MS (2007) Sensitivity of the concussion assessment battery. Neurosurgery 60(6):1050–1058
9. Register-Mihalik JK, Guskiewicz KM, Mihalik JP, Schmidt JD, Kerr ZY, McCrea MA (2013) Reliable change, sensitivity, and specificity of a multidimensional concussion assessment battery: implications for caution in clinical practice. J Head Trauma Rehabil 28(4):274–283
10. Resch JE, Brown CN, Schmidt J, Macciocchi SN, Blueitt D, Cullum CM, Ferrara MS (2016) The sensitivity and specificity of clinical measures of sport concussion: three tests are better than one. BMJ Open Sport Exerc Med 2(1):e000012
11. Henry LC, Elbin R, Collins MW, Marchetti G, Kontos AP (2016) Examining recovery trajectories after sport-related concussion with a multimodal clinical assessment approach. Neurosurgery 78(2):232–241
12. Sufrinko AM, Marchetti GF, Cohen PE, Elbin RJ, Re V, Kontos AP (2017) Using acute performance on a comprehensive neurocognitive, vestibular, and ocular motor assessment battery to predict recovery duration following sport-related concussion (SRC). Am J Sports Med 45(5):1187–1194
13. Duhaime AC, Beckwith JG, Maerlender AC, McAllister TW, Crisco JJ, Duma SM, Brolinson PG, Rowson S, Flashman LA, Chu JJ, Greenwald RM (2012) Spectrum of acute clinical characteristics of diagnosed concussions in college athletes wearing instrumented helmets: clinical article. J Neurosurg 117(6):1092–1099
14. Elbin R, Sufrinko A, Schatz P, French J, Henry L, Burkhart S, Collins MW, Kontos AP (2016) Removal from play after concussion and recovery time. Pediatrics 138(3):e20160910
15. Yengo-Kahn AM, Hale AT, Zalneraitis BH, Zuckerman SL, Sills AK, Solomon GS (2016) The sport concussion assessment tool: a systematic review. Neurosurg Focus 40(4):E6
16. Chin EY, Nelson LD, Barr WB, McCrory P, McCrea MA (2016) Reliability and validity of the sport concussion assessment tool-3 (SCAT3) in high school and collegiate athletes. Am J Sports Med 44(9):2276–2285
17. McCrea M, Guskiewicz KM, Marshall SW, Barr W, Randolph C, Cantu RC, Onate JA, Yang J, Kelly JP (2003) Acute effects and recovery time following concussion in collegiate football players: the NCAA concussion study. JAMA 290(19):2556–2563
18. McCrea M, Kelly JP, Randolph C, Kluge J, Bartolic E, Finn G, Baxter B (1998) Standardized assessment of concussion (SAC): on-site mental status evaluation of the athlete. J Head Trauma Rehabil 13(2):27–35
19. Meehan WP III, Zhang J, Mannix R, Whalen MJ (2012) Increasing recovery time between injuries improves cognitive outcome after repetitive mild concussive brain injuries in mice. Neurosurgery 71(4):885–892
20. Ellis MJ, Leddy JJ, Willer B (2015) Physiological, vestibulo-ocular and cervicogenic post-concussion disorders: an evidence-based classification system with directions for treatment. Brain Inj 29(2):238–248
21. Kontos AP, Elbin R, Schatz P, Covassin T, Henry L, Pardini J, Collins MW (2012) A revised factor structure for the post-concussion symptom scale: baseline and postconcussion factors. Am J Sports Med 40(10):2375–2384
22. Lau BC, Kontos AP, Collins MW, Mucha A, Lovell MR (2011) Which on-field signs/symptoms predict protracted recovery from sport-related concussion among high school football players? Am J Sports Med 39(11):2311–2318
23. Kontos AP, Elbin RJ, Lau B, Simensky S, Freund B, French J, Collins MW (2013) Posttraumatic migraine as a predictor of recovery and cognitive impairment after sport-related concussion. Am J Sports Med 41(7):1497–1504
24. Howell DR, O'brien MJ, Beasley MA, Mannix RC, Meehan WP (2016) Initial somatic symptoms are associated with prolonged symptom duration following concussion in adolescents. Acta Paediatr 105(9):e426–e432
25. Meehan WP, Mannix RC, Stracciolini A, Elbin R, Collins MW (2013) Symptom severity predicts prolonged recovery after sport-related concussion, but age and amnesia do not. J Pediatr 163(3):721–725
26. Leddy JJ, Baker JG, Willer B (2016) Active rehabilitation of concussion and post-concussion syndrome. Phys Med Rehabil Clin N Am 27(2):437–454
27. Cordingley D, Girardin R, Reimer K, Ritchie L, Leiter J, Russell K, Ellis MJ (2016) Graded aerobic treadmill testing in pediatric sports-related concussion: safety, clinical use, and patient outcomes. J Neurosurg Pediatr 18(6):693–702
28. Leddy JJ, Baker JG, Kozlowski K, Bisson L, Willer B (2011) Reliability of a graded exercise test for assessing recovery from concussion. Clin J Sport Med 21(2):89–94
29. Wallace J, Covassin T, Lafevor M (2016) Use of the stepwise progression return-to-play protocol following concussion among practicing athletic trainers. J Sport Health Sci 2016:1–6
30. Iverson G, Brooks B, Lovell M, Collins M (2006) No cumulative effects for one or two previous concussions. Br J Sports Med 40(1):72–75
31. Lovell MR, Pardini JE, Welling J, Collins MW, Bakal J, Lazar N, Roush R, Eddy WF, Becker JT (2007) Functional brain abnormalities are related to clinical recovery and time to return-to-play in athletes. Neurosurgery 61(2):352–360
32. McClincy MP, Lovell MR, Pardini J, Collins MW, Spore MK (2006) Recovery from sports concussion in high school and collegiate athletes. Brain Inj 20(1):33–39

33. Kontos AP, Braithwaite R, Dakan S, Elbin R (2014) Computerized neurocognitive testing within 1 week of sport-related concussion: meta-analytic review and analysis of moderating factors. J Int Neuropsychol Soc 20(3):324
34. De Marco AP, Broshek DK (2016) Computerized cognitive testing in the management of youth sports-related concussion. J Child Neurol 31(1):68–75
35. Echemendia RJ, Iverson GL, McCrea M, Macciocchi SN, Gioia GA, Putukian M, Comper P (2013) Advances in neuropsychological assessment of sport-related concussion. Br J Sports Med 47(5):294–298
36. Iverson GL, Schatz P (2015) Advanced topics in neuropsychological assessment following sport-related concussion. Brain Inj 29(2):263–275
37. Broglio SP, Ferrara MS, Macciocchi SN, Baumgartner TA, Elliott R (2007) Test-retest reliability of computerized concussion assessment programs. J Athl Train 42(4):509
38. Mayers LB, Redick TS (2012) Clinical utility of ImPACT assessment for postconcussion return-to-play counseling: psychometric issues. J Clin Exp Neuropsychol 34(3):235–242
39. Moser RS, Schatz P, Lichtenstein JD (2015) The importance of proper administration and interpretation of neuropsychological baseline and postconcussion computerized testing. Appl Neuropsychol Child 4(1):41–48
40. Lovell MR, Iverson GL, Collins MW, Podell K, Johnston KM, Pardini D, Pardini J, Norwig J, Maroon JC (2006) Measurement of symptoms following sports-related concussion: reliability and normative data for the post-concussion scale. Appl Neuropsychol 13(3):166–174
41. Elbin R, Schatz P, Covassin T (2011) One-year test-retest reliability of the online version of ImPACT in high school athletes. Am J Sports Med 39(11):2319–2324
42. Lau BC, Collins MW, Lovell MR (2012) Cutoff scores in neurocognitive testing and symptom clusters that predict protracted recovery from concussions in high school athletes. Neurosurgery 70(2):371–379
43. Erlanger D, Feldman D, Kutner K (1999) Concussion resolution index. Headminder Inc, New York, NY
44. Erlanger D, Feldman D, Kutner K, Kaushik T, Kroger H, Festa J, Barth J, Freeman J, Broshek D (2003) Development and validation of a web-based neuropsychological test protocol for sports-related return-to-play decision-making. Arch Clin Neuropsychol 18(3):293–316
45. Gualtieri CT, Johnson LG (2006) Reliability and validity of a computerized neurocognitive test battery, CNS vital signs. Arch Clin Neuropsychol 21(7):623–643
46. Lovell MR (2004) Grade 1 or "Ding" concussions in high school athletes. Am J Sports Med 32(1):47–54
47. Alsalaheen BA, Mucha A, Morris LO, Whitney SL, Furman JM, Camiolo-Reddy CE, Collins MW, Lovell MR, Sparto PJ (2010) Vestibular rehabilitation for dizziness and balance disorders after concussion. J Neurol Phys Ther 34(2):87–93
48. Gurley JM, Hujsak BD, Kelly JL (2013) Vestibular rehabilitation following mild traumatic brain injury. Neuro Rehabilitation 32(3):519–528
49. Broglio SP, Tomporowski PD, Ferrara MS (2005) Balance performance with a cognitive task: a dual-task testing paradigm. Med Sci Sports Exerc 37(4):689–695
50. Bell DR, Guskiewicz KM, Clark MA, Padua DA (2011) Systematic review of the balance error scoring system. Sports Health 3(3):287–295
51. McCREA M, Barr WB, Guskiewicz K, Randolph C, Marshall SW, Cantu R, Onate JA, Kelly JP (2005) Standard regression-based methods for measuring recovery after sport-related concussion. J Int Neuropsychol Soc 11(01):58–69
52. Guskiewicz KM, Ross SE, Marshall SW (2001) Postural stability and neuropsychological deficits after concussion in collegiate athletes. J Athl Train 36(3):263–273
53. Bressel E, Yonker JC, Kras J, Heath EM (2007) Comparison of static and dynamic balance in female collegiate soccer, basketball, and gymnastics athletes. J Athl Train 42(1):42–46
54. Kontos AP, Sufrinko A, Elbin RJ, Puskar A, Collins MW (2016) Reliability and associated risk factors for performance on the vestibular/ocular motor screening (VOMS) tool in healthy collegiate athletes. Am J Sports Med 44(6):1400–1406
55. Mucha A, Collins MW, Elbin RJ, Furman JM, Troutman-Enseki C, DeWolf RM, Marchetti G, Kontos AP (2014) A brief vestibular/ocular motor screening (VOMS) assessment to evaluate concussions: preliminary findings. Am J Sports Med 42(10):2479–2486
56. Valovich McLeod TC, Hale TD (2015) Vestibular and balance issues following sport-related concussion. Brain Inj 29(2):175–184
57. Gottshall KR, Hoffer ME (2010) Tracking recovery of vestibular function in individuals with blast-induced head trauma using vestibular-visual-cognitive interaction tests. J Neurol Phys Ther 34(2):94–97
58. Zhou G, Brodsky JR (2015) Objective vestibular testing of children with dizziness and balance complaints following sports-related concussions. Otolaryngol Head Neck Surg 152(6):1133–1139
59. Kaufman DR, Puckett MJ, Smith MJ, Wilson KS, Cheema R, Landers MR (2014) Test-retest reliability and responsiveness of gaze stability and dynamic visual acuity in high school and college football players. Phys Ther Sport 15(3):181–188
60. Ward BK, Mohammad MT, Whitney SL, Marchetti GF, Furman JM (2010) The reliability, stability, and concurrent validity of a test of gaze stabilization. J Vestib Res 20(5):363–372
61. Capó-Aponte JE, Urosevich TG, Temme LA, Tarbett AK, Sanghera NK (2012) Visual dysfunctions and

symptoms during the subacute stage of blast-induced mild traumatic brain injury. Mil Med 177(7):804–813
62. Brahm KD, Wilgenburg HM, Kirby J, Ingalla S, Chang CY, Goodrich GL (2009) Visual impairment and dysfunction in combat-injured servicemembers with traumatic brain injury. Optom Vis Sci 86(7):817–825
63. Ciuffreda KJ, Kapoor N, Rutner D, Suchoff IB, Han ME, Craig S (2007) Occurrence of oculomotor dysfunctions in acquired brain injury: a retrospective analysis. Optometry 78(4):155–161
64. Pearce KL, Sufrinko A, Lau BC, Henry L, Collins MW, Kontos AP (2015) Near point of convergence after a sport-related concussion: measurement reliability and relationship to neurocognitive impairment and symptoms. Am J Sports Med 43(12):3055–3061
65. Galetta KM, Brandes LE, Maki K, Dziemianowicz MS, Laudano E, Allen M, Lawler K, Sennett B, Wiebe D, Devick S, Messner LV, Galetta SL, Balcer LJ (2011) The King-Devick test and sports-related concussion: study of a rapid visual screening tool in a collegiate cohort. J Neurol Sci 309(1–2):34–39
66. King D, Hume P, Gissane C, Clark T (2015) Use of the King-Devick test for sideline concussion screening in junior rugby league. J Neurol Sci 357(1–2):75–79
67. Tjarks BJ, Dorman JC, Valentine VD, Munce TA, Thompson PA, Kindt SL, Bergeron MF (2013) Comparison and utility of King-Devick and ImPACT(R) composite scores in adolescent concussion patients. J Neurol Sci 334(1–2):148–153
68. Anzalone AJ, Blueitt D, Case T, McGuffin T, Pollard K, Garrison JC, Jones MT, Pavur R, Turner S, Oliver JM (2016) A positive vestibular/ocular motor screening (VOMS) is associated with increased recovery time after sports-related concussion in youth and adolescent athletes. Am J Sports Med 45(2):474–479
69. Kontos AP, Deitrick JM, Reynolds E (2016) Mental health implications and consequences following sport-related concussion. Br J Sports Med 50(3):139–140
70. Meares S, Shores EA, Taylor AJ, Batchelor J, Bryant RA, Baguley IJ, Chapman J, Gurka J, Dawson K, Capon L (2008) Mild traumatic brain injury does not predict acute postconcussion syndrome. J Neurol Neurosurg Psychiatry 79(3):300–306
71. Morgan CD, Zuckerman SL, Lee YM, King L, Beaird S, Sills AK, Solomon GS (2015) Predictors of post-concussion syndrome after sports-related concussion in young athletes: a matched case-control study. J Neurosurg Pediatr 15(6):589–598
72. Ponsford J, Cameron P, Fitzgerald M, Grant M, Mikocka-Walus A, Schönberger M (2012) Predictors of postconcussive symptoms 3 months after mild traumatic brain injury. Neuropsychology 26(3):304
73. Wojcik SM (2014) Predicting mild traumatic brain injury patients at risk of persistent symptoms in the Emergency Department. Brain Inj 28(4):422–430
74. Beck AT, Steer RA, Brown GK (1996) Beck depression inventory-II. San Antonio 78(2):490–498
75. Beck A, Steer R (1993) Beck anxiety inventory manual. The Psychological Corporation. Harcourt Brace & Company, San Antonio, TX
76. Morey LC (2007) Personality assessment inventory (PAI): professional manual. PAR (Psychological Assessment Resources), Lutz, FL
77. Heuchert J, McNair D (2012) POMS-2 manual: a profile of mood states. Multi-Health Systems Inc, North Tonawanda, NY
78. Ben-Porath YS, Tellegen A (2008) MMPI-2-RF: manual for administration, scoring and interpretation. University of Minnesota Press, Minneapolis, MN
79. Spielberger CD (1983) Manual for the State-Trait Anxiety Inventory STAI (form Y) ("self-evaluation questionnaire"). Consulting Psychologists Press, Palo Alto, CA

Sport-related Concussion: Experience from the National Football League

52

Michael W. Collins, Natalie Sandel, John A. Norwig, and Sonia Ruef

Contents

52.1 Preseason Baseline Evaluation

Prior to the start of football season, all players are required to review educational materials on concussion and undergo a preseason physical examination. Educational resources assist players in identifying signs and symptoms of concussion and emphasize the importance of removal from play after injury. Preseason physical examinations include a comprehensive interview of past medical and concussion history, neurological examination, and baseline testing [1]. The NFL has adopted a baseline assessment model for managing concussion [2], in which athletes are required to complete mental status testing and neuropsychological baseline testing when noninjured that is used as a "control" should a player sustain a concussion in the future. Baseline testing is particularly important for individuals with a history of a neurodevelopmental disorder such as attention deficit hyperactivity disorder [3, 4] or who have above average intelligence [5] who are not well represented by available normative data [6, 7]. The NFL does not require it, but it is often recommended that all baseline testing includes validity indicators to prevent athletes from "gaming" their baseline testing [8–10].

52.2 Sideline Assessment and Management of Concussion

Players suspected of sustaining a concussion on field must adhere to a strict concussion management protocol outlined by the NFL's Head, Neck, and Spine Committee. The NFL's sideline concussion protocol focuses on (1) detection of the injury and (2) evaluation of the player for concussion or other neurological pathologies [1].

M.W. Collins (✉) • N. Sandel
Sports Medicine Concussion Program, Department of Orthopaedic Surgery, University of Pittsburgh Medical Center, 3200 S. Water St, Pittsburgh, PA 15203, USA
e-mail: collinsmw@upcm.edu

J.A. Norwig • S. Ruef
Pittsburgh Steelers Football Club, Pittsburgh, PA, USA

V. Musahl et al. (eds.), *Return to Play in Football*, https://doi.org/10.1007/978-3-662-55713-6_52

Players suspected of a concussion are immediately removed from play for further evaluation to ensure the safety of the athlete [11–14].

52.2.1 Detection of Concussion

Identification of on-field concussion is executed by the team medical staff, coaches, teammates, and/or player. Given the tendency for athletes to underreport their symptoms of concussion or for a general lack of player awareness [15–18], the NFL has implemented an organized team of medical personnel to watch closely for concussions during games. Personnel required include the team physician, club athletic trainer, booth athletic trainers (also known as the "eyes in the sky"), and an unaffiliated neurotrauma consultant (UNC) [1]. Personnel are trained to monitor players for acute signs and symptoms of concussion, as outlined in Table 52.1, after sustaining a traumatic blow to the head or body. With increasing education around concussion, it is common for coaches and/or teammates to report a suspected concussion as well, especially if the player in question is not exhibiting obvious or outward signs/symptoms.

Fact Box 1
A loss of consciousness is not required for a diagnosis of concussion.

Contrary to popular belief, a loss of consciousness (LOC) is not required for a diagnosis of concussion [13, 19–21], and LOC or posttraumatic amnesia [22–24] at the time of injury does not always equate to a more severe concussion [22, 23, 25–27]. On-field endorsement of dizziness [25, 27] and posttraumatic migraine [28–30] may be better clinical indicators of length of recovery time from concussion. If a player is suspected of sustaining a concussion, the player is immediately removed from play and evaluated by medical personnel. There are six "Go/No-Go" criteria that require immediate removal of the NFL player

Table 52.1 On-field acute signs and symptoms of concussion

Acute (observable) signs of head injury	Concussion symptoms (player report)
Loss of consciousness	Headache
Incoordination/imbalance	Nausea
Dazed	Photosensitivity/ phonosensitivity
Disorientation/confusion	Dizziness
Clutching head	Balance/coordination problems
Physically slow	Tinnitus
Vomiting	Cognitive slowness
	Visual disturbance
	Amnesia (retrograde or anterograde)

from the field without chance of return. They include LOC, confusion, amnesia, new or persistent symptoms (e.g., headache, nausea, dizziness), abnormal neurological findings, and progressive or worsening symptoms [1].

It is important to remove players immediately after a potential injury to rule out critical neurological pathology and prevent from additional blows to the head while the brain is in a vulnerable state of neurometabolic crisis [19, 21] from concussion [31–34]. Football players who continue to play immediately after sustaining a concussion are at an increased risk of a prolonged recovery. In fact, a recent manuscript shows that athletes who continue to play after experiencing concussion symptoms may double their recovery time [35].

Fact Box 2
Athletes who continue to play after sustaining a concussion may double their recovery time from the injury.

52.2.2 Evaluation of the Player for Concussion

Once removed from play for a concussion evaluation, sideline assessment of the athlete includes an evaluation of concussion signs and symp-

Table 52.2 Modified Maddock's questions in NFL concussion checklist

Modified Maddock's questions
1. Where are we?
2. What quarter is it right now?
3. Who scored last in the practice/game?
4. Who did we play last game?
5. Did we win the last game?

toms, a focused neurological examination, and a modified Maddock's questioning [1, 36] for evaluation of orientation and recent memory. Traditional orientation questions (e.g., person, place, and time) have been demonstrated to be unreliable for sideline assessment of sports concussion when compared to recent memory questioning (Table 52.2) [13, 36, 37]. If a player is suspected of having a concussion or there are abnormal findings on the sideline assessment, then the player is taken to the locker room for further evaluation.

The NFL utilizes an NFL-specific tailored version of a standardized sideline assessment tool for concussion, known as the Sideline Concussion Assessment Tool – 3rd Edition (SCAT3), for brief cognitive and mental status testing once an athlete is removed from play [1, 37, 38]. Results of testing are compared with the player's preseason baseline testing. The player is not permitted to return to the same game or practice if suspected of a concussion and is required to enter the NFL concussion protocol for return to football participation. To return to contact football, the player must be cleared by his team physician and an independent concussion specialist in accordance with international guidelines [1, 11–13, 39, 40].

52.3 In-Office Evaluation of Concussion

Initiation of the NFL concussion protocol first results in the player receiving education surrounding the expected signs and symptoms of concussion. Injured players are then managed by their team medical staff and/or in-office by a licensed concussion specialist. The NFL requires concussed players to return to their baseline functioning in terms of their report of symptoms and neurological/neurocognitive exam before re-engaging in physical activity [1]. Aside from the recommendation of serial neuropsychological testing to track players' neurocognitive recovery [1, 2] post-injury, there is little direction provided by the NFL and international concussion consensus statements regarding the in-office management and treatment of concussion to facilitate concussed players' return to baseline functioning [11–14, 39].

Current guidelines requiring a return to baseline status are helpful for preventing a premature return to play. The recommendations vary among team physicians and athletic trainers in the NFL. The role of "active rehabilitation" from concussion is in evolution and being studied. A "one-size-fits-all" approach to concussion management is no longer embraced [41]. In the recent past, to promote recovery post-injury, most players are prescribed physical and some form of cognitive rest until asymptomatic; however, there is sparse evidence to support strict rest for managing concussion [42–45]. A randomized control study [46] demonstrated that strict rest after concussion may actually lead to a slower recovery and worsened symptoms [46–49]. A recent consensus meeting held in Pittsburgh, Pennsylvania, among leading concussion experts, including NFL physicians and concussion consultants, on the "Targeted Evaluation and Active Management (TEAM) Approaches to Treating Concussion," indicated that 97% of experts believed that strict rest may have detrimental effects after concussion and may not be an effective strategy for all concussions. Furthermore, 100% of these experts advocated for an individualized, active treatment approach to concussion, in which treatment was matched to the individual clinical profile of the concussed athlete [41]. To improve treatment approaches, the NFL, in collaboration with other institutions, has launched a $60 million Head Health Initiative to expedite development of better diagnostic tools, improved protective gear, and better treatment techniques for concussion [50].

52.3.1 Diagnostic Assessment of Concussion

To develop an individualized treatment plan for concussion, a comprehensive, multimodal diagnostic assessment is warranted in order to delineate the clinical profile of the concussed player [13, 51–53]. The NFL currently employs a neurological exam with mental status, neuropsychological, and balance testing for their initial assessment [1] and has recently started to implement other cutting-edge measures sensitive to concussion [50]. Traditional neurodiagnostic techniques (e.g., computed tomography, magnetic resonance imaging), although helpful in ruling out intracranial bleeds and/or skull fracture, are not recommended for determining diagnosis of concussion. They are typically not sensitive to concussion and may involve potentially harmful radiation exposure [54, 55]. International guidelines recommend that the in-office assessment of concussion includes a thorough clinical interview, a subjective report of symptoms, and the use of empirically established, objective tools sensitive to concussion [13, 51]. Table 52.3 provides an overview of a multimodal approach to concussion diagnosis and evaluation utilized by concussion consultants for the Pittsburgh Steelers [13, 51, 52, 56, 57]. The multimodal assessment includes a clinical interview, symptom report, cognitive testing, and vestibular-oculomotor screening.

Table 52.3 Multimodal diagnostic assessment of concussion

Assessments	Brief description
Clinical interview	Establish rapport, determine mechanism of injury, acute markers of injury, acute and chronic symptom presentation, detailed personal and family medical history, review of medical records, identify concussion risk factors, psychosocial history
Symptom report	Self-report symptom questionnaires
Cognitive testing	Computerized neurocognitive testing/paper-and-pencil neuropsychological testing
Vestibular-oculomotor screening	Balance testing, vestibular-ocular reflex, visual motion sensitivity, oculomotor screening, near point of convergence

52.3.1.1 Clinical Interview

Establishing a trusting relationship with the player and team organization is important for gaining an understanding of the player and facilitating comprehensive care. Sideline evaluations conducted by the team medical staff are useful in identifying the mechanism of injury, acute signs and symptoms of concussion, and performance on mental status testing in order to gain an appreciation for the severity and nature of the injury. Detailing the personal and family medical history is important for identifying risk factors of concussion. Records from the player's medical history collected in the preseason evaluation by the team medical staff should be utilized when possible for verification of medical history.

A thorough review of concussion risk factors is vital in order to prognosticate recovery time. Most athletes are expected to recover within 1 to 3 weeks of injury; however, 10–20% of athletes in the general population do not recover in this timeframe [23, 53, 58]. The presence of multiple prior concussions [27, 59–61] or a personal or family history of the following preinjury conditions have been identified as potential risk factors for a protracted recovery: neurodevelopmental/neurological condition [27, 62–64], psychiatric condition such as anxiety/depression [65–69], migraine [28–30], and/or sleep disturbance [70, 71]. Other suspected risk factors that have yet to be fully established include a personal or family history of oculomotor dysfunction [72, 73] or motion sensitivity such as vertigo [53, 74–76]. An understanding of these risk factors can set the stage for conceptualizing a player's clinical profile and necessary treatment.

Psychosocial history is also pertinent to conceptualizing the functional challenges and limitations a player may experience after a concussion. Players may endorse different types of symptoms in specific environments (e.g., being in the locker room, riding a bus, and watching film) that can provide useful information about the deficits and functional impairments from the concussion. For instance, a player who experiences a headache while watching film may suggest the presence of oculomotor dysfunction due to the visual demand involved in this task. There may also be environmental stressors that can play a role in the player's response to injury, including a lack of social support in the nearby area, external pressures to return to play quickly, and fears surrounding long-term health. The overall goal of the clinical interview is to establish concussion risk factors, address the player's concerns, and determine specific functional limitations from the injury.

52.3.1.2 Symptom Report

A concussion can result in a myriad of physical, cognitive, sleep, and mood symptoms. Table 52.4 details some of the most common symptoms of concussion that are often reported on post-concussion symptom questionnaires [77–79]. The pattern of symptom reporting can provide useful information regarding the clusters of symptoms most bothersome to the player [30, 51–53, 73]. Athletes who report a higher total symptom score upon initial evaluation tend to take a longer time to recover from concussion [24, 80, 81]. Although evaluating symptoms is an important aspect of the assessment, objective measures should also be utilized in conjunction with self-report data given athletes' tendency to underreport their symptoms of concussion [15, 18, 82–84].

Table 52.4 Common symptoms of concussion

Common symptoms
Headache
Nausea
Vomiting
Balance problems
Dizziness
Fatigue
Trouble falling asleep
Sleeping more than usual
Sleeping less than usual
Drowsiness
Sensitivity to light
Sensitivity to noise
Irritability
Sadness
Feeling more emotional
Numbness or tingling
Feeling slowed down
Feeling mentally "foggy"
Difficulty concentrating
Difficulty remembering
Visual problems

Fact Box 3

Athletes who report a greater number of symptoms upon initial evaluation tend to take longer to recover from concussion.

52.3.1.3 Cognitive Testing

Neuropsychological testing has been recognized by international guidelines as a valid and reliable tool for the objective evaluation of concussion [11–14]. Neuropsychological testing can be administered one on one through paper-and-pencil tests or in a computerized format with all test instructions embedded within the computer program. Computerized neurocognitive testing is recognized as one of the most widely used assessments for concussion management [85, 86], and one tool, ImPACT (Immediate Post-Concussion Assessment and Cognitive Testing), has recently become the first device for concussion assessment approved by the Food and Drug Administration (FDA) [87]. It is sensitive in detecting concussed from non-concussed athletes, can be serially administered to track recovery over time, and has prognostic value in estimating length of recovery time [18, 81, 84, 88]. Athletes who are reportedly asymptomatic can still demonstrate deficits on computerized neurocognitive testing [18, 84].

52.3.1.4 Vestibular-Oculomotor Screening

The vestibular system is a complex sensory system that allows for neural maintenance of balance/postural control and stabilization of vision during movement. When this sensory system is disturbed after a concussion, it can result in subjective complaints of dizziness, vertigo, nausea, light-headedness, unstable vision, imbalance, and motion discomfort [89–93]. Given that nearly 40% of athletes report balance impairment [78] and 50%

Table 52.5 Vestibular/Ocular Motor Screening (VOMS) for concussion

	Headache (1–10)	Dizziness (1–10)	Nausea (1–10)	Fogginess (1–10)
Baseline symptoms (at rest)				
Smooth pursuits				
Saccades – horizontal				
Saccades – vertical				
Convergence (near point)[a]				
Vestibular-ocular reflex (VOR) – horizontal				
Vestibular-ocular reflex (VOR) – vertical				
Visual motion sensitivity test				

[a]Near point of convergence measurements are averaged across three measurement trials

endorse dizziness [80] after a concussion, a thorough evaluation of the vestibular-oculomotor system is recommended [51, 93]. Balance testing is currently utilized by the NFL to assess disturbance of the vestibulospinal tract [1, 91, 94, 95], and some teams have begun to implement screening of dynamic vestibular functions (e.g., vestibular-ocular reflex, visual motion sensitivity) that are involved in the stabilization of vision and tolerance of dynamic movement [50, 93]. Disruption of vestibular reflexes can be a contributor to players' intolerance of exercise post-injury and is associated with increased recovery time following sport-related concussion [74, 89, 90].

Oculomotor abnormalities in which there is a deficit in the neural control of eye movements are also common following concussion. There are multiple oculomotor abnormalities that can occur after a head injury, including abnormal eye movement and function [96]. For example, a convergence insufficiency occurs when there is a reduced ability for the eyes to team toward each other upon near vision. Athletes with a sport-related concussion are 10 times more likely to demonstrate a convergence insufficiency when compared to the general population [72, 73]. Athletes with oculomotor dysfunction often report increased symptoms when engaging in visually demanding tasks such as watching film, engaging in computer work, and reading [72, 73]. Concussion consultants for the Pittsburgh Steelers have developed and validated a brief vestibular-ocular screening tool that can be used for in-office or sideline assessment of vestibular-oculomotor dysfunction; see Table 52.5 [74, 78, 93]. This Vestibular/Ocular Motor Screening (VOMS) tool evaluates multiple vestibular-oculomotor functions and has athletes endorse their experience of headache, dizziness, nausea, and fogginess on a scale from 1 to 10 at rest and with each assessment. The VOMS can be serially administered to track recovery over time.

52.3.2 Individual Clinical Profiles and Targeted Treatment for Concussion

Multimodal assessment of concussion as outlined above facilitates conceptualization of the player's clinical profile and trajectory from the injury. Establishment of the clinical profile allows for targeted, active rehabilitation from concussion rather than a "one-size-fits-all" approach. In the first few days of injury, athletes may demonstrate a global concussion presentation that includes primarily cognitive deficits, fatigue, and migraine symptoms [78]. It is suggested by experts that beyond the acute stage of injury, athletes begin to demonstrate a more delineated clinical profile/s from the concussion [41, 51, 52, 56].

Utilizing information gleaned from sideline assessments, clinical interview, preexisting risk factors, record review, symptom report, cognitive testing, and vestibular-oculomotor screening, a comprehensive and targeted rehabilitation program can be initiated for more active treatment and rehabilitation of concussion. Conceptualization of the clinical profile/s should incorporate a careful consideration of concussion risk factors, mechanism of injury, symptoms, functional deficits, and abnormalities on objective examination. Summarized in Table 52.6 are emerging clinical profiles from concussion. Each profile is associated with specific symptoms, objective test findings, and rehabilitation recommendations [41, 53]. Establishment of these clinical profiles is in its infancy and requires further empirical investigation which is underway by multiple institutions, including studies funded by the NFL [41, 50–53]. Once a player's profile is determined, treatment can begin to actively rehabilitate the player for return to football.

Fact Box 4
Concussion is an individualized injury that has different clinical profiles that require targeted treatment rather than a "one-size-fits-all" approach.

52.3.3 Return to Play Criteria

International return to play (RTP) guidelines are standardized in order to protect athletes from returning to sport participation prematurely. A player is never returned to play on the same day as a concussion is diagnosed. In order to receive full clearance back to contact football, these guidelines require an athlete to be (1) asymptomatic at rest, (2) asymptomatic with noncontact exertion, and (3) at their neurocognitive baseline. These criteria protect and prevent athletes who still demonstrate signs and symptoms of concussion from returning to football while the brain is still recovering from injury [13]. If an athlete has not met these criteria or there is a question of criteria being met, then holding an athlete from RTP is warranted as additional head insult while the player is still concussed can have potentially deleterious outcomes [31, 32].

Fact Box 5
A player is never returned to play on the same day as a concussion is diagnosed. In order to receive full clearance back to play, international guidelines require an athlete to be (1) asymptomatic at rest, (2) asymptomatic with noncontact exertion, and (3) at their neurocognitive baseline.

The NFL's Head, Neck, and Spine Committee's Return to Participation Protocol [1] and International Consensus Statements [13] advocate for a graduated, stepwise return to physical exertion. The NFL exertion protocol is initiated once the player returns to their baseline status in terms of symptoms and neurological examination. Stepwise exertion protocols such as the NFL's often require an athlete to start with low-level physical activity and (suggest but do not require) the athlete remain asymptomatic for 24 h at each stage before progressing to the next level.

This stepwise, homogenous approach for returning to physical activity can be problematic in select athletes. Firstly, as noted in the treatments for different concussion trajectories, some players can tolerate physical activity early after the injury. Participation in exercise may actually expedite some players' recovery time, while players with different concussion trajectories may be highly symptomatic with certain types of exertion [49, 56, 89, 90, 97, 98]. The clinical profile of the athlete plays a role in their tolerance of particular physical activity (e.g., heavy aerobic activity versus dynamic movement). A "one-size-fits-all" approach is again not uniformly successful for prescribing exertion activities and treatment approaches in concussion management given the individualized nature of the injury. Secondly, preventing players from exercising after injury may have deleterious effects on their mood and physical conditioning [47, 99]. Lastly, requiring a player to follow a structured, stepwise exertion protocol when they can tolerate exercise

Table 52.6 Clinical trajectories and targeted treatment for concussion

Clinical trajectory	Common symptoms	Objective findings	Treatment
Cognitive/fatigue	Fatigue Decreased energy Nonspecific headache Sleep disruption Worse symptoms at the end of the day Trouble concentrating	Global deficits on cognitive testing Declines in functional cognition	Behavioral regulation Pharmacological intervention (stimulants, sleep aids) Cognitive therapy if protracted Allow for moderate physical activity
Vestibular	Dizziness Fogginess Nausea Feeling of being detached Anxiety Overstimulation in complex environments Motion sensitivity	Symptom provocation with vestibular-ocular reflex or optokinetic sensitivity Imbalance Processing speed/reaction time deficits on cognitive testing	Vestibular therapy by a neuro-rehabilitation specialist Pharmacological intervention (if mood or migraine overlay)
Oculomotor	Localized, frontal headache Fatigue Distractibility Pressure behind eyes Trouble focusing Headache with visual tasks	Abnormal oculomotor exam Convergence insufficiency Accommodation insufficiency Global deficits on cognitive testing	Neuro-optometry for vision therapy Vestibular-ocular therapy by a neuro-rehabilitation specialist Allow for physical activity
Anxiety/mood	Anxiety Ruminative thinking Hypervigilance Feeling overwhelmed Sadness Hopelessness Sleep disturbance Somatic symptoms with stress	Mild symptom provocation with vestibular screening	Treatment of vestibular dysfunction if present Heavy, dynamic physical activity Behavioral regulation Pharmacological or behavioral treatment of anxiety/mood
Posttraumatic migraine	Unilateral headache Moderate/severe headache Pulsating headache Nausea Photosensitivity Phonosensitivity Dizziness	Verbal or visual memory deficits on cognitive testing	Behavioral regulation Pharmacological therapy (tricyclic antidepressants, anticonvulsants, beta or calcium channel blockers, or triptans) Aerobic, structured physical activity
Cervical	Headache (suboccipital location) Neck pain Numbness/tingling in extremities	Abnormal decreased range of motion, muscle weakness, ligamentous instability, limited musculature flexibility in the neck	Range of motion exercises Manual cervical and thoracic mobilization Soft tissue mobilization Posture reeducation Biofeedback Pain management Trigger point injections Pharmacological therapy if protracted (analgesics, anti-inflammatories, muscle relaxants)

early after injury may potentially delay their return to full health.

Once a player has successfully returned to their baseline status and completed the exertion protocol, clearance is required from multiple members of the NFL concussion management team. The player must have baseline scores returned to normal as interpreted by a team's neuropsychological consultant, receive clearance from the team physician, and receive clearance from an independent neurological consultant with expertise in concussion. Full clearance allows the player to return to full sport participation, including competition and contact activities.

Take-Home Message

The NFL's Head, Neck, and Spine Committee has evolved their guidelines for concussion identification and management to protect the health of players. Standardized protocols designed by the NFL for return to football participation prevent concussed players from being prematurely returned to play. Individualized clinical profiles after concussion have started to emerge and are being studied to potentially allow for targeted treatment from the injury rather than a "one-size-fits-all" approach.

Top Five Evidence Based References

Anzalone AJ, Blueitt D, Case T, McGuffin T, Pollard K, Garrison JC et al (2017) A positive vestibular/ocular motor screening (VOMS) is associated with increased recovery time after sports-related concussion in youth and adolescent athletes. Am J Sports Med 45(2):474–479

Collins MW, Kontos AP, Okonkwo DO, Almquist J, Bailes J, Barisa M et al (2016) Statements of agreement from the targeted evaluation and active management (TEAM) approaches to treating concussion meeting held in Pittsburgh, Oct 15–16, 2015. Neurosurgery 79:912–929

Elbin R, Sufrinko A, Schatz P, French J, Henry L, Burkhart S et al (2016) Removal from play after concussion and recovery time. Pediatrics 2016:e20160910

Collins MW, Kontos AP, Reynolds E, Murawski CD, Fu FH (2014) A comprehensive, targeted approach to the clinical care of athletes following sport-related concussion. Knee Surg Sports Traumatol Arthrosc 22(2):235–246

McCrory P, Meeuwisse W, Dvorak J, Aubry M, Bailes J, Broglio S et al (2017). Consensus statement on concussion in sport: The 5th international conference on concussion in sport held in Berlin, October 2016. Br J Sports Med, https://doi.org/10.1136/bjsports-2017-097699

References

1. NFL Head Neck and Spine Committee (2014) NFL Head, Neck, and Spine Committee's protocols regarding diagnosis and management of concussion
2. Barth JT, Alves W, Ryan T, Macciocchi SN, Rimel RW, Nelson WE (1989) Mild head injury in sports: Neuropsychological sequelae and recovery of function. *Mild Head Injury*. Oxford University Press, New York, NY, pp 257–275
3. Elbin RJ, Kontos AP, Kegel N, Johnson E, Burkhart S, Schatz P (2013) Individual and combined effects of LD and ADHD on computerized neurocognitive concussion test performance: evidence for separate norms. Arch Clin Neuropsychol. https://doi.org/10.1093/arclin/act024
4. Zuckerman SL, Lee YM, Odom MJ, Solomon GS, Sills AK (2013) Baseline neurocognitive scores in athletes with attention deficit-spectrum disorders and/or learning disability. J Neurosurg Pediatr. https://doi.org/10.3171/2013.5.PEDS12524
5. Schatz P, Robertshaw S (2014) Comparing post-concussive neurocognitive test data to normative data presents risks for under-classifying "above average" athletes. Arch Clin Neuropsychol 29:625–632
6. Solomon GS, Haase RF (2008) Biopsychosocial characteristics and neurocognitive test performance in National Football League players: an initial assessment. Arch Clin Neuropsychol 23:563–577
7. Solomon GS, Kuhn A (2014) Relationship between concussion history and neurocognitive test performance in national football league draft picks. Am J Sports Med. https://doi.org/10.1177/0363546513518742
8. Erdal K (2012) Neuropsychological testing for sports-related concussion: how athletes can sandbag their baseline testing without detection. Arch Clin Neuropsychol 27:473–479
9. Schatz P, Glatts C (2013) "Sandbagging" baseline test performance on ImPACT, without detection, is more difficult than it appears. Arch Clin Neuropsychol 28:236–244
10. Szabo AJ, Alosco ML, Fedor A, Gunstad J (2013) Invalid performance and the ImPACT in national collegiate athletic association division I football players. J Athl Train 48:851–855
11. Aubry M, Cantu R, Dvorak J, Graf-Baumann T, Johnston K, Kelly J et al (2002) Summary and agree-

ment statement of the first international conference on concussion in sport, Vienna 2001. Recommendations for the improvement of safety and health of athletes who may suffer concussive injuries. Br J Sports Med 36:6–10
12. McCrory P, Johnston K, Meeuwisse W, Aubry M, Cantu R, Dvorak J et al (2005) Summary and agreement statement of the 2nd international conference on concussion in sport, Prague 2004. Br J Sports Med 39:196–204
13. McCrory P, Meeuwisse W, Aubry M, Cantu B, Dvorak J, Echemendia R et al (2013) Consensus statement on concussion in sport—the 4th international conference on concussion in sport held in Zurich, November 2012. J Sci Med Sport Sports Med Aust 16:178–189
14. McCrory P, Meeuwisse W, Johnston K, Dvorak J, Aubry M, Molloy M et al (2009) Consensus statement on concussion in sport: the 3rd international conference on concussion in sport held in Zurich, November 2008. Br J Sports Med 43(Suppl 1):76–90
15. Delaney JS, Lacroix VJ, Leclerc S, Johnston KM (2002) Concussions among university football and soccer players. Clin J Sport Med 12:331–338
16. McCrea M, Hammeke T, Olsen G, Leo P, Guskiewicz K (2004) Unreported concussion in high school football players: implications for prevention. Clin J Sport Med 14:13–17
17. Meehan WP III, Mannix RC, O'Brien MJ, Collins MW (2013) The prevalence of undiagnosed concussions in athletes. Clin J Sport Med 23:339
18. Schatz P, Sandel N (2012) Sensitivity and specificity of the online version of ImPACT in high school and collegiate athletes. Am J Sports Med. https://doi.org/10.1177/0363546512466038
19. Barkhoudarian G, Hovda DA, Giza CC (2011) The molecular pathophysiology of concussive brain injury. Clin Sports Med 30(33–48):vii–iii
20. Centers for Disease C, Prevention (2014) Concussion in sports. BrainLine, Pretoria
21. Giza CC, Hovda DA (2001) The neurometabolic cascade of concussion. J Athl Train 36:228–235
22. Collins MW, Iverson GL, Lovell MR, McKeag DB, Norwig J, Maroon J (2003) On-field predictors of neuropsychological and symptom deficit following sports-related concussion. Clin J Sport Med 13:222–229
23. McCrea M, Guskiewicz K, Randolph C, Barr WB, Hammeke TA, Marshall SW et al (2013) Incidence, clinical course, and predictors of prolonged recovery time following sport-related concussion in high school and college athletes. J Int Neuropsychol Soc 19:22–33
24. Meehan WP III, Mannix RC, Stracciolini A, Elbin RJ, Collins MW (2013) Symptom severity predicts prolonged recovery after sport-related concussion, but age and amnesia do not. J Pediatr. https://doi.org/10.1016/j.jpeds.2013.03.012
25. Lau BC, Kontos AP, Collins MW, Mucha A, Lovell MR (2011) Which on-field signs/symptoms predict protracted recovery from sport-related concussion among high school football players? Am J Sports Med 39:2311–2318
26. Lovell MR, Iverson GL, Collins MW, McKeag D, Maroon JC (1999) Does loss of consciousness predict neuropsychological decrements after concussion? Clin J Sport Med 9:193–198
27. Zemek RL, Farion KJ, Sampson M, McGahern C (2013) Prognosticators of persistent symptoms following pediatric concussion: a systematic review. JAMA Pediatr 167:259–265
28. Kontos AP, Elbin RJ, Lau B, Simensky S, Freund B, French J et al (2013) Posttraumatic migraine as a predictor of recovery and cognitive impairment after sport-related concussion. Am J Sports Med. https://doi.org/10.1177/0363546513488751
29. Mihalik JP, Register-Mihalik J, Kerr ZY, Marshall SW, McCrea MC, Guskiewicz KM (2013) Recovery of posttraumatic migraine characteristics in patients after mild traumatic brain injury. Am J Sports Med. https://doi.org/10.1177/0363546513487982
30. Mihalik JP, Stump JE, Collins MW, Lovell MR, Field M, Maroon JC (2005) Posttraumatic migraine characteristics in athletes following sports-related concussion. J Neurosurg 102:850–855
31. Cantu RC, Gean AD (2010) Second-impact syndrome and a small subdural hematoma: an uncommon catastrophic result of repetitive head injury with a characteristic imaging appearance. J Neurotrauma 27:1557–1564
32. McCrory P, Davis G, Makdissi M (2012) Second impact syndrome or cerebral swelling after sporting head injury. Curr Sports Med Rep 11:21–23
33. Vagnozzi R, Signoretti S, Cristofori L, Alessandrini F, Floris R, Isgro E et al (2010) Assessment of metabolic brain damage and recovery following mild traumatic brain injury: a multicentre, proton magnetic resonance spectroscopic study in concussed patients. Brain J Neurol 133:3232–3242
34. Vagnozzi R, Tavazzi B, Signoretti S, Amorini AM, Belli A, Cimatti M et al (2007) Temporal window of metabolic brain vulnerability to concussions: mitochondrial-related impairment--part I. Neurosurgery 61:379–388
35. Elbin R, Sufrinko A, Schatz P, French J, Henry L, Burkhart S et al (2016) Removal from play after concussion and recovery time. Pediatrics 2016:e20160910
36. Maddocks DL, Dicker GD, Saling MM (1995) The assessment of orientation following concussion in athletes. Clin J Sport Med 5:32–35
37. McCrea M, Kelly JP, Randolph C, Kluge J, Bartolic E, Finn G et al (1998) Standardized assessment of concussion (SAC): on-site mental status evaluation of the athlete. J Head Trauma Rehabil 13:27–35
38. Concussion in Sport Group (2013) SCAT3: sport concussion assessment tool – 3rd edition. Br J Sports Med 47:259–262
39. Concussion in Sport Consensus statement on concussion in sport: the 5th international conference on concussion in sport held in Berlin, October 2016. Paper

presented at: consensus statement on concussion in sport: the 5th international conference on concussion in sport held in Berlin, Oct 2016; Berlin
40. McCrory P, Meeuwisse W, Johnston K, Dvorak J, Aubry M, Molloy M et al (2009) Consensus statement on concussion in sport–the 3rd international conference on concussion in sport held in Zurich, November 2008. S Afr J Sports Med 21:1613
41. Collins MW, Kontos AP, Okonkwo DO, Almquist J, Bailes J, Barisa M et al (2016) Statements of agreement from the targeted evaluation and active management (TEAM) approaches to treating concussion meeting held in Pittsburgh, Oct 15–16, 2015. Neurosurgery 79:912–929
42. Broglio SP, Collins MW, Williams RM, Mucha A, Kontos AP (2015) Current and emerging rehabilitation for concussion: a review of the evidence. Clin Sports Med 34:213–231
43. Buckley TA, Munkasy BA, Clouse BP (2016) Acute cognitive and physical rest may not improve concussion recovery time. J Head Trauma Rehabil 31:233–241
44. Moser RS, Glatts C, Schatz P (2012) Efficacy of immediate and delayed cognitive and physical rest for treatment of sports-related concussion. J Pediatr. https://doi.org/10.1016/j.jpeds.2012.04.012
45. Moser RS, Schatz P, Glenn M, Kollias KE, Iverson GL (2015) Examining prescribed rest as treatment for adolescents who are slow to recover from concussion. Brain Inj 29:58–63
46. Thomas DG, Apps JN, Hoffmann RG, McCrea M, Hammeke T (2015) Benefits of strict rest after acute concussion: a randomized controlled trial. Pediatrics 135:213–223
47. Berlin AA, Kop WJ, Deuster PA (2006) Depressive mood symptoms and fatigue after exercise withdrawal: the potential role of decreased fitness. Psychosom Med 68:224–230
48. Giza CC, Griesbach GS, Hovda DA (2005) Experience-dependent behavioral plasticity is disturbed following traumatic injury to the immature brain. Behav Brain Res 157:11–22
49. Griesbach GS, Hovda D, Molteni R, Wu A, Gomez-Pinilla F (2004) Voluntary exercise following traumatic brain injury: brain-derived neurotrophic factor upregulation and recovery of function. Neuroscience 125:129–139
50. NFL Communications (2017). NFL partners with CFL on concussion testing. 2015. https://nflcommunications.com/Pages/NFL-Partners-With-CFL-On-Concussion-Testing.aspx. Accessed 12 Jan 2017
51. Collins MW, Kontos AP, Reynolds E, Murawski CD, Fu FH (2014) A comprehensive, targeted approach to the clinical care of athletes following sport-related concussion. Knee Surg Sports Traumatol Arthrosc 22:235–246
52. Ellis MJ, Leddy JJ, Willer B (2015) Physiological, vestibulo-ocular and cervicogenic post-concussion disorders: an evidence-based classification system with directions for treatment. Brain Inj 29:238–248
53. Henry LC, Elbin RJ, Collins MW, Marchetti G, Kontos AP (2016) Examining recovery trajectories after sport-related concussion with a multimodal clinical assessment approach. Neurosurgery 78:232–241
54. Haydel MJ, Preston CA, Mills TJ, Luber S, Blaudeau E, DeBlieux PM (2000) Indications for computed tomography in patients with minor head injury. N Engl J Med 343:100–105
55. Pearce MS, Salotti JA, Little MP, McHugh K, Lee C, Kim KP et al (2012) Radiation exposure from CT scans in childhood and subsequent risk of leukaemia and brain tumours: a retrospective cohort study. Lancet 380:499–505
56. Leddy JJ, Sandhu H, Sodhi V, Baker JG, Willer B (2012) Rehabilitation of concussion and post-concussion syndrome. Sports health 4:147–154
57. Moser RS, Iverson GL, Echemendia RJ, Lovell MR, Schatz P, Webbe FM et al (2007) Neuropsychological evaluation in the diagnosis and management of sports-related concussion. Arch Clin Neuropsychol 22:909–916
58. Collins M, Lovell MR, Iverson GL, Ide T, Maroon J (2006) Examining concussion rates and return to play in high school football players wearing newer helmet technology: a three-year prospective cohort study. Neurosurgery 58:275–286
59. Bruce JM, Echemendia RJ (2004) Concussion history predicts self-reported symptoms before and following a concussive event. Neurology 63:1516–1518
60. Colvin AC, Mullen J, Lovell MR, West RV, Collins MW, Groh M (2009) The role of concussion history and gender in recovery from soccer-related concussion. Am J Sports Med 37:1699–1704
61. Covassin T, Moran R, Wilhelm K (2013) Concussion symptoms and neurocognitive performance of high school and college athletes who incur multiple concussions. Am J Sports Med. https://doi.org/10.1177/0363546513499230
62. Collins MW, Grindel SH, Lovell MR, Dede DE, Moser DJ, Phalin BR et al (1999) Relationship between concussion and neuropsychological performance in college football players. JAMA 282:964–970
63. Fay TB, Yeates KO, Taylor HG, Bangert B, Dietrich A, Nuss KE et al (2010) Cognitive reserve as a moderator of postconcussive symptoms in children with complicated and uncomplicated mild traumatic brain injury. J Int Neuropsychol Soc 16:94–105
64. Nelson LD, Guskiewicz KM, Marshall SW, Hammeke T, Barr W, Randolph C et al (2016) Multiple self-reported concussions are more prevalent in athletes with ADHD and learning disability. Clin J Sport Med 26:120–127
65. Carroll LJ, Cassidy JD, Peloso PM, Borg J, von Holst H, Holm L et al (2004) Prognosis for mild traumatic brain injury: results of the WHO collaborating centre task force on mild traumatic brain injury. J Rehabil Medicine 43(Suppl):84–105

66. Covassin T, Crutcher B, Bleecker A, Heiden EO, Dailey A, Yang J (2014) Postinjury anxiety and social support among collegiate athletes: a comparison between orthopaedic injuries and concussions. J Athl Train 49:462
67. Kontos AP, Covassin T, Elbin RJ, Parker T (2012) Depression and neurocognitive performance after concussion among male and female high school and collegiate athletes. Arch Phys Med Rehabil 93:1751–1756
68. Ponsford J, Cameron P, Fitzgerald M, Grant M, Mikocka-Walus A (2011) Long-term outcomes after uncomplicated mild traumatic brain injury: a comparison with trauma controls. J Neurotrauma 28:937–946
69. Ponsford J, Cameron P, Fitzgerald M, Grant M, Mikocka-Walus A, Schonberger M (2012) Predictors of postconcussive symptoms 3 months after mild traumatic brain injury. Neuropsychology 26:304–313
70. Kostyun RO, Milewski MD, Hafeez I (2014) Sleep disturbance and neurocognitive function during the recovery from a sport-related concussion in adolescents. Am J Sports Med. 0363546514560727
71. Sufrinko A, Johnson EW, Henry LC (2016) The influence of sleep duration and sleep-related symptoms on baseline neurocognitive performance among male and female high school athletes. Neuropsychology 30:484
72. Master CL, Scheiman M, Gallaway M, Goodman A, Robinson RL, Master SR et al (2016) Vision diagnoses are common after concussion in adolescents. Clin Pediatr 55:260–267
73. Pearce KL, Sufrinko A, Lau BC, Henry L, Collins MW, Kontos AP (2015) Near point of convergence after a sport-related concussion: measurement reliability and relationship to neurocognitive impairment and symptoms. Am J Sports Med 43:3055–3061
74. Anzalone AJ, Blueitt D, Case T, McGuffin T, Pollard K, Garrison JC et al (2016) A positive vestibular/ocular motor screening (VOMS) is associated with increased recovery time after sports-related concussion in youth and adolescent athletes. Am J Sports Med 0363546516668624:[pii]
75. Gurley JM, Hujsak BD, Kelly JL (2013) Vestibular rehabilitation following mild traumatic brain injury. NeuroRehabilitation 32:519–528
76. Sosnoff JJ, Broglio SP, Shin S, Ferrara MS (2011) Previous mild traumatic brain injury and postural-control dynamics. J Athl Train 46:85–91
77. King NS, Crawford S, Wenden FJ, Moss NEG, Wade DT (1995) The rivermead post concussion symptoms questionnaire: a measure of symptoms commonly experienced after head injury and its reliability. J Neurol 242:587–592
78. Kontos AP, Elbin RJ, Schatz P, Covassin T, Henry L, Pardini J et al (2012) A revised factor structure for the post-concussion symptom scale: baseline and post-concussion factors. Am J Sports Med 40:2375–2384
79. Pardini D, Stump JE, Lovell M, Collins MW, Moritz K, Fu FH (2004) The post-concussion symptoms scale (PCSS): A factor analysis. Br J Sports Med 38:661
80. Lau B, Lovell MR, Collins MW, Pardini J (2009) Neurocognitive and symptom predictors of recovery in high school athletes. Clin J Sport Med 19:216–221
81. Lau BC, Collins MW, Lovell MR (2012) Cutoff scores in neurocognitive testing and symptom clusters that predict protracted recovery from concussions in high school athletes. Neurosurgery 70:371–379; discussion 379
82. Meehan WP III, Mannix RC, O'Brien MJ, Collins MW (2013) The prevalence of undiagnosed concussions in athletes. Clin J Sport Med. https://doi.org/10.1097/JSM.0b013e318291d3b3
83. Sandel NK, Lovell MR, Kegel NE, Collins MW, Kontos AP (2012) The relationship of symptoms and neurocognitive performance to perceived recovery from sports-related concussion among adolescent athletes. Appl Neuropsychol. 10.1080/21622965.2012.670580; M3: doi:10.1080/21622965.2012.670580; 02 10.1080/21622965.2012.6705801-6
84. Van Kampen DA, Lovell MR, Pardini JE, Collins MW, Fu FH (2006) The "value added" of neurocognitive testing after sports-related concussion. Am J Sports Med 34:1630–1635
85. Kinnaman KA, Mannix RC, Comstock RD, Meehan WP (2013) Management strategies and medication use for treating pediatric patients with concussions. Acta Paediatr (Oslo 1992). https://doi.org/10.1111/apa.12315
86. Kinnaman KA, Mannix RC, Comstock RD, Meehan WP III (2014) Management of pediatric patients with concussion by emergency medicine physicians. Pediatr Emerg Care 30:458–461
87. U.S. Food and Drug Administration (2016) FDA allows marketing of first-of-kind computerized cognitive tests to help assess cognitive skills after a head injury. http://www.fda.gov/NewsEvents/Newsroom/PressAnnouncements/ucm517526.htm
88. Fazio VC, Lovell MR, Pardini JE, Collins MW (2007) The relation between post concussion symptoms and neurocognitive performance in concussed athletes. NeuroRehabilitation 22:207–216
89. Alsalaheen BA, Mucha A, Morris LO, Whitney SL, Furman JM, Camiolo-Reddy CE et al (2010) Vestibular rehabilitation for dizziness and balance disorders after concussion. J Neurol Phys Ther 34:87–93
90. Alsalaheen BA, Whitney SL, Mucha A, Morris LO, Furman JM, Sparto PJ (2013) Exercise prescription patterns in patients treated with vestibular rehabilitation after concussion. Physiother Res Int 18:100–108
91. Goldberg JM (2012) The vestibular system: a sixth sense. OUP USA, New York, NY
92. Hoffer ME, Gottshall KR, Moore R, Balough BJ, Wester D (2004) Characterizing and treating dizziness after mild head trauma. Otol Neurotol 25:135–138
93. Mucha A, Collins MW, Elbin RJ, Furman JM, Troutman-Enseki C, DeWolf RM et al (2014) A brief vestibular/ocular motor screening (VOMS) assessment to evaluate concussions: preliminary findings. Am J Sports Med 42:2479–2486

94. Guskiewicz KM (2001) Postural stability assessment following concussion: one piece of the puzzle. Clin J Sport Med 11:182–189
95. Riemann BL, Guskiewicz KM (2000) Effects of mild head injury on postural stability as measured through clinical balance testing. J Athl Train 35:19–25
96. Ciuffreda KJ, Kapoor N, Rutner D, Suchoff IB, Han ME, Craig S (2007) Occurrence of oculomotor dysfunctions in acquired brain injury: a retrospective analysis. Optometry 78:155–161
97. Leddy JJ, Kozlowski K, Donnelly JP, Pendergast DR, Epstein LH, Willer B (2010) A preliminary study of subsymptom threshold exercise training for refractory post-concussion syndrome. Clin J Sport Med 20:21–27
98. Leddy JJ, Willer B (2013) Use of graded exercise testing in concussion and return-to-activity management. Curr Sports Med Rep 12:370–376
99. Thomas DG, Apps JN, Hoffmann RG, McCrea M, Hammeke T (2015) Benefits of strict rest after acute concussion: a randomized controlled trial. Pediatrics. peds.2014-0966 [pii]

53 Controversy Around Headers

Anthony P. Kontos

Contents

A.P. Kontos, Ph.D.
Department of Orthopaedic Surgery, University of Pittsburgh, Pittsburgh, PA, USA

UPMC Rooney Sports Complex,
3200 South Water Street, Pittsburgh, PA 15203, USA
e-mail: akontos@pitt.edu

53.1 Heading in Football

Football is the most popular sport in the world, with more than 265 million participants across the world [1]. Football is unique compared to other sports in that players use their unprotected heads to purposefully pass, shoot, redirect, and control the ball (Fig. 53.1). Football heading technique is considered an important part of both offensive and defensive play and is frequently implemented by players. Researchers, coaches, and players alike have expressed concerns about the potential adverse effects of purposeful heading in football on cognitive function, postural control, and concussion-related symptoms [2–5]. In an effort to prevent potential acute (i.e., concussion) and chronic (i.e., residual symptoms, cognitive and motor impairment) effects from purposeful heading, mandatory restrictions on heading exposure in youth players have recently been implemented.

53.2 Heading and Concussions

Concussion is a major health concern in football. A concussion results in a variety of symptoms (e.g., headache, dizziness, fogginess) [6] and cognitive (e.g., memory, reaction time, processing speed) [7], psychological (e.g., depression, anxiety) [8], and vestibular/oculomotor (e.g., dizziness, imbalance, gait, vestibuloocular) impairment [9]. The effects of concussions typically last for

V. Musahl et al. (eds.), *Return to Play in Football*, https://doi.org/10.1007/978-3-662-55713-6_53

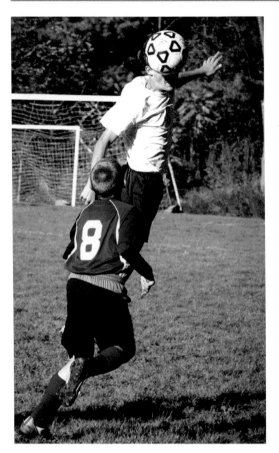

Fig. 53.1 Soccer is unique in that players purposefully head the ball

1–3 weeks but can extend to months or longer [10]. Based on cumulative concussion incidence estimates of approximately 13% for football in the United States (USA) [11], more than 34 million players worldwide will have a concussion playing football. Previously, researchers have reported that heading is involved in 25–30% of concussions in football [11], with 62–78% of concussions resulting from incidental head-to-head contact [12]. Heading-related concussions may result from improper head-to-ball contact, head-to-head contact, and risky behaviors (i.e., attempting to head the ball in a crowd of players). Therefore, efforts to minimize the effect of these head impacts, as well as lower the risk of concussion in the youth football, are critical in protecting the safety of players and the integrity of the game moving forward.

Fact Box 1

The majority of concussions in football do not involve heading.

53.3 Heading and Chronic Effects

For the past four decades, researchers have hypothesized that football heading may negatively affect cognitive function and symptoms. Early studies supported this hypothesis [13, 14], but studies were limited by retrospective research designs, an emphasis on retired professional players, and did not account for concussion history as a confounding variable. More recent studies have reported no relationship between heading exposure and cognitive performance in adolescent football players [15–17]. A recent review of not only the effects of heading but also the incidence of concussions in football, the mechanism of injury, and the neurocognitive implications of concussions in football indicated the long-term effects of heading were similar to those effects seen in athletes with a history of concussion [18]. Many of the studies examined, however, failed to record concussion history of the participants in the study, thus limiting the accuracy of the assessment. Additionally, many of the studies reported conflicting results, again suggesting the need for further exploration as recent literature continues to be inconclusive.

As a result of the inconsistency in the literature and selective nature of the previously discussed systematic review, we conducted the first meta-analytic review of the effects of football heading [19]. The findings from our analyses did not support an overall adverse effect for heading across studies, suggesting that reported effects associated with heading are a product of small sample sizes, inconsistent methodologies, and sampling errors and, at best, are equivocal in the literature. We did find some evidence for age as modifier for any effects of heading. In short, reported effects associated with heading appear to be limited to professional players who have had substantial levels of exposure to heading over long careers. However, the empirical evidence is limited even in this select group of players. There is a clear need for larger-scale, systematic, and longitudinal studies of the purported effects of football heading. In spite of these recent findings to the contrary, researchers and clinicians continue to raise concerns about the potential adverse effects associated with football heading in youth, especially in regard to long-term exposure and concussion (Fig. 53.2).

Heading in football has typically been quantified using self-reported data, which are notoriously wrought with error and bias. Part of the reason for the reliance on self-reported heading data is that football players do not wear protective headgear like in American football and ice hockey. Consequently, accelerometer sensors that measure in vivo head impacts have only recently been developed and tested for use in football players [20]. These newer sensors are affixed via adhesive to the head (typically behind the ear) or contained within soft headbands or special mouth guards. Although these sensors hold promise to assess the frequency, intensity, and accumulation of head impacts in football players [21], there are limitations associated with their use including compliance and false positives. Regardless, accelerometer sensor technology is critical to furthering our understanding of repetitive exposure to heading and concussion in at-risk youth football players.

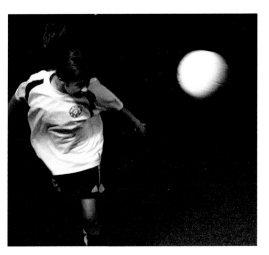

Fig. 53.2 Researchers and clinicians have raised concerns about heading in youth players

53.4 A Lack of Support for Protective Head Gear

Several manufacturers have designed and marketed soft protective headbands that are purported to reduce concussions and impact forces associated with heading in football players (Fig. 53.3). Players are permitted to wear these headbands by most football governing bodies. Several high-profile professional players have begun receiving financial endorsements from manufacturers and subsequently wearing these protective headbands during professional games, lending anecdotal support to their effectiveness. As a result of these endorsements and increased visibility, some parents of youth players have begun outfitting their children with these protective headbands in an attempt to minimize risk of injury. However, the findings on the effectiveness of protective headbands in football in the existent literature are equivocal. For example, some researchers have reported that headbands reduce peak linear forces associated with head-to-ball contact in laboratory dummies [22], whereas other researchers have reported that headbands do *not* reduce these impacts to the head [23].

With regard to the effectiveness of the headbands in actual players, an earlier retrospective study by Delaney and colleagues [24] suggested that players who wore a protective headband reported fewer concussions on a survey than those who did not, but this study did not examine

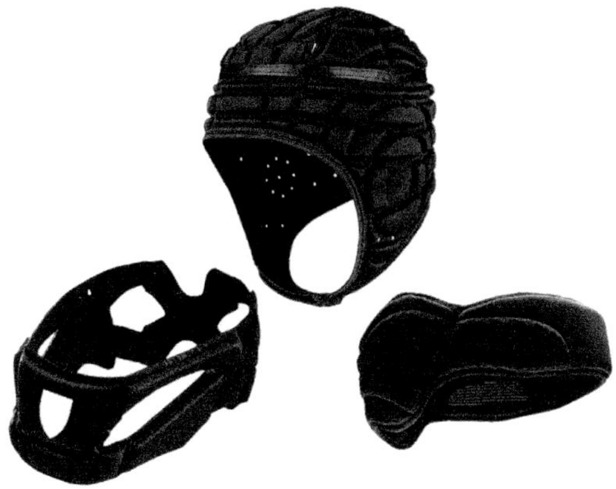

Fig. 53.3 Soft protective headbands have been marketed to soccer players

exposure or player behavior and involved recall of concussions. Moreover, the players were not randomly assigned to the headbands during the study. In a more recent study of the effects (i.e., symptoms, cognitive performance) of an acute bout of heading, collegiate football players in the USA were randomly assigned to wear protective headbands and then exposed to 15 headers over 15 min [25]. The findings from this study were contrary to what was expected, with players who wore the headbands actually performing worse on memory and reaction time than the players who did not wear the headbands. These findings, together with a general lack of support in the literature, suggest that protective headbands have little impact in reducing any effects associated with heading and are unlikely to reduce the risk of concussion. In fact, some researchers, coaches, and players have suggested that wearing protective gear in football may actually increase risk behaviors such as headers in a crowded penalty area or diving headers by the post. Researchers need to examine further the effects of headbands on biomechanical forces to the head, concussion risk, and player behaviors.

Fact Box 2

Protective headbands have little impact in reducing any effects associated with heading and are unlikely to reduce the risk of concussion.

53.5 Concerns About Concussion in Youth Players

Participation in youth (5–19 years) football is at an all-time high with more than 22 million registered participants worldwide and over 3 million in the USA alone [26]. This steady increase in youth football participation has also resulted in an increased concern about concussions. The main reason for concern about concussion in youth football players is that the effects of this injury may be more pronounced in youth sport participants due to ongoing brain development [27, 28]. Although most players with concussions recover within a week to 21 days, symptoms and impairment can extend longer depending on the domain [29]. These extended sequelae and prolonged recoveries can lead to increased costs associated with additional care, as well as adverse impacts on academic and psychosocial functioning.

The cumulative concussion incidence in youth (11–14 years) football is 13%, and the incidence rate is 1.2 concussions/1000 athletic exposures [11]. These data translate to an estimated 2.9 million concussions among youth football players worldwide and 390,000 in the USA. However, these data may represent an underestimation of the incidence of concussion in youth football as the majority of youth leagues lack sufficient and consistent medical oversight for this injury. Consequently, many concussions in youth football may go unreported or unrecognized. In older player age groups in sport (i.e., 15–19 years), with appropriate and consistent medical coverage, as many as 40% of all concussions are unreported [30]. Using this estimate, nearly 9 million concussions may go unreported in youth football.

Fact Box 3

It is estimated that 13% of youth footballers will experience a concussion.

53.6 Sex and Age Differences in Concussion and Heading

The greatest proportional growth in football participation worldwide and in the USA is in female youth players [1]. Researchers report that female football players are at greater risk for concussion compared to males [12, 31, 32]. In addition, a greater percentage of concussions occur from purposeful heading in females (31%) compared to males (12%), and concussions related to purposeful heading have increased significantly over the past 9 years for females [12]. Among the explanations for the increased risk for females sustaining head-to-ball concussive injuries than males are decreased head stability and increased angular acceleration in females [33, 34]. Although female athletes are at a greater risk for concussion, male athletes tend to head the ball more frequently than female athletes [17, 35]. Researchers suggest that male adolescent football players head the ball at a greater frequency than female adolescent players in both practices and games [35]. In a previous study on the effects of football heading in youth, we compared directly males and females and found that males headed the ball nearly two times more than females in games and over three times more in practices [17]. However, males tended to have more years of playing experience, which may be driving sex differences in heading.

Fact Box 4

Males head the ball nearly two times more than females in games and over three times more in practices. Although female football players head the ball less frequently than male players, female players actually have more concussions from heading.

There are few studies that have examined age differences in concussion or heading exposure among football players. Previous research has suggested that younger sport participants (i.e., adolescent) are at a greater risk and take longer to recover from a concussion than older participants (i.e., adult) [36, 37]. Purcell and colleagues [38] reported that early to middle adolescence (i.e., 12–15) was the period of greatest risk for concussion in youth. Youth football players are undergoing rapid brain changes and development during the ages of 11–14 years [39], which may be associated with increased vulnerability to the neurometabolic and pathophysiological events that occur following concussion and heading [40, 41]. However, none of these studies have focused on football players. In regard to the effects associated with heading exposure, findings from our recent meta-analysis suggested age was a potential modifying factor for adverse outcomes associated with football heading. Specifically, older players seemed to be more at risk for negative effects associated with heading. However, this finding is likely a product of older players at higher levels of play having more experience and therefore exposure to heading overall longer period of time.

53.7 Concussion and Heading Guidelines in Football

Unparalleled media focus on concussions in sport has resulted in significant concerns for football governing bodies worldwide. In fact, following a well-publicized concussion involving a German football player during the 2014 FIFA World Cup, the FIFA Medical Committee implemented changes in protocols impacting how concussions in FIFA-sanctioned competitions are managed. Specifically, FIFA recommended that whenever a suspected concussion occurs, the referee should stop the game for 3 min to allow for an on-pitch assessment to determine if a player is concussed. Players are allowed to return to the pitch only if cleared to do so by the team physician. Unfortunately, a 3-min evaluation on the pitch does not allow for a complete assessment of all of the potential signs, symptoms, and impairments (e.g., cognitive, vestibular spinal, vestibular ocular, vision) associated with a concussion. Moreover, pitch side is not an ideal environment in which to conduct an evaluation. Players and team physicians may also feel added pressure to return a player to the pitch, especially in light of FIFA substitution limitations and the realities of professional football. Injuries may also be ignored due to the potential impact of a 3-min absence from the game due to the required assessment. In fact, in 2015, the head coach admonished the head team physician and physiotherapist from an English Premier League team for trying to assess a player for a suspected concussion, even though the referee had waved them on the pitch for that purpose. In addition, players may have delayed onset of concussion-related symptoms and impairment that may not be evident until several hours or even days following injury.

Fact Box 5

Players are allowed to return to the pitch following a suspected concussion only if the team physician clears them.

53.8 Author's Recommendation

The current FIFA recommendations, while a step in the right direction, could be enhanced. A head injury-specific substitution rule would alleviate the pressure experienced by players and team physicians to keep potentially injured players on the pitch. FIFA could also borrow approaches used by the National [American] Football League including the implementation of an independent physician to assess suspected concussions on the pitch, thereby reducing pressure from coaches and players, and a trained "spotter" in the broadcast booth that uses video replay to identify potentially concussed players.

While concussions have been the focus at the professional levels of football, at the youth levels, exposure to football heading has received heightened attention. Consequently, several football governing bodies have developed heading guidelines designed to reduce both concussion risk and exposure to heading in youth players. In November 2015, the US Soccer Federation (US Soccer) released their "Recognize to Recover" program, which is a comprehensive health and safety initiative that promotes safer play in football at the youth level and is focused on limited exposure to heading. As a result of this initiative, US Soccer set forth the following youth football heading guidelines:

1. Players under the age of 10 years should not engage in heading either in practice or in games (this is to include 11-year-olds who may be playing on under-11 [U-11] teams). For members adopting this recommendation, any deliberate attempts to head the ball by players 10 years old and younger will be penalized by allowing an indirect free kick to the opposing team.
2. Players between the ages of 11 and 13 years should have limited heading training, at a weekly maximum of 30 min and no more than 15–20 headers per player. Heading is allowed in games at these ages without restriction or penalty.

Players at younger (i.e., U-11) ages rarely head the ball and when they do it typically involves limited head impact forces. As such, eliminating heading in players under age 11 is both intuitive and will have limited effect on the way in which football is played at these age groups. However, the restriction of heading in players aged 11–13 years is not evidence based and will likely have limited effects on reducing concussion risk, as the majority of concussions in football do *not* involve heading. Moreover, if these early adolescent-aged players are not taught proper heading technique in a safe manner in practice but allowed to perform headers in matches, they are more at risk for injury from heading during matches. In addition, by teaching proper heading technique in practice to these younger players, they will have more time to develop this skill than if they learn it later in their career.

Fact Box 7

Football heading guidelines should be evidence based.

53.9 Improving Heading Skill

In 2016, the National Soccer Coaches Association of America (NSCAA) in conjunction with researchers, players, and coaches developed an online instructional course titled Get aHEAD Safely in Soccer™ (Get aHEAD™). The objective of this instruction course is to educate youth football coaches on the best ways to instruct

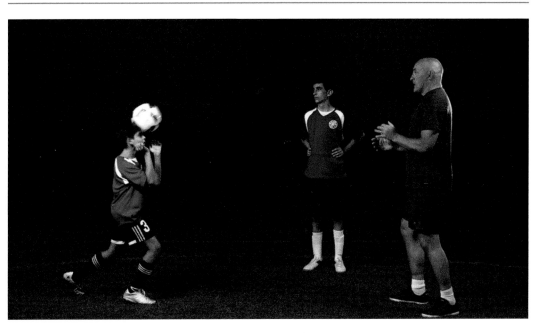

Fig. 53.4 Teaching proper heading technique can help promote safe play in soccer

youth players in proper and safer purposeful heading. The objective of the Get aHEAD™ intervention is to reduce the risk of concussion in youth football players while at the same time teaching safe and effective techniques to head a ball purposefully. The intervention comprises teaching proper heading techniques, strengthening neck and core musculature, avoiding risky situations on the pitch, educating referees, and incorporating lightweight footballs to minimize impacts on the head during practice. The Get aHEAD™ approach represents a paradigm shift away from heading restrictions toward promoting safe play through proper heading instruction. Researchers need to examine empirically the programs such as Get aHEAD™ to determine their effectiveness in improving heading skill and preventing injuries such as concussion (Fig. 53.4).

Take-Home Message

Concussion is a major health concern in football that warrants awareness and attention from researchers and clinicians alike. However, the effects of purposeful heading on players are unclear and warrant additional research. As such, any heading guidelines in football should be evidence based. Instructional programs that focus on teaching proper heading and promote safer play could help reduce concussions and exposure to football headers that are risky, especially among youth players.

Top Five Evidence-Based References

Kontos AP et al (2016) Meta-analytical review of the effects of football heading. Brit J Sports Med 51(15):1118–1124

Maher ME, Hutchison M, Cusimano M, Comper P, Schweizer TA (2014) Concussions and heading in soccer: a review of the evidence of incidence, mechanisms, biomarkers and neurocognitive outcomes. Brain Inj 28(3):271–285

O'Kane JW et al (2014) Concussion among female middle-school soccer players. JAMA Pediatr 168(3):258–264

Chrisman SP, Mac Donald CL, Friedman S, Andre J, Rowhani-Rahbar A, Drescher S, Stein E, Holm M, Evans N, Poliakov AV, Ching RP, Schwien CC, Vavilala MS, Rivara FP (2016) Head impact exposure during a weekend youth soccer tournament. J Child Neurol 31(8):971–978

Elbin RJ, Beatty A, Covassin T, Schatz P, Hydeman A, Kontos AP (2015) A preliminary examination of neurocognitive performance and symptoms following a bout of soccer heading in athletes wearing protective soccer headbands. Res Sports Med 23(2):203–214

References

1. FIFA FIdF (2007) Big count report http://www.fifa.com. Accessed 13 Feb 2017
2. Baroff GS (1998) Is heading a soccer ball injurious to brain function? J Head Trauma Rehabil 13(2):45–52
3. Kirkendall DT, Garrett WE Jr (2001) Heading in soccer: integral skill or grounds for cognitive dysfunction? J Athl Train 36(3):328–333
4. Putukian M (2004) Heading in soccer: is it safe? Curr Sports Med Rep 3(1):9–14
5. Spiotta AM, Bartsch AJ, Benzel EC (2012) Heading in soccer: dangerous play? Neurosurgery 70(1):1–11. discussion 11
6. Kontos AP, Elbin RJ, Fazio-Sumrock VC, Burkhart S, Swindell H, Maroon J, Collins MW (2013) Incidence of sports-related concussion among youth football players aged 8–12 years. J Pediatr 163(3):717–720
7. Lau BC, Kontos AP, Collins MW, Mucha A, Lovell MR (2011) Which on-field signs/symptoms predict protracted recovery from sport-related concussion among high school football players? Am J Sports Med 39(11):2311–2318
8. Kontos APCM, Russo S (2004) An introduction to sport concussion for the sport psychology consultant. Appl Sport Psychol 16(3):220–235
9. Mucha A, Collins MW, Elbin RJ, Furman JM, Troutman-Enseki C, DeWolf RM, Marchetti G, Kontos AP (2014) A brief vestibular/ocular motor screening (VOMS) assessment to evaluate concussions: preliminary findings. Am J Sports Med 42(10):2479–2486
10. Collins MW, Kontos AP, Okonkwo DO, Almquist J, Bailes J, Barisa M, Bazarian J, Bloom OJ, Brody D, Cantu R, Cardenas J, Clugston J, Cohen R, Elbin RJ, Ellenbogen R, Fonseca J, Gioia G, Guskiewicz K, Heyer R, Hotz G, Iverson GL, Jordan B, Manley G, Maroon J, McAllister T, McCrea M, Mucha A, Pieroth E, Podell K, Pombo M, Shetty T, Sills A, Solomon G, Thomas DG, Valovich McLeod TC, Yates T, Zafonte R (2016) Statements of agreement from the targeted evaluation and active management (TEAM) approaches to treating concussion meeting held in Pittsburgh, October 15–16, 2015. Neurosurgery.
11. O'Kane JW, Schiff MA (2014) Concerns about concussion rates in female youth soccer-reply. JAMA Pediatr 168(10):968
12. Comstock RD, Currie DW, Pierpoint LA, Grubenhoff JA, Fields SK (2015) An evidence-based discussion of heading the ball and concussions in high school soccer. JAMA Pediatr 169(9):830–837
13. Kröss R, Ohler K, Barolin G (1983) Effect of heading in soccer on the head--a quantifying EEG study of soccer players. EEG EMG Z Elektroenzephalogr Elektromyogr Verwandte Geb 14(4):209–212
14. Tysvaer A, Storli O (1981) Association football injuries to the brain. A preliminary report. Br J Sports Med 15(3):163–166
15. Dorminy M, Hoogeveen A, Tierney RT, Higgins M, McDevitt JK, Kretzschmar J (2015) Effect of soccer heading ball speed on S100B, sideline concussion assessments and head impact kinematics. Brain Inj 2015:1–7
16. Kaminski TW, Cousino ES, Glutting JJ (2008) Examining the relationship between purposeful heading in soccer and computerized neuropsychological test performance. Res Q Exerc Sport 79(2):235–244
17. Kontos AP, Dolese A, Elbin R III, Covassin T, Warren BL (2011) Relationship of soccer heading to computerized neurocognitive performance and symptoms among female and male youth soccer players. Brain Inj 25(12):1234–1241
18. Maher ME, Hutchison M, Cusimano M, Comper P, Schweizer TA (2014) Concussions and heading in soccer: a review of the evidence of incidence, mechanisms, biomarkers and neurocognitive outcomes. Brain Inj 28(3):271–285
19. Kontos A, Braithwaite R, Chrisman SP, McAllister-Deitrick J, Symington L, Reeves V, Collins M (2016) A meta-analytic review of the effects of soccer heading. Br J Sports Med 51(15):1118–1124
20. Chrisman SP, Mac Donald CL, Friedman S, Andre J, Rowhani-Rahbar A, Drescher S, Stein E, Holm M, Evans N, Poliakov AV, Ching RP, Schwien CC, Vavilala MS, Rivara FP (2016) Head impact exposure during a weekend youth soccer tournament. J Child Neurol 31(8):971–978
21. Catenaccio E, Caccese J, Wakschlag N, Fleysher R, Kim N, Kim M, Buckley TA, Stewart WF, Lipton RB, Kaminski T, Lipton ML (2016) Validation and calibration of HeadCount, a self-report measure for quantifying heading exposure in soccer players. Res Sports Med 24(4):416–425
22. Broglio SP, YY J, Broglio MD, Sell TC (2003) The efficacy of soccer headgear. J Athl Train 38(3):220–224
23. Withnall C, Shewchenko N, Wonnacott M, Dvorak J (2005) Effectiveness of headgear in football. Br J Sports Med 39(Suppl 1):i40–i48. discussion i48
24. Delaney JS, Al-Kashmiri A, Drummond R, Correa JA (2008) The effect of protective headgear on head injuries and concussions in adolescent football (soccer) players. Br J Sports Med 42(2):110–115. discussion 115
25. Elbin RJ, Beatty A, Covassin T, Schatz P, Hydeman A, Kontos AP (2015) A preliminary examination of neurocognitive performance and symptoms following a bout of soccer heading in athletes wearing protective soccer headbands. Res Sports Med 23(2):203–214
26. Soccer UY (2017) Key statistics. http://www.usyouthsoccer.org/media_kit/keystatistics/. Accessed 17 Feb 2017
27. Field M, Collins MW, Lovell MR, Maroon J (2003) Does age play a role in recovery from sports-related

concussion? A comparison of high school and collegiate athletes. J Pediatr 142(5):546–553
28. Giedd JN (2004) Structural magnetic resonance imaging of the adolescent brain. Ann N Y Acad Sci 1021:77–85
29. Henry LC, Burkhart SO, Elbin RJ, Agarwal V, Kontos AP (2015) Traumatic axonal injury and persistent emotional lability in an adolescent following moderate traumatic brain injury: a case study. J Clin Exp Neuropsychol 37(4):439–454
30. McCrea M, Hammeke T, Olsen G, Leo P, Guskiewicz K (2004) Unreported concussion in high school football players: implications for prevention. Clin J Sport Med 14(1):13–17
31. Gessel LM, Fields SK, Collins CL, Dick RW, Comstock RD (2007) Concussions among United States high school and collegiate athletes. J Athl Train 42(4):495–503
32. Lincoln A, Caswell S, Almquist J, Dunn R, Norris J, Hinton R (2011) Trends in concussion incidence in high school sports: a prospective 11-year study. Am J Sports Med 39(5):958–963
33. Mansell J, Tierney R, Sitler M, Swanik K, Stearne D (2005) Resistance training and head-neck segment dynamic stabilization in male and female collegiate soccer players. J Athl Train 40(4):310–319
34. Tierney R, Sitler M, Swanik B, Swanik K, Higgins M, Torg J (2005) Gender differences in head-neck segment dynamic stabilization during head acceleration. Med Sci Sports Exerc 37:272–279
35. Webbe F, Ochs S (2003) Recency and frequency of soccer heading interact to decrease neurocognitive performance. Appl Neuropsychol 10(1):31–41
36. Covassin T, Elbin RJ, Harris W, Parker T, Kontos A (2012) The role of age and sex in symptoms, neurocognitive performance, and postural stability in athletes after concussion. Am J Sports Med 40(6):1303–1312
37. Dompier T, Kerr Z, Marshall S, Hainline B, Snook E, Hayden R, Simon J (2015) Incidence of concussion during practice and games in youth, high school, and collegiate American football players. JAMA Pediatr 169(7):659–665
38. Purcell L, Harvey J, Seabrook JA (2016) Patterns of recovery following sport-related concussion in children and adolescents. Clin Pediatr (Phila) 55(5):452–458
39. Courchesne E, Chisum HJ, Townsend J, Cowles A, Covington J, Egaas B, Harwood M, Hinds S, Press GA (2000) Normal brain development and aging: quantitative analysis at in vivo MR imaging in healthy volunteers. Radiology 216(3):672–682
40. Giza CC, Hovda DA (2014) The new neurometabolic cascade of concussion. Neurosurgery 75(Suppl 4):S24–S33
41. Maugans TA, Farley C, Altaye M, Leach J, Cecil KM (2012) Pediatric sports-related concussion produces cerebral blood flow alterations. Pediatrics 129(1):28–37

Concussion: Predicting Recovery

54

Robert J. Elbin, Nathan D'Amico, Tamara Valovich McLeod, Tracey Covassin, and Morgan Anderson

Contents

R.J. Elbin, Ph.D. (✉) • N. D'Amico, M.S., A.T.C.
M. Anderson, B.S.
Department of Health, Human Performance and Recreation, Office for Sport Concussion Research, University of Arkansas, Fayetteville, AR, USA
e-mail: rjelbin@uark.edu

T.V. McLeod, Ph.D., A.T.C., F.N.A.T.A.
Athletic Training Programs, School of Osteopathic Medicine in Arizona, A.T. Still University, Mesa, AZ, USA

T. Covassin, Ph.D., A.T.C., F.N.A.T.A
Department of Kinesiology, Michigan State University, East Lansing, MI, USA

54.1 Introduction

Determining when an athlete is fully recovered from a sport-related concussion (SRC) can be one of the more difficult decisions for the sports medicine clinician. Sport-related concussion is an injury involving the brain, which is a complex organ that is responsible for many different functions. Moreover, the signs, symptoms, and impairments that are associated with SRC are unique to each athlete and require an individualized and multifaceted assessment approach [1, 2]. The heterogenic presentation of SRC has prompted clinicians and researchers to utilize both objective (e.g., neurocognitive, vestibular, oculomotor, balance) and subjective data (e.g., symptom reports) in conjunction with a thorough clinical examination to identify clinical profiles [3] that subsequently can inform targeted treatment and rehabilitation strategies. The successful completion of prescribed rehabilitation and treatment is then followed by a gradual, stepwise return-to-play (RTP) protocol outlined in recent consensus statements [2, 4]. Despite clinical advances in the assessment, management, and treatment of SRC, estimating time until clinical recovery remains a challenge. Although most athletes will recover from SRC within 3 weeks [5], there are a small percentage of athletes that will exhibit a prolonged recovery longer than this 3-week

V. Musahl et al. (eds.), *Return to Play in Football*, https://doi.org/10.1007/978-3-662-55713-6_54

time period [6]. Identifying these athletes soon after injury may enable earlier interventions.

54.2 Defining Recovery Following Sport-Related Concussion

There is no recognized gold standard for determining recovery from SRC. The multifaceted, serial assessment of symptom reporting, neurocognitive performance, postural stability, and vestibular and ocular motor function provide clinicians with the ability to track the resolution of impairments in the days and weeks following injury. In most clinical settings, the sports medicine clinician periodically gathers and records subjective and objective data from the patient to determine recovery of persistent impairment. Once the athlete is deemed to be within normal limits of function, they are then cleared to begin the recommended graduated RTP protocol [2]. The elapsed time that occurs between SRC and the "return to baseline" or pre-injury levels of functioning is often considered a recovery milestone, and the additional time that it takes the athlete to successfully complete the stepwise RTP protocol may add more time to the recovery process. Although there is great clinical benefit from the comprehensive assessment of multiple domains following SRC, each of these domains resolve at different times following SRC and may not match physiological recovery [5, 7].

54.3 Post-concussion Symptom Recovery

The recovery from a SRC has traditionally been defined as the resolution of self-reported symptoms and often termed as an athlete reporting being "asymptomatic." Symptom resolution is a key determinant for allowing an athlete to begin the RTP process [2]. However, there are limitations to the reliance of self-reported symptoms to determine recovery, as many individuals endorse symptoms at baseline or in an otherwise healthy state [8–10]. In addition, several researchers have reported that self-reported symptoms are often minimized and/or unreported by the concussed athlete in an effort to expedite recovery from SRC [7]. Therefore, some researchers suggest a better estimation of symptom recovery is to redefine asymptomatic as a return to a "normal" symptom presentation for that individual instead of a "zero" endorsement on a post-concussion symptom scale [11]. For example, athletes that suffer from migraine frequently endorse a mild headache when noninjured, and to expect that this athlete will report a "zero" on a post-concussion symptom scale when recovered from concussion may be unrealistic.

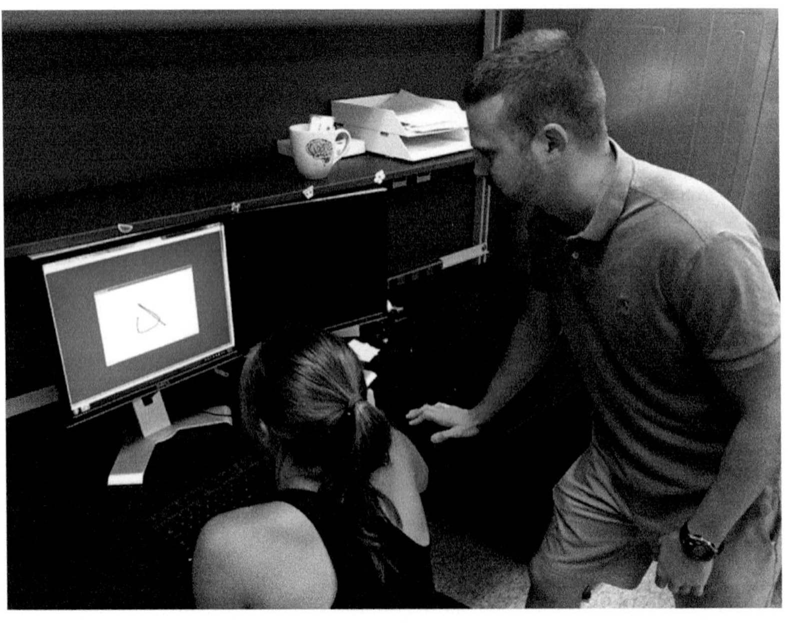

The time course of symptom recovery following SRC is well documented in the literature. Researchers report that [12] the resolution of symptoms was reported to occur around the first week following SRC in a large sample of predominantly male college athletes. Several consensus papers report that the complete (i.e., symptoms, cognitive, balance) recovery following SRC is approximately 7–10 days [2, 4, 13]. Other investigators [14] report post-concussion symptom duration lasting approximately 6 days in a sample of concussed high school and college athletes. These researchers also reported that more than 70% of their sample exhibited symptom recovery within 7 days of SRC. In addition, 93.7% and 99.3% of their sample reported symptom recovery within 14–30 days, respectively [14]. However, other researchers report that symptom recovery may take longer than previously reported, which may be attributable to certain factors that predispose an athlete to reporting symptoms such as somatization [15] and migraine history [1, 16] or continuing to play with their SRC without notifying medical professionals [17, 18]. Although the monitoring of symptoms is a critical piece of SRC management, these reports are subjective and can be minimized by the athlete. As a result of these limitations, it is best practice to supplement subjective symptom reports with more objective assessments to better determine SRC recovery [2, 19].

54.4 Recovery of Neurocognitive Performance, Postural Stability, and Vestibular/ Oculomotor Function

The use of neurocognitive testing and balance assessments increases the objectivity of SRC management [12, 20, 21]. Sports medicine clinicians often administer these testing batteries in a pretest (i.e., baseline)-posttest method that allows for post-injury performance to be compared to pre-injury levels of function. The literature documenting the recovery of neurocognitive function following SRC is mixed. Early studies, using pencil and paper or brief neurocognitive batteries, noted neurocognitive recovery times ranging between 5 and 7 days [12], and more recent evidence suggests that neurocognitive recovery on more widely used computerized neurocognitive batteries ranges from 11 [22] to 28 days [5]. Similarly, researchers examining the recovery of postural stability in athletes with SRC report improvement within the first 3–5 days following injury [12, 23]. In contrast to this short time frame, other studies using more sophisticated gait and dual-task measures report deficits lasting several weeks to months following concussion [24–26].

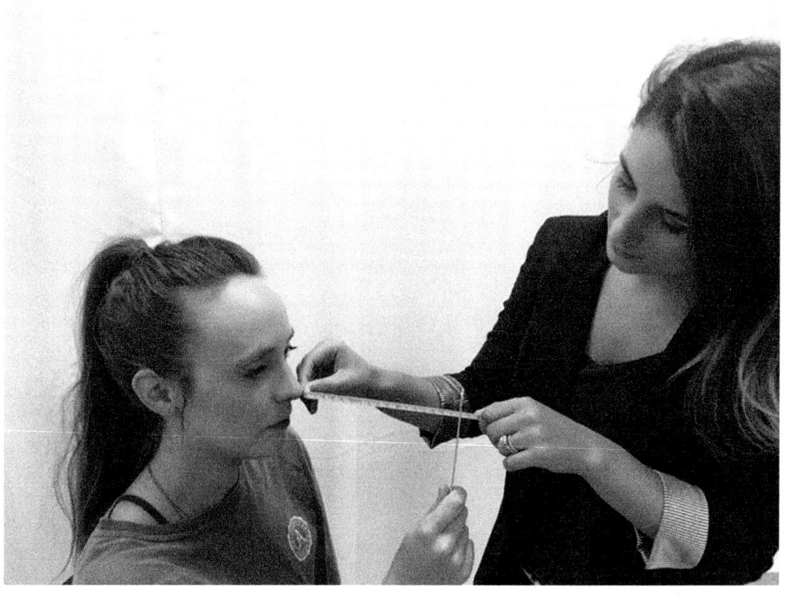

More recently, additional assessments of the vestibular and oculomotor systems have been introduced into clinical practice [27, 28]. Assessment of saccadic eye movement using the King-Devick test has noted significantly slower time on this task following SRC [29]. A more comprehensive assessment of the oculomotor system and the additional evaluation of the vestibular system is the vestibular/ocular motor screening (VOMS). Recent studies reveal that the VOMS is sensitive to detecting vestibular and oculomotor impairments following SRC [28, 30]. The documented recovery times for vestibular and oculomotor impairment following SRC are currently understudied.

54.5 Safely Returning an Athlete to Play Following SRC

Once an athlete reports being asymptomatic and their objective data is within baseline and/or normal levels of function, the sports medicine clinician can begin a graduated RTP protocol [2]. The graduated RTP protocol (Fig. 54.1) is designed to slowly introduce physical exertion that increases the demands placed on the body to determine whether incremental physical exertion results in a return of symptoms. The most often cited progression is the six-step progression endorsed by the International Conference on Concussion in Sport [2] in which the athlete progresses through each step, under supervision, with 24 h between each step. Should symptoms return at any step in the progression, the protocol is halted, and the athlete should resume at the level prior to symptom provocation once symptoms have resolved. This progression typically takes approximately a week to fully progress through each stage without any setbacks. However, recent studies suggest that relying solely on symptom reports to determine progress through this protocol may be faulty, as approximately 16% of athletes demonstrated clinical deficits on objective neurocognitive testing despite reporting asymptomatic following the completion of the RTP protocol [31]. These data support the need for post-exertional objective assessment, such as neurocognitive testing, to more accurately ensure recovery following the RTP protocol.

Rehabilitation Stage	Ex Exercise at Each Stage	Objective at Each Stage
1. No Activity	Physical and cognitive rest	Recovery
2. Light Aerobic Exercise	Walk, swim, stationary bike, <70% of max HR, no resistance training	Increase HR
3. Sport-Specific Exercise	Skating drills (hockey), running (soccer), no head impact activities	Increase HR Add movement
4. Non-contact drills	More complex training drills, may being progressive resistance training	Exercise, coordination, and cognitive load
5. Full-contact practice	Following medial clearance, participate in normal training activities	Restore athlete's confidence; coaching staff assess functional skills
6. Return to play	Normal game play	

Fig. 54.1 Return-to-play progression outlined in concussion in sport group consensus (Adapted from McCrory et al. [2])

54.6 Identifying Athletes at Risk for Protracted SRC Recovery

As previously discussed, the majority of athletes that sustain a SRC will experience a full recovery (e.g., symptoms, neurocognitive, postural stability) within 2–3 weeks [5, 6, 18], and a small percentage of athletes will experience a protracted recovery longer than 21 days [6]. Previous studies estimate that this "miserable minority" is comprised of approximately 20% of concussed athletes [32]. Given these dichotomous "normal" and "protracted" SRC recovery classifications, a new area of research has emerged and focuses on the identification of risk factors for predicting protracted SRC recovery. Researchers have identified several factors that increase the likelihood of an athlete experiencing a protracted recovery, and sports medicine clinicians should screen and document the presence of these secondary risk factors for supporting earlier intervention and treatment for SRC.

54.7 Factors that Influence Recovery from Sport-Related Concussion: Age, Sex, and Concussion History

In the SRC literature, age commonly refers to comparing youth and adolescent athletes (i.e., less than 17 years) to older adult-aged athletes (i.e., college and professional athletes 18 years and older) on SRC recovery. There is a general consensus that younger athletes demonstrate longer recovery compared to older, adult-aged athletes [2, 33, 34]; however, studies directly comparing SRC recovery outcomes between adolescent and adult-aged athletes are scant. The developmental changes that occur during the youth and adolescent years and the increased vulnerability of the developing brain to the neurometabolic changes that accompany mTBI [35] have prompted a conservative approach to SRC management in youth. In short, additional research substantiating age as a risk factor for prolonged SRC recovery is needed.

Fact Box 1

Risk factors that influence recovery time from sport-related concussion:

- Age: younger athletes (i.e., less than 17 years old) demonstrate longer recovery compared to older-aged athletes (i.e., college and professional athletes 18 years and older) following SRC.
- Sex: female athletes report more symptoms and demonstrate greater neurocognitive impairment than male athletes following SRC.
- Concussion history: athletes with history of multiple SRCs are 7.7 times more likely to demonstrate major memory impairments than athletes with no previous history of SRC acutely (i.e., 2 days post-injury) following injury.

The literature documenting differences in SRC recovery outcomes among adolescent and adult athletes is sparse and lacks consistent support [1, 19, 36]. One seminal study [34] reported that post-SRC memory impairment resolved within 3 days following injury in a college-aged cohort, while memory impairment persisted in a high school-aged cohort up to 7 days post-injury. High school athletes also reported more SRC symptoms compared to college athletes at 1, 3, and 5 days following injury. Other researchers [33] documented memory impairment (relative to baseline) during the first week following SRC in both high school and college athletes. Specifically, high school athletes demonstrated significantly lower post-injury memory scores than college athletes that suggest that high school athletes may demonstrate a different recovery trajectory than older, college-aged athletes. However, there were no differences between high school and college athletes on post-concussion symptom reports, reaction time, processing speed, and/or postural stability [33], and these findings were more recently supported by Nelson and colleagues [37]. Other studies by Meehan et al. [38] reported that age was not a significant predictor of protracted recovery, and Lee and colleagues [39] reported similar recovery times among concussed high school and college athletes. Purcell and colleagues [40] compared children to adolescents during recovery from concussion. This retrospective study found that 24.5% of children and 19.3% of adolescents were symptom-free within 7 days post-injury, 18.9% of children and 18.3% of adolescents within 7–10 days, 30.2% of children and 13.8% of adolescents within 2 weeks, and 15.1% of children and 18.3% of adolescents in 3 weeks. Of interest was that both children and adolescents took about 2–4 weeks to become asymptomatic, with adolescents taking significantly longer than children to be symptom-free [40].

Overall, the few available studies directly examining age-related differences in SRC risk and recovery have produced conflicting results. Additional evidence is needed to further solidify this factor as a significant contributor to SRC recovery. Further, a conservative approach for managing SRC in youth athletes remains a critical component of care for younger athletes.

The influence of sex on SRC recovery outcomes is also examined in the literature. The majority of the research conducted on concussion outcomes suggests that female athletes report a greater number of total symptoms and demonstrate greater neurocognitive impairment following SRC than male athletes [41–44]. For example, female athletes with SRC took significantly longer to become asymptomatic compared to male athletes with SRC [41]. Additionally, Zuckerman and colleagues [45] reported that females demonstrated a protracted symptom recovery compared to male athletes. Female athletes may be more symptomatic on some components of vestibular screening as well [46]. Covassin and colleagues [33] examined soccer athletes due to the similar sport environment and equipment in the male and female game and reported that female soccer athletes had higher total symptom scores and lower visual memory function compared to male soccer athletes following SRC. In addition, other studies demonstrate that female athletes exhibit post-SRC declines on visual memory and reaction time compared to males [33, 42]. Broshek et al. [42] reported that female concussed high school and collegiate athletes were impaired 1.7 times more often on neurocognitive testing than concussed male athletes. Other researchers have also reported that female athletes with SRCs demonstrate a longer recovery than male athletes with SRCs [33]. These data emphasize the need for clinicians to be cognizant of differences between male and female athletes in regard to varying recovery outcomes associated with SRC.

In addition to discrepancies on clinical measures and recovery time, sex differences for specialty management and treatment for SRC are documented between male and female athletes. In a sample of concussed adolescent athletes recruited from an SRC specialty clinic [44], female concussed athletes were eight times more likely to be prescribed vestibular therapy, seven times more likely to be prescribed rest, four times more likely to be prescribed medicine (i.e., for headaches or anxiety), and three times more likely to be prescribed academic accommodations compared to males. Moreover, female athletes with SRCs demonstrated a longer recovery than males (75.6 ± 73 days to 49.7 ± 62 days). These data suggest that females not only demonstrate a longer symptom and neurocognitive SRC recovery but are also more likely to receive specialty referral for SRC compared to male athletes.

The literature investigating history of SRC as a secondary risk factor influencing SRC recovery has produced mixed findings. Covassin and colleagues [47] reported that concussed athletes with two previous injuries demonstrated longer neurocognitive recovery of memory and reaction time compared to concussed athletes without history of SRC. A similar study by Iverson et al. [48] also reported that concussed athletes with a history of three or more concussions reported significantly greater memory impairment at 2 days post-injury compared to concussed athletes without a history of concussion (i.e., recovering from their first injury). Athletes with a history of multiple SRCs were also 7.7 times more likely to demonstrate a major decrease in memory performance than athletes with no previous concussion acutely following injury (i.e., 2 days post-injury). These data are in concordance with other studies that report concussed athletes with a history of three or more SRCs present a greater number of post-concussion symptoms [49] and exhibit longer symptom recovery than athletes without a history of concussion.

Although there is empirical evidence suggesting concussion history is associated with worse recovery outcomes, these findings have not been consistently supported for recovery duration. Meehan et al. [38] reported that concussion history was not a significant predictor of prolonged symptomatology beyond 28 days post-injury, and McCrea et al. [12] also reported that concussion history was not associated with a prolonged recovery longer than 7 days post-SRC. The conflicting findings regarding the relationship between concussion history and SRC recovery are likely due to the limitations of utilizing self-reported concussion history. Recent studies indicate that athletes were moderately reliable in self-reporting their concussion history [50] and that athletes' understanding of the current definitions of SRC were not consistent. This lack of reliability and variability in defining SRC may lead to inaccurate self-reported histories of concussion [51]. In order to better determine the influence of concussion history as a risk factor for poor SRC outcome, future research should corroborate these data with medical records and documented injuries.

54.8 On-Field Signs and Symptoms and SRC Recovery

The post-concussion symptom profile of an injured athlete has also been examined as a potential secondary risk factor for prolonged SRC recovery. More specifically, several empirical studies have investigated which specific cognitive impairments and symptom clusters [52, 53] are related to protracted recovery (i.e., >14 days) following SRC [54–57]. Identifying athletes at risk for protracted recovery from SRC is critical to informing early intervention and targeted treatment approaches, and using symptom inventories may be beneficial to understanding different clinical trajectories of SRC [58].

Historically, loss of consciousness (LOC) and post-traumatic amnesia (PTA) were considered key factors in determining the severity of an SRC and determining the length of time an individual should remain out of play following an SRC, making those two symptoms the basis for concussion grading scales [59]. However, since LOC occurs in fewer than 10% [60] and PTA in fewer than 30% [60] of athletes with SRCs, consensus statements recommend not using these antiquated grading scales for SRC management [61]. Moreover, the importance of LOC and PTA as reliable markers of severity has been questioned. Three studies have documented a significant relationship between LOC and SRC recovery persisting longer than 7 days in samples of professional football players [62] and in high school and college athletes [63, 64]. However, other studies have not supported this relationship between LOC and SRC recovery outcomes [56, 65–67].

Similarly, the available literature examining the relationship between PTA and prolonged SRC recovery yields inconsistent results. In professional football athletes, both retrograde and anterograde amnesia were documented in a significantly higher percentage of athletes who missed more than 7 days due to SRC [62]. In addition, retrograde amnesia was also related to prolonged SRC recovery in high school and college athletes [63]. These findings were supported by work analyzing three large databases of high school and college athletes; those who reported both retrograde and post-traumatic amnesia were associated with a prolonged recovery [64]. However, in other studies, amnesia was not associated with a prolonged recovery in collegiate [66] or high school [57] athletes nor was it associated with symptoms lasting longer than 1 week in high school football or non-football athletes [65].

Headache is often mentioned as the primary symptom associated with concussion, reported in up to 90% of injured athletes [60, 66, 67]. While the acute presentation of headache does not nec-

Fact Box 2

Loss of consciousness (LOC), post-traumatic amnesia (PTA), and concussion recovery:

- Less than 10% of athletes that sustain a concussion will experience LOC.
- College and high school athletes that experience LOC demonstrate recovery lasting longer than 7 days.
- Less than 30% of athletes that sustain a concussion will experience PTA.
- College and high school athletes that experience retrograde amnesia demonstrate longer recovery time.
- Professional football athletes that experience retrograde and anterograde amnesia demonstrate recovery lasting longer than 7 days.

essarily correlate to severity or recovery [65], prolonged (i.e., over 7 days) headache has been associated with an increased time to recover and return to sport [63, 67], poorer cognitive test scores [68], and higher overall symptom reports [68]. In addition to headache, some athletes may experience nausea and light and/or noise sensitivity following SRC. This specific cluster of symptoms represents post-traumatic migraine (PTM) and is associated with prolonged SRC recovery [54]. Recent studies reveal that concussed athletes with PTM are 7.3 times more likely to demonstrate a recovery longer than 21 days compared to concussed athletes with headache only and athletes without headache or PTM [54]. In addition, the presence of PTM following SRC has resulted in significantly worse neurocognitive presentation compared to only headache and without PTM or headache [54, 69]. In addition to research examining recovery outcomes and PTM, a recent study by Kontos et al. [70] reported decreased brain network activation in concussed athletes with PTM compared to those without PTM and matched noninjured controls. Although the available data substantiating PTM as a secondary risk factor is sparse, the preliminary findings for this symptom presentation are promising and may have significant clinical value.

Other somatic symptoms, independent of headache, including dizziness, nausea, and sensitivity to light and noise, have also been associated with a prolonged recovery. On-field dizziness was found to result in a sixfold increased risk of a prolonged (i.e., >21 days) recovery in high school athletes [56]. However, dizziness was not reported to be associated with prolonged symptoms (i.e., >7 days) in a separate study of high school football and non-football athletes [65]. An initial clinical presentation that included nausea was associated with a 60% and 80% increased risk in prolonged symptoms in football and non-football athletes, respectively [65]. Similarly, sensitivity to noise and light resulted in a 2.7 times increase in prolonged symptoms in non-football athletes [65], and migraine-related symptoms have also been associated with a longer time to clinical recovery [57].

Cognitive symptoms including drowsiness, concentration, cognitive, or memory problems and fogginess have also been associated with prolonged recovery following concussion. In a study of high school athletes, drowsiness was associated with a two times risk for prolonged symptoms in football and non-football athletes [65]. Similarly, fatigue, tiredness, or fogginess were associated with an increased time until return to activity in Australian rules football athletes [67], and high school athletes with persistent fogginess had significantly higher total symptom score and deficits in the cognitive functioning domains of reaction time, processing speed, and memory [48]. Athletes with an initial SRC presentation within the first week following injury that included concentration problems demonstrated in a twofold increase of prolonged symptoms in both football athletes and non-football athletes [65], while another study [57] found that self-reported cognitive or memory problems were associated with a protracted recovery.

In contrast to the aforementioned studies identifying the predictive value of individual symptoms, other researchers report that an overall symptom burden may best predict protracted SRC recovery [38, 71, 72]. Meehan and colleagues [72] examined predictors of protracted recovery in a sample of adults (>18 years) with concussion and reported that initial symptom burden (i.e., higher symptom total at first clinical visit within 2 weeks of injury) was more predictive of a SRC recovery longer than 28 days than age, sex, concussion history (personal and family), and migraine/headache history. These findings are in concordance with previous studies that also report initial symptom burden predicting recovery in a sample of pediatric patients with concussion [38].

54.9 Continuing to Play with SRC and Recovery

Recent studies have addressed the consequences of immediate removal from play following a suspected SRC. Despite advances for the education of the signs and symptoms of SRC, athletes' reporting behaviors have not changed [73, 74], and unfortunately many athletes continue to play with SRC. The immediate removal of an athlete from play following a suspected SRC is a critical first step in preventing additional trauma and catastrophic outcomes (i.e., chronic impairment or second-impact syndrome) associated with continued exposure to head impacts. Researchers have reported that athletes continuing to play with SRC demonstrate a twofold increase in recovery time compared to athletes that were immediately removed from play [18]. Other researchers report that athletes not immediately reporting SRC symptoms to a medical professional and staying in the game took approximately 5 days longer to recover than athletes that did immediately report their symptoms [17]. In addition, removal from play status (i.e., removed or not removed) was the most robust predictor of prolonged recovery following SRC [18]. The concept that postponing removal from play delays recovery is consistent with research describing the brain's window of vulnerability in the acute stage following SRC [35]. The immediate reporting of symptoms after a suspected SRC may give athletes the best chance to not experience a prolonged recovery [17].

Fact Box 3
Removal from play and sport-related concussion (SRC) recovery:

- Athletes with a SRC that continue to play demonstrate a 2× longer recovery than athletes with SRC that are immediately removed from play.
- Whether or not an athlete with SRC is immediately removed from play is the most robust predictor of prolonged recovery (≥21 days).

Take-Home Message

- Overall, several of the proposed factors influencing SRC recovery lack consistency in the literature or are simply understudied. Many of these discrepancies are due to the wide variability of research designs, sample selection, and instrumentation used to gather data on athletes with SRC.
- Despite the lack of consistent findings in research samples, sports medicine professionals should be aware of risk factors when managing athletes with SRC. Identifying and documenting athletes with presentations of secondary risk factors for SRC will assist in the management decisions and further inform RTP.
- The clinical benefits of successfully identifying secondary risk factors can assist both the clinician and athlete in the navigation of the SRC recovery process, which is often characterized by a path of uncertain and uncontrollable recovery.
- As research into SRC risk factors continues to grow and new technology is developed, the documented influence of currently identified factors will increase, and new factors will emerge. It is important for the clinician to stay up-to-date with the current research, as updates in knowledge further inform accurate clinical presentation of SRC and influence treatment and management practices.

Top Five Evidence-Based References

Elbin RJ, Sufrinko A, Schatz P, French J, Henry L, Burkhart S, Collins MW, Kontos AP (2016) Removal from play after concussion and recovery time. Pediatrics 138(3). https://doi.org/10.1542/peds.2016-0910

Kontos AP, Elbin RJ, Lau B, Simensky S, Freund B, French J, Collins MW (2013) Posttraumatic migraine as a predictor of recovery and cognitive impairment after sport-related concussion. Am J Sports Med 41(7):1497–1504. https://doi.org/10.1177/0363546513488751

Covassin T, Elbin RJ, Harris W, Parker T, Kontos AP (2012) The role of age and sex in symptoms, neurocognitive performance, and postural stability in athletes after concussion. Am J Sports Med 40(6):1303–1312

McGrath N, Dinn WM, Collins MW, Lovell MR, Elbin RJ, Kontos AP (2013) Post-exertion neurocognitive test failure among student-athletes following concussion. Brain Inj 27(1):103–113. https://doi.org/10.3109/02699052.2012.729282

Meehan WP III, Mannix R, Monuteaux MC, Stein CJ, Bachur RG (2014) Early symptom burden predicts recovery after sport-related concussion. Neurology 83(24):2204–2210. https://doi.org/10.1212/WNL.0000000000001073

References

1. Harmon KG, Drezner JA, Gammons M, Guskiewicz KM, Halstead M, Herring SA, Kutcher JS, Pana A, Putukian M, Roberts WO (2013) American Medical Society for Sports Medicine position statement: concussion in sport. Br J Sports Med 47(1):15–26
2. McCrory P, Meeuwisse W, Aubry M, Cantu B, Dvorak J, Echemendia RJ, Engebretsen L, Johnston K, Kutcher JS, Raftery M, Sills A (2013) Consensus statement on concussion in sport-the 4th international conference on concussion in sport held in Zurich, November 2012. Clin J Sport Med 23(2):89–117
3. Collins MW, Kontos AP, Okonkwo DO, Almquist J, Bailes J, Barisa M, Bazarian J, Bloom OJ, Brody DL, Cantu R, Cardenas J, Clugston J, Cohen R, Echemendia R, Elbin RJ, Ellenbogen R, Fonseca J, Gioia G, Guskiewicz K, Heyer R, Hotz G, Iverson GL, Jordan B, Manley G, Maroon J, McAllister T, McCrea M, Mucha A, Pieroth E, Podell K, Pombo M, Shetty T, Sills A, Solomon G, Thomas DG, Valovich McLeod TC, Yates T, Zafonte R (2016) Statements of agreement from the targeted evaluation and active management (TEAM) approaches to treating concussion meeting held in Pittsburgh, October 15–16, 2015. J Neurosurg 79(6):912–929
4. McCrory P, Meeuwisse W, Johnston K, Dvorak J, Aubry M, Molloy M, Cantu R (2009) Consensus statement on concussion in sport—the 3rd international conference on concussion in sport held in Zurich, November 2008. J Sci Med Sport 12(3):340–351
5. Henry LC, Elbin RJ, Collins MW, Marchetti G, Kontos AP (2015) Examining recovery trajectories after sport-related concussion with a multimodal clinical assessment approach. Neurosurgery 78(2):232–241
6. Collins MW, Lovell MR, Iverson GL, Ide T, Maroon J (2006) Examining concussion rates and return to play in high school football players wearing newer helmet technology: a three-year prospective cohort study. Neurosurgery 58(2):275–286. discussion 275–286
7. McCrea M, Hammeke T, Olsen G, Leo P, Guskiewicz KM (2004) Unreported concussion in high school football players: implications for injury prevention. Clin J Sport Med 14:13–17
8. Asken BM, Snyder AR, Smith MS, Zaremski JL, Bauer RM (2017) Concussion-like symptom reporting in non-concussed adolescent athletes. Clin Neuropsychol 2017:1–16
9. Iverson GL, Silverberg ND, Mannix R, Maxwell BA, Atkins JE, Zafonte R, Berkner PD (2015) Factors associated with concussion-like symptom reporting in high school athletes. JAMA Pediatr 169(12):1132–1140
10. Mailer BJ, Valovich-McLeod TC, Bay RC (2008) Healthy youth are reliable in reporting symptoms on a graded symptom scale. J Sport Rehabil 17(1):11–20
11. Alla S, Sullivan SJ, McCrory P (2012) Defining asymptomatic status following sports concussion: fact or fallacy? Br J Sports Med 46(8):562–569
12. McCrea M, Guskiewicz KM, Marshall SW, Barr W, Randolph C, Cantu RC, Onate JA, Yang J, Kelly JP (2003) Acute effects and recovery time following concussion in collegiate football players: the NCAA Concussion Study. JAMA 290(19):2556–2563
13. McCrory P, Johnston KM, Meeuwisse W, Aubry M, Cantu RC, Dvorak J, Graf-Baumann T, Kelly J, Lovell MR, Schamasch P (2005) Summary and agreement statement of the 2nd international conference on concussion in sport, Prague 2004. Clin J Sport Med 15(2):48–55
14. Pfaller AY, Nelson LD, Apps JN, Walter KD, McCrea MA (2016) Frequency and outcomes of a symptom-free waiting period after sport-related concussion. Am J Sports Med 44(11):2941–2946
15. Nelson LD, Tarima S, LaRoche AA, Hammeke TA, Barr WB, Guskiewicz K, Randolph C, McCrea MA (2016) Preinjury somatization symptoms contribute to clinical recovery after sport-related concussion. Neurology 86(20):1856–1863
16. Morgan CD, Zuckerman SL, Lee YM, King L, Beaird S, Sills AK, Solomon GS (2015) Predictors of post-concussion syndrome after sports-related concussion in young athletes: a matched case-control study. J Neurosurg Pediatr 15(6):589–598

17. Asken BM, McCrea MA, Clugston JR, Snyder AR, Houck ZM, Bauer RM (2016) "Playing through it": delayed reporting and removal from athletic activity after concussion predicts prolonged recovery. J Athl Train 51(4):329–335
18. Elbin RJ, Sufrinko A, Schatz P, French J, Henry L, Burkhart S, Collins MW, Kontos AP (2016) Removal from play after concussion and recovery time. Pediatrics 138(3):10
19. Giza CC, Kutcher JS, Ashwal S, Barth J, Getchius TS, Gioia GA, Gronseth GS, Guskiewicz K, Mandel S, Manley G, McKeag DB, Thurman DJ, Zafonte R (2013) Summary of evidence-based guideline update: evaluation and management of concussion in sports: report of the guideline development subcommittee of the American Academy of Neurology. Neurology 80(24):2250–2257
20. Bell DR, Guskiewicz KM, Clark MA, Padua DA (2011) Systematic review of the balance error scoring system. Sports Health 3(3):287–295
21. Van Kampen DA, Lovell MR, Pardini JE, Collins MW, FH F (2006) The "value added" of neurocognitive testing after sports-related concussion. Am J Sports Med 34(10):1630–1635
22. Black AM, Sergio LE, Macpherson AK (2017) The epidemiology of concussions: number and nature of concussions and time to recovery among female and male canadian varsity athletes 2008 to 2011. Clin J Sport Med 27(1):52–56
23. Guskiewicz KM, Ross SE, Marshall SW (2001) Postural stability and neuropsychological deficits after concussion in collegiate athletes. J Athl Train 36(3):263–273
24. Cavanaugh JT, Guskiewicz KM, Giuliani C, Marshall S, Mercer VS, Stergiou N (2006) Recovery of postural control after cerebral concussion: new insights using approximate entropy. J Athl Train 41(3):305–313
25. Fait P, Swaine B, Cantin JF, Leblond J, BJ MF (2013) Altered integrated locomotor and cognitive function in elite athletes 30 days postconcussion: a preliminary study. J Head Trauma Rehabil 28(4):293–301
26. Howell DR, Osternig LR, Chou LS (2013) Dual-task effect on gait balance control in adolescents with concussion. Arch Phys Med Rehabil 94(8):1513–1520
27. Galetta KM, Brandes LE, Maki K, Dziemianowicz MS, Laudano E, Allen M, Lawler K, Sennett B, Wiebe D, Devick S, Messner LV, Galetta SL, Balcer LJ (2011) The King-Devick test and sports-related concussion: study of a rapid visual screening tool in a collegiate cohort. J Neurol Sci 309(1–2):34–39
28. Mucha A, Collins MW, Elbin RJ, Furman JM, Troutman-Enseki C, DeWolf RM, Marchetti G, Kontos AP (2014) A brief vestibular/ocular motor screening (VOMS) assessment to evaluate concussions: preliminary findings. Am J Sports Med 42(10):2479–2486
29. Galetta KM, Morganroth J, Moehringer N, Mueller B, Hasanaj L, Webb N, Civitano C, Cardone DA, Silverio A, Galetta SL, Balcer LJ (2015) Adding vision to concussion testing: a prospective study of sideline testing in youth and collegiate athletes. J Neuroophthalmol 35(3):235–241
30. Kontos AP, Sufrinko A, Elbin RJ, Puskar A, Collins MW (2016) Reliability and associated risk factors for performance on the vestibular/ocular motor screening (VOMS) tool in healthy collegiate athletes. Am J Sports Med 44(6):1400–1406
31. McGrath N, Dinn WM, Collins MW, Lovell MR, Elbin RJ, Kontos AP (2013) Post-exertion neurocognitive test failure among student-athletes following concussion. Brain Inj 27(1):103–113
32. Ruff RM, Camenzuli L, Mueller J (1996) Miserable minority: emotional risk factors that influence the outcome of a mild traumatic brain injury. Brain Inj 10(8):551–565
33. Covassin T, Elbin RJ, Harris W, Parker T, Kontos AP (2012) The role of age and sex in symptoms, neurocognitive performance, and postural stability in athletes after concussion. Am J Sports Med 40(6):1303–1312
34. Field M, Collins MW, Lovell MR, Maroon J (2003) Does age play a role in recovery from sports-related concussion? A comparison of high school and collegiate athletes. J Pediatr 142(5):546–553
35. Giza CC, Hovda DA (2014) The new neurometabolic cascade of concussion. Neurosurgery 75(Suppl 4):S24–S33
36. Broglio SP, Cantu RC, Gioia GA, Guskiewicz KM, Kutcher J, Palm M, Valovich McLeod TC, National Athletic Trainer's A (2014) National Athletic Trainers' Association position statement: management of sport concussion. J Athl Train 49(2):245–265
37. Nelson LD, Guskiewicz KM, Barr WB, Hammeke TA, Randolph C, Ahn KW, Wang Y, McCrea MA (2016) Age differences in recovery after sport-related concussion: a comparison of high school and collegiate athletes. J Athl Train 51(2):142–152
38. Meehan WP III, Mannix RC, Stracciolini A, Elbin RJ, Collins MW (2013) Symptom severity predicts prolonged recovery after sport-related concussion, but age and amnesia do not. J Pediatr 163(3):721–725
39. Lee YM, Odom MJ, Zuckerman SL, Solomon GS, Sills AK (2013) Does age affect symptom recovery after sports-related concussion? A study of high school and college athletes. J Neurosurg Pediatr 12(6):537–544
40. Purcell L, Harvey J, Seabrook JA (2015) Patterns of recovery following sport-related concussion in children and adolescents. Clin Pediatr (Phila) 55(5):452–458
41. Berz K, Divine J, Foss K, Heyl R, Ford K, Myer G (2013) Sex-specific differences in the severity of symptoms and recovery rate following sports-

related concussion in young athletes. Phys Sportsmed 41(2):58–63
42. Broshek DK, Kaushik T, Freeman JR, Erlanger D, Webbe F, Barth JT (2005) Sex differences in outcome following sports-related concussion. J Neurosurg 102(5):856–863
43. Colvin A, Mullen J, Lovell M, West R, Collins M, Groh M (2009) The role of concussion history and gender in recovery from soccer-related concussion. Am J Sports Med 37(9):1699–1704
44. Kostyun R, Hafeez I (2015) Protracted recovery from a concussion a focus on gender and treatment interventions in an adolescent population. Sports Health 7(1):52–57
45. Zuckerman SL, Apple RP, Odom MJ, Lee YM, Solomon GS, Sills AK (2014) Effect of sex on symptoms and return to baseline in sport-related concussion. J Neurosurg Pediatr 13(1):72–81
46. Sufrinko AM, Mucha A, Covassin T, Marchetti G, Elbin RJ, Collins MW, Kontos AP (2016) Sex differences in vestibular/ocular and neurocognitive outcomes after sport-related concussion. Clin J Sport Med 27(2):133–138
47. Covassin T, Stearne D, Elbin RJ (2008) Concussion history and postconcussion neurocognitive performance and symptoms in collegiate athletes. J Athl Train 43(2):119–124
48. Iverson GL, Gaetz M, Lovell MR, Collins MW (2004) Relation between subjective fogginess and neuropsychological testing following concussion. J Int Neuropsychol Soc 10(6):904–906
49. Gaetz M, Goodman D, Weinberg H (2000) Electrophysiological evidence for the cumulative effects of concussion. Brain Inj 14(12):1077–1088
50. Kerr ZY, Marshall SW, Harding HP Jr, Guskiewicz KM (2012) Nine-year risk of depression diagnosis increases with increasing self-reported concussions in retired professional football players. Am J Sports Med 40(10):2206–2212
51. Robbins CA, Daneshvar DH, Picano JD, Gavett BE, Baugh CM, Riley DO, Nowinski CJ, McKee AC, Cantu RC, Stern RA (2014) Self-reported concussion history: impact of providing a definition of concussion. Open access. J Sports Med 5:99–103
52. Kontos AP, Elbin RJ, Schatz P, Covassin T, Henry L, Pardini J, Collins MW (2012) A revised factor structure for the post-concussion symptom scale: baseline and postconcussion factors. Am J Sports Med 40(10):2375–2384
53. Pardini J, Stump JE, Lovell M, Collins MW, Moritz K, FH F (2004) The Post Concussion Symptom Scale (PCSS): a factor analysis [abstract]. Br J Sports Med 38:661–662
54. Kontos AP, Elbin RJ, Lau B, Simensky S, Freund B, French J, Collins MW (2013) Posttraumatic migraine as a predictor of recovery and cognitive impairment after sport-related concussion. Am J Sports Med 41(7):1497–1504
55. Lau BC, Collins MW, Lovell MR (2012) Cutoff scores in neurocognitive testing and symptom clusters that predict protracted recovery from concussions in high school athletes. Neurosurgery 70(2):371–379
56. Lau BC, Kontos AP, Collins CL, Mucha A, Lovell MR (2011) Which on-field signs and symptoms predict protracted recovery from sport-related concussion among high school football players? Am J Sports Med 39(11):2311–2318
57. Lau BC, Lovell MR, Collins MW, Pardini J (2009) Neurocognitive and symptom predictors of recovery in high school athletes. Clin J Sport Med 19(3):216–221
58. Collins MW, Kontos AP, Reynolds E, Murawski CD, FH F (2014) A comprehensive, targeted approach to the clinical care of athletes following sport-related concussion. Knee Surg Sports Traumatol Arthrosc 22(2):235–246
59. Cantu RC (2001) Posttraumatic retrograde and anterograde amnesia: pathophysiology and implications in grading and safe return to play. J Athl Train 36(3):244–248
60. Guskiewicz KM, Weaver NL, Padua DA, Garrett WE (2000) Epidemiology of concussion in collegiate and high school football players. Am J Sports Med 28(5):643–650
61. Aubry M, Cantu RC, Dvorak J, Graf-Baumann T, Johnston KM, Kelly JP, Lovell MR, McCrory PR, Meeuwisse W, Schamasch P (2002) Summary and agreement statement of the 1st international symposium on concussion in sport, Vienna 2001. Clin J Sport Med 12:6–11
62. Pellman EJ, Viano DC, Casson IR, Arfken C, Powell J (2004) Concussion in professional football: injuries involving 7 or more days out—part 5. Neurosurgery 55(5):1100–1119
63. Asplund CA, McKeag DB, Olsen CH (2004) Sport-related concussion: factors associated with prolonged return to play. Clin J Sport Med 14(6):339–343
64. McCrea M, Guskiewicz KM, Randolph C, Barr WB, Hammeke TA, Marshall SW, Powell MR, Woo Ahn K, Wang Y, Kelly JP (2012) Incidence, clinical course, and predictors of prolonged recovery time following sport-related concussion in high school and college athletes. J Int Neuropsychol Soc 2012(18):1–12
65. Chrisman SP, Rivara FP, Schiff MA, Zhou C, Comstock RD (2013) Risk factors for concussive symptoms 1 week or longer in high school athletes. Brain Inj 27(1):1–9
66. Guskiewicz KM, McCrea M, Marshall SW, Cantu RC, Randolph C, Barr W, Onate JA, Kelly JP (2003) Cumulative effects associated with recurrent concussion in collegiate football players: the NCAA concussion study. JAMA 290(19):2549–2555
67. Makdissi M, Darby D, Maruff P, Ugoni A, Brukner P, McCrory PR (2010) Natural history of concussion in sport: markers of severity and implications for management. Am J Sports Med 38(3):464–471
68. Collins MW, Field M, Lovell MR, Iverson GL, Johnston KM, Maroon J, FH F (2003) Relationship

between postconcussion headache and neuropsychological test performance in high school athletes. Am J Sports Med 31(2):168–173
69. Mihalik JP, Stump JE, Collins MW, Lovell MR, Field M, Maroon JC (2005) Posttraumatic migraine characteristics in athletes following sports-related concussion. J Neurosurg 102(5):850–855
70. Kontos AP, Reches A, Elbin RJ, Dickman D, Laufer I, Geva AB, Shacham G, DeWolf R, Collins MW (2015) Preliminary evidence of reduced brain network activation in patients with post-traumatic migraine following concussion. Brain Imaging Behav 10(2):594–603
71. Meehan WP III, Mannix R, Monuteaux MC, Stein CJ, Bachur RG (2014) Early symptom burden predicts recovery after sport-related concussion. Neurology 83(24):2204–2210
72. Meehan WP III, O'Brien MJ, Geminiani E, Mannix R (2016) Initial symptom burden predicts duration of symptoms after concussion. J Sci Med Sport 19(9):722–725
73. Baugh CM, Kroshus E, Daneshvar DH, Filali NA, Hiscox MJ, Glantz LH (2015) Concussion management in United States college sports: compliance with National Collegiate Athletic Association concussion policy and areas for improvement. Am J Sports Med 43(1):47–56
74. Register-Mihalik JK, Guskiewicz KM, McLeod TC, Linnan LA, Mueller FO, Marshall SW (2013) Knowledge, attitude, and concussion-reporting behaviors among high school athletes: a preliminary study. J Athl Train 48(5):645–653

Part VII

Medical Issues and Doping

Return to Play After Cardiac Conditions

55

Mats Börjesson and Jonathan Drezner

Contents

M. Börjesson (✉)
Department of Neuroscience and Physiology, Sahlgrenska Academy, Göteborg University, Göteborg, Sweden

Department of Food, Nutrition and Sport Sciences and Sahlgrenska University Hospital/Östra, Göteborg University, Göteborg, Sweden
e-mail: mats.brjesson@telia.com

J. Drezner
Department of Family Medicine, University of Washington, Washington, DC, USA

55.1 Introduction

Regular physical activity (PA) is associated with numerous health benefits, including lower cardiovascular and total morbidity and mortality [1]. Paradoxically, intense physical activity is associated with an increased risk of serious cardiac events, including sudden cardiac arrest/death (SCA/SCD), especially in subjects with an underlying (also subclinical) cardiovascular disease. In fact, intense PA may act as a trigger of adverse cardiac events. The cause of exercise-related SCD is age dependent, with inherited/congenital diseases, including cardiomyopathies and ion-

V. Musahl et al. (eds.), *Return to Play in Football*, https://doi.org/10.1007/978-3-662-55713-6_55

channel disease, being the major cause in athletes <25 years of age, while coronary artery disease (CAD) is almost exclusively the cause in >35-year-olds [2]. Cardiac screening has therefore globally been routinely recommended, since a number of years for younger athletes [3, 4], as well as for master athletes [5, 6].

After identification of a relevant cardiac condition, and the proper management according to established standards, follows the important clinical decision of return to play (when? and if?). Some cardiac conditions, such as acute myocarditis, may heal and allow return to play, while other cardiac conditions may be lifelong and invariably treatable. Some cardiac conditions are not even compatible with return to play. In the present chapter, we discuss a number of major cardiovascular disorders encountered in athletes and the diagnosis, management, and recommendations on return to sport for the various conditions.

55.2 Clinical Symptoms

The main symptoms flagging serious underlying disease include exercise-related syncope and exercise-related chest pain. The causes of these symptoms are most often benign, but they need to be further evaluated to exclude any relevant cardiovascular abnormality. For instance, syncope could be due to an underlying (primary) arrhythmia or to secondary arrhythmia related to myocardial ischemia (in CAD, cardiomyopathy, myocarditis). Myocardial ischemia is associated with exercise-related chest pain, which is, however, a late and unreliable sign of ischemia. Therefore, exercise testing remains an important evaluation tool, in patients with suspected CAD/risk factors for CAD as well as in suspected structural heart disease, to unravel/provoke any exercise-related ischemia.

Syncope associated with exercise should be characterized as occurring during or after exercise. Syncope occurring during exercise is an ominous sign and warrants a high index of suspicion for underlying cardiac disease. A variety of structural disorders (cardiomyopathies, congenital coronary artery anomalies, aortic stenosis) and primary electrical diseases (Wolff-Parkinson-White (WPW), long QT syndrome (LQTS), and catecholaminergic polymorphic ventricular tachycardia (CPVT)) are all associated with syncope in athletes. Thus, evaluation of syncope occurring during exercise requires a comprehensive evaluation to rule out disorders predisposing to SCD before a return to sport is considered [7]. The diagnostic evaluation of exertional syncope includes an ECG, echocardiogram, stress ECG, and possibly advanced cardiac imaging such as MRI or CT and/or prolonged ECG monitoring.

Arrhythmogenic syncope usually occurs during exercise (not post-exercise) and typically presents with abrupt loss of consciousness without premonitory symptoms. Secondary injury is common as individuals are unconscious before they hit the ground and cannot protect their head. Syncope is typically brief, and upon awakening most individuals feel normal quite quickly, a quality which distinguishes malignant syncope from neurocardiogenic syncope. Syncope during exercise can also occur because of left ventricular outflow tract obstruction from hypertrophic cardiomyopathy or aortic stenosis. Syncope associated with exertional outflow obstruction typically occurs during peak exercise and may have a brief period of light-headedness prior to collapse.

Post-exertional syncope, occurring while standing in a huddle or after the finish line, is typically neurocardiogenic [8–11]. In neurocardiogenic syncope, also known as vasovagal syncope, premonitory symptoms are common and include light-headedness, dizziness, flushing, nausea, tunnel vision, and profuse sweating. The individual typically slumps to the ground, not completely unconscious, and is most often able to avoid injury. Syncope episodes are short-lived; however, following the episode, individuals often have a prolonged period of nausea and fatigue. Athletes with neurocardiogenic syncope should be questioned regarding other cardiovascular symptoms or a relevant family history of cardiac disease and an ECG performed. If the presentation is consistent with neurocardiogenic syncope, the ECG is normal, and there are no other clinical features of concern, additional evaluation is not necessary and prompt return to play is allowed.

55.3 Hypertension

55.3.1 Background

Hypertension is one of the most important modifiable risk factors for cardiovascular morbidity and mortality [12], and blood pressure (BP) measurement is a vital part of cardiac screening recommendations in competitive athletes. Essential hypertension, which is the result of a complex combination of genetic predisposition and lifestyle factors, including physical inactivity, affects most hypertensives. Approximately 5% suffer from secondary hypertension, caused by a variety of disorders, such as coarctation of the aorta (must be ruled out by thorough clinical palpation of femoral pulses), renal artery stenosis, Cushing's syndrome, or pheochromocytoma [13]. Different medications/drugs including nonsteroidal anti-inflammatory drugs (NSAIDs), corticosteroids, and/or erythropoietin (doping) could also increase BP [13, 14]. Importantly, the use of anabolic steroids has also been shown to be associated with increased blood pressure [15] and must be ruled out in young athletes with hypertension. Exercise-induced cardiac adaptation may add to the hypertrophy secondary to hypertension, possibly aggravating negative long-term effects [16].

The prevalence of hypertension in athletes varies greatly, with figures ranging from 7% [17] to 19% [18], or even higher, possibly due to varying study quality [19]. As more and older (master) athletes take part in various competitions, the prevalence will increase [20]. Masked hypertension, being unmasked by ambulatory blood pressure recordings, possibly affects 1/3 of middle-aged runners [21].

55.3.2 Diagnosis

The diagnosis of hypertension requires repeated measurements of >140 mmHg systolic and/or 90 mmHg diastolic blood pressure (BP), performed in a standardized manner, with the patient in a sitting position [13]. Ambulatory blood pressure measurements (24-h blood pressure) use a 5–10 mmHg lower cutoff value as abnormal [13, 22]. Secondary hypertension must be ruled out, and the total risk of CVD of each individual has to be assessed. The total risk of the individual with hypertension is dependent on the actual blood pressure level, on the existence of other cardiovascular risk factors (total risk), and on the presence of any target organ damage (eyes, kidneys, heart; TOD) [23]. Exclusion of TOD is especially important in athletes and includes ophthalmological evaluation, kidney tests (creatinine, albuminuria), and ECG and echocardiography (left ventricular hypertrophy).

55.3.3 Management

Treatment of hypertension in athletes is typically the same as for nonathletes [23]. Specific consideration must be taken, as some of the antihypertensive drugs may interact with physical performance. Beta-blockers, no longer being the first-line treatment for hypertension in the absence of other cardiac disease, are associated with a lowering of maximal pulse during activity, of up to 30 beats/min [24], leading to a lower maximal exercise capacity [24]. In addition, beta-blockers are prohibited in some sports (shooting, archery) by the World Anti-Doping Agency (WADA). Diuretics may lead to dehydration in exercising individuals, especially in warm temperatures, and may lead to hypokalemia (12) and are also included in the WADA prohibited (doping) list. Calcium channel blockers may increase the risk of excessive vasodilation and accompanying hypotension, post-exercise [23]. The ACE inhibitors and angiotensin blockers (ARBs) may have similar effects, especially in a warmer temperature, but are still the preferred treatment in active individuals [23].

At BP follow-ups, the athlete should be reevaluated for any emerging additional risk factors and TOD. Any reversal/aggravation of existing TOD should be assessed by regular kidney testing as well as by ECG/echocardiography. Sports eligibility and medications should be re-reviewed regularly.

	A: Low dynamic	B: Moderate dynamic	C: High dynamic
I. Low static	Bowling, Cricket, Golf, Riflery	Fencing, Table tennis, Tennis (diubles), Volleyball, baseball/softball	Badminton, Race walking, Running (marathon), Cross-country skiing (classic), Squash,
II. Moderate static	Auto racing, Diving, Equestrian, Motorcycling, Gymnastics, Karate/Judo, Sailing, Archering	Field events (jumping), Figure skating, Lacrosse, Running (sprint)	Basketball, Biathlon, Ice hockey, Rugby, Soccer, Cross-country skiing (skating), Running (mid/long), Swimming, Tennis (single), Handball
III. High static	Bobsledding, Field events (throwing), Luge, Rock climbing, Waterskiing, Weight lifting, Windsurfing	Body building, Downhill skiing, Wrestling, Snow boarding	Boxing, Canoeing/Kayaking, Cycling, Decathlon, Rowing, Speed skating, Triathlon

Fig. 55.1 Classification of sports (dynamic a–c and static a–c), adapted and modified after Mitchell [25]. This classification is used to define the dynamic and static components of different sporting disciplines, to aid the clinician regarding eligibility and return to play

Fact Box 1 Return to play—hypertension

- All sports are permitted in athletes with a well-controlled BP (by lifestyle and/or medical treatment), who have no added risk and where no target organ damage (TOD) can be shown [23].
- In athletes with moderate added risk, high static, high dynamic sports (IIIC) (according to Fig. 55.1) is not recommended [23].
- In case of proven kidney, eye, or heart TOD, elite sports activity may not be recommended [23].
- In case of a blood pressure >200/115, sporting activity is contraindicated, and medical therapy should be instigated, before sports is re-considered [23].

55.4 Coronary Artery Disease

55.4.1 Background

Coronary artery disease (CAD) is a progressive, atherosclerotic disease of the coronary arteries [26]. The symptoms include effort-related angina, dyspnea, palpitations, light-headedness, or syncope, but more diffuse symptoms or even subclinical disease is common. Regular physical exercise reduces the risk of developing CAD. However, the risk of sudden cardiac death (SCD) is increased by (could be triggered by) vigorous exertion [27]. Physical activity and competitive sport participation should, therefore, be individually tailored in patients with CAD [28].

55.4.2 Diagnosis

The detection of CAD has traditionally been based on the presence and levels of major risk factors (risk factor profile) and exercise testing, with the diagnosis being confirmed by coronary angiography. During recent years, cardiac biomarkers (e.g., hsCRP, nt-proBNP, troponins) and novel cardiac imaging techniques (e.g., calcium score (CAC), cardiac CT, and cardiac MRI) are increasingly used in assessing the presence of subclinical CAD and the risk of cardiac events. However, the traditional stress tests (e.g., exercise tests, using cycle ergometry or treadmill) or stress echocardiography still plays a central role in diagnosing ischemia. In athletes, exercise testing has the advantage of being widely available and providing additional functional information on maximal exercise capacity, on blood pressure response, and on exercise-induced arrhythmias. However, it has a low sensitivity in less advanced cases of CAD, partially due to the limited diagnostic value of a submaximal exercise test [29–31].

55.4.3 Management

CAD in athletes is managed according to international standards for all patients with CAD, including antianginal and antithrombotic therapy. Regular PA is recommended at an individual level for all subjects [29], while sporting activity may be restricted [32]. Some medications could also be on the WADA list of prohibited drugs (diuretics and beta-blockers for certain sports).

55.4.4 Return to Play

Eligibility is primarily based on the presence or absence of CAD and myocardial ischemia but also on the type and volume of competition/sport, the fitness level of the individual, as well as on the current risk factors, i.e., glucose, blood pressure, and cholesterol [5, 33, 34]. As a general principle, a competitive athlete with suspected, but not confirmed, CAD should be assessed by a truly maximal exercise stress test (Borg > 18, RER > 1.1, Lactate > 8 mmol/l). In those athletes who intend to perform exercise with a high volume and high intensity in training or competition, ischemia should also be ruled out by additional stress imaging.

The risk of patients with CAD can be stratified into having "lower" or "higher" probability of adverse cardiac events, according to criteria, which include coronary angiography, echocardiography/other imaging, and exercise test variables.

In recent years, the development of new eligibility criteria for athletes with CAD has been discussed. In the future, as the scientific knowledge on risk stratification increases, the recommendations may become less limiting and allow for more sporting activity on an individual basis (Fig. 55.1).

Fact Box 2 Return to sport—coronary artery disease (CAD)

- The current recommendations from the European Society of Cardiology are only low static, lowmoderate dynamic type of competitive sports (I A-B) (Fig. 55.1), in patients with established CAD, having a lower probability for adverse events. The American Heart Association may allow all sports in patients with clinically manifest CAD, if the resting ejection fraction is above 50%, they are asymptomatic, and they have no inducible ischemia or electrical instability [35].
- Patients with CAD, having a nornal exercise test, but a diminished left ventricular ejection fraction of 45–55% (higher probability for adverse events), although not eligible for sports participation, may be eligible for low or moderate intensity activities [32]. However, exercise training at a level with no ischemia is recommended [36], with the threshold being self-monitored by the patient, for example with a heart rate monitor or rate of perceived exertion (RPE).
- Eligibility assessment should always include advise on fitness and training and periodical reevaluation. The success of the risk factor modification may influence the frequency of examinations.

55.5 Myocarditis

55.5.1 Background

For many years, myocarditis was considered to be the main cause of sudden cardiac death in athletes. With emerging knowledge, this number is now approximated to 3–6% of SCDs in young athletes [37]. Acute myocarditis is defined as an inflammation of the myocardium (heart muscle), with accompanying necrosis. The cause is mostly viral infection, but myocarditis may also be secondary to a variety of other disorders, including systemic disease, malignancy, kidney disease, and toxicity.

Physical activity during an ongoing infection will increase the risk of acute myocarditis. Different viruses have different propensity to affect the heart, i.e., being more or less cardiotrophic. Coxsackie B, adenovirus, parvovirus (fifth disease), cytomegalovirus, and Epstein-Barr viruses are more prone to cause myocarditis, while the virus causing the "common cold," rhinoviruses, is considerably less prone. This is the reason for variations in clinical recommendations regarding return to play, during infections. Gastroenteritis, for instance, is typically caused by viruses more prone to cause myocarditis, than the ones causing the common cold.

The myocardium is damaged by both direct toxic effects of the virus but also by more chronic inflammatory reactions, including autoimmune necrosis and fibrosis. This may lead to a variety of arrhythmias (supraventricular and/or ventricular), in up to 50% of cases, or even sudden cardiac death. Most often acute myocarditis will heal without any residual symptoms, but around 1/3 will experience scar tissue/fibrosis, with increased risk for arrhythmias [38]. A smaller subset may experience a long-term decrease in cardiac function, i.e., dilated cardiomyopathy.

55.5.2 Diagnosis

The clinical symptoms of acute myocarditis include tiredness/malaise, effort-related dyspnea, palpitations, and/or (diffuse) chest pain. More seldom the initial presentation may be syncope or sudden cardiac arrest, due to arrhythmia [39]. The clinical diagnosis is established by a combination of symptoms, ECG changes, increased biochemical markers, and cardiac echocardiography. Virus serology and/or PCR and additional imaging with multislice CT and cardiac MRI have an increasing role. Myocardial biopsy, however, has a low sensitivity and is invasive and therefore has a limited role.

55.5.3 Management

Acute myocarditis in an athlete is treated in the same way as for any patient, depending on the degree of cardiac dysfunction and on the symptoms. The management includes arrhythmia detection and management, treatment of any cardiac insufficiency, and proper restrictions of sporting activity.

The development of cardiac imaging by MRI, and late gadolinium enhancement, has made it possible to unveil cardiac fibrosis and its extent in a subset of patients with previous acute myocarditis [40]. At present, it is not possible to determine if the sporting activity does contribute to any observed changes by itself, or in combination with a previous myocarditis, and/or a genetic predisposition contributes. The right ventricular dysfunction seen in extreme elite cyclists, for instance, could be an example of acquired heart dysfunction, where the role of acute myocarditis remains unknown. However, independent of the cause, the presence of fibrosis increases the future risk of arrhythmias in these athletes [38].

Fact Box 3 Return to play—acute myocarditis

- The international Cardiac Societies agree on 6 months absence from competitive sports after the diagnosis of myocarditis is established [32].
- After this period the athlete could resume training, provided no symptoms remain, and if no arrhythmias or symptoms on maximal exercise testing and with a normalized cardiac echocardiography.
- Sometimes a long-term ECG (Holter) is required to show the absence of arrhythmias.

55.6 Ventricular Preexcitation/ Wolff-Parkinson-White Syndrome

55.6.1 Background

Ventricular preexcitation occurs when an accessory pathway bypasses the atrioventricular (AV) node resulting in abnormal conduction to the ventricle (preexcitation) with shortening of the PR interval and widening of the QRS. This displays on the electrocardiogram (ECG) as the Wolff-Parkinson-White (WPW) pattern.

The WPW pattern occurs in approximately 1/1000–4/1000 athletes [41–44]. The presence of an accessory pathway can predispose an athlete to sudden death if the athlete also goes into atrial fibrillation as rapid conduction across the accessory pathway can result in ventricular fibrillation (VF). The risk of sudden death associated with asymptomatic WPW in adults is approximately 0.1% per year [45] with children and younger adults having higher risk of sudden death [46–48]. WPW accounted for only 1% of cardiovascular deaths in a long-term registry of sudden death in athletes [49]. However, WPW also may account for a proportion of autopsy-negative sudden unexplained deaths. Athletes with WPW may present with symptoms of palpitations, near-syncope, or syncope. Symptomatic patients found to have WPW pattern on ECG are classified as having "WPW syndrome."

55.6.2 Diagnosis

WPW pattern on ECG is defined as a short PR interval (<120 ms), the presence of a delta wave (slurring of the initial QRS), and a wide QRS (>120 ms) (Fig. 55.2) [50]. In some instances, the QRS duration is <120 ms, but a short PR interval and delta wave are still present and signify WPW pattern. WPW should be differentiated from an ectopic atrial rhythm with a short PR interval (without a delta wave) that is a common finding in athletes.

55.6.3 Management

Asymptomatic athletes with WPW pattern warrant further assessment of the refractory period of the accessory pathway and should be investigated for the presence of a low- or high-risk accessory pathway [51–54]. Intermittent preexcitation during sinus rhythm on a resting ECG is also consistent with a low-risk pathway and may eliminate the need for an exercise test [55].

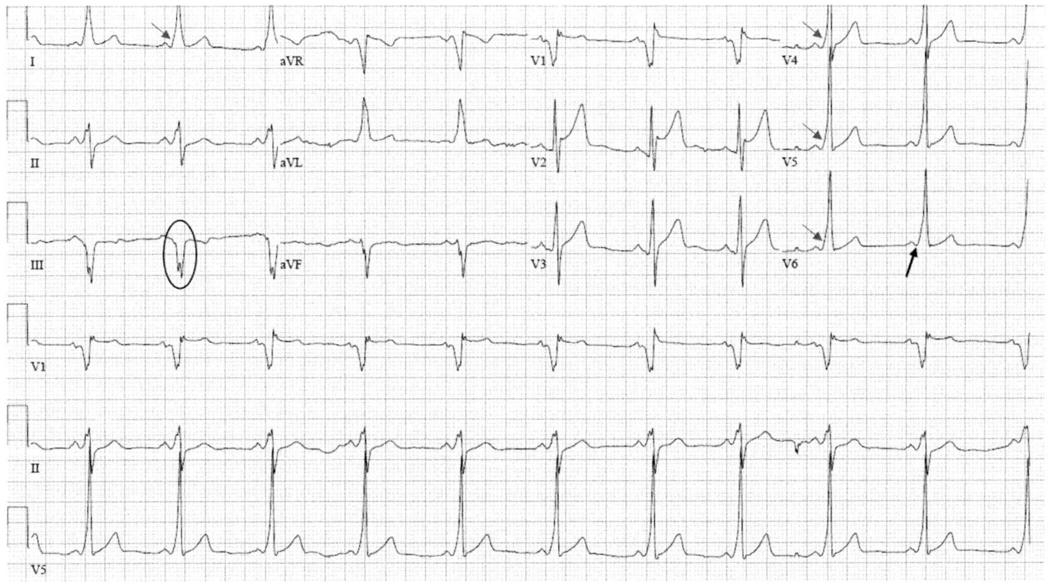

Fig. 55.2 ECG shows WPW pattern (ventricular preexcitation) with the classic findings of a short PR interval (≤120 ms), delta waves (*red arrows*), and wide QRS (≥120 ms). Other associated findings suggestive of WPW pattern include a large Q wave in lead III (*circle*) and lack of a Q wave in V6 (*black arrow*)

If stress testing cannot confirm a low-risk pathway or is inconclusive, electrophysiology testing should be considered. Young athletes with a high-risk pathway should proceed with transcatheter pathway ablation [51, 52]. An echocardiogram is also indicated due to the association of WPW with cardiomyopathy, for example [56].

Some physicians may recommend electrophysiological studies in all competitive athletes with WPW pattern involved in moderate or high intensity sport irrespective of the results of the exercise stress test. This is based on the premise that high catecholamine concentrations during intensive exercise may modify the refractory period of an accessory pathway in a way that cannot be reproduced during stress testing.

Fact Box 4 Return to play—WPW

- Athletes with WPW pattern in which a low risk accessory pathway is determined by stress testing (abrupt and complete loss of preexcitation at higher heart rates) can return to sport without limitations [53, 54].
- Exercise should be restricted for 1 week after catheter ablation, and a repeat ECG performed 1 week after the ablation. If the WPW pattern is still resolved and there are no recurrent symptoms (if previously present), the athlete may return to sport without limitation.

55.7 Long QT Syndrome

55.7.1 Background

Congenital long QT syndrome (LQTS) is a potentially lethal genetic ventricular arrhythmia syndrome with the hallmark ECG feature of QT prolongation. Symptoms if present may include syncope, seizures, or aborted cardiac arrest/sudden death from *torsades de pointes* (type of ventricular tachycardia) and ventricular fibrillation (VF). The pathophysiology of LQTS involves gene mutations that cause delayed ventricular repolarization. LQTS is estimated to affect 1 in 2000 individuals, but this prevalence does not include gene-positive "concealed" LQTS with a normal QT interval [57].

Autopsy-negative sudden unexplained death represents 25–44% of sudden unexpected deaths in persons under the age of 40 years [26, 58–61]. In sudden death cases that lack structural autopsy findings, cardiac ion channelopathies have been implicated by postmortem genetic testing as the probable cause in up to 25–35% of cases in selected cohorts [59, 62–64]. Thus, LQTS may be a more common cause of SCA/SCD than previously thought.

55.7.2 Diagnosis

In asymptomatic athletes, QTc values ≥470 ms in males and ≥480 ms in females define the abnormal cutoff of QT prolongation that warrants further evaluation [52]. It is critical that an athlete with a single screening ECG with QTc values above these thresholds is not given a diagnosis of LQTS but rather referred to further in-depth evaluation.

Accurate measurement and manual confirmation of the computer-derived QT interval corrected for heart rate (QTc) are critical. Most ECG devices utilize Bazett's heart rate correction formula ($QTc = QT/\sqrt{RR}$; RR interval measured in seconds) [65]. Importantly, Bazett's formula loses accuracy at slow and fast heart rates <50 or >90 bpm.

To properly perform a manual QT measurement, leads II and V5 usually provide the best delineation of the end of the T wave, using the "teach-the-tangent" or "avoid-the-tail" method to determine the end of the T wave [66].

55.7.3 Management

Athletes with a prolonged QTc (≥470 ms in males; ≥480 ms in females) should have a repeat resting ECG a few days later. The athlete should be questioned in terms of the use of any QT-prolonging medications, symptoms (exercise-, emotion-, or auditory-triggered syncope or seizure), and family history (unexplained syncope, seizures, sudden cardiac arrest, and unexplained drowning or motor vehicle accident) [52].

Athletes with an abnormally prolonged QTc should be referred to a heart rhythm specialist or sports cardiologist for further evaluation of possible congenital LQTS. A combination of personal symptoms, family history, ECG features, stress-ECG, and genetic testing (summarized in scoring systems), may be needed to [67–69].

Management of LQTS involves an extensive counseling to avoid QT-prolonging medications and ensure proper hydration and electrolyte balance with exercise, use of β-blockers, consideration of an implantable cardioverter defibrillator (ICD) or left cardiac sympathetic denervation, and discussion of safe activity recommendations.

55.7.4 Return to Play

Once a diagnosis in which expert guidelines recommended exclusion from competitive sports for all athletes with LQTS [32, 70], recent studies have demonstrated the safety and effectiveness of individualized management and an informed decision-making model. Return to play decisions should occur within a structure that emphasizes a comprehensive evaluation, extensive patient/family counseling, prudent medical management for risk reduction, and informed decision-making [71].

Fact Box 5 Return to play—long QT syndrome

- For an athlete with LQTS, competitive sports participation may be considered assuming appropriate precautionary measures and disease-specific treatments are in place and the athlete has been asymptomatic on treatment for at least three months [72].
- For asymptomatic athletes who are genotype-positive/phenotype-negative, a return to all competitive sports is allowed assuming appropriate LQTS precautionary measures [72].

55.8 Catecholaminergic Polymorphic Ventricular Tachycardia

55.8.1 Background

Catecholaminergic polymorphic ventricular tachycardia (CPVT) is an inherited arrhythmia disorder characterized by ventricular ectopy induced by exercise or emotional stress. If untreated, approximately 30% of individuals experience cardiac arrest and up to 80% have at least one episode of syncope [73]. The prevalence of CPVT is estimated at 1 in 10,000 persons [74]. The incidence of SCD in athletes related to CPVT is not known.

55.8.2 Diagnosis

CPVT should be considered in any person who experiences syncope during exercise or extreme emotion, particularly in children who experience repeated episodes of syncope with exercise. A resting ECG is typically normal in patients with CPVT. Thus, exercise stress testing is a requisite test for the diagnosis of CPVT [75].

Fact Box 6 Return to play—CPVT

CPVT is the channelopathy most vulnerable to exercise-triggered arrhythmias and breakthrough events despite β-blocker therapy. Thus, vigorous exercise and competitive sports should be approached with caution.

- For an athlete with CPVT, participation in competitive sports is generally not recommended except for class IA sports [72, 79] (Fig. 55.1).

55.8.3 Management

The mainstay of treatment for patients with CPVT is β-blockers which significantly reduce the risk of cardiac events [76, 77]. Other antiarrhythmic may be effective in further reducing ventricular arrhythmias [78]. Consideration of an ICD or left cardiac sympathetic denervation is also common. Genetic testing is recommended in family members with treatment of asymptomatic, genotype-positive relatives.

55.9 Cardiomyopathies

55.9.1 Background

Cardiomyopathies include a number of inherited, progressive heart muscle diseases, hypertrophic cardiomyopathy (HCM), arrhythmogenic right ventricular cardiomyopathy (ARVC), and non-compaction cardiomyopathy, which all are associated with an increased risk of arrhythmia and SCA, in association with exercise [32]:

- The most common of the cardiomyopathies is HCM, with a prevalence of about 1/500 in grown-ups. The absolute annual risk of death in asymptomatic individuals with HCM is approximately 0.5% in adults and 3.5% in children [80]. HCM is the most common cause of SCD in the USA [49] especially in the young athletes. HCM is also the cardiomyopathy most likely to be picked up by screening. Indeed, the decreased mortality in Italian competitive athletes has been in parallel with a decrease in death from HCM, in the same geographic region [81].
- ARVC, typically autosomally dominantly inherited, is more uncommon, with a prevalence of about 1/2500–5000, but remains a significant cause of SCD also in countries with mandatory screening [81].
- Finally, non-compaction cardiomyopathy, with unknown prevalence, has recently been highlighted as a differential diagnosis to athletic adaptation to training [82]. However, established non-compaction cardiomyopathy is considered as having an increased risk of arrhythmias and SCA, in line with the other cardiomyopathies.

55.9.2 Diagnosis

HCM is typically diagnosed by a combination of symptoms, family history, and electrocardiographic changes. The diagnosis is then confirmed by echocardiography, complemented by cardiac MRI if needed.

ARVC is much more difficult to pick up in screening. International recommendations highlight family history, symptoms of palpitations, syncope, or chest pain during exercise and verified arrhythmias, various ECG changes at rest, echocardiographic findings, and cardiac MRI as the key to diagnosis [83]. Genetic testing is useful, to identify the mutation, mainly in established cases of cardiomyopathy.

Non-compaction cardiomyopathy is also identified by echocardiography and MRI and has to be distinguished from the physiologic adaptation to training (and pregnancy) causing hypertrabeculation of the left ventricle [84]. All cases of suspected cardiomyopathy should also be assessed for any associated arrhythmias with exercise test and long-term ECG recordings.

Importantly, physiologic adaptation to long-term intensive exercise, i.e., “athlete’s heart,” may mimic cardiomyopathy [3]. Echocardiography, alone or in combination with cardiac MRI, may

Fact Box 7 Return to play—cardiomyopathies

- As the risk of SCA is increased in individuals with established cardiomyopathy (HCM, ARVC, and non-compaction cardiomyopathy), competitive sports is not recommended, by either American Heart Association (AHA) or European Society of Cardiology (ESC) [4, 32].
- Gene-positive but-phenotype negative athletes with ARVC are also not advised to continue competitive sports at present, while for HCM-gene carriers, without evidence of disease, the current recommendations are divided, with the AHA allowing sports, with continuous follow-up, in individual cases [4].

distinguish between these entities, but a "gray zone" may remain, needing further assessment by family screening, exercise testing, and even deconditioning (stop training) in some cases.

55.9.3 Management

Cardiomyopathies are managed according to international standards, including risk stratification and symptomatic treatment of any associated arrhythmias [83]. Family screening is mandatory, and arrhythmia protection by ICD has to be considered. Exercise typically has to be restricted.

55.10 Summary

While regular physical activity is associated with numerous health benefits, intense physical activity, somewhat paradoxically, is associated with an increased risk of serious cardiac events, including sudden cardiac arrest/death (SCA/SCD), especially in subjects with an underlying (also subclinical) cardiovascular disease.

After identification and management of a relevant cardiac condition follows the important clinical decision of return to play. Some cardiac conditions, such as acute myocarditis, may heal and allow return to play, while other cardiac conditions may be lifelong and invariably treatable. Some cardiac conditions are not even compatible with return to play. The ultimate decision of return to play after cardiac conditions should be made in collaboration with a recognized expert in the field.

Take-Home Message

- While regular physical activity is associated with numerous health effects, high-intensity activity (sports) may act a trigger for serious cardiac events, especially in individuals with underlying (also silent) cardiovascular disease.
- The aim of cardiac screening is to identify athletes at risk, i.e., those having a relevant underlying cardiac condition.
- Treatment and management of cardiac conditions in athletes are according to established protocols, similar to nonathletes. In athletes, the clinician has to take into consideration if the medication is on the WADA list and the possible effect of sporting activity on the progress of the underlying disease.
- Return to play decisions after cardiac conditions should always be taken in association with relevant expertise and according to international recommendations for eligibility.

Top Five Evidence-Based References

Drezner JA, Sharma S, Baggish A, Papadakis M, Wilson MG, Prutkin JM et al (2017) International criteria for electrocardiographic interpretation in athletes: Consensus statement. Br J Sports Med 51:704–731

Harmon KG, Asif IM, Maleszewski JJ, Owens DS, Prutkin JM, Salerno JC et al (2015) Incidence, etiology, and comparative frequency of sudden cardiac death in NCAA athletes: a decade in review. Circulation 132(1):10–19

Kindermann I, Barth C, Mahfoud F, Ukena C, Lenski M, Yilmaz A et al Update on myocarditis (2012). J Am Coll Cardiol 59:779–792

Lim SS, Vos T, Flaxman AD, Danaei G, Shibuya K, Adair-Rohani H et al (2012) A comparative risk assessment of burden of disease and injury attributable to 67 risk factors and risk factor clusters in 21 regions, 1990–2010: a systematic analysis for the Global Burden of Disease Study 2010. Lancet 380:2224–2260

Mancia G, Fagard R, Narkiewicz K, Redon J, Zanchetti A, Bohm M et al (2013) 2013 ESH/ESC guidelines for the management of arterial hypertension: the Task Force for the management of arterial hypertension of the European Society of Hypertension (ESH) and of the European Society of Cardiology (ESC). J Hypertens 31:1281–1357

References

1. Lee DC, Pate RR, Lavie CJ, Sui X, Church TS, Blair SN (2014) Leisure-time running reduces all-cause and cardiovascular mortality risk. J Am Coll Cardiol 64:472–481
2. Borjesson M, Pelliccia A (2009) Incidence and aetiology of sudden cardiac death in young athletes: an international perspective. Br J Sports Med 43:644–648

3. Corrado D, Pelliccia A, Bjornstad HH, Vanhees L, Biffi A, Borjesson M et al (2005) ESC Report: Cardiovascular pre-participation screening of young competitive athletes for prevention of sudden death: proposal for a common European protocol. Consensus statement of the Study Group of Sports Cardiology of the Working Group of Cardiac rehabilitation and exercise physiology and the Working Group of Myocardial and Pericardial diseases of the European Society of Cardiology. Eur Heart J 26:516–524
4. Maron BJ, Levine BD, Washington RL, Baggish AL, Kovacs RJ, Maron MS et al (2015) Eligibility and disqualification recommendations for competitive athletes with cardiovascular abnormalities: task force 2: preparticipation screening for cardiovascular disease in competitive athletes: a scientific statement from the American Heart Association and American College of Cardiology. Circulation 132:e267–e272
5. Börjesson M, Urhausen A, Kouidi E, Dugmore D, Sharma S, Halle M et al (2011) Cardiovascular evaluation of middle-aged/senior individuals engaged in leisure-time sport activities: position stand from the section of exercise physiology and sports cardiology of the European Association of Cardiovascular Prevention and Rehabilitation. Eur J Cardiovasc Prev Rehabil 18:446–458
6. Maron BJ, Araujo CG, Thompson PD, Fletcher GF, deLuna AB, Fleg JL et al (2001) Recommendations for preparticipation screening and the assessment of cardiovascular disease in masters athletes: an advisory for healthcare professionals from the working groups of the World Heart Federation, the International Federation of Sports Medicine, and the American Heart Association Committée on Exercise, Cardiac Rehabilitation, and Prevention. Circulation 103:327–334
7. Colivicchi F, Ammirati F, Santini M (2004) Epidemiology and prognostic implications of syncope in young competing athletes. Eur Heart J 25:1749–1753
8. Calkins H, Seifert M, Morady F (1995) Clinical presentation and long-term follow-up of athletes with exercise-induced vasodepressor syncope. Am Heart J 129:1159–1164
9. Kosinski D, Grubb BP, Kip K, Hahn H (1996) Exercise-induced neurocardiogenic syncope. Am Heart J 132:451–452
10. Sakaguchi S, Shultz JJ, Remole SC, Adler SW, Lurie KG, Benditt DG (1995) Syncope associated with exercise, a manifestation of neurally mediated syncope. Am J Cardiol 75:476–481
11. Sneddon JF, Scalia G, Ward DE, McKenna WJ, Camm AJ, Frenneaux MP (1994) Exercise induced vasodepressor syncope. Br Heart J 71:554–557
12. Lim SS, Vos T, Flaxman AD, Danaei G, Shibuya K, Adair-Rohani H et al (2012) A comparative risk assessment of burden of disease and injury attributable to 67 risk factors and risk factor clusters in 21 regions, 1990–2010: a systematic analysis for the global burden of disease study 2010. Lancet 380:2224–2260
13. Mancia G, Fagard R, Narkiewicz K, Redon J, Zanchetti A, Bohm M et al (2013) 2013 ESH/ESC guidelines for the management of arterial hypertension: the Task Force for the management of arterial hypertension of the European Society of Hypertension (ESH) and of the European Society of Cardiology (ESC). J Hypertens 31:1281–1357
14. Geleijnse JM, Kok FJ, Grobbee DE (2004) Impact of dietary and lifestyle factors on the prevalence of hypertension in Western populations. Eur J Pub Health 14:235–239
15. Grace F, Sculthorpe N, Baker J, Davies B (2003) Blood pressure and rate pressure product response in males using high-dose anabolic androgenic steroids (AAS). J Sci Med Sport 6:307–312
16. Leischik R, Spelsberg N, Niggemann H, Dworrak B, Tiroch K (2014) Exercise-induced arterial hypertension - an independent factor for hypertrophy and a ticking clock for cardiac fatigue or atrial fibrillation in athletes? F1000Res 3:105
17. Berge HM, Andersen TE, Solberg EE, Steine K (2013) High ambulatory blood pressure in male professional football players. Br J Sports Med 47:521–525
18. Karpinos AR, Roumie CL, Nian H, Diamond AB, Rothman RL (2013) High prevalence of hypertension among collegiate football athletes. Circ Cardiovasc Qual Outcomes 6:716–723
19. Berge HM, Isern CB, Berge E (2015) Blood pressure and hypertension in athletes: a systematic review. Br J Sports Med 49:716–723
20. Aagaard P, Sahlen A, Braunschweig F (2012) Performance trends and cardiac biomarkers in a 30-km cross-country race, 1993–2007. Med Sci Sports Exerc 44:894–899
21. Trachsel LD, Carlen F, Brugger N, Seiler C, Wilhelm M (2015) Masked hypertension and cardiac remodeling in middle-aged endurance athletes. J Hypertens 33:1276–1283
22. National Clinical Guideline Centre (2011) Hypertension: clinical management of primary hypertension in adults. Hypertension: clinical management of primary hypertension in adults. National Clinical Guideline Centre, London. http://www.nice.org.uk/Guidance/CG127. Accessed 9 Oct 2014
23. Fagard RH, Bjornstad HH, Borjesson M, Carre F, Deligiannis A, Vanhees L et al (2005) ESC Study Group of Sports Cardiology recommendations for participation in leisure-time physical activities and competitive sports for patients with hypertension. Eur J Cardiovasc Prev Rehabil 12:326–331
24. Gordon NF (1997) Hypertension. In: Durstine JL (ed) ACSM's exercise management for persons with chronic diseases and disabilities. Human Kinetics, Champaign, IL
25. Levine BD, Baggish AL, Kovacs RJ, Link MS, Maron MS, Mitchell JH (2015) Eligibility and disqualification recommendations for competitive athletes with cardiovascular abnormalities: task force 1: classification of sports: dynamic, static, and impact: a scientific statement from the American Heart Association and

American College of Cardiology. J Am Coll Cardiol 66:2350–2355
26. Meyer L, Stubbs B, Fahrenbruch C, Maeda C, Harmon K, Eisenberg M et al (2012) Incidence, causes and survival trends from cardiovascular-related sudden cardiac arrest in children and young adults 0 to 35 years of age: a 30-year review. Circulation 126:1363–1372
27. Mittleman MA, Maclure M, Tofler GH, Sherwood JB, Goldberg RJ, Muller JE (1993) Triggering of acute myocardial infarction by heavy physical exertion. Protection against triggering by regular exercise. N Engl J Med 329:1677–1683
28. Vanhees L, Rauch B, Piepoli M, van BUuren F, Takken T, Borjesson M et al (2012) Importance of characteristics and modalities of physical activity and exercise in the management of cardiovascular health in individuals with cardiovascular disease (part III). Eur J Prev Cardiol 19:1333–1356
29. Börjesson M, Assanelli D, Carré F, Dugmore D, Panhuysen-Goedkoop NM, Seiler C et al (2006) ESC Study Group of Sports Cardiology: recommendations for participation in leisure-time physical activity and competitive sports for patients with ischemic heart disease. Eur J Cardiovasc Prev Rehabil 13:137–149
30. Börjesson M, Dellborg M (2012) The role of exercise testing in the interventional era: a shift of focus. Interv Cardiol 4:577–583
31. Thompson PD, Franklin BA, Balady GJ, Blair SN, Corrado D, Estes NAM III et al (2007) Exercise and acute cardiovascular events. Placing the risks into perspective. A scientific statement from the American heart Association Council on nutrition, physical activity, and metabolism and the Council on Clinical Cardiology. Circulation 115:2358–2368
32. Pelliccia A, Fagard R, Bjornstad H, Anastassakis A, Arbustini E, Assanelli D et al (2005) Recommendations for competitive sports participation in athletes with cardiovascular disease: a consensus document from the Study Group of Sports Cardiology of the Working Group of Cardiac Rehabilitation and Exercise Physiology and the Working Group of Myocardial and Pericardial Diseases of the European Society of Cardiology. Eur Heart J 26:1422–1445
33. Mons U, Hahmann H, Brenner H (2014) A reverse J-shaped association of leisure-time physical activity prognosis in patients with stable coronary heart disease: evidence from a large cohort with repeated measurements. Heart 100:1043–1049
34. Williams PT, Thompson PD (2014) Increased cardiovascular disease mortality associated with excessive exercise in heart attack survivors. Mayo Clin Proc 89:1187–1194
35. Thompson PD, Myerburg RJ, Levine BD, Udelson JE, Kovacs RJ. Eligibility and disqualification recommendations for competitive athletes with cardiovascular abnormalities: Task Force 8: coronary artery disease. A scientific statement from the American Heart Association and the American College of Cardiology
36. NIebauer J, Hambrecht R, Hauer K, Marburger C, Schöppenthau M, Kälberer B et al (1994) Identification of patients at risk during swimming by Holter monitoring. Am J Cardiol 74:651–656
37. Maron BJ, Haas TS, Murphy CJ, Ahluwalia A, Rutten-Ramos S (2014) Incidence and causes of sudden death in U.S. college athletes. J Am Coll Cardiol 63:1636–1643
38. Grun S, Schumm J, Greulich S, Wagner A, Schneider S, Bruder O et al (2012) Long-term follow-up of biopsy-proven viral myocarditis: predictors of mortality and incomplete recovery. J Am Coll Cardiol 59:1604–1615
39. Kindermann I, Barth C, Mahfoud F, Ukena C, Lenski M, Yilmaz A et al (2012) Update on myocarditis. J Am Coll Cardiol 59:779–792
40. Zagrosek A, Abdel-Aty H, Boye P, Wassmuth R, Messroghli D, Utz W et al (2009) Cardiac magnetic resonance monitors reversible and irreversible myocardial injury in myocarditis. JACC Cardiovasc Imaging 2:131–138
41. Drezner JA, Prutkin JM, Harmon KG, O'Kane JW, Pelto HF, Rao AL et al (2015) Cardiovascular screening in college athletes. J Am Coll Cardiol 65:2353–2355
42. Fudge J, Harmon KG, Owens DS, Prutkin JM, Salerno JC, Asif IM et al (2014) Cardiovascular screening in adolescents and young adults: a prospective study comparing the pre-participation physical evaluation monograph 4th edition and ECG. Br J Sports Med 48:1172–1178
43. Marek J, Bufalino V, Davis J, Marek K, Gami A, Stephan W et al (2011) Feasibility and findings of large-scale electrocardiographic screening in young adults: data from 32,561 subjects. Heart Rhythm 8:1555–1559
44. Pelliccia A, Culasso F, Di Paolo FM, Accettura D, Cantore R, Castagna W et al (2007) Prevalence of abnormal electrocardiograms in a large, unselected population undergoing pre-participation cardiovascular screening. Eur Heart J 28:2006–2010
45. Munger TM, Packer DL, Hammill SC, Feldman BJ, Bailey KR, Ballard DJ et al (1993) A population study of the natural history of Wolff-Parkinson-White syndrome in Olmsted County, Minnesota, 1953–1989. Circulation 87:866–873
46. Deal BJ, Beerman L, Silka M, Walsh EP, Klitzner T, Kugler J (1995) Cardiac arrest in young patients with Wolff-Parkinson-White syndrome. PACE 815(a)
47. Klein GJ, Bashore TM, Sellers TD, Pritchett EL, Smith WM, Gallagher JJ (1979) Ventricular fibrillation in the Wolff-Parkinson-White syndrome. N Engl J Med 301:1080–1085
48. Russell MW, Dick MD (1993) Incidence of catastrophic events associated with the Wolff-Parkinson-White syndrome in young patients: diagnostic and therapeutic dilemma. Circulation 484(a)
49. Maron BJ, Doerer JJ, Haas TS, Tierney DM, Mueller FO (2009) Sudden death in young competitive athletes. Analysis of 1866 deaths in the United States, 1980–2006. Circulation 119:1085–1092

50. Surawicz B, Childers R, Deal BJ, Gettes LS, Bailey JJ, Gorgels A et al (2009) AHA/ACCF/HRS recommendations for the standardization and interpretation of the electrocardiogram: part III: intraventricular conduction disturbances: a scientific statement from the American Heart Association Electrocardiography and Arrhythmias Committee, Council on Clinical Cardiology; the American College of Cardiology Foundation; and the Heart Rhythm Society: endorsed by the International Society for Computerized Electrocardiology. Circulation 119:e235–e240
51. Cohen MI, Triedman JK, Cannon BC, Davis AM, Drago F, Janousek J et al (2012) PACES/HRS expert consensus statement on the management of the asymptomatic young patient with a Wolff-Parkinson-White (WPW, ventricular preexcitation) electrocardiographic pattern: developed in partnership between the Pediatric and Congenital Electrophysiology Society (PACES) and the Heart Rhythm Society (HRS). Endorsed by the governing bodies of PACES, HRS, the American College of Cardiology Foundation (ACCF), the American Heart Association (AHA), the American Academy of Pediatrics (AAP), and the Canadian Heart Rhythm Society (CHRS). Heart Rhythm 9:1006–1024
52. Drezner JA, Sharma S, Baggish A, Papadakis M, Wilson MG, Prutkin JM et al (2017) International criteria for electrocardiographic interpretation in athletes: consensus statement. Br J Sports Med 51:704–731
53. Rao AL, Asif IM, Salerno JC, Drezner JA (2014) Evaluation and management of Wolff-Parkinson-White in athletes. Sports Health 6(4):326–332
54. Zipes DP, Link MS, Ackerman MJ, Kovacs RJ, Myerburg RJ, Estes NAM III et al (2015) Eligibility and disqualification recommendations for competitive athletes with cardiovascular abnormalities: task force 9: arrhythmias and conduction defects: a scientific statement from the American Heart Association and American College of Cardiology. Circulation 132:e315–e325
55. Klein GJ, Gulamhusein SS (1983) Intermittent preexcitation in the Wolff-Parkinson-White syndrome. Am J Cardiol 52:292–296
56. Finocchiaro G, Papadakis M, Behr ER, Sharma S, Sheppard M (2017) Sudden cardiac death in pre-excitation and Wolff-Parkinson-White: demographic and clinical features. J Am Coll Cardiol 69:1644–1645
57. Schwartz PJ, Stramba-Badiale M, Crotti L, Pedrazzini M, Besana A, Bosi G et al (2009) Prevalence of the congenital long-QT syndrome. Circulation 120:1761–1767
58. Eckart RE, Shry EA, Burke AP, McNear JA, Appel DA, Castillo-Rojas LM et al (2011) Sudden death in young adults: an autopsy-based series of a population undergoing active surveillance. J Am Coll Cardiol 58:1254–1261
59. Finocchiaro G, Papadakis M, Robertus JL, Dhutia H, Steriotis AK, Tome M et al (2016) Etiology of sudden death in sports: insights from a United Kingdom Regional Registry. J Am Coll Cardiol 67:2108–2115
60. Harmon KG, Asif IM, Maleszewski JJ, Owens DS, Prutkin JM, Salerno JC et al (2015) Incidence, etiology, and comparative frequency of sudden cardiac death in NCAA athletes: a decade in review. Circulation 132(1):10–19
61. Tester DJ, Ackerman MJ (2009) Cardiomyopathic and channelopathic causes of sudden unexplained death in infants and children. Annu Rev Med 60:69–84
62. Behr E, Wood DA, Wright M, Syrris P, Sheppard MN, Casey A et al (2003) Cardiological assessment of first-degree relatives in sudden arrhythmic death syndrome. Lancet 362:1457–1459
63. Tan HL, Hofman N, van Langen IM, van der Wal AC, Wilde AA (2005) Sudden unexplained death: heritability and diagnostic yield of cardiological and genetic examination in surviving relatives. Circulation 112:207–213
64. Tester DJ, Spoon DB, Valdivia HH, Makielski JC, Ackerman MJ (2004) Targeted mutational analysis of the RyR2-encoded cardiac ryanodine receptor in sudden unexplained death: a molecular autopsy of 49 medical examiner/coroner's cases. Mayo Clin Proc 79:1380–1384
65. Bazett HC (1920) An analysis of the time-relations of electrocardiograms. Heart:353–370
66. Postema PG, De Jong JS, Van der Bilt IA, Wilde AA (2008) Accurate electrocardiographic assessment of the QT interval: teach the tangent. Heart Rhythm 5:1015–1018
67. Gollob MH, Redpath CJ, Roberts JD (2011) The short QT syndrome: proposed diagnostic criteria. J Am Coll Cardiol 57:802–812
68. Schwartz PJ, Crotti L (2011) QTc behavior during exercise and genetic testing for the long-QT syndrome. Circulation 124:2181–2184
69. Schwartz PJ, Moss AJ, Vincent GM, Crampton RS (1993) Diagnostic criteria for the long QT syndrome. an update. Circulation 88:782–784
70. Maron BJ, Zipes DP (2005) 36th Bethesda conference: eligibility recommendations for competitive athletes with cardiovascular abnormalities. J Am Coll Cardiol 45:1312–1377
71. Drezner JA (2013) Detect, manage, inform: a paradigm shift in the care of athletes with cardiac disorders? Br J Sports Med 47:4–5
72. Ackerman MJ, Zipes DP, Kovacs RJ, Maron BJ, American Heart Association E, Arrhythmias Committee of Council on Clinical Cardiology CoCDiYCoC, et al. (2015) Eligibility and disqualification recommendations for competitive athletes with cardiovascular abnormalities: task force 10: the cardiac channelopathies: a scientific statement from the American Heart Association and American College of Cardiology. Circulation 132:e326–e329

73. Kontula K, Laitinen PJ, Lehtonen A, Toivonen L, Viitasalo M, Swan H (2005) Catecholaminergic polymorphic ventricular tachycardia: recent mechanistic insights. Cardiovasc Res 67:379–387
74. Napolitano C, Priori SG, Bloise R (2004) Catecholaminergic polymorphic ventricular tachycardia. In: RABT P, Dolan CR, Stephens K, Adam MP (eds) GeneReviews™. National Center for Biotechnology Information, Bethesda, MD. http://www.ncbi.nlm.nih.gov/books/NBK1289/. Accessed 16 Feb 2012
75. Liu N, Ruan Y, Priori SG (2008) Catecholaminergic polymorphic ventricular tachycardia. Prog Cardiovasc Dis 51:23–30
76. Hayashi M, Denjoy I, Extramiana F, Maltret A, Buisson NR, Lupoglazoff JM et al (2009) Incidence and risk factors of arrhythmic events in catecholaminergic polymorphic ventricular tachycardia. Circulation 119:2426–2434
77. Priori SG, Napolitano C, Memmi M, Colombi B, Drago F, Gasparini M et al (2002) Clinical and molecular characterization of patients with catecholaminergic polymorphic ventricular tachycardia. Circulation 106:69–74
78. Kannankeril PJ, Moore JP, Cerrone M et al (2017) Efficacy of flecainide in the treatment of catecholaminergic polymorphic ventricular tachycardia:: a randomized clinical trial. JAMA Cardiol 2(7):759–766
79. Ostby SA, Bos M, Owen HJ et al (2016) Competitive sports participation in patients with catecholaminergic polymorphic ventricular tachycardia: a single center's early experience. JACC Clin Electrophysiol 2:253–262
80. Ostman-Smith I, Wettrell G, Keeton B, Holmgren D, Ergander U, Gould S et al (2008) Age- and gender-specific mortality rates in childhood hypertrophic cardiomyopathy. Eur Heart J 29:1160–1167
81. Corrado D, Basso C, Pavei A, Michieli P, Schiavon M, Thiene G (2006) Trends in sudden cardiovascular death in young competitive athletes after implementation of a preparticipation screening programme. JAMA 296:1593–1601
82. Ganga HV, Thompson PD (2014) Sports participation in non-compaction cardiomyopathy: a systematic review. Br J Sports Med 48:1466–1471
83. Corrado D, Wichter T, Link MS, Hauer R, Marchlinski F, Anastasakis A et al (2015) Treatment of arrhythmogenic right ventricular cardiomyopathy/dysplasia: an international task force consensus statement. Eur Heart J 36:3227–3237
84. Gati S, Chandra N, Bennett RL, Reed M, Kervio G, Panoulas VF et al (2013) Increased left ventricular trabeculation in highly trained athletes: do we need more stringent criteria for the diagnosis of left ventricular non-compaction in athletes? Heart 99:401–408
85. Maron BJ, Udelson JE, Bonow RO, Nishimura RA, Ackerman MJ, NA E 3rd et al (2015) Eligibility and disqualification recommendations for competitive athletes with cardiovascular abnormalities: task force 3: hypertrophic cardiomyopathy, arrhythmogenic right ventricular cardiomyopathy and other cardiomyopathies, and myocarditis: a scientific statement from the American Heart Association and American College of Cardiology. J Am Coll Cardiol 66:2362–2371

56 Return to Play After Infectious Disease

Mats Börjesson, Daniel Arvidsson, Christa Janse Van Rensburg, and Martin Schwellnus

Contents

M. Börjesson (✉)
Department of Food and Nutrition, and Sport Science, Center for Health and Performance (CHP), University of Gothenburg, Gothenburg, Sweden

Department of Neuroscience and Physiology, Sahlgrenska Academy and Sahlgrenska University Hospital/Östra, Göteborg, Sweden
e-mail: mats.brjesson@telia.com

D. Arvidsson
Department of Food and Nutrition, and Sport Science, Center for Health and Performance (CHP), University of Gothenburg, Skånegatan 14b, Box 300, 40530 Gothenburg, Sweden

C.J.V. Rensburg • M. Schwellnus
Faculty of Health Sciences, Section Sports Medicine, Sport, Exercise Medicine and Lifestyle Institute (SEMLI), University of Pretoria, Pretoria, South Africa

56.1 Introduction

Acute illness, specifically infective illness, is a significant health concern for recreational and elite athletes. An acute illness may prevent participation in training sessions or important competitions. Also in the football player, the pathophysiological consequences of an acute infective illness not only reduce exercise performance but also increase the risk of serious medical complications, including sudden death [1–5]. Some recommendations have been produced that can aid the sports medicine physician in return to play (RTP) decisions after illness but also to prepare the athlete to act in a more preventive manner.

V. Musahl et al. (eds.), *Return to Play in Football*, https://doi.org/10.1007/978-3-662-55713-6_56

56.2 Scope of the Problem: Epidemiology

Adults suffer on average from one to six episodes of an acute infection per year. The epidemiology of acute illness in elite level athletes has been studied in a variety of settings, mainly during major tournaments and in different sports including swimming, rugby and football [6]. Six to seventeen percent of registered athletes participating in major international games and tournaments of shorter duration (<4 weeks) are likely to suffer an acute illness episode. There are some data indicating that higher-risk subgroups are (1) female athletes, (2) athletes participating in winter sports (e.g. Olympic and Paralympic Games), (3) athletes with disability [7–9] and (4) athletes participating in more prolonged tournaments or competition [10]. Data from these studies consistently show that the most common system affected by acute illness is the respiratory tract, followed by the gastrointestinal system and the dermatological system [11, 12]. Scarce data exists on the incidence and aetiology of acute illness of athletes outside the major tournaments and competitions, i.e. in their home setting. Studies exclusively in football players show that the respiratory and gastrointestinal tracts are the most common systems affected by illness, during the studied tournaments. During the 2009 Confederations Cup, the incidence of illness was 16.9 per 1000 player days, with the respiratory tract (RT) accounting for over 50% of all illness (the ear, nose and throat = 37%; other respiratory tract = 20%) [12]. Similarly, during the 2010 FIFA World Cup, respiratory illness was the most common medical condition affecting football players (40% of all illness) [11].

56.3 Risk Factors Associated with Acute Illness in Athletes

There are many intrinsic and extrinsic risk factors that are being linked to acute illness in athletes, with varying degree of scientific support. Risk factors for acute illness can differ between different organ systems.

56.3.1 General Intrinsic Risk Factors Associated with Acute Illness in Athletes

56.3.1.1 Immune System Changes

An extensive body of literature describes the relationship between exercise and the immune system. The main theory is that a transient or more prolonged immune depression postexercise may contribute to the pathophysiology and risk of acute illness [13–18]. Indeed, changes in a variety of immune system components following a single intensive exercise session have been observed. Postexercise immune changes may be most pronounced when the exercise session is >90-min long and the intensity is 55–75% of maximum oxygen uptake (VO_2Max) [13], while other data indicate that a session longer than 60 min at an intensity >80% of maximum ability causes a depression in the immune system [19]. Observed changes include an increase in circulating neutrophils [3, 15, 20], a decrease in the lymphocytes [3, 15], a decrease in neutrophil function (oxidative activity and phagocytic capacity) for 1–3 days after the exercise session [3, 15, 17], a reduction in natural killer (NK) cell numbers and cytotoxic activity [3, 13] as well as a decrease in the salivary IgA concentrations [3, 17, 21]. Furthermore, there is an increase in the neutrophil/lymphocyte ratio (used as a predictor of stress to the immune system) for most of the following days after a heavy exercise session [22]. A 20% reduction in plasma glutamine concentration may occur, while there is conflicting evidence regarding T-cell function [3, 23]. The existing studies are typically in endurance type of sports, while strength sports have been less studied, in this regard.

A single bout of exercise thus results in changes in various immune parameters, typically lasting for 3–72 h. This period is known as the “open window” and has been widely proposed to reflect a time of “dysfunction” of the immune system, during which the athlete may be predisposed to viral and bacterial infections [1, 3, 21, 23]. However, the clinical relevance of the observed changes is still debated. Despite evidence that certain immunologic parameters change after strenuous exercise sessions, there is a lack of evidence of a direct link between the altered immune parameters and an increased incidence for URT illness, postexercise [3, 13, 24, 25]. The reason for this lack of evidence may be that some of the observed changes are physiological, as part of the acute-phase (inflammatory) response to training [26]. In addition, it has also been shown that overtraining leads to immune suppression, which may render the athlete susceptible to an acute URT illness [19, 27]. Clinically, reports of elite athletes experiencing repeated colds could also be due to the fact that an elite athlete will be relatively more affected by an ordinary cold than the average person who has less demand on maximal performance in everyday life.

56.3.1.2 A History of a Recent Acute Illness

In one prospective cohort study conducted during the Stockholm Marathon, 33% of athletes who experienced an URT illness in the 3-week period prior to the race developed an URT illness in the 3-week period after the race [28]. This was significantly greater than the 16% of athletes who did not have an acute illness prior to the marathon race. These data suggest that strenuous exercise too soon after an acute illness may be a risk factor to develop a subsequent illness. Alternatively, it may reflect that the athlete may have had a subclinical disease during the race, being aggravated by exercise.

56.3.1.3 Female Gender

Some evidence suggests that female athletes are at higher risk of an acute illness. In one prospective cohort study, 210 endurance athletes (63 females and 147 males) completed a self-reported health questionnaire on a daily basis for 16 weeks [29]. The proportion of participants who experienced one or more periods of URT illness symptoms was 40% in males and 52% in females, with the mean duration of URT illness symptoms being longer in female athletes (15.5 days vs. 11.6 days, $p = 0.024$).

Similarly, in the 2012 Winter Youth Olympic Games ($N = 1021$), the incidence of acute illness was 84.2 per 1000 athletes [30], with 6% of male athletes and 11% of female athletes suffering from an illness ($p = 0.003$). During the 2012 Summer Olympic Games, similar figures were found [8], with an overall illness incidence of 71.7 per 1000 athletes, with females again having a higher incidence (8.6% vs. 5.3%).

56.3.1.4 Body Mass Index

There are limited data to suggest that an increased body mass index (BMI) raises an athlete's risk to develop an acute illness. In one prospective cohort study, illness patterns were studied in 530 runners who completed a monthly log for 12 months. The results of this study showed that a higher BMI was associated with an increased risk to develop an URT illness [31].

56.3.2 General Extrinsic Risk Factors for Acute Illness in Athletes

56.3.2.1 Training Load

Individuals that engage in regular moderate exercise (50–70% of maximum ability, 30–60 min per session, 3–5 sessions per week) have a lower incidence of symptoms of URT illness compared with sedentary individuals [3]. On the other hand, regular, intense and prolonged exercise bouts may result in a chronic depression of the immune system, possibly increasing the risk of illness.

Historically, the relationship between the training load ("dose") of exercise and the risk of acute illness was reported as a "J-shaped" curve [2, 32–35]. However, more recently it has been suggested that the J-shaped relationship between absolute training load and illness is not necessarily applicable to elite athletes [36], as data from a number of recent studies show that high absolute training loads in international-level [37–39] and medal-winning athletes [40] are associated with a lower risk of illness compared with sub-elite or national-level athletes [6].

In 2016, the relationship between illness risk and training and competition load was reviewed [6]. The main findings were that changes in both external (increased volume and intensity of training) and internal training load are associated with an increased risk of illness. However, it is not yet possible to quantify which amount of training load increase is related to increased risk of a specific illness or in a specific sport.

56.3.2.2 Nutritional Factors

In general, immune cells require an adequate amount of glucose, protein, water and electrolytes to maintain normal function. Therefore, a well-balanced diet seems to be important for immune function. In a review of 66 placebo-controlled and/or crossover trials, it was concluded that a poor nutritional status affects almost all aspects of the immune system [15]. More specifically, an unbalanced diet, training in a dehydrated state and excessive use of nutritional supplements may negatively affect immune function.

In addition, glucose is considered to be an important fuel substrate for various immune cells, including macrophages, lymphocytes and neutrophils. There is some evidence that frequent ingestion of a ≥6% carbohydrate solution (1 l/h) during prolonged or high-intensity exercise maintains blood glucose levels, which lead to an attenuated postexercise cortisol level, resulting in a less suppressed immune function [15]. The ingestion of the carbohydrate may also attenuate exercise-induced increases in the total leucocyte count and/or monocytes and neutrophils and cytokine changes, which are associated with a decreased immune function. It has also been documented that the immune function is suppressed during periods of low calorie intake and weight loss [32].

56.3.2.3 Other Extrinsic Risk Factors

If too few resting periods are applied between strenuous exercise sessions, the athlete is at an increased risk to develop an URT illness, as the immune function has insufficient time to recover from the perturbations caused by the strenuous exercise session [2, 3, 41]. Increased risk of illness has also been related to fatigue [20] and overtraining [2, 3, 5]. There is also evidence that other extrinsic factors such as alterations in normal sleep patterns and psychological stress can increase the risk of acute illness [22].

Nowadays the elite football player frequently travels to different locations throughout the world to participate in events lasting from a few days to weeks. These events are characterized by regular strenuous games with training sessions in-between. Matches are also scheduled at night causing sleep disturbances. Data from two studies show that during periods of travelling, players may be exposed to higher risk of acute illness [40, 42]. Different environmental conditions such as extremes of temperature, humidity, adverse atmospheric pollution, aeroallergen exposure and dietary changes may play a role. Travelling between the northern and southern hemispheres, athletes are exposed to different pathogenic organisms including seasonal viral influenza strains, which may increase the risk of developing an illness [42]. In addition, sports physicians travelling with teams to foreign destinations should be aware of general and location-specific vaccination requirements.

Fact Box 1 Risk factors for developing acute illness in athletes

Intrinsic factors	Variable
Immune system	Depression of immune system components
Medical history	History of recent acute illness
Gender	Female
BMI	BMI > 75th percentile
Extrinsic factors	
Training load	High training volume High training intensity
Nutrition	Inadequate carbohydrate intake Inadequate calorie intake Exercise in dehydrated state Exercise without food intake
Other extrinsic factors	International travel Inadequate recovery time between exercise bouts Altered sleeping patterns Psychological stress Overtraining

56.4 Possible Sequelae to Infections

56.4.1 Fever

Fever is the symptom best known to any athlete or team physician, to make them aware of a possible ongoing infection. An infection will result in different degrees of response from the immune system. The hypothalamic thermoregulatory centre integrates afferent information from the periphery to regulate body temperature [43]. The core body temperature is normally kept within a range of 1–36.5–37.5 °C. Clinically, it is important to note that rectal temperatures are slightly higher than oral temperatures, with the difference being about 0.5°C. Women may have cyclic variations in their body temperature, in association with the menstrual phases. Fever is defined as a temperature that exceeds the normal and is accompanied by a shift in the thermoregulatory control. Exogenous pyrogens, such as microbial toxins or viruses, bind to macrophages and trigger the release of endogenous pyrogens (pyrogenic cytokines such as interleukins, TNF, IFN-α) [44]. Both types of pyrogens increase the synthesis of prostaglandin E2 (PGE2), which acts on the hypothalamus, via cyclic AMP, to adjust the thermoregulation upwards. Although fever is a physiologic response to an infection, it could also be the result of other immune stimuli, such as inflammation, malignancy or haemorrhagic stroke.

The potential complications during exercise due to fever are multiple. For several reasons, it may also be beneficial to treat the fever itself and not only the underlying cause. Especially, when the temperature is extremely high, approaching hyperpyrexia (>41.5°C), it is necessary to decrease the temperature by antipyretics, as the risk of complications is increased

56.4.2 Heat Stroke

Fever due to an infectious disease needs to be differentiated from hyperthermia (heat stroke) [45]. Heat stroke is defined as an increased body temperature, not caused by exogenous or endogenous pyrogens. The mechanism is an uncontrolled increase in body temperature due to excessive heat production (i.e. playing in a hot environment, without proper cooling). In this case, heat production may be faster than the combined peripheral loss of heat by sweating and respiration. This condition may be fatal, in extreme cases (>41–43°C) causing multi-organ dysfunction, including rapid liver and kidney failure (due to muscle necrosis) [46, 47], and is therefore important to distinguish from fever/hyperpyrexia. Heat stroke is the most extreme form of heat-related illnesses, which also include heat exhaustion and muscle cramps. Importantly, antipyretics may be ineffective in reducing the temperature in hyperthermia.

Fact Box 2 Complications of fever during exercise

- Fever is associated with systemic symptoms such as headache, myalgia and arthralgia
- The body will be dehydrated – due to sweating and decreased ADH production [17]
- Protein catabolism (amino acids for immune system components), decreased glucose availability and increased peripheral vascular resistance lead to nutritional deficiency and decreased muscle strength. Acute infectious disease may result in 5–15% decrease in isometric muscle strength, compared to bed rest [48]
- Fever reduces stroke volume and cardiac output to an extent depending on the severity of the fever [5]. It also increases oxygen consumption and heart rate: for every 1°C body temperature rise above 37°C, there is a 13% increase in oxygen consumption, and for every 1.5°C increase in body temperature, the heart rate may increase by 2.44 beats per minute [5]. A febrile illness may also decrease the blood volume and total haemoglobin. Together, these changes can lead to as much as a 25% reduction in endurance capacity. Maximal aerobic performance and endurance capacity decreased by 13–18% as a result of illness [49]

56.4.3 Reasons for Not Exercising During Infections

One of the most common clinical situations, in association with infection, is the question of the athlete's availability for training and/or competition. Later we will discuss some specific infections, but there are some general considerations, which may be used in the discussion with the athlete and the coach regarding the reasons for not exercising during infections:

- The infection may be prolonged and/or get worse, as has been shown in animal studies [43]. In humans, there is conflicting clinical evidence. It has been documented that exercising in the presence of an URT illness (with or without the presence of a fever) may aggravate the infection by causing more pronounced symptoms and/or prolonging the length of the illness [1, 2].
- The infection may be transmitted to teammates and colleagues. Depending on the type of infection and the causative agent, different precautions have to be undertaken [43]. See below, for diarrheal disease and dermatological infections.
- Neurologically, the coordination has been shown to decrease during infection/fever. In 1 study, 14 participants with influenza or echovirus infection, all suffering from myalgia, and 9 participants with mumps, in whom this symptom was lacking, were investigated with single-fibre electromyography (EMG) in the acute phase and during convalescence. A possible disturbance in neuromuscular transmission was revealed [1]. Decreased coordination and balance may be associated with an increased injury risk.
- Muscle strength will be negatively affected during an ongoing infection. There is evidence that infection leads to a decrease in muscle protein content (which correlates to a decline in muscle strength and endurance), a reduction in muscle enzyme activity and mitochondrial abnormalities. It might take up to 2 weeks for the muscle protein to be replenished. This is in addition to fever, which in itself may also cause a decrease in muscle strength (see above). The infection will contribute to the decrease in exercise performance experienced by athletes after an URT infection [50]. This is a reason in itself to refrain from training/playing. Furthermore, the decrease in exercise performance after full clinical recovery from an URT illness can last for 2–4 days [3] and in more severe infections (influenza) may be present for several weeks after the infection has subsided, even after the athlete has returned to sport.

Fact Box 3 Influence of acute illness on body systems, which leads to decreased exercise performance

System	Influence
Musculoskeletal	Muscle wasting (decrease in protein content) Decrease in muscle strength (isometric and isotonic) Decrease in muscle endurance Mitochondrial abnormalities
Cardiovascular	Decrease in stroke volume with a reduced cardiac output
Neurological	Impaired motor coordination Decreased neuromuscular transmission
Metabolism	Inability to maintain euglycemia Dehydration

- The risks of severe complications include cardiac complications, such as peri- and myocarditis. Different viruses and bacteria are more or less prone to affect the heart (being more cardiotoxic), with coxsackie B, influenza and parvoviruses being more and the common rhinovirus, less likely to cause myocarditis. Myocarditis is typically associated with general symptoms such as malaise and tiredness. Dyspnoea, palpitations, chest pain or even sudden cardiac arrest, due to malignant arrhythmia, may also be present [51]. Pericarditis is a similarly acquired infection of the pericardium and is also a possible complication to exercise during an ongoing infection [52].

- Rhabdomyolysis is the breakdown of skeletal muscle leading to compromised integrity of the muscle membrane, with subsequent leaking of the contents of the muscle cell into the plasma [4]. The myoglobin released from the muscle cells is filtered through the kidneys and excreted into the urine and can be directly toxic to the renal tubule and can lead to acute renal failure. It has been documented that the risk to develop rhabdomyolysis is increased when exercising during or after a viral illness [4].
- Other potential complications are listed in Fact Box 4.

Fact Box 4 Medical complications and risks associated with exercise training in athletes with an acute URT illness

System	Complication
Cardiovascular	Viral myocarditis Myopericarditis Dysrhythmias Sudden death
Musculoskeletal	Rhabdomyolysis Joint, ligament and tendon injuries due to impaired motor coordination
Respiratory system	Bronchial hyperreactivity
Others	Post-viral fatigue syndrome Increased duration and severity of symptoms of illness Heatstroke

56.5 Return to Play (RTP) After Infection

56.5.1 General Recommendations

Assuming that the athlete follows the recommendations of refraining from intense exercise during the duration of the infection, the key question will arise: When can he/she return to play? Although the specific recommendations vary for various infections, some general recommendations could be made:

- Firstly, and most importantly, return to play should occur only after the infection has cleared. This means that the athlete should have no remaining muscle pain, general malaise, fever or specific symptoms of the disease (diarrhoea, etc.).
- Secondly, RTP is a gradual process. The athlete should be closely monitored and only be allowed to increase training load if he/she is symptom-free. The length of this adjustment period is dependent on the duration and severity of the infection.
- Importantly, the athlete should not be advised to exercise in an alternative fashion, i.e. strength training instead of endurance training, which has sometimes been considered to be a less demanding activity. He or she should abstain from all training during the infection, to give the body a chance to recover fully.

56.5.2 Specific Conditions

56.5.2.1 Upper Respiratory Tract (URT) Infection

The most frequent upper respiratory infection (URI) is the common cold. It usually has a short duration of 2–4 days, typically being caused by rhinovirus, although many more viruses could be involved (Fact Box 5). URT is very common and is the reason for a large part of training interruption for an athlete, possibly several times/year [53]. An increase in the frequency of infections is usually seen in athletes during the years they have small children but also during heavy training periods. The clinically common worry of many athletes with frequent URI that they may have some underlying immune deficiency is typically unfounded. However, as the immune function may be decreased secondary to intense, prolonged and/or increased activity, athletes have to be gradually accustomed to the higher intensity of play/training. This is specifically applicable to new players coming from junior and/or lower football leagues. Repeated infections should therefore be taken as a possible warning sign of overloading (see below).

The return to play after a common cold follows the general recommendations as outlined above, that the athlete should return only after full recovery and gradually resume training. If the URI is caused by bacteria (differential diagnosis), this could both be a primary infection and secondary to a viral infection. Most commonly these infections are caused by the beta-streptococci, causing tonsillitis, impetigo, medial otitis and/or acute bronchitis. Oral antibiotic treatment should be started, and the athlete may return to sport when the infection has subsided and after finishing the antibiotic treatment.

In one prospective study performed on elite athletes, it was shown that pathogens were identified in less than 30% of athletes who reported symptoms of an URT illness [54], reflecting that non-infectious conditions must also be considered.

Fact Box 5 Most common viral causes for upper respiratory tract infection and related infections

Common cold	Rhinovirus Coronavirus Echovirus Coxsackie B
Influenza	Influenza A, B and C
Upper respiratory tract infection	Adenovirus Parainfluenza Coxsackie A Respiratory syncytial virus
Lower respiratory tract infection	Adenovirus Respiratory syncytial virus
Infectious mononucleosis	Epstein-Barr virus

The Clinical Neck Check

As different infections have different propensity for cardiac and other complications, because they are caused by different microbes, the differential diagnosis is important. Simple tests (such as for beta-streptococci in the throat) may be used to differentiate between a viral and bacterial infection. However, other tests, such as C-reactive protein (CRP), leucocyte count and liver enzymes, may also be used to establish the degree of severity of any given infection. Indeed, the most common clinical decision regarding URI is if the infection is viral or bacterial and thus treatable by antibiotics. A sign often used in clinical practice, with little scientific evidence, to determine the athletes' availability for training/playing, is the "neck check". The underlying theory is that infections causing symptoms below the neck contradict exercise, i.e. joint pain, widespread muscle pain, gastrointestinal symptoms and productive cough, while infections causing only symptoms above the neck, such as runny nose in an otherwise unaffected athlete, may be more compatible with exercise (slight cold or allergies). The grey zone will be the athlete presenting solely with a "sore throat". In our clinical experience, such an athlete should be advised to refrain from training/playing during the day in question. On the following day, the infection has become evident or the athlete will possibly have recovered fully to resume training.

Current recommendations for contraindications to exercise participation in athletes with an acute URT illness include [3]:

- Presence of fever
- Presence of myalgia (muscle pain)
- Presence of chest pain
- Resting tachycardia
- Excessive shortness of breath
- Excessive fatigue
- Swollen painful lymphadenopathy

More specifically, it has been suggested that rest should be advised to an athlete with an infection when fever is present (>38 °C) or when the individual's resting temperature has increased by 0.5–1 °C or more and their resting pulse rate has increased by 10 beats per minute or more, in combination with symptoms such as malaise, myalgia, arthralgia or headache [1]. However, an acute onset of general malaise, especially in combination with pains in the muscles or joints, should also prompt the recommendation of rest, even in the absence of fever [1]. Training is gradually resumed after the infection has resolved, and if any symptoms referable to the heart appear (chest pain, chest discomfort, irregular heartbeat, abnormal breathlessness, abnormal fatigue or exertional syncope), the exercise bout should be stopped immediately [1].

56.5.2.2 Infective Mononucleosis (IM)

Mononucleosis is a special case of URIs that is very common in young individuals (i.e. "kissing disease"). The disease is clinically important in sports medicine, because of the possible long lay-off from sports and because of potential serious complications from sporting activity during the infection. IM is caused by the Epstein-Barr virus and typically presents as a URI, with dominating throat pain, fever, headache and malaise. Importantly, a majority of individuals affected by mononucleosis may be asymptomatic (subclinical infection). IM may mimic tonsillitis with swollen cervical lymph nodes and yellow detritus at the tonsils [55]. Treatment with antibiotics is typically not associated with improvement of the clinical picture.

"Tonsillitis", not responding to antibiotics in a young individual, should thus raise the suspicion of IM. To confirm the diagnosis, the physician may use a fast-track antibody test (monospot) or serology. Often the liver may be affected (as shown by increased liver enzymes) and T lymphocytes are increased. The most important complication may be enlargement of the spleen and loss of its architectural stability, increasing the risk of splenic rupture secondary to abdominal trauma [2] or increased intra-abdominal pressure [1, 56]. Data indicate that 50% of splenic ruptures occur without a direct blow to the spleen and the risk of rupture is 0.1–0.5% [3]. The risk for rupture is highest in the first 3 weeks but is very rare after 28 days [2].

Athletes with IM with splenomegaly should refrain from doing sport for at least 3 weeks, but may be out of training for 6–8 weeks, or even longer depending on if and to what extent the spleen is affected. Full fitness is often reached only after 3 months of training [3]. Contact sports are contraindicated until the spleen has returned to its normal size. The size of the spleen has to be followed, clinically or by repeated imaging using ultrasound. In addition, all blood tests should return to normal (leukocytes, liver tests), and the athlete should be symptom-free, before resuming intensive training. In severe cases, IM may put an end to a whole season, while many cases give little symptoms and cause a shorter absence.

56.5.2.3 Dermatological Infections

Secondary to URI, the most common infections in athletes are skin infections, affecting 8–21% of all consultations at US college level [57]. Three main types of microbes typically cause these infections: viruses, bacteria and fungi.

Regarding fungal skin infections, the most common is tinea pedis (athlete's foot), affecting a majority of athletes presenting with skin infections [58], tinea corporis and tinea versicolor. All of these fungal infections may be treated using oral or local antifungal tablets or cream, respectively. The main preventive methods include sufficient hygienic precautions (keep the skin dry between toes) and not to share towels with teammates, for instance. These fungal infections rarely put a barrier to training or play, but tinea corporis should be treated for at least 72 h before play.

The bacterial infections include impetigo, caused by streptococci, and secondary infections such as folliculitis, cellulitis and abscesses. Full body shaving has become popular and may give rise to folliculitis in armpits and groins, often due to *Staphylococcus aureus*. Another common secondary infection is bacterial contamination of an athlete's foot or of a small wound around the toes or foot. Secondary to infections, the local lymph nodes may swell and even be accompanied by fever. This may include the groin lymph nodes secondary to foot infection. The athlete could be treated with antibiotics and should refrain from playing until recovered. If an infection is resistant to treatment, MRSA (methicillin-resistant *Staphylococcus aureus*) should be suspected and evaluated. Treatment includes incision and drainage of a lesion and appropriate covering. Proper antibiotic treatment for up to 10 days and healing of the wound are required for return to sport.

Regarding viral skin infections, the most common type is herpes virus infections, typically herpes labialis, caused by the HSV-1 virus. A special case of herpes infection is herpes gladiatorum, affecting the face and neck of athletes in some close contact sports (25% of wrestlers and rugby players [59]). The transmission is direct contact, and the athlete should not compete with active lesions, having at least 48 h of treatment with antiviral treatment, before returning to competition. All lesions should be covered.

56.5.2.4 Gastrointestinal Infections

Athletes frequently travel to training or competition, thereby having the risk of acquiring gastrointestinal infections, such as gastroenteritis. This ailment is typically caused by viruses (rotavirus or similar enteroviruses). The preventive measures include (oral) vaccination before travel and/or oral treatment by norfloxacin before and after symptoms. Vomiting, fever and diarrhoea are typical symptoms, and the treatment is directed at fluid replacement, as the risk of dehydration is increased. Rest and antipyretics may also be required. The athlete should only return to sport when having no remaining symptoms. A practical guideline is 48 h after the last diarrhoea or bout of vomiting. In the clinical situation, this advice is important to follow, as this will aid to prevent transmission of the infection.

56.6 General Recommendations to Prevent Acute Infective Illness in Team Sports

Due to acute infective illness, players often lose weeks of training each year or will miss an all-important match after months of preparation. Prevention of illness is of utmost importance in elite sports.

56.6.1 Individual Precautions

Personal hygiene is not only the most important but also the most practical and easiest preventative strategy. Most URT infections are transmitted through airborne droplets (sneezing and coughing) and by contact (direct skin contact or indirect contact with sporting equipment) [1]. The most important preventative measure to stop transmission of URT is frequent handwashing [2, 5] and avoiding contact between the hands, eyes and nose, as this is a primary route of introducing viruses into the body [34]. Other measures include covering the mouth and nose with the cubital fossa (elbow pit) when sneezing or coughing [60], avoiding direct skin-to-skin contact [5] and avoiding contact with ill individuals [2, 34]. Sharing of water bottles, towels and sporting equipment should be strongly discouraged [2, 5]. Regarding infections spread by vectors (insects, mots), an additional advice is to wear clothing covering the arms and legs during training sessions when travelling in tropical areas, particularly at dusk and dawn. To wear open footwear when using public showers, swimming pools and locker rooms prevents dermatological infections. Individual strategies that facilitate good quality sleep such as napping during the day and correct sleep hygiene practices at night are recommended. Avoid excessive and binge drinking of alcohol, as this impairs immune function for several hours, particularly after strenuous training or competition. Practice the principles of safe sex and use condoms, to prevent sexually transmitted disease (STD) [6].

56.6.2 The Role of the Medical Staff

The medical and administrative support staff should develop, implement and monitor illness prevention guidelines for athletes and screen for airway inflammation disturbances (asthma, allergy and other inflammatory airway conditions). They should identify high-risk athletes and take preventative precautions during competition periods. This may include arranging single room accommodation during tournaments for athletes with known susceptibility to respiratory tract infections. Consider protecting the airways of athletes from being directly exposed to very cold (<0 °C) and dry air during strenuous exercise by using a facial mask. The medical staff should adopt measures to reduce the risk of illness associated with international travel. Update athletes' vaccines needed at home and for foreign travel and take into consideration that influenza vaccines take 5–7 weeks to take effect. Intramuscular vaccines may have some side effects. It is therefore advised to avoid vaccinating just before competitions or if symptoms of illness are present. Vaccinations during the winter months [1, 2, 5, 34] may reduce respiratory illness by 30–50% [60], although this is somewhat debated.

The use of sensitive measures to monitor an athlete's health can lead to early detection of symptoms and signs of illness, early diagnosis and appropriate intervention. Athletes' tendency to continue to train and compete despite the existence of physical complaints or functional limitations, particularly at the elite level, highlights the pressing need to use appropriate illness monitoring tools.

56.6.3 Management of Combined Stress and Load on the Athlete

It is recommended that coaches and support staff schedule adequate recovery. Particularly after intensive training periods, athletes should have a detailed individualised training and competition planning, including post-event recovery measures (encompassing nutrition and hydration, sleep and psychological recovery) [6]. Sleep disruption has also been linked to immune depression [34], and efforts should thus be made to get adequate sleep [2, 3, 5]. Sports governing bodies have the responsibility to consider the competition load and hence the health of the athletes when planning their event calendars. This requires increased coordination between single- and multisport event organisers and the development of a comprehensive calendar of all international sports events. Psychological load (stressors) such as negative life event stress and daily hassles can significantly increase the risk of illness in athletes. Practical recommendations should be centred on educating athletes, coaches and support staff in proactive stress management [61].

56.6.4 Nutritional Strategies

Inadequate nutrition may contribute to impaired immunity [2, 3, 5, 25, 34]. Compounds, which are discussed as having a role in prevention of disease, are described briefly below. However, none of these strategies are substitutes for eating a well-balanced diet.

56.6.4.1 Vitamin C

In 1 double-blind, placebo-controlled study that was conducted on 92 runners who had entered the 1990 90 km Comrades Ultra-Marathon in South Africa, daily supplementation with 600 mg vitamin C reduced the incidence of postrace URT illness, from 68% to 33% ($p < 0.01$) [62]. A limitation to this study is that the URT illnesses were never proven to be infectious. Furthermore, whether vitamin C supplementation reduces the risk of acute illness during training or in the prerace period has not been studied.

56.6.4.2 Vitamin D

In one prospective cohort study, the influence of vitamin D status on the incidence of respiratory illness and immune function during a 4-month (16-week) winter training period in endurance sport athletes was examined [63]. After 16 weeks, a significantly higher proportion of participants presented with symptoms of an URT illness in the vitamin D-deficient group compared with the optimal vitamin D group (deficient group 67%, optimal 27%, $p = 0.039$) and saliva secretory immunoglobulin A (SIgA) secretion rate was also significantly higher. This study indicating that vitamin D status could influence URT illness has to be confirmed.

56.6.4.3 Glutamine

Several glutamine supplementation intervention studies showed that glutamine supplementation before and after exercise has no detectable effect on exercise-induced changes in immune cell functions [64, 65]. Therefore, the available evidence is thus not strong enough to warrant a recommendation for an athlete to use a glutamine supplement to prevent URT illness.

56.6.4.4 Cystine and Theanine

A small randomised, double-blind, placebo-controlled, parallel-group study in 15 male long-distance runners showed that ingestion of cystine and theanine prevented a reduction in the leucocyte count after a training camp (which was observed in placebo group) and prevented an increase in the neutrophil count and high sensitive CRP after the camp (which was also observed in the placebo group) [66].

56.6.4.5 Carbohydrate Ingestion During Exercise

It has been documented that carbohydrate ingestion by endurance athletes during intensive exercise is associated with an attenuated cortisol, growth hormone, epinephrine response, fewer perturbations in blood immune cell counts, lower granulocyte and monocyte phagocytosis and oxidative burst activity and diminished pro- and anti-inflammatory cytokine response compared to placebo ingestion [67], and this is reviewed by Gunzer [25]. Ingestion of ≥6% carbohydrates during prolonged exercise may maintain the immune function [15], but more research is required to prove that this translates into the reduction of URT illness.

56.6.4.6 Probiotics

There is increasing evidence from a double-blind, randomised, controlled trial and meta-analysis of randomised, placebo-controlled trials that probiotic supplementation can reduce the number, duration and severity of acute infectious diarrhoea and URT infection in the general population [68]. Furthermore, it has been documented that probiotics may reduce gastrointestinal illness in endurance athletes [69].

Take-Home Message

Acute illnesses and infections are the most common medical problem a sport medicine and football team physician will encounter. The recommendations generally stipulate that an athlete can participate in sport when symptoms and signs are only local (blocked nose, runny nose) and with the absence of symptoms and signs of systemic involvement (fever, tachycardia or resting heart rate increase by 10 beats or more, myalgia, malaise, lymphadenopathy, cough, chest pain and shortness of breath). If systemic symptoms are present, rest should be advised until the infection has subsided.

Fact Box 6 Strategies for prevention of illness

Strategy	Action
6.1 Individual precautions	Frequent handwashing Avoiding contacts between the hands, eyes and nose Covering of the mouth and nose when sneezing or coughing Avoiding skin-to-skin contact Avoiding contact with ill individuals
6.2 Medical staff	Develop, implement and monitor illness prevention guidelines Screen for airway inflammation disturbances Identify and manage high-risk athletes
6.3 Management of stress and load	Recovery plan Stress management education (athletes, staff)
6.4 Nutrition	Well-balanced diet with sufficient intake of nutrients (specific nutrients may be targeted)

When the athlete returns from an illness (return to play), exercise should be resumed in successive manner, always considering any symptoms. Special considerations are required for a few conditions. Firstly, no exercise should be allowed when the athlete has gastroenteritis. Secondly, when an athlete has infectious mononucleosis, non-contact sport should only be considered after 3 weeks at the earliest. The athlete may only participate in contact sports once symptoms have abated and the spleen has regressed to its normal size (proven by ultrasonography). The most important steps, however, is to prevent illness/infections by individual preventive measures (hygiene, nutrition, sleep) and by balancing external load (training load, playing load, stress) with adequate recovery.

Top Five Evidence-Based References

Derman W, Schwellnus M, Jordaan E, Blauwet CA, Emery C, Pit-Grosheide P et al (2013) Illness and injury in athletes during the competition period at the London 2012 Paralympic Games: development and implementation of a web-based surveillance system (WEB-IISS) for team medical staff. Br J Sports Med 47:420–425

Haaland DA, Sabljic TF, Baribeau DA, Mukovozov IM, Hart LE (2008) Is regular exercise a friend or foe of the aging immune system? A systematic review. Clin J Sport Med 18:539–548

Malm C (2006) Susceptibility to infections in elite athletes: the S-curve. Scand J Med Sci Sports 16:4–6

Schwellnus MP, Soligard T, Alonso JM, Bahr R, Clarsen B, Dijkstra HP et al (2016) How much is too much? (Part 2) International Olympic Committee consensus statement on load in sport and risk of illness. Br J Sports Med 50:1043–1052

Svendsen IS, Taylor IM, Tønnessen E, Bahr R, Gleeson M (2016) Training-related and competition-related risk factors for respiratory tract and gastrointestinal infections in elite cross-country skiers. Br J Sports Med 50:809–815

References

1. Friman G, Wesslén L (2000) Special feature for the Olympics: effects of exercise on the immune system: infections and exercise in high-performance athletes. Immunol Cell Biol 78:510–522
2. Purcell L (2007) Exercise and febrile illnesses. Paediatr Child Health 12:885–892
3. Schwellnus MP (ed) (2008) The olympic textbook of medicine in sport. In: The encyclopaedia of sports medicine: an IOC commission publication, Vol IXV. Wiley-Blackwell, Hoboken, NJ
4. Tseng GS, Hsieh CY, Hsu CT, Lin JC, Chan JS (2013) Myopericarditis and exertional rhabdomyolysis following an influenza A (H3N2) infection. BMC Infect Dis 13:283
5. Weidner TG, Sevier TL (1996) Sport, exercise, and the common cold. J Athl Train 31:154–159
6. Schwellnus M, Soligard T, Alonso JM, Bahr R, Clarsen B, Dijkstra HP et al (2016) How much is too much? (Part 2) International Olympic Committee consensus statement on load in sport and risk of illness. Br J Sports Med 50:1043–1052
7. Derman W, Schwellnus M, Jordaan E, Blauwet CA, Emery C, Pit-Grosheide P et al (2013) Illness and injury in athletes during the competition period at the London 2012 Paralympic Games: development and implementation of a web-based surveillance system (WEB-IISS) for team medical staff. Br J Sports Med 47:420–425
8. Engebretsen L, Soligard T, Steffen K, Alonso JM, Aubry M, Budgett R et al (2013) Sports injuries and illnesses during the London Summer Olympic Games 2012. Br J Sports Med 47:407–414
9. Soligard T, Steffen K, Palmer-Green D, Aubry M, Grant ME, Meeuwisse W et al (2015) Sports injuries and illnesses in the Sochi 2014 Olympic Winter Games. Br J Sports Med 49:441–447
10. Schwellnus M, Derman W, Page T, Lambert M, Readhead C, Roberts C et al (2012) Illness during the 2010 Super 14 Rugby Union tournament—a prospective study involving 22 676 player days. Br J Sports Med 46:499–504
11. Dvorak J, Junge A, Derman W, Schwellnus M (2011) Injuries and illnesses of football players during the 2010 FIFA World Cup. Br J Sports Med 45:626–630
12. Theron N, Schwellnus M, Derman W, Dvorak J (2013) Illness and injuries in elite football players--a prospective cohort study during the FIFA Confederations Cup 2009. Clin J Sport Med 23:379–383
13. Brolinson PG, Elliott D (2007) Exercise and the immune system. Clin Sports Med 26:311–319
14. Gleeson M, Nieman DC, Pedersen BK (2004) Exercise, nutrition and immune function. J Sports Sci 22:115–125
15. Hackney AC, Koltun KJ (2012) The immune system and overtraining in athletes: clinical implications. Acta Clin Croat 51:633–641
16. Nieman DC (2003) Current perspective on exercise immunology. Curr Sports Med Rep 2:239–242
17. Peters EM (1997) Exercise, immunology and upper respiratory tract infections. Int J Sports Med 18(Suppl 1):S69–S77
18. Peters-Futre EM (1997) Vitamin C, neutrophil function, and upper respiratory tract infection risk in distance runners: the missing link. Exerc Immunol Rev 3:32–52
19. Haaland DA, Sabljic TF, Baribeau DA, Mukovozov IM, Hart LE (2008) Is regular exercise a friend or foe of the aging immune system? A systematic review. Clin J Sport Med 18:539–548
20. Gleeson M (2007) Immune function in sport and exercise. J Appl Physiol (1985) 103:693–699
21. Hughes WT (1997) The athlete: an immunocompromised host. Adv Pediatr Infect Dis 13:79–99
22. Nieman DC (1995) Upper respiratory tract infections and exercise. Thorax 50:1229–1231
23. Mackinnon LT (1997) Immunity in athletes. Int J Sports Med 18(Suppl 1):S62–S68
24. Bonsignore MR, Morici G, Vignola AM, Riccobono L, Bonanno A, Profita M et al (2003) Increased airway inflammatory cells in endurance athletes: what do they mean? Clin Exp Allergy 33:14–21
25. Gunzer W, Konrad M, Pail E (2012) Exercise-induced immunodepression in endurance athletes and nutritional intervention with carbohydrate, protein and fat-what is possible, what is not? Nutrients 4:1187–1212
26. Markanday A (2015) Acute phase reactants in infections: evidence-based review and a guide for clinicians. Open Forum Infect Dis 2:ofv098

27. Calabrese LH, Nieman DC (1996) Exercise, immunity, and infection. J Am Osteopath Assoc 96:166–176
28. Ekblom B, Ekblom O, Malm C (2006) Infectious episodes before and after a marathon race. Scand J Med Sci Sports 16:287–293
29. He CS, Bishop NC, Handzlik MK, Muhamad AS, Gleeson M (2014) Sex differences in upper respiratory symptoms prevalence and oral-respiratory mucosal immunity in endurance athletes. Exerc Immunol Rev 20:8–22
30. Ruedl G, Schobersberger W, Pocecco E, Blank C, Engebretsen L, Soligard T et al (2012) Sport injuries and illnesses during the first Winter Youth Olympic Games 2012 in Innsbruck, Austria. Br J Sports Med 46:1030–1037
31. Heath GW, Ford ES, Craven TE, Macera CA, Jackson KL, Pate RR (1991) Exercise and the incidence of upper respiratory tract infections. Med Sci Sports Exerc 23:152–157
32. Groër M (1995) Exercise and immunity. Image J Nurs Sch 27:90
33. Martin SA, Pence BD, Woods JA (2009) Exercise and respiratory tract viral infections. Exerc Sport Sci Rev 37:157–164
34. Nieman DC (1997) Risk of upper respiratory tract infection in athletes: an epidemiologic and immunologic perspective. J Athl Train 32:344–349
35. Nieman DC (2000) Special feature for the Olympics: effects of exercise on the immune system: exercise effects on systemic immunity. Immunol Cell Biol 78:496–501
36. Malm C (2006) Susceptibility to infections in elite athletes: the S-curve. Scand J Med Sci Sports 16:4–6
37. Hellard P, Avalos M, Guimaraes F, Toussaint JF, Pyne DB (2015) Training-related risk of common illnesses in elite swimmers over a 4-yr period. Med Sci Sports Exerc 47:698–707
38. Mårtensson S, Nordebo K, Malm C (2014) High training volumes are associated with a low number of self-reported sick days in elite endurance athletes. J Sports Sci Med 13:929–933
39. Veugelers KR, Young WB, Fahrner B, Harvey JT (2016) Different methods of training load quantification and their relationship to injury and illness in elite Australian football. J Sci Med Sport 19:24–28
40. Svendsen IS, Taylor IM, Tønnessen E, Bahr R, Gleeson M (2016) Training-related and competition-related risk factors for respiratory tract and gastrointestinal infections in elite cross-country skiers. Br J Sports Med 50:809–815
41. MacKinnon LT (2000) Special feature for the Olympics: effects of exercise on the immune system: overtraining effects on immunity and performance in athletes. Immunol Cell Biol 78:502–509
42. Schwellnus MP, Derman WE, Jordaan E, Page T, Lambert MI, Readhead C et al (2012) Elite athletes travelling to international destinations >5 time zone differences from their home country have a 2–3-fold increased risk of illness. Br J Sports Med 46:816–821
43. Dick NA, Diehl JJ (2014) Febrile illness in the athlete. Sports Health 6:225–231
44. Broom M (2007) Physiology of fever. Paediatr Nurs 19:40–44
45. Yoshizawa T, Omori K, Takeuchi I, Miyoshi Y, Kido H, Takahashi E et al (2016) Heat stroke with bimodal rhabdomyolysis: a case report and review of the literature. J Intensive Care 4:71
46. Smith JE (2004) The pathophysiology of exertional heatstroke. J R Nav Med Serv 90:135–138
47. Sucholeiki R (2005) Heatstroke. Semin Neurol 25:307–314
48. Friman G (1977) Effect of acute infectious disease on isometric muscle strength. Scand J Clin Lab Invest 37:303–308
49. Friman G (1978) Effect of acute infectious disease on human isometric muscle endurance. Ups J Med Sci 83:105–108
50. Roberts JA (1986) Viral illnesses and sports performance. Sports Med 3:298–303
51. Scharhag J, Meyer T (2014) Return to play after acute infectious disease in football players. J Sports Sci 32:1237–1242
52. Tingle LE, Molina D, Calvert CW (2007) Acute pericarditis. Am Fam Physician 76:1509–1514
53. Ahmadinejad Z, Alijani N, Mansori S, Ziaee V (2014) Common sports-related infections: a review on clinical pictures, management and time to return to sports. Asian J Sports Med 5:1–9
54. Spence L, Brown WJ, Pyne DB, Nissen MD, Sloots TP, McCormack JG et al (2007) Incidence, etiology, and symptomatology of upper respiratory illness in elite athletes. Med Sci Sports Exerc 39:577–586
55. Ebell MH, Call M, Shinholser J, Gardner J (2016) Does this patient have infectious mononucleosis? The rational clinical examination systematic review. JAMA 315:1502–1509
56. Barnwell J, Deol PS (2017) Atraumatic splenic rupture secondary to Epstein-Barr virus infection. BMJ Case Rep 2017:pii:bcr2016218405
57. Yard EE, Collins CL, Dick RW, Comstock RD (2008) An epidemiologic comparison of high school and college wrestling injuries. Am J Sports Med 36:57–64
58. Pickup TL, Adams BB (2007) Prevalence of tinea pedis in professional and college soccer players versus non-athletes. Clin J Sport Med 17:52–54
59. Sharp JC (1994) ABC of sports medicine. Infections in sport. BMJ 308:1702–1706
60. Mossad S. Upper respiratory tract infections. 2013. Accessed 17 Dec 2017 (http://www.clevelandclinicmeded.com/medicalpubs/diseasemanagement/infectious-disease/upper-respiratory-tract-infection/).
61. Ivarsson A, Johnson U, Podlog L (2013) Psychological predictors of injury occurrence: a prospective investigation of professional Swedish soccer players. J Sport Rehabil 22:19–26
62. Peters EM, Goetzsche JM, Grobbelaar B, Noakes TD (1993) Vitamin C supplementation reduces the incidence of postrace symptoms of upper-respiratory-

tract infection in ultramarathon runners. Am J Clin Nutr 57:170–174
63. He CS, Handzlik M, Fraser WD, Muhamad A, Preston H, Richardson A et al (2013) Influence of vitamin D status on respiratory infection incidence and immune function during 4 months of winter training in endurance sport athletes. Exerc Immunol Rev 19:86–101
64. Gleeson M (2008) Dosing and efficacy of glutamine supplementation in human exercise and sport training. J Nutr 138:2045S–2049S
65. Krieger JW, Crowe M, Blank SE (2004) Chronic glutamine supplementation increases nasal but not salivary IgA during 9 days of interval training. J Appl Physiol (1985) 97:585–591
66. Murakami S, Kurihara S, Koikawa N, Nakamura A, Aoki K, Yosigi H et al (2009) Effects of oral supplementation with cystine and theanine on the immune function of athletes in endurance exercise: randomized, double-blind, placebo-controlled trial. Biosci Biotechnol Biochem 73:817–821
67. Nieman DC (2001) Exercise immunology: nutritional countermeasures. Can J Appl Physiol 26(Suppl):S45–S55
68. West NP, Pyne DB, Cripps AW, Hopkins WG, Eskesen DC, Jairath A et al (2011) Lactobacillus fermentum (PCC®) supplementation and gastrointestinal and respiratory-tract illness symptoms: a randomised control trial in athletes. Nutr J 10:30
69. Cox AJ, Pyne DB, Saunders PU, Fricker PA (2010) Oral administration of the probiotic Lactobacillus fermentum VRI-003 and mucosal immunity in endurance athletes. Br J Sports Med 44:222–226

57 Return to Play in Asthma and Pulmonary Conditions

David Espinoza, Thomas Sisk, George Chiampas, and Aaron V. Mares

Contents

D. Espinoza, M.D. (✉) • T. Sisk, M.D. • A.V. Mares, M.D.
Department of Orthopaedics, University of Pittsburgh, Pittsburgh, PA 15213, USA
e-mail: Espinozadr@upmc.edu; sisktm2@upmc.edu; Maresav@upmc.edu

G. Chiampas, M.D.
Department of Orthopaedics, Northwestern University, Chicago, IL 60611, USA

57.1 Introduction

Football (soccer) is a sport of tremendous physical demand. The dynamic nature of the sport places great stress on an individual athlete. Those sports-specific demands not only involve the musculoskeletal system but also place a lot of stress on the cardiopulmonary system. In this chapter, we will address the effect of asthma and other pulmonary conditions in the football athlete.

57.1.1 Introduction: Physiologic Demands

The physiologic and strength demands are high, with METs (metabolic equivalents) being in the 5–12 range [1]. The oscillation of low-intensity

V. Musahl et al. (eds.), *Return to Play in Football*, https://doi.org/10.1007/978-3-662-55713-6_57

and high-intensity varies throughout a football match. The body must be able to meet the metabolic needs during those variances.

There are many pathologic conditions that may affect an athlete's ability to inspire, exchange gases, and expire. One of those conditions is asthma.

57.1.2 Introduction: Potential Conditions

Asthma in sports tends to break down into two main categories: exercise-induced asthma (EIA) and exercise-induced bronchospasm (EIB). EIA is exercise causing bronchial obstruction in patients with clinical asthma, while EIB is an airway obstruction in association with exercise without a clinical diagnosis of asthma [2]. Other topics of discussion will include pneumothorax and pulmonary infections. Finally, this chapter will try to address the current dogma and recommendations on return to play in each of those conditions.

57.2 Asthma

Asthma is a chronic pulmonary condition that can negatively affect athletes to varying degrees with regard to airway inflammation, hyperresponsiveness, and reversible obstruction. Asthma affects approximately 25 million people in the United States, 7 million of which are children [3]. The prevalence of asthma in athletes overall is actually higher than the general population ranging from 23% to 55%, with higher rates noted in endurance athletes [4].

57.2.1 Asthma: Pathophysiology

In asthmatics there is a chronic underlying inflammatory state in the lungs with increased levels of cytokines and inflammatory molecules within the epithelium of the bronchial tree. When exposed to certain triggers, such as pollen, mold, allergens, cold air, or exercise, these inflammatory markers induce a cascade of molecular reactions that result in increased mucus production, swelling of the bronchial epithelium, and bronchial muscle tightening.

57.2.2 Asthma: Symptoms and Presentation

The previously discussed changes in asthma lead to airway narrowing and obstruction. Athletes will present with symptoms including cough, wheezing, shortness of breath, or chest tightness—in severe cases, these symptoms can lead to a life-threatening state of hypoxia due to obstruction of the airways. The diagnosis of asthma can typically be made by taking a thorough history with athletes that have had episodes of reversible symptoms. These episodes are typically associated with certain triggers that may also be identified with skilled history taking. Lung function testing with spirometry can be used to diagnose the condition with objective evidence.

57.2.3 Asthma: Diagnosis

Spirometry is a functional test used to diagnose asthma. This test can objectively measure the forced expiratory volume in 1 second (FEV_1) as the athlete forcibly exhales, and if that value is <80% predicted and the FEV_1/forced vital capacity (FVC) ratio is <70%, then asthma is the diagnosis as long as there is reversibility by a FEV_1 increase of >12% from baseline or ≥10% of the predicted FEV_1 after the use of a short-acting beta-agonist inhaler such as albuterol [5]. Based on history and spirometry results, the diagnosis of asthma can be classified into four separate categories that will guide treatment depending on the severity of symptoms as shown in Table 57.1. The diagnosis of asthma can also be made after a 4–6-week trial of controller medication with reassessment to determine if the symptoms have improved or resolved [3].

Table 57.1 Asthma classification and treatment

	Intermittent	Mild persistent	Moderate persistent	Severe persistent
Symptoms	≤2 days/week	>2 days/week	Once daily	Throughout the day
Nighttime awakenings	≤2 events/month	3–4 events/month	>Once/week	Often 7 days/week
Use of SABA	≤2 days/week	>2 days/week and not > once per day	Daily	Several uses daily
Treatment	SABA as needed for symptoms	Low-dose ICS with SABA as needed	Medium-dose ICS with LABA	High-dose ICS with LABA and possible oral corticosteroid

ICS inhaled corticosteroid, *SABA* short-acting beta-agonist, *LABA* long-acting beta-agonist

Fact Box 1 Spirometry Diagnostic Values

FEV_1 < 80%
FEV_1/FVC < 70%
Reversibility of values with inhaled SABA:
 FEV_1 > 12%
 Predicted FEV_1 ≥ 10%

57.2.4 Asthma: Treatment

When it comes to treatment of asthma in footballers, it is important to verify which medications may be prohibited based on the World Anti-Doping Agency. This agency bans all inhaled beta-agonists, except salmeterol, salbutamol (1600 μg maximum over 24 h), and formoterol (54 μg maximum over 24 h) [6]. However one recent study did show that inhaled salbutamol up to 1600 μg did not improve lung exercise performance [7]. The Medical Commission of the International Olympic Committee imposed its ban on inhaled beta-agonists in 1993 due to the growing concern of increased use among elite athletes in order to help improve oxygen uptake and thus lead to an unfair advantage in endurance, speed, and strength. Other organizations have imposed their bans as well, and it is important to be aware of sport governing bodies when it comes to treating asthma and bronchospasm.

Along with the pharmacological treatment of asthma, education and prevention of symptoms is also a key component to maintaining adequate control of the athlete's symptoms. The athlete should attempt to identify triggers for their symptoms, which may vary from seasonal allergies, like pollen to dust mites or even weather changes. For example, cold weather changes can be correlated to the development of asthma symptoms. An individual must demonstrate vigilance to keep their symptoms under control by altering environmental exposures and utilizing controller medication. These environmental changes may include changing practice locations based on the weather, using a humidifier or anti-allergen air filters at home, or even avoiding the use of NSAIDs, as they may predispose athletes to asthma flares [8]. Also, as part of the education process, athletes should be reminded of their asthma action plan that provides them with a step-by-step process of what to do when their symptoms start to become uncontrolled (Fig. 57.1).

The athlete and medical provider should be aware of when the last asthma exacerbation took place, if the athlete was ever hospitalized, and if they ever had to have a breathing tube placed (intubation) due to severe symptoms. Peak flows may also be utilized to monitor asthma symptom severity; however, this may be unfeasible or cumbersome when it comes to its proper and judicious use among the athletic population. Other modifying factors include increasing endurance training as studies have shown that endurance athletes tend to have higher lung volumes by way of strengthening respiratory muscles, reducing resistance through bronchial canals, and increasing lung elasticity and alveolar expansion in order to adapt to the demands brought forth by endurance training [9]. This training may theoretically help reduce incidences of asthma exacerbation and symptoms that can prevent footballers from participating at their highest ability.

Fig. 57.1 Asthma action plan from AAFA

Asthma Action Plan

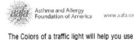

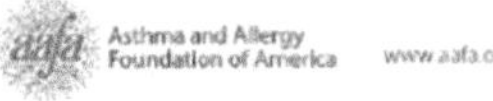

Name	Date
Doctor	Medical Record #
Doctor's Office Phone #: Day	Night/Weekend
Emergency Contact	
Doctor's Signature	

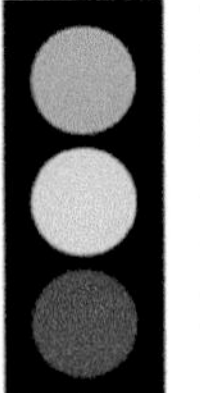

The Colors of a traffic light will help you use your asthma medicines.

Green means **Go Zone!**
Use preventive medicine.

Yellow Means **Caution Zone!**
Add quick-relief medicine.

Red means **Danger Zone!**
Get help from a doctor.

Personal Best Peak Flow ____________

GO

You have *all* of these:
- Breathing is good
- No cough or wheeze
- Sleep through the night
- Can work and play

Peak flow from ______ to ______

Use these daily preventive anti-inflammatory medicines:

MEDICINE	HOW MUCH	HOW OFTEN/WHEN

For asthma with exercise, take:

CAUTION

You have *any* of these:
- First signs of a cold
- Exposure to known trigger
- Cough
- Mild wheeze
- Tight chest
- Coughing at night

Peak flow from ______ to ______

Continue with green zone medicine and add:

MEDICINE	HOW MUCH	HOW OFTEN/WHEN

CALL YOUR PRIMARY CARE PROVIDER.

DANGER

Your asthma is getting worse fast:
- Medicine is not helping
- Breathing is hard and fast
- Nose opens wide
- Ribs show
- Can't talk well

Peak flow reading below ______

Take these medicines and call your doctor now.

MEDICINE	HOW MUCH	HOW OFTEN/WHEN

GET HELP FROM A DOCTOR NOW! Do not be afraid of causing a fuss. Your doctor will want to see you right away. It's important! If you cannot contact your doctor, go directly to the emergency room. DO NOT WAIT.

Make an appointment with your primary care provider within two days of an ER visit or hospitalization.

57.2.5 Asthma: Return to Play

It is generally acceptable to allow an athlete to return to sport once his or her lung function has returned to baseline and is able to participate in all sport-related activities without adverse pulmonary symptoms. Medications have demonstrated quicker improvement in symptoms and may allow for a sooner return to play timeline.

57.3 Exercise-Induced Bronchoconstriction

Exercise-induced bronchoconstriction (EIB) is a pulmonary condition characterized by transient reversible airway narrowing that increases respiratory resistance resulting in coughing, shortness of breath, wheezing, or chest tightness shortly after vigorous exercise. EIB is present in 7–20% of the general population. However, its prevalence in athletes has been found to be much higher with one study finding up to 50% depending on the sport and environmental conditions [10].

57.3.1 Exercise-Induced Bronchoconstriction: Symptoms and Presentation

EIB is a condition outside that of asthma, as these patients have no symptoms while at rest. Symptoms will typically present after

5–10 minutes of vigorous exercise and may last up to 20–30 minutes after exercise has concluded [8]. The key factor is that symptoms are reversible and do not occur at rest. Symptoms may also be influenced by other factors including weather, allergens, and intermittent bursts of exercise intensity during match play [11].

57.3.2 Exercise-Induced Bronchoconstriction: Pathophysiology

The etiology of EIB is centered on the idea of having to warm and condition air that is normally done so by the upper airway prior to the cool air reaching the lower airway and bronchial tree. While at rest, the upper airway's ability to warm the air is adequate secondary to the respiratory rate being slow enough to complete the task. However, when athletes exert themselves and the respiratory rate increases, this allows for the cool environmental air to reach the lower airways, thus giving the distal bronchial tree the task of warming and conditioning the air. It is this alteration in physiologic role that may lead to changes in an individual's symptoms.

There are two main theories as to the pathophysiology of EIB, thermal expenditure and osmotic. The thermal expenditure theory states that the airway cooling from the increased respiratory rate will cause vasoconstriction surrounding the lower airway bronchial tree and that upon the rewarming of the airway, the surrounding vasculature will dilate to engorge and rewarm the bronchial epithelium and leads to vascular leakage and airway edema [10]. The osmotic theory focuses on the water loss mechanisms that the bronchial epithelium and submucosa utilize in an attempt to warm the cool air that reaches the lower airways, which then causes changes in the epithelial pH and creates a hyperosmolar state that then leads to a cascade of molecular changes that release immune-modulators and mediators instigating bronchial constriction [10]. Though no one theory is definitive, it is likely a combination of the two that leads to the manifestation of EIB.

57.3.3 Exercise-Induced Bronchoconstriction: Diagnosis

The diagnosis of EIB is typically made through history and physical exam; however, it must be noted that this can lead to either overdiagnosis or underdiagnosis of the condition given the vast variance of symptom severity and presentation as well as a refractory period that some individuals may have. The refractory period is the time following spontaneous resolution of EIB symptoms where athletes will not experience any further symptoms for the next 1–2 hours, however, may have return of symptoms following this grace period [6]. This period may mask the diagnosis as athletes may not report the issue to their medical staff but then have recurrence of symptoms afterward. To properly diagnose the condition, pulmonary function tests (PFTs) should be conducted while at rest to rule in or out any underlying chronic asthma. Following this, other pathologies should be ruled out including vocal cord dysfunction, gastroesophageal reflux, and cardiac abnormalities.

The diagnosis of EIB can be made with the use of an exercise challenge test, eucapnic voluntary hyperventilation test (EVH), hyperosmolar saline challenge test, mannitol challenge test, or a direct challenge test with the use of methacholine to induce bronchoconstriction. The most commonly used tests are the exercise challenge test and the EVH, which focus on the FEV1 and its decline from baseline following provocation with either exercise or voluntary hyperventilation measured at various time limits following introduction of the stimulus. A decline in FEV1 of >10% in EVH or peak expiratory flow rate (PEFR) of 15% or greater indicates positive results with these tests [8, 11].

57.3.4 Exercise-Induced Bronchoconstriction: Treatment

When it comes to the treatment of EIB, it is important to look at all modifiable factors as well as pharmacologic options to maximize a football player's pulmonary capabilities. The use of gaiters, scarves, or masks can theoretically limit the amount of cool air that reaches the lower respiratory tree, thus limiting the effects of bronchoconstriction. Short warm-ups 15–20 min prior to activity at 80–90% of maximum exertion, calisthenics, and proper cooldown post-workouts have also been shown to limit the EIB response with athletes [4].

Many of the same medications that treat asthma can be utilized. Two to four puffs of a short-acting beta-agonist (SABA) inhaler (Fig. 57.2), 20 min prior to exercise or a match, can help control the onset of symptoms, if exercise is expected to last no more than 6 h. If there is a tournament or the player is expected to exert themselves for a longer period of time, then a long-acting beta-agonist (LABA) can be considered as their effects can last up to 12 h after administration. Leukotriene antagonists and cromolyn can also be utilized for those that cannot tolerate the beta-agonist inhalers; however, these may not be as effective. Inhaled corticosteroids do not play a role in the management and treatment of EIB. The use of these medications has shown improvement of symptoms and have allowed for quicker resolution as well.

57.3.5 Exercise-Induced Bronchoconstriction: Return to Play

A football player experiencing symptoms of EIB should be removed from play and evaluated properly on the sideline. If a baseline PEFR is known, then a repeat at the time of symptom onset should be conducted to assist in the evaluation of symptom severity [9]. If the PEFR is below 15% from baseline, then two puffs of a SABA may be utilized. If symptoms are still present after 5 min, then two more puffs may be administered [9]. Serial PEFR readings can be conducted until the value returns to normal limits or back to baseline. If values do not return to normal or baseline, then the athlete should be evaluated more properly off the sideline in case further treatment modalities are indicated, including emergency options as the condition could progress to a life-threatening state such as status

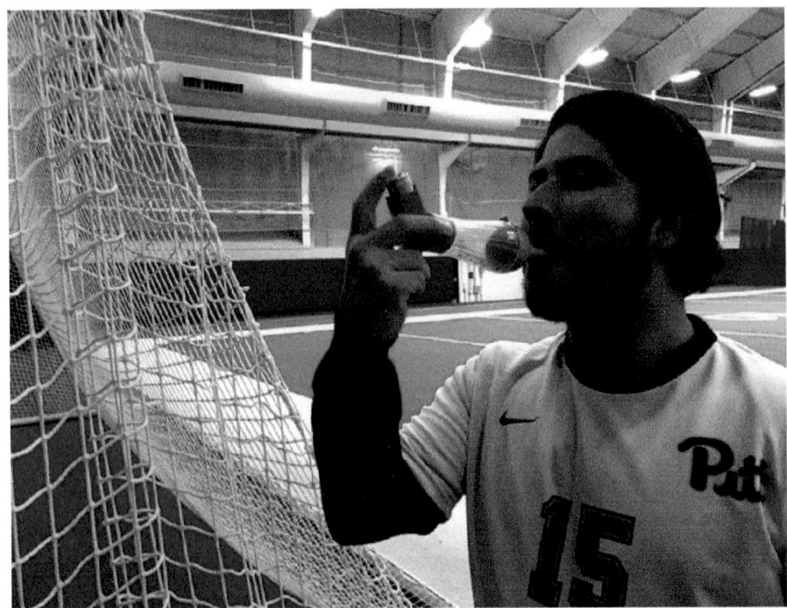

Fig. 57.2 Athlete demonstrating proper inhaler technique with spacer

asthmaticus [9]. Once the athlete's respiratory function has improved and he or she is no longer symptomatic, then he or she may return to the playing field.

57.4 Pneumothorax

A pneumothorax (PTX) is a rare but potentially life-threatening pulmonary condition that requires prompt recognition and expedited treatment and care. The condition is defined as a collection of air within the pleural space between the chest wall and the lung. Due to the intrinsic intrathoracic negative pressure created by inspiration, the accumulation of this air can eventually reach enough pressure to induce collapse of the lung and potentially lead to cardiopulmonary compromise. Only 2% of all adult pneumothoraces are associated with sports and can be spontaneous or tension-related [12].

Spontaneous PTX is found more often in tall, thin, and young individuals. It will occur, as its name suggests, spontaneously from primary or secondary etiology, secondary being in the setting of underlying pulmonary disease including pneumonia, asthma, cystic fibrosis, or interstitial lung disease. Tension PTX is much less common and typically occurs due to blunt or penetrating trauma from a fracture rib that disrupts the pleura. Particular to football, blunt trauma causing tension PTX is typically the result of thoracic collisions at high speed; athletes are more prone to this type of injury during keeper attacks or going for headers.

57.4.1 Pneumothorax: Symptoms and Presentation

Patients can present with difficulty in breathing, pleuritic chest pain with inspiration, rapid respiratory rates, increased heart rate, or even a presence of anxiety. These symptoms will most often develop in a progressive nature, which highlights the importance of serial exams. Associated pathology must be excluded including internal organ injury following blunt trauma as well, including pulmonary contusion, hemothorax, pneumomediastinum, splenic rupture, kidney laceration, rib fracture, or other internal derangement. Examination with a focus on primary assessment that includes airway, breathing, circulation, and frequent vital sign checks is crucial to obtaining rapid treatment in order to avoid progressive lung collapse or potential cardiovascular compromise.

57.4.2 Pneumothorax: Diagnosis

The physical exam plays an essential role in determining the potential concern for a pneumothorax. The pulmonary exam may include diminished breath sounds, rales, hyperresonance on percussion, hypoxia, hypotension, or even tracheal deviation away from the affected side. It is also imperative to assess for thoracic cage injury including rib fractures and potential cardiac involvement with a full cardiovascular exam.

Imaging studies are also useful in making the diagnosis. Chest X-ray (CXR) (Fig. 57.3) and ultrasound are good initial studies; however, helical CT imaging could also be utilized once the patient is stabilized in order to assess for any other associated pathology such as pulmonary contusion, laceration, and rib fractures. Once the diagnosis is even suspected, the transport of the athlete to a nearby emergency department for higher-level care, evaluation, and treatment is necessary if there is concern for respiratory compromise and overall decompensation. Football players will typically have high health reserve that may allow them to compensate for a period of time before becoming limited by PTX symptoms; therefore, a high index of suspicion is required with serial physical exams in order to make the diagnosis. Following blunt trauma that is limiting the player, he or she should be evaluated thoroughly as a missed diagnosis of PTX could result in serious complications.

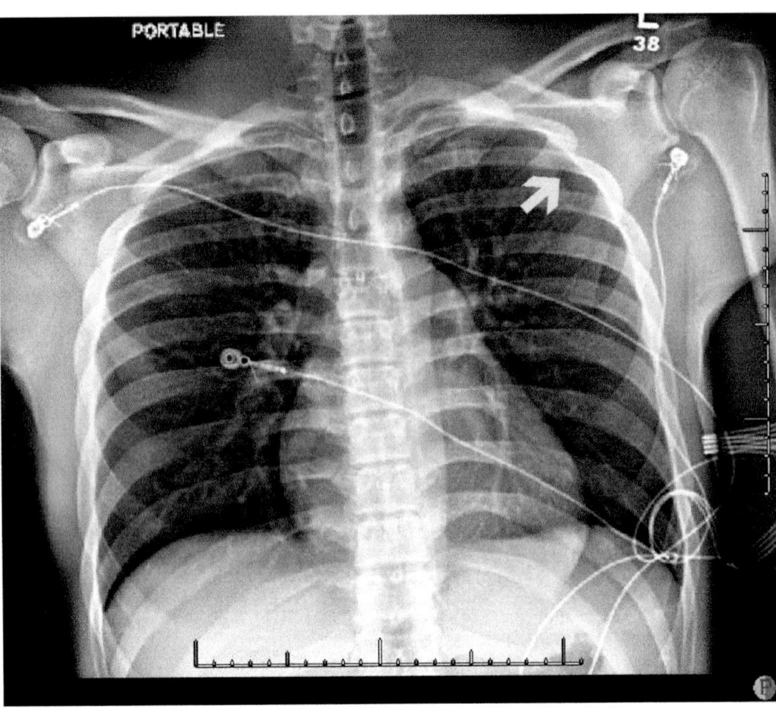

Fig. 57.3 Left-sided pneumothorax after blunt trauma with *yellow arrow* pointing to visceral pleural line

57.4.3 Pneumothorax: Treatment

Treatment for an uncomplicated pneumothorax may be observational depending on size. An example of this would be a non-tension pneumothorax <10%. However, if a tension pneumothorax is suspected, supplemental oxygen and needle decompression with either a 14- or 16-G needle can be performed. The needle is inserted into the second intercostal space in the midclavicular line to relieve the pressure, which may be followed by a rush of air [4, 13]. Following this procedure, the placement of a chest tube to allow for lung re-expansion is needed. Repeat CXR to visualize re-expansion of the lung and ensure proper chest tube placement is recommended (Fig. 57.4). This should be followed up with serial CXRs, a minimum of 2 days later, to ensure stability. If the PTX remains resolved, then the chest tube can be removed after 2–3 days of monitoring in an acute care setting.

With regard to a spontaneous PTX, the American College of Chest Physicians published that a small PTX (<3 cm apex-to-cupola distance) in a hemodynamically stable patient without significant symptoms may be managed by observation alone with close follow-up after the exclusion of progression with 3–6 h of observation and repeat CXR in an emergency setting; larger PTX (>3 cm) should re-expanded with decompression [13].

57.4.4 Pneumothorax: Return to Play

There are no consensus guidelines when it comes to return to play (RTP) from a resolved pneumothorax. Case reports and opinion typically cite return to play ranging anywhere from 2 to 10 weeks, with an average of 3–4 weeks prior to RTP [13]. Air travel should be avoided in the first 1–3 weeks following a pneumothorax as the change in air pressure may result in hypoxemia and gas expansion in a closed parenchymal space. Recommends may differ if an athlete has associated pathology like multiple rib fracture or flail chest. During this time, repeat CXR should be obtained to ensure continued resolution of the PTX, and treatment with a pulmonary toilet including beta-agonists, mucolytics, and cough

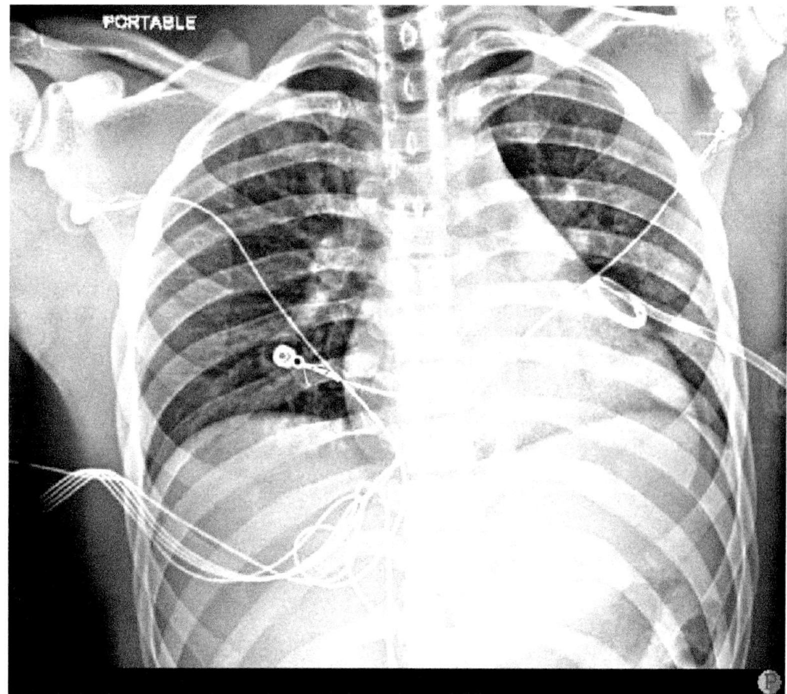

Fig. 57.4 Left-sided pneumothorax with re-expanded lung after chest tube placement

suppressants may be utilized for symptom control. A chest wall protector may also be implemented for extra protection.

Close follow-up should also be implemented to ensure that the development of acute respiratory distress syndrome (ARDS) does not occur. All in all, a slow return to physical activity with using pain as a guide is typically the mainstay of return to play from this pulmonary condition.

57.5 Respiratory Infections

Respiratory infections and their associated symptoms are a very common complaint among the general population as well as the athletic population. Symptoms can present in a variety of ways and in different orders. The most common symptoms are nasal congestion, sore throat, cough, postnasal drip, headache, fatigue, nausea, and fever. Although the symptoms may be similar, it is important to keep a broad differential when determining the etiology, as many ailments could present with those symptoms.

57.5.1 Respiratory Infections: Types of Infection

Types of infection include, among others, viral upper respiratory infection (URI), bacterial or viral pharyngitis, mononucleosis, viral or bacterial sinusitis, peritonsillar abscess, lower respiratory infection (LRI), bronchitis, and/or pneumonia. The athlete diagnosis is made mostly through history and physical exam; however, at times, it may be necessary to rule out other potential causes if red flags exist, and, thus, lab work including a CBC, CMP, EBV titers, or even a CXR may be needed to make the correct diagnosis.

57.5.2 Respiratory Infections: Treatment

Once the etiology of the symptoms is determined, the proper course of treatment can then be initiated. Viral URIs can be treated symptomatically with decongestants, antihistamines, or other over-the-counter medications as indicated based on symptoms. Vitamin C and zinc may also play a role in symptom duration as well. Most viral-induced URIs typically will resolve after 4–5 days. If the etiology for the athlete's symptoms is determined to be bacterial in origin, then the proper antibiotic is indicated with special attention paid to the most likely bacterial culprit, age, medical allergies, or other specific issues that may alter the antibiotic selection (Table 57.2). It is also important to monitor the athlete's hydration status and ensure that they are obtaining the proper nutrient and caloric intake during their illness.

57.5.3 Respiratory Infections: Return to Play

Return to sports decisions should be made in conjunction with close follow-up, as reevaluation and examination may be necessary. One special consideration to be mindful of when it comes to return to play is the presence of a fever greater than 101 °F. If an athlete engages in sports with a fever greater than 101 °F, then he or she does have an increased risk of developing myocarditis, a condition that affects cardiac function and output, and should be held from practice until the fever resolves without the use of antipyretic for 24 h. Also, it is important to ensure that the symptoms are not due to mononucleosis and EBV, as this ailment could lead to splenic enlargement and prohibit a footballer from playing for at least 3 weeks from symptom onset.

There are no clear "return to play" guidelines when it comes to URI or LRI; however, the "above the neck" rule is typically implemented for most athletes, including those in football. This rule refers to that if the symptoms of sore throat, nasal congestion, and others are mainly "above the neck" without other systemic involvement, then the athlete may continue with training uninterrupted. If the symptoms are present "below the neck" or include systemic symptoms such as fever or myalgia, then it may be necessary for the athlete to rest until they improve. Return to play guidelines with pneumonia are limited as well, but typically the athlete should rest for 10–14 days as needed. However, this timeline is variable and depends on the individual athlete and his or her ability to safely play [6].

Fact Box 2 Return to play considerations with URI

Resolution of fever (oral temp. <101 °F)
Euvolemic hydration status
Respiratory capacity to athletically perform
No diagnosis of mononucleosis

Table 57.2 Common respiratory infections and treatment

	Common pathogens	Treatment
Bacterial pneumonia	*S. pneumoniae*, *M. pneumoniae*, *H. influenzae*	Azithromycin, clarithromycin, doxycycline
Bacterial sinusitis	*S. pneumoniae*, *H. influenzae*, *M. catarrhalis*	Augmentin, doxycycline
Bacterial pharyngitis	Group A streptococcus	Penicillin G IM, amoxicillin
Peritonsillar abscess	Group A streptococcus, *S. aureus*, MRSA	Augmentin, clindamycin, drainage
Influenza	Influenza A or B	Tamiflu if within 24–48 h of symptoms onset
Viral etiologies	RSV, rhinovirus, adenovirus, coronavirus, parainfluenza	Antihistamine, decongestant, nasal spray, expectorants, zinc, vitamin C

Conclusions

Take-Home Message: Summary

Pulmonary conditions in football athletes present a diverse spectrum of challenges to a sports medicine team. To adequately diagnose and appropriately manage, a strong understanding of each pathologic entity is necessary. A thorough clinical history accompanied by a systematic physical exam will frequently establish the diagnosis. With respect to non-emergent scenarios, peak flow measurements, environment exposure management, pulmonary conditioning, pharmacological management, and action plans are useful modalities. In emergent scenarios, diligent attention should be placed on assessment of airway, breathing, and circulation as well as prompt diagnosis. It is stressed that return to play criteria should be determined on case-by-case bases and that recommendations may vary depending on an athlete's individual circumstances.

Top Five Evidence-Based References

Boulet LP, Turmel J, Cote A (2017) Asthma and exercise-induced respiratory symptoms in the athlete: New insights. Current Opinion Pulmonary Medicine 23(1):71–77

Feden JP (2013) Closed lung trauma. Clinics in Sports Medicine 32:255–265

Hull JH, Ansley L, Robson-Ansley P, Parsons JP (2012) Managing respiratory problems in athletes. Clinical Medicine 12(4):351–356

O'Connor FG, Casa DJ, Davis BA, Pierrer PS, Sallis RE, Wilder RP (2013) Pulmonary. ACSM's Sports Medicine: A Comprehensive Review 1st edition 38: 248–255

National heart lung and blood institute NIH (2014) What is asthma? https://www.nhlbi.nih.gov. Accessed Dec 2016

References

1. Allen TW (2005) Return to play following exercise-induced bronchoconstriction. Clin J Sports Med 15(6):421–425
2. National heart lung and blood institute NIH (2014) What is asthma? https://www.nhlbi.nih.gov. Accessed Dec 2016
3. Boulet LP, Turmel J, Cote A (2017) Asthma and exercise-induced respiratory symptoms in the athlete: new insights. Curr Opin Pulm Med 23(1):71–77
4. Feden JP (2013) Closed lung trauma. Clin Sports Med 32:255–265
5. Hull JH, Ansley L, Robson-Ansley P, Parsons JP (2012) Managing respiratory problems in athletes. Clin Med 12(4):351–356
6. World Anti-Doping Agency (2016) What is prohibited. https://www.wada-ama.org/en/prohibited-list. Accessed Jan 2017
7. Pongdee T, James TL (2013) Exercise-induced bronchoconstriction. Ann Allergy Asthma Immunol 110:311–315
8. Lazovic B, Mazic S, Suzic-Lazic J, Djelic M, Djordjevic-Saranovic S, Durmic T, Zikic D, Zugic V (2015) Respiratory adaptations in different types of sport. Eur Rev Med Pharmacol Sci 19:2269–2274
9. Mead WF, Harwig R (1981) Fitness evaluation and exercise prescription. J Fam Pract 13(7):1039–1050
10. O'Connor FG, Casa DJ, Davis BA, Pierrer PS, Sallis RE, Wilder RP (2013) ACSM's sports medicine: a comprehensive review 1st edition. Pulmonary 38:248–255
11. Partridge R, Coley A, Bowie R, Woolard RH (1997) Sports-related pneumothorax. Ann Emerg Med 30(4):539–541
12. Weiler JM, Bonini S, Coifman R, Craig T, Delgado L, Capao-Filipe M, Passali D, Randolph C, Storms W, Ad Hoc Committee of Sports Medicine Committee of American Academy of Allergy, Asthma & Immunology (2007) American academy of allergy, asthma and immunology work group report: exercise-induced asthma. J Allergy Clin Immunol 119(6):1349–1358
13. Ansley L, Kippelen P, Dickinson J, Hull JH (2011) Misdiagnosis of exercise-induced bronchoconstriction in professional soccer players. Allergy 67:390–395

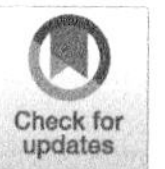

Return to Play After Injury: A Medicolegal Overview

58

Heiko Striegel, Werner Krutsch, and Raymond Best

Contents

H. Striegel, M.D. (✉)
Department of Sports Medicine, University Hospital Tübingen, Hoppe-Seyler-Strasse 6, 72076 Tuebingen, Germany
e-mail: heiko.striegel@med.uni-tuebingen.de

W. Krutsch, M.D.
Department of Trauma Surgery, University Medical Centre Regensburg, Franz-Josef-Strauss-Allee 11, 93053 Regensburg, Germany

R. Best, M.D.
Department of Sports Orthopaedics and Sports Traumatology, Sportklinik Stuttgart, Taubenheimstraße 8, 70372 Stuttgart, Germany

58.1 Introduction

Over the past decades, football has become the number one sport in the world. Similar to handball and basketball, football is a team sports with the highest risk of sustaining an injury. This issue was investigated in a prospective cohort study of 14 team sports during the Summer Olympics in 2004 [1]. The type and location of football injuries have hardly changed over the past three decades, and the body region most affected by football injuries is the lower extremities [2–6]. Most injuries are slight and associated with only a few days away from football. Severe injuries with time away from football of more than 4 weeks only amount to approximately 10–20% of all football injuries [2, 7, 8]. Severe injuries have led to the development of different return-to-play strategies and the determination of various factors and parameters influencing the decision-making process.

Although the time-out in football and return to play after injury have been the subjects of several studies [9], there is a lack of sufficient evidence-based guidelines for decision-making processes and the factors influencing the time point of return to play. This chapter presents the medicolegal aspects of the return-to-play process from the point of view of a team physician and a lawyer. Medicolegal issues include the definition of fitness and completion of the healing process and medical aspect recommendations for team

V. Musahl et al. (eds.), *Return to Play in Football*, https://doi.org/10.1007/978-3-662-55713-6_58

physicians on how to understand and improve the return-to-play process of injured players. The topic "performance improvement" by legal or illegal instruments, such as doping, is also relevant for debates on return to play after injury and hence part of this discussion.

58.2 Definition of the (Un-)fitness to Work or to Do Sports

Both the medical and the legal literature lack a valid definition of fitness to work. Some examples are given in the national directive of the Joint Committee of the Federal Ministry of Health in Germany and in the regulations on assessing the incapacity for work and measures for gradual reintegration (disability regulations) established by insurance companies. According to these regulations, a person is incapable of working if he or she is no longer able to practice their profession on account of illness or if practicing the profession carries the risk of disease aggravation. Moreover, incapacity for work is also present when it is foreseeable that practicing the activity at a certain stage of the disease—which alone does not result in incapacity for work—may have direct injurious effects on health or recovery. In addition, incapacity for work even continues during gradual recovery, which is intended to enable an injured person to return to full work capacity through gradual reintroduction.

Incapacity for work may also exist during stress testing and work therapy. In accordance with the national disability regulations of a country, insurance holders must also take their physical and mental health into account when determining their ability to work. According to the disability regulations, an injured person must be given the same physical, mental, and emotional state of health when their incapacity for work is ascertained. Therefore, incapacity for work should only be determined on the basis of a medical examination, and the same applies to making recommendations for gradual reintegration. In professional football, medical examinations should include sport-specific testing for return to play, whereas recreational football players only require the normal reintegration examinations for return to work.

National health regulations and insurance guidelines may differ significantly among countries. In football, it is essential to differentiate between professional and recreational football. In professional football, the definition of fitness or readiness for the job is the same as participating in football activities. In contrast, injured amateur football players tend to mostly care about how and when to be reintegrated into their job and when to return to football. This difference needs to be observed, and improved evidence or at least a consensus in football medicine would be helpful. Additionally, the time point of confirming a player "fit for football" after injury is still unclear. Is it the time point of the first football-specific exercises, the first time back on the field, the first team training, or the first match? This question also requires an interdisciplinary as well as an international consensus. For German sports professionals, the time point of fitness for sports is the first successfully completed team training, defined and confirmed by the team physician and postulated by the public trauma insurance for professional athletes.

Fact Box 1

- The legal definition of "fit for work" or "fit for sports" has not yet been finalized in detail and needs to differentiate between professional and recreational football.

58.3 Decision-Making Models for Assessing the Fitness to Do Sports

The physical ability of athletes to do sports should be solely determined on the basis of medical findings, completely independent of any other factors that may influence the decision, such as the athletic situation of the player, the ranking of the club, or the importance of the match [10–12]. Approaches to decision-making and simplification mainly refer to high-grade injuries, for which—purely from a medical point of view—clear exclusion criteria from sports participation already exist (e.g., ligament rupture, cardiovascular rhythm disturbances, or concussion).

Such case-oriented approaches refer to independent measurements, such as muscle size, force value, and laboratory parameters, or imaging criteria that help assess the ability to participate in sports [13–18]. However, there is hardly any literature on approaches to the standardized assessment of the predominant number of injuries—mostly of muscular or tendinous nature—with a layoff of less than 4 weeks [19, 20].

In acute injury situations and during subsequent further diagnostic evaluation, physicians and physiotherapists in football have to decide on the optimal treatment regimen, whereas the main concern of the player or the club is usually the earliest possible time of return to play [19, 21]. Particularly in professional football, the choice of treatment procedure favored by the players and their agents is often not primarily based on evidence-based medical knowledge but rather on which therapist promises the shortest layoff. From the athlete's point of view, this attitude is understandable when taking the sporting and sociological aspects and particularly the economic aspects of today's professional sports into account [12, 15].

A three-step "return-to-play" model was developed to structure and objectify the decision-making process of a player's return to sport [15]. This model involves risk-modifying factors, such as the type of sports, the level of play, and the position in the game as well as external factors, for instance, the sporting situation of the player or the team, the importance of the match, or the time point in the season. The advantages and disadvantages of the two options "to be able to play" or "to be not able to play" should be weighed against each other to ensure a comprehensible and moderate decision in each individual case [11, 22].

A multilevel decision model has been developed to simplify the decision process that focuses on clear, quantifiable criteria, such as inflammatory response, restricted ability to move, swelling, or effusion. The model also includes the recommendation that the strength level of the injured limb should be at least 70% of the level before injury. Unfortunately, most of the published recommendations are based on low-level evidence [11, 19]. According to the multilevel decision model, slight injuries such as minor residual swelling of the ankle after ankle joint contusion would be classified as "incapacity for work." However, even a difference in muscular strength of 20% would be acceptable for return to play from a medical point of view, although such a power deficit may be detrimental to some footballers.

Fact Box 2

- Decision-making in return-to-play processes in football is currently not based on scientific evidence, although different approaches have been reported in the literature.

58.4 Principles of Classifying Sports Capability

Because of the missing evidence on return-to-play decisions after football injury, it may be helpful to classify the medical condition and the situation of the injured player. Clear decisions in football are rare, because players may sustain several injuries per season that require different decisions. Classification should be simple, and lay language should be used in discussions between players, team managers, and team physicians (Fig. 58.1). A considerable number of injuries that rank between "capable to play" and "not capable to play" are not classified. Such injuries can be divided into five categories:

Category I: Harmless
Category II: Not harmless
Category III: Not advisable, but acceptable
Category IV: Borderline
Category V: Not justifiable

In category II and III, clear decisions are difficult, and the decision-making process depends on several external factors (Fig. 58.1) [11].

58.4.1 Category I: "Harmless"

The athlete is able to play without any restrictions. Medical diagnostic findings are close to normal. The risk of repeated or recurrent injury is statistically in the normal range and corresponds to that stated in the literature.

58.4.2 Category II: "Not Harmless"

In the presence of minor symptoms or medical anomalies, the player may return to unrestricted sporting activities. In consideration of the above-mentioned cofactors, the physicians, the team of coaches, and the athlete may decide on a reduced training frequency.

58.4.3 Category III: "Not Advisable, but Acceptable"

The athlete's participation in competition is not advisable because of the possible worsening of the medical symptoms. If match participation is acceptable from a medical point of view, it is the physician's responsibility to inform the athlete about the medical findings and discuss the possibility of match participation. Each party should be aware that playing football may worsen the injury.

58.4.4 Category IV: "Borderline"

Participation in a football match is not advisable and only marginally acceptable from the medical perspective. Medical findings and risks posed by continuing to play have to be clarified. Each further exercise is only done at the request by the athlete. The consent discussion should be documented in writing.

58.4.5 Category V: "Not Justifiable"

The clinical diagnosis and medical diagnostics show that further participation in sports exercises poses a high risk of health deterioration or even permanent disability. From a medical point of view, further sports participation is inadvisable, so that the player is declared unfit to play. The athlete and the coaches (after approval by the player) need to be informed of the possible risks. The athlete may act independently of explicit medical advice to not continue sports activity. In this case, the responsible physician should send a written confirmation of the decision "unfit to play" to the athlete and the club [19, 23, 24]. Experiences in elite sports have shown improved decisions if the cooperation between the parties involved is marked by trust.

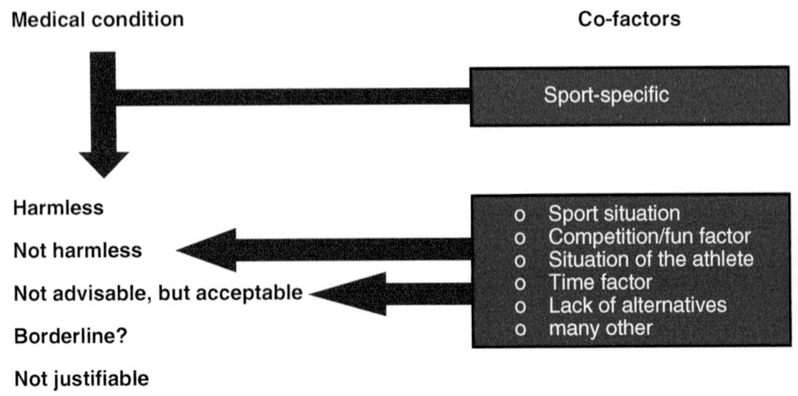

Fig. 58.1 Medical decision-making process in elite sports [34]

Fact Box 3

- A clear classification of return-to-play stages is essential to obtain further evidence on this topic. Discussions between players, team managers, and team physicians should be in lay language.

58.5 Doping and Return to Play

The return-to-play process represents a difficult and vulnerable period in a football player's career [25]. Treatment issues, the hard and long rehabilitation process, and the different stages of the return-to-play process are difficult experiences for injured football players. Because professional football players wish to shorten the return-to-play process, they try to exhaust all possibilities with regard to tissue healing, functional improvements, muscle regeneration or muscle building, as well as athletic skills. The mental situation of a severely injured player may be clouded due to the pressure to return to football quickly. In these difficult situations, players may be open to different types of support and might be tempted to try and receive allowed or even illicit instruments, medications, or strategies to return to football quickly [26–30].

The return-to-play process after injury in professional football is also a period of frequent doping controls. Only in exceptional circumstances and only with the confirmation of the National Anti-Doping Agency (NADA) and the World Anti-Doping Agency (WADA) is it allowed to use medications or substances stated on the anti-doping list. However, the use of legal medications is also increased during injury time, which may represent a problem. The use of painkillers is a general problem in football, and the return-to-play process after injury is likely to be a period of increased painkiller use. Data on this issue are rare [31, 32], but the task of the medical team supporting a football player is to monitor and possibly reduce the use of such medications and adjuncts.

There is no evidence that the use of legal or illegal medications reduces the time away from football. However, in professional football players, it might stretch the biological and legal possibilities to shorten the return-to-play process.

58.6 Summary

In most cases, the decision on an athlete's ability to play is not straightforward "yes" or "no" but rather a decision that increasingly depends on many nonmedical factors. Standardized considerations are difficult, and physicians often have to act on a case-by-case basis. Considering the lack of evidence on the return-to-play decision from the medicolegal point of view, it is important that all parties involved use lay language that can be understood by everyone. Such discussions would benefit from a classification of the return-to-play process.

Compared to exhibition games, an athlete's participation in Olympic Games or the Football World Cup requires special consideration. The ability to participate in sports cannot be determined without consideration of the athlete's medical findings [33]. The task of the team physician is to minimize the risk of far-reaching negative consequences.

It would be useful if all parties involved in the decision-making process balance the sporting abilities of the injured player at the beginning of the return-to-play process between acceptable sport-specific risks and medical exclusion criteria. Medical diagnostics as well as a complete documentation of the medical findings and the decision-making process are indispensable. Physicians are often under great pressure during the decision-making process, and sufficient communication with the team may reduce both pressure as well as the fear of medicolegal consequences. Consequent documentation of all medical decisions and communication between the parties may be exhausting, but such documentation is the key to clear decisions that may additionally reduce medicolegal consequences for the medical staff, particularly in professional football. Economic, political, or media-associated stress situations should not dilute evidence-based medical recommendations. Therefore, the ability of an injured athlete to return to play might need to be classified at the beginning of the decision-making process, i.e., as harmless, not harmless, not advisable but acceptable, borderline, and not justifiable (Fig. 58.1) [34].

Take-Home Message

Diseases or injuries in professional high-performance football are special situations for athletes and physicians. Returning to highly stressful sports as quickly as possible is often more important to athletes than optimal treatment. Rehabilitation time is sometimes insufficient for professional athletes, which would pose a higher risk of recurring injuries or questionable treatment decisions. High-performance sports such as football involve situations that not only comprise medical aspects but also external factors, such as the athlete's current athletic situation or the importance of upcoming matches that may play a role in deciding on the further procedure. The physician's dilemma between responsible medical treatment and athletic stress situations makes it necessary to follow a straight, transparent treatment regime and decision-making process.

Top Five Evidence-Based References

Anderson BR, Vetter VL (2009) Return to play? Practical considerations for young athletes with cardiovascular disease. Br J Sports Med 43:690–695

Clover J, Wall J (2010) Return to play criteria following sports injury. Clin Sports Med 29:169–175

Creighton DW, Shrier I, Shultz R et al (2010) Return-to-play in sport: a decision based model. Clin J Sports Med 20:379–385

Maron BJ, Brown RW, McGrew CA et al (1994) Ethical, legal and practical considerations affecting medical decision-making in competitive athletes. JACC 24:845–899

Best R, Bauer G, Niess A, Striegel H (2011) Return to play decisions in professional soccer: a decision algorithm from a team physician's viewpoint. Z Orthop Unfall 149(5):582–587. https://doi.org/10.1055/s-0031-1280160

References

1. Junge A, Langevoort G, Pipe A et al (2006) Injuries in team sport tournaments during the 2004 Olympic Games. Am J Sports Med 34:565–576
2. Dupont G, Nedelec M, McCall A et al (2010) Effect of 2 soccer matches in a week on physical performance and injury rate. Am J Sports Med 38:1749–1751
3. Hawkins RD, Hulse MA, Wilkinson C et al (2001) The association football medical research programme: an audit of injuries in professional football. Br J Sports Med 35:43–47
4. Inklaar H (1994) Soccer injuries. I: incidence and severity. Sports Med 18:55–73
5. Inklaar H (1994) Soccer injuries. I: aetiology and prevention. Sports Med 18:81–93
6. Junge A, Dvorak J (2004) Soccer injuries: a review on incidence and prevention. Sports Med 34:929–938
7. Chomiak J, Junge A, Peterson L et al (2000) Severe injuries in football players. Am J Sports Med 28:S58–S68
8. Hägglund M, Walden M, Ekstrand J (2003) Exposure and injury risk in Swedish elite football: a comparison between seasons 1982 and 2001. Scand J Med Sci Sports 13:364–370
9. Petersen W, Taheri P, Forkel P, Zantop T (2014) Return to play following ACL reconstruction: a systematic review about strength deficits. Arch Orthop Trauma Surg 134(10):1417–1428
10. Baumann J (2005) Returning to play: the mind does matter. Clin J Sports Med 15:432–435
11. Creighton DW, Shrier I, Shultz R et al (2010) Return-to-in sport: a decision based model. Clin J Sports Med 20:379–385
12. McFarland EG (2004) Return to play. Clin J Sports Med 23:xv–xxiii
13. Anderson BR, Vetter VL (2009) Return to play? Practical considerations for young athletes with cardiovascular disease. Br J Sports Med 43:690–695
14. Cascio BM, Culp L, Coscarea AJ (2004) Return to play after anterior cruciate ligament reconstruction. Clin Sports Med 23:395–408
15. Clover J, Wall J (2010) Return to play criteria following sports injury. Clin Sports Med 29:169–175
16. Drake DF, Nadler SF, Chou LH et al (2004) Sports and performing arts medicine. 4. Traumatic injuries in sports. Arch Phys Med Rehabil 85:S67–S71
17. Lam MH, Fong DT, Yung P et al (2009) Knee stability assessment on anterior cruciate ligament injury: clinical and biomechanical approaches. Sports Med Arthrosc Rehabil Ther Technol 1:20
18. Myklebust G, Bahr R (2005) Return to play guidelines after anterior cruciate ligament surgery. Br J Sports Med 39:127–131
19. Best TM, Brolinson PG (2005) Return to play: the sideline dilemma. Clin J Sports Med 15:403–404
20. Orchard J, Best TM (2002) The management of muscle strain injuries: an early return versus the risk of occurrence. Clin J Sports Med 12:3–5
21. Verrall G, Brukner PD, Seward HG (2006) Doctor on the sidelines. Med J Aust 84:244–248
22. Reyna VF, Rivers SE (2008) Current theories of risk and rational decision making. Dev Rev 28:1–11
23. Maron BJ, Brown RW, McGrew CA et al (1994) Ethical, legal and practical considerations affecting medical decision-making in competitive athletes. J Am College Cardiol 24:845–899

24. Mitten MJ (1996) When is disqualification from sports justified? Medical judgement vs. patients' rights. Phys Sportsmed 24:75–78
25. Dunn WR, George MS, Churchill L et al (2007) Ethics in sports medicine. Am J Sports Med 35: 840–844
26. Baume N, Geyer H, Vouillamoz M, Grisdale R, Earl M, Aguilera R, Cowan DA, Ericsson M, Gmeiner G, Kwiatkowska D, Kioukia-Fougia N, Molina A, Ruivo J, Segura J, Van Eenoo P, Jan N, Robinson N, Saugy M (2016) Evaluation of longitudinal steroid profiles from male football players in UEFA competitions between 2008 and 2013. Drug Test Anal 8(7):603–612
27. Dietzel DP, Hedlund EC (2005) Injections and return to play. Curr Pain Headache Rep 9:11–16
28. Giraldi G, Unim B, Masala D, Miccoli S, La Torre G (2015) Knowledge, attitudes and behaviours on doping and supplements in young football players in Italy. Public Health 129(7):1007–1009
29. Orchard JW (2004) Is it safe to use local anaesthetic painkilling injections in professional football? Sports Med 34:209–219
30. Seif Barghi T, Halabchi F, Dvorak J, Hosseinnejad H (2015) How the Iranian football coaches and players know about doping? Asian J Sports Med 6(2):e24392
31. Tscholl PM, Dvorak J (2012) Abuse of medication during international football competition in 2010 – lesson not learned. Br J Sports Med 46(16):1140–1141
32. Vaso M, Weber A, Tscholl PM, Junge A, Dvorak J (2015) Use and abuse of medication during 2014 FIFA World Cup Brazil: a retrospective survey. BMJ Open 5(9):e007608
33. Junge A (2000) The influence of psychological factors on sports injuries. Am J Sports Med 28:S10–S15
34. Best R, Bauer G, Niess A, Striegel H (2011) Return to play decisions in professional soccer: a decision algorithm from a team physician's viewpoint. Z Orthop Unfall 149(5):582–587. https://doi.org/10.1055/s-0031-1280160

Part VIII

Ethical Issues in Return to Play: The Role of Clinical Judgment

59 Expectations and Responsibilities of Players and Team Coaches in the Return-to-Play Process

Werner Krutsch, Frank Wormuth, and Tobias Schweinsteiger

Contents

W. Krutsch, M.D. (✉)
Department of Trauma Surgery, FIFA Medical Centre of Excellence, University Medical Centre Regensburg, Franz-Josef-Strauss-Allee 11, 93053 Regensburg, Germany
e-mail: werner.krutsch@ukr.de

F. Wormuth
Deutscher Fußball-Bund, Otto-Fleck-Schneise 6, 60528 Frankfurt am Main, Germany
e-mail: dfb.wormuth@t-online.de

T. Schweinsteiger
FC Bayern München e.V., Säbener Str. 51-57, 81547 Munich, Germany
e-mail: tobias.schweinsteiger@fcb.de

59.1 Introduction

Long lay-off of football players from competitive matches is often caused by traumatic and overuse injuries. Particularly severe injuries resulting in absence from football of more than 3 months are an important factor for an interruption in or even the end of a football career. Long lay-off from sports is frequently caused by traumatic injuries, for instance, to the anterior cruciate ligament (ACL) injury of the knee [1] or by overuse injuries such as pubic overload associated with groin pain [2]. After such injuries, football players have to resume physical activities and training and gain match experience, which requires a lot

V. Musahl et al. (eds.), *Return to Play in Football*, https://doi.org/10.1007/978-3-662-55713-6_59

of time, well-planned rehabilitation and patience. The duration of the return-to-play process is generally well documented for ACL injuries, but little evidence is available for other typical football injuries. After minor injuries, only few team members are generally involved in the decision-making process, while severe injuries or surgical treatments require an increased number of medical staff such as surgeons. The return-to-play process with its different stages represents a challenge to all experts and staff supporting the injured football player. Team coaches, the football players themselves or—in the case of junior players—their parents are the main group of people to improve and change prevention strategies [3]. Particularly the team coach is well-accepted as a key player to implement and improve prevention steps in a football team, a fact that is highlighted in both the scientific literature and in daily football routine [4–6]. The performance of football players and team coaches with regard to medical issues highly depends on their individual experience and education [7], which is the focus of this chapter. To better understand the group of persons supporting football players not only requires close communication but also knowledge about the different points of view of players and team coaches [8].

59.2 The 'Injury Problem' in Football

59.2.1 The View of Players

Injuries not only affect the football activity but also the daily personal life of football players. Particularly severe injuries resulting in lay-off from football of more than 6 months considerably disrupt the daily life of both amateur and professional players. Injuries of professional athletes and elite (under contract and with salary for playing football) amateur football players jeopardise participation in the running season and subsequently to be successful in their profession. Severe injuries also carry a risk of a premature end to one's football career and may prompt football players to stop or change their professional type of sports. Injuries of amateur football players may also have a negative effect on their occupation due to long lay-off after surgery or rehabilitation.

The high incidence of football injuries [1, 9] is a well-established fact. Nearly every player in professional and amateur football with a career of more than 10 years has sustained at least one injury. Therefore, football players are usually experienced with regular medical services in the context of such injuries. Even amateur football clubs tend to have a physiotherapist supporting training sessions and matches. Little is known, however, about the general knowledge of football players at different skill levels on medical issues such as first aid on the field, injury prevention, regeneration, rehabilitation or return to play after injury. Generally, football players are advised by their team coaches and rely on their own experiences or that of their team colleagues. These facts have to be considered in any discussion about the knowledge of football players on medical issues. No scientific analysis is yet available related to football players on medical issues and their return-to-play expectations. The authors of this chapter describe internal investigations in amateur and professional football that show a generally sufficient knowledge of players about injury problems in football [10]. Football injuries mainly affect knees, ankles and thighs. Most serious injuries are to the ACL, PCL or cartilage. The main concern in terms of the severity of an injury from a player's point of view is not lay-off from football, which is part of the scientific injury definition and data collection [11], but persistent long-term changes in the injured body part.

Because of the possible consequences of football injuries, football players need to be aware of injury prevention measures. Such measures have become more and more important during the last years. Active injury prevention strategies carried out by players themselves are a common method for ensuring continuous sports activity at all skill levels and particularly in professional football. The major problem is the generally low rate of compliance and perseverance to participate in injury prevention strategies. Injury prevention should ideally already start in junior football but is unfortunately still rather uncommon at that level. From a player's point of view, injury prevention over one's entire football career might be considered an impossible task. The only chance for football players to stay fit and healthy is to do everything possible to prevent injury. Frequently, football players only start to participate in active prevention strategies many years after the beginning of their football career and/or after a severe injury.

General expectations of football players are to 'play football', to 'proceed playing football' or to 'return to play football after injury' as quickly and safely as possible. After an injury or another health complaint, players only want to return to play football and expect support from their team and medical staff to achieve this aim. This expectation is identical in both amateur and professional football.

59.2.2 The View of Team Coaches

The view of team coaches on medical issues is influenced by many different factors. Team coaches are often former football players who had a long career and are thus automatically experienced in training load, regeneration, warm-up, match preparation, injury prevention or injury recovery. Different skill levels in football involve different situations for medical issues in football [12]. The best precondition for team coaches to understand the quality and quantity of medical support provided at a given football skill level is if they played at the same level themselves. For example, team coaches who used to play at a higher skill level may expect more medical support and quality than available at a lower football level. This situation may create a conflict between the team coach and the players or the medical staff with negative effects on the entire football team. However, all members of a football team may learn from the experience and knowledge obtained at higher skill levels and thus benefit from team coaches with such experience. On the other hand, to expect too little with regard to the quality of medical services provided in a team may also cause problems. In conclusion, all staff members and particularly the team coach should understand the quality and quantity of services needed and services provided by the medical team at the respective skill level.

Team coaches expect high compliance in terms of preventive health behaviour and injury prevention strategies from their players, which is not easily accomplished by a team of 20-odd players. Experienced players and players who already have sustained a severe injury can and should guide the other players of the team in active prevention strategies. Independent of the football level, muscle injuries are not only the most annoying type of injury over the course of a season but also the most difficult injuries to avoid in modern football. Team coaches are now becoming educated on the impact of particular training exercises on muscles as well as on the influence of their play and regeneration concept on the occurrence of muscular injury. Consequently, team coaches should analyse their concepts with regard to muscular complaints and injuries of their players. Team coaches should also realise that football players themselves have a high potential for active injury prevention. Thus, team coaches should introduce their players to injury prevention measures and supervise their continuous participation in these strategies.

Team coaches at different skill or educational levels vary in their skills and knowledge on football and consequently also on medical issues such as warm-up, injury prevention measures or regeneration. The so far unpublished data obtained by the chapter authors from professional football in Germany include information on the expectations of football players and team coaches [10]. In this investigation of professional football teams as part of a German injury prevention study, the team coaches reported on deficits in and the necessity of injury prevention strategies in professional football, mainly with regard to ACL and PCL injuries as well as ankle and muscle injuries. The team coaches themselves had mainly finished their football career after one single severe injury or after a several minor injuries, mainly of the knee and ankle. Furthermore, team coaches describe the increasing problem, particularly in junior football, that children and adolescents are nowadays less exposed to athletic training at school than in the past. Particularly junior football players may enhance their athletic abilities and neuromotor skills by being exposed to many different types of sports.

Fact Box 1

- Injuries of football players are an important reason for the lack of success of football teams and therefore a vital issue for the management of a football team.
- Football injuries represent an important reason for less successful results as well as declining fitness levels and physical integrity of the players.
- Players and team coaches know their responsibilities in terms of injury prevention strategies but may have different approach on football injuries.

59.3 Team Coaches in Football: The Perspective of a Former Football Player

59.3.1 The Main Responsibilities of Football Coaches

The main responsibilities of a football coach do not include medical issues. For both players and the medical staff, it is essential to know the main responsibilities of a team coach. Details on coaching practice have been described rarely in the literature [13], but Kaß [14] described the main responsibilities of a team coach in German professional football (Table 59.1).

To fulfil these multifold responsibilities, a team coach requires many different skills, for instance, long experience as a football player and sufficient sports education. To adequately fulfil all these responsibilities is a time-consuming task, so that additional responsibilities such as medical issues may overextend the capacity of a team coach. Accordingly, professional football clubs employ medical experts, so that team coaches only have to communicate their expectations on the medical service and stay in contact with the respective members of staff. In amateur football, coaches need to be educated in at least the basics of the most important medical issues.

Table 59.1 Responsibilities of team coaches in professional football

Regulation and supervision of training sessions
Planning of training sessions
Technical training
Tactical training
Athletic and fitness training
Team planning
Analysis of the opponent team (next game)
Team leadership
Team organisation and administration
Management of resources
Media and public management
Supervision of the staff around the team
Exchange with the club officials
Junior and talent promotion
Exchange with the medical team

59.3.2 Education of Football Coaches in Medical Issues

Topics of the education of team coaches depend on the quality and quantity of a team's football level. Team coach licences for lower football levels mainly include issues such as training and tactics, whereas licences for the highest level, the UEFA Pro Licence, also include detailed medical issues. Thus, awareness of a team coach's level of football education by all members of a football team helps to better understand any decisions made by the coach. The main issues of team coach education defined and implemented in the German Pro Licence curriculum are defined in Table 59.2.

The curriculum of the Pro Licence includes also medical topics. These medical topics present a multifaceted job profile for a team coach in professional football (Table 59.3).

Several medical topics for team coaches have been well-described in the literature as well as the often important role of team coaches in the prevention of injuries [4, 6]. Particularly well-documented are level I studies for the primary prevention of

Table 59.2 Main issues of the team coach education in the German Pro Licence

Software tools for match analysis and presentations	Legal issues for team coaches
Rhetoric and communication	Public relations and interviews
Team building practice	Match analysis
Role, competence and requirements of team coach	Match rules
Football science	Physiology
Training principles	Warm-ups
Current situation of modern professional football	Team members and staff
Goal shooting and goal situations	Motivation
Team tactics, position tactics and player's tactics	Season preparation
Time management during the week and over the season	Match coaching
Defensive and offensive strategies	Perception and concentration
Mental aspects and stress management	Free kicks and penalties
Speed, endurance and strength	To form team
Special consideration of goalkeepers and in women's football	Junior football aspects
Traineeships in football teams	

Table 59.3 Medical topics for football coaches in the German Pro Licence

Physical stress on players
Anatomy of human beings
Energy metabolism
Sports medical care
Screening examinations and performance diagnostics
Muscular functional tests and FMS
Flexibility and strength exercises
Head injuries in football
Injury prevention and management
Nutrition
Consultation of a dentist
Fatigue and regeneration
Anti-doping
Sports psychology, burnout and depression

injuries through team training [6, 15] and, as a secondary prevention step, coach-controlled training programmes during the rehabilitation period after injuries to prevent reinjury [4].

Table 59.4 Eleven for coaches Medical recommendations for coaches (11 for coaches)

1. Respect your medical team, understand each other and communicate consistently
2. Organise at the beginning of the season: prevention, first aid, treatment *and* rehab management in your team
3. Customise your training sessions and consider environmental factors (heat/cold)
4. Allow players time to recover (consider different age group regeneration)
5. Implement prevention programmes like the 11+
6. Offer education in active ways for how to avoid injuries
7. Encourage balanced nutrition and avoid supplements and drugs (consider the World Anti-Doping Code)
8. Respect mental and psychological status of the players
9. Help build consensus within the players, coaches, medical staff and athletic trainers
10. Promote safe and effective return to play after injuries and illness
11. Be fair and open for changes and improvement in football medicine and science

After some disagreements between football coaches and team physicians in some UEFA Champions League teams, a group of F-MARC established 11 recommendations for football coaches to better understand medical issues. This list of recommendations illustrating team coach responsibilities from the medical point of view was developed by an interdisciplinary group of experts [16]. These recommendations are called "11 for coaches" (Table 59.4).

By now, the instruction in medical issues is a firmly established part of the education of football coaches that has shown to be effective in injury prevention [5–7, 17, 18]. The most scientifically investigated football injuries that show the success of team coach education are concussion [7, 19–22] and other head injuries [23]. Apart from medical issues, both team coaches and football players should be instructed in adequate stress management, which may also facilitate the prevention of injuries [24].

59.3.3 Medical Issues in Daily Football Routine

Despite sufficient knowledge of football players and team coaches about medical issues, the implementation of this knowledge in daily routine is often inadequate. Knowledge about the most important medical issues in football differs at the different skill levels [12]. All experts and football players agree that certain medical topics are essential for football teams, irrespective of the skill level [8]. These medical topics are first aid on the field, anti-doping, injury prevention, training and endurance control, regeneration, reintegration after injury and individual personal management. Each of these medical topics should be focussed on for players and team coaches (Table 59.5). The job of team coaches in professional football is managing and leading different members of a team and the medical experts around the team while encouraging active and open communication, which is easier for coaches with own football career and own experiences in a football team. Team coaches in amateur and junior football are often less well educated in but responsible for the majority of medical issues [3, 8, 12]. Because the practical performance depends on the medical knowledge and skills available in a football team, team coaches in junior football must study these medical issues on a private basis or by attending professional courses [12].

Fact Box 2

- Team coaches and football players are familiar with general injury prevention strategies because of their training, but the implementation of this knowledge in daily routine is often inadequate.
- At any skill level, team coaches are the leaders of football teams and responsible not only for a team's success but also for training standards and medical issues.
- Team coaches significantly influence medical issues, such as first aid on the field, injury prevention, regeneration and rehabilitation after injury; however, these topics are only a small part of a team coach's education and therefore often insufficiently implemented in daily practice.

59.4 Responsibilities of Football Coaches and Players in Basic Primary Injury Prevention

In terms of injury prevention strategies, integrating new scientific knowledge or successful experiences from other sports into football has been shown to be difficult. Team sports typically have their own specific culture that is difficult to change [25]. In future, all members of a football team need to learn from other sports regarding topics such as injury prevention or to increase strength and endurance. Although members of football teams are familiar with the main aspects of injury prevention, implementation of such knowledge into daily routine is often difficult [5]. Orr et al. [26] reported that the knowledge of team coaches and the parents of young players on injury prevention strategies in football was better than that of the football players themselves. The education of football players in terms of medical issues has been successful in several countries with regard to concussion; here, comprehensive instruction resulted in the reporting of detailed symptoms and subsequently in confirmation of the suspected diagnosis [19, 27, 28]. Other issues that should be reported to psychologists are depression and anxiety because these medical conditions tend to be underestimated in modern football [29].

59.4.1 Injury Prevention Strategies for Players

As participants in a team sport, football players are not entirely free in their decisions on what kind of medical service or prevention programme to use. Especially players of professional football clubs have access to a medical team associated with the club that includes a physiotherapist and often a team physician, who are always present on the field. Permission to use other medical services is officially allowed by public law, and football clubs have frequently obtained an additional medical opinion of a second medical doctor as external consultant for specific injuries in the past few years. Football players at an interna-

Table 59.5 Possible persons responsible for medical issues

Topics	Junior + recreational football	Elite amateur football	Professional football
First aid on field	Team coach	Physical therapist	Physician
Medical equipment	Team coach	Physical therapist	Physician
Injury prevention	Team coach	Team coach	Athletic coach
Training/endurance control	Team coach	Team coach	Co-coach
Regeneration	Team coach	Team coach	Co-coach
Mental support	Team coach	Team coach	Sports psychologist
Return to play	Team coach	Team coach/physical therapist	Medical staff

tional level frequently employ private physiotherapists in addition to the team physiotherapists, which emphasises the importance of physiotherapy for football players.

Besides the many strategies for injury prevention included in warm-ups and training sessions as the main responsibility of the team coach, football players themselves may use preventive measures (Table 59.6) [30, 31].

One of the most important preventive steps for football players is obligatory screening examinations of the cardiovascular and musculoskeletal systems according to international and national guidelines for professional football as well as for junior elite football. These examinations should be extended to the lower football levels. Other examinations are less common in football, even in professional football, but essential for successful football playing. Regular dental examinations are important to exclude oral infections as a principle cause of muscular imbalance or muscular injuries of the back and lower extremities. Other advisable examinations for football players to reduce injuries are ophthalmologic examinations. Players may not realise any visual impairment, but unrestricted vision is essential, particularly during evening matches where floodlight is used. Smaller foot injuries and complaints such as callused skin on the sole of the foot, ingrown or broken toenails, blisters or other inflammations on the feet may stress the musculoskeletal balance of the body and lead to severe injuries of the joints of the lower extremities [1], which may be prevented by regular visits to a podiatrist. Particularly professional football players should regularly undergo such examinations as well as frequent blood screenings to avoid easily preventable injuries and illness. Fair play is also important because aggressive behaviour on the field facilitates the occurrence of injuries [31, 32].

To protect their health status, football players should also try to avoid colds, influenza and other infections, particularly during winter. Specific vaccinations should be mandatory for football players. Wearing appropriate clothing during and after playing football not only reduces illness but also muscular complaints that are often caused by rapid changes between warm and cold temperatures. Additionally, the lifestyle of football

Table 59.6 Preventive measures of football players

1. Compliance in obligatory and optional screening examinations
2. Frequent training sessions during the season without any long absence from football practice
3. Complete recovery after previous injuries
4. Knowledge about and consideration of previous injuries and participation in an adapted additional training programme to prevent recurrent injury
5. Sufficient compliance with warm-ups and prevention exercises during team training
6. Active regeneration and cool down after training sessions and matches
7. Sufficient communication with the team coach about endurance and regeneration
8. Sufficient sleep before and after matches
9. No drugs, alcohol or doping
10. Balanced nutrition
11. Adequate fluid substitution
12. Adequate behaviour on the field and fair play
13. Compliance with the treatment and rehabilitation of football injuries
14. Communication and decision-making during the return-to-play process after injuries

players should be adapted to the requirements of their sports activity and their expectations with regard to a successful career in football. Particularly professional football players should have sufficient rest after and between matches and training sessions. Further factors are well-balanced nutrition, avoidance of alcohol and good sleeping habits. Amateur football players may find it harder to adapt their daily living patterns to the requirements of a successful football career because of the demands of their occupational job on their physical capacity, particularly during weekday training sessions. Therefore, matches on working days, which mainly take place in the evening, may lead to increased risk of overstressing. Thus, amateur players may benefit from a change in their work responsibilities on match days.

59.4.2 Injury Prevention Strategies for Team Coaches

Team coaches are some of the most important persons for implementing adequate injury prevention strategies for football players [30, 31, 33–35]. Additionally, team coaches also play a key role in the mental support of football players. Scientific literature reports have described the influence of team coaches on team atmosphere and on the individual expectations of players in terms of medical issues such as injury prevention [17, 36, 37].

The importance of team coaches is also well documented in relation to building the confidence of their team and that of individual players, which may represent an important mental basis for injury prevention and for playing football successfully [38]. To detect symptoms of mental problems in a player is difficult, although mental afflictions are a frequent problem in professional football. To help prevent severe consequences such as depression is an important responsibility of team coaches [29].

The following medical prevention strategies are closely associated with team coaches in football (Table 59.7) [30, 31]:

Table 59.7 Prevention strategies of team coaches

1. Physical preparation of the players before the start of a football season
2. Mental fitness and team building over the entire season
3. Supervision and management of the training programme and endurance over the entire season
4. Performing adequate training sessions including injury-preventing measures such as neuromotorical exercises, exercises for facilitating trunk stability and agility and stretching on a regular basis
5. Conducting warm-ups for the team before training sessions and matches
6. Conducting cool-down programmes after training sessions and matches
7. Planning of recovery time for the team and individual players over the entire season
8. Reasonable reintegration and return-to-play decisions for injured players
9. Exemplification of 'fair play on the field'
10. Attention with regard to wearing protection equipment during training sessions and matches (e.g. shin guards in training sessions)

Because implementation of all these medical issues by just one person such as the team coach is impossible, professional football clubs employ several different members of medical staff to manage the various medical tasks. In contrast, team coaches in amateur and junior football have to cover most of these preventive measures in addition to their main responsibility, i.e. football-specific preparation of the players and the team [3, 12, 30]. To take care of appropriate training sessions and warm-ups is the team coach's main responsibility to prevent injuries [15]. For the success of such preventive measures, team coaches not only need to know the most important aspects of injury prevention but also how to transfer this knowledge onto the field. For example, injury prevention exercises could be integrated in both warm-ups and training sessions, thus becoming part of the respective programme. An important new development of the past years has been neuromotorical screening examinations of a team before and over the football season. Focussed on the preparation period before the season, these screening tests may show any weakness in the strength or athletic and neuromotorical capacity of a player, and findings can be appropriately addressed in the training schedule, regeneration and activation process over the season. One important aspect that all team coaches should understand is that injured player requires specific exercises because regular training sessions do not address the individual needs of a player after injury to prevent reinjury. As a result, individual exercises need to be implemented for players who are returning to play after injury.

Fact Box 3

- Injury prevention in football is highly associated with the compliance of football players and the performance of team coaches.
- Both football player and team coaches have specific duties in the prevention of injuries.
- After recurrent injuries, intensive collaboration and communication between the injured player and the coach as well as implementation of a well-adapted training programme are essential to avoid recurrent or new injury.

59.5 The Responsibilities of Coaches and Players in Basic Secondary Injury Prevention and RTP

59.5.1 Return to Play from a Player's Point of View

Sufficient communication between players, medical staff and team members is necessary during the entire return-to-play process. Football players may have one main contact person responsible for all return-to-play stages. In the period after injury, physicians and surgeons are mainly responsible for the treatment programme and the decision if a player is ready to advance to the next return-to-play stage. At the beginning of the rehabilitation programme, the main responsible person for supervising the healing and recovery process of all functions of the injured extremity is the physiotherapist. The subsequent rehabilitation period requires the cooperation of the athletic and the rehabilitation coach and the intensive support of the physiotherapist. In many amateur football clubs, only one person, i.e. the physiotherapist, is responsible for all these aspects of the rehabilitation process. The advantage in this case is the improved communication situation, but the physiotherapist has to provide expertise in many different fields that are covered by several members of staff in professional football. Frequent communications between staff members and the team coach are necessary for the successful recovery of a football player, who has to advance to the different return-to-play stages, i.e. from return to activity to return to sports to return to individual training to return to team training [39]. The team coach is the most important person to make the decision about a player's return to play on the field. The occurrence of any complaints or problems after the reintegration of a player after injury requires continuous support by the medical staff, also after the return-to-play process.

The important role of the team coach in improving the reintegration process of players after injury through well-adapted exercises and rehabilitation training programmes to prevent reinjury is well established [4]. In modern professional football, the return-to-play process is more and more influenced by the agents of football players, who often request a second opinion by another medical doctor or employ a different physiotherapist. In this case, the player has to keep control of such external influences to avoid further communication problems and information chaos.

59.5.2 Return to Play from a Team Coach's Point of View

The team coach has several responsibilities during the entire return-to-play process of a football player after injury. A team coach is responsible for the general planning and performance of the entire team and also needs to be informed about the recovery process of every injured player throughout the entire return-to-play period.

1. Directly after the injury of a player, the team coach has to adapt his intended system of play for the team for the running match and the subsequent matches. The first step for a team coach is the immediate substitution of the injured player to ensure successful continuation of the running match or the training session.
2. In amateur or junior football, the team coach also has to provide first aid on the field. This is the same as is provided by medical staff in professional football [3, 12].
3. After the end of the match or training session, the team coach needs to be informed if the injured player will be available for the next match. For planning the next match, the team physician should inform the team coach as soon as possible about the severity of the injury and the expected lay-off time. Generally, such information is only available after adequate diagnostics by the team physician. In professional football, however, team physicians frequently give a prognosis on the injury directly after the match. Once this information is provided, the team coach may plan for the next match (with or without the injured player).
4. Having decided on the team available for the next match, the team coach may plan for the rest of the half season or the entire season. If the injured player is included in the planning usually depends on the result of the clinical and imaging diagnostics. A correct diagnosis is essential for the team coach, because the absence of a specific player will influence team planning and may even require the signing of a new player.
5. After the start of the treatment, the team coach has to stay in contact with the injured player to help ensure a smooth healing process. Some players may also require mental support during the recovery period [40]. Direct contact between the team coach and medical staff is not necessary, only in case of complications and only with the consent of the player. From a legal point of view, exchange of medical information between the team coach and the team physician is only allowed if football players give their consent. It should be born on mind that written consents are rather uncommon in football [3].
6. Over the entire rehabilitation period, the team coach should be involved in the progress of a player from one return-to-play stage to the next, i.e. from the start of the running programme to athletic exercises to sports activity and football-specific activity. At the end of return-to-play process, the first prognoses about the actual return to playing football on the field may be made.
7. Before a player proceeds to the team training stage, the team coach should be continuously informed about the progress of the rehabilitation programme and the player's fitness level and football skills. Close communication with the player but also with the physiotherapist and the athletic and rehabilitation coach is necessary. Specific screening tests to assess the player's neuromotorical capability, strength and athletic skills may help the staff and team coach in their decision that the player may rejoin the team training sessions.
8. During the step-by-step integration of the recovered player into team training, additional individual training sessions are necessary to guarantee sufficient preventive exercises and regeneration. Typical situations for the partial integration of a player after injury involve warm-ups or running exercises and non-contact match simulations. Other possible exercises in this context are ball playing/shooting, positional play exercises and tactical exercises. At this stage, the main supervisor of the recovered player is the assistant coach, who helps the player step-by-step to return to full team training.
9. After the reintegration into team training is completed, the team coach should continue to check on the player to assess any problems that may occur after return to the field.
10. After the first official matches, the team coach has to adapt endurance and regeneration of the player to the actual situation, which requires close communication with the player.

11. After completion of the return-to-play process, the team coach has to know that the recovered player is at risk for injury to the same body location [4, 41] or another body part [1]. Appropriate warm-ups and training programmes including exercises for neuromotorical adaption, trunk stability, jumping and landing as well as agility performance may prevent players and hence the team from future injuries [4].

Team coaches generally assess the return-to-play process of their injured players on an individual basis. Besides objective screening tests as 'return-to-play test battery', it is also important to subjectively monitor players with regard to their body movements and behaviour. Many team coaches know their players well and also meet with them outside the football field. Therefore, team coaches are able to recognise and understand individual behavioural patterns, for instance, if a player is willing to take risks or if a player is being oversensitive. Such knowledge may also influence decisions related to the time point of reintegration.

Fact Box 4

- The return-to-play process is influenced by the level of compliance of the injured player.
- Close communication between the player, medical staff and team staff is fundamental.
- The team coach is the most important person for a player during the return-to-training and return-to-competition periods.
- After reintegration of the player in official matches, the team coach is also an important factor for secondary and tertiary prevention.
- To make an adequate decision on the reintegration of a recovered player into team training, the team coach requires objective information such as return-to-play screenings tests but also an individual assessment of the player.

59.6 Expectations of Injured Players During the Return-to-Play Process

After sustaining an injury, the main goal of football players is to participate in the next official match. The road to this goal is often difficult and requires perseverance and compliance with the requirements of the rehabilitation process. The expectations of football players on the medical staff and the return-to-play process are as follows:

- An exact diagnosis by the team physician. The diagnosis may be correlated with scientific [42] and individual experiences regarding the expected time of return to play on the field.
- An exact football-specific explanation of the indicated treatment of the injury, particularly with regard to the fastest possible return to play, long-term changes and continuation of the football career and also in terms of possible complications and problems as a potential risk to the football career.
- Players require a quick and safe return-to-play process and expect adequate and individualised support from their medical team and other staff.
- Football players expect to be included in the season planning of team coaches. Thus, detailed communication of the injured player with the team coach related the time point of return to play is essential. The behaviour of the team coach towards the injured player may influence the expectation and the recovery of the player [40, 43].
- After the return to team training, football players expect their team coach to provide them with a well-adapted training programme in order to avoid reinjury. Injury prevention measures are considered an essential part of team training, especially for players recovering from injury [4].

The medical staff should understand the expectations of injured players in terms of the return-to-play process. Before starting the treatment process, the football-specific goals of the player for the season, the near future or the general football career should be assessed in detail. A typical example for this important evaluation is a traumatic rupture of the meniscus, which includes the potential indication of a meniscus suture. Because of the long lay-off from football after arthroscopically meniscal repair (suture), many professional football players expect an alternative treatment option such as partial resection to be able to return to play more quickly.

Another important aspect is that the decision of football players on the time point of return to play is highly subjective. Older players are more experienced in listening to their body and in assessing their readiness to return to play than younger players. Both the objective criteria for the return-to-play process and also the subjective feeling of the football players themselves have to be considered when deciding on the time point of return to play. Thus, the team physician should be open to the opinion of the recovered player to avoid decisions made against doctor's recommendations. In junior football, a player's successful return to play after injury depends on sufficient communication between the parents and the team coach. Junior players who have not sufficiently recovered from their injury should not be enticed by family members or the team coach to return to play football. On the other hand, team coaches should be aware if players with minor injuries are overprotected by their parents. At a first glance, this aspect does not appear to be relevant; however, young football players may only advance to the elite junior level when pushing the limits in several aspects.

59.7 Expectations of Team Coaches During the Return-to-Play Process of Injured Players

After the injury of a player, team coaches have specific expectations on the player and the medical staff. As the main responsible person in a football team, the team coach has to supervise all processes concerning training sessions and matches. General rules for both players and medical staff are therefore essential:

- Team coaches need to be in close communication with the injured player and the medical staff about the healing and recovery process.
- Team coaches expect the medical staff to conduct every step of the return-to-play process according to current scientific knowledge. Moreover, team coaches expect to be informed about any complication or delay in the time point of return to play to be able to restructure seasonal planning.
- During the last stages of the return-to-play process, team coaches expect to be informed in detail about athletic, neuromotorical and football-specific skills by both medical staff and the players themselves, which is important for making decisions on players' reintegration into team training.
- Team coaches expect their players to adapt their daily routine to the specific requirements of the rehabilitation period, for instance, additional training sessions, well-balanced nutrition and learning from past mistakes. The goal for all players is come back stronger!
- Team coaches further expect players to immediately report any minor complaints and injuries during or after reintegration into team training or competition. Well-adapted return-to-play training sessions are only possible, if players regularly inform the team coach about their well-being or the occurrence of any new problems, which might increase the risk of recurrent injury. Because the majority of football coaches are former players, they are usually rather experienced with injuries. Non-verbal communication with players and subjective assessment during the training sessions are also helpful tools.

A recent study has shown that team coaches are able to provide detailed insight into ongoing return-to-play processes [10]. In the above investigation, almost all team coaches knew the neuromotorical and athletic measurements of their players, which enabled them to make decisions on the time points of return to training or return to competition. Moreover, the investigation showed that preseasonal screening tests are conducted in only approximately 50% of all elite amateur football teams.

Fact Box 5

- The team coach is the most important decision-maker in the return-to-play process after injury, once the player returns to team training.
- To understand decisions made by the team coach, injured players, medical and other staff need to know the expectations and knowledge of the team coach on the return-to-play process after injuries.
- Return-to-play decisions of team coaches are highly influenced by their own experience with injuries during their own football career.
- Football players have specific expectations on the return-to-play process, and it is the responsibility of physicians to inquire and consider the expectations of the players.
- The football-specific aims of an injured player are essential for the development of a well-adapted treatment and rehabilitation programme to reach the targeted football level.
- Medical anamnesis directly after injury is necessary to understand a player's expectations on the healing process.
- Return-to-play decisions may be influenced by the pressure of professional players to return to play football as early as possible as well as by the natural desire to play football of both professional and amateur players, which may result in premature return to play.

59.8 Decision-Making at the Different Stages of the Return-to-Play Period

The return-to-play process consists of specific stages [39], which are differently organised and managed at the various skill levels in football. Professional football clubs with their large financial power are not only able to provide a large group of experts for the return-to-play process of injured players but also high-quality medical equipment, which represents a major contrast to services available at amateur football clubs. Negative aspects of return-to-play processes in professional football are time pressure, missing or insufficient communication and the expected high physical and psychological demands on the injured player after return to play.

From football players and team coaches' point of views, return-to-play processes involve several responsibilities but also some pitfalls. To avoid problems during the return-to-play process, football teams need a structured system. While most professional football clubs have already established such a system that includes several experts who know their responsibilities in the return-to-play process, such structures are lacking in amateur football. The following figure shows the different responsibilities of football players, team coaches and medical staff in the different stages of the return-to-play process (Fig. 59.1). While medical staff, particularly the medical doctor, dominate the decision-making for the treatment, the rehabilitation period until the return to team training is dominated by medical staff members like physical therapists or athletic coaches. At the end of the return to play process, the team coach has to decide, if the former injured player is fit enough for competition.

At the end of each return-to-play stage, the decision to proceed to the next stage needs to be made. The popular phrase 'return-to-play decisions after football injuries are a team decision' is correct; however, it does often not reflect reality. The decision only represents a team decision if agreed upon by all experts. But different experts may have different points of view and suggestions at each stage of the return-to-play process.

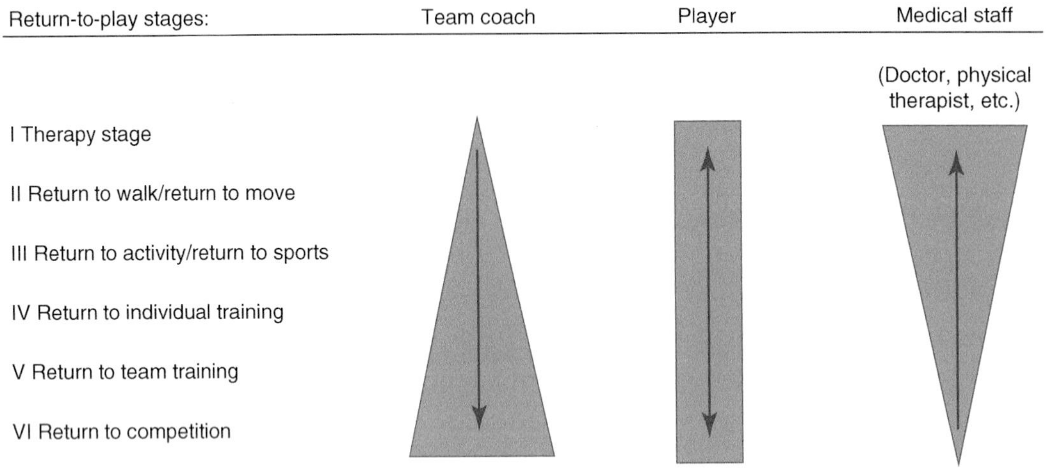

Return-to-play stages:	Team coach	Player	Medical staff
			(Doctor, physical therapist, etc.)
I Therapy stage			
II Return to walk/return to move			
III Return to activity/return to sports			
IV Return to individual training			
V Return to team training			
VI Return to competition			

Fig. 59.1 Compilation of responsibilities and main decision-making authority of the team coach and player at the different return-to-play stages

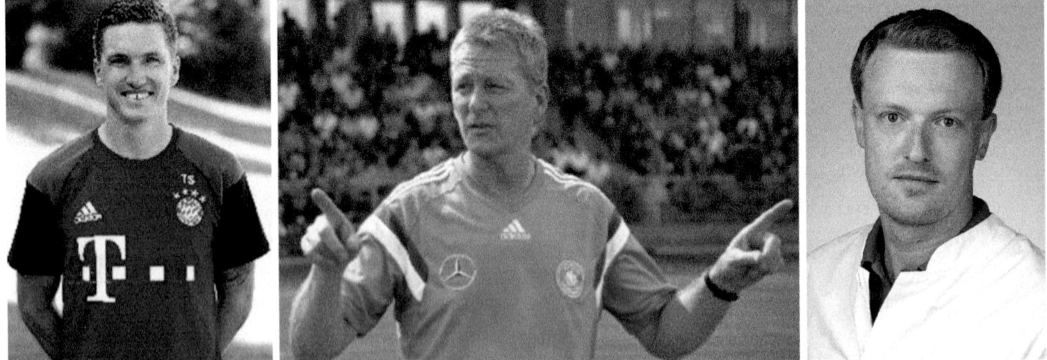

Fig. 59.2 Team coaches in amateur and professional football are head of the team (*mid picture*, FW) with closed communication to players (*left picture*, TS) and medical doctors (*right picture*, WK) regarding return-to-play decisions

In this case, the injured player needs to know who the best expert is for the different stages of the return-to-play process and who will make the final decision. The last stage, the return to competition stage is decided at all football skill levels mainly by the team coach.

At the end of any discussions about decision-making and theoretical structures, it must be clearly determined who will have the authority to make the final decision on the time point of return to play. Apart from the last decision on return-to-competition that is made by the team coach, all decisions are ultimately made by the football players themselves and all other persons just act as consultants. Only the team physician may disagree with the decision made by the team coach or the player in the case of any risk to the player's health. In such situations, the team coach should accept the professional opinion of the team physician and discuss the best decision for the player and the team with the player and the physician (Fig. 59.2). Such situations are potentially difficult with regard to team building and authority. In the case of concussion, for instance, players and team coaches have been known to press medical doctors for an earlier return to play [44]. Thus, mutual respect is absolutely essential for any discussions and decisions. Members of the medical staff need to use simple and football-adapted language to ensure that players and team coaches are able to understand the medical terms. Moreover, players and team coaches can expect team physicians and other medical staff to be familiar with the specific requirements of football. Players and team coaches should understand that the rule of medical doctors is to 'play safe' with a kind of 'fear to make mistakes'. On the other hand, physicians have to accept that always doing the right thing in terms of the return-to-play decision is not always possible and suitable in football [25]. Only close communication with players will enable medical doctors to accept a higher risk by the players for an early return to play.

Fact Box 6

- Decision-making is a team responsibility that should be based on frequent communication between the different members of the team.
- In football, responsibilities for the return-to-play process differ at the different skill levels.
- In professional football clubs with their large financial resources, all steps of the return-to-play process are conducted by an interdisciplinary group of experts in contrast to amateur football team which usually employ a team coach and a physiotherapist.
- The return-to-play decision is therefore made differently at amateur and professional football levels.
- From a practical point of view, the decision on each return-to-play stage is made by the players themselves with all experts acting as consultants.
- Only the last decision on the return-to-competition is made by the team coach.
- Players and coaches have specific expectations on medical staff, particularly at the professional football level.
- Return-to-play tests are currently under-represented in professional football and completely missing in amateur football.

Take-Home Message

In general, the phrase 'return-to-play decisions after injuries in football are team decisions' is correct. Thus, the different stages of a return-to-play process involve different experts who decide if the injured player is able to proceed to the next return-to-play stage. Football teams require clear agreements about the respective responsibilities of each member of staff and close communication among team members to guarantee a smooth return-to-play process, particularly over the course of the different return-to-play stages. Hardly any scientific evidence is available on this topic. Future scientific work in this field should include the view of team coaches and football players on the return-to-play process. Good understanding of the different professions in a football team requires simple non-technical language, a team coach knowledgeable in general medical issues and medical staff familiar with football-specific requirements.

Top Five Evidence Based References

Krutsch W, Voss A, Gerling S, Grechenig S, Nerlich M, Angele P (2014) First aid on field management in youth football. Arch Orthop Trauma Surg 134(9):1301–1309

Cunningham A (2002) An audit of first aid qualifications and knowledge among team officials in two English youth football leagues: a preliminary study. Br J Sports Med 36(4):295–300

Hägglund M, Waldén M, Ekstrand J (2007) Lower reinjury rate with a coach-controlled rehabilitation program in amateur male soccer: a randomized controlled trial. Am J Sports Med 35(9):1433–1442

Steffen K, Meeuwisse WH, Romiti M, Kang J, McKay C, Bizzini M, Dvorak J, Finch C, Myklebust G, Emery CA (2013) Evaluation of how different implementation strategies of an injury prevention programme (FIFA 11+) impact team adherence and injury risk in Canadian female youth football players: a cluster-randomised trial. Br J Sports Med 47(8):480–487

McKay CD, Steffen K, Romiti M, Finch CF, Emery CA (2014) The effect of coach and player injury knowledge, attitudes and beliefs on adherence to the FIFA 11+ programme in female youth soccer. Br J Sports Med 48(17):1281–1286

References

1. Krutsch W, Zeman F, Zellner J, Pfeifer C, Nerlich M, Angele P (2016) Increase in ACL and PCL injuries after implementation of a new professional foot-

ball league. Knee Surg Sports Traumatol Arthrosc 24(7):2271–2279
2. Schöberl M, Prantl L, Loose O, Zellner J, Angele P, Zeman F, Spreitzer M, Nerlich M, Krutsch W (2017) Non-surgical treatment of pubic overload and groin pain in amateur football players: a prospective double-blinded randomised controlled study. Knee Surg Sports Traumatol Arthrosc 25(6):1958–1966
3. Cunningham A (2002) An audit of first aid qualifications and knowledge among team officials in two English youth football leagues: a preliminary study. Br J Sports Med 36(4):295–300
4. Hägglund M, Waldén M, Ekstrand J (2007) Lower reinjury rate with a coach-controlled rehabilitation program in amateur male soccer: a randomized controlled trial. Am J Sports Med 35(9):1433–1442
5. McKay CD, Steffen K, Romiti M, Finch CF, Emery CA (2014) The effect of coach and player injury knowledge, attitudes and beliefs on adherence to the FIFA 11+ programme in female youth soccer. Br J Sports Med 48(17):1281–1286
6. Steffen K, Meeuwisse WH, Romiti M, Kang J, McKay C, Bizzini M, Dvorak J, Finch C, Myklebust G, Emery CA (2013) Evaluation of how different implementation strategies of an injury prevention programme (FIFA 11+) impact team adherence and injury risk in Canadian female youth football players: a cluster-randomised trial. Br J Sports Med 47(8):480–487
7. Chrisman SP, Schiff MA, Chung SK, Herring SA, Rivara FP (2014) Implementation of concussion legislation and extent of concussion education for athletes, parents, and coaches in Washington State. Am J Sports Med 42(5):1190–1196
8. Chung KC, Lark ME, Cederna PS (2017) Treating the football athlete: coaches' perspective from the University of Michigan. Hand Clin 33(1):1–8
9. Koch M, Zellner J, Berner A, Grechenig S, Krutsch V, Nerlich M, Angele P, Krutsch W (2015) Influence of preparation and football skill level on injury incidence during an amateur football tournament. Arch Orthop Trauma Surg 136(3):353–360
10. Loose O, Krutsch W (2017) Team coach expectations in elite football. Oral communication presented at the isokinetics conference 2016. Football medicine strategies – return to play. London, 9th–11th April 2016
11. Fuller CW, Ekstrand J, Junge A, Andersen TE, Bahr R, Dvorak J, Hägglund M, McCrory P, Meeuwisse WH (2006) Consensus statement on injury definitions and data collection procedures in studies of football (soccer) injuries. Br J Sports Med 40(3):193–201
12. Krutsch W, Voss A, Gerling S, Grechenig S, Nerlich M, Angele P (2014) First aid on field management in youth football. Arch Orthop Trauma Surg 134(9):1301–1309
13. Hall ET, Gray S, Sproule J (2015) The microstructure of coaching practice: behaviours and activities of an elite rugby union head coach during preparation and competition. J Sports Sci 34(10):896–905
14. Kaß P (2013) Die Trainertätigkeit im Profifußball – Eine multimethodale Anforderungsanalyse zur Optimierung des Fußball-Lehrer-Lehrgangs. Dissertation, Deutsche Sporthochschule Köln
15. Soligard T, Myklebust G, Steffen K, Holme I, Silvers H, Bizzini M, Junge A, Dvorak J, Bahr R, Andersen TE (2008) Comprehensive warm-up programme to prevent injuries in young female footballers: cluster randomised controlled trial. BMJ 337:a2469
16. Dvorak J (2016) 11 for coaches. Oral communication presented at the isokinetics conference 2016. Football medicine strategies – return to play. London, 9th–11th April 2016
17. Brown JC, Gardner-Lubbe S, Lambert MI, van Mechelen W, Verhagen E (2016) Coach-directed education is associated with injury-prevention behaviour in players: an ecological cross-sectional study. Br J Sports Med pii:bjsports-2016-096757
18. Gianotti S, Hume PA, Tunstall H (2010) Efficacy of injury prevention related coach education within netball and soccer. J Sci Med Sport 13(1):32–35
19. Broglio SP, Vagnozzi R, Sabin M, Signoretti S, Tavazzi B, Lazzarino G (2010) Concussion occurrence and knowledge in italian football (soccer). J Sports Sci Med 9(3):418–430
20. Kurowski B, Pomerantz WJ, Schaiper C, Gittelman MA (2014) Factors that influence concussion knowledge and self-reported attitudes in high school athletes. J Trauma Acute Care Surg 77(3 Suppl 1):S12–S17
21. Kurowski BG, Pomerantz WJ, Schaiper C, Ho M, Gittelman MA (2015) Impact of preseason concussion education on knowledge, attitudes, and behaviors of high school athletes. J Trauma Acute Care Surg 79(3 Suppl 1):S21–S28
22. Rivara FP, Schiff MA, Chrisman SP, Chung SK, Ellenbogen RG, Herring SA (2014) The effect of coach education on reporting of concussions among high school athletes after passage of a concussion law. Am J Sports Med 42(5):1197–1203
23. Onyeaso CO, Adegbesan OA (2003) Knowledge and attitudes of coaches of secondary school athletes in Ibadan, Nigeria regarding oro-facial injuries and mouthguard use by the athletes. Dent Traumatol 119(4):204–208
24. Ivarsson A, Johnson U, Podlog L (2013) Psychological predictors of injury occurrence: a prospective investigation of professional Swedish soccer players. J Sport Rehabil 22(1):19–26
25. McKinney R Jr (2016) Being right isn't always enough: NFL culture and team physicians' conflict of interest. Hast Cent Rep 46(Suppl 2):S33–S34
26. Orr B, Brown C, Hemsing J, McCormick T, Pound S, Otto D, Emery CA, Beaupre LA (2013) Female soccer knee injury: observed knowledge gaps in injury prevention among players/parents/coaches and current evidence (the KNOW study). Scand J Med Sci Sports 23(3):271–280

27. Baker JF, Devitt BM, Green J, McCarthy C (2012) Concussion among under 20 rugby union players in Ireland: incidence, attitudes and knowledge. Ir J Med Sci 182(1):121–125
28. Bramley H, Patrick K, Lehman E, Silvis M (2012) High school soccer players with concussion education are more likely to notify their coach of a suspected concussion. Clin Pediatr (Phila) 51(4):332–336
29. Junge A, Feddermann-Demont N (2016) Prevalence of depression and anxiety in top-level male and female football players. BMJ Open Sport Exerc Med 2(1):e000087
30. Angele P, Hoffmann H, Williams A, Jones M, Krutsch W (2016) Specific aspects of football in recreational and competitive sport. In: Mary HO, Zaffagnini S et al (eds) Prevention of injuries and overuse in sports. Directionary for physicians, physiotherapists, sports scientists and coaches. Springer, London, pp 117–136
31. Dvorak J, Junge A, Grimm K (2009) F-Marc-football medicine manual, 2nd edn. RVA Druck und Medien AG, Altstätten
32. Traclet A, Moret O, Ohl F, Clémence A (2015) Moral disengagement in the legitimation and realization of aggressive behavior in soccer and ice hockey. Aggress Behav 41(2):123–133
33. Hampson R, Jowett S (2012) Effects of coach leadership and coach-athlete relationship on collective efficacy. Scand J Med Sci Sports 24(2):454–460
34. Norcross MF, Johnson ST, Bovbjerg VE, Koester MC, Hoffman MA (2016) Factors influencing high school coaches' adoption of injury prevention programs. J Sci Med Sport 19(4):299–304
35. O'Brien J, Finch CF (2016) Injury prevention exercise programmes in professional youth soccer: understanding the perceptions of programme deliverers. BMJ Open Sport Exerc Med 2(1):e000075
36. Balduck AL, Jowett S (2010) Psychometric properties of the Belgian coach version of the coach-athlete relationship questionnaire (CART-Q). Scand J Med Sci Sports 20(5):779–786
37. De Backer M, Boen F, De Cuyper B, Høigaard R, VandeBroek G (2015) A team fares well with a fair coach: Predictors of social loafing in interactive female sport teams. Scand J Med Sci Sports 25(6):897–908
38. Fransen K, Vanbeselaere N, De Cuyper B, VandeBroek G, Boen F (2015) Perceived sources of team confidence in soccer and basketball. Med Sci Sports Exerc 47(7):1470–1484
39. Krutsch W, Hoffmann H (2016) Return to play nach Kreuzbandverletzungen im Fußball. Sportärztezeitung 2. Thesportgroup GmbH, Mainz, pp 28–35
40. Podlog L, Dionigi R (2010) Coach strategies for addressing psychosocial challenges during the return to sport from injury. J Sports Sci 28(11):1197–1208
41. Walden M, Hägglund M, Magnusson H et al (2011) Anterior cruciate ligament injury in elite football: a prospective three-cohort study. Knee Surg Sports Traumatol Arthrosc 19:11–19
42. Ekstrand J, Hägglund M, Törnqvist H, Kristenson K, Bengtsson H, Magnusson H, Waldén M (2013) Upper extremity injuries in male elite football players. Knee Surg Sports Traumatol Arthrosc 21(7):1626–1632
43. Manley AJ, Greenlees IA, Smith MJ, Batten J, Birch PD (2014) The influence of coach reputation on the behavioral responses of male soccer players. Scand J Med Sci Sports 24(2):e111–e120
44. Kroshus E, Baugh CM, Daneshvar DH, Stamm JM, Laursen RM, Austin SB (2015) Pressure on sports medicine clinicians to prematurely return collegiate athletes to play after concussion. J Athl Train 50(9):944–951

Return to Play: Team Doctor Roles and Ethics

60

Ricard Pruna, Matilda Lundblad, and Khatija Bahdur

Contents

R. Pruna, M.D., Ph.D. (✉)
FC Barcelona Medical Services, FIFA Medical Excellence Center,
Av Once de setembre S/N, St Joan Despi, 07980 Barcelona, Spain
e-mail: ricard.pruna@fcbarcelona.cat

M. Lundblad
Department of Orthopaedics, Sahlgrenska University, Gothenburg, Sweden
e-mail: matildalundblad@gmail.com

K. Bahdur
Department of Human Movement Science, University of Zululand, Kwadlangezwa, South Africa
e-mail: bahdurk@unizulu.ac.za

60.1 Introduction

Injury management is a vital aspect of football medicine. The final stage of the process where it is determined when players should return to training and more importantly when they are able to return to play is a key stage in the process. Players are required to return as early as possible to enable them to contribute to the team performance. At the same time, it is important that the return is not premature as this can result in setbacks in the recovery process, recurrence of the injury, and increased likelihood of further injuries.

So where are we going? It is not and may not be a guessing game. Taking into account the latest scientific publications, the study of the RTP has made limited progress [1–3]. Today only few studies are addressing the situation properly and are focusing on the reality of football [4].

This leads to two key questions:

1. In what way do we assess RTP today?
2. How should we understand the RTP process?

Is RTP merely used as a static step composed of a series of issues that must be fulfilled when the injured player has reached the final recovery stage, or is it a constant decision-making process? Every decision starting with those made at the beginning of the injury process affects the final RTP criteria [5]. The first decision leads to the next, and they turn into a network of deci-

V. Musahl et al. (eds.), *Return to Play in Football*, https://doi.org/10.1007/978-3-662-55713-6_60

sions that imply a long process where the different variables interact. But, which are the variables?

1. A correct diagnosis
2. A strict control of the physical loading during the recovery process
3. A well-planned management of the sport risk modifiers and decision modifiers

In order to fully understand and explain these variables in depth, it is important to stress that RTP has to be understood as a dynamic and personalized process. The main objective is to reduce the risk of reinjuries and not to exactly predict the RTP in terms of time. It is important to note that this is not a guessing game. During a dynamic process, there are lots of different factors that interact and modify the final result.

60.2 A Correct Diagnosis

A common and serious mistake in the RTP is incorrect diagnosis. It is related to incorrect and badly planned decisions about the injury and has influence on the final results [6]. Accordingly, it is important to understand that RTP is influenced from the beginning of the recovery process.

A correct diagnosis is the most relevant step in RTP; it is in fact the cornerstone in this process. We cannot rely only on the MRI, or GPS alone, but must consider all parts together with clinical symptoms, and we must understand that all those are an important part in the decision-making process.

In reference to the diagnosis, many variables must be taken into account when dealing with football-related. Anatomical variability and different healing capacity of connective tissues, such as tendon, muscles, and fasciae [7–9], are important to define when dealing with a muscle injury [10]. Thus, it must be born in mind that tendon healing [11] is much different compared with muscle repair. It is also important to differentiate between first-time injury and reinjury up to the point where the player may have a chronic problem.

Fact Box 1

What is the role of MRI in RTP?

It is agreed that MRI is not a useful tool in the final criteria of RTP (Reurink, 2015; Reurink, 2014), but it is very useful in the diagnostic evaluation (Petersen, 2014). Several injuries must be treated by surgery without delay immediately, and if the clinicians are not skilled in interpreting the MRI and clinical symptoms, the final RTP prediction will be inaccurate (Moen, 2014).

The following three topics need to be carefully monitored:

- Early weight-bearing
- ROM exercises
- Quadriceps and hamstring muscle strengthening

Return to play should be considered when quadriceps and hamstring strength has reached 90% or more of the contralateral side, physical examination demonstrates a stable ligament with a firm endpoint, and the player has regained physical function and psychological readiness to return.

It is important to differentiate the recovery process based on the exact needs of the injured player and carefully monitor the progress of rehabilitation and the impact an injury may have had on the overall fitness and mobility but also to provide lifestyle and dietary advice that may enhance the recovery process. It is also the responsibility of the medical team to ensure that players do not take harmful or banned substances in their quest to facilitate RTP.

60.3 Strict Controls of Tissue Load

RTP is determined by several issues. While the range of definitions of RTP is wide, the most appropriate concept in RTP definition [12] is full availability to train and participate in matches. Also, the training phase has to be understood as a part of the recovery process. There are several goals to consider before making the decision that it is time to return to play. These include:

- Reaching a pre-injury level
- Completion of a rehabilitation program
- Full activity and availability for training sessions

These concepts require further definition.

What does the pre-injury level mean? Is it a point where the player is always 100% healthy?

Who can state that the player at the pre-injury level was healthy and free of injuries [13–15]?

Taking the pre-injury level into account, it is important to understand whether the pre-injury level was a possible risk factor for injury. This is in most cases more relevant for noncontact injuries. Often the pre-injury level was a part of an incomplete adaptation to a complete injury recovery, which might indicate that the player was already at risk. Would the player have been less likely to suffer the injury if his/her pre-injury condition was better? Was there an indication that the player was at risk for a specific injury? Was the injury related to a loss of strength? And if the player had deficits in terms of muscle strength, what was the cause? There are many possible factors that can result in a player ending up with an increased risk of injury. The type of injury and reason for strength deficits and loss of flexibility are key factors in determining RTP [13]. Some of the points to consider are found in Table 60.1.

Customizing training loads is the second key component in RTP [16]. Football has become more scientific requiring players and coaches to adapt to the "new sport" quickly. Some strategies and coaching methods are obviously outdated. Most of the exercises, included as a secondary prevention, don't have any preventive effect and most of the time just overload the muscles. Therefore, it is imperative to discuss changing the concept of prevention. The goal should not be seen as prevention per se, but instead the concept of "adaptation" should be introduced.

Table 60.1 Possible causes of increased injury risk

Question to ask	Example
Training deficit	During the training sessions, certain muscles were not loaded appropriately
Wrong periodization based on competition schedules	Were players given enough time to recover following high- intensity training sessions or match-days?
Preventive exercises causing overloading	• Prescribing resistance training exercises that are too intense or not appropriate when considering other training • Creating an imbalance in contralateral muscles

Muscle strain injury should not be understood as a mechanical disruption of healthy tissue, but as series of aberrant adaptive responses that, over time, will not allow the tissue to adapt to increased loads and stress. There have been numerous advances in the understanding of the human body functioning. This has led to new methods and ideologies in terms of structure, type, and intensity of training, with the aim of maximizing football performance but at the same time also maintaining player health.

Medical teams should do what is possible to enhance their functioning and create an understanding for some of the decisions taken by educating players and technical teams. They should simplify concepts and communicate both short- and long-term goals and also the risks that might be the result of the decisions they make [17]. Educating all other stakeholders related to the development of rehabilitation of a specific player highlights the practical implications, and a benefit for them is important.

A static assessment of a player's skills, regardless of the specific sport environment, is a new challenge that sports physicians must face. Important information is no longer only derived from the medical room. Apart from clinical examination and MRI, attesting on the training field, for instance, using GPS [18–20], is considered important by many medical and technical teams in personalizing the progress of the injury and obtaining a solid framework to validate the

RTP and in the assessment, monitoring, and management of soft tissue loading. Technology to control workloads provides a lot of data, and physicians must validate what might be useful in determining the fit profile, which is the profile obtained by collecting data from every training and match when the player is absolutely healthy and in an optimal physical state.

There are different profiles within a team: with predominant acceleration, deceleration, or combination of both. This implies that different RTPs depend on the specific skills of the player. The variables collected daily from trainings and matches will help to shape the state of the player, where the most important are acceleration, deceleration, high-speed running (HSR), HML, sprints, and step balance. In this way, we are able to know what the individual player's characteristics are and then enhance the individual fit profile.

60.4 Individual Fit Profile (Fig. 60.1)

Tracking these variables long-term creates a full profile of each individual player based on his/her individual characteristics and can help identify the state where they are most vulnerable to injuries, burnout, or overtraining and help to understand the recovery progress better. During the recovery process, adapted circuits are focused on the objective that is needed to reach. They are different depending on whether the objective is speed or strength.

The use of on-field technology enables assessments of whether the player is ready not only for intense physical activity but also for intense activity against an opponent and can provide psychological input by analyzing hesitation on the part of the player and whether they are willing to push the body to the maximum. This could indicate fear of reinjury and lack of confidence to be able to last through the competition. These psychological variables could become manifest in physical symptoms, such as slower reaction times and increased muscle tension, which could also act as an injury risk in itself (Fig. 60.2).

60.5 Intelligent Management of Modifiers

The rules of different sports affect the return to play to a large extent; in football you need to be fully recovered from an injury, whereas in handball or basketball, you could start playing earlier because these sports allow frequent changes of players during the competition [21, 22].

Return to play does not necessarily dictate that a player must begin and end their first match after return. The laws of football enable the use of substitutions, which gives teams the opportunity to introduce a player gradually back into play and ensure that the strain and load is not too high, too soon.

For this reason we can assume that RTP criteria could evolve in parallel with possible new rules in the future. Physicians must be involved in the sport and have a deep knowledge of the environment to be able to manage intelligently the decisions made together with a player, technical staff, and coaches, and the physician's acquired experience will increasingly depend on this knowledge.

Already there is attention to immediate care of injuries sustained during matches. Referees must be educated to identify immediate risks and know when to stop the play and give the medical team immediate access to an injured player on the field. There are guidelines that decide how to handle players who may have suffered a concussion, but further input is required from doctors to ensure that player safety is always included as part of the laws of the game and tournament rules.

60.6 Ethics Aspects Related to RTP

Medical teams are employed by the football club to meet the requirements and needs of the club but at the same time are required to fulfill their obligations and to act in the interest of the player. These interests are sometimes not exactly the same. This means ensuring both the short- and the long-term welfare of the player in an environ-

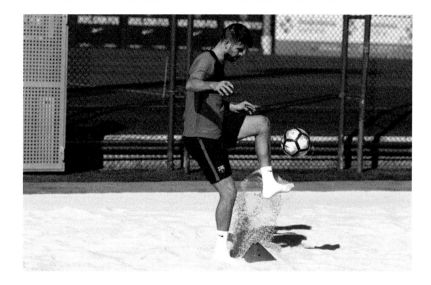

Fig. 60.1 Assessing fit profile within the recovery process

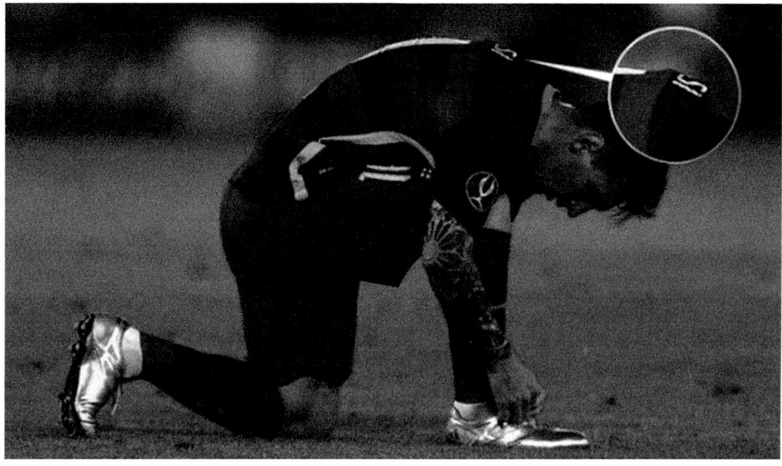

Fig. 60.2 Collecting data from training and competition is key point in the final RTP decision

ment where there is constant pressure from all parties to ensure that the most important players are always available and there might be demand for premature return to play. This can result in a conflict of interest, where the medical team becomes emotionally involved and has the same desire to win trophies and be a part of a successful club, as opposed to where it may be detrimental to the long-term health of the players, even though absence of the player could compromise the team's success. Medical teams must find the best balance and a way to ensure both success and health within the team structure. This can be compromised by the player's desire to return prematurely to play [2, 23–27].

Patient autonomy dictates that the player has the rights over his/her body, and it is his/her decision when to play even if the player is still injured. Autonomy is linked to informed consent and ensures that players are part of the discussion when deciding if they are ready to return. However, players often make their decisions not only from a medical perspective but also influenced by internal and external pressure, the importance of the competition, the opportunity to maintain place in starting lineup, financial benefits, games leading to international call-ups, etc. Autonomy is often balanced by the benefits where a player would be entitled to the best possible medical treatment. This indicates that regardless of the consequences, medical teams must always act in the interest of the player using his/her experience and knowledge to make the best medical decision [2, 23–26, 28].

One of the other key ethical issues in terms of RTP is confidentiality. It is important that the details of the medical conditions of players are known only to those who need the information (such as the technical team) and permission from the player is respected. Given the popularity of football, there will always be a discussion about the relationship with the media and the fans, but it is important that the needs and rights of the player are well respected and that they are in the first place [2, 23–26, 28].

60.7 Club Versus Country

Players who represent their countries at international level can be exposed to two different medical teams who may have different ways of working. This means that the level of care might not be the same. Often international players are required to stay with their international team for 10 days (excluding international tournaments such as World Cup, European Championships, Copa America, AFCON). This can result in international federations being more willing to rush players' return to play to ensure that the national team get the benefit of the player while looking at the fact that should the player have any reinjury or setbacks with his/her recovery, it becomes the problem of the club. It is important that national teams manage the players properly both in terms of training loads and injury management. They should continuously be in contact with the club personnel and inform about injuries, irrespective of minor or major, and the risks to ensure that they manage each individual according to his/her requirements.

60.8 Where to Go Next?

As with other aspects of football, the concept, timing, and principles of RTP will continue to evolve. Research and information sharing will in future play a key role in developing the foundation of RTP at all levels of football. The big data concept is going to help in the future, because physicians will be able to share the medical experience from different environments and different countries and use it to improve the knowledge specially the issues used for RTP criteria [29–32].

Take Home Message

- The RTP decision-making process should be understood as dynamic, focusing on avoiding reinjuries and not on predicting the exact RTP time.
- On-field technology can be very useful as it may personalize the process of decision- making, and will do it even more in the near future, but the clinical experience is valuable and the knowledge of the environment of the football is important as well.
- Decisions in terms of RTP must be ethical and protect the rights and well-being of the player involved.
- It is important to consider possible new rules in football that could influence the RTP decision-making process, in the same way modifiers are considered.

Top Five Evidence Based References

Börjesson M, Karlsson J (2014) Ethical dilemmas faced by the team physician: overlooked in sports medicine education? Br J Sports Med 48:1398–1399

Creighton DW, Shrier I, Shultz R et al (2010) Return to play in sport: a decision-based model. Clin J Sport Med 20(5):379–385

Herring SA, Kibler WB, Putukian M (2012) The team physician and the return-to-play decision: a consensus statement. Med Sci Sports Exerc 44(12):2446–2448

Malcolm D, Scott A (2014) Practical responses to confidentiality dilemmas in elite sport medicine. Br J Sports Med 48:1410–1413

Tenford AS, Fredericson M (2015) Athlete return-to-play decisions in sport medicine. AMA J Ethics 17(6):511–514

References

1. Creighton DW, Shrier I, Shultz R et al (2010) Return to play in sport: a decision-based model. Clin J Sport Med 20(5):379–385

2. Matheson GO, Schultz R, Bido J, Mitten MJ, Meeuwisse WH, Shrier I (2011) Return-to-play decisions: are they the team physician's responsibility? Clin J Sport Med 21(1):25–30
3. Miller MD, Arciero RA, Cooper DE et al (2009) Doc, when can he go back to the game? Instr Course Lect 58:437–443
4. Delvaux F, Rochcongar P, Bruyère O et al (2014) Return to play criteria after hamstring injury: actual medicine practice in professional soccer teams. J Sport Sci Med 13(3):721–723
5. Orchard J, Best TM, Verrall GM (2005) Return to play following muscle strains. Clin J Sport Med 15(6):436–441
6. Heiderscheit BC, Sherry MA, Silder A et al (2010) Hamstring strain injuries: recommendations for diagnosis, rehabilitation, and injury prevention. J Orthop Sport Clin Ther 4:67–81
7. Danna NR, Beutel BG, Campbell KA et al (2014) Therapeutic approaches to skeletal muscle repair and healing. Sport Health 6(4):348–355
8. Järvinen TA, Kääriäinen M, Järvinen M et al (2000) Muscle strain injuries. CurrOpinRheumatol 12(2):155–161
9. Silder A, Heiderscheit BC, Thelen DG et al (2008) MRI observations of long-term musculotendon remodeling following a hamstring strain injury. Skelet Radiol 37:1101–1109
10. Garrett WE Jr (1996) Muscle strain injuries. Am J Sport Med 24(6 Suppl):S2–S8
11. Voleti PB, Buckley MR, Soslowsky LJ (2012) Tendon healing: repair and regeneration. Annu Rev Biomed Eng 14:47–71
12. Hallén A, Ekstrand J (2014) Return to play following muscle injuries in professional footballers. J Sport Sci 32(13):1229–1236
13. Askling C, Saartok T, Thorstensson A (2006) Type of acute hamstring strain affects flexibility, strength, and time to return to pre-injury level. Br J Sport Med 40:40–44
14. Müller U, Krüger-Franke M, Schmidt M et al (2014) Predictive parameters to return to pre-injury level of sport 6 months following anterior cruciate ligament reconstruction surgery. Knee Surg Sports Traumatol Arthrosc 23(12):3623–3631. (Epub ahead of print)
15. Tol JL, Hamilton B, Eirale C et al (2014) At return to play following hamstring injury the majority of professional football players have residual isokinetic deficits. Br J Sports Med 48(18):1364–1369
16. Opar DA, Williams MD, Shield AJ (2012) Hamstring strain injuries: factors that lead to injury and re-injury. Sports Med 42(3):209–226
17. Herring SA, Kibler WB, Putukian M (2012) The team physician and the return-to-play decision: a consensus statement. Med Sci Sports Exerc 44(12):2446–2448
18. Dellaserra CL, Gao Y, Ransdell L (2014) Use of integrated technology in team sports: a review of opportunities, challenges, and future directions for athletes. J Strength Cond Res 28(2):556–573
19. Dogramac SN, Watsford ML, Murphy AJ (2011) The reliability and validity of subjective notational analysis in comparison to global positioning systems tracking to assess athlete movement patterns. J Strength Cond Res 25:852–859
20. Reid LC, Cowman JR, Green BS et al (2013) Return to play in elite rugby union: application of global positioning systems technology in return to play running programs. J Sport Rehabil 22(2):122–129
21. Verstegen M, Falsohne S, Orr R et al (2012) Suggestion from the field for return to sports participation following anterior cruciate ligament reconstruction: American football. J Orthop Sports Phys Ther 42(4):337–344
22. Waters E (2012) Suggestions from the field for return to sports participation following anterior cruciate ligament reconstruction: basketball. J Orthop Sports Phys Ther 42(4):326–336
23. Börjesson M, Karlsson J (2014) Ethical dilemmas faced by the team physician: overlooked in sports medicine education? Br J Sports Med 48:1398–1399
24. Burgess T (2011) Ethical issues in return-to-sport decisions. SAJSM 23(4):138–139
25. Dunn WR, George MS, Churchill L, Spindler KP (2007) Ethics in sports medicine. Am J Sports Med 35(5):840–844
26. Leglise M (2011) Return to competition, medical, legal, and ethical considerations. Available online at http://www.fig-gymnastics.com/site/files/page/editor/files/Medical-Retour%20a%20la%20competition-e.pdf (Accessed 27 July 2016)
27. Malcolm D, Scott A (2014) Practical responses to confidentiality dilemmas in elite sport medicine. Br J Sport Med 48:1410–1413
28. Tenford AS, Fredericson M (2015) Athlete return-to-play decisions in sport medicine. AMA J Ethics 17(6):511–514
29. Moen MH, Reurink G, weir A et al (2014) Predicting return to play after hamstring injuries. Br J Sports Med 48(18):1358–1363
30. Petersen J, Thorborg K, Nielsen MB et al (2014) The diagnostic and prognostic value of ultrasonography in soccer players with acute hamstring injuries. Am J Sports Med 42(2):399–404
31. Reurink G, Brilman EG, de Vos JR et al (2015) Magnetic resonance imaging in acute hamstring injuries: can we provide a return to play prognosis? Sports Med 45(1):133–146
32. Reurink G, Goudswaard GJ, Tol JL et al (2014) MRI observations and return to play of clinically recovered hamstring injuries. Br J Sport Med 48(18):1370–1376

Ethical Issues in Return to Play: RTP in Football: An Evidence-Based Approach

61

Philip Batty

Contents

61.1 Introduction

What do we mean by clinical judgement? Mosby's Medical Dictionary defines clinical judgement as "the application of information based on actual observation of a patient combined with objective and subjective data that lead to a conclusion [1]".

P. Batty
Isokinetic Medical Centre,
11 Harley Street, London, UK

University College, London, UK
e-mail: p.batty@isokinetic.com

The "actual observation" in a consultation consists of a history and clinical examination. There may be additional information from any number of diagnostic tests, such as blood, saliva, urine, imaging, heart rate, physical tests and GPS data.

As science advances with the advent of more diagnostic investigations, there has been a devaluation in the role of clinical judgement [2]. It appears that practitioner experience, history taking and clinical evaluation are valued less than investigations that are of more "scientific value". The practitioner working in football is asked much more infrequently "What is your opinion?" in place of "What does the scan show?"

Fact Box 1
We treat the player, not the scan!

With the exception of a few conditions, such as fracture to the cervical spine without spinal cord injury and abnormal cardiac screening, there is inherent danger in treating the investigation rather than the player. Imaging often reveals incidental findings of no clinical significance (3), and this can lead to unnecessary surgical intervention with increased risk of adverse events [3–5].

Nonetheless, we yearn for scientific clarity regarding the practice of football medicine.

V. Musahl et al. (eds.), *Return to Play in Football*, https://doi.org/10.1007/978-3-662-55713-6_61

Science, when researched correctly, is truth. Science not only confirms a hypothesis, but is robust to attempts to disprove the hypothesis. Patients and practitioners want to benefit from scientific advances to improve health and performance; however, the practice of history taking and clinical evaluation is very difficult to measure and validate. Whilst the sensitivity and specificity of clinical examination is studied and reported, we do not have high-quality scientific measuring tools to evaluate history and clinical evaluation [6].

61.2 Can We Quantify Return to Play Criteria?

Return to play requires a player to have appropriate aerobic and anaerobic fitness, strength, co-ordination and the ability to tackle, head, land, pass, shoot and move at high speed in multiple directions, with additional diving, catching and landing for goalkeepers. There is no single investigation or combination of investigations that can scientifically assess all these demands. These movements are performed on a field and need to be evaluated in the same environment in order to be valid [7]. Clinical judgement for return to play cannot be performed in the confines of a clinic or office.

Return to play decisions depend on where the injury was sustained and can be time dependent:

1. During a match
   The only tools a medical team will have at this time are observing the mechanism of injury (occasionally with the benefit of video feedback), the history from the player (if he or she is conscious) or other observers together with the clinical examination. The decision here is whether the player can continue to play. The decision is often time critical in a competitive environment because the team is weakened by the loss of a player if the assessment is protracted.
2. During training
   Any injury during training is usually away from medical diagnostic services, and a decision to resume training is dependent on history and clinical evaluation, as with a match; however, this is less time critical and the medical practitioner can take longer to perform their assessment.
3. Return from injury
   A player may have an injury that requires absence from training and possibly matches, of either short- or long-term duration. There is opportunity for the use of diagnostics to assist clinical assessment.

In the first two scenarios, the decision to return to play has to be entirely clinical. There are no investigations available, and a decision has to be made in a short period.

The third scenario affords the opportunity to perform diagnostic investigations. The importance of the diagnostic tests regarding the management will depend on the education and experience of the practitioner, but also there are external factors that can influence. It can be difficult to justify a plan based on history and clinical examination if the diagnostic investigations do not offer concordance. The first principle in a return to play decision requires an accurate diagnosis or diagnostic hypothesis, and if other members of the multidisciplinary medical team are not behind the plan, this can cause problems. The player should be at the centre of a multidisciplinary medical team with good clear communication around him. If there are any weaknesses in the communication around the player, this can cause lack of confidence from the player and coaching team, with potential adverse effects.

61.3 The Rehabilitation Ladder and Decision-Making Model

The rehabilitation principles for return to play are defined [7]. For the large majority of injuries that are musculoskeletal, these are (Fig. 61.1):

1. Reduction of pain and swelling
2. Restoration of joint mobility and range of motion
3. Recovery of muscle strength and endurance
4. Recovery of co-ordination
5. Recovery of football-specific skills and movement

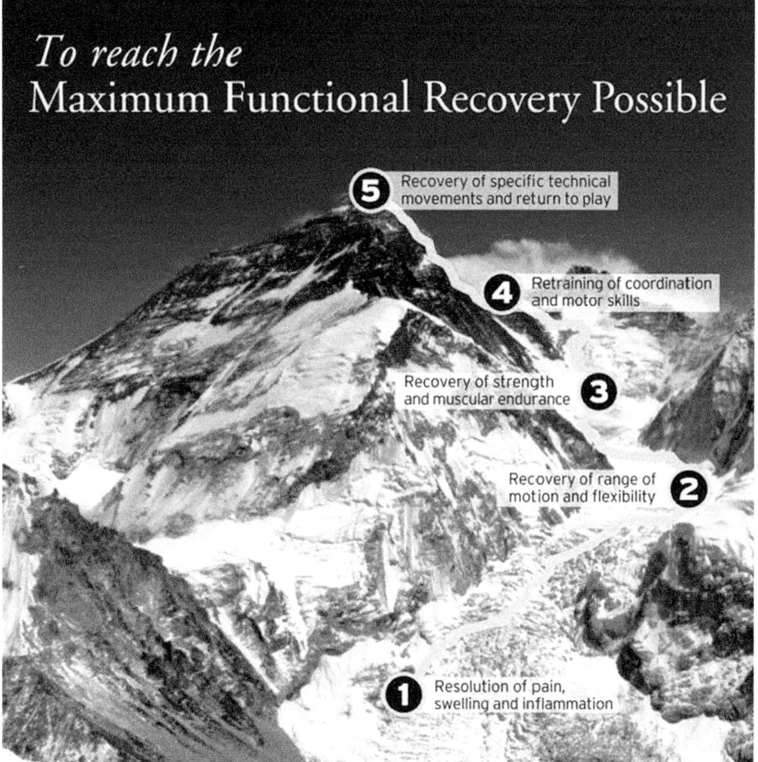

Fig. 61.1 Five phases of rehabilitation leading to maximal functional recovery possible

There are decision-making models for return to play [8, 9]. Creighton outlines the competing factors that can affect a decision on return to play [8] (Fig. 61.2).

61.4 Is Return to Play Science or Art?

Whilst scientific validation is desirable and should be our ultimate goal, this model highlights the limitations of our current scientific method on the decisions required. Any scientific study with such a range of competing interests and potential for bias would be quickly discredited. The great majority of the decision-making model is based on clinical judgement, with value-driven modifiers.

We should, therefore, consider how much of the decision on return to play is science? Cosmacini states that: "Medicine is not a science, but a practice based on science that operates in a world of values [10]". This is consistent with the approach required for return to play. Kelly et al. state "Values infuse evidence (in all sciences) at many levels [11]. Evidence based medicine (EBM), like all science, is necessarily value-laden. Not only is eliminating values from the scientific method—in general and the EBM process in particular—impossible, but in trying to do so, researchers may introduce new (mostly covert and unacknowledged) biases".

The problem with values, however, is that from an individual (practitioner, player, coach, board member) or team (organisational) perspective, this is different from person to person or team to team, and this has an effect on clinical judgement.

There are ethical challenges for the doctor working in a professional environment that are outlined in a previous section. This can affect clinical judgement, which is open to interpretation and can also vary from person to person depending on experience, training, knowledge, pressure and values. In the absence of a good scientific tool to validate the clinical judgement, it is

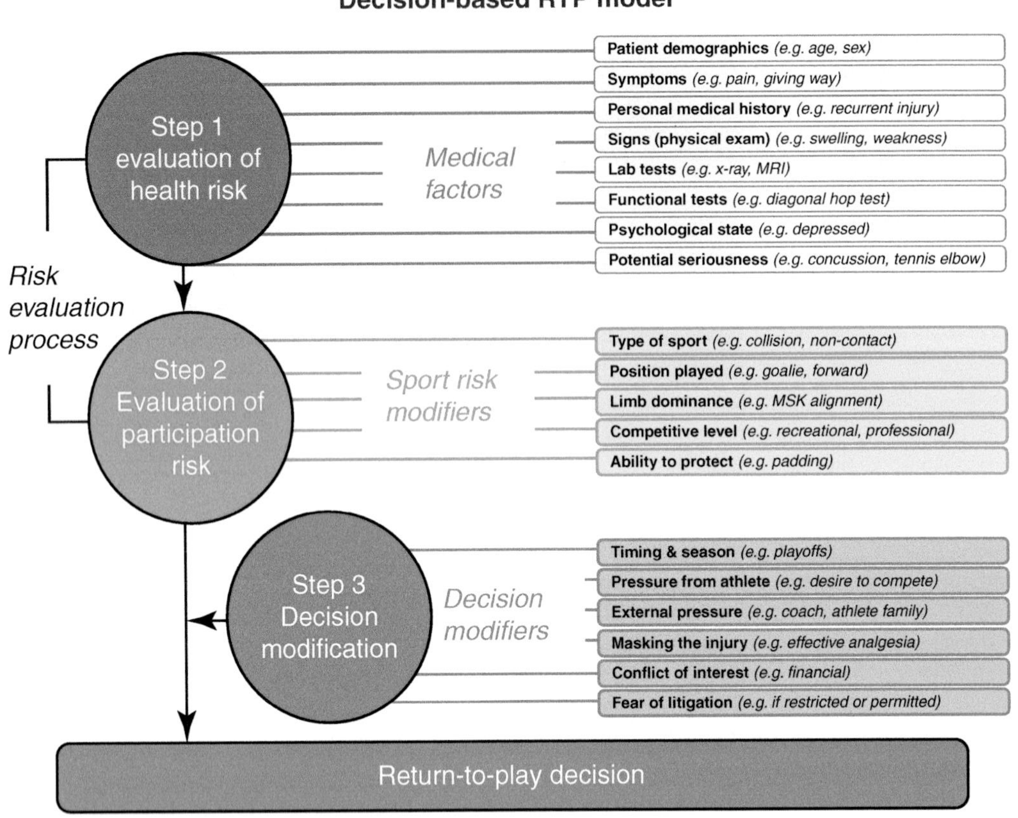

Fig. 61.2 Return to play decision-making model (Adapted from Creighton et al. [8])

legitimate to try to validate that decision with an investigation such as imaging. This can often assist with the communication and commitment to the recovery plan by the player and coach by providing additional information. There is, however, an important distinction between requesting imaging to support a clinical hypothesis and requesting an investigation blindly. It is imperative to assist any radiologist by asking appropriate questions and offering appropriate clinical findings in order to confirm the clinical hypothesis [2–4]. The usefulness of a radiological examination can be reduced if the clinical background and the specific problem to be answered are not provided with the request [12].

There needs to be a renaissance in accepting clinical judgement on return to play, as ultimately the decision is almost entirely clinical [2]. Whilst the evidence for orthopaedic surgery and sports medicine is so poor, there needs to be much more scientific scrutiny and research to support clinical judgement [4, 13]. Practitioners employed by professional clubs may be open to "employer bias", in much the same way as researchers can be affected by funding from the pharmaceutical industry. The practitioner's first duty is to the patient; however, clinical judgement is open to error and mistakes justified by cognitive dissonance [14]. It is, therefore, imperative that the player (patient) is fully informed of any medical treatment and rehabilitation goals and is involved in all decisions unless they lack mental capacity to do so, such as with concussion [15].

The management of concussion over the years is an example where clinical judgement has been possibly suppressed even with scientific evidence of the potential for long-term harm due to chronic traumatic encephalopathy [16]. The management of concussion is an example of the need for clinical judgement operating within scientific validated protocols for player safety. There are a number of investigations that may become more useful in the confirmation of the diagnosis of concussion and possibly the degree of concussion; however, the diagnosis and management is currently based on clinical observations and findings [15].

61.5 Mitigating Against Clinical Judgement Bias

How can the practitioner mitigate against the potential inherent bias of clinical judgement? This involves putting the player at the centre of the decision-making process regarding his injury management and a multidisciplinary medical and science team approach. Shared decision making is consistent with good medical practice [17].

This model of care can challenge previous perceived need for surgery for injury and reduce the time to return to play [18]. Albeit that the practice of shared decision-making is difficult to fully validate scientifically from a patient outcome perspective, it is still considered good practice [19, 20].

At the professional level, a player may trust his or her agent (without medical training) as their advocate more than the medical team employed by the club. It may be helpful to therefore consult a respected opinion more independent of the club to ensure consistency of information and risk assessment.

Where a multidisciplinary medical and science team are available for the player, there should be mutual respect and co-operation. The team should be focussed on clinical and performance issues. This involves shared decision-making between the team, so there is a consistent message, method and approach. All members should agree that the player is fit to return, together with any external consultant (such as a surgeon if recovering from surgery). Whilst clubs employ more medical and science staff, the scientific evidence of return to play remains very poor [13, 21].

Ultimately the final decision on return to play should rest with the player when he or she is confident that they have recovered and completed the five phases of rehabilitation, including on-field activities to test appropriate football-specific movements and skills before resuming competitive action. When the player is available for selection, the coach is responsible for team selection but may require advice on load management.

61.6 The Future

We face a dichotomy. We wish to offer the best care to players by offering up-to-date evidence-based medicine to support return to play at the optimum time. This discourages practice based on impressions, arrogance or exclusively economic consideration. The practice of return to play has poor scientific validation, and we should all encourage and support more research in this area for the benefit of players. Nonetheless, to use bad science to usurp the power of clinical judgement is counterproductive to the best interests of patients.

Fanos uses a formula to suggest the future of medicine:

FM = EBM + MBE + OBM + NBM

where FM is the future of medicine, EBM is evidence-based medicine, MBM is medicine-based evidence (evidence based on clinical experience, what has been learned by practice from patient and case exposure), OBM is omics-based medicine (medicine based on the omics technologies) and NBM is narrative-based medicine (the importance of communication and medical humanities) [10].

Current practices regarding decisions on return to play are largely dominated by the least scientific numerators of Fanos' formula, namely, medicine-based evidence (eminent-based evidence) and narrative-based medicine, which are the major features of clinical judgement. It is to be hoped this proportion will reduce with advances in evidence-based medicine and omics-based medicine.

Take-Home Message

The scientific evidence for return to play is poor. More research is needed.

Clinical judgement is undervalued, but remains the major decision-making process of return to play.

Practitioners should be wary of devaluing clinical judgement in place of poor scientifically validated investigations or tools.

Top Five Evidence Based References

Creighton DW, Shrier I, Shultz R, Meeuwisse WH, Matheson GO (2010) Return-to-play in sport: a decision-based model. Clin J Sport Med 20(5): 379–385

Dijkstra HP, Pollock N, Chakraverty R, Alonso JM (2014) Managing the health of the elite athlete: a new integrated performance health management and coaching model. Br J Sports Med 48(7):523–531

Kelly MP, Heath I, Howick J, Greenhalgh T (2015) The importance of values in evidence-based medicine. BMC Med Ethics 16(1):69

Kienle GS, Kiene H (2011) Clinical judgement and the medical profession. J Eval Clin Pract 17(4):621–627

McCartney M, Treadwell J, Maskrey N, Lehman R (2016) Making evidence based medicine work for individual patients. BMJ 353:i2452. https://doi.org/10.1136/bmj.i2452

References

1. Mosby, Inc (2009) Mosby's medical dictionary, 8th edn. Mosby, Edinburgh
2. Kienle GS, Kiene H (2011) Clinical judgement and the medical profession. J Eval Clin Pract 17(4):621–627
3. Brinjikji W, Luetmer PH, Comstock B, Bresnahan BW, Chen LE, Deyo RA, Halabi S, Turner JA, Avins AL, James K, Wald JT, Kallmes DF, Jarvik JG (2015) Systematic literature review of imaging features of spinal degeneration in asymptomatic populations. AJNR Am J Neuroradiol 36(4):811–816
4. Harris IA (2016) Surgery, the ultimate placebo: a surgeon cuts through the evidence. NewSouth, Sydney
5. Roos EM, Thorlund JB (2017) It is time to stop meniscectomy. Br J Sports Med 51(6):490–491
6. Reiman MP, Goode AP, Hegedus EJ, Cook CE, Wright AA (2013) Diagnostic accuracy of clinical tests of the hip: a systematic review with meta-analysis. Br J Sports Med 47(14):893–902
7. Della Villa S, Boldrini L, Ricci M, Danelon F, Snyder-Mackler L, Nanni G, Roi GS (2012) Clinical outcomes and return-to-sports participation of 50 soccer players after anterior cruciate ligament reconstruction through a sport-specific rehabilitation protocol. Sports Health 4(1):17–24
8. Creighton DW, Shrier I, Shultz R, Meeuwisse WH, Matheson GO (2010) Return-to-play in sport: a decision-based model. Clin J Sport Med 20(5):379–385
9. Dijkstra HP, Pollock N, Chakraverty R, Alonso JM (2014) Managing the health of the elite athlete: a new integrated performance health management and coaching model. Br J Sports Med 48(7):523–531
10. Fanos V (2016) Metabolomics and microbiomics : personalized medicine from the fetus to the adult, 1st edn. Academic Press, London
11. Kelly MP, Heath I, Howick J, Greenhalgh T (2015) The importance of values in evidence-based medicine. BMC Med Ethics 16(1):69
12. Davis A (2007) Making the best use of clinical radiology services: referral guidelines, 6th edn. Royal College of Radiologists, London
13. Lohmander LS, Roos EM (2016) The evidence base for orthopaedics and sports medicine: scandalously poor in parts. Br J Sports Med 50(9):564–565
14. Tavris C, Aronson E (2015) Mistakes were made (but not by me): why we justify foolish beliefs, bad decisions, and hurtful acts. Mariner Books, Boston
15. McCrory P, Meeuwisse WH, Aubry M, Cantu B, Dvorak J, Echemendia RJ, Engebretsen L, Johnston K, Kutcher JS, Raftery M, Sills A, Benson BW, Davis GA, Ellenbogen RG, Guskiewicz K, Herring SA, Iverson GL, Jordan BD, Kissick J, McCrea M, McIntosh AS, Maddocks D, Makdissi M, Purcell L, Putukian M, Schneider K, Tator CH, Turner M (2013) Consensus statement on concussion in sport: the 4th international conference on concussion in sport held in Zurich, November 2012. Br J Sports Med 47(5):250–258
16. Fainaru-Wada M, Fainaru S (2014) League of denial: the NFL, concussions, and the battle for truth, 1st edn. Three Rivers Press, New York
17. McCartney M, Treadwell J, Maskrey N, Lehman R (2016) Making evidence based medicine work for individual patients. BMJ 353:i2452. https://doi.org/10.1136/bmj.i2452
18. Weiler R, Monte-Colombo M, Mitchell A, Haddad F (2015, 2015) Non-operative management of a complete anterior cruciate ligament injury in an English premier league football player with return to play in less than 8 weeks: applying common sense in the absence of evidence. BMJ Case Rep. https://doi.org/10.1136/bcr-2014-208012
19. Shay LA, Lafata JE (2015) Where is the evidence? A systematic review of shared decision making and patient outcomes. Med Decis Mak 35(1):114–131
20. Elwyn G, Frosch D, Thomson R, Joseph-Williams N, Lloyd A, Kinnersley P, Cording E, Tomson D, Dodd C, Rollnick S, Edwards A, Barry M (2012) Shared decision making: a model for clinical practice. J Gen Intern Med 27(10):1361–1367
21. Hegedus EJ, Cook CE (2015) Return to play and physical performance tests: evidence-based, rough guess or charade? Br J Sports Med 49(20):1288–1289

Ethical Issues in Return to Play: Surgical Implications for Return to Play

62

Matthew A. Tao, Dean Wang, and Riley J. Williams

Contents

62.1 Introduction

The role of the surgeon as it relates to return to play (RTP) is a unique and, at times, challenging position. Team sports, particularly at an elite level, invariably have a complex political landscape that requires attention by the orthopedic surgeon to ensure the best possible outcome for the athlete. But regardless of the intricate nature of RTP, we hold our role as a privileged one with the chance to have a truly meaningful impact on an athlete's present situation as well as their future well-being.

The following chapter details our approach to RTP and particularly how the consultant surgeon comes into play. An appropriate diagnosis and understanding of a player's physical and mental fitness are prerequisite to postoperative success. An honest and detailed discussion of goals and expectations is critical to have with the player and their surrounding sphere of influence prior to embarking on the road to recovery—this ensures that all involved parties have an appropriate understanding. Where there are questions, either from the player or team, these should be addressed candidly with every effort to create a unified plan preoperatively. And while high-caliber surgical technique is important, this merely lays the framework for the rehabilitation process to come. Both quantitative and qualitative metrics help drive the RTP algorithm, and ultimately, the definitive decision is a multidisciplinary one with the surgeon at the helm.

62.2 Team Approach

At all high levels of play, the injured athlete is surrounded by a host of individuals who have a role in their RTP algorithm. And while we advo-

M.A. Tao, M.D. • D. Wang, M.D.
R.J. Williams, M.D. (✉)
Hospital for Special Surgery, New York, NY, USA
e-mail: williamsr@hss.edu

V. Musahl et al. (eds.), *Return to Play in Football*, https://doi.org/10.1007/978-3-662-55713-6_62

cate for the surgeon holding the key position as it relates to the medical well-being of the player, the entire decision pathway necessarily involves multiple people. From the medical standpoint alone, each team will typically have a head surgeon, primary care sports physician, athletic trainer, physical therapist, strength and conditioning coaches, nutritionist, and possibly other affiliates. And while this represents the typical scenario for elite teams, medical representation is often more sparse for lower-level athletics. Additionally, the coaches, the front office staff, and the player's agent are all intimately involved even if not from a medical perspective. This creates a complex environment with which to approach RTP, and certainly, each player and organization represents a unique situation.

One of the reasons the surgeon plays such a vital role is not just for the operative expertise but perhaps more so for the ability to globally direct the care of the injured athlete. As with all our patients, it should be born in mind that the primary allegiance is to the player—not the coaches, organization, or any outside voices that may be present. Indeed, all of the aforementioned parties are important in the discussion surrounding injury, but the surgeon is ultimately responsible to the athlete and for their recovery process. Although historical, the Hippocratic oath still sets the ethical framework for sports medicine interactions in modern times.

Figure 62.1 depicts the interplay between all such parties, and open lines of communication with all involved are emphasized. While the surgeon is directing the process, reliance on trainers for functional demands, therapists for strength/movement assessments, and coaches for understanding expectations is all vital to a successful road to RTP.

Interestingly, consultant surgeons are commonly utilized either at the player's request or the behest of their agents or families; however, the role of the consultant specifically is rarely discussed in forums such as this. The involvement of the consulting surgeon automatically inserts him or her into the operative and RTP equations and subsequently places them in a unique position. Much of the onus is on the consultant to navigate the dynamic of the surrounding team and communicate appropriately. Coordinating specifically with the head team physician and head trainer [and, at times, coach/administration] is part of the duty of the consultant to ensure an athlete's successful reintegration to the team. Although one's own RTP protocol sets the framework, flexibility and appropriate adaptations are important given that the actual rehabilitation rarely occurs in geographic proximity to the consulting surgeon. As such, listening to the thoughts and advise of those working directly with the player should influence the RTP process.

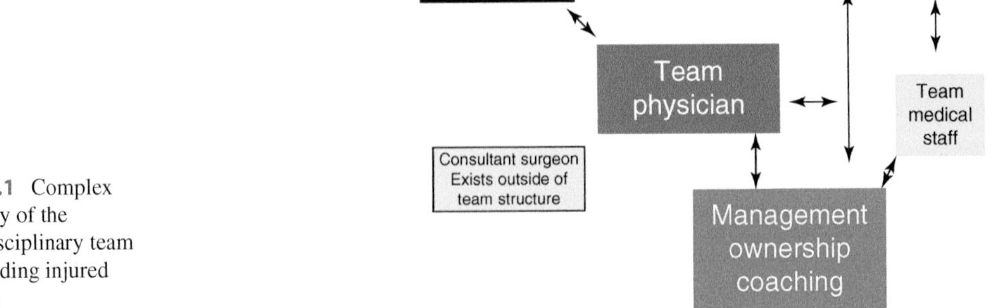

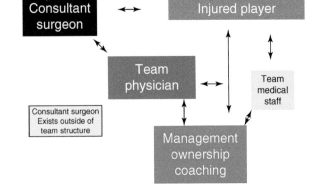

Fig. 62.1 Complex interplay of the multidisciplinary team surrounding injured athletes

62.3 Accurate Diagnosis and Best Treatment

While seemingly an obvious point, obtaining a correct diagnosis is not a foregone conclusion, and its implications to the life and career of any athlete are profound. Discussing the nature of the injury with the patient and those present at the time is helpful along with any photographic or video evidence to provide a context for injury mechanism. Even with the advent of modern diagnostic tools, an accurate history and meticulous physical exam remain the mainstays of diagnosis. Regardless of the condition, imaging is invariably obtained, and it can be helpful to delineate etiology as well as alter or direct the treatment algorithm. Given the implications injuries can have for a player's livelihood, the consultant should take care to avoid rendering a hasty diagnostic conclusion. A thoughtful consideration of the player's anatomic abnormality, mind-set, and team status is a must. It is important to keep in mind that the player may have had multiple consults and explanations regarding their particular malady. As such, how the consultant's impression and plan may not necessarily conform or agree with what the player has been told. Ultimately, an honest discussion of the player's diagnosis and plan is advocated; be concise, rational, and clear. If language, cultural, or educational barriers exist, these should be addressed as best as possible to allow the athlete to gain full understanding of their condition and make a maximally informed decision.

Following the determination of an accurate diagnosis, the consultant should be prepared to administer individualized treatment to the affected athlete. This requires that surgeons stay up-to-date with the most recent literature [best practice] and pair it with their experience and skill set. As an example, Fact Box 1 highlights the variability of RTP and timeline with various cartilage repair techniques. The consultant need be well aware of these studies as they should drive the discussion of RTP expectation and duration. Additionally, and particularly as it relates to chondral defects, the network of options continues to grow; it is the job of the surgeon to help the player wade through what may or may not be viable options. Although cost is often not an obstacle for professional athletes and organizations, prudency and safety still warrant consideration. Ultimately, the best operation is the one that has a durable track record and can be performed well in the hands of the surgeon.

Fact Box 1 RTP rate and timeline with various cartilage repair techniques

Technique	RTP rate (%)	Timeline (months)
Microfracture [1, 2]	44–66	8
Autologous chondrocyte implantation [1, 3]	67–73	18
Osteochondral allograft [4]	88	10
Osteochondral autograft [1]	91	7

62.4 Well-Being

One of the often neglected aspects to injury is the psychological well-being of patients. Hall-of-fame basketball player, Earvin "Magic" Johnson, once spoke of the difficulty of RTP following a serious injury: "I had lost a lot of confidence during the long lay-off. And for a long time after I returned, I still held back. All I could think about was protecting my knee from another injury" [5]. Like a pilot with bad eyes or a surgeon with a lame hand, a serious sports-related injury to an elite athlete has the potential to be both physically and mentally devastating. And while surgeons tend to ignore the psychological aspect of recovery as the softer side of medicine, it would be foolish not to recognize the significant effect it has on RTP, particularly at the highest levels of sport.

A recent consensus statement highlights the importance that a more holistic biopsychosocial view plays in understanding athletic injuries [6]. The risk of injury is certainly more than physical factors alone as detailed in Fig. 62.2, and a solid appreciation of this can influence the recovery process. In fact, a recent study yet to be published out of our own institution [Benedict Nwachukwu & RJW] evaluated a variety of preoperative out-

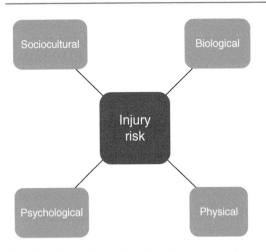

Fig. 62.2 Injury risk profile as it relates to biopsychosocial factors. Figure adapted from text within Wiese-Bjornstal DM. Psychology and socioculture affect injury risk, response, and recovery in high-intensity athletes: a consensus statement. Scandinavian Journal of Medicine & Science in Sports. 2010;20(s2):103–11

come scores and found that only the SF-12 correlated to RTP. Low scores on the mental [and physical] components of the SF-12 significantly predicted failure to RTP, which has potential implications for setting expectations and counseling athletes preoperatively.

Outcomes [and ultimately RTP] are mated to a player's cognition, affect, and behavior as it relates to their injury. Likewise, gaining an appreciation for the motivations behind RTP may not always be so simple. For professional athletes, their career is at stake, and perhaps their incentives are more transparent. But one study of elite and sub-elite athletes found that intrinsic motivations were associated with a positive psychological outcome, while extrinsic provocations led to a negative psychological outcome [7]. Accordingly, attempts have been made to quantify this with scales such as the Injury-Psychological Readiness to Return to Sport (I-PRRS) scale [8] although this has not yet been widely adopted. Regardless, the guiding principle is acknowledging the effect biopsychosocial factors have on outcome [as well as the potential for reinjury] and allowing that to impact an individual's RTP protocol.

62.5 Goals and Expectations

As it relates to the discussion of goals and expectations surrounding an operative injury, surgeons often address this in two separate but intertwined conversations. The first [and most important] is a face-to-face discussion with the player. It is then important to have a similar conversation with the team to provide information and also learn their perspective on the player's future.

62.5.1 Player

As previously mentioned, the primary duty of both the head team physician and consultant surgeon is to the player, and that must always remain in the forefront. A concerted effort to explain the nature of the injury is made, the surgical options and plan required to address it and the anticipated recovery and timeline—often in the presence of the family and/or agent. At times, this is a relatively straightforward conversation depending on the player and situation; however, it can be a fairly lengthy process and accommodations must be made to provide appropriate education and time for a decision. There are many factors that play into an athlete's decision, and the surgeon must make an effort to be aware of these as well.

Assuming that operative intervention is chosen, expectations should be very clearly delineated. The surgeon must gain an understanding of the player's short- and long-term goals as it relates to his/her career and then tailor the ensuing discussion accordingly. As opposed to providing generalized numbers like 55% RTP rate across all sports following anterior cruciate ligament (ACL) reconstruction [9], it is important to provide specific data as it relates to each individual as demonstrated in Fact Box 2. Physicians and others involved in the treatment should never seek to remove hope from the equation; laying out an honest, forthright set of expectations from a medical and functional standpoint is critical even if the prognosis is poor.

Fact Box 2 RTP rate and timeline following ACL reconstruction by sport

	RTP rate (%)	Timeline (months)
NFL [10]	63	10.8
WNBA [11]	78	11.8
NBA [12]	86	11.6
UEFA [13]	89	12

62.5.2 Team

In discussing the injury situation with organization, it is integral to gain an understanding of their view on the player's current status and future role. While this should not alter the treatment plan of the surgeon, it does provide a useful perspective on the more global situation. Although most teams work in concert with the medical staff, one should be prepared to defend the indication for surgery as well as the rationale for the necessary rehabilitation and timeline, especially if prolonged. For the consultant surgeon, many players elect to recover either at home or near the team, both of which are usually geographically removed from the surgeon—as such, the rehabilitation process should be rooted in one's own protocol but not so rigidly as to not adapt to the needs of the athlete and the culture of the team. There should be "hard stops" that must be met, but acknowledge areas of flexibility that can be altered along the way. Regardless of proximity to the player, the onus is on the surgeon to stay engaged throughout the entire rehabilitation process, communicate regularly with the team's medical staff, and manage the recovery journey.

62.6 Rehabilitation

One of the guiding principles of RTP is that the timeline should not outpace the physiology of the surgical repair. Certainly, some athletes' constitution and symptomatology will allow for an accelerated course, but this should not be at the expense of the healing process. For instance, our anecdotal experience is that shorter footballers often feel better faster in comparison with their basketball counterparts following ACL reconstruction, which may well stem from an easier functional recovery given significantly lower weight and shorter limb and trunk length. These athletes often push to get back to running, cutting, and pivoting far sooner than their biology will support. Until true ligamentization occurs (approximately 6–12 months) [14], RTP places the graft and the patient at significantly increased risk for reinjury, e.g., after an ACL reconstruction. Such caution should be held for all situations in which an accelerated course is the goal.

Fitness is often well addressed by trainers and therapists but tends to be overlooked by surgeons. Mental fitness has already been discussed and remains a key component that may require special attention from a sports psychologist or similar specialist. Cardiovascular fitness should also not be ignored as it can usually be built up concomitantly during the rehabilitation process, and without the requisite endurance, effective RTP is a foolish endeavor. Similarly, neuromuscular fitness requires the critical eye of therapists and trainers along the way. Focusing on a functional recovery of the injured limb is the primary goal; however, this postoperative period provides an excellent opportunity to address poor movement patterns, many of which predated the injury [15]. To that end, using the contralateral side as the benchmark for success may be flawed in certain individuals, and the surgeon must be in tune with the therapists so as to not make a premature RTP decision.

Our preference during this process has been to utilize both quantitative and qualitative assessments to track progress as well as make the final RTP determination. Postoperative imaging modalities, isokinetics, and testing such as KT-1000 all provide objective, quantitative measurements that speak to the state and rate of healing. Surgeons also rely heavily on the training staff for their qualitative assessment of functional movement analysis. The so-called performance pyramid [16] is depicted in Fig. 62.3 and provides an easy framework for understanding the progression that must be

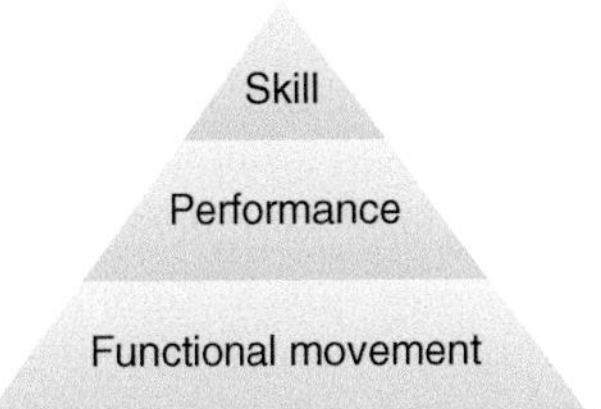

Fig. 62.3 Performance pyramid during the rehab process. Adapted from Cook G. Movement: Functional movement systems: Screening, assessment, corrective strategies: On Target Publications; 2010

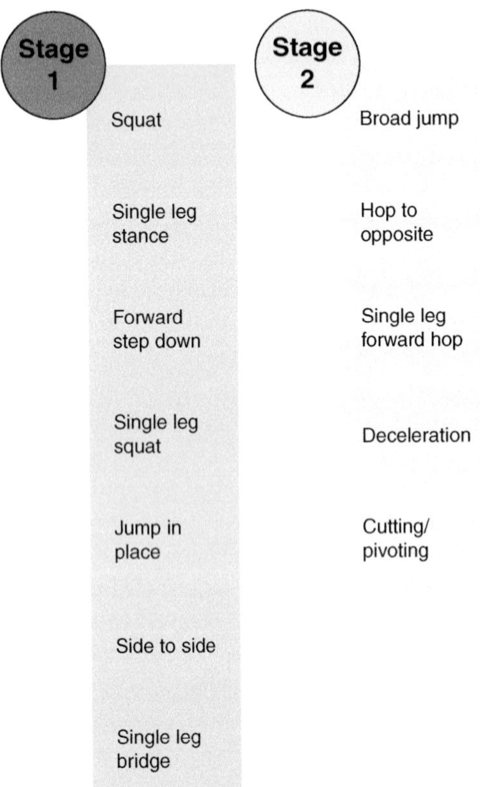

Fig. 62.4 Quality of movement assessment—our basic framework for functional movement analysis

achieved by athletes en route to RTP. Essentially, foundational movement patterns must be established prior to addressing higher-level performance and eventually position-specific skills necessary to play the game. Figure 62.4 demonstrates an example of the basic framework for analyzing the quality of movement specifically as it relates to recovery from ACL reconstruction. Addressing contralateral deficiencies has been mentioned, but in an even broader sense, the importance of the entire kinetic chain cannot be overstated—there is limited utility for a strong, stable knee in the setting of weak hips and poor truncal control. Ultimately, a functional recovery requires an astute physical therapist, diligent trainers, and open lines of communication with a surgeon willing to listen and make adjustments as needed.

62.7 Case Examples

62.7.1 Case #1

A 17-year-old senior is his high school team's star defensive midfielder and his being recruited by top college programs. During an early-season game, he sustains an acute patellar dislocation to his right knee after tripping over an opponent. Physical examination and MRI reveal a tear of the medial patellofemoral ligament (MPFL) with a large full-thickness chondral defect of the patella (Fig. 62.5). After consulting with the player and his family, you decide to perform an MPFL reconstruction and cartilage restoration

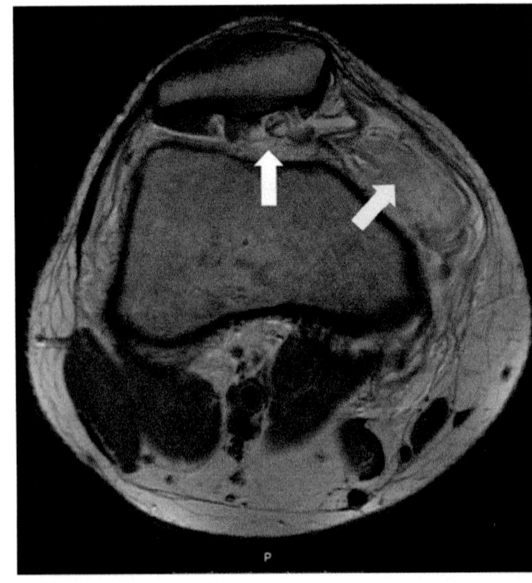

Fig. 62.5 Axial magnetic resonance image of the knee demonstrates medial patellofemoral ligament tear (*yellow arrow*) and large full-thickness chondral defect of the patella (*white arrow*)

procedure using particulated juvenile cartilage allograft. Three months after surgery, the player feels that his rehabilitation is lagging and is worried that his recovery process coincides with the recruitment period for collegiate athletics. Top college programs are becoming increasingly inquisitive about his knee.

The question now is, how should the player be counseled in terms of the goals and expectations surrounding this type of injury and surgery?

Prior to surgery, several issues should be discussed with the player, his family, and his current coach. This includes the severity of the injury, the rehabilitation timeline of approximately 7–10 months, and how the injury will potentially impact the player's college recruitment process and ability to play in the future. Although the player is being pressured by colleges and is eager to resume playing football, it is the primary duty of the surgeon to offer appropriate medical treatment and guidance to ensure the player's safe return to sports participation. Doing so follows the principle of beneficence.

62.7.2 Case #2

A 28-year-old striker experiences a sharp pain to his right posterior upper leg while running during a game. Physical examination and MRI reveal a grade 2 hamstring tear at the proximal biceps femoris (Fig. 62.6). After discussion with the player and team staff, an ultrasound-guided aspiration and platelet-rich plasma (PRP) injection at the proximal myotendinous junction are given in an attempt to accelerate healing and RTP. You estimate a 4-week recovery for RTP based on resolution of soreness, return of leg strength, and fitness. At the 4-week reevaluation, the player reports improvement but has noticeable strength deficits and pain with eccentric contraction. You decide to withhold the player from returning to competition and reevaluate in another week. One week later, the player demonstrates full strength without pain, but cannot replicate sport-specific movements at competition speed. Again, you decide to withhold the player from returning to competition. The player and coach cannot understand why you continue to restrict play.

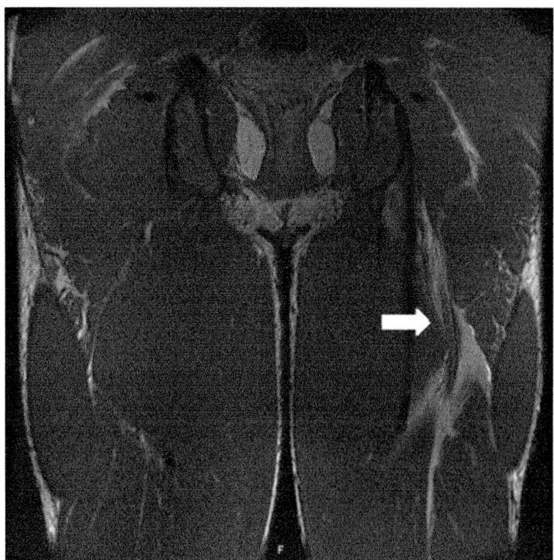

Fig. 62.6 Coronal magnetic resonance image of the thigh demonstrates a partial tear (grade 2) of the proximal biceps femoris (*white arrow*)

The question now is, what should you tell the player and coach?

Team physicians must be knowledgeable of current guidelines and be proficient in educating players and coaches. In this case, the potential immediate and long-term consequences of premature RTP should be thoroughly explained. Consulting with the team trainers and therapists, who are often more in tune with the neuromuscular fitness and functional recovery of the athlete, can help fortify the decision to the players and coaches. Predetermined benchmarks on quantitative functional movement tests can also serve as an objective measure on when athlete can safely RTP.

Take-Home Message

The ethics involved in postoperative RTP can be challenging and at times based on the political landscape of the situation. However, the surgeon stands in a privileged and critical position to maximize an athlete's success, and Fact Box 3 offers information how to success that has been garnered over time. Ultimately, RTP is a multidisciplinary effort that must be owned by the player, driven by the surgeon, and rely on the support of family, medical staff, and the organization as a whole.

Fact Box 3 Pearls for RTP success

- Always keep open lines of communication.
- Avoid prolonged immobilization.
- Strive for early load bearing.
- Be mindful of the physiology of your repair and tailor the rehab accordingly.
- Medical clearance ≠ readiness to play.
- Couple preoperative objective criteria ("hard stops") with flexible progression based on individual and team factors.

Top Five Evidence Based References

Cook G (2010) Movement: functional movement systems: screening, assessment, corrective strategies. On Target Publications, Mumbai

Falconiero RP, DiStefano VJ, Cook TM (1998) Revascularization and ligamentization of autogenous anterior cruciate ligament grafts in humans. Arthroscopy 14:197–205

Hewett TE, Paterno MV, Myer GD (2002) Strategies for enhancing proprioception and neuromuscular control of the knee. Clin Orthop Relat Res 402:76–94

Krych AJ, Robertson CM, Williams RJ, Group CS (2012) Return to athletic activity after osteochondral allograft transplantation in the knee. Am J Sports Med 40:1053–1059

Mithoefer K, Williams RJ, Warren RF, Wickiewicz TL, Marx RG (2006) High-impact athletics after knee articular cartilage repair a prospective evaluation of the microfracture technique. Am J Sports Med 34:1413–1418

References

1. Mithoefer K, Hambly K, Della Villa S, Silvers H, Mandelbaum BR (2009) Return to sports participation after articular cartilage repair in the knee scientific evidence. Am J Sports Med 37:167S–176S
2. Mithoefer K, Williams RJ, Warren RF, Wickiewicz TL, Marx RG (2006) High-impact athletics after knee articular cartilage repair a prospective evaluation of the microfracture technique. Am J Sports Med 34:1413–1418
3. Pestka JM, Feucht MJ, Porichis S, Bode G, Südkamp NP, Niemeyer P (2016) Return to sports activity and work after autologous chondrocyte implantation of the knee which factors influence outcomes? Am J Sports Med 44:370–377
4. Krych AJ, Robertson CM, Williams RJ, Group CS (2012) Return to athletic activity after osteochondral allograft transplantation in the knee. Am J Sports Med 40:1053–1059
5. Johnson E, Novak W (1992) My life. Fawcett Books, Minnesota
6. Wiese-Bjornstal DM (2010) Psychology and socioculture affect injury risk, response, and recovery in high-intensity athletes: a consensus statement. Scand J Med Sci Sports 20:103–111
7. Podlog L, Eklund RC (2005) Return to sport after serious injury: a retrospective examination of motivation and psychological outcomes. J Sport Rehabil 14:20–34
8. Meyerding H (1932) Spondylolisthesis. Surg Gyencol Obstet 54:371–377
9. Ardern CL, Taylor NF, Feller JA, Webster KE (2014) Fifty-five per cent return to competitive sport following anterior cruciate ligament reconstruction surgery: an updated systematic review and meta-analysis including aspects of physical functioning and contextual factors. Br J Sports Med 48(21):1543–1552
10. Shah VM, Andrews JR, Fleisig GS, McMichael CS, Lemak LJ (2010) Return to play after anterior cruciate ligament reconstruction in national football league athletes. Am J Sports Med 38:2233–2239
11. Namdari S, Scott K, Milby A, Baldwin K, Lee G-C (2011) Athletic performance after ACL reconstruction in the women's national basketball association. Phys Sportsmed 39:36–41
12. Harris JD, Erickson BJ, Bach BR, Abrams GD, Cvetanovich GL, Forsythe B et al (2013) Return-to-sport and performance after anterior cruciate ligament reconstruction in national basketball association players. Sports Health 5(6):562–568
13. Waldén M, Hägglund M, Magnusson H, Ekstrand J (2011) Anterior cruciate ligament injury in elite football: a prospective three-cohort study. Knee Surg Sports Traumatol Arthrosc 19:11–19
14. Falconiero RP, DiStefano VJ, Cook TM (1998) Revascularization and ligamentization of autogenous anterior cruciate ligament grafts in humans. Arthroscopy 14:197–205
15. Hewett TE, Paterno MV, Myer GD (2002) Strategies for enhancing proprioception and neuromuscular control of the knee. Clin Orthop Relat Res 402:76–94
16. Cook G (2010) Movement: functional movement systems: screening, assessment, corrective strategies. On Target Publications, Mumbai

How to Work with Agents: Medical and Ethical Aspects—Today's Practice, Questions, Reality and Solutions

63

José F. Huylebroek, Francis Lemmens, and Kristof Sas

Contents

63.1 Outline

- Between 1900 and 1930, football players were not allowed to receive money for "playing".
- Later on, the players became the "property" of the club they were playing for.
- The club decided about the future of the player.
- Then the "Bosman ruling" arrived in December of 1995
- The transfer money remained the same if the player changed club during the contract period.
- But, if the club who wanted the player could not show the bank warrant, the club, owner of the player, could block the transfer.
- After the Bosman decree, clubs could not afford to work out decent networks, but they still engaged in buying new and, if possible, exceptional players.
- So, the work of the "agent" became interesting, necessary and profitable.
- The relations between agents, players, clubs and physicians are discussed.

63.2 How to Work with Agents: Medical and Ethical Aspects

63.2.1 Today's Reality

The sports agent has emerged as an increasingly important person in the negotiation of contracts for professional athletes.

With respect to an agents' background, attorneys now comprise more than 50% of all agents representing professional athletes, particularly in the Anglo-American sports world. Therefore, one must contemplate ethical considerations related to agents' fees and to the medical situation of a player [1].

J.F. Huylebroek, M.D.
Sportsmed Orthopaedic Centre, Parc Leopold, Rue Froissart 38, 1040 Brussels, Belgium
e-mail: jose@sportsmedchirec.be

F. Lemmens, M.D.
Paediatrics ZOL, Genk, Belgium

K. Sas, M.D.
Urgentist AZ Glorieux, Ronse, Belgium

V. Musahl et al. (eds.), *Return to Play in Football*, https://doi.org/10.1007/978-3-662-55713-6_63

The goal of the agent is to maximize the athlete's salary for as long as possible.

This requires that the agent understand a multitude of issues, including the long-term effects of common sports injuries.

The arrangement of medical consultations is becoming more and more a function of the sports agent.

During the negotiation process, there are many variables that are likely to come into play in the determination of the athlete's value.

The medical history is one such variable, and the agent will have some role in determining that value: his/her representation will be even more competent if (s)he proves to handle the medical business of their client as competent as handling the athlete's financial business.

In order to explore this complex relationship among the agent-player-doctor club, three (important) agents were interviewed (C.H., M.B., P.S.).

Interestingly, the three very "competitive" agents, representing a total of hundreds of millions of Euros and hundreds of players, did not differ much when discussing medical matters.

The most reported item remains the confidence: the club and the player should trust the agent.

If the player loses faith in the team physician, the agent will never be able to repair that crisis of confidence.

Of course, the body of the player belongs to himself, not to the club nor to the agent. But, most contracts between clubs and players mention the (medical) rights and responsibilities of the club.

Most clubs have, by contract, the right to decide about the choice of surgeons, the hospital or even the treatment of the player.

Nowadays, most clubs have competent medical teams, even with international experience in one way or another.

The hot topics today in sports medicine, often career-ending problems in the past (hamstring injuries, ligament tears or cartilage problems), are taken care of by specialists who are well recognised by players, clubs and agents.

The moment of the return to sport can be a discussion point where "the doctor of the agent" can help to advise the player. The doctor of the agent is the agents' confidant who has a medical/surgical background.

The point of final interest remains the same for the team physician, the player, the club and the agent: return to play at the same (or even a better) level than before the injury. However, by disclosing a conflict about a diagnosis or treatment, the agent risks losing a valuable player in an extremely competitive market. For instance, the team physician diagnoses an ankle ligament injury, but does not include more specific exams to exclude a cartilage problem in the ankle even though the player keeps complaining about pain and swelling in the ankle.

Another problem is that the player and even the agent may not be knowledgeable or sophisticated enough regarding the impact of the conflict with the club or the medical staff; and some players/agents may be incapable of appreciating the risks.

Additionally, as athletes begin to play professional sports at younger age, situations surrounding conflicts will become more numerous.

Today we are confronted with people, circulating around youngsters of 10, 11 and 12 years old.

A young player at that age should just enjoy the game, relax in a stable family environment, enjoy the friends at school and go to a training centre where (s)he can show his/her talents. From the U13 and onward, there are often more agents than parents at a game.

Education at home remains the most important factor for young players.

If the parents of a talented player start pushing in the same direction as the agent, then a dangerous situation may be created: some parents lose all sense of reality.

Today, in the world of sports agents, players and team physicians, all parties are confronted with the "negotiation of injury settlements", particularly in the USA [2].

Injury settlements are agreements between players and clubs, spelling out compensation and other terms in which the two parties will immediately part ways. Components of an injury settlement are:

- The agent and the player release the club, doctor and coaches from all liability associated with the injury.
- Clubs will be responsible for the cost of all second medical opinions, rehabilitation, medical and related expenses.
- A player (or his agent) may choose to rehabilitate his injury at a place of his/her own choice.
- The applicable workers' compensation laws of the different states/countries may play a (major) role.
- Offset language preventing a player from "double dipping", which can be described as a practice that means receiving more than one income or collecting double benefits from the same employer.

If the agent or the player is not interested in an injury settlement, it is the clubs' obligation to provide rehabilitation for the player and provide the player with medical treatment.

Team physicians can also be confronted with a player who the doctor would like to release from the injured list, while at the same time the player feels that (s)he is still injured. Here, the doctor of the agent can play a major role, either in discussing the case with the medical staff of the club or in proposing an independent arbitrator [3].

In fact, agents usually stipulate in the players' contract that the player has the right to file an injury grievance against the club.

In most cases, agents will argue on behalf of the player for a time beyond the predicted recovery table, to avoid short changing their client.

Negotiating an injury settlement can be tricky and can be an exhaustive and emotional process.

For example, a player suffers from a hamstring injury, clearly documented on MRI, and the team doctor proposes a 6-week time period until full recovery of the injury.

The player obtains a second opinion, and this doctor foresees a 12-week time period for full recovery.

The doctor of the agent or the agent himself may choose for the longer recovery time prediction to protect the health of the player.

In today's world, sophisticated and structured test batteries with repeated MRI's and second opinions by radiologists and orthopaedists help to settle the problem.

The role of the agent was developed to protect the athletes' interest in relation to that of the clubs (president, owner, sponsor). According to Melissa Neiman, the problem now, to some degree, has become the protection of the athletes' interests in relation to those of the agents. Melissa Neiman is an MD (Texas Medical Branch) and JD (University of Houston Law Center), who published an important paper about ethical considerations in negotiating by sports agents.

The best outcome for the player will depend on a good relationship between the medical team of the club and the medical team of the agent. The bottom line is that both teams (the medical team of the club and the medical team of the agent) are looking for the best therapeutic solution for the injured player.

63.3 Potential Solutions to Ethical Dilemmas

Previously independent agents are forming conglomerates and larger agencies, operating as full-service organisations and taking care of all of the athlete's needs.

This consolidation has created large agencies like Creative Artists Agency (CAA, Los Angeles, CA, USA), Excel (New York, NY, USA), Boras Corp. (basketball) (Newport Beach, CA, USA), Wasserman Media Group (Los Angeles, CA, USA), Octagon (Norwalk, CT, USA), Independent Sports & Entertainment (ISE, New York, NY, USA).

These big six agencies represent more than 30% of all professional athletes and serve as financial manager, accountant, public relations agent, tasks and estate planner, attorney, health advisor and if necessary even as coach. This situation may create conflicts of interest, with important ethical consequences [4].

From an athlete's perspective, having the right agent, the right coach and the right medical entourage is crucial to success.

The athlete must take into consideration personal ties, long-term health issues and ethical considerations.

The job of the team physician also changed.

Modern sports medicine has emerged as an important anchor of the athlete's performance, and ethics in sports medicine are driven by the always glooming tension between its two components: sport and medicine.

Medicine aims for health and sports aims for victory.

If the pursuit of victory and the pursuit of health sometimes mean following opposite directions, this tension may result in an ethical problem, where the team, the athlete and the agent can play a crucial role facing possible ethical dilemmas [5].

In an attempt to identify the ethical challenges on different levels, some possible solutions are outlined below.

Conflicts of interest created by the consolidation in sports agencies and the increase in different services offered pose the biggest problems.

Some examples are:

- Agencies representing multiple players in the same league
- Agencies representing multiple players on the same team
- Agencies representing players and coaches
- Agencies representing events and athletes
- Agencies providing the attorney to assist the athlete in signing contracts, where the agency is an involved party
- Agencies providing medical advice to the athlete by a physician who is paid by the agency

In an attempt to meet ethical challenges, some initiatives are taken by big sports federations, some large agencies and some governments [6].

63.3.1 Federations

- Federation Internationale De Football Association (FIFA) Player's Agents Regulations (2008): licence issued by each national federation following an exam. Requirements for operating as an agent are subject to control and sanction by FIFA.
- International Association Of Athletics Federations (IAAF): (2009) competition rules Rule 7: athletes' representatives (agents), authorisation issued by national federations
- International Olympic Committee (IOC) Guidelines for the conduct of the athletes' entourage (Durban, 2011 July 4):
  The entourage (all the people associated with the athlete, including agents, coaches and medical staff) must respect and promote ethical principles contained in the Olympic Charter, the IOC Code of Ethics and the World Anti-Doping Agency (WADA) code and must, in accordance with such principles, always act in the best interest of the athletes. The entourage shall demonstrate the highest level of integrity in particular respecting the following principles:
  - Avoid conflicts of interest.
  - Fight against any form of bribery and cheating or corruption.
  - Reject any form of doping.
  - Refrain from any form of betting activity on the athlete's sport.

The entourage shall also respect confidentiality, protecting personal and inside information [7].

The entourage must be transparent, responsible and accountable.

63.3.2 Countries (Governments)

- USA: the agents are subject to regulation by the federal government, some state governments and the players' association [8].
  - Sports Agent Responsibility and Trust Act (SPARTA), 2004
  - Uniform Athlete Agents Act (UAAA)
- Europe: the licensing system is regularly updated.

Five EU countries (Bulgaria, France, Greece, Hungary, Portugal) have a licensing system with terms and conditions for exercising the profession (most detailed in France with control and sanctions).

63.3.3 Agencies

Several solutions are proposed to overcome conflict of interest problems.

The most pragmatic solution would be full disclosure by the agent of all possible issues and asking the athlete for his/her consent.

Unanimity on this subject however seems still far away: not all sports associations agree about strict regulations for agents.

The players do not find unanimity about the different regulations and disclosures of agents.

On top of the conflicts of interest, created by the evolution in agencies, medical ethical issues exist. In the past decade an increasing amount of articles have been published in different journals {7} {3} {2}{8}.

Particular areas of medical ethics that present unique challenges in sports medicine are informed consent, third-party influences, advertising, confidentiality, drug use and innovative technology.

The ethics of the doctor-patient relationship is evolving around the above discussed parties, athlete, doctor, club and agent.

The team's priorities or agent's priorities can sometimes equal or even replace those of the athlete.

Medical risks sometimes have to be balanced with non- medical benefits of an overwhelming size.

Let's take, for example, X, a professional soccer player who sustains a potentially repairable meniscal tear 6 weeks before the start of the World Cup, at the very moment his agent is about to arrange a transfer to the Premier League.

An excision of the tear (partial meniscectomy) would require minimal rehabilitation and would permit participation in the World Cup but would also increase the long-term risk of arthritis.

A meniscal repair offers the chance at pain-free function in the near term and would probably avoid articular degeneration but would exclude participation in the World Cup.

The athlete wants to play but has some doubts about the consequences for his future career. His agent tells him that absence in the World Cup could jeopardise his transfer.

The World Cup coach pressures the team physician to ensure the player can make the selection of the World Cup team.

The story is covered extensively by the media and the fans voice that X must play. What is the ethical decision to be made by the team physician, and do we believe ethics will prevail in this kind of situation?

The pressure by the player on the team physician was too high: the player underwent an arthroscopic partial meniscectomy and not a meniscal repair.

Sometimes the influence of agents can be positive. Agents can surround the athlete with a well-balanced medical team that secures optimal physical condition while preventing injuries as much as possible.

Agents can provide the team physician and the athlete with additional medical information to make the right decisions.

Agents can also use their connections around the globe to provide first-class treatment in case of serious injuries.

Sometimes however the influence of agents can be negative.

Agents can "prepare" their athlete for medical tests preceding a transfer to mask (upcoming) injuries as much as possible, even at the risk of the athlete's future health.

Agents conversely could instruct their athletes to not optimally treat or even fake an injury to create better financial conditions for a transfer.

Agents can cause a conflict of interest in well-known "experts" by involving (and paying) experts in the medical care of their athletes, thus compromising their role in later "expert advice".

Agents can cause a conflict of decision-making in athletes and team physicians by providing them with second opinions of well-known experts, picked by the agencies because their general opinion favours the solution that fits the agencies' interest.

There is a growing fear for conflicts of interest potentially ruining the essence of sports.

In the authors' opinion, a solution could be to safeguard the new services an agency can offer to the athlete but to instal a "confidant" or "trustworthy friend" as an ombudsmen between the agency and the athlete.

In a sense this would reintroduce proximity and loyalty of the agent to the athlete.

The qualities of such a "confidant" can be found in the description of "the personal advisor" in the IOC manifest on agents, agencies and personal advisors.

The role of the personal advisors would be a trusted voice and a sounding board for the athlete.

Personal advisors often act as a liaison between athlete and agents.

Personal advisors may have legal, medical or other useful skills, but their key characteristic is the close personal relationship with the athlete.

Not usually paid, personal advisors would have the athlete's best interest at heart and no financial or other motivation of their own.

Such a confidant, if properly skilled, should make it possible that the athlete's best interest and autonomy prevails in an environment where third-party influence is imminent. Alternatively, the agencies could come up with their own "independent" personal advisor (or lawyer), who should be protected against conflicts of interest because, by contract, the personal advisor would be due to serve only the best interest of the athlete.

It is the authors' opinion that agents and agencies should address the ethical problems and conflicts of interest they face.

Integrity, transparency, full disclosure of all conflicting issues and full priority to the athlete's best interest can provide the base to build on.

Medical and ethical experts should lead the way by avoiding conflicts of interest themselves and coming forward with expert opinions, also in the digital and social media. "Big money", news media and the "entourage" of elite athletes will continue to dictate the evolution in sports. Agencies and agents play a critical role in all of these areas [9].

In the meantime medical and ethical experts should assist in a better communication.

Fact Box (Definitions)

A/Agent

A specific person (might be a lawyer, old player, manager, etc.) who represents a professional player or group of players, as a link between the player and the club.

He also may be in charge of reorienting the career of the player; he intervenes in case of professional conflicts and particularly discusses the contracts between the player, the club and third parties.

B/Player

A sportsperson who is involved (in this context) in football, a team sport played between two teams of eleven players. A professional football player signed a contract with the club, is payed and insured by that club and can only play in competition for that club (apart from his national team).

C/Team Physician

A professional doctor, usually specialised in sports medicine, who has been engaged by a club, to take care of the players and staff.

He meets with the trainer/physical coach/etc. to prepare the players for the game in the best physical condition. During the game he has his place on the bench and goes on the pitch to help an injured player.

D/Doctor of the Agent

A sports physician (or an orthopaedic surgeon in some cases) who has been engaged, in most cases part-time, to check the physical condition or injury of players who have a contract with a particular agent. This can be a routine check or a second opinion requested by the player and/ or his agent.

F/Medical Team of Agent

Every medical doctor who has a professional relationship with a football agent and who can be contacted in case of second opinion or dispute between the player and the medical staff of the club. This can be a cardiologist, a dentist or any other specialist, related to the specific problem but asked/payed by the agent.

G/Bosman

Jean-Marc Bosman was a player of RFC Liege, Belgium, whose contract had expired in 1990: he wanted to move to Dunkerque, France. However, Dunkerque refused to meet his Belgians' club transfer fee demand, so Liège refused to let him go.

Bosman took his case to the European Court of Justice and sued for "restraint of trade" citing FIFA's rules regarding football. On the 15th of December 1995, the court ruled that the system placed a restriction on the free movement of workers and was prohibited by Article 39(1) of the EC Treaty.

Bosman and all were given the right to a *free transfer* at the end of their contracts, within the EU.

Significance: players (or their agents) became able to negotiate deals according to their market value when their contracts expired!

Before the Bosman ruling, a player could not leave at the end of their deal unless that club agreed to let him go on a free or that club received an agreed fee from a buying club.

H/Sports Agency

An organised (usually international) football management that offers solutions and proposals able to overcome the most demanding needs of players. The legal representation negotiates employment and endorsement contracts for the athlete or coach they represent.

They can handle public relation matters, business management and financial and risk analysis.

And via the agent's doctor, the agency can intervene in the case of medical discussions or second opinions. Agents and agencies are now licenced by their association.

References

1. Matthias MB (2004) The competing demands of sport and health: an essay on the history of ethics in sports medicine. Clin Sports Med 23(2):195–214
2. Rossner S (2004) Conflicts of interest and the shifting paradigme of athlete representation. UCLA Ent Law Rev 193:194–245
3. Tucker AM (2004) Ethics and the professional team physician. Clin Sports Med 23(2):227–241
4. Forbes sports money magazine (2016)
5. Bernstein J, Perlis C, Bartolozzi AR (2004) Normative ethics in sports medicine. Clin Orthop Relat Res 420:308–318
6. Devitt BM (2016) Fundamental ethical principles in sports medicine. Clin Sports Med 35(2):195–204
7. IOC executive board Durban guidelines for the conduct of the athlete's entourage (2011, July 4)
8. Testoni D, Hornik CP, Smith PB, Benjamin DKJR, Mckinney REJR (2013) Sports medicine and ethics. Am J Bioeth 13(10):4–12
9. Dunn WR, George MS, Churchill L, Spindler KP (2007) Ethics in sports medicine. Am J Sports Med 35(5):840–844

Ethical Issues in Return to Play: How to Deal with Parents and Coaches

64

Jeremy M. Burnham, Greg Gasbarro, Justin Arner, Thomas Pfeiffer, and Volker Musahl

Contents

64.1 Introduction

The field of sports medicine is unique in that the sports medicine professional is not only tasked with treating and interacting with the patient but must also skillfully navigate potentially complex relationships with an athlete's parents and coaches. While the underlying principle of "first, do no harm" still applies in sports medicine, medical decision-making and treatment algorithms are oftentimes made more complex by the temporal nature of sports seasons and the societal and economic pressures related to missed sports participation. For these reasons, it is crucial that sports medicine physicians have a clear understanding of sound return-to-play (RTP) principles and adhere to strict ethical standards. By communicating these guidelines early in the treatment process with the player, parents, therapists, athletic trainers, and coaches, all involved entities will be on the same page, and RTP conflicts are less likely to occur.

64.2 Principles of Return to Play

Decision-making in terms of RTP following injury is a collaborative effort among the athlete, parents, guardians, coaches, physical therapist, athletic trainers, and team physician [1, 2]. Successful outcome is predicated on clear communication and goal-oriented rehabilitation. There is considerable empirical evidence that both parents and coaches influence psychosocial well-being of youth athletes [3]. As such, there are multiple stakeholders involved in team sports that challenge the traditional notion of confidentiality and autonomy. Ultimately, it is the respon-

J.M. Burnham • G. Gasbarro • J. Arner
V. Musahl, M.D. (✉)
Department of Orthopaedic Surgery, UPMC Center for Sports Medicine, University of Pittsburgh, 3200 S Water St, Pittsburgh, PA 15203, USA
e-mail: musahlv@upmc.edu

T. Pfeiffer
Department of Orthopaedic Surgery, Traumatology, and Sports Medicine, Kliniken der StadtKoelngGmbH, Köln, Germany

V. Musahl et al. (eds.), *Return to Play in Football*, https://doi.org/10.1007/978-3-662-55713-6_64

sibility of the physician to ensure no harm to the athlete during this process while enabling participation at the highest possible level [1].

Establishing guidelines prior to the outset of the season among all stakeholders can pay dividends as injuries occur throughout the year. While specifics may not be included, informing others of who makes decisions, under what circumstances, and how the safety of the athletes takes priority can minimize unrealistic or harmful expectations [1]. This may help alleviate parents from "doctor shopping" until they find RTP criteria that they believe best suits their youth athletes' interest [1]. The role of the parent must not be underestimated. Parental support is fundamental to initial participation and ongoing success in team sports. Overly engaged parents might play a disruptive role, however, with regard to medical decision-making.

RTP considerations for musculoskeletal injuries should establish an athlete's range of motion, strength, and functional athletic ability [1]. Evaluation should be conducted out of plain sight of the crowd attending the sporting event, but in the presence of the coach and/or parent if possible. This may be advantageous so all stakeholders witness the ability or inability of the athlete to perform a task [1]. With regard to concussion, change in baseline psychometric characteristics after injury and clinical practice guidelines for graduated return to play has been established and should be followed [4, 5]. Other factors include but are not limited to the type of sport in which the athlete participates, the timing in the season, the level of competition, the position played, the athlete's limb dominance, and the efficacy of bracing, taping, or padding.

Goal-oriented rehabilitation includes objective performance parameters in the gym and on the playing field as well as psychological issues. The role of the athletic trainer to this regard is paramount. Given the time spent together during preseason, practice, and regular season games, athletic trainers have unique insight into the cognitive aspect and personality traits of each athlete. This may have benefits as it relates to understanding the athlete's level of pain threshold, normal demeanor, and other personality traits. One common behavior seen is the athlete who sustains an injury and then hides from the athletic training staff for fear of being taken out of competition. In some cases, this behavior may be promoted by the coaches or parents of the athlete. Despite resistance after initial evaluation, the best way to demonstrate that the athlete is unable to return to competition is by adhering to preestablished RTP guidelines and criteria. In other circumstances, athletes may exhibit a lack of emotional preparedness or mental readiness required to RTP safely. These traits must be identified, especially in contact sports, as RTP may predispose the athlete for risk of further injury [1].

Fact Box 1 Importance of patient confidentiality

- Physicians are obligated to maintain their patient's confidentiality.
- Maintaining patient confidentiality is challenging in a team setting.
- Physicians serving as a team physician should be educated about ethical obligations and challenges, including patient confidentiality, in this unique environment.

64.3 Ethical Considerations

Due to conflicts of interest, the team physician faces a unique situation related to ethical principles of autonomy and confidentiality [6]. Confidentiality regarding medical decisions in the traditional sense is an obligation that physicians owe to their patients [7]. In addition, state and federal laws mandate healthcare professionals to uphold these standards. Numerous occasions in sports medicine challenge this framework. As such, it is suggested that prior to any examination or care of an athlete, the team physician has a duty to clarify the nature of the relationship with the athlete indicating the importance of confidentiality and that the physician will strive to maintain that confidentiality, despite the challenges associated with patient care in a team setting [8]. Most healthcare professionals balance ethical principles of the patient's right to autonomy, with fairness, and their obligation to first do no harm. To achieve this goal, it was advocated that physicians pursue team coverage to gain education in the basic principles and concepts of applied ethics [9]. Physicians should also be familiar with current management guidelines, particularly as it relates to sports-related concussion [10].

Fact Box 2 Common ethical considerations among a sports medicine team

- Understanding each persons' role
- Conflict of interest due to divided loyalties
- Acting in the athlete's best interest, despite return-to-play pressure from coaches, parents, or athletes

The myriad of ethical considerations in sports medicine have been well described in the literature. For example, a group of athletic trainers was surveyed and qualitative examination of 154 ethical issues revealed seven common themes [11]. These include miscommunication about roles, conflicts of interest due to divided loyalties, conflicts in acting on the athlete's best interest, and pressure to RTP from the coach, parent, supervisor, administrator, or athlete [11]. Another study reviewed the relationship between management of professional sports teams and team doctors. The researchers reported that team management often places pressure on physicians to return an athlete quickly to competition [12]. Although most sports organizations have the best interest of the athlete in mind, some promote shortened recovery through substandard treatment protocols. Despite pressures by team management, it is pertinent that medical staff on the sidelines during games remove an athlete from competition if assessment is concerning for further injury. If initial evaluation permits RTP deemed by preestablished guidelines, ongoing close observation of the athlete is necessary to confirm that decision and ensure the athlete's safety. The outcome of a game should never have an effect on RTP decisions despite the culture among athletes, coaches, and parents in some sports that playing through the pain is a sign of toughness [1].

RTP guidelines are multifactorial, and decision-making in terms of long-term goals is best conducted away from the playing field in the office setting. Topics and conversations may vary depending on the current level of participation of the athlete and ultimate goals regarding level of competition. RTP decisions should not be influenced by parents of high school athletes' who pressure RTP based on the potential for earning or losing college athletic scholarship [6]. Furthermore, there is often a discrepancy between patient-reported health status and parent-reported health status, further underscoring the importance of limiting parental influence in the setting of younger athletes [13]. At the collegiate level, judgment cannot be altered by high-salaried coaches and athletic administrators who are under pressure from students, fans, boosters, and politicians to succeed [2]. Perhaps ethical decision-making is most challenged at the professional sports level. Athletes stand to gain economic benefit from their athletic ability, but so do agents, family members, sponsors, team owners, and many others, requiring vigilance by physicians to adhere to RTP guidelines and ethical standards in medical decision-making [1]. The impact of missed games can have a significant impact on the earning capacity of professional athletes. These financial concerns must be weighed against the risk of early RTP to the athlete's current and future health. Despite attempts to uphold ethical standards, studies have shown that there is great variability among team physicians in RTP decisions.

64.4 Psychological Aspects of Return to Play

Numerous studies have shown that psychological characteristics and mental health play a significant role in outcomes after musculoskeletal injury [14–17], and monitoring of these levels may provide insight into readiness for RTP [18]. Moreover, adolescents often respond differently to injury and surgery than adults [19, 20]. For example, one group of researchers found that identification of oneself as an athlete was more important than general self-motivation in adherence to a home rehabilitation program in adolescents, but not in adults [19]. Another study reported greater pain catastrophizing in adolescent patients compared to adult patients [20]. These findings underscore the need for an individualized approach that is focused on treating the patient according to their specific physical, emotional, and mental needs. These needs may differ from parents' and coaches' expectations or understanding, and consideration must be given to bridging these knowledge gaps. Ultimately, effective communication among physicians, coaches, parents, therapists, and athletic trainers is key to optimizing the mental health of the injured athlete.

64.4.1 Psychological Health of the Athlete

Pain catastrophizing is arguably one of the most important psychological characteristics affecting RTP outcomes, especially in the short term. Catastrophizing can be described as a sense of helplessness in controlling or responding to pain and is associated with negative outcomes [20]. Tripp et al. demonstrated that adolescents had significantly higher levels of pain catastrophizing at 24-h post-ACL reconstruction than adult patients [20]. Although further research is needed, this suggests that adolescent athletes should receive focused postoperative interventions aimed at controlling these negative emotions. Interestingly, while verbalizing and communicating emotions related to the injury is associated with better outcomes, many athletes are hesitant to express these feelings to avoid any perception of being "weak" by parents, coaches, or teammates. This is more common in athletes with a poor social support system, and they often express inauthentic "positive" emotions while failing to adequately address their psychological health. A large body of research has shown that these athletes have poor outcomes and a higher rate of reinjury [21]. RTP programs should be tailored according to the psychological needs of the athlete, and adequate buy-in from coaches, parents, and athletic trainers is crucial to optimizing outcomes.

64.4.2 Role of the Parents

Parents play a critical role in athletes' psychological well-being. Both mothers and fathers can facilitate athletic success and reduce emotional stress when involved in the appropriate manner. In fact, parental encouragement of sports participation could potentially help to increase their children's activity levels and decrease the rates of childhood obesity. As these children age, their earlier parental involvement may help to improve the chances that they remain physically active as adults [22]. It is important, however, that parents assess the specific psychological, social, and emotional needs of their child and adjust their involvement accordingly [23–25]. In fact, studies have provided specific guidelines on how athletes prefer their parents behave before, during, and after sports competitions [26]. Notably, athletes reported a preference that their parents encourage them and the rest of the team to focus on effort rather than outcomes, maintain control of their own emotions, and provide positive and realistic feedback [27]. Although this data was collected in the setting of athletic competition and not specifically RTP after injury, the general findings likely translate across athletic settings. Further data supported these findings and demonstrated that structured parental involvement increased youth's perceived enjoyment and decreased stress levels associated with sports participation [23], and positive parental involvement has been correlated with improved mastery of sport [28].

On the other hand, it is critical to identify parent motivations or perceptions that may be detrimental to the athlete and redirect these to have a more positive impact on the athlete's performance and recovery from injury. There is significant potential for inappropriate parental involvement to result in negative consequences. In many cases, parents encourage or force sports participation past the level that the child is interested or capable of. This type of negative parental involvement results in increased anxiety, higher likelihood of a negative sports experience, and a greater chance of injury [22].

Some parents are overprotective, which has been shown to hamper athlete growth and development. The term "helicopter parent" was first published in 1990 to refer to parents that hover over their children, never allowing them to succeed or fail on their own [29, 30]. Parents must strike a balance between providing protection and security and encouraging their children to learn from experience and gain skills necessary for independent living in the future. Being overprotective in the form of helicopter parenting leads to poorer functioning and worse emotional decision-making [30]. In fact, this hyper-parenting can lead to reduced physical activity in younger children [31].

The nature of parent-athlete involvement becomes even more complicated as the patient reaches the age legal independence (18 years of age in most countries). While the parents are legal guardians of younger children, this relationship changes rather quickly when the adolescent reaches the age of legal independence. However, many parents remain heavily involved in their child's athletic participation and health care even past this age. It is important to realize the legal and medical distinction between a teenager legally under the care of their parents, and a child who may only be days, weeks, or months older, but is legally independent. In many cases, it is necessary for the 18-year-old patient to provide either a verbal or written consent before medical professionals can discuss personal health information with the parents. Similarly, the 18-year-old athlete, not the parent(s), has the ultimate say in medical treatment and return-to-play decisions [32]. This may be difficult for the parents, athlete, and coaches to accept in athletes that recently were under the care of their parents. While the preservation of true informed consent is difficult in sports medicine at any age [32], it is even more challenging in the case of a young but legally independent athlete, who may be under even more pressure from their parents than older athletes, in addition to that from their coaches, agents, and teammates. In these settings, sports medicine professionals must remember that true informed consent and patient autonomy are cornerstones in medicine, and outside pressures to dilute these principles must be guarded against.

64.4.3 Role of the Coaches

Coaches also play a crucial role in young athletes' sports careers. Their actions, words, and even nonverbal communication can have dramatic effects on the psychological well-being of their players. In fact, studies have reported that the manner in which a coach delivers verbal feedback can have as significant of an effect as the actual words that were spoken. Additional studies have suggested that optimal coach-player communication could decrease the number of sports injuries, or at least those that are attributable to poor technique [33], and that even basic communication training for coaches can improve young athletes' performance and psychological health [3, 33]. While most coaches are not medical professionals, they play an arguably equal, or perhaps even more important, role in guiding the injured athlete's psychological health than the treating physician. As such, the coach should be considered an important part of the sports medicine team, and discussions regarding the emotional and mental well-being of the patient should ideally include the coach (with proper patient permissions).

64.4.4 Role of the Athletic Trainers and Physical Therapists

During the road to recovery, athletic trainers and/or physical therapists will likely spend more time with the athlete than any other medical professional. Perhaps no one in the sports medicine team will be more qualified to gauge the athlete's psychological status and provide appropriate feedback than their athletic trainer or therapist. Furthermore, the athletic trainer provides a critical link between the coaches and the sports medicine physician. For these reasons, optimal psychological rehabilitation and successful RTP will revolve around the athletic trainer or therapist.

64.5 Objective Return-to-Play Criteria for Soccer: Injury-Specific Examples

As return-to-play decisions become increasingly more complex, objective return-to-play criteria help to provide unbiased and consistent guidelines in assessing injured athletes. These guidelines help to assure patient readiness and prevent potentially risky premature return to sport.

64.5.1 Concussion

Likely the most complex return-to-play decision and most concerning for all parties is head injuries. Understandably, much anxiety can exist among the parents as recovery and severity are difficult to predict and visualize. Involving parents in all aspects of evaluation and treatment is key to educate and ease anxiety among loved ones. Although less common, education is also key for parents pushing for quick return to play. This can be difficult to address as symptoms are not as easily definable or observed. Comprehensive evaluation and buy-in by all, including the athlete, parents, and coaching and medical staff, is paramount in proper treatment of concussion.

Concussions commonly can have serious effects on young athletes including irritability, memory loss, confusion, and difficulty with concentration. This is obviously problematic in school-aged children. Any athlete with concern for a concussion should be removed from play immediately and be evaluated by a medical professional. If the player is found to have signs or symptoms of concussion such as dizziness, headache, confusion, or memory loss, they must be removed from play for the entirety of the day, and if any question exists, one should err on the side of caution. If the athlete sustains a second event, they are at risk for second-impact syndrome which carries risk of prolonged recovered and worsened symptoms. Further evaluation regarding symptoms must be continually done, and gradual return to play is recommended only after these symptoms cease [34]. It is key to involve parents, particularly in this aspect of data gathering and treatment, as they can provide accurate assessments of their child's symptoms and behavior which helps the physician to treat the child more appropriately.

Currently, it is recommended that the student athlete slowly returns to normal daily activates without prolonged absence. This typically begins with a walk a few times a day and slow return to school activities. Return to sport is handled in the same manner with gradual return in a stepwise progression without advancing to the next level until the previous activity is successfully completed without symptoms [34]. Many societies have published return to activity guidelines. However, practitioners must realize one size does not fit all, and concussion treatments must take an individualized approach, with involvement of the parents being key [34].

Current consensus guidelines, clinical examination, and objective testing are used in concert to determine safe return to play after concussion. Neurocognitive tests such as Immediate Post-Concussion Assessment and Cognitive Test (ImPACT™) and Standardized Concussion Assessment Tool (SCAT™) are useful when used in conjunction with clinical evaluation to provide a score which can be compared to the patient's baseline and allow object measures of head injury. Again, in the increased pressure with return to play in many environments, these objective measures allow medical professionals to provide hard data to parents and coaches [34, 35].

Anyone with persistent symptoms and deficits should be referred to a concussion specialist who can provide multimodal therapies such ocular, vestibular, and cognitive treatments. A multidisciplinary approach should be utilized in the treatment of concussion, and parents must be included, updated, and consulted to provide accurate assessments of their child's recovery [34].

64.5.2 Anterior Cruciate Ligament (ACL)

Knee ligament and ankle sprains are the most common injuries in adolescent football [36]. Proper education of the parents and realistic return-to-play estimates should be discussed with the understanding that continued evaluation may change the return-to-play timing. Many parents, athletes, and media seem to equate earlier return to play after ACL reconstruction to a better surgeon and technique. However, the surgeon must resist being influenced by this notion. Return to play too early may lead to higher graft rupture rates due to insufficient healing and lack of psychological and physiologic readiness [18].

Like concussions, objective measures can assist the therapist, surgeon, and athlete, and parent agree on a safe return to play. Close correlation with a trusted physical therapist can be beneficial for the athlete, parent, and physician. More standardized techniques such as biometric testing can be useful and should be discussed with the athlete and parents so both are aware of the required milestones that must be reached to move on to the next level rehabilitation. This can be helpful in athletes and parents who push for earlier return to play as well as in patients who require more confidence in their reconstructed knee. If a well-outlined play is discussed pre- and postoperatively, return to play is less likely to be questioned until milestones are met. A trusted physical therapist can aid and provide helpful input in this process. Specific football-based return-to-play guidelines and milestones also exist and can be helpful [37].

Psychological readiness and confidence in return to play is important and must be assessed. This can be done by private conversation between the athlete and surgeon outlining that commonly after ACL reconstruction, patients may not feel mentally prepared for return to play even after the medical team determines they may return. After discussion of the athlete's thoughts, a conversation with the physical therapist can be helpful as they spend more time evaluating the athlete's physiologic preparedness and clues related to their psychological preparedness can be observed, all in a less threatening atmosphere. The importance of physiological preparedness should be discussed with the parents as well as an unprepared athlete could lead to further injury and inferior performance. When athletes are determined not to be ready either psychologically or physiologically, the physician must be the athlete's liaison if parents and coaches are anxious for their return to sport [18].

64.5.3 Ankle Injuries

Although usually less severe than ACL reconstruction, ankle injuries are very common in football. Less controversy typically exists in return-to-play timing; however, due to their incidence, it is important to be well versed in their treatment and return to play. Like most injuries, successful sport-specific activities must be performed before return to play is allowed after a proper physical exam and, if indicated, imaging [1]. Rest, ice, compression, and taping or bracing can be effective. In young athletes with recurrent ankle sprains, potential causes must be ruled out so long-term ligamentous laxity and cartilage damage do not occur leading to early ankle dysfunction from injury at a young age. Like all injuries in young athletes, expected outcome and the process to get there, including return to play, must be discussed realistically with the patient and their parents.

Concussion, ACL injury, and ankle injuries are common in football with differing incidences, severities, and therefore controversies in return to play. Education of the athlete, parents, and coaches is key, and buy-in of the process is essential for the safety of the player. This may require more time from the surgeon, but is imperative for optimal outcome.

Fact Box 3 Key factors to successful return to play

- The entire sports medicine team is needed to ensure successful and appropriate return to play.
- Objective criteria help to provide accurate return-to-play assessments and limit emotional or self-serving influences.
- Effective communication with the athlete, parents, and coaches is crucial.

Take-Home Message

A comprehensive RTP program involves engagement and collaboration by the sports medicine physician, coaches, athletic trainers and therapists, and—in the setting of younger athletes—parents. While there are many societal and economic pressures associated with RTP decisions after sports injury, objective RTP criteria and effective communication help to minimize conflict and ensure athlete well-being. Not only should parents and coaches understand RTP criteria, but they should also be actively engaged in providing psychological and emotional support to the rehabilitating athlete. Keys to success include setting realistic expectations early, encouraging a culture that facilitates open athlete discussion with constructive feedback, and always placing the athlete's well-being first, regardless of external economic or societal pressures.

Top Five Evidence Based References

Cahill PJ, Refakis C, Storey E, Warner WC Jr (2016) Concussion in sports: what do orthopaedic surgeons need to know? J Am Acad Orthop Surg 24(12):e193–e201

Dunn WR, George MS, Churchill L, Spindler KP (2007) Ethics in sports medicine. Am J Sports Med 35(5):840–844

Tripp DA, Stanish WD, Reardon G, Coady C, Sullivan MJ (2003) Comparing postoperative pain experiences of the adolescent and adult athlete after anterior cruciate ligament surgery. J Athl Train 38(2):154–157

O'Rourke D, Smith R, Smoll F, Cumming S (2014) Relations of parent and coach initiated motivational climates to young athletes self esteem performance anxiety and autonomous motivation who is more. J Appl Sport Psychol 26:395–408

Luebbe AM, Mancini KJ, Kiel EJ, Spangler BR, Semlak JL, Fussner LM (2016) Dimensionality of helicopter parenting and relations to emotional, decision-making, and academic functioning in emerging adults. Assessment. https://doi.org/10.1177/1073191116665907

References

1. Clover J, Wall J (2010) Return-to-play criteria following sports injury. Clin Sports Med 29(1):169–175. table of contents
2. Greenfield BH, West CR (2012) Ethical issues in sports medicine: a review and justification for ethical decision making and reasoning. Sports Health 4(6):475–479
3. O'Rourke D, Smith R, Smoll F, Cumming S (2014) Relations of parent and coach initiated motivational climates to young athletes self esteem performance anxiety and autonomous motivation who is more. J Appl Sport Psychol 26:395–408
4. Iverson GL, Lovell MR, Collins MW (2003) Interpreting change on ImPACT following sport concussion. Clin Neuropsychol 17(4):460–467
5. Kirschen MP, Tsou A, Nelson SB, Russell JA, Larriviere D, Ethics L, Humanities Committee aJCotAAoNANA, Child Neurology S (2014) Legal and ethical implications in the evaluation and management of sports-related concussion. Neurology 83(4):352–358
6. Attarian DE (2001) The team physician: ethics and enterprise. J Bone Joint Surg Am 83-A(2):293
7. Dunn WR, George MS, Churchill L, Spindler KP (2007) Ethics in sports medicine. Am J Sports Med 35(5):840–844
8. Bernstein J, Perlis C, Bartolozzi AR (2004) Normative ethics in sports medicine. Clin Orthop Relat Res 420:309–318
9. Beauchamp TL, Childress JF (2013) Principles of biomedical ethics, 7th edn. Oxford University Press, New York
10. Giza CC, Kutcher JS, Ashwal S, Barth J, Getchius TS, Gioia GA, Gronseth GS, Guskiewicz K, Mandel S, Manley G, McKeag DB, Thurman DJ, Zafonte R (2013) Summary of evidence-based guideline update: evaluation and management of concussion in sports: report of the guideline development subcommittee of the American academy of neurology. Neurology 80(24):2250–2257

11. Barnum M, Swisher LL, Nyland J, Klossner D, Beckstead J (2009) Ethical issues in athletic training: a foundational descriptive investigation. Athl Ther Today 14(2):3–9
12. Polsky S (1998) Winning medicine: professional sports team doctors' conflicts of interest. J Contemp Health Law Policy 14(2):503–529
13. Sundblad GM, Saartok T, Engstrom LM (2006) Child-parent agreement on reports of disease, injury and pain. BMC Public Health 6:276
14. Hamdan TA (2008) Psychiatric aspects of orthopaedics. J Am Acad Orthop Surg 16(1):41–46
15. Mercado RC, Wiltsey-Stirman S, Iverson KM (2015) Impact of childhood abuse on physical and mental health status and health care utilization among female veterans. Mil Med 180(10):1065–1074
16. Schalet BD, Rothrock NE, Hays RD, Kazis LE, Cook KF, Rutsohn JP, Cella D (2015) Linking physical and mental health summary scores from the veterans RAND 12-item health survey (VR-12) to the PROMIS((R)) global health scale. J Gen Intern Med 30(10):1524–1530
17. Wylie JD, Suter T, Potter MQ, Granger EK, Tashjian RZ (2016) Mental health has a stronger association with patient-reported shoulder pain and function than tear size in patients with full-thickness rotator cuff tears. J Bone Joint Surg Am 98(4):251–256
18. Hartigan EH, Lynch AD, Logerstedt DS, Chmielewski TL, Snyder-Mackler L (2013) Kinesiophobia after anterior cruciate ligament rupture and reconstruction: noncopers versus potential copers. J Orthop Sports Phys Ther 43(11):821–832
19. Brewer BW, Cornelius AE, Van Raalte JL, Petitpas AJ, Sklar JH, Pohlman MH, Krushell RJ, Ditmar TD (2003) Age-related differences in predictors of adherence to rehabilitation after anterior cruciate ligament reconstruction. J Athl Train 38(2):158–162
20. Tripp DA, Stanish WD, Reardon G, Coady C, Sullivan MJ (2003) Comparing postoperative pain experiences of the adolescent and adult athlete after anterior cruciate ligament surgery. J Athl Train 38(2):154–157
21. Salim J, Wadey R, Diss C (2015) Examining hardiness coping and stress related growth following sport injury. J Appl Sport Psychol 28(2):154–169
22. Merkel DL (2013) Youth sport: positive and negative impact on young athletes. Open Access J Sports Med 4:151–160
23. Dorsch TE, King MQ, Dunn CR, Osai KV, Tulane S (2016) The impact of evidence based parent education in organized youth sport: a pilot study. J Appl Sport Psychol 29(2):199–214 ref.51. Online
24. Lin AC, Salzman GA, Bachman SL, Burke RV, Zaslow T, Piasek CZ, Edison BR, Hamilton A, Upperman JS (2015) Assessment of parental knowledge and attitudes toward pediatric sports-related concussions. Sports Health 7(2):124–129
25. Wuerth S, Lee MJ, Alfermann D (2004) Parental involvement and athletes career in youth sport. Psychol Sport Exerc 5:21–33
26. Knight C, Dorsch TE, Osai KV, Haderlie K, Sellars PA (2016) Influences on parental involvement in youth sport. Sport Exerc Perform Psychol 5(2): 161–178
27. Kinight CJ, Neely CC, Holt N (2011) Parental behaviors in team sports: how do female athletes want parents to behave? J Appl Sport Psychol 23(1): 76–92
28. Jowett S, Lavallee D (2007) Social psychology in sport. Human Kinetics, Champaign, IL
29. Cline F, Fay J (2006) Parenting with love and logic : teaching children responsibility, Updated and expanded edn. Piñon Press, Colorado Springs, CO
30. Luebbe AM, Mancini KJ, Kiel EJ, Spangler BR, Semlak JL, Fussner LM (2016) Dimensionality of helicopter parenting and relations to emotional, decision-making, and academic functioning in emerging adults. Assessment. https://doi.org/10.1177/1073191116665907
31. Janssen I (2015) Hyper-parenting is negatively associated with physical activity among 7-12year olds. Prev Med 73:55–59
32. Bunch WH, Dvonch VM (2004) Informed consent in sports medicine. Clin Sports Med 23(2):183–193
33. Koester MC (2000) Youth sports: a pediatrician's perspective on coaching and injury prevention. J Athl Train 35(4):466–470
34. Cahill PJ, Refakis C, Storey E, Warner WC Jr (2016) Concussion in sports: what do orthopaedic surgeons need to know? J Am Acad Orthop Surg 24(12):e193–e201
35. Provance AJ, Engelman GH, Terhune EB, Coel RA (2016) Management of sport-related concussion in the pediatric and adolescent population. Orthopedics 39(1):24–30
36. Emery CA, Meeuwisse WH, Hartmann SE (2005) Evaluation of risk factors for injury in adolescent soccer: implementation and validation of an injury surveillance system. Am J Sports Med 33(12): 1882–1891
37. Della Villa S, Boldrini L, Ricci M, Danelon F, Snyder-Mackler L, Nanni G, Roi GS (2012) Clinical outcomes and return-to-sports participation of 50 soccer players after anterior cruciate ligament reconstruction through a sport-specific rehabilitation protocol. Sports Health 4(1):17–24

65 Mental Health in Professional Football Players

Vincent Gouttebarge and Gino M.M.J. Kerkhoffs

Contents

V. Gouttebarge (✉)
World Players' Union (FIFPro), Hoofddorp, The Netherlands

Academic Center for Evidence based Sports Medicine (ACES), Academic Medical Center, Amsterdam, The Netherlands

Department of Orthopaedic Surgery, Academic Medical Center, University of Amsterdam, Amsterdam Movement Sciences, Amsterdam, The Netherlands
e-mail: v.gouttebarge@fifpro.org

G.M.M.J. Kerkhoffs
Academic Center for Evidence based Sports Medicine (ACES), Academic Medical Center, Amsterdam, The Netherlands

Department of Orthopaedic Surgery, Academic Medical Center, University of Amsterdam, Amsterdam Movement Sciences, Amsterdam, The Netherlands

65.1 Introduction

In professional football, most of the epidemiological studies have been directed towards the physical health of players, principally towards the occurrence of musculoskeletal injuries and more recently towards the prevention of these injuries. By contrast, scientific information about the mental health of professional footballers remains scarce. This is surprising because players are (cumulatively) exposed during their career to specific and non-specific stressors that might lead to symptoms of common mental disorders (CMD). These symptoms of CMD are likely to influence the performances of players but also their quality of life negatively.

This chapter focuses on the symptoms of CMD (self-reported and not clinically diagnosed) that might occur during a career in professional football. After its definition, the magnitude of the symptoms of CMD among professional footballers is presented. Subsequently, the non-specific and football-specific stressors that play a role in the occurrence of symptoms of CMD are

V. Musahl et al. (eds.), *Return to Play in Football*, https://doi.org/10.1007/978-3-662-55713-6_65

presented. Finally, a concise overview of the symptoms of CMD that are most frequently reported by players is given.

65.2 Definition of Symptoms of Common Mental Disorders

Someone suffers from symptoms of CMD when he or she experiences adverse feelings or thoughts or when he or she shows some abnormal or maladaptive behaviour that impair his or her activities either in daily life, work or sport (Fact Box 1). Examples of symptoms of CMD are related to distress, burnout, anxiety, depression or sleep disturbance. In contrast to symptoms of CMD that are self-reported, mental disorders are clinically diagnosed and refer to the combination of more severe symptoms. In accordance with the standard classification of mental disorders used by mental health professionals in the USA (Diagnostic and Statistical Manual of Mental Disorders), mental disorders are divided into different categories such as depressive disorders (e.g. major depressive disorder), anxiety disorders (excessive fear and anxiety and related behavioural disturbances), sleep-wake disorders (e.g. insomnia disorder, hypersomnolence disorder), substance-related and addictive disorders (e.g. alcohol, caffeine, cannabis) and feeding and eating disorders (anorexia nervosa, bulimia nervosa) [1]. Symptoms of CMD are often comorbid (several symptoms occurring simultaneously).

Fact Box 1
Symptoms of common mental disorders include feelings and thoughts of psychological disturbance—such as feelings and thoughts of distress, anxiety, depression or sleep disturbance—and describe a mental and emotional state that affects significantly the way of thinking, feeling and behaving to such an extent that important areas of life such as learning, living, working, exercising and socialising are impaired.

65.3 Prevalence and Incidence of Symptoms of Common Mental Disorders in Professional Football

In recent years, several studies have been conducted about the occurrence of symptoms of CMD among professional footballers [2–7]. In 2013, a preliminary study on symptoms of CMD was conducted in a sample of 149 male professional footballers (mean age of 27 years; mean career duration of 9 years; 60% playing in the highest professional league) from Australia, Ireland, the Netherlands, New Zealand, Scotland and the USA [2]. In this cross-sectional study, the 4-week prevalence of symptoms of CMD was 10% for distress, 26% for anxiety/depression and 19% for adverse alcohol use [2]. Subsequently to this preliminary study, a 12-month prospective cohort study on symptoms of CMD was conducted among 607 male professional players (mean age of 27 years; mean career duration of 8 years; 55% playing in the highest professional league) recruited in 11 countries [3]. In that study, the same scales for measuring symptoms of CMD were used as in the preliminary study. The 4-week prevalence of symptoms of CMD found at baseline was 15% for distress, 38% for anxiety/depression, 23% for sleep disturbance and 9% for adverse alcohol use [3]. A sub-analysis of these baseline data showed that the prevalence rates of symptoms of CMD were quite similar across five European countries, ranging from 6% in Sweden for adverse alcohol use to 43% in Norway for anxiety/depression [4]. Based on the longitudinal data collected during the 12-month follow-up period (follow-up rate of 68%), incidence of symptoms of CMD among professional footballers was 12% for distress, 37% for anxiety/depression, 19% for sleep disturbance and 14% for adverse alcohol use [5]. A study among 471 top-level football players from Switzerland found a prevalence of 8% for mild to moderate depression, 3% for major depression and around 1% for an at least moderate anxiety disorder [7]. In that study (using different scales for measuring depression and anxiety than those used the studies aforementioned), male players had a lower prevalence of depression and anxiety than female players [7].

Table 65.1 Prevalence of symptoms of common mental disorders among professional footballers and professional athletes from other sport disciplines

	Distress	Anxiety/depression	Sleep disturbance	Adverse alcohol use
Footballers	*10–15*	*26–38*	*23*	*9–19*
Cricketers	38	37	38	26
Dutch athletes	27	45	22	6
Gaelic athletes	38	48	33	23
Handball	20	26	22	3
Ice hockey	9	17	9	6
Rugby players	17	30	13	15

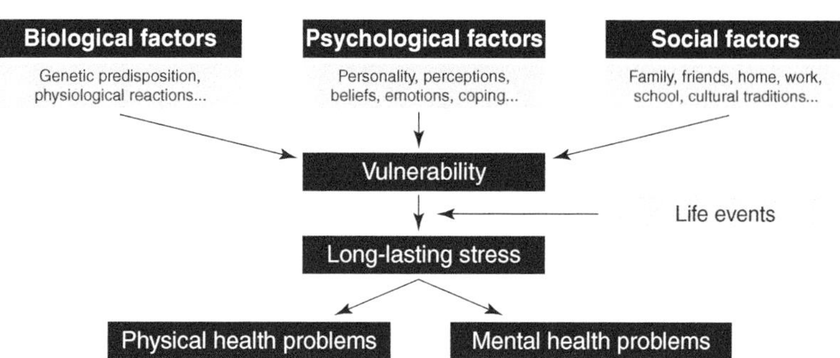

Fig. 65.1 Biopsychosocial model

In other professional sports, recent studies found similar prevalence rates than those among football players (Table 65.1). In 2015, a cross-sectional study involving 224 Australian elite athletes showed that 45% of them had experienced symptoms of at least one mental health problem such as anxiety, depression or distress in the previous few weeks [8]. In another recent study involving more than 2000 young and adult French Olympics athletes, 17% of them reported having encountered mental problems in the past [9]. Among 203 Dutch elite athletes, 4-week prevalence of symptoms of CMD ranged from 6% for adverse alcohol use to 45% for anxiety/depression, while 17% reported two simultaneous symptoms of CMD [10]. Among 204 elite Gaelic athletes, a prospective cohort study (2016) showed a 4-week prevalence of symptoms of CMD reaching up to 48% for anxiety/depression, while around 24% and 16% reported two and three simultaneous symptoms of CMD, respectively [11]. In South African professional cricket ($N = 78$), 4-week prevalence of symptoms of CMD ranged from 26% for adverse alcohol use to 38% for distress and anxiety/depression [12]. Among 990 (semi-)professional rugby players, 4-week prevalence of symptoms of CMD was 18% for distress, 30% for anxiety/depression, 13% for sleep disturbance, 23% for eating disorders and 15% for adverse alcohol use [13].

65.4 Aetiology of Symptoms of Common Mental Disorders

The occurrence of symptoms of CMD is not caused by a single stressor but is usually multifactorial. Among professional footballers, symptoms of CMD can occur as a consequence of the interaction between psychosocial, sport-specific and career-related stressors.

65.4.1 Psychosocial Stressors

As indicated in the biopsychosocial model (Fig. 65.1), biological (genetic, biochemical, etc.), psychological (mood, personality, behaviour, etc.) and social (cultural, familial, socioeconomic, medical, etc.) stressors play a role in the occurrence of symptoms of CMD (as well as physical health problems) [14]. The biopsychosocial model is a general framework arguing that the complex and dynamic interaction between these three types of stressors determines the course of health-related outcomes, and not one type of stressors in isolation.

Especially, vulnerability due to potential predisposition, combined with environmental stressors or life events, can lead to symptoms of CMD. Because of the exposure to many life changes and related stressors between the 18th and 25th year of someone's life, symptoms of CMD occur especially in young adulthood, with some symptoms being clearly gender related [15]. As any human being, professional footballers are likely to develop symptoms of CMD as a consequence of potential biological, psychological and social stressors. In addition, professional footballers are also exposed during their career to sport-specific stressors.

65.4.2 Sport-Specific Stressors

Recently, the scientific literature has shown that professional footballers as well as competitive athletes might be confronted during their career (including transitioning out of sport) with up to 640 distinct stressors that could induce symptoms of CMD (Fact Box 2) [16].

Fact Box 2
Four main categories of sport-specific stressors:

- Leadership and personnel issues: adverse coach's behaviour and attitudes, conflict with coach, dealing with media and spectators, governing bodies, etc.
- Logistical and environmental issues: poor travel and accommodation arrangements, adverse weather conditions, poor facilities and equipment, etc.
- Cultural and team issues: adverse teammates' behaviour and attitudes, lack of support, poor communication, etc.
- Performance and personal issues: decreased performances, injuries, etc.

These sport-specific stressors are divided into four main categories: (1) leadership and personnel issues (adverse coach's behaviour and attitudes, conflict with coach, dealing with media and spectators, governing bodies, etc.), (2) logistical and environmental issues (poor travel and accommodation arrangements, adverse weather conditions, poor facilities and equipment, etc.), (3) cultural and team issues (adverse teammates' behaviour and attitudes, lack of support, poor communication, etc.) and (4) performance and personal issues (decreased performances, injuries, etc.) [16].

Especially injuries that lead to a long layoff period can be considered as a major stressor that might induce symptoms of CMD. Cross-sectional analyses within the aforementioned 12-month prospective cohort study showed that the total number of severe time-loss (28 days or more) injuries during a football career was positively correlated with distress, anxiety and sleeping disturbance (Fact Box 3) [6]. These analyses showed that professional footballers who had sustained one or more severe time-loss injuries during their career were 2–4 times more likely to report symptoms of CMD than professional footballers who had not suffered from severe time-loss injuries [6].

Fact Box 3
The number of severe musculoskeletal injuries during a football career is correlated with distress, anxiety and sleeping disturbance. Professional footballers who have sustained one or more severe musculoskeletal injuries (time-loss >4 weeks) during their career are two to nearly four times more likely to report symptoms of common mental disorders than professional footballers who have not suffered from severe musculoskeletal injuries.

These sport-specific stressors, combined with more traditional biological, psychological and social stressors, form a complex dynamic to which professional footballers are exposed from their young adulthood until the end of their career. The interaction between all these stressors can lead to symptoms of CMD among professional footballers but can also impair their development as players [17].

65.4.3 Developmental Model of Transitions

The developmental model of transitions (Fig. 65.2) shows that the development of an athlete (such as a professional footballer) can be characterised by different developmental transitions that occur on four levels [17]: (1) stages and transitions related to sport development (for instance from the years within the academy of a football club to the transition out of competitive football), (2) stages and transitions occurring at psychological level (childhood, adolescence and (young) adulthood), (3) stages and transitions occurring in the athlete's psychosocial development relative to her or his sport involvement (athlete family, peer relationships, coach-player relationships, marital relationships and other interpersonal relationships significant to players) and (4) stages and transitions related to the academic and vocational level (primary education/elementary school, secondary education/high school, higher education (college/university), vocational training and/or an professional occupation).

To continue to develop and thus continue to achieve the required level of performance, athletes should be able to successfully cope with these stages and transitions within and across all four developmental levels. Inadequate coping, for example, when there is insufficient social support within the athlete's environment or when an athlete does not concur with the requirements of a first-year senior athlete (being no longer the strongest, competing with mature and experienced athletes), can lead to a transitional crisis that might be associated with symptoms of CMD. The developmental model of transitions (Fig. 65.2) underlines not only the interactive nature of transitions in different domains of life of athletes but also that nonathletic transition may affect, aside their mental health, the development of athletes' sports career.

Age	10	15	20	25	30	35
Athletic level	Initiation	Development		Mastery	Discontinuation	
Psychological level	Childhood	Adolescence			Adulthood	
Psychosocial level	Parents Siblings peers	Peers Coaches Parents		Partner Coach	Family (Coach)	
Academic vocational level	Primary education	Secondary education	Higher education		Vocational training Professional occupation	

Note: A dotted line indicates that the age at which the transition occurs is an approximation

Fig. 65.2 The developmental model of transitions

65.5 Prevalent Mental Health Problems in Professional Football

The next sections present some basic information (definition, symptoms and signs, assessment and screening, treatment approach) about the symptoms of CMD being prevalent among professional footballers, namely, anxiety/depression (prevalence up to 38%), sleep disturbance (prevalence up to 23%) and adverse alcohol use (prevalence of up to 19%) [1, 18]. These symptoms can have some negative influence for the performances of players but also for their return-to-play process.

65.5.1 Depression

Depression is a common, but often serious, mood disorder causing severe symptoms that affect how you feel, think and handle activities of daily life, work and/or sport. Depression is characterised by persistent and long-lasting symptoms such as:

- Low or sad moods, often with crying episodes
- Irritability and anger
- Thinking negatively and feeling worthless, helpless and hopeless
- Appetite and sleeping disturbance
- Decrease in energy and activity levels with feelings of fatigue or tiredness
- Decreases in concentration, interest and motivation
- Social withdrawal or avoidance
- Unexplained aches and pains (increased in physical complaints such as headaches, back pain, aching muscles and stomach pain)
- In severe cases: thoughts of death or suicide

To be diagnosed with depression, a person must have experienced during more than 2 weeks a major depressive episode including a combination of symptoms. To establish such a diagnosis, information is collected through medical history about the presence of symptoms and the level of impairment (daily life, work and/or sport). In addition, reproducible and valid screening instruments can be used such as Hospital Anxiety and Depression Scale (HADS), General Health Questionnaire (GHQ) and Profile of Mood States (POMS). While a short depressive episode can resolve naturally, treatment is warranted when the depression becomes more severe, lasts longer, occurs more frequently and impairs functioning significantly (Fact Box 4).

65.5.2 Anxiety

Anxiety is a normal part of everyday life: everyone is likely from time to time to experience symptoms of anxiety, either in the cognitive (e.g. worries), emotional (e.g. feelings of nervousness), behavioural (e.g. pacing) or physiological (e.g. muscle tension) domain. Anxiety is characterised by feelings of abnormal, e.g. extreme fear, panic and/or worry, that lead to sustainable irrational or to impairment in social context. Difference should be made between panic disorder, social anxiety disorder, generalised anxiety disorders and phobias.

Being often comorbid with depression, anxiety includes symptoms such as:

- Feelings of panic, fear and uneasiness
- Sleeping disturbance
- Cold or sweaty hands or feet
- Shortness of breath
- Heart palpitations
- Not being able to be still and calm
- Dry mouth
- Numbness or tingling in the hands or feet
- Nausea
- Muscle tension
- Dizziness

Anxiety can be diagnosed using structured and semi-structured interviews (Diagnostic Interview Schedule, Anxiety Disorders Interview Schedule) as well as with (behavioural) observations. In addition, reproducible and valid screening instruments can be used such as Symptom Checklist-90

(SCL-90), Hospital Anxiety and Depression Scale (HADS), General Health Questionnaire (GHQ) and Profile of Mood States (POMS). Depending on the type of anxiety disorder, several therapy strategies can be applied (Fact Box 4).

Fact Box 4

Treatment strategies for depression (depending on duration and severity):

- Self-management and education (with minimal support) or counselling
- Forms of physical activity such as walking, running, cycling or swimming
- Evidence-based psychotherapy approach such as cognitive behavioural therapy, interpersonal therapy and problem-solving therapy
- e-Health interventions
- Medication including especially (modern) antidepressants

65.5.3 Sleep Disturbance

Sleep disturbance includes complaints that affect the ability to sleep well on a regular basis. While occasionally experiencing difficulties to sleep is normal, it is abnormal to regularly have problems getting to sleep at night, to wake up feeling exhausted or to feel sleepy during the day. Insomnia might be the most known type of sleep disturbance, being defined as having poor sleep at least three times a week that may lead to daily life impairments (e.g. fatigue, irritability, decreased concentration). Depending on its severity and type, sleep disturbance includes symptoms such as:

- Difficulty falling or staying asleep
- Daytime fatigue
- Strong urge to take naps during the day
- Irritability or anxiety
- Lack of concentration
- Depression

Information collected through medical history is generally sufficient to establish the diagnosis of sleep disturbance. During the anamnesis, several issues need to be addressed, among which (1) nature, duration, course and frequency of the symptoms, (2) impairments in daily living, (3) potential causes, (4) sleep patterns (including evening activities disturbing sleep) and (5) physical symptoms and disorders (pain, cough, dyspnoea, nasal congestion, night sweats, palpitations). Physical examination is not often necessary, only in case of the presence of physical symptoms and disorders. In addition to the use of a sleep diary, reproducible and valid screening instruments can be used such as Sleep Disorders Questionnaire (SDQ), Epworth Sleepiness Scale (ESS) and Holland Sleep Disorders Questionnaire.

Depending on the type and underlying cause, the treatment for sleep disturbance generally includes a combination of medical treatments and lifestyle adjustments. Medical treatments might include sleeping pills, melatonin supplements, medications for any underlying health problems, breathing device and a dental guard. Lifestyle adjustments aim at improving the quality of sleep, for instance, by reducing stress and anxiety through exercising, having a regular sleeping schedule, limiting the consumption of caffeine, decreasing tobacco and alcohol use and eating smaller meals before bedtime.

65.5.4 Adverse Alcohol Use

Adverse alcohol use and alcohol dependence are characterised by either a persistent pattern of inappropriate alcohol use or of adverse consequences. While alcohol dependence is typically considered to be synonymous with alcoholism, adverse alcohol use can be defined as a recurring pattern of high-risk drinking that results in adverse outcomes such as personal problems (e.g. memory and cognition, job, family and friends), problems to others (e.g. injuries, violence) and problems for society (e.g. underage drinking, health care costs). Depending on the type and amount of alcohol consumed and an individual's personality, several (physical) signs might occur as a consequence of adverse alcohol use, for instance, decreased involvement and interest in social activities, work or school, lack of interest in family or friends, depression, restlessness, erratic and violent behaviour and redness of the face during or after periods of consumption.

Moderate drinking can be defined as consuming (1) up to one drink (10 g of alcohol, which is around 100 ml of wine) per day for women and (2) up to two drinks per day for men. Excessive (binge) drinking can be defined as consuming (1) four or more drinks during a single occasion for women and (2) five or more drinks during a single occasion for men. *Heavy drinking* can be defined as consuming (1) 8 or more drinks per week for women and (2) 15 or more drinks per week for men. Adverse alcohol use (and dependence) can be screened with the following reproducible and valid instruments: Michigan Alcoholism Screening Test (MAST), Alcohol Use Disorders Identification Test (AUDIT), Cut down, Annoyed by criticism, Guilty about drinking, Eye-opener (CAGE-test).

The first step of any treatment is to go through detoxification, being the process of removing alcohol from the body and eliminate any physical dependency to the substance. Such a process is associated with developing withdrawal symptoms such as nausea, trembling and sweating. In addition to medication (such as benzodiazepines or naltrexone), various interventions can be used such as motivational interviewing, cognitive behavioural therapy, teaching social skills and self-control training.

65.6 Potential Influence on Performances and Return to Play

Symptoms of CMD reported by professional footballers are likely to influence negatively their performances. Most of professional footballers believe that symptoms of CMD influence football performances negatively, while a large majority (65%) mentioned that they had been impaired during their own career because of symptoms of CMD. Because of their nature and consequences, a logical assumption is that symptoms of CMD are likely to interfere within the return-to-play process, especially with regard to the following aspects:

- Concentration and focus
- Coordination
- Power
- Emotion
- Reaction time
- Strength
- Endurance

Take-Home Message

- Four-week prevalence of symptoms of common mental disorders among professional footballers ranges from 9% for adverse alcohol use to 38% for anxiety/depression and 12-month incidence from 12% for distress to 37% for anxiety/depression.
- Professional footballers who have sustained one or more severe time-loss injuries during their career are two to four to nearly four times more likely to report symptoms of a mental disorder than professional footballers who have not suffered from similar time-loss injuries.
- Symptoms of common mental disorders are likely to influence football performance negatively and to interfere with return to play.

Top Five Evidence-Based References

Gouttebarge V, Aoki H, Kerkhoffs G (2015) Symptoms of common mental disorders and adverse health behaviours in male professional soccer players. J Hum Kinet 49:277–286

Gouttebarge V, Backx F, Aoki H et al (2015) Symptoms of common mental disorders in professional football (soccer) across five European countries. J Sports Sci Med 14:811–818

Gouttebarge V, Aoki H, Verhagen EA et al (2017) A 12-month prospective cohort study of symptoms of common mental disorders among European professional footballers. Clin J Sport Med 27:487–492

Gouttebarge V, Aoki H, Ekstrand J et al (2016) Are severe joint and muscle injuries related to symptoms of common mental disorders among male European professional footballers? Knee Surg Sports Traumatol Arthrosc 24:3934–3942

Junge A, Eddermann-Demont N (2016) Prevalence of depression and anxiety in top-level male and female football players. BMJ Open Sport Exerc Med 2:e000087. https://doi.org/10.1136/bmjsem-2015-000087

References

1. American Psychiatric Association (2013) Diagnostic and statistical manual of mental disorders, Fifth Edition (Dsm-5). American Psychiatric Publishing, Arlington
2. Gouttebarge V, Frings-Dresen MHW, Sluiter JK (2015) Mental and psychosocial health among current and former professional football players. Occup Med 65:190–196
3. Gouttebarge V, Aoki H, Kerkhoffs G (2015) Symptoms of common mental disorders and adverse health behaviours in male professional soccer players. J Hum Kinet 49:277–286
4. Gouttebarge V, Backx F, Aoki H et al (2015) Symptoms of common mental disorders in professional football (soccer) across five European countries. J Sports Sci Med 14:811–818
5. Gouttebarge V, Aoki H, Verhagen EA et al (2017) A 12-month prospective cohort study of symptoms of common mental disorders among European professional footballers. Clin J Sport Med 27:487–492
6. Gouttebarge V, Aoki H, Ekstrand J et al (2016) Are severe joint and muscle injuries related to symptoms of common mental disorders among male European professional footballers? Knee Surg Sports Traumatol Arthrosc 24:3934–3942
7. Junge A, Eddermann-Demont N (2016) Prevalence of depression and anxiety in top-level male and female football players. BMJ Open Sport Exerc Med 2:e000087. https://doi.org/10.1136/bmjsem-2015-000087
8. Gulliver A, Griffiths KM, Mackinnon A et al (2015) The mental health of Australian elite athletes. J Sci Med Sport 18:255–261
9. Schaal K, Tafflet M, Nassif H et al (2011) Psychological balance in high level athletes: gender-based differences and sport-specific patterns. PLoS One 6:e19007
10. Gouttebarge V, Jonkers R, Moen M et al (2017) The prevalence and risk indicators of symptoms of common mental disorders among current and former Dutch elite athletes. J Sports Sci 35(21):2148–2156. https://doi.org/10.1080/02640414.2016.1258485
11. Gouttebarge V, Tol J, Kerkhoffs G (2016) Epidemiology of symptoms of common mental disorders among elite Gaelic athletes: a prospective cohort study. Phys Sportsmed 44:283–289. https://doi.org/10.1080/00913847.2016.1185385
12. Schuring N, Kerkhoffs, G, Gray J et al (2017) The mental wellbeing of current and retired professional cricketers: an observational prospective cohort study. Phys Sportsmed, pp. 1–7. https://doi.org/10.1080/00913847.2017.1386069
13. Gouttebarge V, opley P, Kerkhoffs G et al (2017) Symptoms of common mental disorders in professional rugby: an international observational descriptive study. Int J Sports Med 38:864–870
14. Engel GL (1977) The need for a new medical model: a challenge for biomedicine. Science 196:129–136
15. Krueger RF, Caspi A, Moffit TE et al (1998) The structure and stability of common mental disorders (DSM-III-R): a longitudinal – epidemiological study. J Abnorm Psychol 107:216–227
16. Arnold R, Fletcher D (2012) A research synthesis and taxonomic classification of the organizational stressors encountered by sport performers. J Sport Exerc Psychol 34:397–429
17. Wylleman P, Reints A, De Knop P (2013) A developmental and holistic perspective on athletic career development. In: Sotiaradou P, De Bosscher V (eds) Managing high performance sport. Routledge, New York
18. Barlow DH (2008) Clinical handbook of psychological disorders. The Guilford Press, New York

Part IX

Injury and Reinjury Prevention

66 The 11+ Injury Prevention Programme (2008–2016)

Mario Bizzini

Contents

M. Bizzini, Ph.D., P.T.
Schulthess Clinic, Lengghalde 2,
8008 Zurich, Switzerland
e-mail: Mario.Bizzini@kws.ch

66.1 Introduction

Football is the most popular sport worldwide and is played on amateur or recreational level by almost 300 million people. While football can be considered a healthy leisure activity, football, as a contact team sport, entails also a certain risk of injury. The medical treatment of football-related injuries can have a significant socio-economic impact in terms of related healthcare costs [1]. In 1994 FIFA realised their responsibility towards player's health and safety and founded its FIFA Medical Assessment and Research Centre (F-MARC) in order to create and disseminate scientific knowledge on various medical topics in football, to reduce football injuries and, thus, to promote football as a health-enhancing leisure activity [2]. The chapter presents the theoretical background, development, scientific evaluation, implementation and dissemination strategies of FIFA's injury prevention programmes ("The 11, The 11+ or FIFA 11+"), under the leadership of F-MARC (1994–2016), in order to provide a role model of how an international sports governing body can make its sport safer.

66.2 Development of Injury Prevention Programmes

The first scientific study on injury prevention in football was published in 1983 [3]. In the next 20 years, only few authors reported stud-

V. Musahl et al. (eds.), *Return to Play in Football*, https://doi.org/10.1007/978-3-662-55713-6_66

ies on prevention of football injuries. In 2000 F-MARC conducted its first study on prevention of football injury in male Swiss youth teams, showing 21% fewer injuries in the intervention compared to the control group [4]. The interventions were focused on improving the structure and content of the training by educating and supervising the coaches and players. The prevention program included general interventions such as improvement of warm-up, regular cool-down, taping of unstable ankles, adequate rehabilitation, promotion of the spirit of fair play and ten sets of exercises designed to improve coordination, stability of ankle and knee, flexibility and strength of trunk, hip and leg muscles. Based on the experiences with this pilot study and in cooperation with international experts, F-MARC developed in 2003 a simple injury prevention programme for amateur football players called "The 11".

"The 11" comprises ten evidence-based or best-practice exercises (core stability, balance, dynamic stabilisation and eccentric hamstring strength) and the promotion of Fair Play. The programme was designed to reduce the most common football injuries (ankle and knee sprains, hamstring and groin strains). It can be completed in 10–15 min and requires no equipment other than a ball. "The 11" was implemented in two countrywide campaigns (Switzerland and New Zealand) in cooperation with the national accident insurance company and the national football association [1].

In Switzerland, the implementation of "The 11" and its effects on the injury rates were evaluated by an independent research institute. Four years after the launch of the programme, teams that included "The 11" as a part of their warm-up had 11.5% fewer match injuries and 25.3% fewer training injuries than team that warmed-up as usual [5]. In New Zealand the implementation of "The 11" resulted in an 8.2 dollars of return of investment (per invested dollar) for the national accident insurance company after 7 years [1].

In two controlled randomised studies (RCTs) on "The 11", no statistical significant effects were found in terms of injury prevention in male and female players. Compliance issues and exercise dosage were discussed as the main points of concern [1]. Based on experiences with "The 11", "PEP" (Prevent Injury and Enhance Performance) Programme [6] and other exercised-based programmes to prevent football injuries, an advanced version ("The 11+, later called FIFA 11+") was developed in 2006 together with the OSTRC and the Santa Monica Orthopaedic and Sports Medicine Research Foundation. "The 11+" is a complete warm-up programme with running exercises in the beginning and at the end to activate the cardiovascular system and specific preventive exercises focussing on core and leg strength, balance and agility, each of three levels of increasing difficulty (to providing variation and progression). It takes about 20–25 min to be completed and requires a minimum of equipment (a set of cones and balls) (Fig. 66.1). "The 11+" should replace the usual warm-up few times a week [1].

As from 2007, different research groups worldwide evaluated the preventive and performance effects of this basic prevention programme [7].

66.3 Evidence of Injury Prevention for 11+ in Female and Male Players

The efficacy of the 11+ was first proven in young female players, which was similar for "PEP" (Prevent Injury and Enhance Performance), a non-contact ACL prevention programme. A significant reduction (up to 50%) of injuries was found in young female players in large RCTs, when the warm-up exercises were performed at least twice a week [8, 9]. In both studies the role of compliance was documented, showing a further reduction of injury risk in those players with higher adherence to the programme. Recently a similar impact of the 11+ was reported in two RCTs involving male players [10, 11]. Owoeye

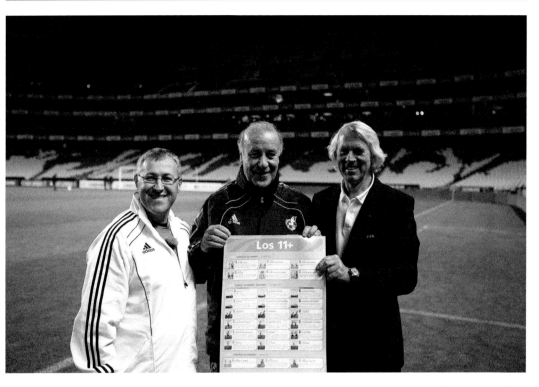

Fig. 66.1 Vicente del Bosque, coach of the Spanish national football team (World Cup winner 2010), promoting "Los 11+" together with Mario Bizzini (*left*) and Jiri Dvorak (*right*), Madrid, December 2010

et al. [10] found a significantly lower (ca. 40%) incidence of injuries in young Nigerian male players, and Silvers-Granelli et al. [11] reported similar results in American male NCAA Division I–II players—when performing the programme regularly (2–3×/week). These four RCTs impressively showed how a basic injury prevention programme, with proper player compliance, significantly reduces injuries both in female and male amateur football. Two recent systematic reviews on structured neuromuscular warm-up programmes underline the evidence behind the preventive effects of the 11+ in youth amateur football [7]. A recent systematic review and meta-analysis concluded that the 11+ has a substantial injury-preventing effect by reducing football injuries in recreational/subelite football by 39% [12].

In other age groups, especially in children (below 14 years of age), there is a paucity of research in injuries and their prevention [13]. Researchers [14] formulated the basis for preventive strategies in children playing football, and after developing an adapted "11+ Kids" programme [15], F-MARC conducted a large multicentre intervention study (four European countries), which showed an impressive overall reduction (by ca. 50%) of injuries in children performing the 11+ Kids exercises [16] (Fig. 66.2).

Fact Box 1

The 11+ prevention programme reduces the top four most prevalent football injuries: hamstring by 60%, hip/groin by 41%, knee by 48% and ankle by 32% (level 1 evidence-based information form the last systematic review and meta-analysis) [12].

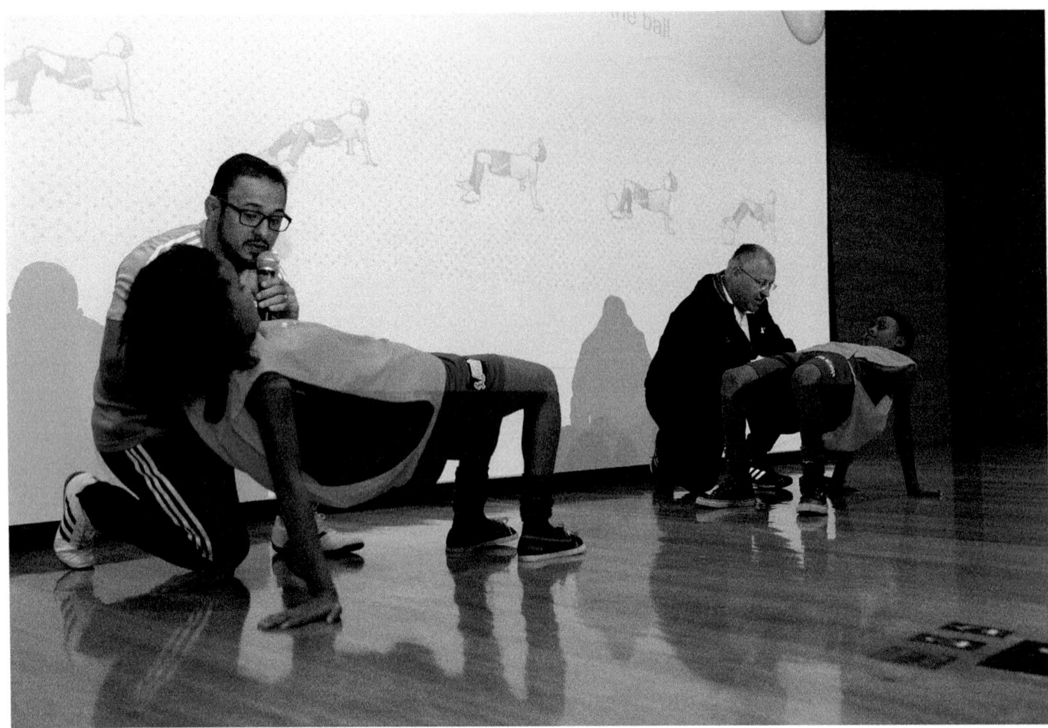

Fig. 66.2 Demonstration of 11+ KIDS exercises at the CBF (Confederacao Brasileira de Futebol) headquarters, Rio de Janeiro, August 11, 2016

66.4 The Referees

The match officials are an important but often unrecognised part in football. In modern football, referees (especially at elite level) are exposed to considerable amounts of match and training loads. While several (but to a lesser extent than in players) studies have addressed different aspects of performance and training, recently the associated injury risk in referees has been investigated. Based on the their specific injury profile and on the successful 11+, a "11+ Referee" injury prevention programme for referees and assistant referees has been developed and pilot tested [17]. The programme is being distributed worldwide (since 2013) within the FIFA refereeing courses and can be accessed online (http://fifamedicinediploma.com/courses/referee/).

66.5 Performance and Warm-Up Effects of FIFA 11+

"Which are the performance benefits of such exercises?" is one of the most common questions by football coaches, when exposed to a so-called "injury prevention programme". Various studies have investigated the performance effects of the 11+ in male and female players. A RCT found significantly better neuromuscular control (quicker stabilisation time of lower extremity and core) in Italian amateur male players after 9 weeks of FIFA 11+ practice [18]. Others [19] showed significant better functional balance in Canadian young female players performing the 11+ during a season in another RCT. Other studies found improved knee strength ratios, static/dynamic balance and agility skills in Asian male players after performing the 11+ warm-up for an average time of 2 months. A pre-post study in Italian male amateur players showed how 11+ induces similar physiological responses as other published warm-ups [20]. Recently two studies showed how 11+ exercises can trigger core and hip musculature activation, therefore improving neuromuscular control (Fig. 66.2). Other studies have found positive performance enhancement effects of the 11+ in male futsal players [20].

While epidemiological data are available in professional football, almost no prevention studies in elite-level players have been published so far. Recent published surveys on the preventative strategies in premier league clubs and national teams showed that some most of the rated preventive exercises were components of the 11+ programme [21, 22].

66.6 Development of an Implementation Strategy

From the beginning of F-MARC activities in injury prevention, the coach—especially at lower levels—was identified as the key instigator in performing injury prevention programmes with her/his players. The successful countrywide campaign in Switzerland was the first example demonstrating how a basic injury prevention programme can be disseminated and implemented at large scale in amateur football through coaching education [5]. For the countrywide campaign in Switzerland, "The 11" was integrated in the coach education of the Swiss Football Association (Schweizerischer Fussballverband (SFV)) using a "teach the teacher" strategy or "cascade approach". All instructor coaches of the SFV were educated by sports physical therapists on how to deliver the programme to the coaches in their licencing or refresher courses. During a period of 3 years, 5000 licenced amateur coaches were subsequently instructed on performing "The 11" with their teams and received the information material [5]. The same strategy was used in New Zealand, where "The 11" was implemented as part of the "Soccer Smart Program". In Belgium, the introduction of the 11+ (via coaching courses by the National Football Federation) together with other preventive policies (i.e. no matches if weather conditions are bad) has led to an overall reduction of football-related injuries [7].

In a RCT evaluating different delivery methods of the 11+ found that a pre-season coaching workshop was more effective (than unsupervised delivery, additional on-field supervision) in terms of adherence and even reduced injury risk in teams performing the injury prevention programme [9]. Delivery strategies should be further tailored to coaches (and players), as other factors (knowledge, beliefs, experience) may also influence their behaviour towards endorsing injury prevention programmes.

"The 11+" is best taught to coaches in a workshop that includes theoretical background knowledge and practical demonstration of the exercises (Fig. 66.3). After raising the coach motivation and awareness of injury prevention, the exercises should be briefly explained and demonstrated. It is helpful to select a participant to perform the exercise, while the instructor highlights the correct execution of the exercises. The participants should then perform the exercises and be corrected by the instructor(s). The participants should get "a feel" for the exercises and appreciated the challenges behind each exercises. In the second half of the workshop, each of the participants should teach at least one of the exercises to the group and get feedback on this from the instructor [1].

Fact Box 2

Information material on "The 11+" was developed, produced and made available for coaches and players. The material includes a detailed manual, an instructional DVD, posters and promotional booklet/clips. All material is available in various languages and can be accessed on http://fifamedicinediploma.com/courses/injury-prevention/.

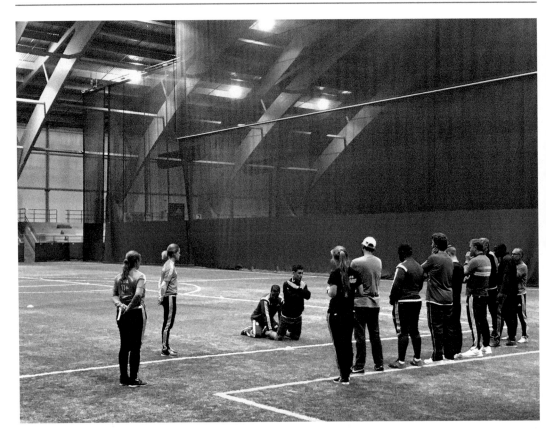

Fig. 66.3 11+ Instructor coaching course with the Canadian Soccer Association (CSA), Montreal-Laval, October 2016

66.7 Worldwide Dissemination of "The 11+"

In 2009 FIFA started the dissemination of the programme in its 209 Member Associations (MAs). Based on the experience with the countrywide implementation in Switzerland and New Zealand, a guideline on how to implement the "The 11+" injury prevention programme at large scale in amateur football was developed. The implementation is conducted either in close cooperation with MAs or via FIFA Coaching Instructor courses coaching courses. F-MARC supports the MAs in the preparation of the educational material in the local language and the workshops for the first group of instructor in initiate the cascade training [1].

Various important national football associations (such as Germany, Brazil, Italy, Japan) integrated "The 11+" in their basis coaching curriculum or their physical training/education curriculum. Despite implementation problems, other countries followed these role models, and in general the interest towards injury prevention in football has increased over the years [1].

66.8 Implementation of 11+: The Example of Germany

The German Football Association (DFB, Deutscher Fussball-Bund), the four-time FIFA World Cup winner, is the largest MA worldwide. The DFB has for many years had a state-of-the-art organisation and knowledge at all levels of football: nevertheless, the Association (at its highest levels) decided in 2011 to promote 11+ among its nearly seven million registered amateur players. Following the cooperation with one of the German national insurance companies (Verwaltungs-Berufsgenossenschaft; VBG) and

F_MARC, the 11+ was first presented to executives and representatives of the DFB Amateur Football at a congress in Kassel (February 2012). The dissemination plan was then finalised, with the financial costs (material, course organisation, others) divided by DFB (50%) and VBG (50%). The position of a dedicated manager within the DFB was crucial to ensure the realisation of this project. F-MARC provided full support in realising the first two instructor's courses, targeting the DFB head regional coaches and the DFB head talent coordinators (October 2012). During 2013 and 2015, 45 courses were conducted in the 21 regions of the DFB, and a total of 1300 coaches were certified as 11+ instructors. This cascade training ("teach the teacher" strategy, as outlined by Junge et al. [5]) allowed the 26,000 registered clubs in DFB amateur football to be subsequently targeted (for ratio of approx. 1 instructor per 23 teams), thus making the outreach of the programme to all clubs easier.

66.9 Challenges

While the scientific evidence has proven that 11+ can prevent non-contact football injuries, its implementation in the field (as for other injury prevention programmes) remains a challenging task. FIFA has included the programme in all official coaching courses and presented this concept of prevention at several occasions in all continents. Despite numerous promotional activities in more than 80 countries and 3 FIFA Medical Conferences (Zürich 2009, Budapest 2012, Zürich 2015), so far the 11+ has been endorsed by only 20 MAs (ca. 10% of all MAs) of FIFA [7]. Current and past World Cup Champions such as Germany, Brazil and Japan (to cite only three) symbolise that the (political) willingness at MA executive levels is crucial in order to strongly support the message of prevention (Fig. 66.4). Therefore, the firm commitment by a MA to realise a given implementation plan, allocating persons and resources for the 11+ "project", is

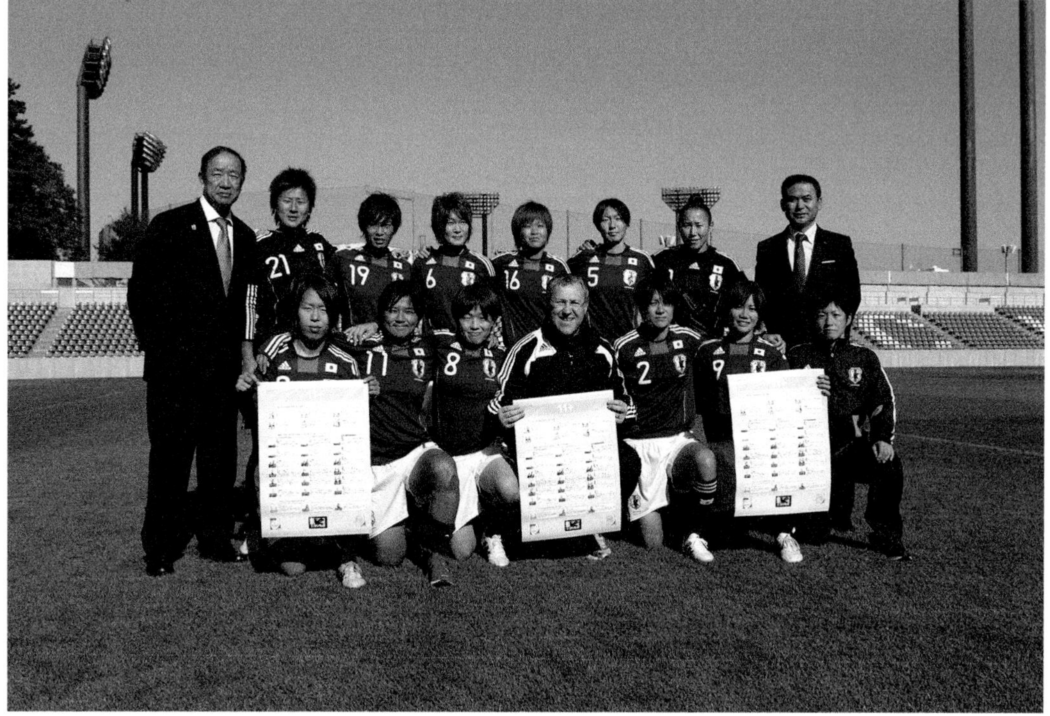

Fig. 66.4 The Japan Football Association (JFA) was the first MA to endorse 11+. The JFA women national football team (winner of the 2011 Women's World Cup) promoting 11+, Tokyo, November 2011

fundamental. The example by the DFB in Germany, as outlined above, shows that this is also feasible in a large country. Furthermore, implementation strategies at various levels, as illustrated by the RE-AIM Sports Setting Matrix [23], and implementation drivers are needed to plan programme adoption, implementation and sustainability.

Fact Box 3

The political willingness at the National Football/Soccer Associations executive levels is crucial in order to strongly support the message of prevention. Therefore, firm commitment to execute a given dissemination and implementation plan, allocating persons and resources for the 11+ project, is fundamental.

Conclusion

Since the introduction of the 11+ (or FIFA 11+), research studies and implementation campaigns with this programme have been conducted in four continents (Europe, North America, Africa and Asia). While some areas are still being investigated (i.e. children), substantial scientific evidence supports the dissemination and implementation of the 11+ as a basic injury prevention programme in amateur football. Although important results have been achieved, a lot still remains to be done, especially in prioritising "injury prevention" in the overall enhancement of the health of football players within the MA's responsibilities. The two countrywide campaigns in Switzerland and New Zealand represent successful examples of injury prevention in amateur football: not only the incidence of football injuries can be reduced, but also the health-related costs can be impressively diminished.

Take Home Message

- The 11+ programme can effectively reduce soccer injuries (non-contact) by 39% in recreational and subelite soccer players.
- Reduction of the four most prevalent soccer injuries—hamstring, hip/groin, knee and ankle injury: 60%, 41%, 48%, 32%, respectively.
- Regular performance of the programme is the key to ensure its preventive effects.
- Injury prevention should be an important piece of the overall soccer training.
- Coaching and players education is crucial.
- Dissemination and implementation should be further facilitated by all relevant parties in football (clubs, academies, associations, confederations).

Top Five Evidence-Based References

Thorborg K, Krommes KK, Esteve E, Clausen MB, Bartels EM, Rathleff MS (2017) Effect of specific exercise-based football injury prevention programmes on the overall injury rate in football: a systematic review and meta-analysis of the FIFA 11 and 11+ programmes. Br J Sports Med 51(7):562–571

Bizzini M, Dvorak J (2015) FIFA 11+: an effective programme to prevent football injuries in various player groups worldwide-a narrative review. Br J Sports Med 49(9):577–579

Silvers-Granelli H, Mandelbaum B, Adeniji O, Insler S, Bizzini M, Pohlig R et al (2015) Efficacy of the FIFA 11+ injury prevention program in the collegiate male soccer player. Am J Sports Med 43(11):2628–2637

Soligard T, Myklebust G, Steffen K, Holme I, Silvers H, Bizzini M et al (2008) Comprehensive warm-up programme to prevent injuries in young female footballers: cluster randomised controlled trial. BMJ 337:a2469

Junge A, Lamprecht M, Stamm H, Hasler H, Bizzini M, Tschopp M et al (2011) Countrywide campaign to prevent soccer injuries in Swiss amateur players. Am J Sports Med 39(1):57–63

References

1. Bizzini M, Junge A, Dvorak J (2013) Implementation of the FIFA 11+ football warm up program: how to approach and convince the Football associations to invest in prevention. Br J Sports Med 47(12):803–806
2. Dvorak J (2009) Give Hippocrates a jersey: promoting health through football/sport. Br J Sports Med 43(5):317–322
3. Ekstrand J, Gillquist J, Liljedahl SO (1983) Prevention of soccer injuries. Supervision by doctor and physiotherapist. Am J Sports Med 11(3):116–120

4. Junge A, Rosch D, Peterson L, Graf-Baumann T, Dvorak J (2002) Prevention of soccer injuries: a prospective intervention study in youth amateur players. Am J Sports Med 30(5):652–659
5. Junge A, Lamprecht M, Stamm H, Hasler H, Bizzini M, Tschopp M et al (2011) Countrywide campaign to prevent soccer injuries in Swiss amateur players. Am J Sports Med 39(1):57–63
6. Gilchrist J, Mandelbaum BR, Melancon H, Ryan GW, Silvers HJ, Griffin LY et al (2008) A randomized controlled trial to prevent noncontact anterior cruciate ligament injury in female collegiate soccer players. Am J Sports Med 36(8):1476–1483
7. Bizzini M, Dvorak J (2015) FIFA 11+: an effective programme to prevent football injuries in various player groups worldwide-a narrative review. Br J Sports Med 49(9):577–579
8. Soligard T, Myklebust G, Steffen K, Holme I, Silvers H, Bizzini M et al (2008) Comprehensive warm-up programme to prevent injuries in young female footballers: cluster randomised controlled trial. BMJ 337:a2469
9. Steffen K, Emery CA, Romiti M, Kang J, Bizzini M, Dvorak J et al (2013) High adherence to a neuromuscular injury prevention programme (FIFA 11+) improves functional balance and reduces injury risk in Canadian youth female football players: a cluster randomised trial. Br J Sports Med 47(12):794–802
10. Owoeye OB, Akinbo SR, Tella BA, Olawale OA (2014) Efficacy of the FIFA 11+ warm-up programme in male youth football: a cluster randomised controlled trial. J Sports Sci Med 13(2):321–328
11. Silvers-Granelli H, Mandelbaum B, Adeniji O, Insler S, Bizzini M, Pohlig R et al (2015) Efficacy of the FIFA 11+ injury prevention program in the collegiate male soccer player. Am J Sports Med 43(11):2628–2637
12. Thorborg K, Krommes KK, Esteve E, Clausen MB, Bartels EM, Rathleff MS (2017) Effect of specific exercise-based football injury prevention programmes on the overall injury rate in football: a systematic review and meta-analysis of the FIFA 11 and 11+ programmes. Br J Sports Med 51(7):562–571. https://doi.org/10.1136/bjsports-2016-097066
13. Faude O, Rossler R, Junge A (2013) Football injuries in children and adolescent players: are there clues for prevention? Sports Med 43(9):819–837
14. Rossler R, Donath L, Verhagen E, Junge A, Schweizer T, Faude O (2014) Exercise-based injury prevention in child and adolescent sport: a systematic review and meta-analysis. Sports Med 44(12):1733–1748
15. Rossler R, Donath L, Bizzini M, Faude O (2016) A new injury prevention programme for children's football -FIFA 11+ KIDS- can improve motor performance: a cluster-randomized controlled trial. J Sports Sci 34(6):549–556
16. Rossler R, Bizzini M; Dvorak J, Chomiak J, Aus der Fünten K, Verhagen E, Lichtenstein E, Beaudouin F, Junge A, Faude O (2016) FIFA 11+ KIDS. A warm up programme to prevent injuries in children's football: cluster-randomized controlled trial. Paper presented at the 21th Annual Congress of the European College of Sports Sciences, Vienna, 6–9 July 2016
17. Weston M, Castagna C, Impellizzeri FM, Bizzini M, Williams AM, Gregson W (2012) Science and medicine applied to soccer refereeing: an update. Sports Med 42(7):615–631
18. Impellizzeri FM, Bizzini M, Dvorak J, Pellegrini B, Schena F, Junge A (2013) Physiological and performance responses to the FIFA 11+ (part 2): a randomised controlled trial on the training effects. J Sports Sci 31(13):1491–1502
19. Bizzini M, Impellizzeri FM, Dvorak J, Bortolan L, Schena F, Modena R et al (2013) Physiological and performance responses to the "FIFA 11+" (part 1): is it an appropriate warm-up? J Sports Sci 31(13):1481–1490
20. McCall A, Carling C, Nedelec M, Davison M, Le Gall F, Berthoin S et al (2014) Risk factors, testing and preventative strategies for non-contact injuries in professional football: current perceptions and practices of 44 teams from various premier leagues. Br J Sports Med 48(18):1352–1357
21. McCall A, Davison M, Andersen TE, Beasley I, Bizzini M, Dupont G et al (2015) Injury prevention strategies at the FIFA 2014 World Cup: perceptions and practices of the physicians from the 32 participating national teams. Br J Sports Med 49(9):603–608
22. Steffen K, Meeuwisse WH, Romiti M, Kang J, McKay C, Bizzini M et al (2013) Evaluation of how different implementation strategies of an injury prevention programme (FIFA 11+) impact team adherence and injury risk in Canadian female youth football players: a cluster-randomised trial. Br J Sports Med 47(8):480–487
23. Finch CF, Donaldson A (2010) A sports setting matrix for understanding the implementation context for community sport. Br J Sports Med 44(13):973–978

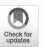

67 Training Load and Injury Risk

Peter Angele, Helmut Hoffmann, and Leonard Achenbach

Contents

67.1 Introduction

Football is a dynamic and physically demanding sport, has an intermittent character, and switches between short high-intensity phases with or without ball such as sprints, jumps, and side-cutting movements and low-intensity phases, such as tactical built-up and game interruptions. To be able to participate on the highest level, players will have to withstand the continuously increasing high athletic demands.

Due to increases in game speed, numbers of matches, and athleticism, the musculoskeletal system has a high demand and therefore a potential high risk of injuries. In an analysis of the national statutory accident insurance company, the first national football league in Germany showed a distribution of 38.3% match injuries and 61.7% training session injuries in the season 2014/2015 [1]. Comparing the distribution of sustained injuries for each month of the season, injuries during training sessions occurred to a higher number during the classic preseason times in July and January in which players have a higher training exposition than in other months,

P. Angele, M.D.
Department of Trauma Surgery, University Medical Centre Regensburg, Franz-Josef-Strauss Allee 11, 93053 Regensburg, Germany

Sporthopaedicum Regensburg, Regensburg, Germany

H. Hoffmann, M.Ed./M.B.A.
Eden Reha, Private Clinic for Orthopaedic/Traumatologic Rehabilitation, Donaustauf, Germany

L. Achenbach, M.D. (✉)
Department of Trauma Surgery, University Medical Centre Regensburg, Franz-Josef-Strauss Allee 11, 93053 Regensburg, Germany
e-mail: leonard.achenbach@ukr.de

V. Musahl et al. (eds.), *Return to Play in Football*, https://doi.org/10.1007/978-3-662-55713-6_67

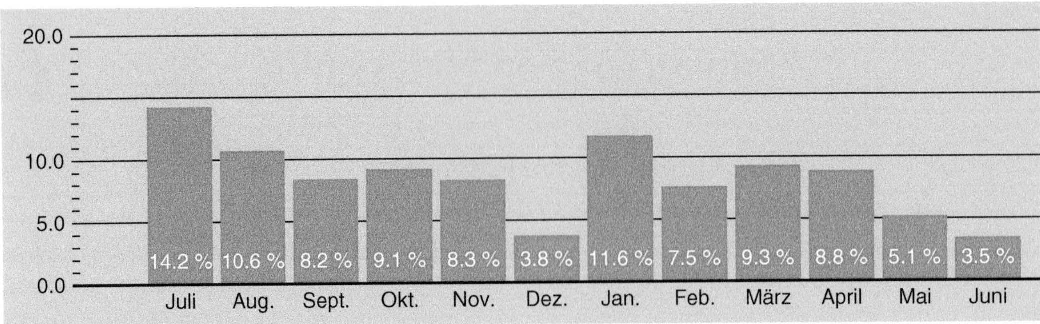

Fig. 67.1 Distribution of training session injuries for each month in the season 2014/2015 in the highest two national football leagues in Germany. Injuries during training sessions occurred to a higher number during the classic preseason times in July and January, from Verwaltungsberufsgenossenschaft-Sportreport 2016 [1]

but evidence is yet inconclusive if increased training volume and increased training intensity may play a role. This chapter will help to provide available evidence to show data connecting football training load and injury risk in elite football players. Injury aetiology models have evolved over the previous two decades highlighting multiple factors which contribute to injury of athletes. These models include internal risk factors, exposure to external risk factors, and an inciting event, wherein biomechanical breakdown and injury occurs (Fig. 67.1).

67.2 Internal and External Risk Factors for ACL Injury

Injury is not a circumstance of destiny. A multifactorial influence of internal and external risk factors modifies the injury risk in a certain unique situation. In the following some of these risk factors will be described in detail. For further information, Chap. 19 will highlight further modifying risk factors.

67.2.1 Internal Risk Factors for ACL Injury

Over 40 million women play football today [2]. Considering the total number of both genders, the incidence of ACL injury is two to three times higher compared to male football [3–5]. Generally, women have a higher incidence in team sports compared to males [3, 6]. Certain differences between men and women as a cause for anterior cruciate ligament injuries have already been established. Women have more often noncontact ACL injuries than male football players. In men, cruciate ligament tears occur more often in their shooting leg compared to the standing leg in women [7]. During an ACL disruption, the bodyweight is shifted over the injured body side, especially in women. Hewett presents different causes on why women have a higher rate of cruciate ligament tears [8]. "Ligament dominance" refers to a neuromuscular imbalance that ends in a knee valgus collapse in certain movements, for example, landing after a jump. Muscles cannot cushion the impact sufficiently enough, and joints and ligaments therefore need to absorb higher-energy peaks.

After a jump, women tend to land in a more extended knee position than males [8]. The dominant muscle for the stabilization of the knee joint while landing is the quadriceps muscle. Its activation results in an extended knee position while landing and to a strain of the ACL through an anterior shift of the tibia. An imbalance between the quadriceps muscle and its antagonist, the hamstring muscles, has been called "quadriceps dominance." A further risk factor for anterior cruciate ligament tears is "leg dominance." Here, muscle power and muscle control present a higher side-to-side difference in females [9]. Athletes that do not possess a sufficient sense of positioning of the body trunk in a three-dimensional space and have need of greater corrective movements are assumed to have a predisposition for an ACL tear [9]. "Trunk dominance" suggests that males typically exhibit greater control of the trunk in performance situations. Rapid growth in pubescence may be a possible trigger for trunk control decrements.

Most injuries of the anterior cruciate ligament occur in young age. Injuries are sustained especially in phases of alterations of anthropometric composition, and resulting biomechanical alteration of lever arms is often not sufficiently stabilized by the musculoskeletal system. This occurs most often during growth spurt. Hormonal changes may also have a great impact on players during a whole season, especially in women. Estrogen levels play an important role and influence muscles and ligaments, which are more loose in women [10]. This fact tends to result in one of the major reasons for injuries of the lower extremity in female football [2, 11, 12].

Another important risk factor for an ACL tear are previous ACL tears or knee injuries [3–5, 13]. An ACL tear of one side is an increased risk for an ACL injury of the other side. Previous knee injuries lead to a persistent disturbance of proprioception. Eighty percent of football players with ACL tears showed a previous injury in a short period before the incident. Most of these injuries were minor injuries, such as muscle injuries on the thigh, ankle injuries, or even blisters on heel or toes. These disturbing factors lead to a disbalance in the coordination of the musculature in the lower extremity [8] and thereby to a vulnerability of the anterior cruciate ligament.

Different sports are characterized by a multitude of highly specific, stereotypical patterns of movement. When the movements are performed at sufficient magnitudes for a long period of time, these sport-specific motor stimuli evoke specific responses in which certain biological structures undergo adaptations that enable the athlete to adequately "process" the loads. These sport-specific adaptions affect bones, ligaments, and musculoskeletal and myofascial structures and are characterized in all sports by an asymmetrical distribution of loads between the right and left sides of the athlete's body (e.g., football with normally dominant kicking and standing leg). Generally the adaptations heighten the quality of the sport-specific movement patterns and thus have a positive effect on the athlete's performance in that particular sport. On the other hand, many of these adaptations cause changes in muscular loads and can sometimes lead to the overuse or unphysiologic loading of certain musculoskeletal structures and in so far could create an additional risk factor, exceeding the stress tolerance of the structures and resulting in injury [14, 15].

Further risk factors include an adequate fitness of the players, fluctuations in weight, and psychological aspects such as match experience, motivation, or performance pressure.

67.2.2 External Risk Factors for ACL Injury

Artificial turf is a typical example for scientific studies being able to assess initially assumed risk factors as harmless. It could be shown that artificial turf of the third and fourth generation that possesses a FIFA license does not increase the risk of injury in football players [16]. Despite these results, the utilization of artificial turf for matches is still controversely discussed in European amateur and professional football. This may be influenced by possible negative results of switching between artificial and natural turf. For this reason, players are supposed to perform their training session on the respective surface their upcoming match will be played.

The data for the influence of football shoes and shoe profile on ACL tears is not yet conclusive. The different interactions between surface of the turf and shoe make influences on injury mechanisms theoretically possible. Yet no scientific study could show connections between different shoe brands or shoe cleats and ACL injury. For example, long cleats do not increase the likelihood of ACL injury [17]. Sport scientists and sport brand manufacturers are very active in the analysis of possible risk factors and optimization of shoe design to reduce the likelihood of injury.

Environmental conditions may influence the likelihood of injury as dry weather increased the rate of ACL injury [18]. But data is yet inconclusive as most data has been published from the Australian Football League.

67.3 Phases with Increased Risk of ACL Injury

Specific phases of a football season or football career are assumed to have an increased risk of ACL injury. The preseason period and the first match days of a new season have an increased risk of ACL injury in amateur and professional football. The series of summer break with loss of fitness, muscle force, and coordination and sudden physical overexertion at the beginning of the new season are assumed to let this time window appear more prone to ACL injuries. In phases of neuromuscular fatigue during preseason, the players have a decreased proprioception which results in increased load of the joints of the lower extremities. Countermovements from full sprint, rotational, or valgus movements may then result in overload of the knee joint and subsequent ACL tear.

The transition from junior football to senior football also appears to present a dangerous age phase. Söderman et al. found an increased risk for ACL tears in female junior football players participating in senior football [19]. The same could be established for male adolescents by our own data (not published). This topic is especially important for permits for junior players that want to play in professional senior football. No scientific data has been established, but young players should be treated with caution to enable neuromuscular adaption and sufficient regeneration.

The increase of physical load in a football player may arise if a player changes its football team, especially if this new team plays in a more professional and demanding level, for example, in a higher-performing league. A promotion of a team into a higher league also increases the demands of the player. Krutsch could show that implementing a new professional third national football league increases the rate of ACL and PCL tears in this league in the first season [20]. The same could be shown in handball, where after restructuring the second league two-division system into one single national second league, Luig et al. (submitted) showed an increase of injury incidence in the second national division to almost the same level of the first national division within the first two seasons.

67.4 Training Load

In addition to the interplay of risk factors or inciting time phase, every athletic injury is sustained while athletes are exposed to training and competition workloads. Match workloads are due to the competitive demands of the sport, while training workloads are applied to athletes with the goal of inducing positive physiological changes and maximizing performance. The various biological adaptations induced by (appropriate) training increase athletes' capacity to accept and withstand load and may thus provide protection from injuries.

67.4.1 External and Internal Training Load

An external training load refers to any external stimulus applied to the athlete, whereas the individual biological response to this external load is called internal load [21, 22]. In football, the former refers to the quality, quantity, organization, and content of physical exercises prescribed by the coach, and the latter is of physiological and psychological nature.

67.4.2 Biological Response

The external load stimulates a biological response and eventually adaptation of the human body's systems. The stimulus for training-induced adaptions is the actual physiological stress, i.e., the internal load, imposed on the football players by the external load [23, 24]. Training results in temporary decrements in physical performance and induces fatigue [25]. These decrements are typically derived from increased muscle damage, impairment of the immune system, imbalances in anabolic-catabolic homeostasis, alteration in mood, and reduction in neuromuscular function [26–32]. Gender differences have not much taken into consideration yet since, for example, estrogens have been shown to protect against reactive oxygen species [33].

The resultant fatigue after a training load can take up to 4–5 days to return to baseline values after the respective training. This fatigue follows a supercompensation phase, whereby the body adapts to increase the specific capabilities affected by the initial stressor [34]. In sports that have frequent training and competition, such as football, fatigue may accumulate over time [35].

Periodization was developed with the aim of manipulating these adaptive processes and effects. Football athletes and coaches push their training to the limits by means of volume and intensity to maximize their performance. The aim of load management is to optimally configure training, competition, and other loads to maximize adaptation and performance with a minimal risk of injury [36]. Load management therefore comprises the appropriate prescription, monitoring, and adjustment of external and internal loads. But limited information exists on the training dose-response relationship in elite football athletes (Fig. 67.2).

67.5 Monitoring Training Load

Warm-up or training programs are created by the football coach in amateur and professional football and present good and simple influencing tools with which the rate for ACL tears can be reduced [11, 38]. Coaches therefore have a decisive share of the responsibility to reduce and prevent injuries. A direct connection between any certain training program and an increase of ACL tears has not been shown, but it is recommended to select exercises for the warm-up and training in such a manner to not only succeed in matches but to prevent injuries. The relationship between training programs and health outcomes can be discussed by monitoring the training load and injury. Assessment of football training load involves measuring external and internal loads, where tools to measure the former can be general or football specific and, for the latter, objective or subjective (Fig. 67.3).

67.5.1 Monitoring External Training Load

To gain an understanding of external training load, a number of tools and technologies are available to athletes, coaches, and medical staff [21]. Measuring single exercises such as lifted weight or distance covered in a certain time may help to

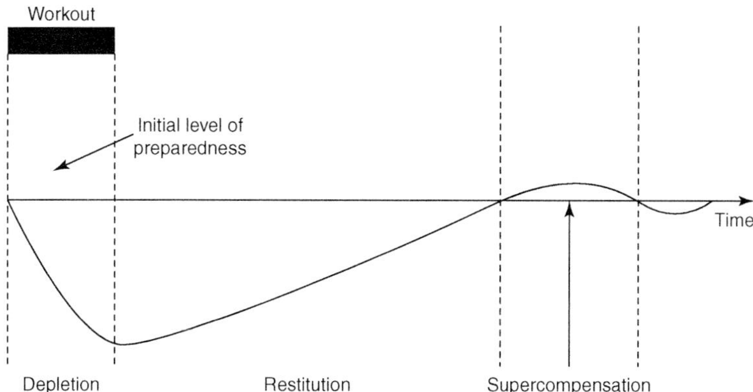

Fig. 67.2 Time course of the restoration process and athlete's preparedness after a workout according to the supercompensation theory. After any given sufficient training stimulus, an athlete's preparedness first declines, then recovers, and is followed by a supercompensation phase, from Zatsiorsky [37]

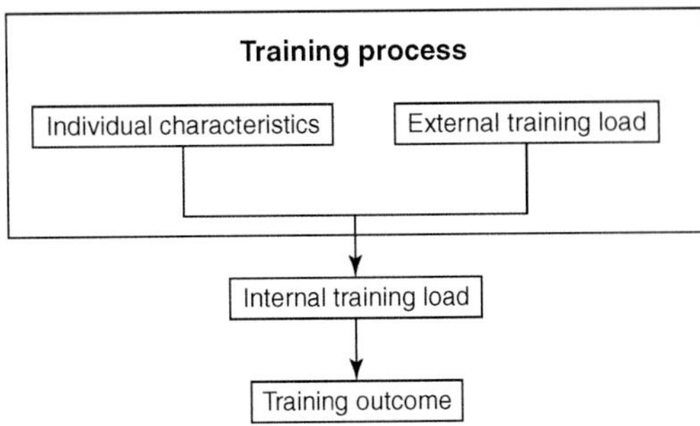

Fig. 67.3 Training outcome is the consequence of internal training load determined by (1) individual characteristics and (2) quality, quantity, and organization of external training load, adapted from Impellizzeri [39]

quantify power output. Training can be recorded to provide information on a number of parameters, including power, speed, and accelerations. Time-motion analysis, such as global positioning system (GPS) tracking, and movement pattern analysis via digital video are popular measuring tools. The reliability of GPS for monitoring movement is influenced by factors such as sample rate, velocity, and duration and type of task. From the available literature, it appears that the higher the velocity of movement, the lower the GPS reliability [40]. Measures of neuromuscular function such as jump tests (squat jump, drop jump), sprint performance, and isokinetic and isoinertial dynamometry are often utilized in team sports due to the simplicity and minimal amount of fatigue induced [41]. To perform, for instance, a drop jump, the athlete drops off a box, hits the ground, and immediately jumps vertically as high as possible at ground contact [42]. Equipment requirements may include contact mats, portable or non-portable force platforms, and rotatory encoders [21]. Common variables from jump tests include mean power, peak velocity, peak force, jump height, flight time, contact time, and rate of force development [41, 43, 44].

67.5.2 Monitoring Internal Training Load

The use of rating of perceived exertion (RPE) is based on the notion that an athlete can monitor their physiological stress during exercise as well as retrospectively provide information regarding their perceived effort post training or competition [21]. The most commonly used scale is introduced by Gunnar Borg and rates exertion on a scale of 6–20. The range is to follow the general heart rate of a healthy young adult by multiplying by 10. For instance, a perceived exertion of 14 would be expected to coincide with a heart rate of roughly 120 beats per minute. Evidence suggests that RPE correlates with heart rate during steady-state exercise and high-intensity interval cycling training, but not as well during short-duration high-intensity soccer drills [45]. RPE is therefore often combined with other variables to provide additional insights into the internal load experienced by the athlete.

Foster developed the “session rating of perceived exertion” method of quantifying a training load unit, which involves multiplying the athlete’s RPE on a 1–10 scale by the duration of the session in minutes [46, 47]. This simple method has been shown to be valid and reliable, with individual correlations between session RPE and summated heart rate (HR) zone scores. Subsequent research in football training has identified individual correlations between RPE and HR zones [48]. The session RPE method was developed to eliminate the need to utilize HR monitors or other methods of assessing exercise intensity. While the session RPE method may be simple, valid, and reliable, the addition of heart rate monitoring may aid in understanding some of the variance that it does not explain [21].

The use of heart rate monitoring during exercise is based on the linear relationship between the heart rate and the rate of oxygen consumption during steady-state exercise [49]. Percentage of maximum heart rate can be used to monitor intensity; heart rate recovery is the rate at which heart rate declines at the cessation of exercise and is suggested to improve with increased training status [50]. Daily variation in heart rate makes individual responses and interpretation difficult and controlling factors such as hydration, environment, and medication important.

Training impulse (TRIMP) is a term coined by Eric Banister to describe the exercise dose as a single number with an integration of time, intensity, and relative weighting of the intensity of the exercise [51]. The mean heart rate is weighted according to the relationship between heart rate and blood lactate as observed during incremental exercise and then multiplied by the session duration. The modeling conducted has focused on endurance training and is limited for use in intermittent sports such as football, mainly because the use of mean heart rate may not reflect the fluctuations that occur during intermittent exercise.

Psychomotor speed tests are often computerized tests and assess reaction time and rapid visual information processing tasks. Overtrained athletes regularly report symptoms such as concentration problems, cognitive complaints, and memory problems [52].

Research in the area of biochemical, hormonal, and immunological assessment is limited, and no definitive marker to monitor internal load, measure fatigue, and minimize excess fatigue has been identified as markers have high inter- and intraindividual difference and are dependent on multiple other factors, such as temperature, hydration, environment, diet, and prescribed exercise. The most popular measure is blood lactate concentration due to the simplicity of sample collection and analysis and is sensitive to changes in exercise intensity and duration [53].

Monitoring sleep quality and quantity can be useful for early detection of performance and health decrements. Athletes can use diaries to indicate hours of sleep and perceived sleep quality. Actigraphy, wristwatch devices utilizing accelerometry, may provide more detailed information, such as bedtime, wake time, sleep onset latency, wake during sleep, sleep efficiency, and sleep routines [21].

67.5.3 Monitoring Athletes

Monitoring athletes may help provide essential data to understand the athlete's response to a prescribed training program, with the goal of minimizing fatigue and injury and examining the effectiveness. Monitoring is incorporated differently, depending on the familiarity of athletes and staff with each monitoring tool, but it appears self-reported measures and sport-specific performance assessment are most commonly used. A recent systematic review on internal load monitoring concluded that subjective measures were more sensitive and consistent than objective measures in determining acute and chronic changes in athlete well-being in response to load [54]. However, the nature of load monitoring required varies greatly between team sport and individual sport athletes. Monitoring in team sports is more challenging due to the diverse range of training activities and number of players. Athletes usually train in groups which leads to the situation that the intensity of the training will not be similar to all the athletes. Players respond differently to given stimuli, and the load required for optimal adaptation therefore differs from one athlete to another. Team sports like football, in which interindividual differences exist, makes prescription of training exercises extremely difficult. Interindividual adjustments to training therefore have to be taken into account. This emphasizes the importance of monitoring the individual athlete, rather than the team as an average, as it may help to ensure the prescribed load by the coach has been applied. Players have to be monitored directly, as the coach's perceptions of the training intensity and the athlete evaluation of the training load might not always be the same. Heinsoo et al. could demonstrate differences between the perception of training intensity in adolescent cross-country skiers and coaches with a 10-point intensity scale. Further, the measurement of cognitive performance and "cognitive load" that influences decision making is important and poses many challenges for accurate assessment.

67.6 Training Load and Injury Risk

In football, players may participate in 50–80 games during a season. In many European top leagues, top teams compete in two games per week during several periods within a season [55]. During these congested periods, players have only 3–4 days of recovery between successive international and national games, which may be insufficient to restore normal homeostasis [27, 56]. Without sufficient regeneration after a match, players will begin their next match with a certain amount of fatigue with the potential of causing performance impairment and injuries in the short and long term [57–59].

67.6.1 Absolute Training Load and Injury Risk

The majority of studies on the relationship between training load and injury risk in team sport have used assessment of absolute load, irrespective of the present or past rate of load application. Absolute training load is the total of all training sessions performed within a specified period, such as a single day or 1 week. Both low and very high acute training loads have been associated with increased risk of injury in Australian football, rugby union, and football [60–65].

Owen monitored maximal heart rate of 23 elite-level professional football players over two consecutive seasons and found significant correlations between training volume and injury incidence [66]. Further analysis revealed how players achieving more time in zones of maximal heart rate of >90% increased the odds of sustaining a match injury but did not for sustaining a training injury. The studies associating low absolute loads with an increased risk of injury suggest the finding the players are not prepared enough for the training and match volume and intensity.

Gabbet proposed the idea of a player's threshold, i.e., the amount of training load that could be sustained before an injury occurred [64]. He suggested this threshold decreased during the season, potentially as players became fatigued when compared to preseason thresholds. In this sense, low acute training loads may be beneficial for players, as some studies indicate. At present knowledge, moderate-to-high workloads can protect best against injury [67].

Fact Box

- High absolute training loads are associated with greater injury risk.
- Moderate-to-high workloads can protect best against injury.

67.6.2 Relative Training Load and Injury Risk

Series completed in cricket, rugby league, and Australian football have shown that if an athlete's training and playing load for a given week (acute load) spikes above the chronic load over the past 4 weeks in average, they are more likely to be injured [68]. The findings demonstrate a strong predictive relationship between acute-chronic load ratio and injury likelihood. In the elite team setting, quantifying the loads the athlete's staff is expecting may help in the return-to-play decision (Fig. 67.4).

Training loads can be achieved in multiple different ways. Volume, intensity, frequency, and training content are unlikely to carry all the identical injury risk. Further research has to elaborate which type of high training load may be an important predictor of injury or injury protecting factor.

Fact Box

- The ratio of acute to chronic training load is a better predictor of injury than acute or chronic loads in isolation.
- To minimize the risk of injury, do not exceed weekly load increases dramatically.

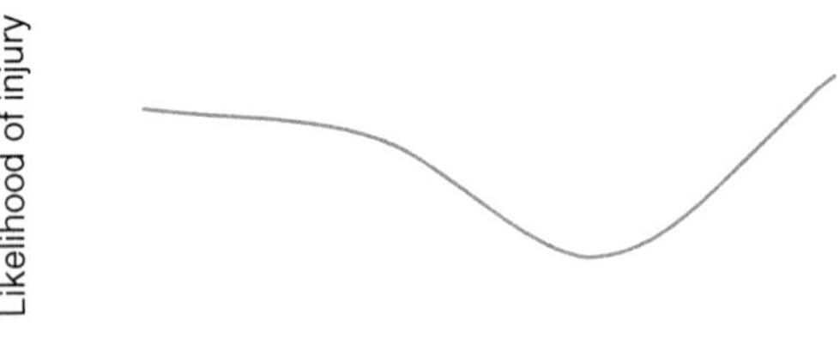

Fig. 67.4 Acute-chronic workload ratio and likelihood of subsequent injury from studies of three different sports. The data indicates that if an athlete's training and playing load for a given week (acute load) spikes above the chronic load over the past 4 weeks in average, they are more likely to be injured, adapted from Blanch P, Gabbett TJ [68]

67.6.3 Training Load and Match Injury Risk

No evidence has yet been established to show a link between training content and injury risk in matches in football. For amateur players, little evidence exist to prove this question as data acquirement has been shown difficult with non-professional players. Further research may answer these questions with the help of databases, for example, national and international ACL injury registers.

Take-Home Message

There is limited evidence at present on training load and injury risk in football. High absolute training loads are associated with greater injury risk while moderate-to-high workloads can protect best against injury at current knowledge. Here, the ratio of acute to chronic training load is a better predictor of injury than acute or chronic loads in isolation. Therefore, to minimize the risk of injury, weekly load should not increase dramatically. More research in the future has to elaborate and identify risk factors associated with training load.

Top Five Evidence-Based References

Halson SL (2014) Monitoring training load to understand fatigue in athletes. Sports Med 44(Suppl 2): S139–S147

Soligard T, Schwellnus M, Alonso J-M, Bahr R, Clarsen B, Dijkstra HP, Gabbett T, Gleeson M, Haegglund M, Hutchinson MR, van Rensburg CJ, Khan Karim M, Meeusen R, Orchard JW, Pluim BM, Raftery M, Budgett R, Engebretsen L (2016) How much is too much? (Part 1) International Olympic Committee consensus statement on load in sport and risk of injury. Br J Sports Med 50:1030–1041

Gabbett TJ, Whyte DG, Hartwig TB, Wescombe H, Naughton GA (2014) The relationship between workloads, physical performance, injury and illness in adolescent male football players. Sports Med 44:989–1003

Malonea S, Owen A, Newton M, Mendes B, Collins KD, Gabbett TJ (2016) The acute:chonic workload ratio in relation to injury risk in professional soccer. Sports Med 44(7):989–1003

Gabbett TJ (2016) The training—injury prevention paradox: should athletes be training smarter and harder? Br J Sports Med 50(5):273–280

References

1. VBG- Sportreport – 2016 (2016) Analyse des Unfallgeschehens in den zwei höchsten Ligen der Männer: Basketball, Eishockey, Fußball & Handball. Verwaltungs-Berufsgenossenschaft. Jedermann-Verlag GmbH, Artikelnummer: 24-05-5458-7
2. Tegnander A, Olsen OE, Moholdt TT, Engebretsen L, Bahr R (2008) Injuries in Norwegian female elite soccer: a prospective one-season cohort study. Knee Surg Sports Traumatol Arthrosc 16(2):194–198
3. Walden M, Hägglund M, Ekstrand J (2006) High risk of new knee injury in elite football players with previous anterior cruciate ligament injury. Br J Sports Med 40:158–162
4. Walden M, Hägglund M, Magnusson H, Ekstrand J (2011) Anterior cruciate ligament injury in elite football: a prospective three-cohort study. Knee Surg Sports Traumatol Arthrosc 19:11–19
5. Walden M, Hägglund M, Werner J, Ekstrand J (2011) The epidemiology of anterior cruciate ligament injury in football (soccer): a review of the literature from gender-related perspective. Knee Surg Sports Traumatol Arthrosc 19:3–10
6. Mandelbaum BR, Silvers HJ, Watnabe DS, Knarr JF, Thomas SD, Griffin LY, Kirkendall DT, Garrett W Jr (2005) Effectiveness of a neuromuscular and proprioceptive training program in preventing anterior cruciate ligament injuries in female athletes: 2-year follow-up. Am J Sports Med 33:1003–1010
7. Brophy R, Silvers HJ, Gonzales T, Mandelbaum BR (2010) Gender influences: the role of leg dominance in ACL injury among soccer players. Br J Sports Med 44:694–697
8. Hewett TE, Ford KR, Hoogenboom BJ, Myer GD (2010) Understanding and preventing ACL injuries: current biomechanical and epidemiologic considerations – update 2010. N Am J Sports Phys Ther 5:234–251
9. Hewett TE, Myer GD, Ford KR, Heidt RS Jr, Colosimo AJ, McLean SG, van den Bogert AJ, Paterno MV, Succop P (2005) Biomechanical measures of neuromuscular control and valgus loading of the knee predict anterior cruciate ligament injury risk in female athletes: a prospective study. Am J Sports Med 33:492–501
10. Grimm K (2007) Fragen und Antworten zum Frauenfussball. In: Grimm K, Kirkendall D (eds) Gesundheit und Fitness für Frauenfussballerinnen – Ein Leitfaden für Spielerinnen und Trainer. Rva Druck und Medien AG, Altstätten, Switzerland
11. Dvorak J, Junge A, Grimm K (2009) F-Marc-football medicine manual, 2nd edn. RVA Druck und Medien AG, Altstätten, Switzerland
12. Junge A, Dvorak J (2003) Injury surveillance in the World Football Tournaments 1998–2012. Br J Sports Med 47:782–788
13. Hägglund M, Walden M, Ekstrand J (2006) Previous injury as a risk factor for injury in elite football: a

prospective study over two consecutive seasons. Br J Sports Med 40:767–772
14. Eder K, Hoffmann H, Schlumberger A, Schwarz S (2016) Verletzungen im Fußball: vermeiden – behandeln - therapieren, 2nd edn. Munich, Germany, Urban&Fischer Verlag. Elsevier GmbH
15. Mayr HO, Zaffagnini S (2016) Prevention of injuries and overuse in sports. Directory for physicians, physiotherapists, sport scientists and coaches. Springer, Heidelberg
16. Williams S, Hume PA, Kara S (2011) A review of football injuries on third and fourth generation artificial turfs compared with natural turf. Sports Med 41(11):903–923
17. Gehring D, Rott F, Stapelfeldt B, Gollhofer A (2007) Effect of soccer shoe cleats on knee joint loads. Int J Sports Med 28:1030–1034
18. Alentorn-Geli E, Myer GD, Silvers HJ, Samitier G, Romero D, Lazaro-Haro C, Cugat R (2009) Prevention of non-contact anterior cruciate ligament injuries in soccer players. Part 1: Mechanism of injury and underlying risk factors. Knee Surg Sports Traumatol Arthrosc 17:705–729
19. Söderman K, Pietilä T, Alfredson H, Werner S (2002) Anterior cruciate ligament injuries in young female playing soccer at senior levels. Scand J Med Sci Sports 12:65–68
20. Krutsch W, Zeman F, Zellner J, Pfeifer C, Nerlich M, Angele P (2016) Increase in ACL and PCL injuries after implementation of a new professional football league. Knee Surg Sports Traumatol Arthrosc 24(7):2271–2279
21. Halson SL (2014) Monitoring training load to understand fatigue in athletes. Sports Med 44(Suppl 2):S139–S147
22. Wallace LK, Slattery KM, Coutts AJ (2009) The ecological validity and application of the session-RPE method for quantifying training loads in swimming. J Strength Cond Res 23:33–38
23. Booth FW, Thomason DB (1991) Molecular and cellular adaptation of muscle in response to exercise: perspectives of various models. Physiol Rev 71:541–585
24. Viru A, Viru M (2000) Nature of training effects. In: Garrett W, Kirkendall D (eds) Exercise and sport science. Lippincott Williams & Williams, Philadelphia, PA, pp 67–95
25. Bangsbo J (1994) The physiology of soccer-with special reference to intense intermittent exercise. Acta Physiol Scand Suppl 619:1–155
26. Gunnarsson TP, Bendiksen M, Bischoff R, Christensen PM, Lesivig B, Madsen K, Stephens F, Greenhaff P, Krustrup P, Bangsbo J (2013) Effect of whey protein-and carbohydrate-enriched diet on glycogen resynthesis during the first 48 h after a soccer game. Scand J Med Sci Sports 23(4):508–515
27. Ispirlidis I, Fatouros IG, Jamurtas AZ et al (2008) Time course of changes in inflammatory and performance responses following a soccer game. Clin J Sports Med 18:428–431
28. Krustrup P, Ortenblad N, Nielsen J, Nybo L, Gunnarsson TP, Iaia FM, Madsen K, Stephens F, Greenhaff P, Bangsbo J (2011) Maximal voluntary contraction force, SR function and glycogen resynthesis during the first 72 h after a high-level competitive soccer game. Eur J Appl Physiol 111(12):2987–2995
29. Mohr M, Draganidis D, Chatzinikolaou A et al (2016) Muscle damage, inflammatory, immune and performance responses to three football games in 1 week in competitive male players. Eur J Appl Physiol 116:179
30. Nedelec M, McCall A, Carling C, Legall F, Berthoin S, Dupont G (2012) Recovery in soccer: Part I - Postmatch fatigue and time course of recovery. Sports Med 42(12):997–1015
31. Russel M, Sparkes W, Northeast J, Cook CJ, Bracken RM, Kilduff LP (2016) Relationships between match activities and peak power output and Creatine Kinase responses to professional reserve team soccer matchplay. Hum Mov Sci 45:96–101
32. Tsubakihara T, Umeda T, Takahashi I, Matsuzaka M, Iwane K, Tanaka M, Matsuda M, Oyamada K, Aruga R, Nakaji S (2013) Effects of soccer matches on neutrophil and lymphocyte functions in female university soccer players. Luminescence 28(2):129–135
33. Akova B, Surmen-Gur E, Gur H, Dirican M, Sarandol E, Kucukoqlu S (2001) Exercise-induced oxidative stress and muscle performance in healthy women: role of vitamin E supplementation and endogenous oestradiol. Eur J Appl Physiol 84(1–2):141–147
34. Wathen D, Baechle TR, Earle RW (2000) Training variation: periodization. In: Baechle TR, Earle RW (eds) Essentials of strength training & conditioning, 2nd edn. Human Kinetics, Champaign, IL, pp 513–527
35. Chiu LZ, Barnes JL (2003) The fitness-fatigue model revisited: implications for planning short-and long-term training. Strength Cond J 25(6):42–51
36. Hoffmann H, Krutsch W (2016) Return to Play nach Kreuzbandverletzungen im Fußball. Sportärztezeitung 1(2):28–35
37. Zatsiorksy V, Kraemer W (2006) Science and practice of strength training, 2nd edn. Human Kinetics, Champaigne, IL
38. Dvorak J, Junge A, Chomiak J, Graf-Baumann T, Peterson L, Ršsch D, Hodgson R (2000) Risk factor analysis for injuries in football players. Possibilities for a prevention program. Am J Sports Med 28:S69–S74
39. Impellizzeri FM, Rampinini E, Marcora SM (2005) Physiological assessment of aerobic training in soccer. J Sports Sci 23:583–592
40. Aughey RJ (2011) Applications of GPS technologies to field sports. Int J Sports Physiol Perform 6:295–310
41. Twist C, Highton J (2013) Monitoring fatigue and recovery in rugby league players. Int J Sports Physiol Perform 8(5):467–474

42. Young WB, Bilby GE (1993) The effect of voluntary effort to influence speed of contraction on strength, muscular power, and hypertrophy development. J Strength Cond Res 7(3):172–178
43. Varley MC, Aughey RJ (2013) Acceleration profiles in elite Australian soccer. Int J Sports Med 34(1):34–39
44. Taylor K (2012) Fatigue monitoring in high performance sport: a survey of current trends. J Aus Strength Cond 20:12–23
45. Borresen J, Lambert MI (2009) The quantification of training load, the training response and the effect on performance. Sports Med 39:779–795
46. Foster C, Daines E, Hector L, Snyder AC, Welsh R (1996) Athletic performance in relation to training load. Wis Med J 95(6):370–374
47. Foster C (1998) Monitoring training in athletes with reference to overtraining syndrome. Med Sci Sports Exerc 30:1164–1168
48. Borresen J, Lambert MI (2008) Quantifying training load: a comparison of subjective and objective methods. Int J Sports Physiol Perform 3:16–30
49. Hopkins WG (1991) Quantification of training in competitive sports. Methods and applications. Sports Med 12:161–183
50. Daanen HA, Lamberts RP, Kallen VL, Jin A, van Meeteren NL (2012) A systematic review on heart-rate recovery to monitor changes in training status in athletes. Int J Sports Physiol Perform 7:251–260
51. Banister EW (1991) Modeling elite athletic performance. In: MacDougall JD, Wenger HA, Green HJ (eds) Physiological testing of elite athletes. Human Kinetics, Champaign, IL
52. Nederhof E, Lemmink KAPM, Visscher C, Meeusen R, Mulder T (2006) Psychomotor speed possibly a new marker for overtraining syndrome. Sports Med 36(10):817–828
53. Beneke R, Leithauser RM, Ochentel O (2011) Blood lactate diagnostics in exercise testing and training. Int J Sports Physiol Perform 6:8–24
54. Saw AE, Main LC, Gastin PB (2016) Monitoring the athlete training response: subjective self-reported measures trump commonly used objective measures: a systematic review. Br J Sports Med 50:281–291
55. Hägglund M, Walden M, Magnusson H, Kristenson K, Bengtsson H, Ekstrand J (2013) Injuries affect team performance negatively in professional football: an 11-year follow-up of the UEFA Champions League injury study. Br J Sports Med 47(12):738–742
56. Fatouros IG, Chatzinikolaou A, Douroudos II, Nikolaidis MG, Kyparos A, Michailidis Y, Vantarakis A, Taxildaris K, Katrabasas I, Mandaladis D, Kouretas D, Jamurtas AZ (2010) Time-course of changes in oxidative stress and antioxidant status responses following a soccer game. J Strength Cond Res 24(12):3278–3286
57. Soligard T, Schwellnus M, Alonso J-M, Bahr R, Clarsen B, Dijkstra HP, Gabbett T, Gleeson M, Haegglund M, Hutchinson MR, van Rensburg CJ, Khan Karim M, Meeusen R, Orchard JW, Pluim BM, Raftery M, Budgett R, Engebretsen L (2016) How much is too much? (Part 1) International Olympic Committee consensus statement on load in sport and risk of injury. Br J Sports Med 50:1030–1041
58. Dupont G, Nedelec M, McCall A, McCormack D, Berthoin S, Wisloff U (2010) Effect of 2 soccer matches in a week on physical performance and injury rate. Am J Sports Med 38(9):1752–1758
59. Ekstand J, Walden M, Hagglund M (2004) A congested football calendar and the wellbeing of players: correlation between match exposure of European footballers before the World Cup 2002 and their injuries and performances during that World Cup. Br J Sports Med 38(4):493–497
60. Orchard JW, Blanch P, Paoloni J, Alex K, Sims K, Orchard JJ, Brukner P (2015) Cricket fast bowling workload patterns as risk factors for tendon, muscle, bone and joint injuries. Br J Sports Med 49:1064–1068
61. Rogalski B, Dawson B, Heasman J, Gabbett TJ (2013) Training and game loads and injury risk in elite Australian footballers. J Sci Med Sport 16(6):499–503
62. Brink MS, Visscher C, Arends S, Zwerver J, Post WJ, Lemmink KA (2010) Monitoring stress and recovery: new insights for the prevention of injuries and illnesses in elite youth soccer players. Br J Sports Med 44:809–815
63. Cross MJ, Williams S, Trewartha G, Kemp SP, Stokes KA (2016) The influence of in-season training loads on injury risk in professional rugby union. Int J Sports Physiol Perform 11:350–355
64. Gabbett TJ, Whyte DG, Hartwig TB, Wescombe H, Naughton GA (2014) The relationship between workloads, physical performance, injury and illness in adolescent male football players. Sports Med 44:989–1003
65. Gabbett TJ (2010) The development and application of an injury prediction model for noncontact, soft-tissue injuries in elite collision sport athletes. J Strength Cond Res 24(10):2593–2603
66. Owen AL, Forsyth JJ, Wong DP, Dellal A, Connelly SP, Chamari K (2015) Heart rate-based training intensity and its impact on injury incidence among elite-level professional soccer players. J Strength Cond Res 29:1705–1712
67. Hulin BT, Gabbett TJ, Lawson DW, Caputi P, Sampson JA (2016) The acute:chronic workload ratio predicts injury: high chronic workload may decrease injury risk in elite rugby league players. Br J Sports Med 50(4):231–236
68. Blanch P, Gabbett TJ (2015) Has the athlete trained enough to return to play safely? The acute:chronic workload ratio permits clinicians to quantify a player's risk of subsequent injury. Br J Sports Med 50(8):471–475

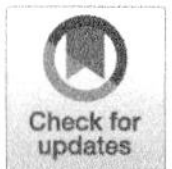

The Experience from the Oslo Sports Trauma Research Center: Injury Prevention

68

Thor Einar Andersen and John Bjørneboe

Contents

68.1 Background

The Oslo Sports Trauma Research Center was established at the Norwegian School of Sport Sciences in May 2000 as a research collaboration between the Department of Orthopaedic Surgery, Oslo University Hospital, Ullevaal, and the Department of Sports Medicine, Norwegian School of Sport Sciences, based on grants from the Royal Norwegian Ministry of Culture, the Norwegian Olympic and Paralympic Committee, and the Confederation of Sports and Pfizer AS. Since 2005, the activity has been expanded based on a grant from the Eastern Norway Regional Health Authority as well as multiple project grants. The main objective has been to develop a long-term research program on sports injury prevention (including studies on epidemiology, risk factors, injury mechanisms, and interventions). The program focuses mainly on three sports (football, team handball, and alpine skiing/snowboarding), as these account for more than 50% of all sports-related injuries treated in Norwegian hospitals. We have addressed the most common (e.g., ankle, hamstrings) and the most serious (e.g., ACL, concussions) injuries seen in these sports. The Oslo Sports Trauma Research Center has aimed to take advantage of novel methodology to identify and rigorously test new methods to prevent injuries, with a particular focus on children and youth sports. We have also applied the approach we used to reduce "acute injuries" (i.e., lower limb acute injuries) to the societal problem of overuse injuries (such as repetitive strain injuries of tendons). The emphasis has not only been on the production of new knowledge but also the translation of research findings into improvements in the health of Norwegian athletes and the Norwegian healthcare system. In 2009, the Oslo Sports Trauma Research Center was inaugurated as a FIFA Medical Center of Excellence and also selected as one of four IOC Research Center for Prevention of Injury and Protection of Athlete Health.

In Table 68.1, selected intervention studies conducted by the OSTRC team are summarized.

T.E. Andersen, M.D., Ph.D. (✉) •
J. Bjørneboe, M.D., Ph.D.
Oslo Sports Trauma Research Center,
Department of Sports Medicine,
Norwegian School of Sport Sciences,
P.O. Box 4014, Ullevaal Stadion, 0806 Oslo, Norway
e-mail: thor.einar.andersen@nih.no

V. Musahl et al. (eds.), *Return to Play in Football*, https://doi.org/10.1007/978-3-662-55713-6_68

Table 68.1 Summary of the injury intervention studies from the Oslo Sports Trauma Research Center (OSTRC)

Reference	Sport	*N*	Study design	Preventive measure	Main finding
Myklebust et al. [1]	Handball	170	Prospective cohort study	Neuromuscular training	No overall reduction of ACL injuries, reduction in ACL injuries in elite players
Olsen et al. [2]	Handball	1837	RCT	Warm-up program	Reduction in ACL injuries
Andersson et al. [3]	Handball	660	RCT	Exercise program	28% lower risk of shoulder problems and 22% lower risk of substantial shoulder problems
Árnason et al. [4]	Football	271	RCT	Video-based awareness program	No difference in injury risk
Árnason et al. [5]	Football	NA[a]	Prospective cohort study	Eccentric training (Nordic hamstring lowers) Flexibility training	Reduced risk of hamstring injuries in the Nordic hamstring group No difference in the flexibility group
Engebretsen et al. [6]	Football	525	RCT	Neuromuscular training Nordic hamstring Groin strength training	No difference in injury risk
Steffen et al. [7]	Football	2100	RCT	Neuromuscular training Strength training	No difference in injury risk
Soligard et al. [8]	Football	1892	RCT	Warm-up program	Reduction in overall, severe, and overuse injuries
Bjørneboe et al. [9]	Football	32 teams	Prospective cohort study	Stricter rule enforcement	Reduction in arm-to-head incidents. No difference in injury risk
Rønning et al. [10]	Snowboard	5029	Prospective cohort study	Wrist protection	Reduction in wrist injuries
Visnes et al. [11]	Volleyball	29	RCT	Eccentric training program	No significant reduction in knee function

[a]Not applicable

68.2 Handball

Prior to the 1999 handball season, a neuromuscular training program was implemented in female handball in order to reduce the risk of anterior cruciate ligament (ACL) injuries [1]. A pre-/post-intervention design was implemented, where the 1998 season served as baseline and the intervention program was included in the two subsequent seasons and served as intervention seasons. The 15-min program constituted of neuromuscular training with increasing difficulty in order to increase knee control and awareness. Three sets of exercises, one on the floor, one on a balance mat, and one on a wobble board, were included. The players were assigned to conduct the intervention program three times a week for 5–7 weeks and then once a week for the rest of the season. The authors found a reduced risk of ACL injuries in the elite division; no overall difference was detected, but a large per-protocol effect was found [1].

Fact Box 1

- Neuromuscular training reduces the risk of injury in adolescent handball with approximately 50%.
- A structured shoulder program reduced the prevalence of shoulder injuries with 28% in female and male elite handball.

Based on these findings, and the conviction that injuries are preventable, a cluster randomized controlled trial introduced a structured warm-up program in adolescent handball for 8 months in the 2002–2003 season [2]. The program included running exercises, cutting and planting technique, landing technique, balance training, and strength training. The risk of injury was almost halved in the intervention group [2].

Studies have showed that the prevalence of shoulder injuries is high in throwing sports, including handball. Based on the understanding of risk factors, a cluster randomized controlled trial was conducted in female and male elite handball [3]. The intervention program aimed to increase the internal rotation in the glenohumeral joint, external rotation strength, and scapular muscle strength. In addition, it sought to improve the kinetic chain and thoracic mobility. The program was conducted three times per week as part of the warm-up program. The overall prevalence of shoulder problems was reduced by 28% in the intervention group; the substantial shoulder injury prevalence was reduced by 22%.

68.3 Football

The first injury prevention study in football from the OSTRC was conducted in the 2000 season [4]. In order to reduce the risk of injury, players were informed about the injury risk and injury mechanisms, and the players were assigned to develop strategies to avoid situations with a high injury risk. Based on previous studies, a 15-min presentation with information regarding the risk of injury and injury mechanisms was presented to seven intervention teams. The players then worked in pairs to develop prevention strategies. Injuries were collected prospectively during the 2000 season and compared with a control group. The control group was not informed about either the risk or the mechanisms of injury. The authors were not able to detect any differences in injury incident between the groups [4].

The rate of hamstring injuries in football is high; thus, hamstring injuries have been the focus of several prevention studies. A study group at OSTRC [12] found that a 10-week training program with Nordic hamstrings (eccentric training) was more effective in increasing eccentric hamstring strength, the hamstrings/quadriceps strength ratio, and isometric hamstring strength, than traditional hamstring curl training (concentric training). The authors therefore suggested that performing Nordic hamstring (NH) regularly might prevent injuries. Thus, a study evaluating the injury preventive effect of NH was conducted [5]. In a prospective study in Norwegian and Icelandic football, two seasons served as baseline, while intervention programs consisting of warm-up stretching, flexibility, and/or eccentric strength training were introduced for (elite) teams in the Icelandic elite division. During the intervention seasons, 48% of the teams used the intervention programs. They found that the incidence of hamstring injuries was lower in teams who used Nordic hamstring combined with warm-up stretching compared to the Norwegian teams in the control group and compared to baseline seasons. No difference was found when performing flexibility training alone [5].

In 2004, a study aimed to identify amateur players with an increased risk of injury based on injury history and reduced function through a questionnaire [6]. The players identified as having a high risk of injury were randomized to an intervention group or a control group. The players in the intervention group were provided with an exercise program based on their injury history and asked to complete it three times a week for 10 weeks during preseason. The screening was able to identify the players with an increased risk of injury through the questionnaire; however, they found no effect of the intervention program on the risk of injury [6]. It should be noted though that compliance was low, with less than 30% of the players at risk completing their prescribed training programs.

The Oslo Sports Trauma Research Center and FIFA collaborated to develop "The FIFA 11" to prevent injuries in football. The effect of this program was evaluated through a large cluster randomized controlled intervention study including over 2000 female adolescent football players in

2005, in order to reduce the overall risk of injury. The intervention group performed the "The FIFA 11" injury prevention program, which included neuromuscular training, lower extremity strength, agility, and core stability throughout the season. No significant difference between the intervention group and control group was observed. However, a compliance study found that only 52% of the intervention teams conducted the program as planned. It should also be noted that a per-protocol analysis found no significant difference in injury risk between the clubs with high and low compliance [7].

Fact Box 2

- The 11+ reduces football injuries with 39% in female and male adolescent and senior football.
- The Nordic hamstrings exercise program lowers and reduces the risk of hamstring injuries in male football.

Then OSTRC and FIFA decided to improve the content of "The FIFA 11" to achieve both better preventive effect and better adherence to the program and hence developed "The 11+." We improved the program by introducing not only evidence-based strength exercises but also implemented best practice warm-up exercises known from and used by top-level clubs and academies. This revised program was named "The 11+" with a focus on core stability, neuromuscular control, balance, hip control, and knee alignment avoiding knee valgus during both static and dynamic movements and was conducted in 2007 [8]. It also included strength exercises, such as the "Nordic hamstring lower," which has been shown to increase eccentric hamstring muscle strength and decrease the rate of hamstring injuries [5, 12]. In addition, "The 11+" included both partner exercises, variation, and progression in order to increase the compliance. In addition, new running exercises were included to make "The 11+" suited as a warm-up program for both training and match. The exercises included in the two programs are found in Figs. 68.1 and 68.2. A recent systematic review from Thorborg et al. [13] found that the "FIFA 11" had no significant effect on injury risk. However, "The 11+" reduced the risk of injury with 39% when pooling results from four different RCTs in different cohorts.

The intervention group conducting "The 11+" reduced the overall risk of injury and severe injuries by 32% and 45%, respectively. "The 11+" had a higher compliance compared to "11", and players with high compliance had a lower risk of injury compared to the group with intermediate compliance [14]. The effectiveness of "The 11+" has later been evaluated in other cohorts, with similar effect on injury reduction [15–17].

Since the 2000 season injuries in Norwegian professional football have been recorded by OSTRC, throughout this continuously injury recording system, it was detected that the injury incidence increased over a 10-year period [18]. Thus, a video analysis comparing incidents with a high risk of injuries between the 2000 and 2010 season was conducted. This study found an increased risk of high-risk incidents in the 2010 season [19]. During the fall of 2010, the Football Association of Norway (NFF) and the Norwegian Professional League Association (NTF) met with the project group from the Oslo Sports Trauma Research Center (OSTRC) and members of FIFA Medical Committee to discuss the implementation of stricter rule enforcement in 2011 in the Norwegian male professional league (Tippeligaen). This involved sanctioning of two-foot tackles as well as tackles with excessive force and intentional high elbow with an automatic red card. The plans for stricter rule enforcement were introduced to each of the teams in meetings with professional league referees appointed for the 2011 season. No significant difference in the overall rate of high-risk incidents or injury incidence was found after the implementation of stricter rule enforcement. However, we found a reduced frequency of contact head

FIFA 11 prevention programme 10-15 min duration in total after familiarization	
Exercises	Repetitions (reps) Seconds (s)
Core stability	
The bench	4 × 15 s
Sideways bench	2 × 15 s each side
Balance	
Cross-country skiing	2 × 15 s each side
Chest pass in single-leg stance	3 × 15 s each side
Forward bend in single-leg stance	3 × 15 s each side
Figure-of-eights in single-leg stance	3 × 15 s each side
Plyometrics	
Line jumps	15 jumps of each type
Zigzag shuffle (20 m)	2 reps in each direction
Bounding (20m)	3 × 10–15 jumps
Strength	
Nordic hamstring	5 reps

FIFA 11+ prevention programme 20 min duration in total after familiarization	
Exercises	Repetitions (reps) Seconds (s)
Running exercises	
Running, straight ahead	2 reps
Running, hip out	2 reps
Running, hip in	2 reps
Running, circling	2 reps
Running and jumping	2 reps
Running, quick run	2 reps
Strength, plyometrics, balance	
The plank (The bench):	
Level 1: both legs	3 × 20–30 s
Level 2: alternate legs	3 × 20–30 s
Level 3: one leg lift	3 × 20–30 s
Side plank (Sideways bench):	
Level 1: static	3 × 20–30 s each side
Level 2: dynamic	3 × 20–30 s each side
Level 3: with leg lift	3 × 20–30 s each side
Nordic hamstring:	
Level 1	3–5 reps
Level 2	7–10 reps
Level 3	12–15 reps
Single leg balance:	
Level 1: holding ball	2 × 30 s each leg
Level 2: throwing ball with pertner	2 × 30 s each leg
Level 3: testing partner	2 × 30 s each leg
Squats:	
Level 1: with heels raised	2 × 30 s
Level 2: walking lunges	2 × 30 s
Level 3: one leg squats	2 × 10 s each leg
Jumping:	
Level 1: vertical jumps	2 × 30 s
Level 2: lateral jumps	2 × 30 s
Level 3: box jumps	2 × 10 s
Running exercises	
Running over pitch	2 reps
Bounding run	2 reps
Running and cutting	2 reps

Fig. 68.1 Characteristics and differences of the FIFA 11 and the 11+ (with permission from Kristian Thorborg)

incidents and subsequently a lower incidence of arm-to-head contact incidents after the implementation of stricter rule enforcement [9].

68.4 Other Sports

Wrist injuries are common among snowboarders; thus, wrist protectors have been developed in order to reduce the risk of injury. A team from OSTRC conducted a prospective, randomized, clinical study where the use of such wrist protectors was evaluated [10]. Snowboarders were randomized to either protection group or control group when arriving at the ski resort. All injuries were recorded at the end of the day at the resort. They found a significant reduction of wrist injuries in the group using wrist protectors [10].

Patellar tendinopathy is a major problem in volleyball. Thus, a RCT including players with patellar tendinopathy from male and female elite volleyball teams in Norway was conducted [11]. Players were randomized to a 12-week intervention eccentric training program or control group. The authors were not able to detect any significant difference in knee function after the 12-week training period or at follow-up at 6 weeks and 6 months [11].

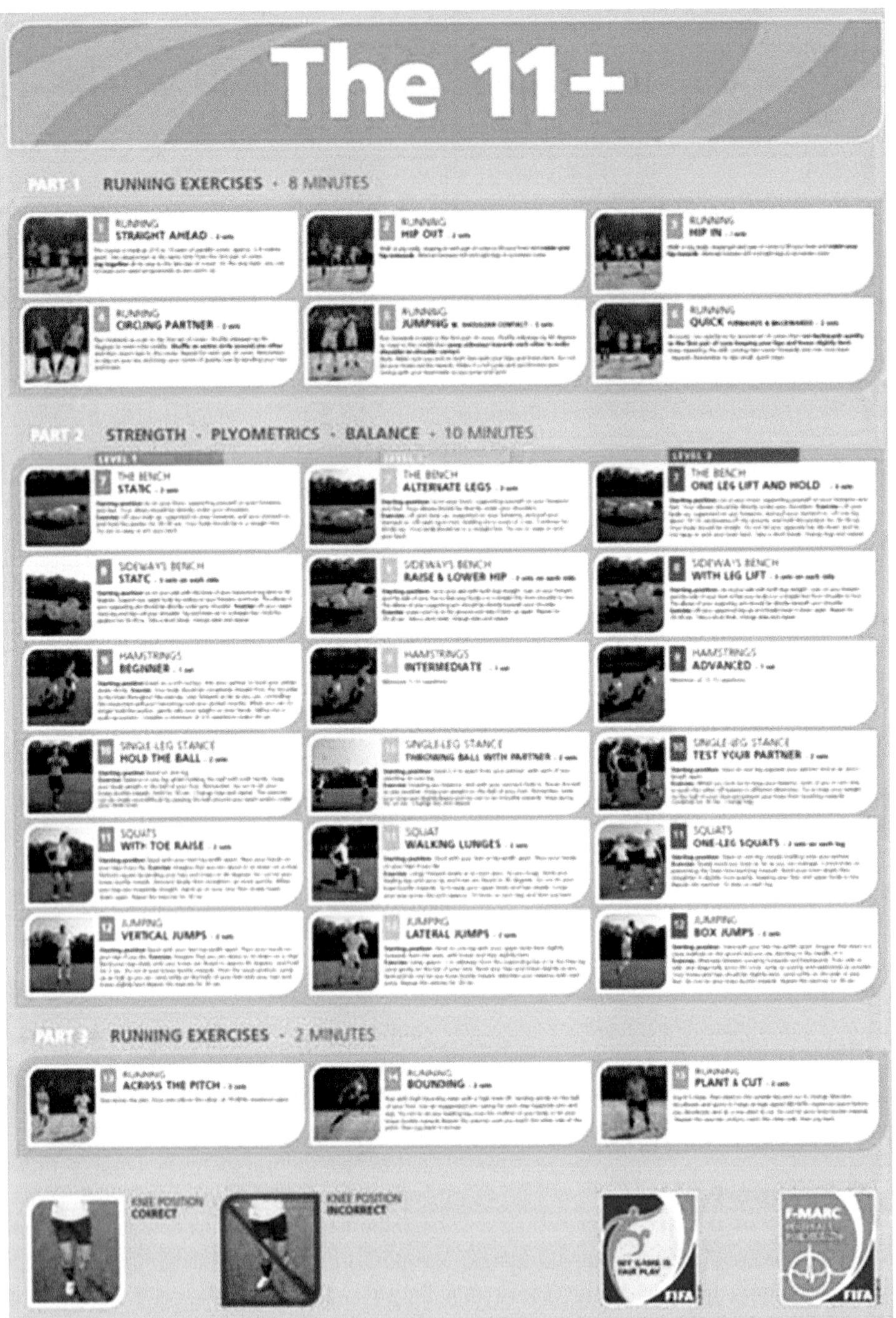
The 11+
PART 1 RUNNING EXERCISES · 8 MINUTES
RUNNING STRAIGHT AHEAD
RUNNING HIP OUT
RUNNING HIP IN
RUNNING CIRCLING PARTNER
RUNNING JUMPING
RUNNING QUICK
PART 2 STRENGTH · PLYOMETRICS · BALANCE · 10 MINUTES
THE BENCH STATIC
THE BENCH ALTERNATE LEGS
THE BENCH ONE LEG LIFT AND HOLD
SIDEWAYS BENCH STATIC
SIDEWAYS BENCH RAISE & LOWER HIP
SIDEWAYS BENCH WITH LEG LIFT
HAMSTRINGS BEGINNER
HAMSTRINGS INTERMEDIATE
HAMSTRINGS ADVANCED
SINGLE-LEG STANCE HOLD THE BALL
SINGLE-LEG STANCE THROWING BALL WITH PARTNER
SINGLE-LEG STANCE TEST YOUR PARTNER
SQUATS WITH TOE RAISE
SQUAT WALKING LUNGES
SQUATS ONE-LEG SQUATS
JUMPING VERTICAL JUMPS
JUMPING LATERAL JUMPS
JUMPING BOX JUMPS
PART 3 RUNNING EXERCISES · 2 MINUTES
RUNNING ACROSS THE PITCH
RUNNING BOUNDING
RUNNING PLANT & CUT
KNEE POSITION CORRECT
KNEE POSITION INCORRECT
F-MARC
FIFA
FIFA

Fig. 68.2 The FIFA 11+ injury prevention program

68.5 New Research Methodology

In 2006, FIFA Medical Committee hosted a group of experts involved in the study of football injuries. The result was a consensus statement that aimed at establishing definitions and methodology, implementation, and reporting standards for studies of injuries in football [20].

The consensus statement defines an injury as "any physical complaint sustained by a player that results from a football match or football training," irrespective of the need of medical attention or time loss from football activity. An injury that results in a player being unable to take a full part in future football training or match is referred to as a "time-loss" injury; an injury that results in a player receiving medical attention is referred to as a "medical-attention" injury [20]. After the consensus article, most studies evaluating the risk of injury both in football and other sports have used a "time-loss" definition. However, a significant proportion of overuse injuries do not lead to time loss from sports participation; players often continue training and playing matches even when limited by pain and reduced function. Thus, overuse injuries are therefore underestimated in most injury surveillance studies [21]. Based on these observations, OSTRC developed and validated a new overuse injury questionnaire, where the athletes on a weekly basis registered problems that were suffered [22]. They found that of 419 recorded overuse problems resulting in reduced performance or participation, however, only 142 (34%) resulted in absence from activity. However, no such studies targeting specifically overuse injuries have been conducted in football; thus, the prevalence of playing with pain, reduced function, and performance limitations has not been explored fully in football. Thus, no injury preventive measures have aimed to reduce the prevalence of overuse injuries in football.

Take-Home Message

Implementation of prevention exercises demonstrated successful decrease of injury as shown in multiple RCTs. "The 11+! reduces the risk of injury by one third and severe injury by as much as one half in female football. Future studies and initiatives should focus on the dissemination of preventive measures to athletes, coaches, and key stakeholders within the sporting community.

Top Five Evidence-Based References

Andersson SH et al (2016) Preventing overuse shoulder injuries among throwing athletes: a cluster-randomized controlled trial in 660 elite handball players. Br J Sports Med. https://doi.org/10.1136/bjsports-2016-09622

Árnason A et al (2008) Prevention of hamstring strains in elite soccer: an intervention study. Scand J Med Sci Sports 18:40–48

Clarsen B et al (2013) Development and validation of a new method for the registration of overuse injuries in sports epidemiology. Br J Sports Med 47(8):495–502

Olsen OE et al (2005) Exercises to prevent lower limb injuries in youth sports: cluster randomized controlled trial. BMJ 330:449

Soligard T et al (2008) Comprehensive warm-up programme to prevent injuries in young female footballers: cluster randomized controlled trial. BMJ 337:a2469

References

1. Myklebust G, Engebretsen L, Braekken IH, Skjolberg A, Olsen OE, Bahr R (2003) Prevention of anterior cruciate ligament injuries in female team handball players: a prospective intervention study over three seasons. Clin J Sport Med 13(2):71–78
2. Olsen OE, Myklebust G, Engebretsen L, Holme I, Bahr R (2005) Exercises to prevent lower limb injuries in youth sports: cluster randomised controlled trial. BMJ 330(7489):449
3. Andersson SH, Bahr R, Clarsen B, Myklebust G (2016) Preventing overuse shoulder injuries among throwing athletes: a cluster-randomised controlled trial in 660 elite handball players. Br J Sports Med. https://doi.org/10.1136/bjsports-2016-09622
4. Arnason A, Engebretsen L, Bahr R (2005) No effect of a video-based awareness program on the rate of soccer injuries. Am J Sports Med 33(1):77–84
5. Arnason A, Andersen TE, Holme I, Engebretsen L, Bahr R (2008) Prevention of hamstring strains in elite soccer: an intervention study. Scand J Med Sci Sports 18(1):40–48
6. Engebretsen AH, Myklebust G, Holme I, Engebretsen L, Bahr R (2008) Prevention of injuries among male soccer players: a prospective, randomized intervention study targeting players with previous injuries or reduced function. Am J Sports Med 36(6):1052–1060
7. Steffen K, Myklebust G, Olsen OE, Holme I, Bahr R (2008) Preventing injuries in female youth football—a cluster-randomized controlled trial. Scand J Med Sci Sports 18(5):605–614
8. Soligard T, Myklebust G, Steffen K, Holme I, Silvers H, Bizzini M et al (2008) Comprehensive warm-up programme to prevent injuries in young female footballers: cluster randomised controlled trial. BMJ 337:a2469

9. Bjørneboe J, Bahr R, Dvorak J, Andersen TE (2013) Lower incidence of arm-to-head contact incidents with stricter interpretation of the Laws of the Game in Norwegian male professional football. Br J Sports Med 47(8):508–514
10. Ronning R, Ronning I, Gerner T, Engebretsen L (2001) The efficacy of wrist protectors in preventing snowboarding injuries. Am J Sports Med 29(5):581–585
11. Visnes H, Hoksrud A, Cook J, Bahr R (2005) No effect of eccentric training on jumper's knee in volleyball players during the competitive season: a randomized clinical trial. Clin J Sport Med 15(4):227–234
12. Mjolsnes R, Arnason A, Osthagen T, Raastad T, Bahr R (2004) A 10-week randomized trial comparing eccentric vs. concentric hamstring strength training in well-trained soccer players. Scand J Med Sci Sports 14(5):311–317
13. Thorborg K, Krommes KK, Esteve E, Clausen MB, Bartels EM, Rathleff MS (2017) Effect of specific exercise-based football injury prevention programmes on the overall injury rate in football: a systematic review and meta-analysis of the FIFA 11 and 11+ programmes. Br J Sports Med. https://doi.org/10.1136/bjsports-2016-097066
14. Soligard T, Nilstad A, Steffen K, Myklebust G, Holme I, Dvorak J et al (2010) Compliance with a comprehensive warm-up programme to prevent injuries in youth football. Br J Sports Med 44(11):787–793
15. Hammes D, Aus Der FK, Kaiser S, Frisen E, Bizzini M, Meyer T (2015) Injury prevention in male veteran football players - a randomised controlled trial using "FIFA 11+". J Sports Sci 33(9):873–881
16. Owoeye OB, Akinbo SR, Tella BA, Olawale OA (2014) Efficacy of the FIFA 11+ warm-up programme in male youth football: a cluster randomised controlled trial. J Sports Sci Med 13(2):321–328
17. Silvers-Granelli H, Mandelbaum B, Adeniji O, Insler S, Bizzini M, Pohlig R et al (2015) Efficacy of the FIFA 11+ injury prevention program in the collegiate male soccer player. Am J Sports Med 43(11):2628–2637
18. Bjørneboe J, Bahr R, Andersen TE (2014) Gradual increase in risk of match injury in Norwegian male professional football - a six-year prospective study. Scand J Med Sci Sports 24(1):189–196
19. Bjørneboe J, Bahr R, Andersen TE (2014) Video analysis of situations with a high-risk for injury in Norwegian male professional football; a comparison between 2000 and 2010. Br J Sports Med 48(9):774–778
20. Fuller CW, Ekstrand J, Junge A, Andersen TE, Bahr R, Dvorak J et al (2006) Consensus statement on injury definitions and data collection procedures in studies of football (soccer) injuries. Clin J Sport Med 16(2):97–106
21. Bahr R (2009) No injuries, but plenty of pain? On the methodology for recording overuse symptoms in sports. Br J Sports Med 43(13):966–972
22. Clarsen B, Myklebust G, Bahr R (2013) Development and validation of a new method for the registration of overuse injuries in sports injury epidemiology. Br J Sports Med 47(8):495–502

Special Considerations of Return to Play in Football Goalkeepers

69

Volker Krutsch, Michael Fuchs, and Werner Krutsch

Contents

V. Krutsch, M.D. (✉)
Department of Otorhinolaryngology, Nuremberg General Hospital, Paracelsus Medical University, Prof.-Ernst-Nathan-Str. 1, 90419 Nürnberg, Germany
e-mail: volker.krutsch@klinikum-nuernberg.de

M. Fuchs
1.FC Nürnberg, Valznerweiherstr. 200, 90480 Nürnberg, Germany
e-mail: mixfux@gmx.de

W. Krutsch, M.D.
Department of Trauma Surgery, University Medical Centre Regensburg, FIFA Medical Centre of Excellence, Franz-Josef-Strauss-Allee 11, 93053 Regensburg, Germany
e-mail: werner.krutsch@ukr.de

69.1 Introduction

Goalkeepers represent an important and unique part of a football team. It is the only position that has the advantage to touch the ball with the hand inside the penalty box. Moreover, goalkeepers have not only the challenge to prevent the own team from conceding a goal, but in modern football, they are also responsible to start the offensive attacks. Goalkeepers show consequently specific requirement on technical and tactical skills in football, which were developed and increasing in the last years. Depending on these specific requirements on the goalkeepers in football, a specific injury profile results during match and training. The "Medline" search about goalkeeping topics in football and the influence on injuries showed weak evidence and a low rate of publications, particularly regarding injury prevention and return to play process after injuries in

V. Musahl et al. (eds.), *Return to Play in Football*, https://doi.org/10.1007/978-3-662-55713-6_69

football goalkeepers [1–3]. To understand and practise a goalkeeping-specific RTP after injuries, a multidisciplinary approach with inclusion of medical staff, football coaches, goalkeepers and goalkeeping coaches is necessary.

69.2 Sport-Specific Requirements on Goalkeepers in Football

69.2.1 Physical Requirements

The primary duty of a goalkeeper in football is the prevention to conceding a goal. In modern football, the function for goalkeepers' activities is principally not restricted. To satisfy the main requirements of the goalkeeping position, it is necessary for a goalkeeper to dominate the penalty box. The latest developments of modern goalkeepers show also the necessity for excellent skills outside of the penalty box, which includes technical skills with the ball like shooting, passing and stopping the ball with the dominant and non-dominant leg, but also in substitute defenders in specific tactical situations [4]. The goalkeepers' duties during match and training result in specific physical requirements and sufficient preparations. Basic physical requirements in general are strength and speed and particularly reaction skills. The goalkeeper has to be trained in all skills as sufficient as outfielders [4]. To achieve the additional and specific skills, which are essential for a successful goalkeeping performance, it is essential to perform a specific goalkeeping training as add on. For this training, a high percentage of football teams in professional and amateur football have a goalkeeping coach with own experiences as goalkeeper. In these add-on trainings, the goalkeepers and their goalkeeping coaches perform also preventive aspects to reduce injuries or to integrate injured goalkeeper into the team training.

The body proportions of football goalkeepers show in general significant differences compared with outfield players. Goalkeepers are in all age groups the tallest and heaviest players of a team [5, 6], and the discrimination to outfielders is getting higher in elite football [7]. An adequate body height is useful in catching high shoots or in controlling the penalty box in case of flanks. Thus, a low height or other weak anatomical body proportions are principally not an exclusion criteria for getting a goalkeeper, but otherwise they are useful to have success. In modern elite and professional football exists a screening system for junior football that includes mainly football goalkeepers with a superior height. In part, it is common in youth elite centres to welcome only junior goalkeeper to their teams, if parents and player allow a medical examination regarding height expectations as adults, which sometimes includes a radiograph or MRI examination of the epiphyseal plate of the distal radius [8].

The typical requirements of goalkeeper result also in different muscular requirements, which have been measured in studies on specific blood marker as a sign of muscle damage [5]. Thus, goalkeepers present well-trained muscles around the lower extremity and the peak torque in extensor and flexor muscles of the thigh and superiority compared with other positions [9]. The running abilities in goalkeepers show generally different profiles compared to outfielders and superiorities in short sprints [10], explosive movements and fast agility runs [6]. Goalkeepers of higher skill levels show superiorities in speed and reaction movements for short distances as typical goalkeeper requirement during matches [11] but also superiorities in testings like Yo-Yo endurance test, squat jumps, countermovement jumps and sprint and agility tests compared to outfield positions [7]. The overall activity distance of a goalkeeper during matches depends also on the skill level and is in professional football approximately 5.5–5.6 km per match, mainly performed as walking and jogging activity. Activities with higher speed showed a high variance in the goalkeepers and depend on individual skills and tactics. The high-intensity runs are a mean of 56 m per match and sprints of 11 m. Low-intensity walking represents 73% of goalkeepers' activity during matches, while high-intensity movements represent 2% of all activities. The first and second half show similar activity distances [12, 13]. The speed and reaction of goalkeepers is also a decision for football coaches to choose their first goalkeeper in a team. The goalkeeper with better reaction and speed tests is more frequently chosen as first goalkeeper of a team, than the goalkeeper with weaker results [14]. Body strength, particularly the trunk, is also essential for goalkeepers, because body contacts of other players in the penalty box occur frequently, and to tolerate these contacts without injury or ball loss, a well-trained trunk stability is necessary [15]. The controlled and uncontrolled diving performance of football goalkeeper shows also a typical situation, where goalkeeper needs trunk controlling and a well-coordinated body activation, but this also represents a situation for potential injuries [16]. Nevertheless, well-developed techniques of typical goalkeeping skills such as catching, saving and throwing the ball are necessary, as well as positional play [17]. Good skilled and frequently trained catching techniques are essential to prepare the hand for incoming forces of a powerfully kicked ball. The downfall, landing and rolling up techniques after jumps and diving are essential and need frequent training performance over many years. Goalkeepers are trained to protect their body against contacts and fouls of other players on the field and are highly prepared for landing techniques on all localisations of the body. Additionally, to the specific movements and duties on field, goalkeepers learn and train to save the ball after a shoot with every single body part. The main aim of all football goalkeepers is to protect the goal with their hands and feet, but if the shoots come from a short distance, all other body parts may need to be in use. In contrast to hands and feet, other body parts are more vulnerable against the ball and shoots with high energy. These body parts are the head and neck and the abdomen and pelvis. In these body regions, hard shoots may result in injuries [18].

Other necessary skills are visual search and anticipation. Particularly the anticipation of movements and actions of other players of the own or the opponent team are one essential part for a goalkeeper, which decides about the success of the goalkeeper and their team. These skills have been trained during the career as football goalkeepers, but should be renewed, if a longer time out period in football occurs, typically after injuries [19–21]. Also, one-on-one duels are for goalkeeper important situations, where specific perceptions of the individual goalkeepers' audio-visual system are decisive for success [22].

69.2.2 Psychological Requirements

Football goalkeepers present specific mental skills during match and training. The typical situations with high necessity of concentration and psychological pressure on the goalkeeper during competition are, for instance, penalty kicks, free kicks and corner kicks [23–27]. A high demand on goalkeeper is to keep concentrated over the complete match and training, without continuously being involved in all match situations. Typical other psychological skills are high motivation, durability against external psychological pressure and durability against fear for making errors. Additional mental skills are, general confidence and the transmission of this to other players on field, skills to guide the other players on the field, to have an overview on the complete match and to keep cool or aggressive, as match situations indicate. The situation of goalkeepers to be the "last man standing" results in a specifically skilled and demanded player on the field. Goalkeepers encounter several situations per match, where they are one-on-one against opponent players. The goalkeeper should support other players of the team but must in a few situations accept that they have to manage the situation on their own. The mid- and long-term results of these specific psychological situations can produce periods of depression during a goalkeeper's football career. The problem is that psychological problems may be misdiagnosed and insufficiently treated. The scientific literature has reported about depression in football goalkeepers and resulting in catastrophic outcome and even suicides [28, 29].

69.2.3 Influence of Match Rules in Football

Goalkeepers are protected inside the penalty by the match laws. No other player is allowed to attack the goalkeeper when they are in control or possession of the ball. The goalkeeper is in control of the ball while the ball is between his hands or between his hands or any surface, while holding the ball in his outstretched open hand and while in the act of bouncing it on the ground or tossing it into the air. Additionally it is an offence by the laws when the goalkeeper is restricted in the movement by unfairly impeding by an opponent player [30]. Unfortunately, there are cases, for example, at a corner kick or long passes where the goalkeeper gets into unexpected collisions with the opponent player. The striker is focused on the ball and may not note the position of the goalkeeper. These situations lead to a high injury risk for the goalkeeper.

Fact Box 1

- Football goalkeepers represent unique and specific physical and psychological requirements on the field, with improved technical skill in the last years.
- Match rules, specific duties and separate goalkeeping coach make the goalkeeper position special in football, with special demands on medical issues.

69.3 Specific Injury Profile in Football Goalkeepers

Goalkeepers have a specific injury profile, which is different from players in other positions on the football field. The goalkeeping position is frequently used as reference mark for the calculation of injury risks in different positions [31, 32]. The goalkeeper position represents in these calculations as "1.0", and other positions show a generally higher-risk like outfielders with a risk between 1.45 and 1.7 [31–34]. Goalkeepers in professional football show higher injury rates than amateur goalkeepers [35]. Generally, the frequent hamstring injuries in football are not a goalkeeper' problem [34]. Joint injuries of the lower extremity [32, 36] and injuries of the upper extremity are the most frequent injuries in football goalkeeper [32, 37]. The majority of goalkeeper injuries occur as non-contact injury.

69.3.1 Injuries to the Upper Extremity

Goalkeepers have a special risk for injuries to the upper extremity [1]. Specific injury analysis related to football goalkeepers in football are rare [1–3], and the most information about goalkeepers' injuries in football are present as secondary to the results about football players in general, irrespective of the position. Studies have shown that most injuries in football players are to the lower extremity [38–40]. The position of the goalkeeper has a five times higher risk for injuries of the upper extremity compared with outfield players [37]. Injuries to the upper extremity in goalkeepers are between 3 and 23% [37, 39, 41]. Particularly, the fingers and the hand are at risk [18, 37, 42]. Injury mechanism for injuries to the hand and fingers occurs mainly as contact injury or due to landing from a fall [43]. The longest lay-off times are related to rotator cuff tear with a mean of 144 days and dislocation of the shoulder with a mean of 100 days [37]. Shoulder injuries usually lead to longer lay-off period than elbow injuries or hand injuries.

69.3.1.1 Hand and Wrist Injuries

The hand and fingers with their multiple small bones, joints, ligaments and tendons are the biological working equipment of football goalkeeper. The contact with the ball, sometimes accidentally with the teammate or the opponent player, is the reason for injury mechanism on the hands [44]. The contact of high ball forces with the fingers may result in hyperextension or axial trauma to the fingertip [41, 45, 46]. This may lead to sprain of the small joints; rupture of joint capsule, ligaments and tendons; or even joint dislocation or fractures. Finger joint sprains are the most common injuries and they result in partial or complete rupture of the capsule [1, 47, 48]. Dislocation of a finger is the second most common injury, mainly the proximal interphalangeal joint handoff the fifth finger. This can lead to capsular injury or an injury to the collateral ligaments [44, 47]. Finger fractures are the most common fractures in goalkeepers. The injury mechanism is twisting or bending the involved fingers [44]. If the keeper tries to safe the ball with both hands and stretched arms, the fingers and hand are in risk of a trauma against the shoe or foot of opponent players. Especially the metacarpal bones of the hand are at risk [18]. In general, the index, middle and ring finger are most frequently injured when the goalkeeper tries to catch or safe the ball, because they absorb the main part of the impacted forces with or without correct catching technique [18]. Even using correct catching technique, the fingers may suffer great forces, and impacts on the proximal phalanx of the thumb may result in subluxation of the metacarpophalangeal joint with rupture of the ulnar collateral ligament (UCL) or fracture of the first metacarpal bone. This injury combination is called "goalkeepers thumb" [18, 49]. Thus, kicks and hits on the hand represent the most frequent injury mechanism with particular risk for the thumb, index finger and little finger [50].

Additional to injuries of the hand and fingers, injuries to the wrist and forearm with the same injury mechanism as described for the finger injuries are common. Also, fractures such as scaphoid bone fractures with long-term complications like scaphoid pseudarthrosis are not uncommon [18, 46]. Distal radius fractures are also relatively frequent in football goalkeepers [46, 51]. The mean lay-off after hand injuries varies markedly. Some injuries on the fingers do not lead to any lay-off. They lay-off for metacarpal fractures is reported as approximately 55 days and finger fractures 26 days [37].

69.3.1.2 Shoulder

The shoulders and arms are one of the most stressed body regions in goalkeepers [2]. The goalkeeper has a higher risk for a shoulder injury than players in other positions on the field. Typical trauma mechanisms are the downfall after a jump directly on the shoulder or on the elbow or hyperextension and overstretched arm by holding a shoot. These mechanisms may result in acute dislocations of the glenohumeral joint, AC joint tear, capsule and ligament ruptures of the shoulder or a rupture of the rotator cuff [37]. The injury severity measured by lay-off time is as follows, published by Ekstrand et al. (2013) for elite football players [37]:

1. Rotator cuff tear (144 days out in football)
2. Shoulder dislocation (100 days out in football)
3. AC joint dislocation (42 days out in football)
4. AC joint sprain (25 days out in football)

A spontaneous rupture of the extensor pollicis longus tendon in a professional youth football goalkeeper may be reported as partial musculotendinous rupture of the distal biceps brachii or as an isolated rupture of the teres major muscle [48, 52, 53]. Other rare injuries are bilateral stress fractures of the carpal scaphoid in a junior goalkeeper [54], multiple simultaneous bilateral mallet fingers of the three and four fingers [1] or a simultaneous double interphalangeal dislocation of one single finger, when an outfielder trots on the little finger [55].

Other rare cases are a true aneurysm of ulnar artery after goalkeeping activity [56] or an isolated latissimus dorsi tear [57]. Special risks in football are lime burns or allergic reactions as a result of chemical substance on the football field.

69.3.2 Injuries to the Trunk and Head

Injuries to the trunk and head are less frequent in football players compared with injuries of the extremities, especially in goalkeepers [39, 40, 58, 59]. However, these injuries may result in severe consequences, particularly after head trauma [60, 61] with neurological and neuropsychological sequelae [62, 63]. Goalkeepers are frequently exposed to situations, with consequently injuries like concussions or facial injuries [64, 65]. Mainly elbow-to-head or head-to-head trauma is the injury mechanism [62, 64, 66, 67]. The most frequent injuries of head injuries are contusions and lacerations. Care must be taken after a hit on the head to recognise symptoms of concussion or mild traumatic brain injuries and not to overlook injuries to the cervical spine [67, 68]. Cervical spine injuries are potentially accompanied with severe neurological outcome [69]. Besides the brain injuries and the neurological consequences, also midfacial fractures like nasal bone, orbital floor, zygomatic bone and zygomatic arch fractures, as well as mandible fractures or fractures of the teeth, are possible as a result of direct contact to the opponent [65]. These fracture types can lead in individual cases to permanent changes of the facial appearance and functional disorders in breathing, vision, smelling and sensation [70, 71]. Injuries to the skull base with liquorrhea, anosmia, vision disorders, meningitis or intracerebral haemorrhage are rare [70, 72].

Injuries to the trunk occur also mainly in the duels in the penalty box. The typical injuries are contusions of the abdomen or thorax by elbows and knees of other players and contusions on the spine during downfall after a jump. Severe injuries on the trunk in goalkeepers are fractures on the ribs or vertebral bodies of the spine. Another serious injury is caused by the ball, shot on the goalkeepers' abdomen form a short distance. The potential consequences are in rare cases a splenic rupture or other injuries to the abdomen [73]. The majority of goalkeepers learn specific techniques to protect their head and the trunk against impact of the ball and other players.

69.3.3 Injuries to the Lower Extremity

Goalkeepers have similar injury mechanism for injuries to the lower extremity compared with other players but with lower frequency. Beside the typical injuries of football players and other team sports like ankle sprains, muscle strains, meniscus lesions or ACL ruptures, goalkeepers also sustain other rare but typical injuries. Because of the jumping and landing movements of a goalkeeper in football, landing on knees and hips are common and may lead to contusions and skin abrasions as a result of the diving [3, 74, 75]. One typical intraarticular knee injury in football goalkeepers is the PCL injury by direct contact of the proximal tibia plateau. During uncontrolled landing, a hard hit on the tibia plateau may result in PCL ruptures [59]. Other intraarticular joint injuries frequently encountered in goalkeepers are ankle sprains and typically as non-contact injury [36]. Contact injuries occur particularly to the hips and mainly during diving movements to catch the ball. While the injury risk for hip injuries in amateur football is significantly higher than in professional football, particularly severe injuries like fractures, professional goalkeepers have a higher rate of bursitis of the hip. In general, hip injuries like contusions and abrasions occur more frequently in training than in match exposure [75].

69.3.4 Overuse Injuries

In addition to traumatic injuries, goalkeepers may also sustain overuse injuries. The fingers have a high stress by frequently catching the ball. Frequent microtrauma may injure the cartilage of the finger joint as well as the ligaments and tendons and result in degenerative changes of the joints [41]. Swelling persists sometimes over months and indicates a chronic problem of the affected joints [45]. PIP joints are the most affected joints and show frequently the typical symptoms in football goalkeepers like persistent pain, chronic joint swelling or impaired movement.

Other overuse complaints on the upper extremity in football goalkeepers may also affect the shoulder joint [76], mainly due to hyperextension and stretching of the capsule and ligaments during throwing the ball or by holding the ball after a shoot. Other typical overuse injuries of the upper extremity with similar injury mechanism are epicondylitis (on the ulnar side) and tendinitis of the extensor tendons of the forearm [37]. Ekstrand et al. reported on lay-off with mean of 5 days in shoulder impingement syndrome and subacromial bursitis, 6 days in elbow olecranon bursitis and 8 days for medial collateral ligament sprain of the elbow.

Other overuse complaints to the hip with typical femoroacetabular impingement [77] are caused by frequent hyperabduction and hyperflexion of the hip. Also, low back pain is frequently present in goalkeepers and a result of during the jumping, flying and landing movements in match and training [78]. Achilles tendinitis is another typical goalkeeping problem. This overuse injury is caused by the frequent change of running forward, sidewards and backwards and a typical result of goalkeepers' requirements [79].

Fact Box 2

- Football goalkeepers present a specific injury profile well documented in the scientific literature.
- Typical traumatic injuries of goalkeepers affect mainly the upper extremity, especially the hand and shoulder.
- Overuse injuries in goalkeepers are mostly related to the shoulder, elbow, hip, Achilles tendon and spine. These injuries show the need for a specific injury prevention strategy in goalkeepers and a detailed return to play process after goalkeepers' injuries.

69.4 Basic Injury Prevention Strategies in Football Goalkeepers

69.4.1 Training and Warm-Up

Recently published studies have reported on the lack in goalkeeper-specific injury prevention program in football [2]. The goalkeeper in football needs a specific strategy for injury prevention to address the specific goalkeeping requirements during match and training. A recently published recommendation for goalkeeper to prevent injuries is called "11+ S" [2]:

- General warm-up exercises
- Strength balance exercises for the shoulder, elbow, wrist and fingers
- Muscle control and core stability exercises

The following exercise topics of "11+ S" are recommended for football goalkeepers:

1. Walking and running
2. Throwing the ball
3. Spinning movements of the hand
4. Shoulder movement exercises (e.g. external and internal rotation)
5. Bench exercises
6. Upper and lower back strength exercise
7. Wrist and finger exercises for extension and flexion
8. Throwing exercises with the ball in jumping position, standing position and sideward movements

Further exercise groups have also been recommended for a training and warm-up program [4]:

- Running to activate the circulation
- Stretching of the lower extremity, upper extremity and the trunk to achieve flexibility
- Exercises for the lower extremity and trunk with trunk stability, jumping and landing, neuromotorical adaption, agility (e.g. FIFA 11+)
- Exercises for the upper extremity; strength training (e.g. in part: 11+ S)
- Ball play with stopping and passing, shooting and long passes. Additional shoot-outs and throw-outs are possible
- Ball play with catching the ball
- General jumping, landing and diving exercises with the ball
- Ball play against the keeper with one-on-one duels, flanks and shootings of the team

Because of the wide range of exercises needed for an adequate preparation of goalkeepers, it is recommended that the goalkeeper should start their warm-up program 10–15 min earlier than outfielders. Besides the normal athletic warm-up with other goalkeepers, the individual exercises with the goalkeeping coach and the exercises with the rest of the team are essential. Generally, goalkeepers have to consider that the complete warm-up must fulfil several functions:

- Physical preparation for the match
- Mental preparation for the match
- Injury prevention
- Matching with the rest of the team

For the configuration of a well-adapted training or warm-up, it is necessary to consider that every movement in the match and training and every kind of contact with the ball should be trained and practised in the warm-up period before every training and match.

69.4.2 Equipment

As important part of injury prevention in football [80], the protection equipment for goalkeepers represents a crucial role. Goalkeepers' gloves are an important feature to improve the possibility of catching and saving the shootened ball and to reduce the impacting forces to the hand and fingers at the same time. But the gloves have an additional indispensable role, to protect goalkeepers hand and fingers against the ball and the foot or other body parts of an opponent player. For this protection of fingers, new developments of the last years provide goalkeepers the use of gloves with "finger-safe" technology. One other important step to protect the fingers of the goalkeeper is to undress rings on the finger, which may lead to severe finger avulsions [50].

The protection of the shank and the compliance for wearing shin guards in training and match are essential for goalkeepers. Other common protection equipment are hip pads in goalkeeper shorts. Padded shorts for football goalkeepers are commonly used in junior football but show only a low evidence for injury preventing effects. The most available products show weak effect and only viscoelastic foam fulfilled essential effects of a protection wear [75]. Other frequently worn pads to protect a joint in the goalkeeper are seen on the elbow, included in the shirt and on the knee. The evidence of the preventive effect of this equipment is low. Typical other protection equipment are warming shorts to prevent groin pain and compressions socks to avoid muscle cramps. This equipment is less reported in the scientific literature but very effective for football goalkeepers to address the different weather situations and in different seasons.

69.4.3 Prevention Behaviour

Considering match rules, the goalkeeper has to respect the fair play character in football, which is an important step and part of prevention of injuries. The goalkeeper has a higher risk for contact injuries of the upper extremity and head and trunk, but by learning protection behaviour in duels with opponent players, they can protect themselves. A typical situation, where goalkeepers protect their body against contact injuries, is by holding their hands before the face when catching the ball or lifting their knee, when jumping in the air to catch the ball. A further important step to prevent injuries in contact situations with opponents are the pretension of the trunk muscle strength. Further skills to prevent injuries on all body regions are practising landing techniques after jumps or divings.

During the protective behaviours of goalkeepers in the penalty box, other players are endangered to be injured by the foot or knee of goalkeepers in the head, the thorax or the abdomen. Rarely, this may result in severe injuries, like pneumothorax, rip fractures or ruptures of the liver or spleen [81] or a direct injury of the larynx [82]. Goalkeepers have to consider that the injuries of opponents are possible.

69.5 Return to Play Testing and Decision-Making After Football Goalkeepers' Injuries

The RTP after injuries in goalkeepers should be adapted to the specific training program and the specific requirements on the field. In general, the literature describes specific goalkeepers' testings such as vertical jumps, lateral shuffle test, accelerations of 5 and 10 m and goalkeeping-specific techniques. A high number of exercises for are available, but a specific and well-planned RTP program is necessary to consider all parts of the goalkeeping play. To illustrate a typical RTP injury the following is recommended.

69.5.1 Return to Play After Upper Extremity Injuries

Injuries of the upper extremities are common in goalkeepers. Quite often these injuries prohibit RTP, although they are not very serious. Principles for a return to play process after upper extremity injuries are:

I. *Therapy stage*
  - Acute phase injury treatment
  - Tactical and mental training
  - Light activity of contralateral upper extremity
  - Active mobilisation and exercises of the lower extremity and trunk

II. *Return to walk/return to move*
  - Light exercises of the affected extremity by movements of the wrist, the elbow and the shoulder
  - Running exercises and general strength exercises
  - Ball exercises with both legs (shooting, passing)
  - Ball exercises with the contralateral upper extremity

III. *Return to activity/return to sports movement*
  - Specific exercises for the specific body region. Specific movements of the small finger joints (passive, active, against resistance)
  - Goalkeeper-specific movements and exercises (jumping techniques, landing techniques)
  - Specific first catching and boxing techniques:
    - With a soft ball
    - With tape and protection devices on the fingers
    - With gloves with finger-safe technology
    - With reduced power
  - Complete athletic and football-specific training for the legs (non-contact)

IV. *Return to full goalkeeper training/return to team training*
  - All aspects of goalkeeper's individual training

V. *Return to competition*
  - After complete integration of the goalkeeper in the team training and unrestricted goalkeeping training, RTP is recommended.

69.5.2 Return to Play After Trunk and Head Injuries

After head injuries, individual return to play is necessary. In general, if goalkeeper suffers a concussion or traumatic brain injury, the graduated return to play protocol with different stages developed by the Consensus Statement on Concussion in Sport (2012) should be applicated [60]:

I. No activity, recovery, tactical and mental education.
II. After the period of no activity, the goalkeeper is allowed to start with light exercises like walking, swimming or stationary cycling. In this step, the goalkeeper should start with light ball-specific exercises like catching or boxing, e.g. with a softball or a balloon and stretching and mobility exercises.
III. In the next step, the goalkeeper can start with sport-specific exercises like running and catching and light throwing techniques. During this activity, the goalkeeper should take care to avoid head impacts.
IV. The next step should be non-contact training drills like passing and throwing exercises, with more and more to complex exercises. In this step, the goalkeeper can start with diving and landing techniques.
V. The goalkeeper can at this stage start with full-contact exercises and training after medical clearance. Headgears are used only by few players in professional football.
VI. Normal match play and practise protection behaviour to avoid a second impact on the head.

69.5.3 Return to Play After Lower Extremity Injuries

Injuries to the lower extremity principally allow very early exercises for the upper extremity, and maintenance of the upper extremity training is possible. Knee injuries need specific return to play:

I. *Therapy stage*
   - Injury treatment and avoidance of moving the affected extremity
   - Performance of tactical and mental education
   - Light activity of contralateral lower extremity
   - Active mobilisation and exercises of the upper extremity and the trunk

II. *Return to walk/return to move*
   - Light exercises to the affected extremity by movements of the ankle and hip
   - Cycling and walking exercises and general strength exercises
   - Ball exercises for the upper extremity (catching, throwing)
   - Movement and strength for the upper extremity

III. *Return to activity/return to sports movement*
   - Specific exercises for the recovered body region and the contralateral side
   - Goalkeeper-specific movements and exercises for the upper extremity
   - Complete athletic and football-specific training for the lower extremity (non-contact)

IV. *Return to full goalkeeper training/return to team training*
   - All aspects of a goalkeeper's individual training (jumping, landing, diving, contact play, ball play)

V. *Return to competition*
   - After complete integration of the goalkeeper in the team training and unrestricted goalkeeping training, return to play in competitions when possible reasonable.

69.5.4 Return to Play Tests

In the different stages of the return to play process, the athletic trainer in collaboration with the goalkeeping coach should perform goalkeeping-specific tests. In contrast to the return to play tests on outfielders, the goalkeeper needs additional goalkeeping tests after stage III (return to activity) up until stage V (return to competition). If one of the tests shows negative results, for example, in comparison to results of the contralateral not injured side or to pre-injury test results, the goalkeeper should improve the specific skills and a new test be performed. Following tests for return to play process of a goalkeeper are useful during the different stages:

- *Return to activity/return to normal sports* (stage III)
  - Jumping and landing tests
  - Agility and sprint tests
  - Catching and throwing the ball
- *Return to full training/return to team training* (stage IV)
  - Repeat the test form stage III
  - Start to reach the same training level as before the injury
  - Shooting and passing the ball
  - Offence and defence play and zone control
  - Crossing, shooting and tactics with the team
  - Individual conversation between team coach and goalkeeper to check the mental status
- *Return to competition* (stage V)
  - Frequent tests of athletic and neuromotorical skills depending on physical strain

The decision-making for a goalkeeper is completely different to outfielders. Form the beginning of the rehabilitations protocol after goalkeepers' injuries; the goalkeeping coach should train specific exercises with the goalkeeper. The goalkeeping coach is an essential part of the return to play process in goalkeeper injuries and must also be involved in the return to play decisions of all stages.

Take-Home Message

Return to play for a football goalkeeper is unique and shows several specific requirements compared with other football positions. These requirements and the transfer to the return to play process after goalkeepers' injuries are represented in scientific literature in limited manner only and the scientific evidence is low. An important perspective for the future should focus on the goalkeeping-specific problems and requirements in the prevention of injuries and the return to play process after injuries.

Fact Box 3

1. Return to play strategies after injuries for goalkeepers should include all stages of goalkeeping practice:
   (a) General physical and psychological fitness
   (b) Specific football skills and exercises
   (c) Goalkeeping-specific training details
   (d) Reintegration decisions
2. Return to play decisions after injuries in football goalkeepers are based on specific testings related to neuromotoric adaption, trunk stability, jumping and landing exercises, agility and reaction training and typical goalkeeping skills using the ball.
3. The decision-making after goalkeeping injuries is a team decision between the goalkeeper, team coaches, goalkeeping coach, athletic coach and medical staff.
4. Because goalkeepers in football rarely are substituted during competitive matches, the substitution of an injured goalkeeper should guarantee a complete preparedness of the goalkeeper for 90 min play without any complaints. Therefore, goalkeepers do not return to play early, which may be different to players of other positions such as forwards, who may have a step-by-step return to play with possible short-term participations in a match.

Top Five Evidence-Based References

Ekstrand J, Hägglund M, Törnqvist H, Kristenson K, Bengtsson H, Magnusson H, Waldén M (2013) Upper extremity injuries in male elite football players. Knee Surg Sports Traumatol Arthrosc 21:1626–1632

Krutsch W, Zeman F, Zellner J, Pfeifer C, Nerlich M, Angele P (2016) Increase in ACL and PCL injuries after implementation of a new professional football league. Knee Surg Sports Traumatol Arthrosc 24:2271–2279

Hunt M, Fulford S (1990) Amateur soccer: injuries in relation to field position. Br J Sports Med 24:265

Kristenson K, Waldén M, Ekstrand J, Hägglund M (2013) Lower injury rates for newcomers to professional soccer: a prospective cohort study over 9 consecutive seasons. Am J Sports Med 41:1419–1425

Ejnisman B, Barbosa G, Andreoli CV, de Castro Pochini A, Lobo T, Zogaib R, Cohen M, Bizzini M, Dvorak J (2016) Shoulder injuries in goalkeepers: review and development of a FIFA 11+ shoulder injury prevention program. Open Access J Sports Med 7:75–80

References

1. Degreef I, De Smet L (2009) Multiple simultaneous mallet fingers in goalkeeper. Hand Surg 14:143–144
2. Ejnisman B, Barbosa G, Andreoli CV, de Castro Pochini A, Lobo T, Zogaib R, Cohen M, Bizzini M, Dvorak J (2016) Shoulder injuries in goalkeepers: review and development of a FIFA 11+ shoulder injury prevention program. Open Access J Sports Med 7:75–80
3. Schmitt KU, Nusser M, Boesiger P (2008) Hip injuries in professional and amateur soccer goalkeepers. Sportverletz Sportschaden 22:159–163
4. Fuchs M, Thomforde K, Ziegler M, Rottenberg S (2016) Leitfaden Torwartspiel. Deutscher Fußball-Bund, Germany
5. de Moura NR, Borges LS, Santos VC, Joel GB, Bortolon JR, Hirabara SM, Cury-Boaventura MF, Pithon-Curi TC, Curi R, Hatanaka E (2013) Muscle lesions and inflammation in futsal players according to their tactical positions. J Strength Cond Res 27:2612–2618
6. Deprez D, Fransen J, Boone J, Lenoir M, Philippaerts R, Vaeyens R (2015) Characteristics of high-level youth soccer players: variation by playing position. J Sports Sci 33:243–254
7. Rebelo A, Brito J, Maia J, Coelho-e-Silva MJ, Figueiredo AJ, Bangsbo J, Malina RM, Seabra A (2013) Anthropometric characteristics, physical fitness and technical performance of under-19 soccer players by competitive level and field position. Int J Sports Med 34:312–317

8. Dvorak J, George J, Junge A, Hodler J (2007) Age determination by magnetic resonance imaging of the wrist in adolescent male football players. Br J Sports Med 41:45–52
9. Bona CC, Tourinho Filho H, Izquierdo M, Pires Ferraz RM, Marques M (2016) Peak torque and muscle balance in the knees of young U-15 and U-17 soccer athletes playing various tactical positions. J Sports Med Phys Fitness 57(7–8):923–929
10. Aziz AR, Mukherjee S, Chia MY, Teh KC (2008) Validity of the running repeated sprint ability test among playing positions and level of competitiveness in trained soccer players. Int J Sports Med 29:833–838
11. Padulo J, Haddad M, Ardigò LP, Chamari K, Pizzolato F (2015) High frequency performance analysis of professional soccer goalkeepers: a pilot study. J Sports Med Phys Fitness 55:557–562
12. Di Salvo V, Benito PJ, Calderón FJ, Di Salvo M, Pigozzi F (2008) Activity profile of elite goalkeepers during football match-play. J Sports Med Phys Fitness 48:443–446
13. Ziv G, Lidor R (2011) Physical characteristics, physiological attributes, and on-field performances of soccer goalkeepers. Int J Sports Physiol Perform 6:509–524
14. Knoop M, Fernandez-Fernandez J, Ferrauti A (2013) Evaluation of a specific reaction and action speed test for the soccer goalkeeper. J Strength Cond Res 27:2141–2148
15. Fuller CW, Smith GL, Junge A, Dvorak J (2004) The influence of tackle parameters on the propensity for injury in international football. Am J Sports Med 32(Suppl 1):43–53
16. Spratford W, Mellifont R, Burkett B (2009) The influence of dive direction on the movement characteristics for elite football goalkeepers. Sports Biomech 8:235–244
17. Piringe K (1999) Zur Sonderstellung des Torhüters im Fußball. GRIN, München
18. Volpi P (2006) Upper extremity injuries. In: Volpi P (ed) Football traumatology: current concepts: from prevention to treatment. Springer, Berlin, pp 123–126
19. Diaz GJ, Fajen BR, Phillips F (2012) Anticipation from biological motion: the goalkeeper problem. J Exp Psychol Hum Percept Perform 38:848–864
20. McMorris T, Hauxwell B (1997) Improving anticipation of goalkeepers using video observation. In: Reilly T, Bangsbo J, Hughes M (eds) Science and football III. Taylor & Francis, London, pp 290–294
21. Savelsbergh GJP, Van der Kamp J, Williams AM, Ward P (2005) Anticipation and visual search behavior in expert soccer goalkeepers. Ergonomics 48:1686–1697
22. Shafizadeh M, Davids K, Correia V, Wheat J, Hizan H (2016) Informational constraints on interceptive actions of elite football goalkeepers in 1v1 dyads during competitive performance. J Sports Sci 34:1596–1601
23. Bar-Eli M, Azar OH, Ritov I, Keidar-Levin Y, Schein G (2007) Action bias among elite soccer goalkeepers: the case of penalty kicks. J Econ Psychol 28:606–621
24. Dessing JC, Craig CM (2010) Bending it like Beckham: how to visually fool the goalkeeper. PLoS One 5:e13161
25. Misirlisoy E, Haggard P (2014) Asymmetric predictability and cognitive competition in football penalty shootouts. Curr Biol 24:1918–1922
26. Noel B, van der Kamp J, Memmert D (2015) Implicit goalkeeper influences on goal side selection in representative penalty kicking tasks. PLoS One 10:e0135423
27. Wood G, Jordet G, Wilson MR (2015) On winning the "lottery": psychological preparation for football penalty shoot-outs. J Sports Sci 33:1758–1765
28. Hegerl U, Koburger N, Rummel-Kluge C, Gravert C, Walden M, Mergl R (2013) One followed by many? - Long-term effects of a celebrity suicide on the number of suicidal acts on the German railway net. J Affect Disord 146:39–44
29. Ladwig KH, Kunrath S, Lukaschek K, Baumert J (2012) The railway suicide death of a famous German football player: impact on the subsequent frequency of railway suicide acts in Germany. J Affect Disord 136:194–198
30. Federation Internationale de Football Association (2015) Laws of the game 2015/2016. Federation Internationale de Football Association, Zürich
31. Deehan DJ, Bell K, McCaskie AW (2007) Adolescent musculoskeletal injuries in a football academy. J Bone Joint Surg Br 89:5–8
32. Kristenson K, Waldén M, Ekstrand J, Hägglund M (2013) Lower injury rates for newcomers to professional soccer: a prospective cohort study over 9 consecutive seasons. Am J Sports Med 41:1419–1425
33. Arnason A, Tenga A, Engebretsen L, Bahr R (2004) A prospective video-based analysis of injury situations in elite male football: football incident analysis. Am J Sports Med 32:1459–1465
34. Woods C, Hawkins RD, Maltby S, Hulse M, Thomas A, Hodson A (2004) Football Association Medical Research Programme. The Football Association Medical Research Programme: an audit of injuries in professional football—analysis of hamstring injuries. Br J Sports Med 38:36–41
35. Hawkins RD, Fuller CW (1998) An examination of the frequency and severity of injuries and incidents at three levels of professional football. Br J Sports Med 32:326–332
36. Woods C, Hawkins R, Hulse M, Hodson A (2003) The Football Association Medical Research Programme: an audit of injuries in professional football: an analysis of ankle sprains. Br J Sports Med 37:233–238
37. Ekstrand J, Hägglund M, Törnqvist H, Kristenson K, Bengtsson H, Magnusson H, Waldén M (2013) Upper extremity injuries in male elite football players. Knee Surg Sports Traumatol Arthrosc 21:1626–1632

38. Dvorak J, Junge A, Derman W, Schwellnus M (2011) Injuries and illnesses of football players during the 2010 FIFA World Cup. Br J Sports Med 45:626–630
39. Junge A, Dvořák J (2015) Football injuries during the 2014 FIFA World Cup. Br J Sports Med 49:599–602
40. Koch M, Zellner J, Berner A, Grechenig S, Krutsch V, Nerlich M, Angele P, Krutsch W (2016) Influence of preparation and football skill level on injury incidence during an amateur football tournament. Arch Orthop Trauma Surg 136:353–360
41. Pförringer W, Ullmann C (1989) Risiken und Gefahren für die Gesundheit. In: Pförringer W, Ullmann C (eds) Fußball: Risiken erkennen, Unfälle vermeiden, Verletzungen heilen. Südwest, München, pp 21–84
42. Hunt M, Fulford S (1990) Amateur soccer: injuries in relation to field position. Br J Sports Med 24:265
43. Sousa P, Rebelo A, Brito J (2013) Injuries in amateur soccer players on artificial turf: a one-season prospective study. Phys Ther Sport 14:146–151
44. Rettig AC (2004) Athletic injuries of the wrist and hand: Part II: Overuse injuries of the wrist and traumatic injuries to the hand. Am J Sports Med 32:262–273
45. Combs JA (2000) It's not "just a finger". J Athl Train 35:168–178
46. Kraus R, Szalay G, Meyer C, Kilian O, Schnettler R (2007) Die distale Radiusfraktur-Eine Torwartverletzung bei Kindern und Jugendlichen. Sportverletz Sportschaden 21:177–179
47. Biener K, Berbig R (1985) Sportunfälle bei Fußballtorhütern (Sport injuries in soccer goalkeepers). In: Biener K, Berbig R (eds) Fußball Sportmedizin, Sporternährung, Sportunfälle. Habegger, Derendingen, pp 73–88
48. Perugia D, Ciurluini M, Ferretti A (2009) Spontaneous rupture of the extensor pollicis longus tendon in a young goalkeeper: a case report. Scand J Med Sci Sports 19:257–259
49. Bowers WH, Hurst LC (1977) Gamekeeper's thumb. Evaluation by arthrography and stress roentgenography. J Bone Joint Surg Am 59:519–524
50. Scerri GV, Ratcliffe RJ (1994) The goalkeeper's fear of the nets. J Hand Surg Br 19:459–460
51. Boyd KT, Brownson P, Hunter JB (2001) Distal radial fractures in young goalkeepers: a case for an appropriately sized soccer ball. Br J Sports Med 35:409–411
52. López-Zabala I, Fernández-Valencia JA (2013) Nonoperative treatment of distal biceps brachii musculotendinous partial rupture: a report of two cases. Case Rep Orthop 2013:970512
53. Maciel RA, Zogaib RK, Pochini Ade C, Ejnisman B (2015) Isolated rupture of teres major in a goalkeeper. BMJ Case Rep. https://doi.org/10.1136/bcr-2015-210524
54. Pidemunt G, Torres-Claramunt R, Ginés A, de Zabala S, Cebamanos J (2012) Bilateral stress fracture of the carpal scaphoid: report in a child and review of the literature. Clin J Sport Med 22:511–513
55. Tomcovcík L, Kubasovský J, Kitka M (2003) Simultaneous double interphalangeal dislocation on a single finger. Acta Chir Orthop Traumatol Cechoslov 70:309–310
56. Galati G, Cosenza UM, Sammartino F, Benvenuto E, Caporale A (2003) True aneurysm of the ulnar artery in a soccer goalkeeper: a case report and surgical considerations. Am J Sports Med 31:457–458
57. Fysentzou C (2016) Rehabilitation after a grade III latissimus dorsi tear of a soccer player: a case report. J Back Musculoskelet Rehabil 29:905–916
58. Faude O, Federspiel B, Kindermann W (2009) Injuries in elite German football-a media based analysis. Dtsch Z Sportmed 60:139–144
59. Krutsch W, Zeman F, Zellner J, Pfeifer C, Nerlich M, Angele P (2016) Increase in ACL and PCL injuries after implementation of a new professional football league. Knee Surg Sports Traumatol Arthrosc 24:2271–2279
60. McCrory P, Meeuwisse WH, Aubry M, Cantu RC, Dvořák J, Echemendia RJ, Engebretsen L, Johnston K, Kutcher JS, Raftery M, Sills A, Benson BW, Davis GA, Ellenbogen R, Guskiewicz KM, Herring SA, Iverson GL, Jordan BD, Kissick J, McCrea M, McIntosh AS, Maddocks D, Makdissi M, Purcell L, Putukian M, Schneider K, Tator CH, Turner M (2013) Consensus statement on concussion in sport: the 4th International Conference on Concussion in Sport, Zurich, November 2012. J Athl Train 48:554–575
61. McCrory P, Meeuwisse W, Johnston K, Dvorak J, Aubry M, Molloy M, Cantu R (2009) Consensus statement on concussion in sport: the 3rd International Conference on Concussion in Sport held in Zurich, November 2008. J Athl Train 44:434–448
62. Straume-Naesheim TM, Andersen TE, Bahr R (2005) Reproducibility of computer based neuropsychological testing among Norwegian elite football players. Br J Sports Med 39(Suppl 1):64–69
63. Straume-Naesheim TM, Andersen TE, Dvorak J, Bahr R (2005) Effects of heading exposure and previous concussions on neuropsychological performance among Norwegian elite footballers. Br J Sports Med 39(Suppl 1):70–77
64. Krutsch V, Gesslein M, Loose O, Weber J, Nerlich M, Gaensslein A, Bonkowsky V, Krutsch W (2017) Injury mechanism of midfacial fractures in football cause in over 40% typical neurological symptoms of minor brain injuries. Knee Surg Sports Traumatol Arthrosc. https://doi.org/10.1007/s00167-017-4431-z
65. Mihalik JP, Myers JB, Sell TC, Anish EJ (2005) Maxillofacial fractures and dental trauma in a high school soccer goalkeeper: a case report. J Athl Train 40:116–119
66. Delaney JS, Puni V, Rouah F (2006) Mechanisms of injury for concussions in university football, ice hockey, and soccer: a pilot study. Clin J Sport Med 16:162–165

67. Dvorak J, Junge A, Grimm K (2009) Head and brain injuries. In: Dvorak J, Junge A, Grimm K (eds) Football medicine manual. Federation Internationale de Football Association, Zürich
68. Fuller CW, Junge A, Dvorak J (2005) A six-year prospective study of the incidence and causes of head and neck injuries in international football. Br J Sports Med 39(Suppl 1):3–9
69. Silva P, Vaidyanathan S, Kumar BN, Soni BM, Sett P (2006) Two case reports of cervical spinal cord injury in football (soccer) players. Spinal Cord 44:383–385
70. Hardt N, Kuttenberger J (2010) Craniofacial trauma: diagnosis and management. Springer, Berlin
71. Higuera S, Lee EI, Cole P, Hollier LH Jr, Stal S (2007) Nasal trauma and the deviated nose. Plast Reconstr Surg 120(Suppl 2):64–75
72. Pappachan B, Alexander M (2006) Correlating facial fractures and cranial injuries. J Oral Maxillofac Surg 64:1023–1029
73. Wan J, Corvino TF, Greenfield SP, DiScala C (2003) Kidney and testicle injuries in team and individual sports: data from the national pediatric trauma registry. J Urol 170:1528–1533
74. Dunsmuir RA, Barnes SJ, McGarrity G (2006) "Goalkeeper's hip": acute haematogenous osteomyelitis secondary to apophyseal fractures. Br J Sports Med 40:808–809
75. Schmitt KU, Nusser M, Derler S, Boesiger P (2010) Analysing the protective potential of padded soccer goalkeeper shorts. Br J Sports Med 44:426–439
76. Marotti F, Polacco A (1983) Chronic lesions of the upper limb in the soccer goal-keeper. Acta Orthop Belg 49:203–212
77. Griffin DR, Dickenson EJ, O'Donnel J, Agricola R, Awan T, Beck M, Clohisy JC, Dijkstra HP, Falvey E, Gimpel M, Hinman RS, Hölmich P, Kassarjian A, Martin HD, Martin R, Mather RC, Philippon MJ, Reiman MP, Takla A, Thorborg K, Walker S, Weir A, Bennell KL (2016) The Warwick Agreement on femoroacetabular impingement syndrome (FAI syndrome): an international consensus statement. Br J Sports Med 50:1169–1176
78. Oztürk A, Ozkan Y, Ozdemir RM, Yalçin N, Akgöz S, Saraç V, Aykut S (2008) Radiographic changes in the lumbar spine in former professional football players: a comparative and matched controlled study. Eur Spine J 17:136–141
79. Gajhede-Knudsen M, Ekstrand J, Magnusson H, Maffulli N (2013) Recurrence of Achilles tendon injuries in elite male football players is more common after early return to play: an 11-year follow-up of the UEFA Champions League injury study. Br J Sports Med 47:763–768
80. Klügl M, Shrier I, McBain K, Shultz R, Meeuwisse WH, Garza D, Matheson GO (2010) The prevention of sport injury: an analysis of 12,000 published manuscripts. Clin J Sport Med 20:407–412
81. Bouwman LH, Ploeg AJ (2007) A man with dyspnoea after a soccer accident. Ned Tijdschr Geneeskd 151:242
82. Varga M, Takács P (1990) A fatal accident on the football field. Int J Legal Med 104:47–48
83. Rebelo-Gonçalves R, Figueiredo AJ, Coelho-E-Silva MJ, Tessitore A (2016) Assessment of technical skills in young soccer goalkeepers: reliability and validity of two goalkeeper-specific tests. J Sports Sci Med 15:516–523

70 Injury Prevention in Football: The Santa Monica Experience

Holly J. Silvers-Granelli, Robert H. Brophy, and Bert R. Mandelbaum

Contents

H.J. Silvers-Granelli, M.P.T., Ph.D. (✉)
Biomechanics and Movement Science, University of Delaware, Newark, DE, USA

Velocity Physical Therapy, 11611 San Vicente Blvd. GF-1, Los Angeles, CA 90049, USA
e-mail: hollysilverspt@gmail.com

R.H. Brophy, M.D.
Department of Orthopaedic Surgery, Washington University School of Medicine, St. Louis, MO, USA

B.R. Mandelbaum, M.D.
Santa Monica Orthopaedic Group, Santa Monica, CA, USA

70.1 Introduction

Soccer-related injuries are a relatively common occurrence across sex, age, and level of competition. The high prevalence of soccer-related injury has been well documented in the literature [1–10]. The impact of sports-related injury is complex and far-reaching, inflicting potential long-term physical, emotional, and financial consequences for the athlete to contend with long after their athletic career has finished. The rate of injury in soccer depends on several factors: age, level of competition, position on the field, field type, timing of injury, and sex [11]. Injuries incurred during soccer most commonly involve the lower extremity and most commonly occur in a game situation [12–15]. In studies analyzing the injury rates of professional male soccer athletes, overall injury rate (IR) ranged from 6.2 to 13.2 injuries per 1000 athletic exposures (AE) [16]. The National Collegiate Athletic Association (NCAA) has long recognized the high rate of injury in men's and women's soccer. Men's game IR ranked third (18.8) and women's game IR ranked fourth overall (16.4), respectively, for all NCAA sports per 1000 athletic exposures (AEs). When the data was stratified by gender, women's soccer had the highest game IR overall. The IR for practices was equally high, with women ranking fourth (5.2/1000 AEs) and men ranking fifth (4.3/1000 AEs) compared to 13 other NCAA collegiate sports [17]. Furthermore, the male IR is

V. Musahl et al. (eds.), *Return to Play in Football*, https://doi.org/10.1007/978-3-662-55713-6_70

four times higher in games compared with practices [16], and women's collegiate IR is three times higher in games than in practices. Approximately 70% of game and practice injuries affected the lower extremities [18]. The sheer magnitude of these injury rates, coupled with the increasing number of athletes participating in collegiate soccer, served as a meaningful impetus to actively intervene and attempt to reduce the current rate of injury, the severity of injury, and time loss associated with injury.

The earlier injury prevention programs primarily focused specifically on anterior cruciate ligament (ACL) injury reduction and prevention, namely, in the female athlete, due to the high rate of injury in this specific cohort [19–23]. Most of these neuromuscular training programs included a variety of strengthening, plyometric, and agility-based drills that addressed the major deficits most commonly associated with the female athlete that had sustained an ACL injury [24–26]. Several programs have been designed as dynamic warm-up programs in order to increase implementation fidelity and compliance, as well as to capitalize on the advantages associated with improved joint position sense found as a component in well-designed neuromuscular training warm-up programs [21, 23, 27]. Despite the development and the evolution of the aforementioned programs, there is a continued and implicit need to address soccer-related injury in totality and for an enhanced understanding of the most common mechanisms of injury in soccer. Recent studies have analyzed injury mechanisms in male and female soccer players to further delineate the specific kinetics and kinematics directly involved in the mechanism of injury [13, 28]. After analyzing videos of male and female athletes incurring a soccer-related injury, the authors have begun to establish the high-risk positioning most commonly associated with the sport, namely, defensive play with the involved player at or near full hip and knee extension [13, 28]. The continued delineation of the risk factors associated with sports-related injury will further the clinicians' ability to elucidate and refine a comprehensive intervention program to effectively decrease the injury rate in sport. Furthermore, the cohesive and consistent implementation of injury prevention and reduction protocols may be considered a very viable and cost-effective option to reducing the rate of soccer injury [29]. This knowledge can provide critical insight to help improve existing injury prevention protocols and secondary prevention strategies. Understanding the epidemiology and the mechanism of injury will allow researchers to refine and expound upon the current gold standard for injury prevention, thus decreasing the long-term deleterious sequelae commonly endured after incurring an injury [30].

70.2 The PEP Program

In the year 2000, the Santa Monica Sports Medicine Foundation created the PEP Program: Prevent Injury and Enhance Performance Program. It is an injury prevention program originally designed to address the high incidence of ACL injuries that were occurring, primarily, in the female soccer player. It is a 20-min dynamic warm-up program that directly replaces the team's traditional warm-up program. It is performed on the field and does not require any additional equipment. It focuses on instructing the athlete to anticipate external forces or loads in order to stabilize the hip and knee joints and subsequently decrease the propensity for ACL injury. Similar to previous prevention programs, PEP focused on proper landing, cutting, and decelerating techniques. It emphasized landing softly on the forefoot; engaging knee and hip flexion on landing; avoiding excessive genu valgus at the knee on landing, cutting, and decelerating; and increasing hamstring, gluteus medius, and hip abductor strength and activation. This soccer-specific study held large implications as it addressed an athletic community of over 300 million players, the largest in the world and at high risk for injuring the ACL relative to other sports [31].

70.2.1 Methodology

The PEP program was initially implemented using two age cohorts: 14–18-year-old and 18–23-year-old female football (soccer) players.

The PEP Program: prevent injury and enhance performance

1. **Warm-up:**
   a. Jog line to line (cone to cone)
   b. Shuttle run (side to side)
   c. Backward running
2. **Strengthening:**
   a. Walking Lunges
   b. Russian hamstring
   c. Single toe raises
3. **Plyometrics**
   a. Lateral hops over cone
   b. Forward/backward hops over cone
   c. Single leg hops over cone
   d. Vertical jumps with headers
   e. Scissors jump
4. **Agilities**
   a. Shuttle run with forward/backward running
   b. Diagonal runs (3 passes)
   c. Bounding run (44 yds)

Training Session per your Coaching staff — approximately 1–1.5 h

5. **Stretching:**
   This portion of the program is to be completed at the end of your regular training session.
   a. Calf stretch
   b. Quadriceps stretch
   c. Figure Four-Piriformis stretch
   d. Hamstring stretch
   e. Inner thigh adductor stretch
   f. Hip flexor stretch

Fig. 70.1 The Santa Monica Orthopaedic and Sports Medicine Research Foundation

It consists of a 20-min dynamic warm-up that preceded the normal training sessions or games and required only cones and a ball to perform. Each team in the intervention group was mailed an educational video depicting the warm-up program and a supplemental literature packet. In addition, each coach attended a mandatory league meeting in which the PEP program was introduced and the parameters were described. The instructional video provided education on three basic warm-up activities, five stretching techniques for the trunk and lower extremity, three strengthening exercises, five plyometric activities, and three soccer-specific agility drills as well as a demonstration on how to perform these activities with proper biomechanical technique (Fig. 70.1) [21].

70.2.2 Results

The first year of the study was conducted in a competitive youth female soccer league (14–18-year-old players). Over the course of the season, two ACL tears were reported for the intervention group (IG) (IR = 0.05 ACL injuries/1000 athletic exposures (AEs)). Thirty-two ACL tears were reported for the control group (CG) (0.47 ACLs/1000 AEs), resulting in an 88% overall reduction in ACL injury. In year 2 of the study, 4 ACL tears were reported in the IG (IR = 0.13/1000 AEs) compared to 35 ACLs in the CG (IR = 0.51/1000 AEs), corresponding to an overall reduction of 74% in ACL tears [21].

70.2.3 Additional Studies Using the PEP Program

Following the initial intervention, a randomized controlled trial was conducted using division I NCAA women's soccer teams (18–23-year-old players). Sixty-one teams with 1429 athletes completed the study: 854 athletes participated in 35 control teams and 575 athletes participated in 26 intervention teams. After the use of the PEP injury prevention program for one season, there were 7 ACL injuries in the IG (IR = 0.14/1000 AEs) and 18 in CG (IR = 0.25/1000 AEs) ($p = 0.15$). A 100% reduction in practice contact and noncontact ACL injuries occurred with no injuries reported in the IG compared with six in the CG (IR = 0.10/1000 AEs) ($p = 0.01$). Noncontact ACL injuries occurred at over three times the rate in control athletes ($n = 10$; 0.14) compared with intervention athletes ($n = 2$; IR = 0.04; $p = 0.06$). Control athletes with a previous history of ACL injury had a recurrence five times more often than those in the intervention group (IR = 0.10 vs. 0.02; $p = 0.06$); this difference reached significance when limited to noncontact ACL injuries during the season (IR = 0.06 vs. 0.00; $p < 0.05$). There was a significant difference in the rate of ACL injuries in the last 6 weeks of the season with a 100% reduction in contact and noncontact ACL injuries (intervention 0.00 vs. control 0.18; $p < 0.05$). This supports the concept that it takes 6–8 weeks for a biomechanical intervention program to have a neuromuscular effect [32].

70.2.4 Conclusions

The results of this study indicated that a neuromuscular training program, such as the PEP program, might significantly reduce the incidence of severe ACL injuries in the female athlete. Based on its findings, SMSMF contended that a prophylactic training program focusing on developing neuromuscular control of the lower extremity through strengthening exercises, plyometrics, and sports-specific agilities may address the proprioceptive and biomechanical deficits that are demonstrated in the high-risk female athletic population. This initial study laid the groundwork for the foundation's next steps: studying the biomechanical implications of instituting neuromuscular training programs via kinetic and kinematic analysis, identifying the mechanism of ACL injury, and, finally, determining a precise neuromuscular intervention program that would specifically counteract the unopposed forces around the trunk and lower extremity to further decrease the incidence of severe ligamentous injury.

Fact Box 1
Neuromuscular training programs that are performed consistently can significantly reduce an athlete's injury risk to ACL injury while playing soccer.

70.3 The 11+ Neuromuscular Training Program

Over the last decade, as researchers continued to unravel the mechanism of injury and pathokinematics surrounding ACL injury, prevention programs garnered serious support in the field of sports med. Both the International Olympic Committee and the Féderation Internationale de Football Association (FIFA) emphasize the protection of athletes' health as a major objective, and, in 1994, FIFA established its own Medical Assessment and Research Center (F-MARC) in order "to prevent football injuries and to promote football as a health-enhancing leisure activity, improving social behavior" [33]. On the basis of previous prevention programs including PEP, F-MARC attempted to create a simple and time-efficient preventive program to reduce the most common football injuries including ankle sprains, hamstring and groin strains, and ligament injuries in the knee. As a result, in 2003, an international group of experts under the tutelage of F-MARC created The 11, a program that was comprised of ten evidence-based or best-practiced exercises, and required no equipment other than a ball, that could be completed within

10–15 min as a matter of routine (F-MARC, 2009). However, in a randomized controlled trial, the Oslo Sports Trauma and Research Center (OSTRC) examined the effect of "The 11" over one season among 2000 female players aged 13–17 and found no difference in injury risk between the intervention group and the control group. Furthermore, OSTRC found that the compliance of the intervention group was too poor in order to identify a statistically significant effect of the program [34].

To improve upon both the preventive impact of The 11 and the compliance of the program, OSTRC, F-MARC, and SMSMF reconvened and developed a new program: the FIFA 11+ in 2006. This program was predicated on key exercises from the PEP program and The 11 that have been shown to have statistically significant impact in previous studies [21, 32]. FIFA 11+ is a comprehensive program encompassing cardiovascular and preventive exercises that focus on core and leg strength, balance, and agility and has a progression of three levels with increasing difficulty to provide variation and increases in difficulty. It takes approximately 20 min to complete and requires a minimum of equipment (a set of cones and soccer balls). Similar to the PEP program, the FIFA 11+ is time-efficient and inherently promotes compliance because it directly replaces the customary warm-up [23, 33, 35].

The FIFA 11+ is an injury prevention program designed as an alternative warm-up program to address lower extremity injury incurred in the sport of soccer for athletes over the age of 14 [23, 35]. It consists of 15 exercises divided into three separate components: running exercises (8 min) that encompass cutting, change of direction, decelerating, and proper landing techniques; strength, plyometric, and balance exercises (10 min) that focus on core strength, eccentric control, and proprioception; and, lastly, running exercise (2 min) to conclude the warm-up and prepare the athlete for athletic participation. There are three levels for each specific exercise (level 1, level 2, level 3) that increase the difficulty for each respective exercise. This allows for both individual and team progression throughout the course of the competitive season (Fig. 70.2). In this specific study, the FIFA 11+ program served as the intervention program over the course of one competitive collegiate soccer season. The warm-up was suggested to be utilized three times per week for the duration of the season.

70.3.1 Results

The average utilization of the FIFA 11+ in the IG was 32.8 ± 12.1 doses over the course of the season. There was no significant difference between the age of the injured athletes (20.4 ± 1.6 IG and 20.7 ± 1.5 CG) nor was there a difference in the number of injured athletes based on player position.

There was a significantly higher proportion of athletes injured in the CG, 665 (70%, IR = 15.04/1000 AEs) than in the IG, 285 (30%, IR = 8.09/1000 AEs), $p < 0.001$). The CG had a significantly higher average number of injuries per team ($M = 19.56$, SD = 11.01) than the IG ($M = 10.56$, SD = 3.64), $t(59) = 4.07$, $p < 0.001$.

There was a significantly higher number of days missed due to injury in the CG ($M = 13.02$, SD = 26.82) than in the IG ($M = 9.31$, SD = 14.83), SE = 0.12 $p = 0.007$, for each day missed in the IG 1.4 days were missed in the CG, OR = 1.40. Total days missed secondary to injury was 8776 in the CG compared to 2824 in the IG. There was no difference in either group for days missed based on field type, Wald $\chi^2(2) = 0.91$, $b = 0.13$, SE = 0.14, OR = 1.15, $p = 0.341$.

A second Poisson regression was used for those who were in the IG to compare the number of days missed if the injury occurred on a day where the intervention was used. The model was significant, LR $\chi^2(2) = 6.02$, $p < 0.049$. There was a significantly higher number of days missed when the intervention was not used on day of injury ($M = 10.65$, SD = 15.35) than when it was used ($M = 6.56$, SD = 10.44), Wald $\chi^2(1) = 4.26$, $b = 4.08$, SE = 1.98, $p = 0.039$. There was no difference on the number of days missed in the intervention group based on field type, Wald $\chi^2(1) = 0.90$, $b = 2.10$, SE = 2.21, $p = 0.343$.

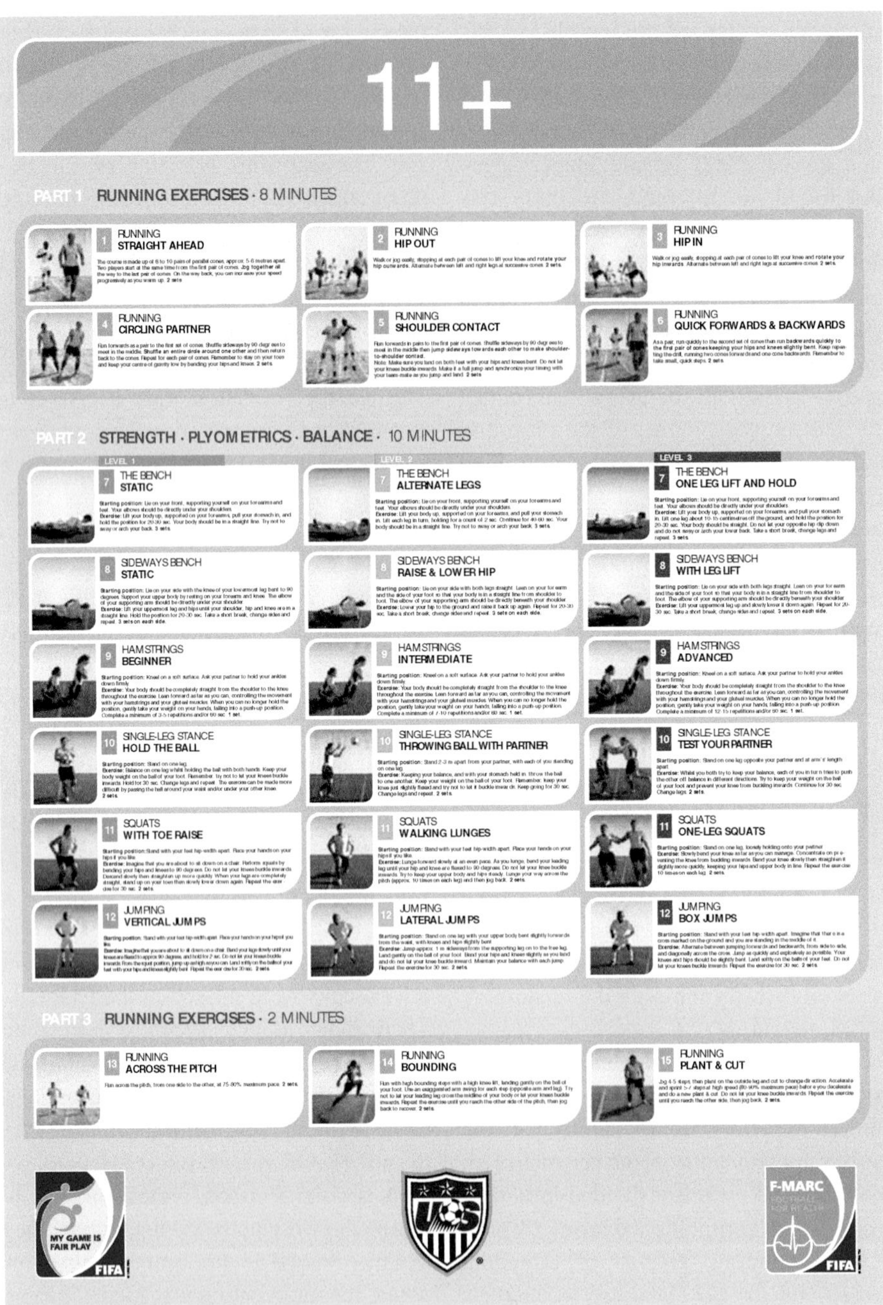
11+
PART 1 RUNNING EXERCISES · 8 MINUTES
1 RUNNING STRAIGHT AHEAD
2 RUNNING HIP OUT
3 RUNNING HIP IN
4 RUNNING CIRCLING PARTNER
5 RUNNING SHOULDER CONTACT
6 RUNNING QUICK FORWARDS & BACKWARDS
PART 2 STRENGTH · PLYOMETRICS · BALANCE · 10 MINUTES
LEVEL 1
LEVEL 2
LEVEL 3
7 THE BENCH STATIC
7 THE BENCH ALTERNATE LEGS
7 THE BENCH ONE LEG LIFT AND HOLD
8 SIDEWAYS BENCH STATIC
8 SIDEWAYS BENCH RAISE & LOWER HIP
8 SIDEWAYS BENCH WITH LEG LIFT
9 HAMSTRINGS BEGINNER
9 HAMSTRINGS INTERMEDIATE
9 HAMSTRINGS ADVANCED
10 SINGLE-LEG STANCE HOLD THE BALL
10 SINGLE-LEG STANCE THROWING BALL WITH PARTNER
10 SINGLE-LEG STANCE TEST YOUR PARTNER
11 SQUATS WITH TOE RAISE
11 SQUATS WALKING LUNGES
11 SQUATS ONE-LEG SQUATS
12 JUMPING VERTICAL JUMPS
12 JUMPING LATERAL JUMPS
12 JUMPING BOX JUMPS
PART 3 RUNNING EXERCISES · 2 MINUTES
13 RUNNING ACROSS THE PITCH
14 RUNNING BOUNDING
15 RUNNING PLANT & CUT
MY GAME IS FAIR PLAY
FIFA
US
F-MARC
FIFA

Fig. 70.2 The 11+ injury prevention program

70.3.2 Conclusions

The results suggest that consistent utilization of a neuromuscular training program, such as the FIFA 11+, may impart a protective benefit to the soccer athlete by achieving an optimal state of physiological preparedness for soccer competition and sufficient biomechanical training to offset the risk of injury associated with soccer participation.

Fact Box 2

The 11+ program has demonstrated the ability to decrease overall injury rate in soccer players and decrease time loss due to injury, a proxy for injury severity.

70.4 Video-Based Analysis

As research continued to confirm a discrepancy between the ACL injury rates of males and females, experts from SMSMF and Washington University Orthopedics next undertook a gender-based study to elucidate the mechanism of injury using video analysis. While there had been video analyses of ACL injuries in basketball, handball, Australian football, and alpine skiing, no such study existed at the time for soccer [36–38]. Video analysis, however, offered a way to accurately describe the game situation and biomechanics of injury and provide a fuller understanding of the underlying risk factors that may be amenable to prevention efforts. The researchers used this tool to test the hypothesis that these risk factors differ between male and female soccer athletes.

70.4.1 Methodology

Fifty-five videos of ACL injuries in 32 male and 23 female soccer players were collected and analyzed. Most injuries were incurred by professionals (22 males, 4 females) or collegiate-level players (8 males, 14 females), with the remainder of the injuries occurring in high school and youth players. Visual analysis of each case was performed to describe the injury mechanisms in detail (game situation, player behavior, lower extremity alignment, and kinematics). The goal was to identify the most frequent game situation in which the injury occurs and to determine the most common mechanisms by which ACL tears occur. Videos had to clearly delineate the position of the injured player on the field along with position of the ball and the events preceding the injury. Videos analyzed for mechanism of injury were of high enough quality to calculate the joint angles and determine the position of the lower extremity at the time of injury.

Each video was analyzed for the game situation immediately prior or during the occurrence of injury. The analysis for game situation included whether the player was playing an offensive or defensive role, the athletic action of the player (heading, passing, receiving the ball, tackling, etc.), whether the player was in control of the ball, and the location on the field where the injury occurred.

The mechanics of the ACL injury were studied in a systematic approach. The side of the injury and whether the injury was via contact or noncontact were recorded. Contact injuries were further divided into two separate subcategories revealing whether the injury was caused by direct contact to the lower extremity or indirect contact to other parts of the body, which influenced the injury by adding perturbation. Noncontact injuries were also examined to determine whether there was an opponent or another player in close proximity (within 1 m of the injured player) during the injury [13].

70.4.2 Results

The majority of ACL injuries occurred when the opposing team had the ball and the injured athlete was defending (73%). Females were more likely to be defending when they injured their ACL (87%) than males (63%) ($p = 0.045$). The most common playing action was tackling (51%), followed by cutting (15%). More than half of injuries occurred due to a contact mechanism (56%). There was a trend toward a greater percentage of ACL injuries occurring via contact in females (61%) compared with males (53%) ($p = 0.06$). ACL injuries that occurred when tackling usually involved contact (79%). In females, 80% of ACL injuries while tackling involved contact compared with 54% in males, but the difference was not significant ($p = 0.13$). For the vast majority of noncontact injuries (83%), an opposing player was within 1 or 2 yards of the injured athlete, but no direct contact occurred. Females (54%) were more likely than males (33%) to suffer a noncontact injury to their left lower extremity ($p = 0.05$).

In addition to game situation results, biomechanical results were also collected. Injuries occurred during a variety of motions, including planting, landing, cutting, and decelerating. Athletes were usually moving forward or changing direction at the time of injury. The majority of contact injuries occurred with the athlete moving forward (80%). There were no significant differences between male and female athletes. Noncontact ACL injuries occurred most often with the hip flexed (88%) and abducted (83%), the knee in valgus (58%) and within 30° of full extension (71%), and the foot flat (58%). Similar patterns of joint position were seen with the contact injuries. There were no significant differences between male and female athletes.

70.4.3 Conclusion

These results demonstrated that soccer players most often injure their ACLs when defending, specifically tackling, and females are more likely to injure their ACLs while defending than are males. Overall, slightly more than half of the injuries occurred via a contact mechanism, although a significant proportion of noncontact injuries occurred with an opponent in close proximity. Because tackling is a reactive maneuver that can require last-minute adjustments in body position and technique, female athletes with poor neuromuscular control and suboptimal biomechanics may be more likely to react in a way that puts the ACL at risk for injury. Although a number of the ACL injuries that occurred during tackling were noncontact, the majority (79%) were contact in nature. Nevertheless, this could be an important finding with regard to potential injury prevention efforts, as proper tackling technique should be addressed during player development and training.

This study also confirmed results obtained previously by SMSMF and the Washington University research team: females have higher involvement of the non-dominant lower extremity in ACL tears compared to males [39]. Additionally, video analysis confirmed past studies suggesting that the ACL is the most vulnerable and most often injured when the knee is at near extension. This evidence was corroborated by a recent study conducting analyzing European soccer injuries [28]. Knee rotational moments combined with near knee extension are often described as the most common situation in which ACLs are injured in observational and retrospective analyses. Other studies have shown knee abduction and flat-footedness as possible mechanisms for ACL injury during tackling. Although this study did not provide ways to improve tackling techniques, it suggests that female soccer players may especially benefit from training focused on safe techniques for defending and tackling.

Fact Box 3
Video analysis of injury mechanism provides important clinical insight into thoroughly understanding how injuries occur during athletic participation. Furthermore, this analysis provides critical information on how we can improve upon existing injury reduction efforts.

70.5 Compliance and Program Adherence to Injury Prevention Programs

The role of compliance in injury prevention protocols has been well documented in the literature [40–42]. Current research has demonstrated an inverse correlation of injury rate and time loss due to injury with the compliance of effective injury prevention protocols [23, 42]. The scientific medical community continues to struggle with consistency in implementation, program fidelity, and therapeutic compliance across all levels of competitive soccer play. The manner in which the program is delivered may impact the rate or program adoption. Studies have analyzed how different program delivery systems impact compliance, and, furthermore, the rate of injury [43]. Nations such as the United States, Canada, and many regions of Asia and Africa are confronted by a large geographic expanse when it comes to efficient and feasible medical delivery and public health messaging. The concept of using instructional DVDs, online streaming resources, and smartphone applications may offer a cost-effective alternate delivery system for injury prevention protocols in the event that a skilled medical professional is unable to be present [43].

It is critical to understand the rationale of why coaches, teams, players, and parents choose to implement a scientifically vetted injury prevention program or not too. Even though intervention programs have been shown to successfully reduce the rate of injury in competitive sport, the potential public health benefit and impact will not be realized if such interventions are not utilized consistently. Therefore, encouraging coaching and player motivation toward implementing injury prevention methodology into their training repertoire could have important public health ramifications and positive socioeconomic impacts on the aforementioned cohorts.

Team performance has been closely linked to player health and availability [44–48]. Careful attention is paid to match scheduling, training loads, minutes played, and overall exposure in order to mitigate risk to the individual athlete. Researchers in a variety of sports have demonstrated a significant association between injury rates and playing performance [49–51]. Including the analysis of team performance is an integral component in the effort to increase compliance rates [52–54]. Coaches, managers, and athletes are often more concerned about individual or team performance outcomes as opposed to actual injury reduction. If researchers can draw a correlation between compliance to an injury prevention program and improved team performance measured in a higher number of wins and fewer losses, this concept may resonate with coaching staffs and ultimately increase overall compliance rates.

Conclusions

The overarching theme of this chapter was to establish the relevance of the PEP and the FIFA 11+ programs and to further highlight the biomechanical mechanism that allow these programs to be successful. These programs have demonstrated their ability to reduce injury rates and severity of injury. Program compliance is paramount; the more consistently the program was utilized, the greater the injury prevention benefit was imparted onto the athlete. Furthermore, the ability for the athlete to stay healthy and available for selection throughout the competitive season seemingly allowed teams to perform more favorably. The benefits of sport participation are numerous and far outweigh the risks. The likelihood of incurring an injury by virtue of participating in soccer should not be underestimated. As clinicians and researchers, we must collectively recognize the risks associated with sport and implement the prevention protocols that have published to date. The information provided may help reduce the incidence of soccer-related injuries. We recognize the need for optimal program adherence and additional randomized controlled trials to continue to elucidate the etiology, mechanism of injury, and the need for continued biomechanical analysis of athletes to address the deficits that may inhibit their overall athletic performance and their ability to enjoy a functional, healthy, and active lifestyle.

Take-Home Message

The PEP and the FIFA 11+ programs have demonstrated its ability to decrease injury rate, including ACL injury rate, and improve overall team performance. The neuromuscular training programs support the importance of the consistent implementation of injury prevention protocols in sport. Compliance is a critical component to the overall impact of the program; teams utilizing the program more consistently demonstrated lower injury rates and more success with respect to team performance.

By prospectively analyzing changes in soccer-specific movement patterns during competition, we are now able to more fully understand mechanism of injury and how the programs may be improved with respect to injury reduction and how the program imparts' a protective benefit. This information will guide future researcher on how to optimize injury prevention efforts, to improve the content and efficiency of therapeutic prevention interventions, and to potentially identify high-risk athletes prospectively prior to a deleterious injury occurring. If these methods are implemented with optimal compliance and consistency early in an athlete's career, the overall risk of injury may be significantly reduced and the long-term health and athletic career longevity may be extended through the later decades of life. Furthermore, the physical and financial longitudinal impact(s) of many sports-related injuries may be significantly mitigated, thus improving overall quality of life of the athlete, extending well past the tenure of a collegiate athletic career.

Top Five Evidence-Based References

Alentorn-Geli E, Mendiguchía J, Samuelsson K, Musahl V, Karlsson J, Cugat R, Myer GD (2014) Prevention of anterior cruciate ligament injuries in sports. Part I: Systematic review of risk factors in male athletes. Knee Surg Sports Traumatol Arthrosc 22(1):3–15

Bizzini M et al (2013) Implementation of the FIFA 11+ football warm up program: how to approach and convince the Football associations to invest in prevention. Br J Sports Med 47(12):803–806

Gilchrist J et al (2008) A randomized controlled trial to prevent noncontact anterior cruciate ligament injury in female collegiate soccer players. Am J Sports Med 36(8):1476–1483

Owoeye OB et al (2014) Efficacy of the FIFA 11+ warm-up programme in male youth football: a cluster randomised controlled trial. J Sports Sci Med 13(2):321–328

Walden M et al (2015) Three distinct mechanisms predominate in non-contact anterior cruciate ligament injuries in male professional football players: a systematic video analysis of 39 cases. Br J Sports Med 49(22):1452–1460

References

1. Arnason A, Andersen TE, Holme I, Engebretsen L, Bahr R (2008) Prevention of hamstring strains in elite soccer: an intervention study. Scand J Med Sci Sports 18:40–48
2. Arnason A, Gudmundsson A, Dahl HA, Johannsson E (1996) Soccer injuries in Iceland. Scand J Med Sci Sports 6:40–45
3. Croisier J (2004) Factors associated with recurrent hamstring injuries. Sports Med 34:681–695
4. Ekstrand J, Gillquist J, Moller M, Oberg B, Liljedahl SO (1983) Incidence of soccer injuries and their relation to training and team success. Am J Sports Med 11:63–67
5. Ekstrand J, Hagglund M, Walden M (2011) Epidemiology of muscle injuries in professional football (soccer). Am J Sports Med 39:1226–1232
6. Engebretsen AH, Myklebust G, Holme I, Engebretsen L, Bahr R (2010) Intrinsic risk factors for groin injuries among male soccer players: a prospective cohort study. Am J Sports Med 38:2051–2057
7. Engebretsen AH, Myklebust G, Holme I, Engebretsen L, Bahr R (2010) Intrinsic risk factors for hamstring injuries among male soccer players: a prospective cohort study. Am J Sports Med 38:1147–1153
8. Giza E, Mithofer K, Farrell L, Zarins B, Gill T (2005) Injuries in women's professional soccer. Br J Sports Med 39:212–216
9. Hagglund M, Walden M, Bahr R, Ekstrand J (2005) Methods for epidemiological study of injuries to professional football players: developing the UEFA model. Br J Sports Med 39:340–346
10. Kristenson K, Bjorneboe J, Walden M, Andersen TE, Ekstrand J, Hagglund M (2013) The Nordic Football Injury Audit: higher injury rates for professional football clubs with third-generation artificial turf at their home venue. Br J Sports Med 47:775–781
11. Alentorn-Geli E, Mendiguchía J, Samuelsson K, Musahl V, Karlsson J, Cugat R, Myer GD (2014) Prevention of anterior cruciate ligament injuries in sports. Part I: Systematic review of risk factors in male athletes. Knee Surg Sports Traumatol Arthrosc 22:3–15
12. Brophy RH, Backus S, Kraszewski AP, Steele BC, Ma Y, Osei D et al (2010) Differences between sexes in lower extremity alignment and muscle activation during soccer kick. J Bone Joint Surg Am 92:2050–2058
13. Brophy RH, Stepan JG, Silvers HJ, Mandelbaum BR (2015) Defending puts the anterior cruciate ligament at risk during soccer: a gender-based analysis. Sports Health 7:244–249
14. Ekstrand J, Gillquist J (1983) Soccer injuries and their mechanisms: a prospective study. Med Sci Sports Exerc 15:267–270

15. Ekstrand J, Hagglund M, Walden M (2011) Injury incidence and injury patterns in professional football: the UEFA injury study. Br J Sports Med 45:553–558
16. Agel J, Evans TA, Dick R (2007) Descriptive epidemiology of collegiate men's soccer injuries: National Collegiate Athletic Association Injury Surveillance System,1988–1989 through 2002–2003. J Athl Train 42:270–277
17. Hootman JM, Dick R, Agel J (2007) Epidemiology of collegiate injuries for 15 sports: summary and recommendations for injury prevention initiatives. J Athl Train 42:311–319
18. Dick R, Agel J, Marshall SW (2007) National Collegiate Athletic Association Injury Surveillance System commentaries: introduction and methods. J Athl Train 42:173–182
19. Hewett TE, Lindenfeld TN, Riccobene JV, Noyes FR (1999) The effect of neuromuscular training on the incidence of knee injury in female athletes. A prospective study. Am J Sports Med 27:699–706
20. Junge A, Rosch D, Peterson L, Graf-Baumann T, Dvorak J (2002) Prevention of soccer injuries: a prospective intervention study in youth amateur players. Am J Sports Med 30:652–659
21. Mandelbaum B, Silvers H, Watanabe D, Knarr J, Thomas S, Griffin L et al (2005) Effectiveness of a neuromuscular and proprioceptive training program in preventing anterior cruciate ligament injuries in female athletes - 2-year follow-up. Am J Sports Med 33:1003–1010
22. Myklebust G, Engebretsen L, Braekken IH, Skjolberg A, Olsen OE, Bahr R (2003) Prevention of anterior cruciate ligament injuries in female team handball players: a prospective intervention study over three seasons. Clin J Sport Med 13:71–78
23. Soligard T, Myklebust G, Steffen K, Holme I, Silvers H, Bizzini M et al (2008) Comprehensive warm-up programme to prevent injuries in young female footballers: cluster randomised controlled trial. BMJ 337:a2469
24. Faude O, Junge A, Kindermann W, Dvorak J (2006) Risk factors for injuries in elite female soccer players. Br J Sports Med 40:785–790
25. Giza E, Silvers HJ, Mandelbaum BR (2005) Anterior cruciate ligament tear prevention in the female athlete. Curr Sports Med Rep 4:109–111
26. Griffin LY, Albohm MJ, Arendt EA, Bahr R, Beynnon BD, Demaio M et al (2006) Understanding and preventing noncontact anterior cruciate ligament injuries: a review of the Hunt Valley II meeting, January 2005. Am J Sports Med 34:1512–1532
27. Salgado E, Ribeiro F, Oliveira J (2015) Joint-position sense is altered by football pre-participation warm-up exercise and match induced fatigue. Knee 22:243–248
28. Walden M, Krosshaug T, Bjorneboe J, Andersen TE, Faul O, Hagglund M (2015) Three distinct mechanisms predominate in non-contact anterior cruciate ligament injuries in male professional football players: a systematic video analysis of 39 cases. Br J Sports Med 49:1452–1460
29. Junge A, Lamprecht M, Stamm H, Hasler H, Bizzini M, Tschopp M et al (2011) Countrywide campaign to prevent soccer injuries in Swiss amateur players. Am J Sports Med 39:57–63
30. Lohmander LS, Ostenberg A, Englund M, Roos H (2004) High prevalence of knee osteoarthritis, pain, and functional limitations in female soccer players twelve years after anterior cruciate ligament injury. Arthritis Rheum 50:3145–3152
31. Alentorn-Geli E, Myer GD, Silvers HJ, Samitier G, Romero D, Lazaro-Haro C et al (2009) Prevention of non-contact anterior cruciate ligament injuries in soccer players. Part 2: A review of prevention programs aimed to modify risk factors and to reduce injury rates. Knee Surg Sports Traumatol Arthrosc 17:859–879
32. Gilchrist J, Mandelbaum BR, Melancon H, Ryan GW, Silvers HJ, Griffin LY et al (2008) A randomized controlled trial to prevent noncontact anterior cruciate ligament injury in female collegiate soccer players. Am J Sports Med 36:1476–1483
33. Bizzini M, Dvorak J (2015) FIFA 11+: an effective programme to prevent football injuries in various player groups worldwide-a narrative review. Br J Sports Med 49:577–579
34. Steffen K, Myklebust G, Olsen OE, Holme I, Bahr R (2008) Preventing injuries in female youth football—a cluster-randomized controlled trial. Scand J Med Sci Sports 18:605–614
35. Bizzini M, Junge A, Dvorak J (2013) Implementation of the FIFA 11+ football warm up program: how to approach and convince the Football associations to invest in prevention. Br J Sports Med 47:803–806
36. Bere T, Florenes TW, Krosshaug T, Koga H, Nordsletten L, Irving C et al (2011) Mechanisms of anterior cruciate ligament injury in World Cup alpine skiing: a systematic video analysis of 20 cases. Am J Sports Med 39:1421–1429
37. Myklebust G, Engebretsen L, Braekken IH, Skjolberg A, Olsen OE, Bahr R (2007) Prevention of noncontact anterior cruciate ligament injuries in elite and adolescent female team handball athletes. Instr Course Lect 56:407–418
38. Wedderkopp N, Kaltoft M, Lundgaard B, Rosendahl M, Froberg K (1999) Prevention of injuries in young female players in European team handball. A prospective intervention study. Scand J Med Sci Sports 9:41–47
39. Brophy R, Silvers HJ, Gonzales T, Mandelbaum BR (2010) Gender influences: the role of leg dominance in ACL injury among soccer players. Br J Sports Med 44:694–697
40. Silvers-Granelli H, Mandelbaum B, Adeniji O, Insler S, Bizzini M, Pohlig R et al (2015) Efficacy of the FIFA 11+ injury prevention program in the collegiate male soccer player. Am J Sports Med. https://doi.org/10.1177/0363546515602009

41. Soligard T, Nilstad A, Steffen K, Myklebust G, Holme I, Dvorak J et al (2010) Compliance with a comprehensive warm-up programme to prevent injuries in youth football. Br J Sports Med 44:787–793
42. Steffen K, Emery CA, Romiti M, Kang J, Bizzini M, Dvorak J et al (2013) High adherence to a neuromuscular injury prevention programme (FIFA 11+) improves functional balance and reduces injury risk in Canadian youth female football players: a cluster randomised trial. Br J Sports Med 47:794–802
43. Steffen K, Meeuwisse WH, Romiti M, Kang J, McKay C, Bizzini M et al (2013) Evaluation of how different implementation strategies of an injury prevention programme (FIFA 11+) impact team adherence and injury risk in Canadian female youth football players: a cluster-randomised trial. Br J Sports Med 47:480–487
44. Carling C, Le Gall F, Dupont G (2012) Are physical performance and injury risk in a professional soccer team in match-play affected over a prolonged period of fixture congestion? Int J Sports Med 33:36–42
45. Dellal A, Lago-Penas C, Rey E, Chamari K, Orhant E (2015) The effects of a congested fixture period on physical performance, technical activity and injury rate during matches in a professional soccer team. Br J Sports Med 49:390–394
46. Frank BS, Register-Mihalik J, Padua DA (2015) High levels of coach intent to integrate a ACL injury prevention program into training does not translate to effective implementation. J Sci Med Sport 18:400–406
47. Gabbett TJ (2016) The training-injury prevention paradox: should athletes be training smarter and harder? Br J Sports Med 50:273–280
48. Gatterer H, Ruedl G, Faulhaber M, Regele M, Burtscher M (2012) Effects of the performance level and the FIFA "11" injury prevention program on the injury rate in Italian male amateur soccer players. J Sports Med Phys Fitness 52:80–84
49. Emery CA, Kang J, Schneider KJ, Meeuwisse WH (2011) Risk of injury and concussion associated with team performance and penalty minutes in competitive youth ice hockey. Br J Sports Med 45:1289–1293
50. Gabbett TJ (2004) Influence of injuries on team playing performance in Rugby League. J Sci Med Sport 7:340–346
51. Otten MP, Miller TJ (2015) A balanced team wins championships: 66 years of data from the National Basketball Association and the National Football League. Percept Mot Skills 121:654–665
52. Inklaar H, Bol E, Schmikli SL, Mosterd WL (1996) Injuries in male soccer players: team risk analysis. Int J Sports Med 17:229–234
53. McCall A, Carling C, Davison M, Nedelec M, Le Gall F, Berthoin S et al (2015) Injury risk factors, screening tests and preventative strategies: a systematic review of the evidence that underpins the perceptions and practices of 44 football (soccer) teams from various premier leagues. Br J Sports Med 49:583–589
54. McCall A, Carling C, Nedelec M, Davison M, Le Gall F, Berthoin S et al (2014) Risk factors, testing and preventative strategies for non-contact injuries in professional football: current perceptions and practices of 44 teams from various premier leagues. Br J Sports Med 48:1352–1357

The Knee Control Prevention Programme

71

Hanna Lindblom, Markus Waldén, Isam Atroshi, Annica Näsmark, and Martin Hägglund

Contents

H. Lindblom (✉)
Division of Physiotherapy, Department of Medical and Health Sciences, Linköping University, Linköping, Sweden
e-mail: hanna.lindblom@liu.se

M. Waldén
Football Research Group, Division of Community Medicine, Department of Medical and Health Sciences, Linköping University, Linköping, Sweden
e-mail: markus.walden@telia.com

I. Atroshi
Department of Clinical Sciences—Orthopaedics, Lund University, Lund, Sweden
e-mail: isam.atroshi@med.lu.se

A. Näsmark
Capio Artro Clinic, Swedish Football Association, Stockholm, Sweden
e-mail: annica.nasmark@capio.se

M. Hägglund
Football Research Group, Division of Physiotherapy, Department of Medical and Health Sciences, Linköping University, Linköping, Sweden
e-mail: martin.hagglund@liu.se

71.1 Injury Prevention in Youth Sports

Football is the most popular sport in Sweden, with approximately 440,000 registered players (total population of ten million) (Fig. 71.1). Given the inherent risk of injury during football play, the sport is the most frequent cause of sports injuries requiring acute medical treatment at hospitals in Sweden [11]. Football also contributes with the highest number of injury insurance claims (42% of all injury claims including data from 35 different sports) based on Swedish national insurance registry data [1]. Lower limb injuries predominate, with the knee and ankle as the most frequent areas of acute injuries in youth players. Severe acute knee injuries, e.g. anterior cruciate ligament (ACL) injury, sustained at a young age may

V. Musahl et al. (eds.), *Return to Play in Football*, https://doi.org/10.1007/978-3-662-55713-6_71

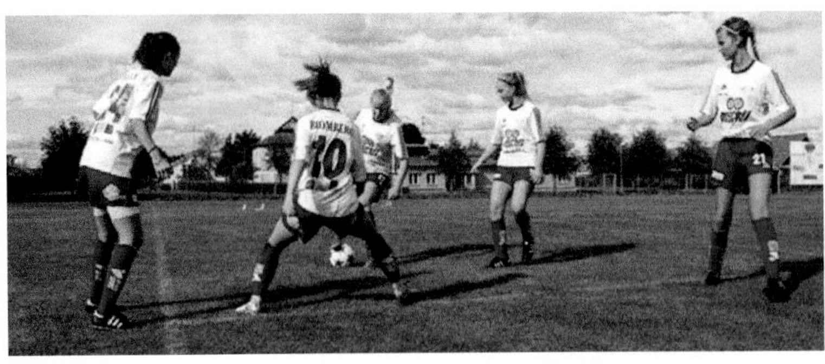

Fig. 71.1 Football is the most popular sport in Sweden. Photo: Emma Busk Winquist with permission

have life-long negative impact on health-related quality of life and physical function [3] and may thus constitute a considerable economic burden to society. Female football players are more prone to suffer an ACL injury, with a two to three times higher risk compared with their male counterparts [10, 14]. To reduce the risk of injury and their long-term consequences, various injury prevention exercise programmes (IPEP) have been developed for use in different sporting populations. These have been found efficacious in reducing lower limb injury risk in high-quality randomised controlled trials (RCT) [9, 13]. Such programmes commonly include exercises focusing on proper technique during landing, cutting and deceleration, core and lower limb strength, hip and knee control and lower limb alignment.

71.2 The Knee Control Project in Swedish Football

Injury insurance claims data have shown a high rate of severe knee injuries, including ACL injuries, in female football in Sweden [12]. In 2008, the Swedish Football Association (FA) and the insurance company Folksam (all football players in Sweden from the age of 15 years have an insurance in Folksam via their mandatory playing license) initiated a project aiming to reduce the burden of severe knee injuries. The aim was to evaluate and distribute a structured IPEP called Knee Control in Swedish football nationwide through coach and player educational workshops.

71.2.1 The Knee Control Injury Prevention Exercise Programme

The Knee Control IPEP (in Swedish Knäkontroll) was developed in 2005 for adolescent team sports, through an initiative from various stakeholders such as the Swedish Sports Confederation, the Swedish School of Sports and Health Sciences and the Swedish Rheumatism Association, in collaboration with the Swedish FA, the Swedish Handball Federation, the Swedish Basketball Federation and the Swedish Floorball Federation. An educational material was commercially available (SISU Idrottsböcker©, Sweden, 2005) including a CD-ROM and a corresponding leaflet describing the IPEP. Films describing all exercises are available on the CD-ROM for the four different sports (football, handball, basketball and floorball).

The programme contains six different principal exercises focusing on neuromuscular control, landing and cutting technique, core and lower limb strength and lower limb alignment (Fig. 71.2). All exercises have four levels of difficulty and an additional pair exercise to allow for progression and variation of exercises (Table 71.1). The programme is led and individually progressed by a coach or other team designate and takes about 10–15 min to complete after familiarisation. The six principal exercises are the same regardless of sport. Some adaptation has, however, been made to make exercises more sports specific (e.g. use of a football in the football version). One of the authors (AN) was responsible for the development of the football-specific parts of the Knee Control IPEP.

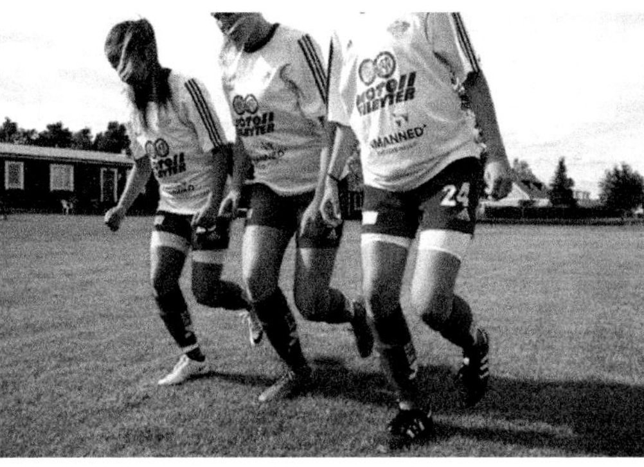

Fig. 71.2 Football girls performing the one-legged knee squat. Photo: Emma Busk Winquist with permission

Table 71.1 The Knee Control injury prevention exercise programme

Exercise/level	*Instructions*: All exercises are performed over three sets with 8–15 repetitions, or 15–30 s for exercise 4 the bench
1. One-legged knee squat	
A	Hands on the hips
B	With a ball over the head
C	Mark the 12-02-04-06 o'clock positions with the nonsupporting foot
D	Diagonal movement holding a ball
Pair exercise	Teammates press a ball between the lateral sides of their feet
2. Pelvic lift	
A	Both feet on the ground
B	One foot on the ground
C	One foot on a football
D	Explosive movement with quick push off from the ground
Pair exercise	Teammate supports the heel of the foot in his/her hands
3. Two-legged knee squat	
A	With a ball in front of the body with straight arms
B	Hands on the hips
C	With a ball over the head
D	Same as level C but continue the upward movement and rise up on the toes
Pair exercise	Teammates face opposite directions holding a ball between them
4. The bench	
A	Prone position. Support on the knees and lower arms
B	Support on the tip of the feet
C	Same as level B but move the foot to the side and back. Alternate sides
D	Sideways bench. Dynamic movement lifting the hip off the ground and back
Pair exercise	The wheelbarrow
5. Lunges	
A	Walking lunges. Hands on the hips
B	Walking lunges holding a ball in front of the body and rotating the upper body
C	Forward lunge holding a ball over the head, pushing back with the front leg to return to the starting position
D	Sideways lunges holding a ball in front of the body
Pair exercise	Teammates stand facing each other 5–10 m apart. One performs a forward lunge while making a throw-in with a ball
6. Jump/landing	
A	Single-leg forward and backward jumps, landing on the same foot
B	Sideways jump landing on one foot and alternating sides
C	A few quick steps on the same spot, then jump forward and land on one foot
D	Same as level C but change of direction during the jump (90° turn)
Pair exercise	Two-legged jump while heading a football and land on two legs

The Knee Control programme (Knäkontroll, SISU Idrottsböcker©, Sverige, 2005) is available as a DVD/leaflet via www.idrottsbokhandeln.se and as a free downloadable mobile phone application via App Store, https://itunes.apple.com and Google Play, https://play.google.com

71.2.2 Evaluating the Preventive Efficacy on Acute Knee Injuries

As a first step, the preventive efficacy of the IPEP was evaluated in a cluster RCT in girls' adolescent football (12–17 years) in 2009 [5, 15]. The primary focus of the trial was on prevention of ACL injuries and, as a secondary outcome, acute knee injuries in total. The study is the largest sports injury prevention RCT to date, with 230 clubs and 4564 players enrolled, and was carried out in eight regional football districts in Sweden. Clubs were randomised into an intervention group (Knee Control IPEP) or control group (training according to usual routines), with all teams from the same club (different age groups) randomised into the same group. In total 2479 players were randomised to the intervention group and 2085 players to the control group. All coaches in the intervention group received theoretical and practical education about the IPEP before the study and were provided with the CD-ROM and leaflet describing the exercises. They were instructed to use the IPEP twice per week throughout the season. Data about individual and team exposure for training and match play in both groups were reported by the team coaches throughout the competitive season of 2009 (7 months). Additionally, the intervention group coaches recorded all training sessions during which the IPEP was carried out over the season. All teams had a designated physiotherapist to assist with data collection and document any acute knee injuries that occurred during scheduled football training or match play. All players with acute knee injuries were examined by the team physiotherapist. If an ACL injury was suspected, or in unclear cases, a study designated orthopaedic surgeon (one for each district) was consulted for further examination and referral to MRI if deemed necessary.

The main results of the RCT are summarised in Table 71.2. During the season 96 acute knee injuries in 92 players were reported, including 21 ACL injuries in 21 players (0.46% of players). This shows that although a considerable problem, acute knee injuries, and ACL injuries in particular, are not an epidemic in girls' football. When evaluating IPEP effect, the rate of ACL injury was 64% lower in the intervention group compared to the control group (Fig. 71.3). A significant reduction in the rates of severe knee injury (more than 4 weeks absence from play) and any acute knee injury, by

Table 71.2 Main results of the Knee Control RCT in girls' football

Number of players with an acute knee injury (%)	Intervention group	Control group	Injury rate ratio (95% CI)
Intention to treat analysis			
ACL injury	7 (0.28)	14 (0.67)	0.36 (0.15–0.85)*
Severe knee injury (>4 weeks)	26 (1.05)	31 (1.49)	0.70 (0.42–1.18)
Any acute knee injury	48 (1.94)	44 (2.11)	0.92 (0.61–1.40)
Sub-group analysis of compliant players			
ACL injury	2 (0.15)	14 (0.67)	0.17 (0.05–0.57)*
Severe knee injury (>4 weeks)	5 (0.38)	31 (1.49)	0.18 (0.07–0.45)*
Any acute knee injury	18 (1.38)	44 (2.11)	0.53 (0.30–0.94)*

ACL anterior cruciate ligament, *CI* confidence interval, *RCT* randomised controlled trial
*Statistically significant at $p < 0.05$

82% and 47%, respectively, was seen in players who had completed the IPEP at least once a week.

71.2.3 Compliance Is Key for Successful Injury Reduction

The association between team and player compliance with the IPEP and injury rate reductions was also evaluated [6]. All intervention group coaches registered team and player execution of the IPEP throughout the season. Based on their number of executed IPEP sessions, teams and players were stratified into tertiles of compliance (low, intermediate and high), and injury rates were then compared between the three groups.

Overall, intervention group teams completed the IPEP in 79% of all training sessions, or an average of 1.4 IPEP sessions per week (recommended weekly dosage two sessions). Teams in the low-, intermediate- and high-compliance

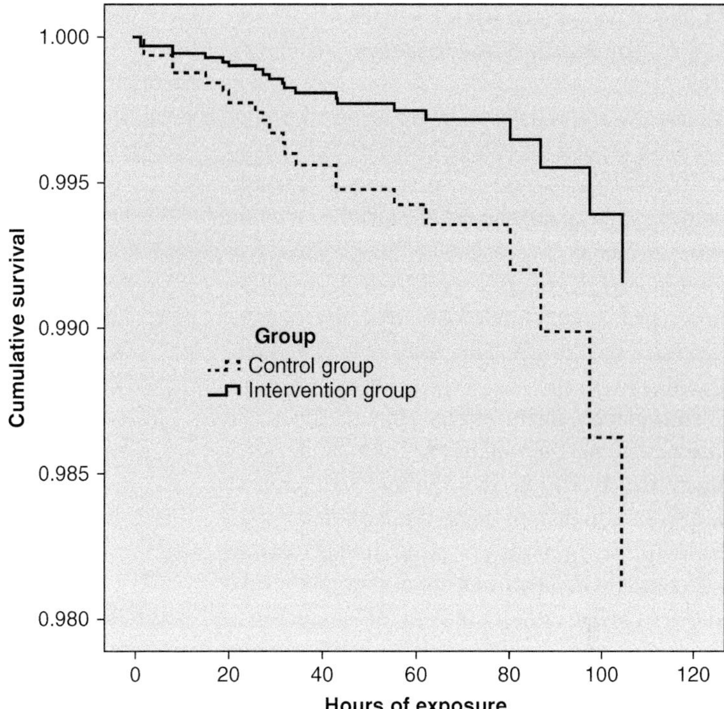

Fig. 71.3 Cumulative survival curve showing a 64% lower ACL injury rate in the intervention group compared with the control group

groups used the IPEP in 63%, 82% and 89% of their training sessions, respectively.

When studying associations with injury rates, the low-compliance group was used as reference, and in comparison, players in the high-compliance group had an 88% reduction in ACL injury rate. Compared with players in the low-compliance group, the high-compliance and intermediate-compliance groups also had significantly lower rates of severe knee injuries (90% and 83%, respectively) and acute knee injuries in total (72% and 74%, respectively). Worth noting is that there were no differences in injury rates between players in the low-compliance group compared with those in the control group. This indicates that sporadic use of the IPEP does not provide an injury-preventive effect.

A noteworthy finding was that compliance with the IPEP deteriorated over the season, on average by 3% each month on team level. At the same time, player attendance at training also deteriorated, by 2% each month, which means that the individual player was even less likely to achieve a sufficient number of IPEP sessions to gain a preventive effect. This raises questions about how to improve compliance with and maintenance of the IPEP throughout the entire season. It also shows the importance of not only frequent use of the IPEP by team coaches but also enhancing player attendance at training sessions, to increase the overall injury reduction effect.

Fact Box 1 Injury preventive effect

- Teams that used the Knee Control IPEP during a season had a 64% reduction of ACL injuries.
- The most diligent players had the largest risk reduction, whereas players who only used the programme sporadically had no preventive effect.
- The rates of severe knee and any acute knee injury decreased in players who had completed the IPEP at least once a week.

71.2.4 Analysis of Risk Factors for Acute Knee Injuries

We also evaluated risk factors for acute knee injuries in the same RCT cohort, covering both intrinsic (player-related) and extrinsic (environmental) factors [4]. A questionnaire designed to capture intrinsic factors was filled in by all players at baseline. Team coaches registered player attendance and football exposure and the various extrinsic factors (playing surface, individual playing time).

In summary, the most important extrinsic risk factor was playing matches, with acute knee injury and ACL injury rates in matches being 15 and 9 times higher, respectively, than in training. Furthermore, girls who played additional matches with teams with older players in their club had a threefold higher risk of injury in those matches as compared with playing with their own team. Only 16% of all acute knee injuries occurred in training, which shows that football practice in these age groups is fairly safe from a knee-injury perspective (Fig. 71.4). We evaluated the influence of playing surface on acute knee injuries and found no difference in injury rates when playing on natural grass compared to artificial turf. As for intrinsic risk factors, higher age (>14 years) and menarche were associated with an increased knee injury rate. Both histories of previous acute knee injury and current knee injury (ongoing knee complaints at the start of the season) increased the risk of sustaining a new acute knee injury during the season. The strongest risk factor for ACL injury was familial disposition; players with a parent or sibling with ACL injury had a fourfold increased ACL injury rate. Other player-related factors such as stature and body mass had no association with knee injury occurrence.

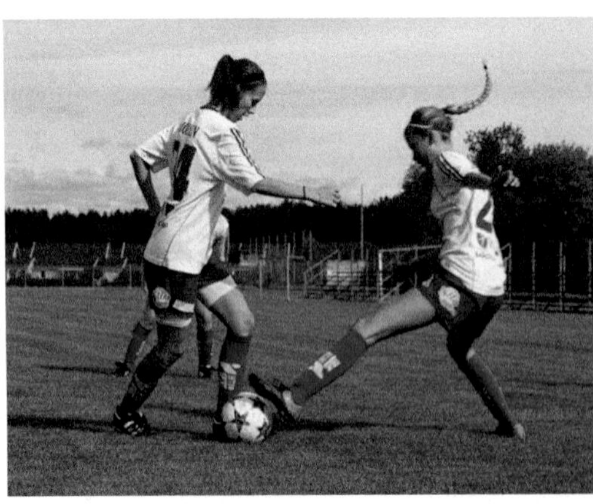

Fig. 71.4 Girls' football practice is fairly safe from a knee-injury perspective. Photo: Emma Busk Winquist with permission

Fact Box 2 Risk factors for acute knee injuries

- Football training is fairly safe from a knee-injury perspective.
- The risk of injury is 10–15 times higher during matches.
- Girls who played additional matches with older teams in their club had a threefold increased risk of injury in those games.

71.2.5 Evaluating Effects on Performance

If we can show effects on performance in addition to injury-preventive effects, coach and player buy-in of IPEPs may improve. Accordingly, the effect of knee control on football-relevant performance was studied in an RCT with four girls' adolescent football teams (41 players) [7]. The two intervention teams used the IPEP twice weekly for 11 weeks, and the control teams followed their usual practice routines. At baseline and follow-up, players were tested using a battery of performance tests covering balance (star excursion balance test), jump ability (triple-hop for distance and countermovement jump tests), agility performance (modified Illinois agility test) and sprint ability (10 and 20 m sprints). No significant effect of training with the IPEP was found on any of the performance tests. One possible reason for the absence of performance effects is that this IPEP focuses on proper technique and slow controlled movements, which might not have provided sufficient stimulus to induce training effects as measured with the current performance tests, mostly requiring explosive muscle actions. Another possible explanation is that even though teams used the IPEP as per recommendation, the individual player only performed one IPEP session per week on average due to a low training attendance. We did not evaluate qualitative aspects of movement control, muscle activation patterns, etc., and any IPEP effects on such measures are unknown. Nonetheless, the most important performance-enhancing effect of the IPEP is probably the reduction of acute knee injury risk.

71.3 Dissemination Efforts After the Randomised Controlled Trial

Following the results from the RCT showing the preventive efficacy of the IPEP, the Swedish FA and the Folksam insurance company together initiated a nationwide implementation of the Knee Control programme in Swedish football in 2010. Efforts to disseminate the IPEP included information spread via the webpages of the Swedish FA and Folksam and development of a freely downloadable smartphone application (app) to facilitate IPEP spread and ease of use. The app (Knäkontroll, SISU Idrottsböcker©) is available for free at App Store, https://itunes.apple.com, and Google Play, https://play.google.com. The app has been downloaded more than 120,000 times over the last 4 years since its launch in October 2012. In the app suggestions for general warm-up before the IPEP were added to the programme to increase player and coach buy-in. Additionally, physiotherapists within national sports physiotherapy organisations and networks were recruited to engage in educational workshops for coaches and football teams in all 24 regional districts in Sweden. Financial and logistical support to arrange educational workshops for coaches and football

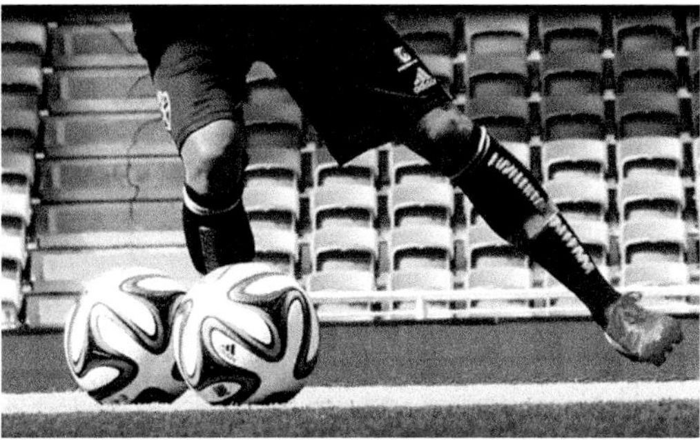

Fig. 71.5 The Swedish women's national football team performing the Knee Control programme. Photo: Onside TV productions with permission

teams nationwide was offered. Educational workshops were also held in conjunction with national team football games (Fig. 71.5). Usually coaches and two or three players from each team have participated in the workshops. Recently the Knee Control IPEP was also incorporated in the Swedish FA coach education curriculum.

71.3.1 Evaluating the Implementation of the IPEP

In 2012 we followed up on the RCT to evaluate the implementation of the IPEP 3 years after the trial [8]. Web-based questionnaires were sent to all coaches of girls' adolescent football teams in the eight districts that had participated in the RCT, as well as to representatives from the Swedish FA and the eight districts' FAs. The questionnaires were based on the Reach Effectiveness Adoption Implementation and Maintenance Sports Setting Matrix (RE-AIM SSM) [2] and covered *reach* (how well spread the IPEP was), perceived *effectiveness* (regarding injury prevention and performance enhancement), *adoption* (whether the coaches used the IPEP), *implementation* (how the IPEP was used) and *maintenance* (continued usage over time) of the IPEP. Representatives for the FAs answered questions about the maintenance of the IPEP and their efforts to disseminate the programme in the football community.

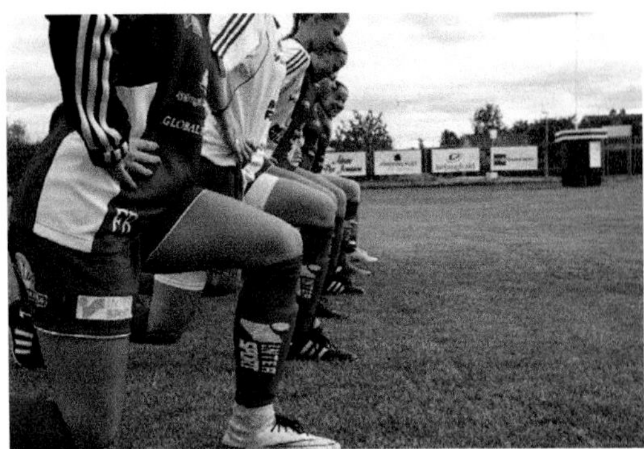

Fig. 71.6 A girls' football team using the Knee Control programme. Photo: Emma Busk Winquist with permission

The survey showed promising results regarding IPEP spread and usage, and perceived effectiveness, among the coaches. Almost all coaches were aware of the IPEP (reach 91–99%) and also used it to a high extent (adopted by 58–74% of all coaches). Furthermore, they reported high perceived effectiveness regarding the IPEP's injury-preventive and performance-enhancing effects, rating both at a median of 8 on a 0–10 numerical rating scale (10 representing the most favourable rating). Worth noting, however, is that IPEP fidelity according to recommendations was low, with three out of four coaches reported having modified the programme. Common modifications included omitting or changing some of the exercises or changing the dosage or frequency of use. As mentioned under Sect. 3, the Swedish FA had formal policies and ongoing IPEP implementation work. However, in the regional district FAs, as well as within the clubs, there was a lack of formal policies for IPEP implementation and education, showing that there is still work to be done to facilitate effective adoption and maintenance of the IPEP in Swedish football (Fig. 71.6).

71.3.2 Coaches Are Key Players for Successful Implementation

Some modification of the IPEP could be positive if it facilitates higher adoption and maintenance over time. However, too big modifications might compromise the injury-preventive effect shown in the RCT. To learn more about coaches' experiences of the IPEP and reasons for programme modifications, we conducted interviews of girls' football coaches. We found that the coach is absolutely vital for IPEP use since he or she must be motivated and prioritise the IPEP for the training to take place. From an ecological point of view, external factors may, however, affect the coach and facilitate or hinder his or her use of the IPEP. If the coach feels support from other coaches, players, the club and FAs IPEP usage is facilitated. Enough resources within the team in terms of economy, manpower, facilities and time for training also affect the possibilities for IPEP usage. Many coaches report low player buy-in and lack of support from both players and other coaches in their teams. Hence, many coaches modify the programme to improve its fit and to improve player buy-in, which probably facilitates long-term maintenance of the IPEP within the team, but may risk limiting the injury-preventive effect. Supporting the coaches and giving suggestions for appropriate modifications or exercise progressions that do not compromise the preventive effect but improve programme fit may be one way to address this issue.

Fact Box 3 Increasing compliance and fidelity for the best possible preventive effect

- Improve player attendance at training.
- Make IPEP usage a coach priority.
- Facilitate IPEP usage through external support (other coaches, players, clubs, football associations, resources).
- Give suggestions for appropriate programme modifications to improve programme fit without compromising the preventive effect.

Take-Home Message

In summary, the experiences from the Knee Control project in Swedish football clearly show that it is possible to reduce the rates of severe knee injuries in girls' football. A simple low-cost IPEP, taking no more than 10–15 min to complete, reduced the rate of ACL injuries by 64%—bang for your buck right there! Compliance with the exercises is key, with large injury rate reductions seen in the most diligent players, while players who only used the programme sporadically experienced no preventive effect. Increasing team compliance as well as player attendance at training is necessary to achieve a full effect. Efforts made to disseminate the IPEP in Swedish football have shown promising results. An excellent spread and good adoption of the IPEP among girls' football coaches were evident in our follow-up 3 years after the intervention trial. Further, the IPEP mobile app is increasing in popularity with more than 120,000 downloads over 4 years. Continuous efforts with coach education and IPEP dissemination are necessary to ensure long-term maintenance and adoption of the preventive training programme among new coaches in the future.

Top Five Evidence Based References

Hägglund M, Atroshi I, Wagner P, Waldén M (2013) Superior compliance with a neuromuscular training programme is associated with fewer ACL injuries and fewer acute knee injuries in female adolescent football players: secondary analysis of an RCT. Br J Sports Med 47:974–979

Hägglund M, Waldén M (2016) Risk factors for acute knee injury in female youth football. Knee Surg Sports Traumatol Arthrosc 24:737–746

Lindblom H, Waldén M, Hägglund M (2012) No effect on performance tests from a neuromuscular warm-up programme in youth female football: a randomised controlled trial. Knee Surg Sports Traumatol Arthrosc 20:2116–2123

Lindblom H, Waldén M, Carlfjord S, Hägglund M (2014) Implementation of a neuromuscular training programme in female adolescent football: 3-year follow-up study after a randomised controlled trial. Br J Sports Med 48:1425–1430

Waldén M, Atroshi I, Magnusson H, Wagner P, Hägglund M (2012) Prevention of acute knee injuries in adolescent female football players: cluster randomised controlled trial. BMJ 344:e3042

References

1. Åman M, Forssblad M, Henriksson-Larsén K (2016) Incidence and severity of reported acute sports injuries in 35 sports using insurance registry data. Scand J Med Sci Sports 26:451–462
2. Finch CF, Donaldson A (2010) A sports setting matrix for understanding the implementation context for community sport. Br J Sports Med 44:973–978
3. Frobell RB, Roos HP, Roos EM, Roemer FW, Ranstam J, Lohmander S (2013) Treatment for acute anterior cruciate ligament tear. BMJ 346:f232
4. Hägglund M, Waldén M (2016) Risk factors for acute knee injury in female youth football. Knee Surg Sports Traumatol Arthrosc 24:737–746
5. Hägglund M, Waldén M, Atroshi I (2009) Preventing knee injuries in adolescent female football players – design of a cluster randomized controlled trial [NCT00894595]. BMC Muskuloskelet Disord 10:75
6. Hägglund M, Atroshi I, Wagner P, Waldén M (2013) Superior compliance with a neuromuscular training programme is associated with fewer ACL injuries and fewer acute knee injuries in female adolescent football players: secondary analysis of an RCT. Br J Sports Med 47:974–979
7. Lindblom H, Waldén M, Hägglund M (2012) No effect on performance tests from a neuromuscular warm-up programme in youth female football: a randomised controlled trial. Knee Surg Sports Traumatol Arthrosc 20:2116–2123
8. Lindblom H, Waldén M, Carlfjord S, Hägglund M (2014) Implementation of a neuromuscular training programme in female adolescent football: 3-year follow-up study after a randomised controlled trial. Br J Sports Med 48:1425–1430
9. Olsen OE, Myklebust G, Engebretsen L, Holme I, Bahr R (2005) Exercises to prevent lower limb injuries in youth sports: cluster randomised controlled trial. BMJ 330(7489):449
10. Prodromos CC, Han Y, Rogowski J, Joyce B, Shi K (2007) A meta-analysis of the incidence of anterior cruciate ligament tears as a function of gender, sport, and a knee injury-reduction regimen. Arthroscopy 23:1320–1325
11. Socialstyrelsen (National Board of Health and Welfare) (2010) Skadehändelser som föranlett läkarbesök vid akutmottagning. Statistik från Socialstyrelsens Injury Database (IDB) Sverige. No. 2011-11-18. http://www.socialstyrelsen.se/Lists/Artikelkatalog/Attachments/18491/2011-11-18.pdf. Accessed 4 Jan 2017
12. Söderman K, Pietilä T, Alfredson H, Werner S (2002) Anterior cruciate ligament injuries in young females playing soccer at senior levels. Scand J Med Sci Sports 12:65–68
13. Soligard T, Myklebust G, Steffen K, Holme I, Silvers H, Bizzini M, Junge A, Dvorak J, Bahr R, Andersen TE (2008) Comprehensive warm-up programme to prevent injuries in young female footballers: cluster randomised controlled trial. BMJ 337:a2469
14. Waldén M, Hägglund M, Werner J, Ekstrand J (2011) The epidemiology of anterior cruciate ligament injury in football (soccer): a review of the literature from a gender-related perspective. Knee Surg Sports Traumatol Arthrosc 19:3–10
15. Waldén M, Atroshi I, Magnusson H, Wagner P, Hägglund M (2012) Prevention of acute knee injuries in adolescent female football players: cluster randomised controlled trial. BMJ 344:e3042

The Female Player: Special Considerations

72

Markus Waldén, Mariann Gajhede Knudsen, Matilda Lundblad, Jan Ekstrand, and Martin Hägglund

Contents

M. Waldén (✉) • J. Ekstrand
Football Research Group, Division of Community Medicine, Department of Medical and Health Sciences, Linköping University, Linköping, Sweden
e-mail: markus.walden@telia.com; jan.ekstrand@telia.com

M.G. Knudsen
Football Research Group, Linköping, Sweden
e-mail: mariannknudsen@hotmail.com

M. Lundblad
Football Research Group, Institute of Clinical Sciences, Sahlgrenska Academy, Gothenburg, Sweden
e-mail: matildalundblad@gmail.com

M. Hägglund
Football Research Group, Division of Physiotherapy, Department of Medical and Health Sciences, Linköping University, Linköping, Sweden
e-mail: martin.hagglund@liu.se

72.1 The History of Women's Football

Although not as old as men's football, women's football is not a new thing. Women played football already in the nineteenth century, but the sport was officially and unofficially counteracted for a long time. The breakthrough for organized women's football came as late as during the 1970s, and to date it is the most popular team sport for women worldwide and is growing rapidly (Fig. 72.1). Early pioneers in organizing women's football were the Nordic countries, followed by the rest of Europe and North America. The first official European Championship was held in 1984 and the first official World Cup in 1991. Finally, women's football has been an Olympic sport since Atlanta 1996.

V. Musahl et al. (eds.), *Return to Play in Football*, https://doi.org/10.1007/978-3-662-55713-6_72

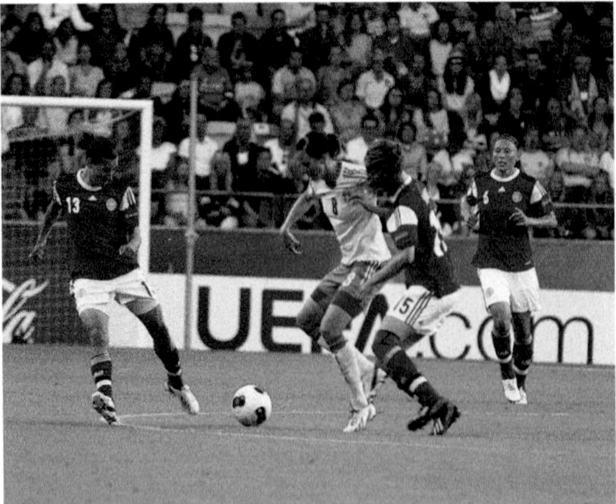

Fig. 72.1 Female football is growing rapidly. Photo: Lennart Weber with permission

72.2 The Menstrual Cycle

The menstrual cycle has repeatedly been discussed as a potential factor involved in injury causation in female athletes.

72.2.1 Menstrual Cycle Phases

Each menstrual cycle can be divided into three phases based on events in the ovary (ovarian cycle) or in the uterus (uterine cycle). There are some inconsistencies in the terminology used, but usually the ovarian cycle is divided into the follicular phase, ovulation, and the luteal phase, whereas the uterine cycle is divided into the menstruation phase (menses), the proliferative phase, and the secretory phase. The menstruation phase always starts the first day of the menstrual bleeding and goes on for the next 7 days. The luteal/secretory phase is sometimes further divided into the postovulatory (secretory) phase and the premenstrual phase (Fig. 72.2). The luteal phase is most often of the same length (14 days), but the follicular phase tends to show more variability. The typical length of the menstrual cycle in adults thus varies between 21 and 35 days (the average cycle length being 28 days).

72.2.2 Menstrual Cycle Regulation

The menstrual cycle is regulated by the hypothalamus, and some of the hormones involved are gonadotrophin-releasing hormone (GnRH), follicle-stimulating hormone (FSH), luteinizing hormone (LH), estradiol (the most potent estrogen), and progesterone (Fig. 72.2). The female sex hormone levels are low at cycle day 1, but then FSH begins to increase and stimulates the development of a group of follicles which produce estradiol. Estradiol inhibits further production of FSH and stimulates LH secretion which results in a large peak the day before ovulation, the LH surge. The empty follicle creates the corpus luteum which produces both progesterone and estradiol resulting in peaks in the middle of the luteal phase. If fertilization does not occur, the hormone levels fall, and this initiates the breakdown of the endometrium which leads to the next menstrual bleeding. A normal blood loss should be below 80 ml, whereas females with larger blood losses, metrorrhagia, is at risk of developing iron deficiency. Since low iron levels, and sometimes even anemia, is not uncommon in female football players [1], it is important to include blood tests for iron deficiency in the annual pre-participation health examination of the players.

72.2.3 Female Sex Hormones and Injuries

Several studies have investigated or discussed the potential association between the peri-pubertal hormonal influx and the hormonal variations during the menstrual cycle and the risk of injury in sports.

72.2.3.1 Mechanical Properties of Ligaments

A frequently discussed factor in the injury causation of ligament injuries, such as anterior cruciate ligament (ACL) tears, is changes in the mechanical properties of ligaments as a consequence of

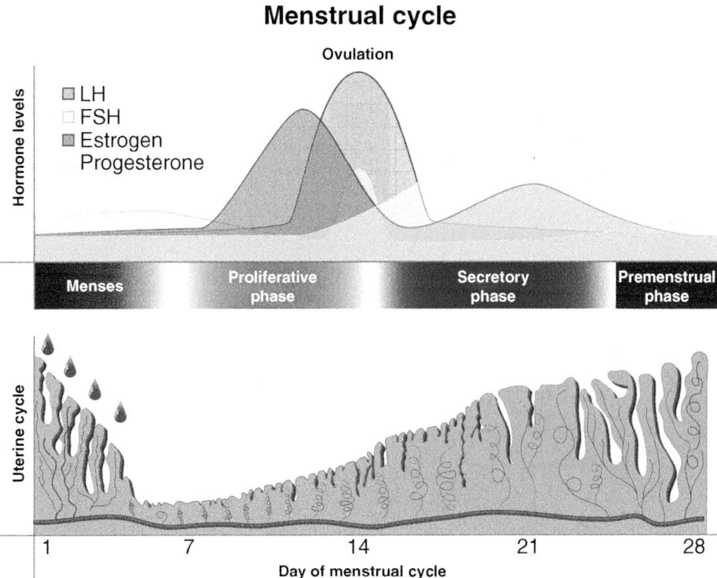

Fig. 72.2 Phases of the menstrual cycle (uterine) with corresponding hormone levels. Figure used with permission

rising or high estrogen levels during and after puberty in females [2]. Collagen forms the major load-bearing structure of ligaments and is produced by fibroblasts which are known to express estrogen receptors in both women and men. Although controversial, there is some evidence that estrogen affects the metabolic and mechanical properties of the ACL negatively which can lead to decreased tensile strength and stiffness in the ligament and in turn lower ability to withstand high loading [2].

Moreover, the role of laxity as a risk factor for knee ligament injuries is still debated, but some studies have identified increased anterior knee laxity during the ovulatory and luteal phases which might be of importance in injury causation [3, 4]. Any increased laxity during the second half of the menstrual cycle is likely mediated by relaxin, which is a peptide hormone produced by the corpus luteum in the nonpregnant woman [5]. Relaxin receptors are found on the human ACL in women, but not in men, but the exact mechanism by which relaxin alters the mechanical properties of the ACL has yet to be elucidated. The most plausible mechanism is a long-term exposure effect of high relaxin levels in some women which leads to decreased ligament integrity and failure [5].

72.2.3.2 Menstrual Cycle Phase and Risk of Injury

The pioneer study in this field was carried out on 86 football players in the three highest divisions in Sweden in 1984 [6]. In that study, the risk of traumatic injury was found to be significantly higher during the premenstrual and menstrual phases. In contrast, no difference in the risk of low back pain was seen between the menstrual cycle phases in a questionnaire study on 261 players in the three highest divisions in Sweden [7]. Thereafter, most research has focused on sports-related ACL injuries, and although several studies have identified a periodicity in ACL injuries during the menstrual cycle, especially for noncontact injuries, findings are equivocal with little consensus on the association between menstrual cycle phase and injury risk. In a systematic review on seven studies published between 1998 and 2003 on different sports such as football, basketball, handball, and skiing, some evidence for an increased injury rate during the preovulatory first half of the menstrual cycle was identified [8]. Most of the included studies were, however, associated with severe methodological limitations such as small cohorts, lack of stratification between females using oral contraceptive (OC) or not, inadequate methods of determining the cycle day, and lack of control groups. In addition, it has been assumed that the included women have regular 28-day menstrual cycles despite the fact that inter- and intra-woman cycle variability is large [9]. Menstrual dysfunction such as anovulatory cycles and luteal phase defects in spite of regular bleedings are also not taken into consideration [9]. Taken together, no definitive conclusions can be drawn in terms of the association between menstrual cycle phase and ACL injury based on current knowledge.

72.2.3.3 Oral Contraceptives and Risk of Injury

The traditionally combined OC contains both estrogen and progesterone and acts mainly through negative feedback on the secretion of GnRH, FSH, and LH. Whereas continuous estrogen has a strong inhibitory effect on the follicle development and ovulation, there is a dose-response relationship for progesterone where low doses inhibit ovulation in about 50% of cycles, intermediate doses inhibit ovulation in close to 100% of cycles, and high doses completely inhibit follicular development and ovulation. In traditional combined OCs and in high-dose progesterone-only OCs, the cycles are anovulatory without any hormonal fluctuations, and any possible effect of the menstrual cycle phase on the risk of injury is therefore dissociated since no periodicity is present. In the aforementioned Swedish study, players who used OCs had fewer injuries than those who did not use OCs [6]. Moreover, there was no increased risk of injury in OC users during the premenstrual and menstrual phases as seen for players without OCs [6]. The main dilemma here is, however, that these findings have not been reproduced in other studies and that most studies that include data on OC use have not registered or not reported on the different types of OCs used.

72.2.3.4 Premenstrual Symptoms

Premenstrual symptoms (PMS) is defined as physical and psychological discomforts during the premenstrual phase that disappears at the time of menstruation. The vast majority of women in fertile age experience at least one premenstrual symptom such as tender breasts, tiredness, irritability, and mood changes. Women with PMS have shown to suffer from impaired motor control during the premenstrual phase compared with women without PMS [10]. Similarly, women with PMS have displayed increased postural sway on an ankle disc and higher threshold to detection of passive motion (kinesthesia) of the knee joint [11]. The inferior knee kinesthesia was especially shown to be present in the premenstrual phase [12]. Using OCs may therefore theoretically be advantageous for females who are negatively affected by their menstrual cycle as they may provide a stable and controllable hormonal milieu [13].

72.2.3.5 The Female Athlete Triad

The term female athlete triad consists of disordered eating, menstrual dysfunction, and low bone mass [14]. Although prevalent in some sports, it appears to be less frequent in women's football. In a study on Norwegian elite athletes, the frequency of self-reported eating disorder among the 69 female football players was 5.9% and of menstrual dysfunction 9.3%, but no player fulfilled all criteria for the triad [14, 15]. Both these numbers were lower than among endurance athletes and controls. Menstrual dysfunction also seems to be less associated with low bone mass in football players as compared with endurance athletes and controls [14].

Fact Box 1

The menstrual cycle is a basic difference between men and women and has repeatedly been discussed as a potential factor involved in injury causation in female athletes.

Currently, the findings in the literature are equivocal with little consensus on the association between menstrual cycle phase and injuries.

72.3 Aspects on Anthropometry and Physiology

In many sports, men and women compete under different conditions. For example, women play fewer sets in tennis, they need fewer points to win a set in badminton, and in athletics less weight is used for females in disciplines such as javelin, discus, and shot put. Similarly, the ball is lighter and smaller for women in popular team sports such as handball and basketball, whereas men and women use the same size football.

In a recent review, the anthropometry of female elite players was on average 161–170 cm and 57–65 kg [16]. In addition, female players have lower maximum oxygen uptake and perform less high-intensity running activities than their male counterparts [16, 17]. Interestingly, it has been suggested that because of inferior technical abilities in women (i.e., they lose the ball more often and display lower pass completion rates), they are forced to work less efficiently than men, which in turn may result in greater accumulated fatigue [18]. It is, however, unclear from the literature if these sex-related differences influence the risk of injury and return to play (RTP) issues, especially since men and women do not compete against each other.

72.4 Injury Rate in Women's Football

The injury rate has been studied extensively in men's football, but to a lesser degree in women's football. It is difficult to compare injury rates between women and men from the existing literature due to differences in study design, injury definition, and populations. Some studies, however, provide injury rate estimates from both women's and men's football using identical injury surveillance methods (Table 72.1).

Table 72.1 Injury rates in adult women's versus men's football from studies comparing injury rates between sexes using the same injury surveillance method

	Setting	Injury definition	Injury rate	F/M ratio
International tournaments				
Junge and Dvorak [19]	WC 1998–2012 OG 1998–2012	Medical attention	F: 1.94/match; M: 2.34/match F: 2.46/match; M: 2.32/match	0.83 1.06
Hägglund et al. [20] Waldén et al. [21]	EC 2004–2008	Time loss	F: 2.5/1000 h training; M: 2.4/1000 h training F: 36.0/1000 h match; M: 38.9/1000 h match	1.05 0.92
Club football				
Hägglund et al. [22]	Premier division Sweden 2005 (1 season)	Time loss	F: 3.8/1000 h training; M: 4.7/1000 h training F: 16.1/1000 h match; M: 28.1/1000 h match	0.81 0.57
Lion et al. [23]	Premier division Luxembourg 2013/2014 (1 season)	Time loss[a]	F: 0.7/1000 h; M: 0.6/1000 h	1.17
Mufty et al. [24]	Royal Belgian FA database 1999/2000 and 2009/2010 (2 seasons)	Insurance claims	F: 5.23/100 players; M 6.83/100 players	0.77
College football				
Agel et al. [25] Dick et al. [26]	NCAA schools 1988–2003 (15 years)	Time loss	F: 5.23/1000 AEs training; M: 4.34/1000 AEs training F: 16.44/1000 AEs match; M: 18.75/1000 AEs match	1.21 0.88
Chandran et al. [27]	NCAA schools 2004–2009 (6 years)	Time loss	F: 5.01/1000 AEs training; M: 5.06/1000 AEs training F: 14.36/1000 AEs match; M: 17.18/1000 AEs match	0.99 0.84
Roos et al. [28]	NCAA schools 2009–2015 (6 years)	Medical attention	F: 5.69/1000 AEs training; M: 5.47/1000 AEs training F: 17.04/1000 AEs match; M: 17.53/1000 AEs match	1.04 0.97

AE athlete exposure, *EC* European Championship, *F* female, *FA* Football Association, *M* male, *NCAA* National Collegiate Athletic Association, *OG* Olympic Games, *WC* World Cup

[a]>15 days absence

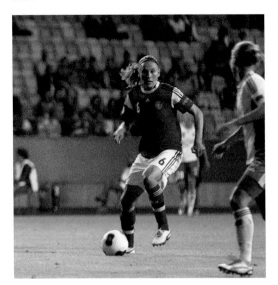

Fig. 72.3 The injury rate in women's football is similar to that in men's football. Photo: Lennart Weber with permission

72.4.1 International Tournaments

Injury surveillance has been implemented as a matter of routine during major international tournaments such as the World Cups, Olympic Games, and European Championships over the last two decades [19–21]. As seen in Table 72.1, the injury rates in these tournaments appear to be fairly even between the sexes, with the female-to-male ratio being 1.05 in training and ranging from 0.83 to 1.06 in matches (Fig. 72.3).

72.4.2 Club Level Football

Comparisons for club level football were possible in two prospective studies from Sweden and Luxembourg and one from the Royal Belgian Football Association database. This yielded somewhat conflicting results with the Swedish study reporting 19–43% lower injury rates in women [22] and the Belgian study a 23% lower injury rate in women [24]. In contrast, the study from Luxembourg, including only moderate and severe injuries, reported a 17% higher injury rate in women [23]. Worth noting is that in the aforementioned Swedish study, no difference in the rate of severe injuries was found between the sexes [22].

72.4.3 Collegiate Football

The most comprehensive comparable injury surveillance dataset comes from collegiate football in the United States, where in total 27 years of National Collegiate Athletic Association (NCAA) injury surveillance data were available [25–28]. The NCAA data also indicate fairly similar injury rates between the sexes; the female-to-male rate ratios ranging from 0.99 to 1.21 in training and from 0.84 to 0.97 in matches.

72.5 Injury Pattern in Women's Football

Hamstring injury has recently been shown to be the most common injury in both men's and women's elite football without any apparent sex-related differences in terms of injury rates [22]. However, some other injury types such as concussions, ACL injuries, and stress fractures are more frequent in female players, whereas groin injuries on the other hand is more frequently encountered in males.

72.5.1 Concussion

A review on potential sex-related differences in concussion rates concluded that female football players were more prone to concussion than males in three out of four included studies [29]. One of the studies in that review, conducted on 20 international tournaments such as the World Cup and Olympic Games, quantified the concussion rate to be 2.4 times higher among female players [30]. A subsequent study on 191 reported concussions among US intercollegiate football players between 2009 and 2014 confirmed an approximately doubled concussion rate in female players [31].

In addition to a higher concussion rate, female youth and senior players perform worse than male players on neurocognitive testing after a concussion [32]. Moreover, some cognitive factors were still impaired in female university players 6–8 months after a concussion [33]. These findings are supported by the results in a meta-analysis of eight studies investigating traumatic brain injury among women and men showing worse outcomes in women for 17 out of 20 measured variables [34].

72.5.2 ACL Injury

Female athletes participating in jumping, cutting, and pivoting sports have historically been attributed to be four to six times more susceptible to ACL injury compared with males [35]. Most of the studies comparing injury characteristics between sexes have been carried out on college athletes in the United States in different sports [36–42]. From these studies, however, the risk increase among the female football players in this age group, typically 18–22 years, appears to be lower than the often cited four to six times higher risk (Table 72.2). In another cohort from collegiate football 2005–2006, in which the ACL injury rate is reported for playing hours instead of athlete exposures [43, 44], there was a 3.1–3.5 higher ACL match injury rate in female players on both natural grass and artificial turf, whereas there was a threefold higher ACL training injury rate on natural grass with no sex-related difference on artificial turf. Similarly, a female-to-male rate ratio of 2.6 was reported among Swedish senior elite players between 2001 and 2009 [45]. Taken together, female football players appear to be a two to three times more susceptible to ACL injury than male players, and this is also in line with what has been calculated in two independent reviews [46, 47].

The underlying causes and mechanisms involved in the increased risk of ACL injury in female football players (Fig. 72.4) are not clear [35, 48, 49]. Potential risk factors are often categorized as being anatomical (e.g., femoral notch size, joint laxity, familiar predisposition, previous ACL injury, etc.), developmental/hormonal (e.g., female sex, maturation status, menstrual status, etc.), and biomechanical/neuromuscular (e.g., knee abduction, hamstring recruitment, etc.). In studies involving football players, female players have shown greater joint laxity [50], and they tear the ACL in the nondominant (supporting) leg more often than male players [51]. The strongest risk factor, however, appears to be a previous injury. In a study on 143 female elite players in Germany, 19 players (13%) had a history of

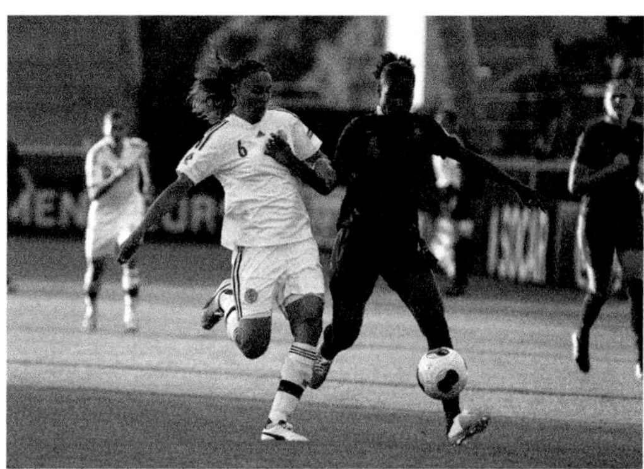

Fig. 72.4 Female football players are more susceptible to anterior cruciate ligament injuries. Photo: Lennart Weber with permission

Table 72.2 ACL injury rates per 1000 AEs among female and male collegiate football players

	Setting	No. of ACL injuries	ACL injuries/1000 AEs	F/M ratio
Agel et al. [36]	NCAA schools 1990–2002	F: 394; M: 192	F: 0.31; M: 0.11	2.8
Agel et al. [37]	NCAA schools 2004–2013	F: 71; M: 26	F: 0.10; M: 0.04	2.6
Arendt and Dick [38]	NCAA schools 1989–1993	F: 178; M: 81	F: 0.31; M: 0.13	2.4
Arendt et al. [39]	NCAA schools 1994–1998	F: 158; M: 77	F: 0.33; M: 0.12	2.8
Beynnon et al. [40]	Vermont colleges 2008–2012	F: 11; M: 6	F: 0.39; M: 0.19	2.1
Harmon and Dick [41]	NCAA schools 1989–1997	F: 194; M: 123	F: 0.32; M: 0.12	2.6
Mihata et al. [42]	NCAA schools 1989–2004[a]	F: 457; M: 212	F: 0.32; M: 0.12	2.7

ACL anterior cruciate ligament, *AE* athlete exposure, *F* female, *M* male, *NCAA* National Collegiate Athletic Association
[a]The 1996–1997 season was not included

previous ACL injury, and these players were five times more likely to tear the ACL compared with the previously uninjured players [52].

72.5.3 Stress Fracture

A stress fracture represents the ultimate failure of the bony skeleton to absorb and withstand repetitive bouts of mechanical loading. In general, it is believed that women are more susceptible to stress fractures of the lower extremities than men [53]. There are, however, no comparative studies between sexes in football, but a few studies on female players have reported the prevalence of having a history of football-related stress fracture. In a large questionnaire study from Norway, 13% of the female football players reported a history of stress fractures [14]. This finding was later supported by another study on a subset of 64 female college and professional players where 11% reported a history of lower extremity stress fracture [54].

72.5.4 Groin Injury

Injury to the hip and groin area is one of the "big four" in male footballers, but constitutes a substantially smaller problem in female players. Regardless of the injury definition, study design, setting, and playing level, the groin injury rate appears to be more than doubled in male players [55]. Possible reasons for this sex-related difference in groin injury rate might include both internal factors (e.g., differences in pelvic anatomy, inherent occurrence of abdominal wall weakness in men, etc.) and external factors (e.g., working load, playing style, playing intensity, etc.).

Fact Box 2

The overall injury rate in women's football players is similar to that in men's football players in most comparing studies.

Concussions, ACL injuries, and stress fractures are, however, more commonly reported in females than in males, whereas the reverse trend is seen for groin injuries.

72.6 Financial Resources and Medical Support

Women's and men's football are two completely different sports from a resource point of view, especially at the higher playing levels in club level football. In the big international tournaments, the medical support is similar, but at the elite and sub-elite club level in women's football, it is less developed compared with men's football.

72.6.1 Financial Resources

The professional status and the financial resources in women's football are very different compared with the men's game. In 2015, the Union of European Football Associations (UEFA) had 2219 registered professional female players in Europe [56]. In that report, the top five women countries (Germany, France, England, Sweden, and Norway) had each an average of 175 professional female players and approximately ten clubs that could sign professional contracts. Consequently, many elite players need to work at least part time to earn enough money for their daily living. Similarly, it is also important for women to secure an education since most players are far from obtaining an income that provide them with financial security for a lengthy period after the playing career. Because of the working obligations or school-related activities, many high-level female players thus have a tight daily schedule with limited time for recovery and increased propensity for fatigue. This combination can negatively affect the players both mentally [57, 58] and physically [58].

It should, however, be acknowledged that the financial situation nowadays is good in some of the top-level women teams in Europe, often as an effect of being supported by the men's team in the same club. Many of these clubs invest in an essentially full-time professional squad also on the women's side and thereby increase the chances for proper recovery and less fatigue. Still, however, the salaries in women's elite players are not comparable to the men's.

72.6.2 Medical Support

Today, the biggest men's professional football clubs have a whole department in the "team behind the team" with managers, coaches, medical practitioners, sports scientists, nutritionists, psychologists, kit managers, etc. The medical team employed by the club usually consists of at least one part-time or full-time doctor and several full-time physiotherapists and sports masseurs. In contrast, many/most women's elite clubs may have access to only part-time physiotherapists (or masseurs) some days per week, with the doctor usually being present at the home matches and perhaps at one to two training sessions a week. This means that there is not always a qualified medical practitioner present who is able to take care of and establish the diagnosis of the injury immediately which in turn might influence the expected time being on the sidelines and the RTP decision. Similarly, lower club medical support in the last rehabilitation phase and in the first critical phase after RTP means that the player needs to rely much on herself and on advice from the coaches. Consequently, the level of medical support around the elite clubs in women's football needs to be improved to resemble the organization in men's elite clubs.

72.7 Safe Return to Play

The responsible medical practitioner always need to be prepared for the "when can I play again?" question from the injured player [59]. Ideally, and regardless of what type of injury, a safe RTP with a low subsequent risk of reinjury is most often in the best interest of the club, the coach, and the player. It is, however, well known that release for RTP after injury/surgery is a complex process depending on both medical and nonmedical factors [60]. It is therefore imperative that a qualified and experienced medical practitioner rule the decision about when releasing a player for RTP, but preferably he/she does this in collaboration with, e.g., the player and the coach [59]. Theoretically, there could be a higher risk of compromises in this respect in women's football because of, e.g., smaller and more heterogeneous squads in which the team is more dependent on its key players.

Taking *the* female football injury, ACL injury, as an example why a safe RTP is important, we know that a previous ACL injury is the strongest risk factor for incurring a new ACL injury [52]. Unfortunately, this risk of subsequent ACL injury after ACL reconstruction seems to be higher among female football players compared with other female athletes [61]. Also, the risk of subsequent ACL injury appears to be higher among female football players compared with males [62, 63]. The risk of reinjury is highest within the first 24 months after ACL reconstruction, and the average release for RTP after approximately 6 months as reported in a few studies involving female players might be riskful in this respect [45, 64]. Interestingly, there is recent evidence against the traditional time-based RTP algorithm of 6 months in football and other similar team sports [65]. In that study on 100 ACL-reconstructed athletes (approximately half of them being football players), the reinjury rate was significantly reduced by 51% for each month RTP was delayed until 9 months after surgery, after which no further reduction was noted.

Finally, ACL injury is a severe injury for a footballer, and not all players do, or should, return to the pitch after ACL injury [45, 61–63]. This information, including the effects on the long-term knee prospects, should therefore always be included in the proper counseling of an ACL-injured football player. In addition, of those football players who choose to undergo ACL reconstruction, fewer women than men return to the pitch [45, 62, 63]. The underlying reasons for this sex-related discrepancy are essentially unknown and need to be investigated further in future research.

Fact Box 3

Release for RTP after injury or surgery is known to be a difficult and complex process depending on both medical and nonmedical factors.

A safe RTP after ACL injury is a main treatment goal because of the high risk of further ipsilateral and contralateral knee injury.

Take-Home Message
Female football is rapidly growing worldwide, but as a physically demanding contact sport, it has a high inherent risk of injury. The overall injury rate in women's football appears to be comparable to that in men's football, but the injury pattern differs somewhat. Concussions, ACL injuries, and stress fractures are more frequent among female players, whereas groin injuries are less frequently encountered.

The release for RTP after injury is a complex process which is reflected by an unacceptably high risk of subsequent injury for some injuries such as ACL injury in female players. There is also some evidence that female players perform worse on neurocognitive testing after a concussion and that they can suffer from prolonged cognitive impairments. It could thus for these events be wise to practice a "better safe than quick" algorithm instead of meeting the frequent wish of the player and coach to go back to pitch as early as possible.

Top Five Evidence Based References

Ardern C, Glasgow P, Schneiders A, Witvrouw E, Clarsen B, Cools A, Gojanovic B, Griffin S, Khan KM, Moksnes H, Mutch SA, Phillips N, Reurink G, Sadler R, Silbernagel KG, Thorborg K, Wangensteen A, Wilk KE, Bizzini M (2016) 2016 Consensus statement on return to sport from the First World Congress in Sports Physical Therapy, Bern. Br J Sports Med 50:853–864

Allen MA, Pareek A, Krych AJ, Hewett T, Levy BA, Stuart MJ, Dahm DL (2016) Are female soccer players at an increased risk of second anterior cruciate ligament injury compared with their athletic peers? Am J Sports Med 44:2492–2498

Dick RW (2009) Is there a gender difference in concussion incidence and outcomes? Br J Sports Med 43(Suppl 1):i46–i50

Waldén M, Hägglund M, Werner J, Ekstrand J (2011) The epidemiology of anterior cruciate ligament injury in football (soccer): a review of the literature from a gender-related perspective. Knee Surg Sports Traumatol Arthrosc 19:3–10

Waldén M, Hägglund M, Magnusson H, Ekstrand J (2011) Anterior cruciate ligament injury in elite football: a prospective three-cohort study. Knee Surg Sports Traumatol Arthrosc 19:11–19

References

1. Landahl G, Adolfsson P, Börjesson M, Mannheimer C, Rödjer S (2005) Iron deficiency and anemia; a common problem in female elite soccer players. Int J Sport Nutr Metab 15:689–694
2. Wild CY, Steele JR, Munro BJ (2012) Why do girls sustain more anterior cruciate ligament injuries than boys? A review of the changes in estrogen and musculoskeletal structure and function during puberty. Sports Med 42:733–749
3. Park SK, Stefanyshyn DJ, Loitz-Ramage B, Hart DA, Ronsky JL (2009) Changing hormone levels during the menstrual cycle affect knee laxity and stiffness in healthy female subjects. Am J Sports Med 37:588–598
4. Zazulak BT, Paterno M, Myer GD, Romani WA, Hewett TE (2006) The effects of the menstrual cycle on anterior knee laxity: a systematic review. Sports Med 36:847–862
5. Dragoo JL, Castillo TN, Braun HJ, Ridley BA, Kennedy AC, Golish R (2011) Prospective correlation between serum relaxin concentration and anterior cruciate ligament tears among elite collegiate female athletes. Am J Sports Med 39:2175–2180
6. Möller-Nielsen J, Hammar M (1989) Women's soccer injuries in relation to the menstrual cycle and oral contraceptive use. Med Sci Sports Exerc 21:126–129
7. Brynhildsen JO, Hammar J, Hammar ML (1997) Does the menstrual cycle and use of oral contraceptives influence the risk of low back pain? A prospective study among female soccer players. Scand J Med Sci Sports 7:348–353
8. Hewett TE, Zazulak BT, Myer GD (2007) Effects of the menstrual cycle on anterior cruciate ligament injury risk: a systematic review. Am J Sports Med 35:659–668
9. Vescovi JD (2011) The menstrual cycle and anterior cruciate ligament injury risk: implications of menstrual cycle variability. Sports Med 41:91–101
10. Möller-Nielsen J, Hammar M (1991) Sports injuries and oral contraceptive use. Is there a relationship? Sports Med 12:152–160
11. Fridén C, Hirschberg AL, Saartok T, Bäckström T, Leanderson J, Renström P (2003) The influence of premenstrual symptoms on postural balance and kinesthesia during the menstrual cycle. Gynecol Endocrinol 17:433–439
12. Fridén C, Hirschberg AL, Saartok T, Renström P (2006) Knee joint kinaesthesia and neuromuscular coordination during three phases of the menstrual cycle in moderately active women. Knee Surg Sports Traumatol Arthrosc 14:383–389
13. Constantini NW, Dubnov G, Lebrun CM (2005) The menstrual cycle and sport performance. Clin Sports Med 24:e51–e82

14. Sundgot-Borgen J, Torstveit MK (2007) The female football player, disordered eating, menstrual function and bone health. Br J Sports Med 41(Suppl 1):i68–i72
15. Torstveit MK, Sundgot-Borgen J (2005) The female athlete triad exists in both elite athletes and controls. Med Sci Sports Exerc 37:1449–1459
16. Datson N, Hulton A, Andersson H, Lewis T, Weston M, Drust B, Gregson W (2014) Applied physiology of female soccer: an update. Sports Med 44:1225–1240
17. Krustrup P, Mohr M, Ellingsgaard H, Bangsbo J (2005) Physical demands during an elite female soccer game: importance of training status. Med Sci Sports Exerc 37:1242–1248
18. Bradley PS, Dellal A, Mohr M, Castellano J, Wilkie A (2014) Gender differences in match performance characteristics of soccer players competing in the UEFA Champions League. Hum Mov Sci 33:159–171
19. Junge A, Dvorak J (2013) Injury surveillance in the World Football Tournaments 1998–2012. Br J Sports Med 47:782–788
20. Hägglund M, Waldén M, Ekstrand J (2009) UEFA injury study - an injury audit of European Championships 2006 to 2008. Br J Sports Med 43:483–489
21. Waldén M, Hägglund M, Ekstrand J (2007) Football injuries during European Championships 2004–2005. Knee Surg Sports Traumatol Arthrosc 15:1155–1162
22. Hägglund M, Waldén M, Ekstrand J (2009) Injuries among male and female elite football players. Scand J Med Sci Sports 19:819–827
23. Lion A, Theisen D, Windal T, Malisoux L, Nührenbörger C, Huberty R, Urhausen A, Seil R (2014) Moderate to severe injuries in football: a one-year prospective study of twenty-four female and male amateur teams. Bull Soc Sci Med Grand Duche Luxemb 3:43–55
24. Mufty S, Bollars P, Vanlommel L, Van Crombrugge K, Corten K, Bellemans J (2015) Injuries in male versus female soccer players: epidemiology of a nationwide study. Acta Orthop Belg 81:289–295
25. Agel J, Evans TA, Dick R, Putukian M, Marshall SW (2007) Descriptive epidemiology of collegiate men's soccer injuries: National Collegiate Athletic Association Injury Surveillance System, 1988–1989 through 2002–2003. J Athl Train 42:270–277
26. Dick R, Putukian M, Agel J, Evans TA, Marshall SW (2007) Descriptive epidemiology of collegiate women's soccer injuries: National Collegiate Athletic Association Injury Surveillance System, 1988–1989 through 2002–2003. J Athl Train 42:278–285
27. Chandran A, Barron MJ, Westerman BJ, DiPietro L (2016) Time trends in incidence and severity of injury among collegiate soccer players in the United States: NCAA injury surveillance system, 1990–1996 and 2004–2009. Am J Sports Med 44:3237–3242
28. Roos KG, Wasserman EB, Dalton SL, Gray A, Djoko A, Dompier TP, Kerr ZY (2017) Epidemiology of 3825 injuries sustained in six seasons of National Collegiate Athletic Association men's and women's soccer (2009/2010–2014/2015). Br J Sports Med 51:1029–1034
29. Dick RW (2009) Is there a gender difference in concussion incidence and outcomes? Br J Sports Med 43(Suppl 1):i46–i50
30. Fuller CW, Junge A, Dvorak J (2005) A six year prospective study of the incidence and causes of head and neck injuries in international football. Br J Sports Med 39(Suppl 1):i3–i9
31. Zuckerman SL, Kerr ZY, Yengo-Kahn A, Wasserman E, Covassin T, Solomon GS (2015) Epidemiology of sports-related concussion in NCAA athletes from 2009–2010 to 2013–2014: incidence, recurrence, and mechanisms. Am J Sports Med 43:2654–2662
32. Chiang Colvin A, Mullen J, Lovell MR (2009) The role of concussion history and gender in recovery from soccer-related concussion. Am J Sports Med 37:1699–1704
33. Ellemberg D, Leclerc S, Couture S, Daigle C (2007) Prolonged neuropsychological impairments following a first concussion in female university soccer athletes. Clin J Sport Med 17:369–374
34. Farace E, Alves WM (2000) Do women fare worse? A metaanalysis of gender differences in outcome after traumatic brain injury. Neurosurg Focus 8:1–8
35. Hewett TE (2000) Neuromuscular and hormonal factors associated with knee injuries in female athletes. Strategies for intervention. Sports Med 29:313–327
36. Agel J, Arendt EA, Bershadsky B (2005) Anterior cruciate ligament injury in national collegiate athletic association basketball and soccer. Am J Sports Med 33:524–531
37. Agel J, Rockwood T, Klossner D (2016) Collegiate ACL injury rates across 15 sports: National Collegiate Athletic Association Injury Surveillance System data update (2004–2005 through 2012–2013). Clin J Sport Med 26:518–523
38. Arendt E, Dick R (1995) Knee injury among men and women in collegiate basketball and soccer: NCAA data and review of literature. Am J Sports Med 23:694–701
39. Arendt EA, Agel J, Randall D (1999) Anterior cruciate ligament injury patterns among collegiate men and women. J Athl Train 34:86–92
40. Beynnon BD, Vacek PM, Newell MK, Tourville TW, Smith HC, Shultz SJ, Slauterbeck JR, Johnson RJ (2014) The effects of level of competition, sport, and sex on the incidence of first-time noncontact anterior cruciate ligament injury. Am J Sports Med 42:1806–1812
41. Harmon KG, Dick R (1998) The relationship of skill level to anterior cruciate ligament injury. Clin J Sport Med 8:260–265
42. Mihata LCS, Beutler AI, Boden BP (2006) Comparing the incidence of anterior cruciate ligament injury in collegiate lacrosse, soccer, and basketball players:

implications for anterior cruciate ligament mechanism and prevention. Am J Sports Med 34:899–904
43. Fuller CW, Dick RW, Corlette J, Schmalz R (2007) Comparison of the incidence, nature and cause of injuries sustained on grass and new generation artificial turf by male and female football players. Part 1: Match injuries. Br J Sports Med 41(Suppl 1):i20–i26
44. Fuller CW, Dick RW, Corlette J, Schmalz R (2007) Comparison of the incidence, nature and cause of injuries sustained on grass and new generation artificial turf by male and female football players. Part 2: Training injuries. Br J Sports Med 41(Suppl 1):i27–i32
45. Waldén M, Hägglund M, Magnusson H, Ekstrand J (2011) Anterior cruciate ligament injury in elite football: a prospective three-cohort study. Knee Surg Sports Traumatol Arthrosc 19:11–19
46. Prodromos CC, Han Y, Rogowski J, Joyce B, Shi K (2007) A meta-analysis of the incidence of anterior cruciate ligament tears as a function of gender, sport, and a knee injury-reduction regimen. Arthroscopy 23:1320–1325
47. Waldén M, Hägglund M, Werner J, Ekstrand J (2011) The epidemiology of anterior cruciate ligament injury in football (soccer): a review of the literature from a gender-related perspective. Knee Surg Sports Traumatol Arthrosc 19:3–10
48. Alentorn-Geli E, Myer GD, Silvers HJ, Samitier G, Romero D, Lázaro-Haro C, Cugat R (2009) Prevention of non-contact anterior cruciate ligament injuries in soccer players. Part 1: Mechanisms of injury and underlying risk factors. Knee Surg Sports Traumatol Arthrosc 17:705–729
49. Renström P, Ljungqvist A, Arendt E, Beynnon B, Fukubayashi T, Garrett W, Georgoulis T, Hewett TE, Johnson R, Krosshaug T, Mandelbaum B, Micheli L, Myklebust G, Roos E, Roos H, Schamasch P, Shultz S, Werner S, Wojtys E, Engebretsen L (2008) Non-contact ACL injuries in female athletes: an International Olympic Committee current concepts statement. Br J Sports Med 42:394–412
50. Rozzi SL, Lephart SM, Gear WS, Fu FH (1999) Knee joint laxity and neuromuscular characteristics of male and female soccer and basketball players. Am J Sports Med 27:312–319
51. Brophy R, Silvers HJ, Gonzales T, Mandelbaum BR (2010) Gender influences: the role of leg dominance in ACL injury among soccer players. Br J Sports Med 44:694–697
52. Faude O, Junge A, Kindermann W, Dvorak J (2006) Risk factors for injuries in elite female soccer players. Br J Sports Med 40:785–790
53. Warden SJ, Creaby MW, Bryant AL, Crossley KM (2007) Stress fracture risk factors in female football players and their clinical implications. Br J Sports Med 41(Suppl 1):i38–i43
54. Prather H, Hunt D, McKeon K, Simpson S, Meyer EB, Yemm T, Brophy R (2016) Are elite female soccer athletes at risk for disordered eating attitudes, menstrual dysfunction, and stress fractures? PM R 8:208–213
55. Waldén M, Hägglund M, Ekstrand J (2015) The epidemiology of groin injury in senior football: a systematic review of prospective studies. Br J Sports Med 49:792–797
56. UEFA (2015) Women's football across the national associations 2015–2016. http://www.uefa.org/MultimediaFiles/Download/OfficialDocument/uefaorg/Women'sfootball/02/30/93/30/2309330_DOWNLOAD.pdf . Accessed 12 Dec 2016
57. Lorist MM, Boksem MA, Ridderinkhof KR (2005) Impaired cognitive control and reduced cingulate activity during mental fatigue. Brain Res Cogn Brain Res 24:199–205
58. Nédélec M, McCall A, Carling C, Legall F, Berthoin S, Dupont G (2012) Recovery in soccer: Part I - Post-match fatigue and time course of recovery. Sports Med 42:997–1015
59. Ardern C, Glasgow P, Schneiders A, Witvrouw E, Clarsen B, Cools A, Gojanovic B, Griffin S, Khan KM, Moksnes H, Mutch SA, Phillips N, Reurink G, Sadler R, Silbernagel KG, Thorborg K, Wangensteen A, Wilk KE, Bizzini M (2016) 2016 Consensus statement on return to sport from the First World Congress in Sports Physical Therapy, Bern. Br J Sports Med 50:853–864
60. Creighton DW, Shrier I, Shultz R, Meeuwisse WH, Matheson GO (2010) Return-to-play in sport: a decision-based model. Clin J Sport Med 20:379–385
61. Allen MA, Pareek A, Krych AJ, Hewett T, Levy BA, Stuart MJ, Dahm DL (2016) Are female soccer players at an increased risk of second anterior cruciate ligament injury compared with their athletic peers? Am J Sports Med 44:2492–2498
62. Brophy RH, Schmitz L, Wright RW, Dunn WR, Parker RD, Andrish JT, McCarty EC, Spindler K (2012) Return to play and future ACL injury risk after ACL reconstruction in soccer athletes from the Multicenter Orthopedic Outcomes Network (MOON) Group. Am J Sports Med 40:2517–2522
63. Sandon A, Werner S, Forssblad M (2015) Factors associated with returning to football after anterior cruciate ligament reconstruction. Knee Surg Sports Traumatol Arthrosc 23:2514–2521
64. Howard JS, Lembach ML, Metzler AV, Johnson DL (2015) Rates and determinants of return to play after anterior cruciate ligament reconstruction in National Collegiate Athletic Association Division 1 soccer athletes: a study of the Southeastern Conference. Am J Sports Med 44:433–439
65. Grindem H, Snyder-Mackler L, Moksnes H, Engebretsen L, Risberg MA (2016) Simple decision rules can reduce reinjury risk by 84% after ACL reconstruction: the Delawere-Oslo ACL cohort study. Br J Sports Med 50:804–808

73 The Young Player: Special Considerations

Jonas Werner, Martin Hägglund, Mariann Gajhede Knudsen, Jan Ekstrand, and Markus Waldén

Contents

J. Werner (✉)
Football Research Group, Department of Orthopaedics, Vrinnevisjukhuset, Norrköping, Sweden
e-mail: jonas.werner@regionostergotland.se

M. Hägglund
Football Research Group, Division of Physiotherapy, Department of Medical and Health Sciences, Linköping University, Linköping, Sweden
e-mail: martin.hagglund@liu.se

M.G. Knudsen
Football Research Group, Linköping, Sweden
e-mail: mariannknudsen@hotmail.com

J. Ekstrand • M. Waldén
Football Research Group, Division of Community Medicine, Department of Medical and Health Sciences, Linköping University, Linköping, Sweden
e-mail: jan.ekstrand@telia.com; markus.walden@telia.com

73.1 Introduction

Football is the most popular team sport worldwide. According to the Federation of International Football Associations (FIFA) Big Count in 2007 [1], it was estimated that almost 60% of all registered players in the world were under the age of 18 (Fig. 73.1). The number of registered players increased by 7% from 2000 to 2006 in this survey. In general, this trend is positive because playing football is a health-promoting activity, but there is also an inherent risk of injury due to its physical nature.

73.1.1 Ball Size

The ball is lighter and smaller for female adolescent and senior players in other popular team sports such as handball and basketball, but male and female football players, regardless of age, play with the same ball. The ball is spherical and made of leather or other suitable material, and the characteristics such as circumference, weight and inflation pressure are regulated by the Laws of

V. Musahl et al. (eds.), *Return to Play in Football*, https://doi.org/10.1007/978-3-662-55713-6_73

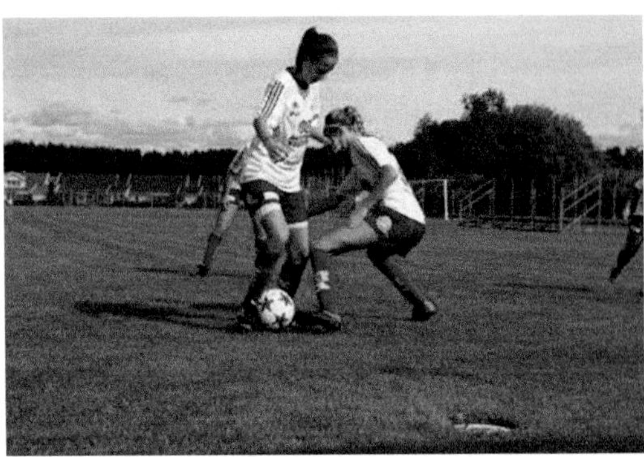

Fig. 73.1 More than half of all registered football players in the world are below 18 years (Photo: Emma Busk Winquist with permission)

the Game. The youngest players (<8 years) use a size 3 ball with a circumference of 58–61 cm, a weight of 310–340 g and a pressure as suggested by the manufacturer. Players aged 8–12 years commonly play with a size 4 ball having a circumference of 64–66 cm, a weight of 350–390 g and also here a pressure as suggested by the manufacturer. Adolescent players from 13 to 15 years (varies slightly from country to country) use a size 5 ball, as in senior players, with a circumference of 68–70 cm, a weight of 410–450 g and a pressure of 59–108 kPa.

73.2 Childhood and Adolescence

Participation in sports and physical activity as a child and adolescent is important for several reasons such as social development, learning in school, gaining high bone mass and avoiding overweight and other lifestyle-related disorders.

73.2.1 Childhood

Childhood is the age span from birth to adolescence beginning with the toddlerhood stage where the child becomes familiar with playing ball as part of the natural development. Thereafter, during the early childhood stage, many children start playing organised football in school or in a club between the ages of 5 and 7 years. Before puberty, girls and boys have similar anthropometry, and there are almost no sex-related differences in the fat and muscle distribution.

73.2.2 Adolescence

Even if a precise definition is difficult to find, the adolescence represents a transitional stage of physical and psychological development that lasts from approximately the start of puberty to adulthood. Puberty is a period of several years in which the rapid physical growth occurs. The average age of onset of puberty is 10–11 years for girls and 12–13 years for boys. The major landmark of puberty in girls is menarche, which usually occurs between 12 and 13 years in developed countries [2].

During the peak height velocity, which typically occurs approximately half a year before menarche in girls, adolescents can grow up to 10 cm in a year. The head and distal extremities are the first locations to grow, followed by the rest of the arms and legs, and finally the torso and shoulders. Consequently, this non-uniform growth contributes to why an adolescent body may seem out of proportion. In addition to the rapid changes in height, adolescents also experience a significant increase in weight during the growth spurt. Briefly, boys grow muscle more and faster, whereas the increase in body fat is more significant for girls. Girls have usually reached full physical development with closed physes of the long bones by 14 years, while boys usually need another 1-2 years.

73.3 Injury Rate in Youth Football

Compared with the scientific literature on injuries in senior football, studies on injuries in youth football are scarce, especially in players younger than 12 years. In general, it is difficult to compare injury rates between youth and senior players from the existing literature due to substantial methodological differences between studies and, likely, in the way players report an injury or time loss from play.

Table 73.1 Injury rates in male youth and senior players from studies using the same surveillance method

	Setting	Participants[a]	Injury definition	Injury rate/1000 h
Hawkins and Fuller [3]	4 professional clubs in England (1994–1997)	108 seniors[b] 30 youths[b]	Time loss	25.9 match; 3.4 training (seniors) 37.2 match; 4.1 training (youths)
Inklaar et al. [4]	2 amateur clubs in the Netherlands (1987)	245 seniors (>18 years) 232 youths (13–18 years)	Combined[b]	15.8 match (>18 years) 28.3 match (17–18 years) 16.1 match (15–16 years) 12.8 match (13–14 years)
Latella et al. [5]	1 professional club in Italy (1980–1991)	190 seniors (>18 years) 642 youths (13–17 years)	Time loss	4.0 match (>18 years) 0.4 match (13–18 years)
McNoe and Chalmers [6]	2 domestic federations in New Zealand (2006)	880 seniors and youths (>12 years)	Medical attention or time loss	62.0 match; 14.3 training (>17 years) 36.8 match; 6.8 training (<17 years)
Nielsen and Yde [7]	1 amateur club in Denmark (1986)	93 seniors (>18 years) 30 youths (16–18 years)	Time loss	18.5 match; 2.3 training (seniors division II) 11.9 match; 5.6 training (seniors series) 14.4 match; 3.6 training (youths)
Peterson et al. [8]	20 clubs of variable levels in the Czech Republic (1998)	84 seniors (>18 years) 180 youths (14–18 years)	Tissue damage	10.2–29.7 (>18 years) 18.9–42.5 (16–18 years) 15.8–37.8 (14–16 years)

[a]Player ages not reported in the study
[b]Injury defined as resulting in at least one of the following: a reduction in the amount of football activity, a need for advice or treatment or adverse social or economic effects

Only a limited number of studies have provided injury rate estimates from both youth and senior players in a club setting, using identical injury definition and surveillance methods (Table 73.1). All of these studies except one included male players exclusively; the study with players of both sexes found an injury rate of 80.1/1000 match hours and 11.9/1000 training hours in females older than 17 years and 51.7/1000 match hours and 7.0/1000 training hours in females younger than 17 years, respectively [6].

73.3.1 Injury Rate in Children

In general, children's football is a safe sport characterised by a low overall injury rate without any apparent sex-related differences. It has been shown that the injury rate among 6- to 12-year-old players was lower than in players aged 13–16 years (1.6 vs. 2.6 injuries per 1000 h) [9]. Increasing injury rate with increasing age was also found in a more recent study on injuries in players up to 12 years, the lowest rate being noted in the 7- to 8-year-old players and the highest in the 11- to 12-year-old players [10].

Fact Box 1
The risk of injury in children's football is low but increases with age and is similar in skeletally mature adolescent players to that in senior players.

73.3.2 Injury Rate in Adolescents

The injury rate in 13- to 19-year-old adolescents appears to be essentially constant during training with rates reported to be between 1 and 5 injuries/1000 h. The injury rate during match play is higher than during training, 15–20 injuries/1000 h, and seems to increase slightly with increasing age [11].

73.3.2.1 International Tournaments

In a study on 12 different European Championships between 2006 and 2008, the time-loss match injury rates were similar for the men's U-17, men's U-19 and women's U-19 tournaments (20.5–23.3/1000 h), whereas it was higher in the senior tournaments of men's U-21 and men's EURO (33.9–41.6/1000 h) [12]. In another study on 53 different tournaments, such as the Olympic Games and World Cups, between 1998 and 2012, the lowest injury rates were found in the women's and men's U-17 World Championships (on average 0.7–0.9 time-loss injuries/match), whereas the highest injury rate was identified for the men's World Cups (on average 1.5 time-loss injuries/match) [13].

73.3.2.2 The Influence of Ball Size

Because of sex-related differences in, e.g. anthropometry, muscle mass and feet size, it has been suggested that female adolescent players should use a smaller and lighter ball than their male counterparts. A few studies have investigated this (ball circumference 64 cm, 95% of standard size 5 ball, weight 360 g) from both performance and injury perspectives in female adolescent players [14, 15].

With this new ball, it was found that the kicking speed among female adolescent players was higher, but there were no differences in technical-tactical and physical performance. The players, however, experienced a lower perceived exertion after playing with the new ball than with a standard ball [14]. This could theoretically influence the risk for fatigue-related injuries, such as muscle injuries that often occur at the end of match halves. However, another study from Denmark found no differences in the risk of injury among 15- to 18-year-old girls playing with the smaller and lighter ball compared with a standard ball [15]. Further studies in this area are thus needed.

73.4 Injury Pattern in Youth Football

Approximately three-quarter of all injuries in youth players have been categorised as being traumatic in their nature, and the same proportion of injuries are located to the lower extremities [11]. Injuries to the upper extremities are relatively more frequent in players younger than 15 years, mainly attributed to fractures. Moreover, players younger than 15 years suffer more head/face injuries and fewer ligament sprains and muscle strains than senior players, whereas older adolescent players have about the same injury characteristics as senior players (Fig. 73.2).

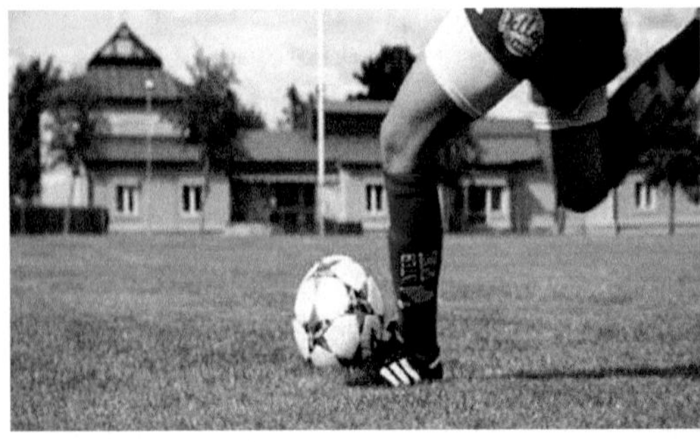

Fig. 73.2 Youth players older than 15 years have similar injury characteristics as senior players (Photo: Emma Busk Winquist with permission)

73.4.1 Concussions

In a review on injuries in youth football, head/face injuries accounted for about 4% of all injuries [11]. In a more recent prospective study, 6% of all football injuries were inflicted to the head/face, and these injuries were twice as common in 7- to 10-year-old players compared with 11- to 12-year-old players [10].

Concussion is a common injury for youth athletes who participate in contact and collision sports, accounting for 3–8% of all injuries presenting to the emergency departments [16]. Specifically in football, as studied among US high school players, the concussion rate has been reported to be higher among female players than in male players [17]. Nevertheless, under-reporting is probably an issue in the young player since concussion symptoms may be hard to recognise for both players and coaches. Players may also be unwilling to report them due to anxiety of being taken out of the game. A high level of suspicion is therefore advised when a young player sustains any direct or indirect trauma to the head and displays somatic, cognitive or emotional symptoms afterwards (Table 73.2). Fortunately, it appears that educational activities have the potential of increasing the number of players who would always notify their coach of concussion symptoms [18].

Table 73.2 Possible concussion symptoms and signs in youth football players

Symptoms	Signs
Headache	Appears dazed or stunned
Nausea or vomiting	Forgets an instruction
Balance problems or dizziness	Is unsure of game, score or opponent
Double or blurry vision	Slowed reaction times
Sensitivity to light or noise	Moves clumsily Answers questions slowly
Feeling dizzy, sluggish or foggy	
Concentration or memory problems	Loss of consciousness (*even briefly*)
Does not "feel right" or is "feeling down"	Shows mood, behaviour or personality changes
Sleep disturbance	Antegrade or retrograde amnesia

73.4.1.1 Head-to-Ball Impact

It has been suggested that children are more prone to suffer concussion than adults because of their smaller heads which leads to greater head acceleration after impact. In addition, the neck muscle strength in children is not as developed as in adults, and it could therefore be more difficult for them to control the mass of the head which is larger relative to body size in children [19].

Currently, however, there is little evidence to support that purposeful heading, even in children, can lead to concussion or subconcussive neurological impairments in the long term [19]. In contrast, unanticipated head-to-ball impact, especially when the player has not pre-tensioned the neck muscles, can lead to sufficient head acceleration to cause concussion. In these situations, the mass and the inflation pressure of the ball might be important factors to consider since a reduction of head acceleration has been identified both for balls with decreased mass and for balls with decreased pressure [19]. Since head acceleration is lowered when impacting a football with a lower mass (derived from Newton's second law), it might be concluded that the aforementioned smaller and lighter football would reduce the risk for head injuries in adolescent players [15]. It should, however, be clearly stated that the vast majority of football-related concussions have been attributed to head-to-hard surface impacts such as head-to-head clashes, head-to-arm duels, head-to-ground falls, etc. rather than head-to-ball impacts.

73.4.1.2 Acute Management

A player with a suspected concussion should always be removed from play and evaluated by a trained healthcare provider as soon as possible using standard emergency management principles. Suspicion of concomitant cervical spine injury and skull fracture is advocated. The use of the Sport Concussion Assessment Tool 5th edition (SCAT5©) for players aged 13 years and older, and Child-SCAT5© for players aged from 5 to 12 years is highly recommended [20]. It is also important to recognise that a player can be seemingly alert and "symptom-free" directly after the impact but can develop concussive symptoms later on. It is therefore advised to carefully watch all players having suffered head impact. In this respect, "when in doubt, sit them out" should be taught to all coaches, parents and other adults around the team.

73.4.1.3 Return to Play Considerations in the Young Player

Historically, the compliance to published return to play (RTP) guidelines after concussion has been poor as, for instance, shown among US high school players [17]. There is nowadays, however, wide consensus that a player with diagnosed concussion should not be allowed to return to play on the day of injury [21].

Limiting physical and cognitive stimuli is key in the early management of concussion; this usually also means staying home from school 1–2 days if a concussion has been diagnosed. Hereafter, a stepwise supervised programme, with stages of progression (Table 73.3), is advised [20]. Each stage should last approximately 24 h (or longer), and the child should drop back to the previous asymptomatic level if any post-concussive symptoms occur. Resistance training should only be added in the later stages. The child should not return to play or sport until he/she has successfully returned to school/learning, without worsening of symptoms. Medical clearance should be given before RTP. If the child is symptomatic for more than 10 days, review by a health practitioner with expertise in the management of concussion is recommended.

The age of the player should be considered in the RTP decision-making after a concussion. It is known that high school athletes take longer time to recover cognitive function than collegiate athletes, with cognitive testing being back to baseline after 10–14 days in the first-named group compared with 5–7 days in the latter [22]. Moreover, clinical experience shows that it takes even longer for children under the age of 12 years to reach baseline values than for high school-aged athletes. Consequently, the minimum time of 6 days before RTP, as outlined in the consensus statement for sport-related concussion in athletes 13 years or older, is probably too short in most occasions for children younger than 13 years [20].

Table 73.3 Graduated return to play protocol in youth football players

Exercise step	Functional exercise at each stage of rehabilitation	Objective of each stage
1. Symptom-limited activity	Daily activities that do not provoke symptoms	Gradual reintroduction of work/school activities
2. Light aerobic exercise	Walking or stationary cycling at slow to medium pace. No resistance training	Increase heart rate
3. Sport-specific exercise	Running drills in football, but no head impact activities	Add movement
4. Non-contact training drills	Harder training drills, e.g. passing drills in football. May start progressive resistance training	Exercise, coordination and cognitive load
5. Full-contact practice	Normal training activities following medical clearance	Restore confidence and assess functional skills by coaching staff
6. Return to play	Normal match play	

Fact Box 2

A conservative approach with longer time frame for the symptom-free phase and until introducing heading and full return to play after concussion is recommended in children.

73.4.1.4 Headgear Is Not Recommended

Considering the current knowledge on concussion, would protective headgear upon RTP decrease the risk of recurrent injury? Several different types of headgear are marketed, all with the aim of protecting the brain during football-related head impact. Common to all headgears is an absorbing foam layer which mitigates head-to-hard surface impacts and could thus possibly decrease the head acceleration in these situations [19]. However, during head-to-ball impact, regardless of wearing a headgear or not, the ball usually deforms more than the skull or the headgear which implies that there is no significant reduction in head acceleration. There is also a risk that the headgear itself might give players a false sense of security which in turn may cause them to play more recklessly and thereby increases the risk of injury [19]. Consequently, it is not recommended to use a headgear in order to clear the young football player for a quick RTP after sustaining a concussion.

73.4.2 Anterior Cruciate Ligament Injuries

ACL injury is a rare injury in football before 11 years of age with no reported sex differences but is thereafter increasing in both sexes up to 18 years [23]. This increase is most pronounced among teenage girls who are believed to be most prone to sustain an ACL injury [24–28]. Unfortunately, there are reasons to believe that paediatric and adolescent intrasubstance ACL injuries are increasing in frequency [29]. Early sport specialisation with increasing demands on performance and year-round high-intensity training has been argued as possible reasons. However, improved magnetic resonance imaging (MRI) diagnostics and increased awareness that this injury also exists in the young population may also contribute to a higher frequency of diagnosing and reporting.

73.4.2.1 The Best Treatment Is Still to Be Elucidated

Treatment of ACL injuries in the young player is often even more challenging than in adults. Treatment strategies for skeletally immature children are continuously debated, and the methodological quality of published studies in this field is limited [30]. As a general rule, non-surgical treatment is usually implemented for at least 3 months if there are no associated injuries, followed by a gradual RTP as long as the child does not experience giving-way symptoms. The younger the player is, the more successful nonoperative treatment can be expected [31]. Some healthcare professionals advocate the use of bracing during physical activity as part of the nonoperative treatment regime, but there are no high-quality studies supporting this.

The general indications for surgery in the young player include instability at the desired activity level, associated repairable meniscal injury or associated high-grade ligament injuries. If secondary injuries to the menisci and joint cartilage can be avoided, bracing and physical activity modification followed by delayed ACL reconstruction (if needed) when the growth plates are closed is probably the safest approach. If surgery is indicated before the closure of the growth plates, there are three principally different ACL reconstruction options: (1) extraphyseal surgery, (2) all-epiphyseal surgery and (3) transphyseal surgery [32]. The extraphyseal and all-epiphyseal reconstructions are both physeal-sparing techniques and are most commonly used in prepubertal or early pubertal children. The transphyseal ACL reconstruction has been used regardless of pubertal development, and this technique is essentially the same as for adults. The transphyseal ACL reconstruction can be complete (used in both the femoral and tibial sides) or partial (used in only one of the femoral and tibial sides). Historically, transphyseal surgery has been debated since it involves drilling over open growth plates and can thereby cause iatrogenic growth disturbances [33]. More recent findings have, however, shown transphyseal drilling to be a safe method if meticulous care is taken to drill small-diameter tunnels perpendicular to the growth plate and fill the tunnels with soft tendon graft and not a hard bone plug or hardware [34].

73.4.2.2 Rehabilitation and Return to Play

The main treatment goal, regardless of the treatment approach, is to allow a high physical activity level and to avoid subsequent ipsi- and contralateral knee injuries such as meniscal and cartilage injuries but also instability episodes and graft failures. The literature is, however, scarce on explicit descriptions of rehabilitation protocols after ACL injury in children, and there is little consensus between existing protocols [35]. In addition, many of the protocols are based on time frame exclusively as the most important RTP criterion [35]. This differs to the current trend in ACL rehabilitation in older adolescents and adults, where a minimum time usually is combined with several functional milestones and discharge criteria.

Taken together, the risk of sustaining a new ipsilateral or contralateral ACL injury is substantially increased in young athletes who are going back to high-level sports after an index ACL injury [36, 37]. Clearly, more research is therefore needed on the specific components of ACL rehabilitation in the young patients and on which criteria to apply in order to facilitate a safe RTP without subsequent knee injuries. Meeting specific functional test criteria and delaying RTP times may reduce reinjury risk substantially [38]. Therefore, in line with the guidelines for concussion, it might be wise to use a more conservative approach than in adults when deciding RTP after ACL injury. Provided that the player also passes a discharge test battery, up to 12 months of rehabilitation before full RTP is proposed.

Fact Box 3

The risk of sustaining a new anterior cruciate ligament injury after returning to play is unacceptably high, and more research on discharge tests and on secondary and tertiary prevention is warranted.

73.4.3 Fractures

There are several skeletal differences between the growing individual and the skeletally mature adult, e.g. the existence of the growth plates between the epiphysis and the metaphysis of the long bones and the apophyses of the tendon insertions. The growing areas (growth plates) are the relatively weak parts of the developing skeleton, and younger players are therefore more susceptible to sustain fractures than adults, but poor falling technique, undeveloped neuromuscular coordination and less developed playing skill have also been suggested to contribute to this high fracture risk [10].

Fractures constitute up to 15% of the reported injuries among young players [11], and the risk of sustaining a fracture is higher during match play compared with training [39]. Whereas adults sustain complete, and potentially unstable, fractures, children have a relatively higher proportion of incomplete fractures such as greenstick fractures in the metaphysis of the distal radius. Other unique fractures not seen in adults are compression fractures, plastic bowing and apophyseal avulsions.

Acute bony injuries to the growth plate areas are also common in children. These physeal fractures are classified according to Salter and Harris [40] and describe if there is involvement of the epiphysis and the joint line. Types I and II normally heal without any long-term sequelae. In contrast, types III and IV involve the joint surface and have a higher risk of disturbing the growth plate which can result in limb length discrepancy, angular deformity and impaired function.

73.4.3.1 The Healing Process

The different phases of fracture healing are the same as in adults: (1) inflammation (hours-days), (2) reparation (days-weeks), and (3) remodelling (months-years). The greater subperiosteal hematoma and the thicker periosteum contribute, however, to a formation of callus that is strong enough to render the fracture healed more rapidly than in adults [41]. Additionally, as a general rule, the younger the child is and the closer the fracture is to the growth plate, the shorter the healing time and the better the remodelling potential is.

73.4.3.2 Return to Play After Fractures

RTP is dependent on, for instance, player position, player age, residual growth, fracture location, fracture type and the chosen treatment. Many fractures in young players are stable and without significant displacement. Non-surgical treatment with a period of casting/bracing and partial or total unloading of the injury site is therefore often successful. The treating physician decides when the fracture can be loaded.

Because of the great diversity in the fracture panorama, it is difficult to suggest general rules or criteria for safe RTP. Player position is, however, important to consider since an outfield player might be able to RTP with a soft cast splint or a brace for a finger fracture or a "buckle fracture" of the wrist (provided that the referee approves the cast or brace). Importantly, RTP should only be allowed if the physician judges the risk for worsening as minimal if, for instance, the player falls on the injured arm. On the other hand, when it comes to fractures in the lower extremities, the player usually needs to be sidelined regardless of whether being immobilised or not. In these occasions, it is advised that full range of motion, neuromuscular coordination and strength are regained before sport-specific training starts. A rule of thumb is that it takes about as long time to regain full fitness to participate in sport as the injured limb has been immobilised, that is, if a player was treated with partial weightbearing in a below-knee cast for 3 weeks after an undisplaced Salter-Harris type I fracture of the distal fibula, the player usually needs another 3 weeks of rehabilitation at minimum before RTP. Meeting functional test discharge criteria and having regained psychological confidence is likewise important.

73.4.4 Apophysitis and Chronic Growth Plate Injuries

Similar symptoms as in insertional tendinopathy among adults can be seen in adolescent players with so-called traction apophysitis or osteochondrosis of the spine or lower extremities. Common examples of these conditions are the Sinding-Larsen-Johansson and Osgood-Schlatter diseases around the knee and the Sever disease in the heel.

73.4.4.1 Apophysitis

All these conditions are characterised by prominent and painful tendon insertions, and pain occurs during running and jumping. These conditions are usually self-limiting with symptoms resolving within 1–2 years or until skeletal maturity is almost completed. Treatment is therefore symptomatic and consists of relieving traction and pressure on the affected apophysis as well as to avoid excessive running, jumping and kicking. A customised knee brace or an insole/heel cup might also help to unload the painful apophysis.

In general, there is no reason to sit the young player out from football for a longer period, but the overall training load might need to be reduced. The player is usually allowed to participate in match play. Treatment usually consists of physiotherapy and painkillers after activity if needed, together with bracing or taping of the patella tendon for the knee conditions and the use of a heel cup or customised insole for the foot problems.

73.4.4.2 Chronic Growth Plate Injuries

The growth plate can also incur injury due to repetitive loading, which is thought to disturb the metaphyseal perfusion and disrupt the endochondral bone formation with widening of the physis in the hypertrophic zone. Normally this process is self-limiting, but in some cases, growth disturbance of the physis can occur [42].

Symptoms of growth plate injury include pain and inability to load the affected extremity as well as swelling and tenderness around the physis. Radiological widening of the physis may be seen, whereas physeal cartilage extension into the metaphysis (another indirect sign of chronic growth plate overload) has been shown with MRI [43].

The principal treatment of chronic growth plate injury is to refrain from further loading of the affected extremity. If appropriate, bracing could be opted for in the initial treatment phase. In parallel, a range of motion exercises are started early, and successively neuromuscular coordination and strength training is introduced. The rehabilitation period required varies from case to case but usually spans over 4–6 weeks. Most commonly these injuries will resolve without any growth disturbance, but there are reports of stress-related premature partial or complete physeal closure [44].

While most commonly described for upper extremity problems in overhead sports, an increasing number of reports describe chronic growth plate problems also in the lower extremity. For example, it has recently been shown in a prospective study on adolescent male football players that the cam deformity of the hip is gradually acquired during skeletal maturation combined with intense physical loading [45]. Considering these findings, it is advised that players entering skeletal maturity pay close attention to symptoms from the groin area and that load is monitored and adjusted. Furthermore, cam and pincer are to be considered as morphological variants of the femur and acetabulum and do not automatically imply pathology in the form of femoroacetabular impingement syndrome (FAI) [46].

73.5 Safe Return to Play

A safe RTP after injury with a low subsequent risk of reinjury is the ultimate goal, regardless of what type of injury, in the young football player. The main dilemma is, however, that the decision for RTP often lies in the hands of coaches, parents and perhaps the player him/herself who rarely have sufficient medical qualifications. It might therefore be wise to recommend a "better safe than quick" attitude towards most injuries and not only severe injuries such as concussions, ACL injuries and fractures. Unfortunately, there is very limited knowledge on valid RTP criteria to be used in youth football without any access to club medical support, and this needs to be addressed in future research. As a minimum, following a stepwise programme with gradually increased stress on the injured limb before returning the player to match play is recommended [47].

Take-Home Message
Football is a popular and safe physical activity for children and adolescents all over the world, contributing to improved physical health and an active lifestyle in adulthood. Injury rate in youth football is generally low but will increase with age and is about the same in late adolescence as in adults. The injury panorama in children is somewhat different from adults. Children under 15 years of age will suffer more injuries to the upper extremity than adults but less strains and sprains in general. Any influence of ball size on injury rate in adolescent football has not been verified to date.

Specific injuries like concussion, ACL injury and growth plate-related injuries require specific caution and knowledge for optimal treatment and safe RTP for the young player. Considering the common lack of medical support in youth football, it is important to educate and involve, for example, parents and coaches on how to prevent injuries, acutely treat common injuries on and adjacent to the field as well as collaborate with sports medicine practitioners on safe RTP. A cautious approach to most injuries in children is therefore advised.

Top Five Evidence Based References

Caccese JB, Kaminski TW (2016) Minimizing head acceleration in soccer: a review of the literature. Sports Med 46:1591–1604

Faude O, Rössler R, Junge A (2013) Football injuries in children and adolescent players: are there clues for prevention? Sports Med 43:819–837

Froholdt A, Olsen OE, Bahr R (2009) Low risk of injuries among children playing organized soccer: a prospective cohort study. Am J Sports Med 37:1155–1160

Rössler R, Junge A, Chomiak J, Dvorak J, Faude O (2015) Soccer injuries in players aged 7–12 years. Am J Sports Med 44:309–317

Shea KG, Pfeiffer R, Wang JH, Curtin M, Apel PJ (2004) Anterior cruciate ligament injury in pediatric and adolescent soccer players: an analysis of insurance data. J Pediatr Orthop 24:623–628

References

1. FIFA Communications Division (2007) FIFA big count 2006: 270 million people active in football. FIFA, Zurich, Switzerland
2. Karapanou O, Papadimitriou A (2010) Determinants of menarche. Rep Biol Endocrinol 8:115
3. Hawkins RD, Fuller CW (1999) A prospective epidemiological study of injuries in four English professional football clubs. Br J Sports Med 33:196–203
4. Inklaar H, Bol E, Schmikli SL, Mosterd WL (1996) Injuries in male soccer players: team risk analysis. Int J Sports Med 17:229–234
5. Latella F, Serni G, Aglietti P, Zaccherotti G, De Biase P (1992) The epidemiology and mechanisms of soccer injuries. J Sports Traumatol 14:107–117
6. McNoe BM, Chalmers DJ (2010) Injury in community-level soccer: development of an injury surveillance system. Am J Sports Med 38:2542–2551
7. Nielsen AB, Yde J (1989) Epidemiology and traumatology of injuries in soccer. Am J Sports Med 17:803–807
8. Peterson L, Junge A, Chomiak J, Graf-Baumann T, Dvorak J (2000) Incidence of football injuries and complaints in different age groups and skill-level groups. Am J Sports Med 28:S51–S57
9. Froholdt A, Olsen OE, Bahr R (2009) Low risk of injuries among children playing organized soccer: a prospective cohort study. Am J Sports Med 37:1155–1160
10. Rössler R, Junge A, Chomiak J, Dvorak J, Faude O (2015) Soccer injuries in players aged 7–12 years. Am J Sports Med 44:309–317
11. Faude O, Rössler R, Junge A (2013) Football injuries in children and adolescent players: are there clues for prevention? Sports Med 43:819–837
12. Hägglund M, Waldén M, Ekstrand J (2009) UEFA injury study – an injury audit of European Championships 2006 to 2008. Br J Sports Med 43:483–489
13. Junge A, Dvorak J (2013) Injury surveillance in the World Football Tournaments 1998–2012. Br J Sports Med 47:782–788
14. Andersen TB, Bendiksen M, Pedersen JM, Ørntoft C, Brito J, Jackman SR, Williams CA, Krustrup P (2012) Kicking velocity and physical, technical, tactical match performance for U18 female football players - effect of a new ball. Hum Mov Sci 31:1624–1638
15. Zebis MK, Thorborg K, Andersen LL, Møller M, Christensen KB, Clausen MB, Hölmich P, Wedderkopp N, Andersen TB, Krustrup P (in press) Effects of a lighter, smaller football on acute match injuries in adolescent female football: a pilot cluster-randomised controlled trial. J Sports Med Phys Fitness
16. Kelly KD, Lissel HL, Rowe BH, Vincenten JA, Voaklander DC (2001) Sport and recreation-related head injuries treated in the emergency department. Clin J Sport Med 11:77–81
17. Yard EE, Comstock RD (2009) Compliance with return to play guidelines following concussion in US high school athletes, 2005–2008. Brain Inj 23:888–898
18. Bramley H, Patrick K, Lehman E, Silvis M (2012) High school soccer players with concussion education are more likely to notify their coach of a suspected concussion. Clin Pediatr (Phil) 51:332–336
19. Caccese JB, Kaminski TW (2016) Minimizing head acceleration in soccer: a review of the literature. Sports Med 46:1591–1604
20. McCrory P, Meeuwisse WH, Dvořák J, Aubry M, Bailes J, Broglio S, Cantu RC, Cassidy D, Echemendia RJ, Castellani RJ, Davis GA, Ellenbogen RG, Emery C, Engebretsen L, Fedderman-Demont N, Giza CC, Guskiewicz K, Herring S, Iverson GL, Johnston KM, Kissick J, Kutcher J, Leddy JJ, Maddocks D, Makdissi M, Manley GT, McCrea M, Meehan WP, Nagahiro S, Patricios J, Putukian M, Schneider KJ, Sills A, Tator CH, Turner M, Vos PE (2017) Consensus statement on concussion in sport: the 5th International Conference on Concussion in Sport held in Berlin, October 2016. Br J Sports Med 51:838–847
21. McClincy MP, Lovell MR, Pardini J, Collins MW, Spore MK (2006) Recovery from sports concussion in high school and collegiate athletes. Brain Inj 20:33–39
22. Reddy CC, Collins MW (2009) Sports concussion: management and predictors of outcome. Curr Sports Med Rep 8:10–15
23. Shea KG, Grimm NL, Ewin CK, Aoki SK (2011) Youth sports anterior cruciate ligament and knee injury epidemiology: who is getting injured? In what sports? When? Clin Sports Med 30:691–706
24. Beynnon BD, Vacek PM, Newell MK, Tourville TW, Smith HC, Shultz SJ, Slauterbeck JR, Johnson RJ (2014) The effects of level of competition, sport, and sex on the incidence of first-time noncontact anterior cruciate ligament injury. Am J Sports Med 42:1806–1812
25. Joseph AM, Collins CL, Henke NM, Yard EE, Fields SK, Comstock RD (2013) A multisport epidemiologic comparison of anterior cruciate ligament injuries in high school athletics. J Athl Train 48:810–817
26. Roos H, Ornell M, Gärdsell P, Lohmander LS, Lindstrand A (1995) Soccer after anterior cruciate ligament injury – an incompatible combination? A national survey of incidence and risk factors and a 7-year follow-up of 310 players. Acta Orthop Scand 66:107–112
27. Swenson DM, Collins CL, Best TM, Flanigan DC, Fields SK, Comstock RD (2013) Epidemiology of knee injuries among US high school athletes, 2005/2006–2010/2011. Med Sci Sports Exerc 45:462–469
28. Waldén M, Atroshi I, Magnusson H, Wagner P, Hägglund M (2012) Prevention of acute knee injuries

in adolescent female football players: cluster randomised controlled trial. BMJ 344:e3042
29. Shea KG, Pfeiffer R, Wang JH, Curtin M, Apel PJ (2004) Anterior cruciate ligament injury in pediatric and adolescent soccer players: an analysis of insurance data. J Pediatr Orthop 24:623–628
30. Moksnes H, Engebretsen L, Eitzen I, Risberg MA (2013) Functional outcomes following a non-operative treatment algorithm for anterior cruciate ligament injuries in skeletally immature children 12 years and younger. A prospective cohort with 2 years follow-up. Br J Sports Med 47:488–494
31. Frosch KH, Stengel D, Brodhun T (2010) Outcomes and risks of operative treatment of rupture of the anterior cruciate ligament in children and adolescents. Arthroscopy 26:1539–1550
32. Fabricant PD, Jones KJ, Delos D, Cordasco FA, Marx RG, Pearle AD, Warren RF, Green DW (2013) Reconstruction of the anterior cruciate ligament in the skelettaly immature athlete: a review of current concepts: AAOS exhibit selection. J Bone Joint Surg Am 95:e28
33. Kocher MS, Saxon JS, Hovis WD, Hawkins RJ (2002) Management and complications of anterior cruciate ligament injuries in skeletally immature patients: survey of the Herodicus Society and The ACL Study Group. J Pediatr Orthop 22:452–457
34. Courvoisier A, Grimaldi M, Plaweski S (2011) Good surgical outcome of transphyseal ACL reconstruction in skeletally immature patients using four-strand hamstring graft. Knee Surg Sports Traumatol Arthrosc 19:588–591
35. Yellin JL, Fabricant PD, Gornitzky A, Greenberg EM, Conrad S, Dyke JA, Ganley TJ (2016) Rehabilitation following anterior cruciate ligament tears in children: a systematic review. JBJS Rev 4(1). pii: 01874474-201601000-00004
36. Fältström A, Hägglund M, Magnusson H, Forssblad M, Kvist J (2016) Predictors for additional anterior cruciate ligament reconstruction: data from the Swedish national ACL register. Knee Surg Sports Traumatol Arthrosc 24:885–894
37. Wiggins AJ, Grandhi RK, Schneider DK, Stanfield D, Webster KE, Myer GD (2016) Risk of secondary injury in younger athletes after anterior cruciate ligament reconstruction: a systematic review and meta-analysis. Am J Sports Med 44:1861–1876
38. Grindem H, Snyder-Mackler L, Moksnes H, Engebretsen L, Risberg MA (2016) Simple decision rules can reduce reinjury risk by 84% after ACL reconstruction; the Delaware-Oslo ACL cohort study. Br J Sports Med 50:804–808
39. Yard EE, Schroeder MJ, Fields SK, Collins CL, Comstock RD (2008) The epidemiology of United States high school soccer injuries, 2005–2007. Am J Sports Med 36:1930–1937
40. Salter R, Harris WR (1963) Injuries involving the epiphyseal plate. J Bone Joint Surg Am 45:587–622
41. Lindaman LM (2001) Bone healing in children. Clin Podiatr Med Surg 18:97–108
42. DiFiori J, Caine D, Malina R (2006) Wrist pain, distal radial growth plate injury, and ulnar variance in the young gymnast. Am J Sports Med 34:840–849
43. Dwek JR, Cardoso F, Chung CR (2009) MR imaging of overuse injuries in the skeletally immature gymnast: spectrum of soft-tissue and osseous lesions in the hand and wrist. Pediatr Radiol 39:1310–1316
44. Caine D, DiFiori J, Mafulli N (2006) Physeal injuries in children's and youth sports: reasons for concern? Br J Sports Med 40:749–760
45. Agricola R, Heijboer MP, Ginai AZ, Roels P, Zadpoor AA, Verhaar JA, Weinans H, Waarsing JH (2014) A cam deformity is gradually acquired during skeletal maturation in adolescent and young male soccer players: a prospective study with minimum 2-year follow-up. Am J Sports Med 42:798–806
46. Griffin DR, Dickenson EJ, O'Donnell J, Agricola R, Awan T, Beck M, Clohisy JC, Dijkstra HP, Falvey E, Gimpel M, Hinman RS, Hölmich P, Kassarjian A, Martin HD, Martin R, Mather RC, Philippon MJ, Reiman MP, Takla A, Thorborg K, Walker S, Weir A, Bennell KL (2016) The Warwick Agreement on femoroacetabular impingement syndrome (FAI syndrome): an international consensus statement. Br J Sports Med 50:1169–1176
47. Hägglund M, Waldén M, Ekstrand J (2007) Lower reinjury rate with a coach-controlled rehabilitation program in amateur male soccer: a randomized controlled trial. Am J Sports Med 35(9):1433–1442

Re-injuries in Professional Football: The UEFA Elite Club Injury Study

74

Martin Hägglund, Markus Waldén, Håkan Bengtsson, and Jan Ekstrand

Contents

M. Hägglund (✉) • H. Bengtsson
Football Research Group, Division of Physiotherapy, Department of Medical and Health Sciences, Linköping University, Linköping, Sweden
e-mail: martin.hagglund@liu.se; info.frg@telia.com

M. Waldén • J. Ekstrand
Football Research Group, Division of Community Medicine, Department of Medical and Health Sciences, Linköping University, Linköping, Sweden
e-mail: markus.walden@telia.com; jan.ekstrand@telia.com

74.1 The UEFA Elite Club Injury Study

The Union of European Football Associations (UEFA) Elite Club Injury Study (ECIS) was launched in 2001 with the aim to study the injury burden for professional football players in Europe [1]. The study is funded by UEFA and coordinated by Professor Jan Ekstrand, former UEFA Medical Committee vice chairman and chair of the Football Research Group (FRG). FRG is an international research group based in Linköping, Sweden, responsible for running the study.

At present, UEFA invites all 32 clubs qualifying for the Champions League group stage to participate in the study (Fig. 74.1). In addition, clubs that have previously participated in the ECIS and stay on the UEFA top 50 club ranking may continue in the study. In 2016 the data set included more than 260 club seasons from nearly 50 professional football clubs representing the highest league level in 17 different countries. Between 2001 and 2016, approximately 13,000 injuries have been registered during 1.8 million hours of football and other physical training exposure.

74.1.1 Study Methodology

To briefly summarise the study methodology, all players with a first team contract are eligible for inclusion. Clubs register individual player

V. Musahl et al. (eds.), *Return to Play in Football*, https://doi.org/10.1007/978-3-662-55713-6_74

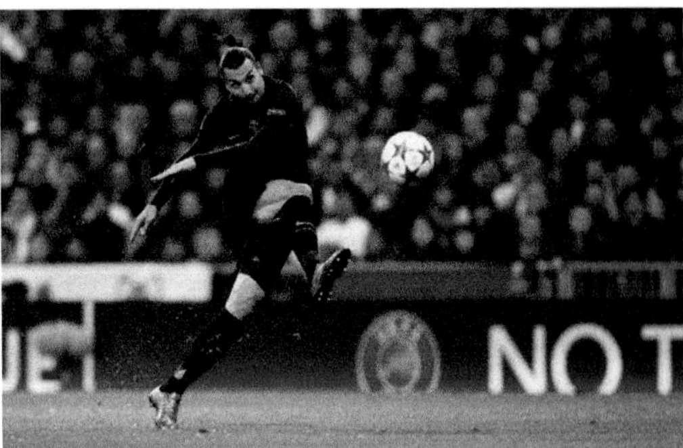

Fig. 74.1 Each season all 32 clubs qualifying for the Champions League group stage are invited to participate in the UEFA Elite Club Injury Study. Photo: Bildbyrån with permission

exposure hours to training and matches and all football-related injuries that result in the player being unable to take full part in training or match play (i.e. time-loss injury) on standardised forms [2]. An injured player is considered absent due to injury until being cleared by the club medical staff to participate fully in all parts of training and being available for match selection. Injury severity is based on the number of days lay-off from the day of injury to the day of return to play (RTP) and categorised into four severity groups: minimal (0–3 days), mild (4–7 days), moderate (8–28 days) and severe (>28 days) [2].

For further reference in this chapter, a *re-injury* is defined as an injury of the same type and at the same site as an index injury within the preceding year. A re-injury within 2 months after return to full participation from the index injury is defined as an *early recurrence* and after more than 2 months as a *late recurrence*. Contusions, lacerations, abrasions, concussions and dental injuries are not eligible for categorisation into recurrence or not [3].

74.1.2 Injury Burden in Top-Level Football

The top-level players in the UEFA-ECIS cohort will sustain, on average, two injuries leading to time loss each season [4]. For a professional club, this translates to just over 50 injuries per season, with player training attendance and match availability averaging 77% and 86%, respectively. The latter figure has significant impact for the clubs since high player match availability has been found to correlate with team success in both the league play (higher league ranking and more average points per league match) and in European Cups (higher UEFA Season Club coefficient) [5]. Having two or more injuries in a match also correlate with higher odds of losing or drawing that match [6]. Thus, reducing the number as well as the time loss from injuries has significant performance and financial implications for top-level football clubs.

Fact Box 1 The UEFA Elite Club Injury Study

Since the start in 2001, about 50 top-level football clubs from 17 different countries have participated in the study.

Thirteen thousand injuries during 1.8 million hours of football have been registered, making it the biggest database of its kind in professional football.

A professional football club can on average expect just over 50 injuries leading to time loss from play each season.

Clubs with fewer injuries and higher player match availability perform better in the league play and in international cups.

74.2 Burden of Re-injuries in Professional Football

Previous injury is probably the most consistently identified and strongest risk factor for injury in football. Players with previous injury have a severalfold increased risk of new identical injury compared with their peers without such injury history. For instance, for the "big four" injuries in football, studies have shown up to 11-fold increased risk of hamstring injury, 7-fold for groin injury, and 5-fold for knee and ankle sprains among previously injured players [7–13]. Re-injuries can comprise up to every fourth injury in elite football and can often be more severe than the index injury, so it is evident that reducing injury recurrence rates should be a priority for professional clubs to decrease the total injury burden.

74.2.1 Re-injury Rates Lower Among Top-Level Clubs

The overall re-injury rate among the European top-level clubs in the UEFA-ECIS is about 17%, which is lower than that found in a domestic league of lower ranking (25%) and in amateur football teams (35%) [14]. Not surprisingly, recurrence rates thus seem to show an inverse relationship with playing level. High manpower of medical staff with access to qualified medical and physiotherapy personnel working full-time with the team to ensure a quick initial injury assessment and high-level support during the rehabilitation is probably a key factor. Similarly, continuous assessment of the player during a graded RTP, as well as maintaining a sufficient level of training load during the rehabilitation, is important. Finally, with a large competitive squad, the top-level clubs may "afford" to have injured players off the pitch with lesser impact on the club's performance and thus allow sufficient time for rehabilitation.

74.2.2 Decreasing Trend for Re-injury Rates

The overall injury rates in the UEFA-ECIS remained virtually stable over the first decade of the study [4]. In contrast, a recent analysis focusing specifically on re-injuries showed a positive trend with approximately 3% decrease in re-injury rate each year between 2001 and 2015 (Fig. 74.2) [14]. Decreasing trends in re-injury rates were seen also specifically for muscle injuries and ligament injuries, whereas for other injury types with high recurrence rates (e.g. tendon injuries and other overuse injuries), no decreasing trend was evident.

Fact Box 2 Re-injury rates

Re-injuries comprise 17% of all injuries in top-level football.

There is an inverse relationship between playing level and re-injury rates.

A positive trend is seen in the UEFA Elite Club Injury Study with a 3% decrease in the re-injury rate each year between 2001 and 2015.

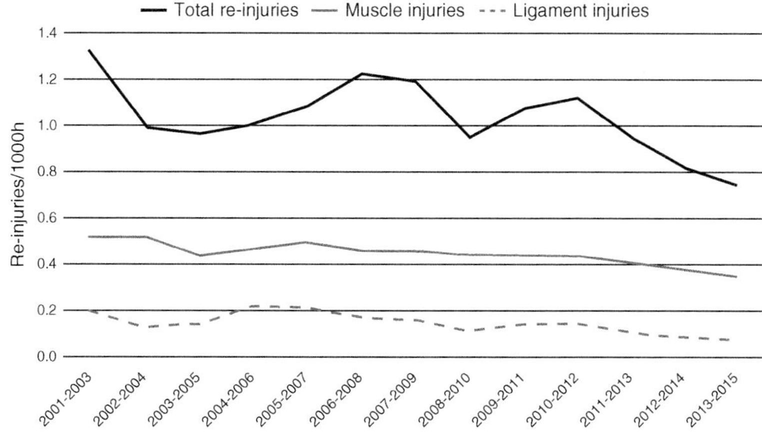

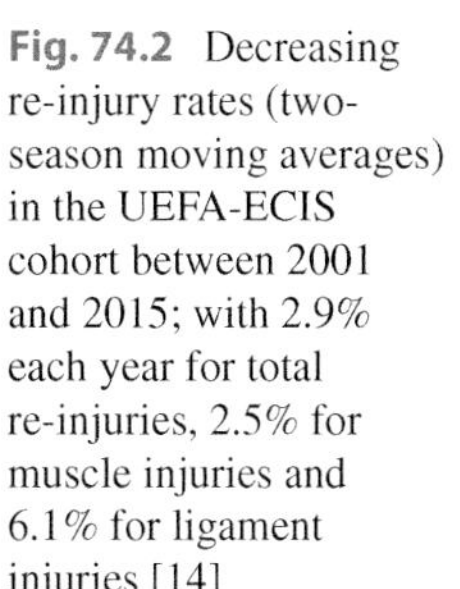
Fig. 74.2 Decreasing re-injury rates (two-season moving averages) in the UEFA-ECIS cohort between 2001 and 2015; with 2.9% each year for total re-injuries, 2.5% for muscle injuries and 6.1% for ligament injuries [14]

74.3 Re-injury Patterns

Re-injury rates are similar between training and match injuries in the UEFA-ECIS cohort, with 17% and 16%, respectively [14]. This is in contrast to amateur level football where higher re-injury rates have been found during matches [15]. In the UEFA-ECIS cohort, re-injury rates are significantly lower during the preseason preparation phase (11%) than during the first half (August–December) and the second half (January–May) of the competitive season, with 15% and 20%, respectively [14]. The fact that recurrence rates are highest towards the end of the season, with conclusion of the league play and the final stages of international cups, could indicate a higher risk acceptance among clubs at this period. That is, players may be allowed to RTP quicker after injury to play important matches or allowed to play with ongoing complaints.

74.3.1 Early Recurrences Are Common

In the UEFA-ECIS, early recurrences (within 2 months) comprise 77% of all within-season re-injuries [14]. The same pattern emerges for many injury types, such as muscle injuries, with a significantly elevated re-injury risk in the first month after RTP (Fig. 74.3). Early recurrent injury indicates premature RTP, irrespective of whether this is reflective of a failure to assess mental and/or physical readiness to RTP or deliberately accepting a high risk (e.g., to allow the player back to an important match). The increased re-injury risk in the early stages after RTP suggests that both intrinsic factors (e.g. residual deficits after the index injury) and extrinsic factors should be monitored at this period. For instance, important extrinsic factors such as match congestion [16] and player workload [17] at RTP should be managed to reduce re-injury risk, especially if the player has had an extended injury absence period.

74.3.2 Common and Time-Costly Re-injuries

Re-injuries are more frequent among overuse-related injuries (21%) than for acute-onset injuries (14%) [14]. The top ten re-injuries with the highest frequency and burden (time loss from play) are shown in Table 74.1. Hamstring injury is by far the most frequent and time-costly re-injury (Fig. 74.4). Other lower extremity muscle injuries to the adductors, quadriceps and calf are also highly represented in the top ten list, as are joint and ligament injuries to the knee and ankle.

74.3.2.1 Muscle Injuries

Muscle injuries represent about one-third of all injuries in top-level football and have remained at a stable high rate over the last decade [12, 18]. Hamstring injuries, the single most common injury in professional football, have even seen a

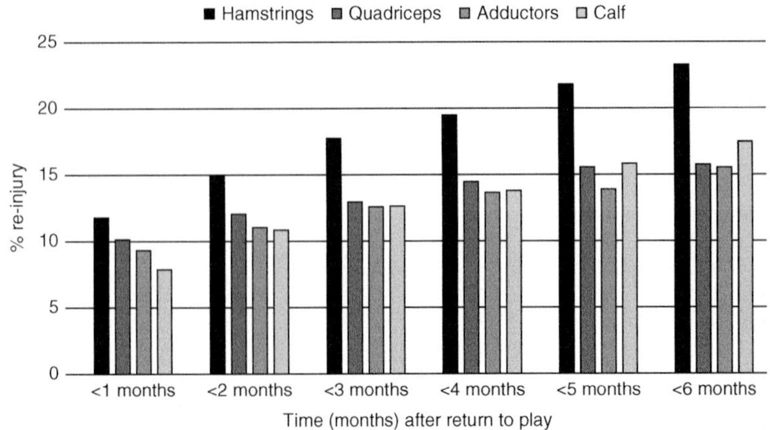

Fig. 74.3 Re-injury risk within 1, 2, 3, 4, 5, and 6 months after return to play from muscle injury

Table 74.1 Ten top recurrent injuries as a function of frequency (% of all re-injuries) and burden (% of all time loss due to re-injury)

Frequency		Burden	
1. Hamstring injury	22.7%	1. Hamstring injury	17.1%
2. Adductor-related injury	11.6%	2. Knee cartilage lesion	8.4%
3. Quadriceps injury	6.4%	3. Adductor-related injury	8.1%
4. Calf muscle injury	6.1%	4. Achilles tendinopathy	6.8%
5. Lateral ankle sprain	6.0%	5. Quadriceps injury	6.5%
6. Achilles tendinopathy	4.3%	6. Calf muscle injury	4.6%
7. Knee synovitis/effusion	4.3%	7. Lateral ankle sprain	3.5%
8. Low back pain	3.3%	8. Knee meniscus tear	3.4%
9. Knee MCL tear	3.2%	9. Knee synovitis/effusion	3.1%
10. Knee cartilage lesion	2.9%	10. Knee MCL tear	3.0%

MCL medial collateral ligament

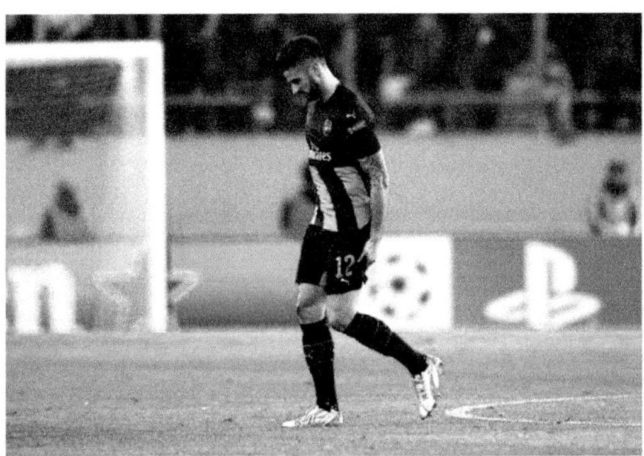

Fig. 74.4 Hamstring injury has the highest frequency and highest burden of all re-injuries in top-level football. Photo: Bildbyrån with permission

2–4% yearly increase over the last 15 years [19]. One could speculate that evolvement of professional football with more match-like training situations (e.g. with more high-sprinting actions), greater match congestion and greater playing intensity in matches might contribute to an increased hamstring injury risk. Furthermore, poor adoption of evidence-based injury preventive exercises such as the Nordic Hamstring Exercise has been reported among professional football teams [20].

Injury severity is often moderate, averaging 2–3 weeks lay-off [18], and with a high risk of recurrence within the season (20–30%) [12]. As seen in Fig. 74.3, the re-injury risk is highest immediately after RTP with about half of all re-injuries to the hamstrings, quadriceps, adductors and calf muscles occurring within the first month. For hamstring injuries, the re-injury risk continues to increase up to 6 months after RTP, whereas for the other three muscle groups, the risk tends to level out at 4–5 months after RTP.

Among hamstring injuries in top-level football, the biceps femoris (BF) muscle is predominately involved (84% of hamstring injuries) and less frequently the semimembranosus (SM) and semitendinosus (ST) muscles with 12% and 4%, respectively [21]. The early recurrence rate is significantly higher among BF injuries (18%) compared with SM/ST injuries (2%) [21] and tends to be lower for injuries with a negative MRI scan (7%) than for injuries with visible pathology (oedema or architectural disruption) on MRI (17–21%) [22].

Adductor-related injuries are more common than iliopsoas-related injuries in the UEFA-ECIS cohort, representing 63% and 8% of all hip/groin injuries, respectively, with a declining trend in incidence seen from 2001 to 2015 [23]. The early recurrence rate is higher for adductor injuries (11–18%) than for iliopsoas injuries (4–6%) [12, 18, 23]. Early recurrence rates for quadriceps and calf muscle injuries ranges 12–17%, with up to 21% of within-season re-injuries [12, 18].

Players who have had an injury to the hamstrings, quadriceps, adductors or calf in the previous season have a two- to threefold increased likelihood of new injury to the same muscle group compared with previously uninjured players [11, 12] and the risk increases with the number of previous injuries [11]. Noteworthy is that previous injury to other lower extremity muscle groups also makes players more prone to new muscle injury [12], and this should be considered in the routine preseason evaluation and signing examination of players.

74.3.2.2 Joint and Ligament Injuries

Joint and ligament injuries have seen a significantly declining trend in the UEFA-ECIS cohort over the last decade [4], including the most frequent ligament injuries: ankle sprains [24] and medial collateral ligament (MCL) injuries of the knee [25]. In contrast, anterior cruciate ligament (ACL) injuries show a stable or even increasing tendency during the same period [26].

Within-season re-injury rates for acute joint injuries such as ligament injuries (11%) and partial/complete joint dislocations (14%) are low to moderate, whereas re-injury among joint overuse injuries, e.g. synovitis (33%), is much more common [14]. Despite a relatively low re-injury rate, ankle sprains and MCL injuries both make it to the top ten list for recurrence frequency and burden (Table 74.1), based on them being both quite common and moderately severe in nature. On the contrary, upper extremity joint injuries are quite rare in football, although more often seen in goalkeepers [27]. A high re-injury rate is seen for shoulder dislocations (32%), whereas for acromioclavicular joint sprains and dislocations, this figure is much lower (<5%).

Similar to the findings for muscle injuries, the re-injury risk for ankle and knee ligament injuries is highest in the first month after RTP, where 50% of all recurrences occur. About 1/10 MCL injuries, and fewer 1/20 ACL injuries, are recurrences [25, 26]. However, following ACL reconstruction, many players experience other complications (e.g. new knee surgery) prior to return to full match play [26], and ACL-reconstructed players are five times more likely to suffer from knee overuse problems than their peers [28]. In line with the findings for muscle injuries, this lends further support that in addition to anatomically directly related re-injuries, other subsequent injuries after RTP are also a problem among joint and ligament injuries.

74.3.2.3 Tendon Injuries and Overuse Injuries

About 30% of all injuries in the UEFA-ECIS are overuse injuries, with a gradual onset and no known macrotrauma [29]. With the time-loss definition used in the study, it is, however, likely that the true burden of overuse injury is underestimated [30], and they thus comprise a significant problem in professional football. Overuse injuries are often associated with extrinsic factors such as training load and volume, and they also peak during the preseason preparation period [29]. Common overuse injuries include low back pain, Achilles and patellar tendinopathies, groin pain and joint synovitis [31]. Overall, one out of five tendon injuries is within-season recurrences, and they show no apparent declining trend over the last 15 years of the UEFA-ECIS [14].

Both Achilles and patellar tendinopathies recur at a high rate, with 27% and 20%, respectively [32, 33]. A high re-injury rate within the first month after RTP (Achilles 15%, patella 7%) probably reflects the recursive nature of tendon-related problems in professional football, as well as management strategies to allow players to RTP with reduced but ongoing symptoms that may flare up again. Many players may suffer from chronic conditions with fluctuating symptoms, and subsequent recovery periods, over the season. Due to their chronic nature, Achilles tendinopathies have the fourth highest injury burden among re-injuries (Table 74.1).

Bone stress injuries are more rarely seen in football but are almost always of severe nature and may result in healing problems and sometimes a career end [34]. Fractures in total represent less than 5% of all injuries in the UEFA-ECIS [4], and traumatic fractures outnumber stress fractures at a rate of 8:1 [35]. Stress fractures, however, cause longer absence from play than traumatic fractures [35]. The most common location for stress fractures is the fifth metatarsal, comprising four out of five stress fractures, followed by the tibia and pelvis [36]. About 20% of all stress fractures are reported as re-injuries [36], with up to one-third of metatarsal five fractures being recurrences [34].

Fact Box 3 Re-injury Patterns
The re-injury risk is elevated in the immediate stages after return to play (RTP), with 50% and 77% of re-injuries occurring within the first and second months, respectively.

Re-injuries are most frequent towards the end of the season, suggesting a higher risk tolerance in the RTP decision.

Muscle injuries to the hamstrings, adductors, quadriceps and calf are among the most common and time-costly re-injuries.

74.4 Better Safe than Quick: Or Is It?

The RTP decision is complex and influenced by many medical (assessment of health risk) and non-medical factors (assessment of activity risk and risk tolerance) [37]. A key element is thus what level of risk the player, medical team, coach, etc. is willing to accept at RTP. This includes not only the risk of a re-injury but may also include risks of poor player performance or poor team results as a consequence of allowing or not allowing RTP [38]. Ideally, the RTP should be as quick *and* as safe as possible. From a strict medical point of view, having the player welfare and safety in focus, it may be tempting to keep all injured players off the pitch a bit longer. By allowing sufficient time for tissue healing, rehabilitation and player recovery both physically and psychologically, the re-injury risk can most certainly be reduced. For instance, a more than doubled re-injury risk was evident for Achilles tendon disorders with a short recovery (<10 days) compared with long recovery (>10 days) [32], and similarly, an association between longer recovery times and lower re-injury rates was reported in a systematic review on RTP after hamstring injury [39]. At youth or amateur levels, a "play it safe" approach is clearly sensible [15], but at the professional level, other factors come into play. A medical team that is overly cautious, i.e. always keeping players off the pitch longer to minimise re-injury risk, may be short lived in the professional football environment. Moreover, from a strict player availability perspective, it may not always pay off.

Figure 74.5 shows a fictive example of two different approaches to RTP decisions and the effect on re-injury risk and player availability. The example shows that both teams suffer ten injuries (average absence 15 days) during a 2-month period, and they are followed for 2 months after RTP. Team 1 has an "aggressive" approach, favouring a quick RTP, and accepts a moderate to high early re-injury risk. In contrast, team 2 has a "play it safe" approach allowing an extra week of rehabilitation for all injuries in order to minimise the re-injury risk. In the "aggressive" team, two of the ten players suffer a re-injury after RTP, whereas the "play it safe" team manages to avoid early re-injuries completely. So, the big question is: Does the "play it safe" approach reduce the total injury burden? The answer is no. Actually the team using the "aggressive" approach has a higher total player availability (85% versus 82%) during the total 4-month period, and the "play it safe" approach results in 22% more days lost to injury. Hence, from player safety and welfare perspectives, the "play it safe" approach (low re-injury risk) is obviously preferable, while from economy (less player absence) and team success (higher player availability) perspectives, the "aggressive" approach might win. We acknowledge that it is a simplified example and not applicable to potentially serious injuries such as concussions. Still it highlights one of the many challenges faced in the RTP decision in professional football. In reality, balancing risk and reward requires a unique judgement for each RTP decision.

Take-Home Message
Re-injuries comprise almost one in five injuries in top-level football, and the re-injury risk is highly elevated in the first month after RTP. Avoiding (early) re-injury is therefore important to reduce the impact of injuries in a club. Valid RTP criteria after injury to reduce re-injury risk are, however, largely lacking and should be a research priority in the future. In the

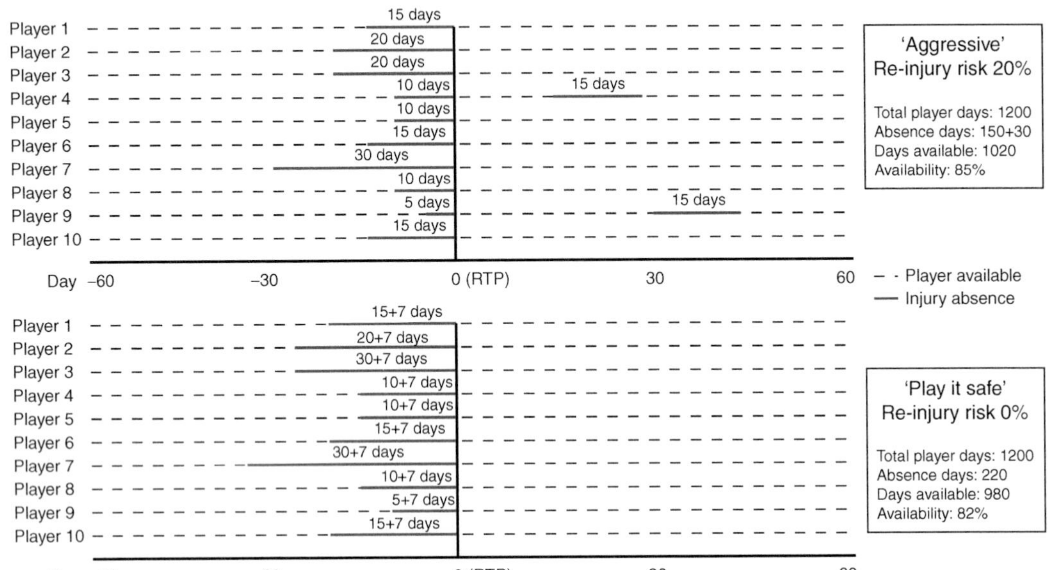

Fig. 74.5 Fictive scenarios of two approaches to return to play decisions. Team 1 has an "aggressive" approach, favouring a quick return, whereas team 2 has a "play it safe" approach allowing an extra week of rehabilitation for all injuries. Even with two re-injuries, the total player availability is higher with the "aggressive" approach

absence of clear evidence, medical practitioners working in the professional football environment are required to make a unique judgement for each RTP decision while balancing the risk and reward of having an accelerated versus prolonged recovery period.

Top Five Evidence Based References.

Ekstrand J, Hägglund M, Kristenson K, Magnusson H, Waldén M (2013) Fewer ligament injuries but no preventive effect on muscle injuries and severe injuries: an 11-year follow-up of the UEFA Champions League injury study. Br J Sports Med 47:732–737

Hägglund M, Waldén M, Ekstrand J (2006) Previous injury as a risk factor for injury in elite football - a prospective study over two consecutive seasons. Br J Sports Med 40:767–772

Hägglund M, Waldén M, Ekstrand J (2007) Lower reinjury rate with a coach-controlled rehabilitation program in amateur male soccer: a randomized controlled trial. Am J Sports Med 35(9):1433–1442

Hägglund M, Waldén M, Ekstrand J (2013) Risk factors for lower extremity muscle injury in professional soccer: the UEFA injury study. Am J Sports Med 41:327–335

Hägglund M, Walden M, Ekstrand J (2016) Injury recurrence is lower at the highest professional football level than at national and amateur levels: does sports medicine & sports physiotherapy deliver? Br J Sports Med 50:751–758

References

1. UEFA website (2016) UEFA club injury study sets the standard. https://wwwuefaorg/protecting-the-game/medical/injury-study/news/newsid=2412835html. Accessed 17 Feb 2017
2. Hägglund M, Waldén M, Bahr R, Ekstrand J (2005) Methods for epidemiological study of injuries to professional football players: developing the UEFA model. Br J Sports Med 39:340–346
3. Fuller CW, Ekstrand J, Junge A, Andersen TE, Bahr R, Dvorak J, Hägglund M, McCrory P, Meeuwisse WH (2006) Consensus statement on injury definitions and data collection procedures in studies of football (soccer) injuries. Br J Sports Med 40(3):193–201
4. Ekstrand J, Hägglund M, Kristenson K, Magnusson H, Waldén M (2013) Fewer ligament injuries but no preventive effect on muscle injuries and severe injuries: an 11-year follow-up of the UEFA Champions League injury study. Br J Sports Med 47:732–737
5. Hägglund M, Waldén M, Magnusson H, Kristenson K, Bengtsson H, Ekstrand J (2013) Injuries affect team performance negatively in professional football: an 11-year follow-up of the UEFA Champions League injury study. Br J Sports Med 47:738–742
6. Bengtsson H, Ekstrand J, Waldén M, Hägglund M (2013) Match injury rates in professional soccer vary

with match result, match venue and type of competition. Am J Sports Med 41:1505–1510
7. Árnason Á, Sigurdsson SB, Gudmundsson A, Holme I, Engebretsen L, Bahr R (2004) Risk factors for injuries in football. Am J Sports Med 32(1 Suppl):5S–16S
8. Engebretsen AH, Myklebust G, Holme I et al (2010) Intrinsic risk factors for hamstring injuries among male soccer players: a prospective cohort study. Am J Sports Med 38:1147–1153
9. Engebretsen AH, Myklebust G, Holme I et al (2010) Intrinsic risk factors for groin injuries among male soccer players: a prospective cohort study. Am J Sports Med 38:2051–2057
10. Engebretsen AH, Myklebust G, Holme I et al (2010) Intrinsic risk factors for acute ankle injuries among male soccer players: a prospective cohort study. Scand J Med Sci Sports 20:403–410
11. Hägglund M, Waldén M, Ekstrand J (2006) Previous injury as a risk factor for injury in elite football - a prospective study over two consecutive seasons. Br J Sports Med 40:767–772
12. Hägglund M, Waldén M, Ekstrand J (2013) Risk factors for lower extremity muscle injury in professional soccer: the UEFA injury study. Am J Sports Med 41:327–335
13. Hölmich P, Thorborg K, Dehlendorff C, Krogsgaard K, Gluud C (2014) Incidence and clinical presentation of groin injuries in sub-elite male soccer. Br J Sports Med 48:1245–1250
14. Hägglund M, Walden M, Ekstrand J (2016) Injury recurrence is lower at the highest professional football level than at national and amateur levels: does sports medicine & sports physiotherapy deliver? Br J Sports Med 50:751–758
15. Hägglund M, Waldén M, Ekstrand J (2007) Lower reinjury rate with a coach-controlled rehabilitation program in amateur male soccer: a randomized controlled trial. Am J Sports Med 35(9):1433–1442
16. Bengtsson H, Ekstrand J, Hägglund M (2013) Muscle injury rates in professional football increase with match congestion - an 11-year follow up of the UEFA Champions League injury study. Br J Sports Med 47:743–747
17. Blanch P, Gabbett TJ (2016) Has the athlete trained enough to return to play safely? The acute:chronic workload ratio permits clinicians to quantify a player's risk of subsequent injury. Br J Sports Med 50:471–475
18. Ekstrand J, Hägglund M, Waldén M (2011) Epidemiology of muscle injuries in professional football (soccer). Am J Sports Med 39:1226–1232
19. Ekstrand J, Waldén M, Hägglund M (2016) Hamstring injuries have increased by 4% annually in men's professional football, since 2001: a 13-year longitudinal analysis of the UEFA Elite Club injury study. Br J Sports Med 50:731–737
20. Bahr R, Thorborg K, Ekstrand J (2015) Evidence-based hamstring injury prevention is not adopted by the majority of Champions League or Norwegian Premier League football teams: the Nordic hamstring survey. Br J Sports Med 49:1466–1471
21. Ekstrand J, Lee JC, Healy JC (2016) MRI findings and return to play in football: a prospective analysis of 255 hamstring injuries in the UEFA Elite Club Injury Study. Br J Sports Med 50:738–743
22. Ekstrand J, Healy JC, Waldén M, Lee JC, English B, Hägglund M (2012) Hamstring muscle injuries in professional football: the correlation of MRI findings with return to play. Br J Sports Med 46:112–117
23. Werner J, Hägglund M, Ekstrand J, Waldén M (2017) Time-loss groin injuries are decreasing in men's professional football: a 15-year prospective survey of the UEFA Elite Club Injury Study. Submitted
24. Waldén M, Hägglund M, Ekstrand J (2013) Time-trends and circumstances surrounding ankle injuries in men's professional football: an 11-year follow-up of the UEFA Champions League injury study. Br J Sports Med 47:748–753
25. Lundblad M, Waldén M, Magnusson H, Karlsson J, Ekstrand J (2013) The UEFA injury study: 11-year data concerning 346 MCL injuries and time to return to play. Br J Sports Med 47:759–762
26. Waldén M, Hägglund M, Magnusson H, Ekstrand J (2016) Anterior cruciate ligament injuries in men's professional football: a 15-year prospective study on time-trends and return to play rates reveals only 65% of players still play at the top level 3 years after ACL rupture. Br J Sports Med 50:744–750
27. Ekstrand J, Hägglund M, Törnqvist H, Kristenson K, Bengtsson H, Magnusson H, Waldén M (2013) Upper extremity injuries in male elite football players. Knee Surg Sports Traumatol Arthrosc 21:1626–1632
28. Waldén M, Hägglund M, Ekstrand J (2006) High risk of new knee injury in elite footballers with previous anterior cruciate ligament injury. Br J Sports Med 40(2):158–162
29. Ekstrand J, Hägglund M, Waldén M (2011) Injury incidence and injury pattern in professional football - the UEFA injury study. Br J Sports Med 45:553–558
30. Bahr R (2009) No injuries, but plenty of pain? On the methodology for recording overuse symptoms in sports. Br J Sports Med 43:966–972
31. Waldén M, Hägglund M, Ekstrand J (2005) UEFA Champions League study: a prospective study of injuries in professional football during the 2001–2002 season. Br J Sports Med 39:542–546
32. Gajhede-Knudsen M, Ekstrand J, Magnusson H, Maffulli N (2013) Recurrence of Achilles tendon injuries in elite male football players is more common after early return to play: an 11-year follow-up of the UEFA Champions League injury study. Br J Sports Med 47:763–768
33. Hägglund M, Zwerver J, Ekstrand J (2011) Epidemiology of patellar tendinopathy in elite male soccer players. Am J Sports Med 39:1906–1911
34. Ekstrand J, van Dijk CN (2013) Fifth metatarsal fractures among male professional footballers: a potential career-ending disease. Br J Sports Med 47:754–758

35. Larsson D, Ekstrand J, Karlsson MK (2016) Fracture epidemiology in male elite football players from 2001 to 2013: 'how long will this fracture keep me out?'. Br J Sports Med 50:759–763
36. Ekstrand J, Torstveit MK (2012) Stress fractures in elite male football players. Scand J Med Sci Sports 22:341–346
37. Shrier I (2015) Strategic Assessment of Risk and Risk Tolerance (StARRT) framework for return-to-play decision-making. Br J Sports Med 49:1311–1315
38. McCall A, Lewin C, O'Driscoll G, Witvrouw E, Ardern C (2016) Return to play: the challenge of balancing research and practice. Br J Sports Med. https://doi.org/10.1136/bjsports-2016-096752
39. Hickey JT, Timmins RG, Maniar N, Williams MD, Opar DA (2016) Criteria for progressing rehabilitation and determining return-to-play clearance following hamstring strain injury: a systematic review. Sports Med. https://doi.org/10.1007/s40279-016-0667-x

Healthy Football Players in Different Playing Situations

Football is the most popular sport in the world. Players are many, spectators many more. There are millions of people watching the big games every weekend all over the world. However, football is not only about the big games, it is also about the vast amount of games played on a lower level. While football is a lot of fun and excitement, there is also the unfortunate backside of injuries and illnesses. We need to pay more attention on how to prevent injuries. In the course after injury we also need to understand much better how and when to return to play. This book is about safe return to play after injury and illness. It covers how to optimize the return and how to avoid the risk of relapse. This is not only relevant for the physical preparations of the players, but also the mental and tactical ones.

We who work with the players' health need to understand their individual needs and requirements. We need to study recent scientific knowledge and understand how to implement it, not only at the clinic but also on the football field.

This book is about football players' health, how to prevent and treat their injuries and when they are fully prepared to return to play. It covers how to make sure that the risk of relapse is minimized, with a long-term good health in focus.

V. Musahl et al. (eds.), *Return to Play in Football*, https://doi.org/10.1007/978-3-662-55713-6

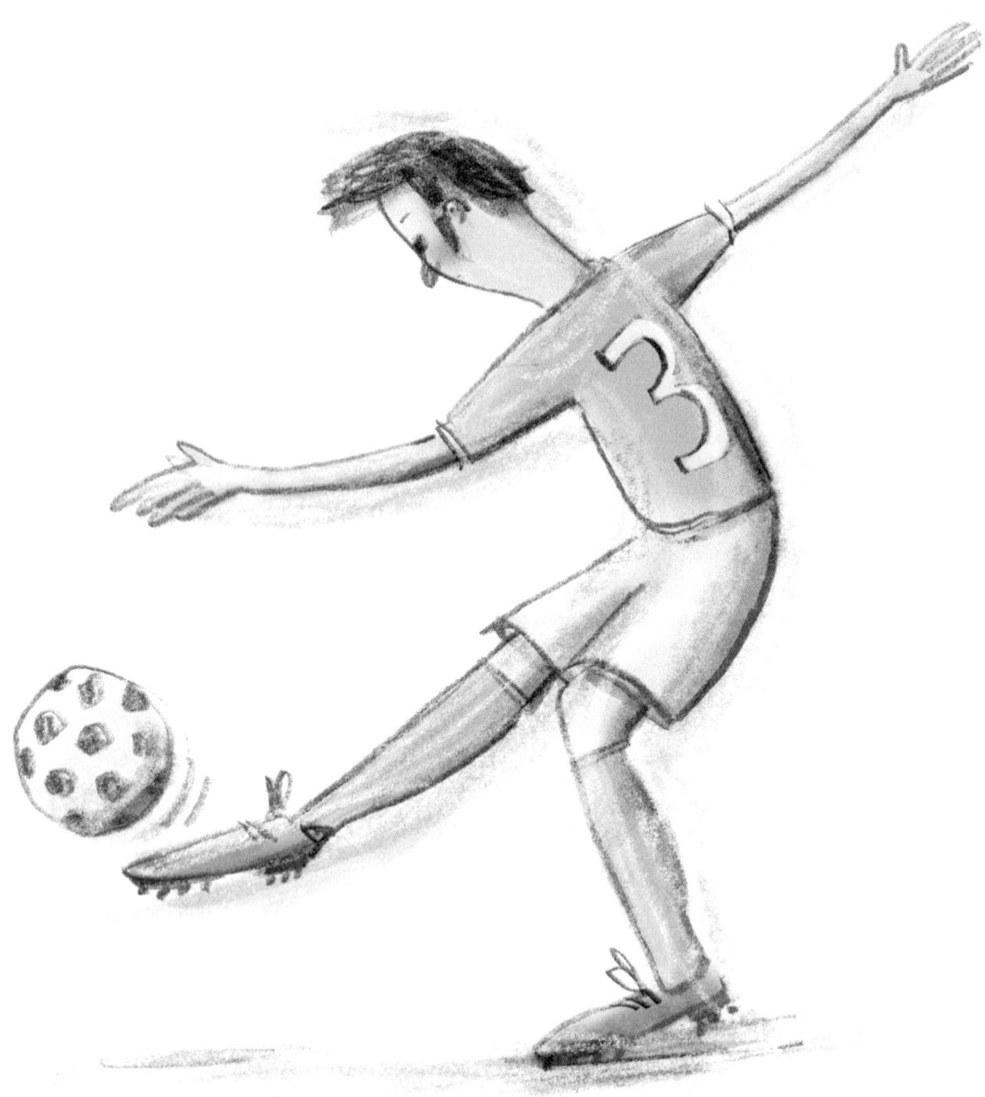
3

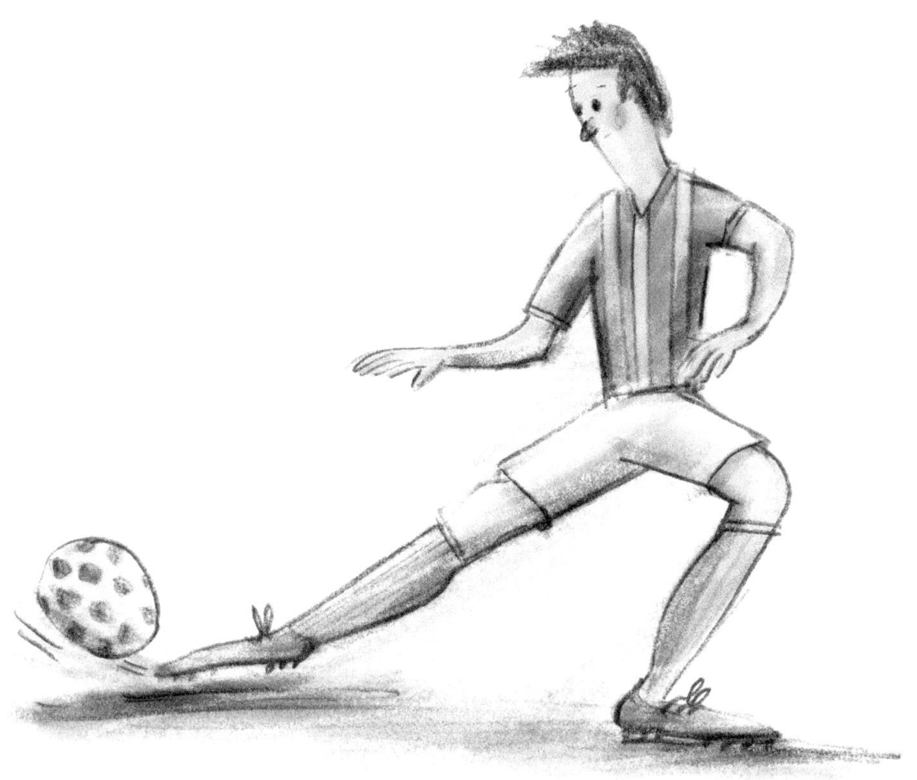

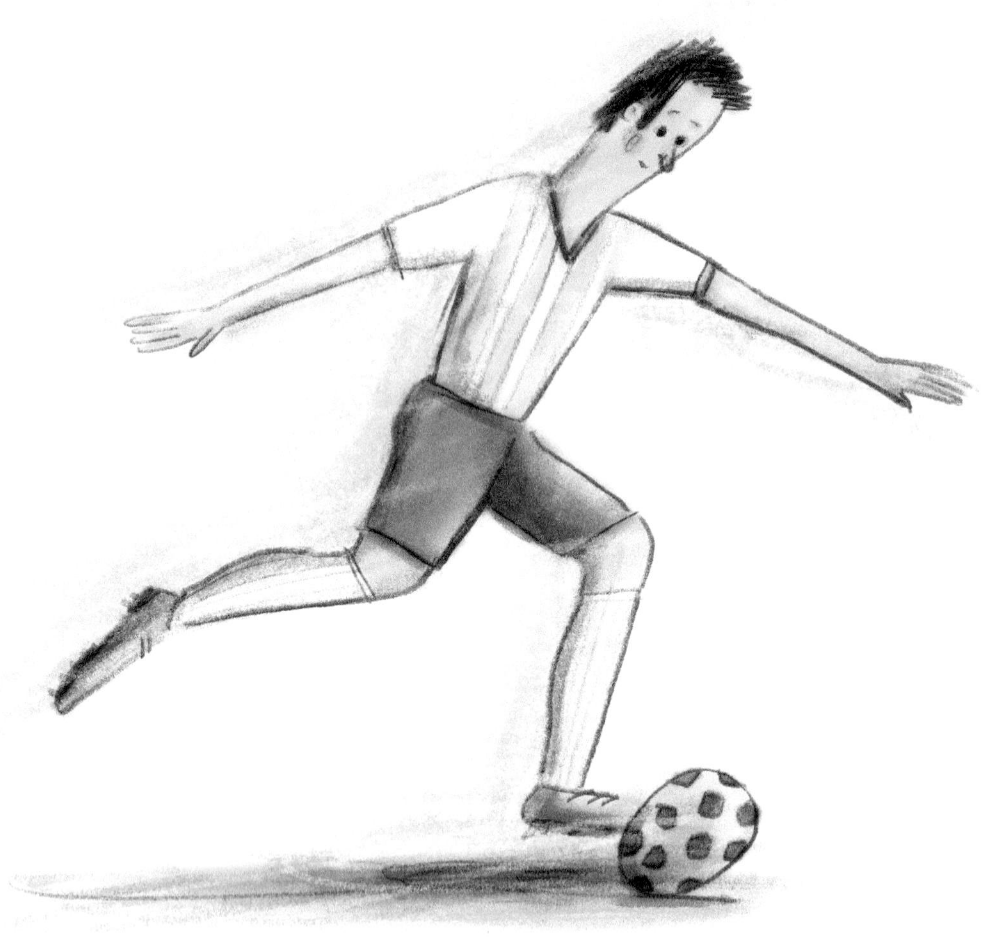

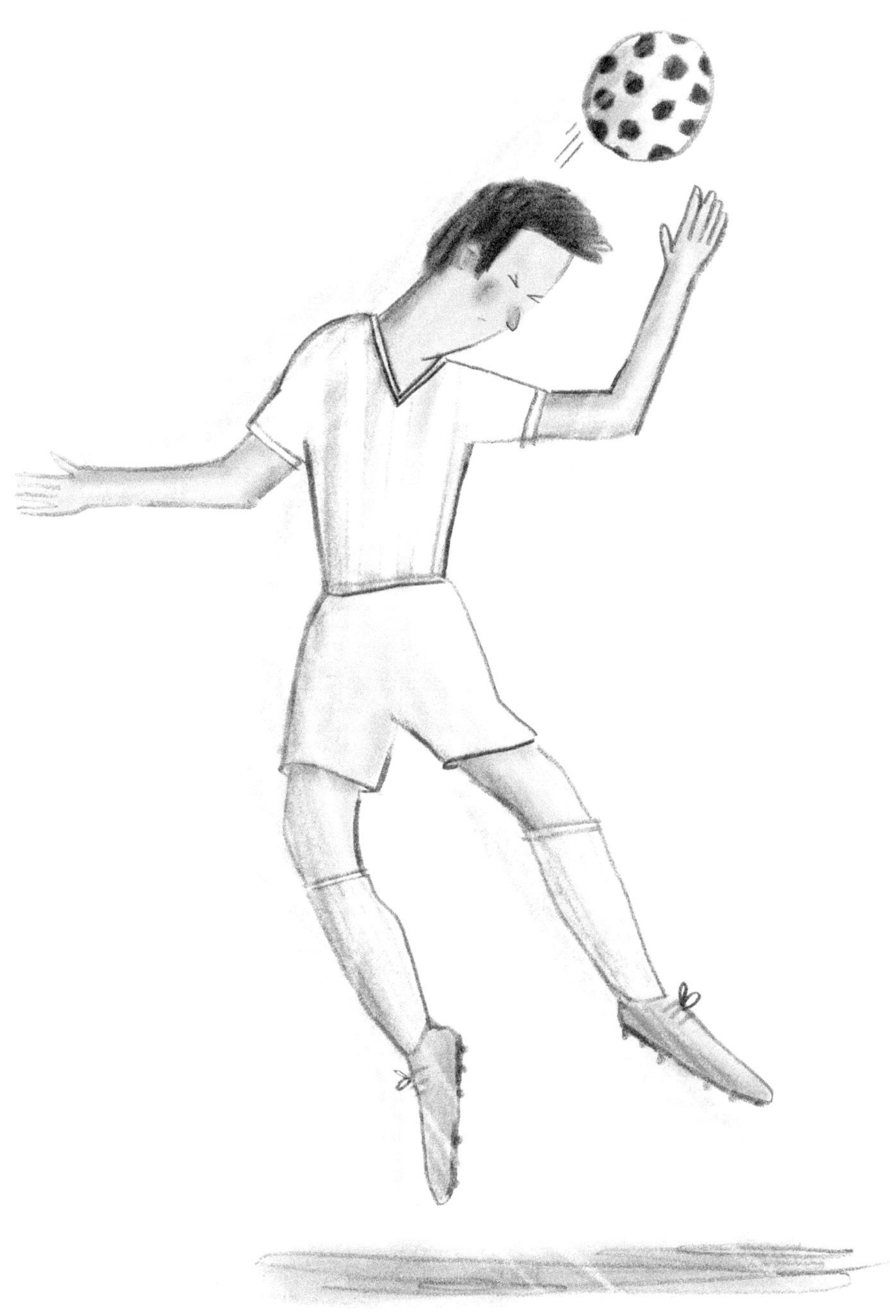

The pictures were created by Artist Birgitta Sif Jónsdóttir

Index

V. Musahl et al. (eds.), *Return to Play in Football*, https://doi.org/10.1007/978-3-662-55713-6

B

J

K

L

M

S

T

Printed by Printforce, the Netherlands